To Dr. Belani,
With best wishes

Susan E. Dorsch...
Orlando, Fl.
October 20, 1998
from Glen...

UNDERSTANDING
ANESTHESIA
EQUIPMENT

EDITION
4

UNDERSTANDING ANESTHESIA EQUIPMENT

Jerry A. Dorsch, M.D.
Associate Professor
Mayo Medical School
Rochester, Minnesota
Mayo Clinic
Jacksonville, Florida

Susan E. Dorsch, M.D.
Jacksonville, Florida

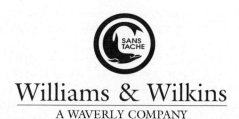

Williams & Wilkins
A WAVERLY COMPANY

BALTIMORE • PHILADELPHIA • LONDON • PARIS • BANGKOK
BUENOS AIRES • HONG KONG • MUNICH • SYDNEY • TOKYO • WROCLAW

Editor: Sharon Zinner
Managing Editor: Tanya Lazar
Marketing Manager: Adam Glazer
Project Editor: Ulita Lushnycky
Copyright © 1999 Williams & Wilkins

351 West Camden Street
Baltimore, Maryland 21201–2436 USA
Rose Tree Corporate Center
1400 North Providence Road
Building II, Suite 5025
Media, Pennsylvania 19063–2043 USA

The publisher is not responsible (as a matter of product liability, negligence or otherwise) for any injury resulting from any material contained herein. This publication contains information relating to general principles of medical care which should not be construed as specific instructions for individual patients. Manufacturers' product information and package inserts should be reviewed for current information, including contraindications, dosages and precautions.

Printed in the United States of America
First Edition, 1975
Second Edition, 1984
Third Edition, 1994

Library of Congress Cataloging-in-Publication Data
Dorsch, Jerry A., 1941–
   Understanding anesthesia equipment / Jerry A. Dorsch, Susan E.
Dorsch.—4th ed.
     p.   cm.
   Includes bibliographical references and index.
   ISBN (invalid) 0-683-30487-9
   1. Anesthesiology—Apparatus and instruments.   I. Dorsch, Susan
E., 1942–   . II. Title.
    [DNLM: 1. Anesthesiology—instrumentation.   WO 240 D717u   1998]
   RD78.8.D67   1998
   617.9'6'028—dc21
   DNLM/DLC
   for Library of Congress   98-15926
                                                        CIP

The publishers have made every effort to trace the copyright holders for borrowed material. If they have inadvertently overlooked any, they will be pleased to make the necessary arrangements at the first opportunity.

To purchase additional copies of this book, call our customer service department at **(800) 638–0672** or fax orders to **(800) 447–8438.** For other book services, including chapter reprints and large quantity sales, ask for the Special Sales department.

Canadian customers should call **(800) 665–1148**, or fax **(800) 665–0103.** For all other calls originating outside of the United States, please call **(410) 528–4223** or fax us at **(410) 528–8550.**

Visit Williams & Wilkins on the Internet: **http://www.wwilkins.com** or contact our customer service department at **custserv@wwilkins.com**. Williams & Wilkins customer service representatives are available from 8:30 am to 6:00 pm, EST, Monday through Friday, for telephone access.

99 00 01 02
1 2 3 4 5 6 7 8 9 10

DEDICATION

This book is dedicated to the many men and women who over the years have worked to develop standards to improve anesthesia equipment.

PREFACE TO THE FOURTH EDITION

Our goals in producing this book were to update subjects found in previous editions and to cover new topics important to anesthesia care providers by bringing together as much of the relevant literature as possible.

When the last edition was sent to the publisher, the laryngeal mask airway was not yet in widespread use in the United States. Since then, a large amount of information on this device has appeared in the literature. We have condensed this knowledge into one chapter.

We have tried to anticipate areas that we believe will become more important in the future. To this end, we have included some new chapters. Oxygen concentrations are coming into widespread use as the source of supply of oxygen for entire pipeline systems. Data management has been included to acquaint the reader with its present status and to aid him/her in making informed decisions when it comes time to consider implementation. Automatic noninvasive blood pressure monitoring has been an integral part of our practice for many years. We have included a chapter that provides a basic overview of this technology. We have added a chapter on design and equipment selection of facilities to aid the practitioner who participates in the construction or remodeling of the operating room facilities. A section dealing with bronchodilator administration was added.

Respiratory pressure and volume measurements have been around for many years. What is new is the addition of gas flow and the integration of these modalities in the form of loops. We have combined previous sections dealing with respirometers and airway pressure monitoring into a new chapter dealing with airway pressures, volumes, and flows.

Alas, it was necessary to say goodbye to some old friends. We deleted information in the book about equipment that is not currently sold or that has outlived its usefulness. Gone are the kettle-type vaporizers and older anesthesia machines that are no longer serviceable or do not meet current standards.

It is our sincere hope that this book will be especially helpful to the anesthesia resident or student nurse anesthetist who faces the daunting challenge of absorbing new knowledge and applying it in practice. We have added board-like questions after each chapter to aid this. It should also be useful to the seasoned practitioner who finds the machine that was a familiar friend has been replaced by one with unfamiliar sounds and computer menus. It is our hope that this edition will help make the transition smoother, resulting in a new level of comfort as well as an improved standard of practice.

ACKNOWLEDGMENTS

The authors have had a great deal of assistance from equipment manufacturers who have supplied pictures and information on their products. Credits have been included with their pictures.

The following individuals were most helpful in reviewing manuscripts: Jim Cicman, and Jay Smith of North American Drager; Gregory A. Clites of De Vilbiss Health Care, Inc.; Stan Gloss of Datex Medical Instrumentation, Inc.; Olli Heinonen of Datex/Engstrom; Barbara Illian of Sterrad; Marilyn M. Lynch of ABTOX, Inc.; Phil Millman of Mercury Medical; David Peel, Frank Primiano, and Robert Spooner of ECRI; and Dennis R. Stone, MD.

Our profound gratitude to Billy Atkins who kept our computers in working order.

We gratefully acknowledge the help of our colleagues at Mayo Clinic Jacksonville.

Literature searches were aided by the Borland Medical Library and the library at St. Luke's Medical Center.

TABLE OF CONTENTS

SECTION IV

MONITORING DEVICES

SECTION V

EQUIPMENT CARE AND PLANNING

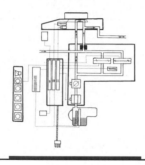

GAS SUPPLY AND DISTRIBUTION SYSTEMS

CHAPTER
1

Medical Gas Cylinders and Containers

I. Definitions
   A. Psia, Psig, Psi
   B. Nonliquefied Compressed Gas
   C. Liquefied Compressed Gas
   D. Cylinder
   E. Container
II. Regulatory Agencies and Industry Standards
III. Medical Gas Cylinders
   A. Components
      1. Body
      2. Valve
         a. Port
         b. Stem
            (1). Packed Valve
            (2). Diaphragm Valve
      3. Handle or Handwheel
      4. Pressure Relief Device
         a. Rupture Disc
         b. Fusible Plug
         c. Combination Rupture Disc/Fusible Plug
         d. Pressure Relief Valve
      5. Conical Depression
      6. Noninterchangeable Safety Systems
         a. Pin Index Safety System
         b. Valve Outlet Connections for Large Cylinders
   B. Sizes
   C. Contents and Pressure
   D. Testing
   E. Filling
   F. Color
   G. Permanent Markings
   H. Labeling
   I. Tags
   J. Rules for Safe Use of Cylinders
      1. General Rules
      2. Storage
      3. Use
      4. After Use
   K. Transfilling
   L. Hazards
      1. Incorrect Cylinder
      2. Incorrect Contents
      3. Incorrect Valve
      4. Incorrect Color
      5. Incorrect Labeling
      6. Inoperable Valve
      7. Damaged Valve
      8. Suffocation
      9. Fires
      10. Explosion
      11. Contamination of Cylinder Contents
      12. Theft of Nitrous Oxide
      13. Overfilled Cylinders
      14. Thermal Injury
IV. Liquid Oxygen Containers
   A. Equipment
   B. Rules for Safe Use of Liquid Oxygen Containers
   C. Storage
   D. Transfilling
   E. Hazards
      1. Fires
      2. High Pressure
      3. Burns
      4. Equipment Freezing
      5. Inaccurate Flows

DEFINITIONS
Psia, Psig, Psi

Psi stands for pounds per square inch. Psig stands for pounds per square inch gauge, which is the difference between the measured pressure and surrounding atmospheric pressure. Most gauges are constructed to read 0 at atmospheric pressure. Psia stands for pounds per square inch absolute. Absolute pressure is based on a reference point of 0 pressure, a perfect vacuum. Psia is psig plus the local atmospheric pressure. For example, at sea level we are at 0 psig, but 14.7 psia. Table 1.1 shows several units of pressure and their conversion factors.

Nonliquefied Compressed Gas

A nonliquefied compressed gas is a gas that does not liquefy at ordinary temperatures and under pressures from 2000 to 2500 psig (13,789 to 17,237 kPa) [1]. Examples include oxygen, nitrogen, air, and helium. These gases become liquids at very low temperatures and are then referred to as cryogenic liquids.

Liquefied Compressed Gas

A liquefied compressed gas is one that becomes liquid to a large extent in containers at ordinary temperatures and at pressures from 25 to 2500

TABLE 1.1. Units of Pressure

kPa - kilopascal
cm H_2O - centimeter of water
psi - pound per square inch
mbar - millibar
mm Hg - millimeter of mercury
100 kPa = 1000 mbar = 760 mm Hg
　　　= 1030 cm H_2O = 14.7 psi = 1 atmosphere
Therefore,

1 kPa = 10.3 cm H_2O	1 cm H_2O = 0.97 kPa
1 kPa = 0.147 psi	1 psi = 6.8 kPa
1 kPa = 7.6 mm Hg	1 mm Hg = 0.13 kPa
1 kPa = 10 mbar	1 mbar = 0.1 kPa
1 mbar = 1.03 cm H_2O	1 cm H_2O = 0.97 mbar
1 mbar = 0.76 mm Hg	1 mm Hg = 1.32 mbar
1 mbar = 0.0147 psi	1 psi = 68 mbar

---

psig (172.4 to 17,237 kPa) [1]. Examples include nitrous oxide and carbon dioxide.

Cylinder

A cylinder is a supply tank containing high-pressure gas or gas mixture at a pressure that can be in excess of 2000 psig (13.8 kPa gauge) [2].

Container

A container is a low-pressure, vacuum-insulated vessel containing gas(es) in liquid form [2].

REGULATORY AGENCIES AND INDUSTRY STANDARDS

All those who produce, supply, transport, or use medical gases must comply with a variety of safety regulations promulgated and enforced by agencies at the federal, state, provincial, and local levels of government.

The purity of medical gases is specified in the United States Pharmacopoeia and enforced by the Food and Drug Administration (FDA).

The Department of Transportation (DOT) and Transport Canada (TC) have published requirements for the manufacturing, marking, labeling, filling, qualification, transportation, storage, handling, maintenance, requalification, and disposition of medical gas cylinders and containers. States and Canadian provinces vary widely in their regulations for compressed gases [1]. In addition, many local governments have regulations that apply to compressed gases.

The United States government regulates matters affecting the safety and health of employees in all industries through the Department of Labor and the Occupational Safety and Health Act (OSHA).

The National Fire Protection Association (NFPA), the Compressed Gas Association (CGA), and the Canadian Standards Association (CSA) have published a number of standards. Although termed *voluntary*, many regulatory agencies have made adherence to these standards mandatory.

MEDICAL GAS CYLINDERS
Components
Body

Most medical gas cylinders (tanks) are constructed of steel, with various alloys added for strength. In recent years cylinders made from aluminum have become available (3, 4). These are especially useful when anesthesia is administered in a magnetic resonance imaging (MRI) environment. Cylinders have flat bases so that they may stand on end. The other end tapers into a neck that is fitted with tapered screw threads for attachment of the valve.

Valve

Cylinders are filled and discharged through a valve (spindle valve) attached to the neck. The valve, which is made of bronze or brass, is an integral part of the cylinder and should be removed only during testing or maintenance of the cylinder.

Port

The port is the point of exit for the gas. It should be protected in transit by a covering. When installing a small cylinder on an anesthesia machine, it is important not to mistake the port for the conical depression on the opposite side of the valve, which is designed to receive the retaining screw on the yoke. Screwing the retaining screw into the port may damage the port and index pins.

Stem

Each valve contains a stem, or shaft, that closes the valve by sealing against the seat. When the valve is opened, the stem moves upward, allowing gas to flow to the port.

Packed valve. Most cylinder valves are of the packed type (Fig. 1.1). In these, the stem is sealed by resilient packing such as Teflon, which prevents leakage around the threads. This type of valve is also called direct acting because turning the stem causes the seat to turn. In the large cylinder valve, the force is transmitted by means of a driver square (Fig. 1.1, right). This type of valve is capable of withstanding high pressures.

Diaphragm valve. In a diaphragm valve (Fig. 1.2), the stem is separated from the seat. A flexible diaphragm seals the opening to the internal parts. Turning the stem raises or lowers the diaphragm. The downward force of the stem is opposed by a spring acting on the seat. Turning the stem clockwise lowers the diaphragm, which in turn lowers the seat and closes the valve. When the stem is turned counterclockwise, the diaphragm is raised and the force of the spring raises the seat, opening the valve. This type of valve has the following advantages (5):

1. It can be opened fully using a one-half to three-quarters turn, whereas the packed valve requires two or three full turns.
2. The seat does not turn and is therefore less likely to leak.

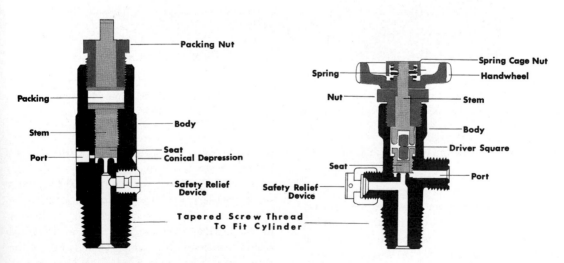

FIGURE 1.1. Small (left) and large (right) packed valves. The packing seals the stem and prevents leaks. Turning the stem on the large cylinder valve counterclockwise causes the seat to turn in its thread, opening the valve. (From drawings furnished by Puritan-Bennett Corp.)

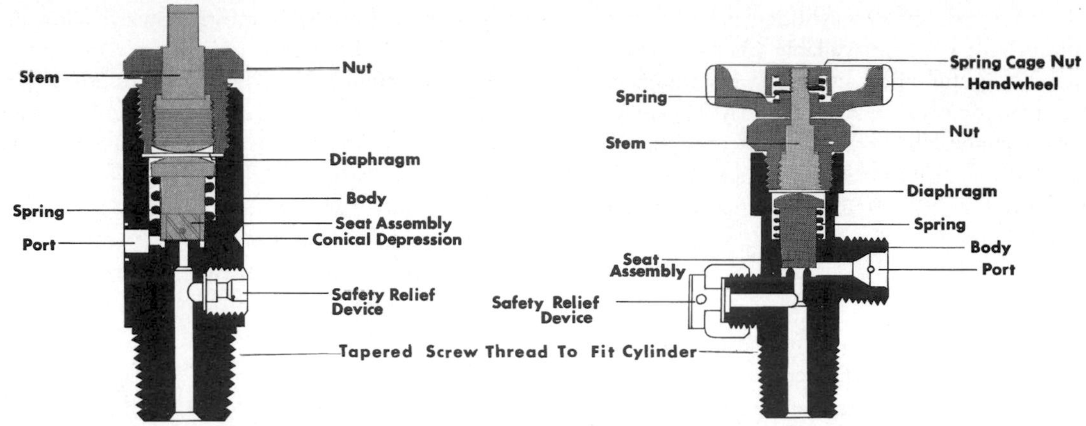

FIGURE 1.2. Small (left) and large (right) diaphragm valves. Turning the handle clockwise forces the diaphragm downward and closes the seat. Upon opening the valve, the upward force of the spring opens the seat. (From drawings furnished by Puritan-Bennett Corp.)

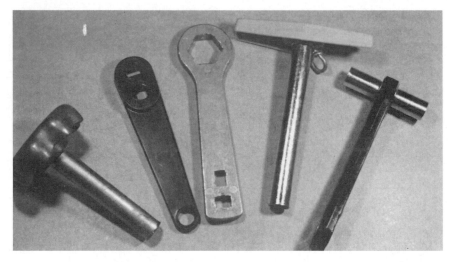

FIGURE 1.3. Small cylinder valve handles. The hexagonal opening at the top of the middle handle can be used to tighten the packing nut on the cylinder valve. A ratchet handle is at the right. After a cylinder has been opened, this handle must be removed, inverted and reapplied to close the cylinder valve.

3. No stem leakage can occur because of the diaphragm.

For these reasons, the diaphragm type is generally preferable when the pressures are relatively low and when no leaks can be allowed, such as with flammable gases. It is somewhat more expensive than the packed type.

Handle or Handwheel

A handle or handwheel is used to open or close a cylinder valve. It is turned counterclockwise to open the valve and clockwise to close it. This causes the stem to turn.

A handle (cylinder wrench) is used to open a small cylinder valve. These come in a variety of shapes (Fig. 1.3). Some handles, such as the one in the middle of Figure 1.3, have a hexagonal opening that fits the packing (gland) nut of the valve (Fig. 1.1). This handle may be used to tighten the nut should it become loose. A hazard associated with this handle is that a person unacquainted with cylinders could loosen the packing nut under the mistaken impression that he or she was opening the valve. This could cause the valve stem and retaining nut to come off the cylinder with great force (6).

A ratchet-type handle is supplied with certain anesthesia machines (Fig. 1.3). After the cylinder is opened, the handle must be removed, inverted, and reapplied to close the cylinder. A burn from nitrous oxide during these maneuvers has been reported (7).

A good practice is to attach a handle to each anesthesia machine or other apparatus for which it may be needed. It is also important to check that the cylinder can be opened before use, as cases where the valve could not be opened have been reported (8).

Each large cylinder valve has a permanently attached handwheel that uses a spring and nut to hold it firmly in place (Figs. 1.1 and 1.2).

Pressure Relief Device

Every cylinder is fitted with a pressure relief device (safety relief device, safety device) whose purpose is to vent the cylinder's contents to the atmosphere if the pressure of the enclosed gas increases to a dangerous level (1).

Rupture Disc

The rupture (frangible, burst) disc is a nonreclosing device with a disc held against an orifice (Fig. 1.4). When the predetermined pressure is reached, the disc ruptures and allows the cylinder contents to be discharged. The pressure opening is the orifice against which the disc functions. The rated burst pressure is the pressure at which the disc is designed to burst. It is determined by the material, thickness, and shape of the disc and the diameter of the pressure opening. This device is used on some air, carbon dioxide, carbon dioxide-oxygen, helium, nitrous oxide, helium-oxygen, nitrogen, and oxygen cylinders. It protects against excess pressure as a result of high temperatures or overfilling.

Fusible Plug

The fusible plug is a thermally operated, nonreclosing pressure-relief device with the plug held against the discharge channel. The plug offers protection from excessive pressure caused by high temperature but not from improper charging practices. The yield temperature is the temperature at which the fusible material becomes sufficiently soft to extrude from its holder so that cylinder contents are discharged. A fusible plug with a yield temperature of 212°F (100°C) is sometimes used on certain nitrogen and air cylinders.

Combination Rupture Disc/Fusible Plug

A combination rupture disc/fusible plug can be used to prevent bursting at a predetermined pressure unless the temperature is high enough to cause yielding of the fusible material. Such a device with a yield temperature of 165°F (74°C) may be found on cylinders of air, oxygen, nitrogen, nitrous oxide, helium, helium-oxygen mixtures, carbon dioxide, and carbon dioxide–oxygen mixtures. Because it functions only in the presence of both excessive heat and excessive pressure, it does not offer protection from high pressures because of overfilling.

Pressure Relief Valve

The pressure relief valve (Fig. 1.5) is a spring-loaded device designed to reclose and prevent discharge of cylinder contents after normal pressures have been restored. The set pressure, at which it will start to discharge, is marked on the valve. A pressure relief valve may be found on air, helium, oxygen, nitrogen, helium-oxygen mixture, carbon dioxide, and carbon dioxide–oxygen mixture cylinders with up to 500 psig charging pressure. Pressure relief valves are generally more susceptible to leakage than rupture discs or fusible plugs (1).

Conical Depression

Above the safety relief device on small cylinders is the conical depression that receives the retaining

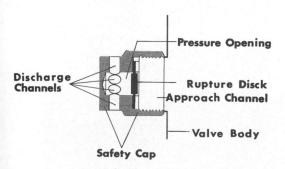

FIGURE 1.4. Rupture disc device. When the rated burst pressure is exceeded, the disc ruptures and gas flows from the approach channel into the pressure opening and to atmosphere through the discharge channels. (Redrawn from Frangible disc safety device assembly. Pamphlet S-3. New York: Compressed Gas Society: 4.)

screw of the yoke (Figs 1.1, 1.2, and 1.6). It must be distinguished from the safety relief device. If the retaining screw is tightened into the safety relief device, the device may be damaged and the cylinder contents escape (9, 10).

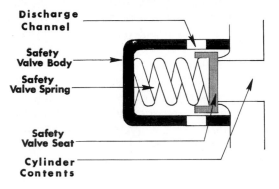

Discharge Channel

Safety Valve Body

Safety Valve Spring

Safety Valve Seat

Cylinder Contents

FIGURE 1.5. Pressure relief valve. When the set pressure is exceeded, the pressure in the cylinder forces the spring to the left and gas flows around the safety valve seat to the discharge channel. (From a drawing furnished by Ohmeda, a division of the BOC Group, Inc.)

Noninterchangeable Safety Systems (1,11)

With widespread use of cylinders containing different gases, a potential hazard is the connection of a cylinder to equipment intended for a different gas. Color coding was developed to help solve this problem; however color coding did not give complete protection against human error. Through the cooperation of the CGA and others, two noninterchangeable systems were developed. Both of these systems are located between the cylinder valve and the regulator and should not be confused with the Diameter Index Safety System, which is on the low pressure side of the regulator and will be discussed in Chapter 2.

Pin Index Safety System

The Pin Index Safety System is used on cylinders of sizes A through E. It consists of holes on the cylinder valve positioned in an arc below the outlet port (Figs. 1.6 and 1.7). Pins on the yoke or regulator are positioned to fit these holes. Pins assigned to gases or gas mixtures used in anesthesia are shown in Table 1.2. Unless the pins and

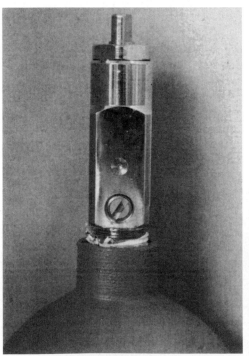

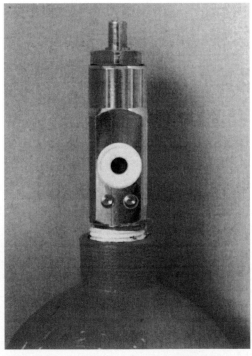

FIGURE 1.6.   Small cylinder valves. Left, the conical depression is above the pressure relief device. Right, the port is above the Pin Index Safety System holes. A washer is over the port.

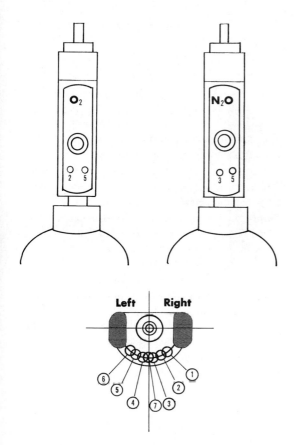

FIGURE 1.7. Pin Index Safety System. The bottom figure shows the six index positions for pins on the yoke. The pins are 4 mm in diameter and 6 mm long, except for pin 7, which is slightly thicker. The seven hole positions are on the circumference of a circle of 9/16 inch radius centered on the port.

TABLE 1.2. **Pin Index System**

Gas	Index Pins
Oxygen	2, 5
Nitrous oxide	3, 5
Cyclopropane	3, 6
O_2-CO_2 (CO_2 < 7.5%)	2, 6
O_2-CO_2 (CO_2 > 7.5%)	1, 6
O_2-He (He > 80.5%)	4, 6
O_2-He (He < 80.5%)	2, 4
Air	1, 5
Nitrogen	1, 4
N_2O-O_2 (N_2O 47.5–52.5%)	7

holes are aligned, the port will not seat. It is possible for a yoke or regulator without pins to receive any cylinder valve, but ordinarily it is not possible for an undrilled cylinder valve to be placed in a yoke or regulator containing pins.

Valve Outlet Connections for Large Cylinders

Size M and larger cylinder valves have threaded outlet connections, as shown in Figure 1.8. When the threads of this outlet mesh with those of the nut, the nut may be tightened by turning it clockwise, causing the nipple to seat against the valve outlet. In this way, the gas channel of the valve is aligned with the channel of the nipple. The outlets and connections are indexed by diameter, thread size, right- and left-handed threading, external and internal threading, and nipple-seat design.

Sizes

Gas suppliers classify cylinders using a letter code, with A being the smallest. Table 1.3 gives the approximate dimensions and capacities for some commonly used cylinders. The volume and pressure of a gas in a cylinder vary, depending upon the gas. However, oxygen and air are similar in volumes and pressures. The same is true for carbon dioxide and nitrous oxide.

Size E is the cylinder most commonly used on anesthesia machines and for patient transport and resuscitation. Size D cylinders are used for limited supplies of gases where size and weight considerations are important. Aluminum cylinders were originally longer than steel cylinders with the same outside diameter (2, 12). Ones manufactured more recently have the same or a shorter length than steel cylinders with a larger outer diameter.

Contents and Pressure

As illustrated in Figure 1.9, the pressure declines steadily as the contents are withdrawn from a cylinder containing a nonliquefied gas. Therefore, the pressure can be used to measure the cylinder contents.

In a cylinder containing a liquefied gas, the pressure depends on the vapor pressure of the liquid and is not an indication of the amount of gas remaining in the cylinder as long as the contents are partly in the liquid phase. The pressure remains nearly constant (with constant temperature) until all the liquid has evaporated, after which the pres-

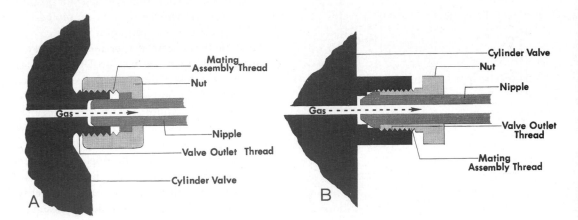

FIGURE 1.8. Valve outlet connections for large cylinders. Left, the valve outlet thread is external—i.e., the threads are on the outside of the cylinder valve outlet and the nut screws over the valve outlet. Right, the valve outlet thread is internal, so that the nut screws into the outlet. The specification for cylinder connections are often shown as in the following example for oxygen:

0.903-14-RH EXT. The first number is the diameter in inches of the cylinder outlet. The next number gives the number of threads per inch. The letters following this indicate whether the threads are right hand or left hand and external or internal. (Redrawn courtesy of the Compressed Gas Association.)

TABLE 1.3. Typical Medical Gas Cylinders, Volumes, Weights, and Pressures

Cylinder Size	Cylinder Dimensions (O.D. × Length in Inches)	Empty Cylinder Weight (lb)	Capacities and Pressures (at 70°F)	Air	Carbon Dioxide	Helium	Nitrous Oxide	Oxygen	Nitrogen	Helium-Oxygen Mixtures[a]	Carbon Dioxide-Oxygen Mixtures[a]
B	3½ × 13	5	liters		370			200			
			psig		838			1,900			
D	4½ × 17	11	liters	375	940	300	940	400	370	300	400
			psig	1,900	838	1,600	745	1,900	1,900	+	+
E	4¼ × 26	14	liters	625	1,590[b]	500	1,590	660	610	500	660
			psig	1,900	838	1,600	745[b]	1,900	1,900	+	+
M	7 × 43	63	liters	2,850	7,570	2,260	7,570	3,450	3,200	2,260	3,000
			psig	1,900	838	1,600	745	2,200	2,200	+	+
G	8½ × 51	97	liters	5,050	12,300	4,000	13,800			4,000	5,300
			psig	1,900	838	1,600	745			+	+
H	9¼ × 51	119	liters	6,550		6,000	15,800	6,900[c]	6,400[c]		
			psig	2,200		2,200	745	2,200[c]	2,200[c]		

[a] The + indicates that the pressures of these mixed gases will vary according to the composition of the mixture.
[b] An E-size cylinder of nitrous oxide contains approximately 250 liters when the pressure begins to decrease below 745 psig.
[c] 7,800-liter cylinders at 2,490 psig are available.

sure declines until the cylinder is exhausted. Weight can be used to determine the amount of liquid in these cylinders. In practice, weighing of cylinders is awkward and rarely performed.

During use, the temperature is not likely to remain constant. Evaporation of the liquid and expansion of a gas require energy in the form of heat, which is supplied mainly by the liquid in the cylinder. This results in cooling. If the outer surface of a cylinder that contains liquefied gas becomes cold as gas is discharged, this is an indication there is residual liquid left in the cylinder (13). As the temperature falls, the vapor pressure of the liquid also falls, so that a progressive fall in pressure accompanies the release of gas from the cylinder (13). If liquid remains when withdrawal stops, cylinder pressure will slowly increase to its original level as the temperature rises.

Testing

A cylinder must be inspected and tested at least every 5 years or, with a special permit, up to every 10 years (1). The test date (month and year) must be permanently stamped on the cylinder.

Each cylinder must pass an internal and external visual check for corrosion and evidence of physical impact or distortion. Cylinders are checked for leaks and retention of structural strength by testing to a minimum of 1.66 (1.5 in Canada) times their service pressures. The service pressure is the maximum pressure to which the cylinder may be filled at 70°F (21°C). Table 1.4 gives the service pressures for gases commonly used in anesthesia.

Filling

If a cylinder containing gas under a safe pressure at normal temperatures is subjected to higher temperatures, the pressure may increase to a dangerous level. To prevent this, the DOT has drawn up regulations limiting the amount of gas a cylinder may contain (1).

1. The pressure in a filled cylinder at 70°F (21°C) may not exceed the service pressure marked on the cylinder except for some nonliquefied, nonflammable gases such as oxygen, helium, carbon dioxide–oxygen mixtures, and helium-oxygen mixtures, which may be allowed an additional 10%.

2. For gases other than nitrous oxide and carbon dioxide, the pressure in the cylinder at 130°F (55°C) may not exceed 1.25 times the maximum permitted filling pressure at 70°F (21°C).

3. As illustrated in Figure 1.9, the pressure will remain nearly constant as long as there is liquid in a cylinder containing a liquefied gas. Thus, if only the pressure was limited, these cylinders could be filled with any amount of liquid. To prevent a cylinder containing a liquefied gas from being overfilled, the maximum amount of gas allowed is defined by a filling density (filling ratio) for each gas. The filling density is the percent ratio of the weight of gas in a cylinder to the weight of water the cylinder would hold at 60°F (16°C) (1). The filling densities of gases commonly used in anesthesia are shown in Table 1.4.

The filling density is not the same as the volume of the full cylinder occupied by the liquid phase. For example, in a full nitrous oxide cylinder, the liquid phase typically occupies 90 to 95% of cylinder volume, whereas the filling density is 68%.

Color

Accidental confusion of cylinders has been a significant cause of mortality. Color can be used to help identify gases (1). The color code used in the United States is shown in Table 1.4. The top and shoulder (the part sloping up to the neck) of each cylinder are painted the color assigned to the gas it contains or the entire cylinder may be covered using a nonfading, durable, water-insoluble paint. In the case of a cylinder containing more than one gas, the colors must be applied in a way that will permit each color to be seen when viewed from the top. This color coding is used on the hoses, connectors, knobs, and gauges on other medical equipment.

An international color code (see Table 1.4) has been adopted by several countries, including Canada (14). This system differs from the one used in the United States in that oxygen's color is white and air is black and white rather than yellow. A number of countries besides the United States use a color code that differs from the international code (15). When people trained in one country

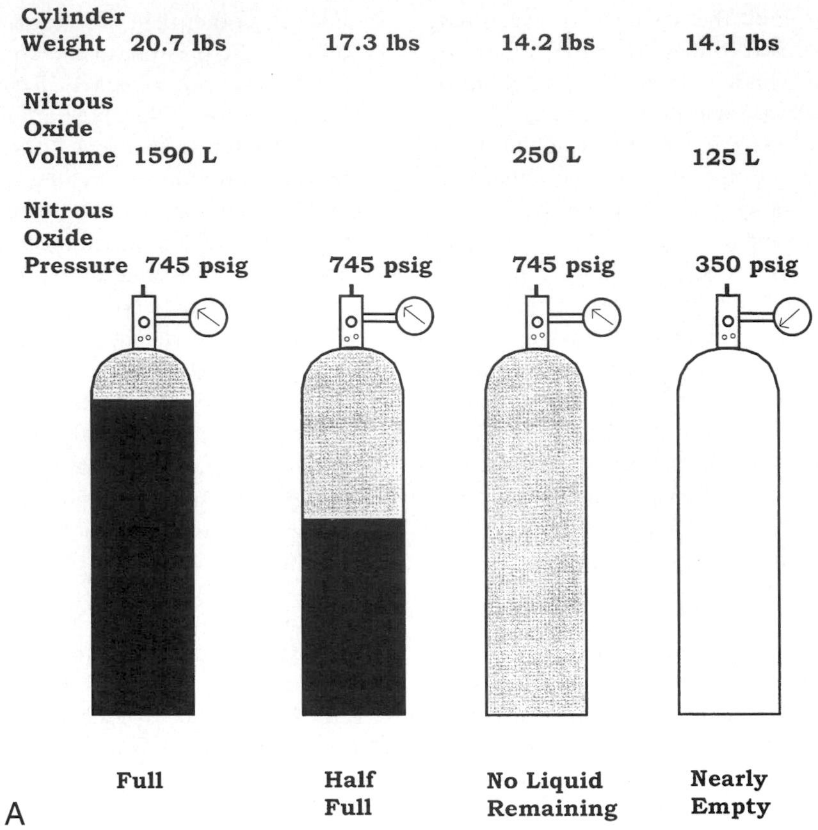

Cylinder Weight	20.7 lbs	17.3 lbs	14.2 lbs	14.1 lbs
Nitrous Oxide Volume	1590 L		250 L	125 L
Nitrous Oxide Pressure	745 psig	745 psig	745 psig	350 psig

| Full | Half Full | No Liquid Remaining | Nearly Empty |

A

FIGURE 1.9. The relationship between cylinder weight, pressure, and contents. A, A gas stored partially in liquid form, such as nitrous oxide, will show a constant pressure (assuming constant temperature) until all the liquid has evaporated, at which time the pressure will drop in direct proportion to the rate at which gas is withdrawn.

work in another country that has a different code, confusion frequently results.

Color should be not be used as the primary means for identification of cylinder contents because of the following: variations in color tones, chemical changes in paint pigments, lighting effects, and differences in color perception by personnel. However, color coding provides a useful check on labeling accuracy.

Markings

DOT and TC regulations require specific markings on each cylinder (1). These are permanently stamped, usually onto the shoulder. Representative markings are shown in Figure 1.10. The first number is the DOT or TC specification number. This indicates the type of material used in manufacture of the cylinder. This is followed by the service pressure for the cylinder in pounds per square inch. Next is a serial number and the identifying symbol of the purchaser, user, or manufacturer.

The initial qualifying test date with an identifying mark for the testing facility between the month and year of the test date may appear last or may be on the opposite side of the shoulder. The retest date and testing facility must appear after the original qualifying date if a cylinder has been retested. A five-pointed star stamped after the most recent test date indicates that the cylinder may be retested every 10 instead of every 5

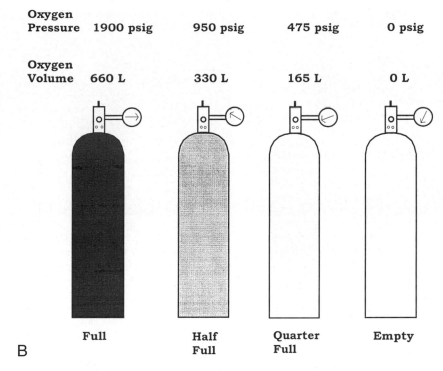

B

FIGURE 1.9. *(continued)* B, A nonliquefied gas such as oxygen will show a steady decline in pressure until the cylinder is evacuated. Each cylinder, however, will show a steady decline in weight as gas is discharged.

TABLE 1.4. **Medical Gases**

Gas	Formula	United States	International	State in Cylinder	Filling Density
Oxygen	O_2	Green	White	Gas[a]	
Carbon dioxide	CO_2	Gray[b]	Gray	Gas + Liquid (below 88°F)	68%
Nitrous oxide	N_2O	Blue	Blue	Gas + Liquid (below 98°F)	68%
Helium	He	Brown[c]	Brown	Gas	
Nitrogen	N_2	Black	Black	Gas	
Air		Yellow[d]	White & black	Gas	

[a] Special containers for liquid oxygen are discussed later in this Chapter.
[b] In carbon dioxide–oxygen mixtures in which the CO_2 is greater than 7%, the cylinder is predominantly gray and the balance is green. If the CO_2 is less than 7%, the predominant color is green.
[c] If helium is greater than 80% in a helium-oxygen mixture, the predominant color is brown and the balance is green.
[d] Air, including oxygen-nitrogen mixtures containing 19.5–23.5% oxygen, is color coded yellow. Cylinders with nitrogen-oxygen mixtures other than those containing 19.5–23.5% oxygen are colored black and green.

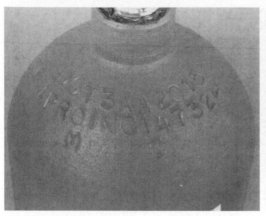 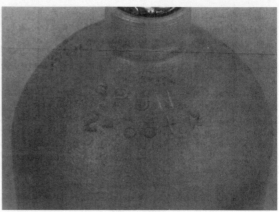

FIGURE 1.10. Cylinder markings. Left, "DOT3AA" is the DOT specification number; "2015" is the service pressure in psig. The next line shows the identifying symbol of the manufacturer and the serial number of the cylinder. Right, "SPUN" indicates that the end of the cylinder was closed by a spinning process. The initial qualifying date is shown with the inspector's mark between the month and year. The plus sign indicates that the cylinder is authorized for charging up to 10% in excess of the marked service pressure. The star indicates that the cylinder may be retested every 10 instead of every 5 years.

years. If a plus sign (+) appears immediately after the test date marking on a cylinder, it means that the cylinder is authorized to be charged up to 10% in excess of the marked service pressure. The word spun or plug must be stamped where an end closure has been made by spinning or by spinning, drilling, and plugging.

Labeling

Each cylinder must bear a label or decal on the side or, when space permits, the shoulder of the cylinder (but may not cover any permanent markings) (1).

Figure 1.11 shows a typical cylinder label. It has a diamond-shaped figure denoting the hazard class of the contained gas and a white panel with the name of the contained gas to the left. The diamond indicates whether the contents contain an oxidizer (yellow), a nonflammable gas (green), or a flammable gas (red). A signal word (DANGER, WARNING, or CAUTION, depending on whether the release of gas would create an immediate, less than immediate, or no immediate hazard to health or property) is present. Following the signal word is the statement of hazard, which gives the dangers with customary or reasonably anticipated handling or use of the gas. A brief pre-cautionary statement giving measures to be taken to avoid injury or damage is usually present.

The label should contain the name and address of the cylinder manufacturer or distributor and a statement as to its content, usually the volume in liters at 70°F (21°C). Other information such as the cylinder weight when empty and full may also be present. DOT regulations permit the use of a combination label-tag—one side of which contains the prescribed wording of the DOT label, while the other side is used as a shipping tag with space for the names and addresses of the shipper and consignee. Medical gas manufacturers usually use these on large cylinders, attached to the cylinder cap. The tag is perforated so that when the cylinder is empty part of the tag may be torn off at the perforation, obliterating the label wording. The part of the tag that remains attached to the cylinder contains the return address of the supplier.

Tags

A typical tag is shown in Figure 1.12. It has three sections labeled FULL, IN USE, and EMPTY connected by perforations. The FULL portion of the tag should be detached when a cylinder is put into service. The IN USE portion

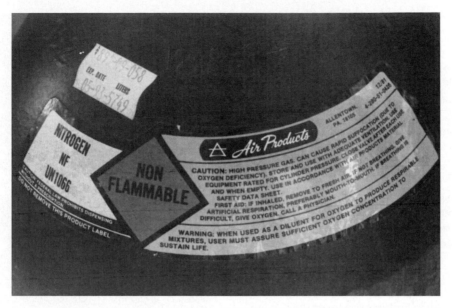

FIGURE 1.11.   Cylinder label, showing the basic Compressed Gas Association (CGA) marking system. The diamond-shaped figure denotes the hazard class of the contained gas (NONFLAMMABLE). To the left is a white panel with the name of contained gas (NITROGEN). The signal word (CAUTION) is to the right, following by a statement of hazards and measures to be taken to avoid injury.

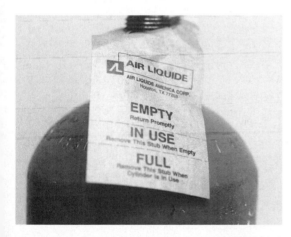

FIGURE 1.12.   Cylinder tag. When the cylinder is first opened, the FULL portion of the tag should be removed. When the cylinder is empty, the IN USE portion should be removed.

should be removed when the cylinder is empty, leaving the EMPTY label. The tag sometimes contains a washer to fit between the small cylinder valve and the yoke or regulator. Tags normally bear the same color as the cylinder. The tag is primarily a means of denoting the amount of cylinder contents and not an identification device.

Rules for Safe Use of Cylinders
General Rules

1. Cylinders should be handled only by personnel trained in safe practices. Frequently personnel involved in the transport, storage, and use of cylinders do not receive adequate instructions regarding their safe handling (16). Even those personnel that receive adequate training may become complacent.
2. Cylinder valves, regulators, gauges, and fittings should never come into contact with oils, greases, organic lubricants, rubber, or other combustible substances. Cylinders or valves should not be handled with hands, rags, or gloves contaminated with oil or grease. Polishing or cleaning agents should not be applied to the valve because they may contain combustible chemicals.
3. No part of any cylinder should ever be subjected to a temperature above 125°F (52°C). A flame, torch, or sparks from any source should never be permitted to come in contact

with any part of a cylinder. A cylinder should not be supported by or placed in proximity to a radiator, steam pipe, or heat duct. If a cylinder is exposed to a high temperature, it should be returned to the manufacturer for testing. Exposure to extremes of cold should also be avoided. Should ice or snow accumulate on a cylinder, it should be thawed at room temperature or with water at a temperature not exceeding 125°F (52°C).

4. Connections to piping, regulators, and other equipment should always be kept tight to prevent leakage. If a hose is used, it should be in good condition.

5. The discharge port of a pressure relief device or the valve outlet must not be obstructed.

6. Regulators, gauges, or other appliances designed for use with one gas should never be used with cylinders containing other gases.

7. Adapters to change the outlet size of a cylinder valve should not be used because this defeats the whole purpose of standardizing valve outlets.

8. The valve should be kept closed except when the cylinder is in use. It should be turned off with no more force than is necessary or damage to the seating may result.

9. The valve is the most easily damaged part of the cylinder. Valve protection caps (metal caps that screw over the valve on large cylinders [Fig. 1.13]) are available. They can protect the valve in case the cylinder topples over and should be kept in place and hand tightened except when the cylinder is connected for use.

10. No part of the cylinder or its valve should be tampered with, painted, altered, repaired, or modified by the user. Cylinders should be repainted only by the supplier.

11. Markings, labels, decals, or tags must not be defaced, altered, or removed.

12. A cylinder should not be used as a roller or support or for any other purpose other than that for which it was intended, even if the cylinder is believed to be empty.

13. A cylinder should not be placed where it may come into contact with electric apparatus or circuits.

14. Cylinders should not be dropped, dragged,

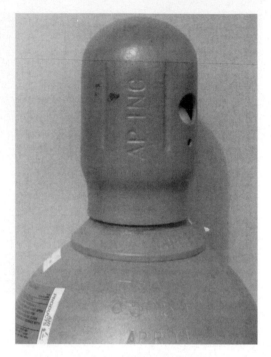

FIGURE 1.13. Large cylinder valve protection cap. This cap should be kept in place at all times, except when the cylinder is connected for use.

slid, or rolled, even for short distances. Cylinders should be transported using a cart or carrier made especially for that purpose (Figs. 1.14 and 1.15).

15. Cylinders should be properly secured at all times to prevent them from falling or being knocked over (Figs. 1.16 and 1.17). Cylinders should not be dropped or permitted to strike each other or other surfaces violently. Cylinders must not be chained to movable apparatus such as beds.

16. Cylinders should never be used where they could become contaminated by other gases or foreign material.

17. The owner of the cylinder must be notified if any damage that might impair its safety is noticed or if any condition that might permit a foreign substance to enter the cylinder or valve has occurred.

18. Disposition of unserviceable cylinders is potentially dangerous and should be done only by qualified personnel (1).

19. Wrappings should be removed and cylinders should be cleaned before being taken into a clean area such as an operating room suite.

Storage

1. A definite area should be designated for storage of cylinders.
2. The storage area should be in a cool, clean room that is constructed of fire-resistant materials. Conductive flooring must be present where flammable gases are stored but is not required where only nonflammable gases are stored. Adequate ventilation should be provided so that if there is a leak in a cylinder, gas will not accumulate in the room. Easily visible signs with texts such as "GAS CYLINDERS. REMOVE TO A SAFE PLACE IN THE EVENT OF FIRE" and "OFF LIM-

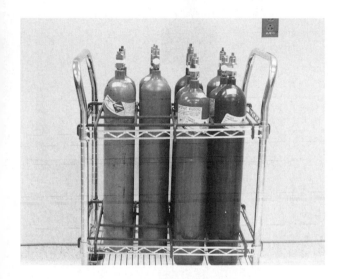

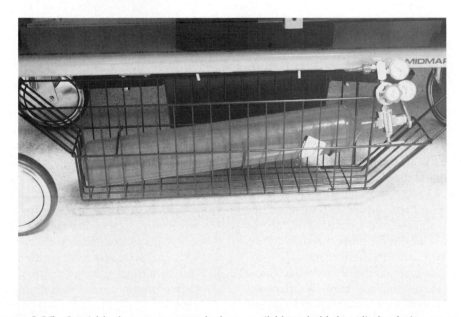

FIGURE 1.14. This cart is designed to store and transport E cylinders in an upright position.

FIGURE 1.15. Special baskets on transport beds are available to hold the cylinder during transport.

FIGURE **1.16.** An unsafe practice. Cylinders should not be allowed to be upright and unsecured.

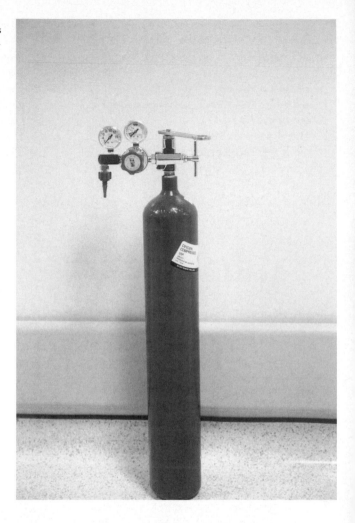

ITS TO UNAUTHORIZED PERSONNEL" should be hung outside the storage area. Signs reading "NO SMOKING," "NO OPEN FLAMES OR SPARKS," "NO OIL OR GREASE," and "NO COMBUSTIBLE MATERIALS" should be posted inside the room and on the door. Cylinders should not be stored in an operating room.

3. Cylinders may be stored in the open but should be protected against extremes of weather and from the ground beneath. During winter, stored cylinders must be protected against accumulations of ice and snow. In summer, cylinders must be screened against continuous exposure to direct rays of the sun in localities where high temperatures prevail. Smoking or open flames should be prohibited in storage areas.

4. Cylinders should be stored in a secure area and subject to removal only by authorized personnel. Cylinders in public areas should be protected from tampering. Deaths have been reported where nitrous oxide has been used for recreational purposes (17).

5. Cylinders of nitrous oxide should be stored where the opportunity for theft and indiscriminate use is minimized. There should be a system for detecting unusually heavy use or loss of nitrous oxide (1). Any theft should be reported promptly to the police and the supplier.

6. Cylinders containing flammable gases should

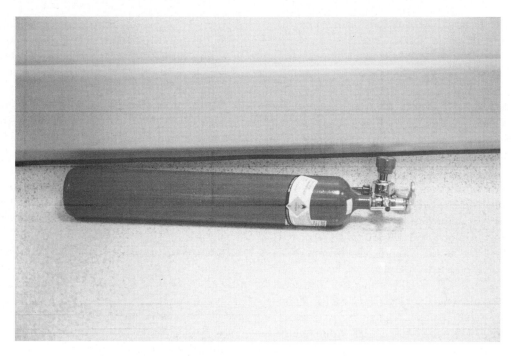

FIGURE 1.17. If there is no means to secure a cylinder upright, it is safer to have it on its side. However, personnel may trip over it or damage it.

not be stored in an enclosure containing oxidizing gases (nitrous oxide, oxygen, or compressed air). Other nonflammable (inert) medical gases may be stored in the same enclosure as oxidizing gases.

7. Combustible materials should not be kept near cylinders containing oxygen or nitrous oxide. An exception to this may be made in the case of cylinder shipping cartons or crates (2). Cylinder storage racks may be made of wood.

8. Sources of heat in storage locations must be protected or located so that cylinders are not heated to the point of activation of integral safety devices. In no case shall the temperature of the cylinder exceed 125°F (52°C).

9. Cylinders should not be exposed to continuous dampness, corrosive chemicals, or fumes because these may damage the cylinders and cause valve protection caps to stick.

10. Cylinders should be protected from mechanical shock. They should not be stored where heavy moving objects may strike them or fall on them.

11. Small cylinders are best stored upright or horizontally in bins or racks constructed of a nonflammable material that will not damage the cylinder surface when it is moved (Fig. 1.14). Large cylinders should be stored upright against a wall and chained in place.

12. Wrappers should be removed from cylinders before storage. Their presence in the storage area is undesirable because they are frequently dirty, provide a combustible medium, and conceal the cylinder labels.

13. A cylinder should not be draped with any material. A combustible mixture may accumulate under the drape, and its removal could provide a spark.

14. Containers should be grouped by contents and by sizes (if different sizes are present) when different types of gases are stored in the same location. Full cylinders should be stored so that they are used in the order they were received from the supplier. Empty cylinders should be marked as such and segregated from full cylinders to avoid confusion and delay.

15. There should be a system of inventory for both empty and full cylinders.

Use

1. Before use, the contents of the cylinder should be identified by the label. The color of a cylinder should not be relied on for identification. The cylinder should be returned to the manufacturer unused if the label is missing, illegible, or altered or if the cylinder color and label do not correspond. The user should also read the precautionary information on the label and follow the recommendations.

2. Only cylinders with the letters DOT or ICC (for Interstate Commerce Commission) should be used. In Canada equivalent cylinders are marked BTC (Board of Transport Commissioners) or CTC (Canadian Transport Commission). A cylinder that does not show evidence of inspection within the required period should not be used. The cylinder valve, especially the pressure relief device, outlet, and pin index holes, should be checked for defects. The valve outlet should be clean and pin indexed or have a proper large valve outlet connection.

3. A pressure-reducing regulator should always be used. The regulator inside the machine performs this function for small cylinders attached to an anesthesia machine.

4. Full small cylinders are usually supplied with a protective cover over the outlet to prevent contamination (Fig. 1.18). This should be removed immediately before fitting the cylinder to the dispensing equipment.

5. The valve protection cap on large cylinders should be removed just before connecting the cylinder for use. Excessive force should not be used.

6. The regulator should be inspected for signs of damage and to ensure it is free of foreign materials before it is connected to a cylinder.

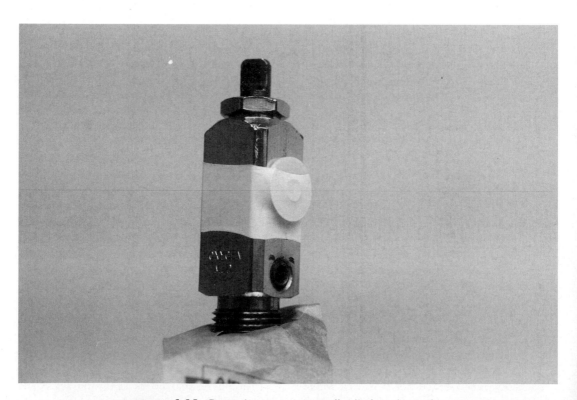

FIGURE 1.18. Protective cover over small cylinder valve outlet.

All wrappings should be removed. Regulators should be kept in good condition and stored in plastic bags to avoid contamination.

7. Before any fitting is applied to the cylinder valve, particles of dust, metal shavings, and other foreign matter should be cleared from the outlet by removing the protective cap or seal and slowly and briefly opening ("cracking") the valve with the port pointed away from the user and any other persons. This reduces the possibility of a flash fire or explosion when the valve is later opened with the fittings in place; also the dust will not be blown into the anesthesia machine or other equipment where it could clog filters or interfere with the internal workings.

8. A sealing washer (gasket) in good condition should always be used with a small cylinder valve. It fits over the port (see Fig. 1.6). Only one washer should be used. If more than one is used, the pins on the yoke or regulator may not extrude far enough to engage the mating holes and the Pin Index Safety System may be negated or a leak may occur (18, 19).

9. The threads on the regulator-to-cylinder valve connection or the pin indexing devices on the yoke-to-cylinder valve connections should mate properly. Connections that do not fit should never be forced.

10. Outlets and connections should be tightened only with wrenches or other tools provided or recommended by the manufacturer. Wrenches with malaligned jaws should not be used because they may damage the equipment or slip and injure personnel. Excessive force should not be used. The handwheel should never be hammered in an attempt to open or close the valve.

11. The valve on a cylinder should be opened before bringing the apparatus to the patient or the patient to the apparatus. If a Bourdon gauge–type regulator is being used, the low-pressure adjustment screw of the regulator should be turned counterclockwise until it turns freely before the cylinder valve is opened. If the cylinder is attached to the yoke of an anesthesia machine or a regulator/flowmeter, the flow control valve for that gas

should be closed before the cylinder valve is opened.

12. The person opening a cylinder valve should position himself or herself and the apparatus so that the valve outlet and the face of the regulator gauge point away from all persons. The user should stand to the side—i.e., not in front and not in back.

13. A cylinder valve should always be opened SLOWLY (16). If gas passes quickly into the space between the valve and the yoke or regulator, the rapid recompression in this space will generate large amounts of heat. Because there is little time for dissipation of this heat, this constitutes an adiabatic process (one in which heat is neither lost nor gained from the environment). Particles of dust, grease, etc., present in this space may be ignited by the heat, causing a flash fire or explosion (16). Opening the valve slowly prolongs the time of recompression and permits some of the heat to dissipate. The cylinder valve should continue to be opened slowly until the pressure on the gauge stabilizes, then opened fully.

14. After the cylinder valve is opened the pressure should be checked. A cylinder with a pressure substantially greater than the service pressure should not be used and should be marked and returned to the supplier. A cylinder arriving with a pressure substantially below the service pressure should be checked for leaks.

15. If a cylinder valve is open but no pressure is registered on the gauge or no gas flows, the cylinder valve should be closed and the cylinder should be disconnected from the dispensing apparatus, marked defective, and returned to the supplier with a note indicating the problem.

16. If a hissing sound is heard when the valve is opened, a large leak exists and the connection should be tightened. If the sound does not disappear, the sealing washer should be replaced (in the case of a small cylinder valve). However, under no circumstances should more than one washer be used. Soapy water, a commercial leak detection fluid, or other suitable solution should be applied to all parts

if the hissing sound persists. Bubbles will appear at the site(s) of the leak(s). A flame should never be used for this purpose. Should a leak be found in the cylinder valve itself, it may be possible to tighten the packing nut by turning it slightly in a clockwise direction (see special handle in Fig. 1.3), unless the manufacturer recommends otherwise. If the leak cannot be remedied by tightening connections without using excessive force, the valve should be closed, and the cylinder should be marked defective and returned to the supplier with a note indicating the fault.

17. Even if no hissing sound is audible when the valve is opened, a slow leak may be present and should be suspected if there is loss of pressure when no gas is being used. These leaks should be located and corrected.

18. When in use, a cylinder must be secured to a cylinder stand or to apparatus of sufficient size to render the entire assembly stable. Cylinders should not be attached to portable objects such as beds or sources of heat.

19. Freestanding cylinders shall be properly chained or supported in a cylinder stand or cart.

20. The valve should always be fully open when a cylinder is in use. Marginal opening may result in failure to deliver adequate gas.

After Use

1. Any time an extended period of nonuse is anticipated, the cylinder valve should be closed completely and all pressure vented (bled) from the system.

2. An empty or near-empty cylinder should not be left on an anesthesia machine. A defective check valve in the yoke could result in accidental filling if the valve is left open. In addition, the presence of an empty cylinder may create a false sense of security. Yokes should not be left empty. If a full cylinder is not available, a yoke plug (see Chapter 4) should be in place. Some gas suppliers prefer that cylinders be returned with enough pressure (e.g., 25 psig) remaining to maintain the integrity of the cylinder.

3. The valve should be closed and all pressure released before removing a cylinder from a regulator or yoke.

4. The lower part of the tag should be removed when a cylinder is empty. A DOT green, yellow, or red label should be covered with an "Empty" label or the lower portion of the combination label-tag should be removed if the cylinder is provided with the combination tag.

5. Valves should be completely closed on all empty cylinders. Often cylinders are not completely empty, and accidents have resulted from release of gas from a supposedly empty cylinder. If the valve is left open on an empty cylinder, debris and contaminants could be sucked into it when the temperature changes.

6. Valve protection caps should be replaced before shipment back to the manufacturer.

Transfilling

Transfilling should not be performed by unskilled, untrained persons (1, 2). It is best performed by a gas manufacturer or distributor. If performed by a user, it should be in accordance with suggested procedures and not in a patient care area. There are several hazards.

1. Transfer of medical gases from one cylinder to another by inexperienced persons may adversely affect purity.

2. When small cylinders are transfilled from large cylinders containing gas at high pressure, rapid recompression of the gas in the small cylinder may cause the temperature to rise sufficiently to ignite combustible materials and oxidize metals.

3. The hazard of overfilling small cylinders is always present. Filling capacities may vary for cylinders even though their sizes appear to be the same. Overfilling may result in damage to the cylinder or dispensing equipment.

4. Cylinders used for one gas may accidentally be charged with a gas other than that originally contained in the cylinder, resulting in a dangerous mixture. If an oxygen cylinder were filled with a gas other than oxygen, hypoxia could occur with use.

5. Safety relief devices and other parts must be inspected at frequent intervals to ensure safe

operation and repairs and to ensure that replacements are made when defects are found. This may not be done if transfilling is performed by users.

Hazards

Incorrect Cylinder

In spite of almost universal use of the Pin Index Safety System, reports of incorrect tanks being connected to yokes or regulators continue to appear (20–31). Yokes or regulators may be incorrectly built or altered. Pins can be bent, broken, sawed off, or forced into the yoke or regulator (32); pin index holes may become worn; and more than one washer may be used. Some lasers have yokes that lack pins (25).

Incorrect Contents

Cylinders may not contain the gas for which they are indexed and labeled (33–36). The gases may not be mixed in cylinders with mixtures (37).

Incorrect Valve

Cylinders may be correctly labeled for the gas contained but have valves for other gases (38–41). This usually will prevent their attachment to the dispensing apparatus. Industrial, rather than medical, gas cylinders are sometimes used to power surgical tools. These may have connections that fit equipment designed for other gases (42).

Incorrect Color

Cylinders may be painted with other than their standard color (39).

Incorrect Labeling

Cylinders with the correct color and valve may have incorrect labels (38, 43).

Inoperable Valve

Cylinders may be delivered with inoperable or blocked valve outlets (8, 39, 44).

Damaged Valve

If the retaining screw of the yoke is screwed into the safety relief device instead of the conical depression, the valve will be damaged. This may result in a leak of cylinder contents (9, 10).

Suffocation

Sudden discharge of large quantities of gas from a cylinder into a closed space could displace the air from that space, creating a dangerous condition. If an oxygen-deficient atmosphere is suspected, the space should be checked with an oxygen monitor. A number of deaths because of inhalation of nitrous oxide has been reported (45, 46).

Fires

Materials that burn in air will burn much more vigorously and at a higher temperature in oxygen at normal pressure and explosively in oxygen under pressure (2). Some materials that do not burn in air will burn in an oxygen-enriched atmosphere, particularly under pressure. Materials that can be ignited in air have lower ignition energies in oxygen. Many materials may be ignited by friction at a valve seat or stem packing or by adiabatic compression produced when oxygen at high pressure is rapidly introduced into a system initially at low pressure. If oxygen equipment is contaminated with grease, oil, paraffin, or other combustible substances, explosive rupture and burning of components may occur (2, 18, 47, 48). Oxygen regulators and cylinders contaminated with oil have been sold (49–51).

Fires can occur if the incorrect gas is used. A fire has been reported during laparoscopy as a result of the incorrect gas being used to inflate the abdomen (52). In this case, a cylinder of carbon dioxide and oxygen rather than one with pure carbon dioxide was used.

Explosion

Because gas in cylinders is under pressure, rapid escape of cylinder contents and rocketing of the cylinder are potential hazards (53–55). Cylinders are sometimes overfilled (38, 39, 56). A cylinder that has been incorrectly filled with the wrong gas may explode if the valve does not have the proper pressure relief device (55).

Improper handling or storage of cylinders can cause them to fall over. If a valve protection cap is not present, the valve could snap off. If the packing nut rather than the stem is loosened, the stem may be ejected when the valve is opened (6). Cylinders with defective valves may be manufactured (57).

Contamination of Cylinder Contents

Medical gases in cylinders may contain contaminants (39, 58–60). Medical-grade oxygen is required to be 99% pure (58, 61). Of the remaining 1% (10,000 ppm), not more than 300 ppm of carbon dioxide, 10 ppm of carbon monoxide, or 5 ppm of oxides of nitrogen can be present. No other contaminants are specifically excluded from the other 9685 ppm. Thus the possibility exists that oxygen or other gases may contain potentially dangerous amounts of other compounds and not be in violation of existing standards (58). An industrial-grade gas may not have the same requirements for purity as a medical-grade gas and may contain relatively large amounts of impurities (42). Accidental use of such gas could cause significant problems. Cases of poisoning by contamination of nitrous oxide cylinders with higher oxides of nitrogen have occurred (59).

There should be no odor from the contents of compressed gas cylinders, and a cylinder should not be used if the gas has an odor. The cylinder should be sequestered, and the appropriate authorities contacted.

Moisture may contaminate a cylinder and flow into the dispensing equipment if the cylinder is inverted (62). Adiabatic expansion of gas as it is released causes cooling, and the moisture could form ice and jam the regulator or yoke. In the past, this has been a significant problem with nitrous oxide.

Traces of methylnitrate, a toxic substance associated with pulmonary complications, has been found in nitrous oxide cylinders (63).

Theft of Nitrous Oxide

Theft of nitrous oxide for substance abuse purposes can be a serious problem. Deaths have been reported (17).

Overfilled Cylinders

Nitrous oxide cylinders that were full of liquid and had excessive pressures have been reported (38, 64, 65).

Thermal Injury

Frostbite injury from nitrous oxide has been reported in patients using the drug recreationally and in anesthesia providers and others handing it occupationally (7, 46, 66, 67, 68).

LIQUID OXYGEN CONTAINERS

Small specially designed containers filled with liquid oxygen have become popular, especially for patient transfer. Another use is when anesthesia is administered outside a health care facility (e.g., by armed forces) (69). Advantages include low pressure, compactness, low weight, and simplicity.

Equipment

A stationary unit (reservoir, supply container) is kept in a suitable area and refilled by the gas supplier as needed (Fig. 1.19). The smaller portable (receiving) units are filled from the stationary unit. The portable unit has a means of regulating oxygen flow. The amount of gas contained can be measured by weighing.

Each container must have a pressure relief device and a means to limit the amount of liquid oxygen contained. When not in use, the pressure in the container is controlled by venting excess gas to atmosphere. This limits the time oxygen can be stored in the portable unit (70).

Liquid gas containers are manufactured, maintained, filled, and transported in accordance with DOT regulations. They are broader and less tall in comparison to cylinders. Required markings include the specification number, service pressure for which the container is designed, an identifying mark of the original container owner, and a serial number. The date of original manufacture and a symbol identifying the inspector are also present.

Rules for Safe Use of Liquid Oxygen Containers

1. A considerable time must be allowed for the liquid oxygen to dissipate if it is spilled.
2. Contact between the skin and liquid oxygen must be avoided.
3. Liquid oxygen equipment must be kept clean of organic or combustible materials. These materials can react violently with liquid oxygen.
4. Cryogenic transfilling devices must be kept free of moisture to prevent accumulation of frost on valves or couplings that may cause them to freeze open or shut.

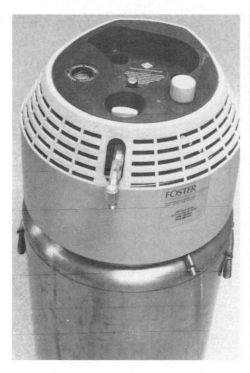
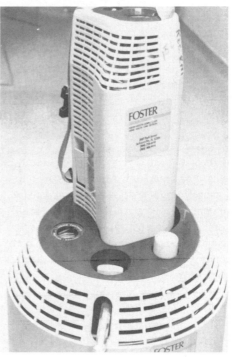

FIGURE 1.19. Liquid oxygen containers. **Left,** The stationary unit, which is refilled by the gas supplier as needed. Note the pressure relief valve at right front. **Right,** the portable unit is attached to the stationary unit for transfilling.

5. Containers should not be subjected to extremes of heat or cold.
6. Containers should be handled so as to avoid physical damage.
7. Markings and labels on containers must be legible and must not be altered.
8. Under no circumstances should any attempt be made to loosen, tighten, or otherwise tamper with the pressure relief device.

Storage

1. Both the stationary and portable units should be kept in open, cool, well-ventilated areas. Containers should not be stored in a closed space such as a closet (2).
2. Liquid oxygen containers should be stored away from any heat source (1).
3. Containers should be protected from corrosive atmospheres.
4. Containers should be stored in an upright position.

Transfilling

Liquid oxygen may be transferred by means of a cryogenic flexible hose assembly or the manufacturer's noninterchangeable direct connection. If a flexible hose assembly is used, its end connections must conform with CGA regulations (1) or the manufacturer's noninterchangeable connections and must have a pressure relief device.

Transfilling must be performed in a well-ventilated location that is remote from patient care areas, has no sources of ignition, and is posted with "NO SMOKING" signs.

Hazards

Fires

Ignition may occur if liquid oxygen equipment becomes contaminated with hydrocarbons such as oil or grease or other combustible materials. Vaporization of spilled liquid oxygen will result in an oxygen-enriched atmosphere, which increases the fire hazard (1).

High Pressure

The large volume of gaseous oxygen resulting from vaporization of liquid oxygen has the potential, if trapped in a closed space not protected by adequate pressure relief devices, to generate pressures high enough to cause danger to life, limb, and property (1).

Burns

Liquid oxygen is at a very low temperature. Contact with cold liquid or frosted valves or couplings may cause cryogenic burns. Physical damage to or failure of liquid oxygen equipment can result in liquid spilling or spraying in an uncontrolled manner. Relief valves on portable containers may open prematurely and vent liquid oxygen during or immediately after filling (1, 71).

Equipment Freezing

Valves or couplings may freeze shut if they are not kept free of moisture (1).

Inaccurate Flows

One study showed a high percentage of portable liquid oxygen devices had flows that differed substantially from those set (1, 72).

REFERENCES

1. Compressed Gas Association. Handbook of compressed gases. 3rd ed. New York: Van Nostrand, Reinhold, 1990.
2. Klein BR. Health care facilities handbook. 5th ed. Quincy, MA: National Fire Protection Association, 1996.
3. Russell WJ. Equipment for anaesthesia and intensive care. Adelaide, Australia: Author, 1997.
4. Petty C. The anesthesia machine. New York: Churchill Livingstone, 1987.
5. McPherson SP. Respiratory therapy equipment. 3rd ed. St. Louis: CV Mosby, 1985.
6. Finch JS. A report on a possible hazard of gas cylinder tanks. Anesthesiology 1970;33:46
7. Yamashita M, Motokawa K, Watanabe S. Do not use the "innovated" cylinder valve handle for cracking the valve. Anesthesiology 1986;64:658.
8. Smith PJB. BOC cylinder valve keys and tight valves. Anaesthesia 1983;38:1232.
9. Fox JWC, Fox EJ. An unusual occurrence with a cyclopropane cylinder. Anesth Analg 1968;47:624–626.
10. Milliken RA. Correspondence. Anesth Analg 1971;50:775.
11. Small medical gas cylinders—Pin-index yoke-type valve connections. Geneva: International Standards Organization, 1991: 407.
12. Andrews JJ, Johnston RV Jr. Not all E cylinders were created equal. Anesth Analg 1992;75:154.
13. Jones PL. Some observations on nitrous oxide cylinders during emptying. Br J Anaesth 1974;46:534–538.
14. Gas cylinders for medical use—Marking for identification of content. Geneva: International Standards Organization, 1997: 32.
15. Kumar P, Mishra LD. Deviation from international colour codes. Anaesthesia 1986;41:1055–1056.
16. Czajka RJ. Cylinder caution: open slowly to minimize recompression heat. Anesthesiology 1978;49:226.
17. Anonymous. Hospital staff death linked to NO_2 inhalation. Biomedical Safety & Standards 1993;23:145–146.
18. Anonymous. Oxygen regulator fire caused by use of two yoke washers. Technology for Anesthesia 1990;11:1–2.
19. Anonymous. Improper connection of laparoscopic insufflators and gas cylinders. Technology for Anesthesia 1992;12:2–3.
20. Anonymous. Patient dies after oxygen tank is replaced with carbon dioxide; investigation clears hospital. Biomedical Safety & Standards 1983;13:5–6.
21. Anonymous. Misconnection of oxygen regulator to nitrogen cylinder could cause death. Biomedical Safety & Standards 1988;18:90–91.
22. Anonymous. Nonstandard user modification of gas cylinder pin indexing. Technology for Anesthesia 1989;10:2.
23. Anonymous. Medical gas cylinders. Technology for Anesthesia 1991;12:12.
24. Goebel WM. Failure of nitrous oxide and oxygen pin-indexing. Anesth Prog 1980;27:188–191.
25. Anonymous. Lack of pin-indexing for laser gas supplies. Technology for Anesthesia 1987;8:1–3.
26. MacMillan RR, Marshall MA. Failure of the pin index system on a Cape Waine Ventilator. Anaesthesia 1981;36:334–335.
27. Mead P. Hazard with cylinder yoke. Anaesthesia and Intensive Care 1981;9:79–80.
28. Euliano TY, Lampotang, Hardcastle JF. Patient simulator identifies faulty H-cylinder. Journal of Clinical Monitoring 1995;11:394–395.
29. Orr IA, Hamilton L. Entonox hazard. Anaesthesia 1985;40:496.
30. Upton LG, Robert EC Jr. Hazard in administering

nitrous oxide analgesia: report of a case. J Am Dent Assoc 1977;94:696–697.

31. Hogg CE. Pin-indexing failures. Anesthesiology 1973; 38:85–87.

32. Chamley D, Trethowen L. Pin index failure. Anaesthesia and Intensive Care 1993;21:128–129.

33. Ward PM, Platt MW. Inappropriate filling of cylinders. Anaesthesia 1992;47:544.

34. Anonymous. Nitrous oxide cylinders found to contain carbon dioxide. Biomedical Safety & Standards 1990; 20:84.

35. Menon MRB, Lett Z. Incorrectly filled cylinders. Anaesthesia 1991;46:155–156.

36. Jawan B, Lee JH. Cardiac arrest caused by an incorrectly filled oxygen cylinder: A case report. Br J Anaesth 1990;64:749–751.

37. Anonymous. Cylinders with unmixed helium/oxygen. Technology for Anesthesia 1990;10:4.

38. Boon PE. C-size cylinders. Anaesthesia and Intensive Care 1990;18:586–587.

39. Feeley TW, Bancroft ML, Brooks RA, et al. Potential hazards of compressed gas cylinders: a review. Anesthesiology 1978;48:72–74.

40. Jayasuriya JP. Another example of Murphy's Law—mix up of pin index valves. Anaesthesia 1986;41:1164.

41. Steward DJ, Sloan IA. Additional pin-indexing failures. Anesthesiology 1973;39:355.

42. Russell WJ. Industrial gas hazard. Anaesthesia and Intensive Care 1985;13:106.

43. Sawhney KK, Yoon YK. Erroneous labeling of a nitrous oxide cylinder. Anesthesiology 1983;59:260.

44. Blogg CE, Colvin MP. Apparently empty oxygen cylinders. Br J Anaesth 1977;49:87.

45. DiMaio VJ, Garriott JC. Four deaths resulting from abuse of nitrous oxide. J Forensic Sci 1978;23:169–172.

46. Garriott J, Petty CS. Death from inhalant abuse: toxicological and pathological evaluation of 34 cases. Clinical Toxicology 1980;16:305–315.

47. Garfield JM, Allen GW, Silverstein P, et al. Flash fire in a reducing valve. Anesthesiology 1971;34:578–579.

48. Ito Y, Horikowa H, Ichiyanagi K. Fires and explosions with compressed gases: report of an accident. Br J Anaesth 1965;37:140–141.

49. Anonymous. Medical gas cylinders. Technology for Anesthesia 1985;6:17.

50. Anonymous. Oxygen regulators may be contaminated with oil. Biomedical Safety & Standards 1990;20:13.

51. Anonymous. Oxygen cylinders recalled because of oil contamination. Biomedical Safety & Standards 1991; 21:20.

52. Greillich PE, Grfeilich NB, Froelich EG. Intraabdominal fire during laparoscopic cholecystectomy. Anesthesiology 1995;83:871–874.

53. Anonymous. Medical Gas Cylinders. Technology for Anesthesia 1987;7:10.

54. Morse HN. Legal case: who is responsible for the oxygen-tank explosion?—manufacturer or user. Med Elect Prod, Dec. 6, 1980, p. 6.

55. Tracey JA, Kennedy J, Magner J. Explosion of carbon dioxide cylinder. Anaesthesia 1984;39:938–939.

56. Gray WM, Richardson W. Filling CO_2 cylinders. Anaesthesia 1985;40:504.

57. Anonymous. Oxygen cylinder valves could "break off." Biomedical Safety & Standards 1997;27:12–13.

58. Bassell GM, Rose DM, Bruce DL. Purity of USP medical oxygen. Anesth Analg 1979;58:441–442.

59. Clutton-Brock J. Two cases of poisoning by contamination of nitrous oxide with higher oxides of nitrogen during anaesthesia. Br J Anaesth 1967;39:388–392.

60. Herlihy WJ. Report: contamination of medical oxygen. Anaesthesia and Intensive Care 1973;1:240–241.

61. Rendell-Baker L. Purity of oxygen, USP. Anesth Analg 1980;59:314–315.

62. Coveler LA, Lester RC. Contaminated oxygen cylinder. Anesth Analg 1989;69:674–676.

63. Barankey MA. Contaminated N_2O is possible toxic etiology. Anesthesia Patient Safety Foundation Newsletter 1994;9:10.

64. Meyer RM, Ferderbar PJ. Liquid full nitrous oxide cylinders. Anesthesiology 1993;78:584–586.

65. Newstead J. Overfull nitrous oxide cylinders. Anaesthesia and Intensive Care 1991;19:473.

66. Svartling N, Ranta S, Vuola J, et al. Life-threatening airway obstruction from nitrous oxide induced frostbite of the oral cavity. Anaesthesia and Intensive Care 1996;24:717–720.

67. Hwang J, Himel H, Edlich R. Frostbite of the face after recreational misuse of nitrous oxide. Burns 1996; 22:152–153.

68. Rowbottom SJ. Nitrous oxide abuse. Anaesthesia and Intensive Care 1988;16:241–242.

69. Bull PT, Merrill SB, Moody RA, et al. Anaesthesia during the Falklands campaign. The experience of the Royal Navy. Anaesthesia 1983;38:770–775.

70. Ramage CMH, Kee SS, Bristow A. A new portable oxygen system using liquid oxygen. Anaesthesia 1991; 46:395–397.

71. Anonymous. Valves may open & release liquid oxygen. Biomedical Safety & Standards 1990;20:20–21.

72. Massey LW, Hussey JD, Albert RK. Inaccurate oxygen delivery in some portable liquid oxygen devices. American Review of Respiratory Disease 1988;137:204–205.

QUESTIONS
FOR THE FOLLOWING QUESTIONS, ANSWER

A if 1, 2, and 3 are correct
B if 1 and 3 are correct
C if 2 and 4 are correct
D if 4 is correct
E if 1, 2, 3, and 4 are correct

1. Liquefied compressed gases at room temperature include the following
   1. Carbon dioxide
   2. Air
   3. Nitrous oxide
   4. Oxygen

2. A typical cylinder label includes
   1. A statement of hazard
   2. The name of the gas in the cylinder
   3. A signal word
   4. The name of the manufacturer or distributor

3. Adiabatic compression
   1. Refers to compression of a gas in a small space
   2. Occurs downstream of a regulator
   3. Can cause a fire
   4. Occurs when a cylinder valve is opened slowly

4. The likelihood of a fire is reduced by the following measures
   1. Cracking the cylinder valve before use
   2. Opening the cylinder valve slowly
   3. Storing regulators in plastic bags
   4. Keeping the cylinder draped during storage

5. Hazards of transfilling cylinder include the following
   1. Flash fires
   2. Overfilling
   3. Contamination of gases
   4. Filling with the wrong gas

6. The filling density is
   1. The ratio of the weight of gas in a container to the weight of water that container would hold
   2. The percentage of a cylinder volume occupied by liquefied gas
   3. A means to limit the amount of a liquefied gas in a cylinder
   4. Proportional to the density of the gas in the cylinder

7. Cracking a cylinder valve
   1. Is momentarily opening it to blow away foreign matter from the outlet
   2. Should be performed before attachment of a dispensing device
   3. Reduces the likelihood of flash fires
   4. Refers to a fracture of the stem of the valve

FOR THE FOLLOWING QUESTIONS, SELECT THE CORRECT ANSWER

8. The government agency responsible for regulating medical gas cylinders and containers in the United States
   A. Food and Drug Administration
   B. Department of Health and Human Services
   C. Department of the Interior
   D. Department of Transportation
   E. Department of Labor

9. An E cylinder of oxygen contains approximately how many liters?
   A. 500
   B. 650
   C. 750
   D. 900
   E. 1200

10. All of the following are required permanent makings on a cylinder except
    A. The service pressure
    B. The serial number
    C. The name of the contained gas
    D. The test date
    E. The symbol of the producer, user, or manufacturer

11. The best means for identifying the contents of a cylinder is the
    A. Color
    B. Label
    C. Tag

D. Markings on the cylinder shoulder
E. Pin index holes

12. The size cylinder most commonly used on anesthesia machines and for patient transport
A. A
B. B
C. C
D. D
E. E

13. If an empty oxygen cylinder is found on an anesthesia machine, the best action to take is to
A. Remove the empty cylinder and leave the yoke empty
B. Remove the cylinder and replace it with a yoke plug
C. Mark the cylinder empty and leave it in place
D. Remove the empty cylinder and replace it with a full cylinder
E. Open the adjacent cylinder valve fully

14. 1 kPa is approximately equivalent to
A. 10 cm H_2O
B. 14.7 psi

C. 0.76 mm Hg
D. 100 mbar
E. 1.47 psi

ANSWERS

1. B. Although both oxygen and air can be liquefied at very low temperatures, they are gases at room temperature.
2. E.
3. B. Adiabatic compression occurs upstream of the regulator and is associated with rapid opening of a cylinder valve.
4. A. Gas may accumulate under a drape and be ignited when the cover is removed.
5. E
6. B
7. A
8. D
9. B
10. C
11. B. Color should not be used because of the following: color codes differ in various countries, fading problems, differences in lighting, and variable color perception by personnel.
12. E
13. D
14. A

Medical Gas Pipeline Systems

MOST HEALTHCARE FACILITIES use a pipeline system to deliver nonflammable gases such as oxygen, nitrous oxide, air, carbon dioxide, and nitrogen to anesthetizing locations and other areas where they are used for administration to patients and to power (pneumatically drive) ventilators or surgical tools. Special care areas where patients depend on oxygen or medical air may be equipped with an alternate local source of supply that is readily available for use in the event of a failure of the medical gas pipeline system (1, 2).

Usually, central piping systems are installed by mechanical contractors and maintained by the engineering or maintenance department with little input from the anesthesia providers. This not only neglects a potentially valuable contribution but also leaves those who use the gases uninformed as to how the system works. Because the system is mostly out of sight and as a rule functions well, the system often does not attract attention until a problem occurs.

Anesthesia personnel should play a key role in designing the piping system when a new facility or addition is being planned (see Chapter 28). Input from the anesthesia personnel is important in sizing the system and locating outlets (including remote parts of the facility where patients undergo diagnostic studies or various types of therapy). Careful planning may avoid expense and inconvenience at a later date.

STANDARDS AND SOURCES OF INFORMATION

The National Fire Protection Association (NFPA), the Compressed Gas Association (CGA), the Canadian Standards Association (CSA), and the International Standards Organization (ISO) have published a number of documents related to piping systems (2–9). Many of their provisions are incorporated into law in many locations. There are also many state and local codes that preempt and sometimes exceed these standards. Compliance with these standards is one of the bases for accreditation by the Joint Commission on the Accreditation of Healthcare Organizations (JCAHO). These organizations do not approve, inspect, or certify any installations, procedures, equipment, or materials. In most cases, compliance with standards is left to the individual gas supplier and facility. Although most medical gas pipeline systems in the United States and Canada are designed to conform to the recommendations of the NFPA and CGA, failure to adhere to existing regulations is widespread (10).

COMPONENTS

A medical gas distribution system consists of a central supply, piping extending to locations where gas may be required, and terminal units at each point of use. Hoses that extend from terminal units to the anesthesia machine or other equipment, although not part of the piped system, are included here because of their importance to anesthesia.

Sources of Supply

A central supply system may be located outdoors (with the control panel protected from the weather) in an enclosure used only for this purpose or in a room or enclosure used only for this purpose that is situated within a building that is used for other purposes. Access to the central supply area should be restricted to individuals familiar with and responsible for the system to prevent unauthorized persons from creating a hazard or harming themselves. The maximum amount of oxygen that can be stored inside a health care facility is 20,000 cubic feet (3).

A common type of central supply for a small facility is shown in Figure 2.1. Two banks (units) of cylinders are present (Fig. 2.2). Each bank must have its own pressure-reducing regulator and must contain a minimum of two cylinders or an average day's supply. Larger amounts may be necessary in areas remote from suppliers. The cylinders are connected to a common manifold (header), which converts them into one continuous supply. A check (nonreturn) valve is placed between each cylinder lead and the header to prevent loss of gas from the manifolded cylinders if there is a leak in an individual cylinder or lead. The primary (duty, running) supply is the portion actually supplying the system at any time, while the other bank is the secondary (standby) supply. The secondary supply automatically becomes the primary supply when the primary supply is unable to supply the system. This is a normal operating procedure. The switch over is accomplished by a

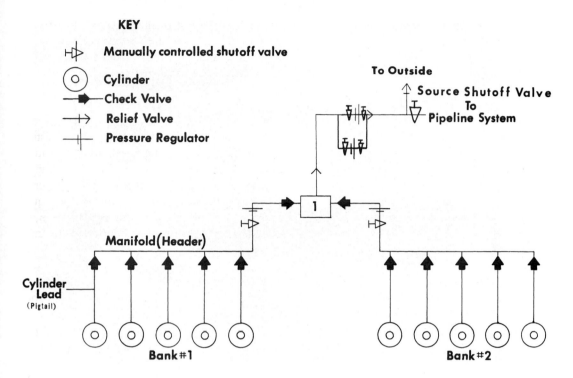

1. Manifold Changeover Device

FIGURE 2.1.   Cylinder supply system without reserve supply. This is known as an alternating supply system. The manual shutoff (on-off) valves permit isolation of either bank of cylinders. Fluctuations in the distribution pressure can be decreased by reducing the pressure in two stages, so a regulator is installed in the outgoing pipe. A manual shutoff valve must be located upstream of and a shutoff or check valve downstream of each regulator. This arrangement, plus having two regulators, makes it possible to service a regulator without shutting down the entire piped system. An actuating switch connected to the master signal panels must be present to indicate when, or just before, the changeover to the secondary bank occurs. Supply systems with different arrangements of valves and regulators are permissible if they provide equivalent safeguards. (Redrawn from a figure in National Fire Protection Association. Standard for Health Care Facilities [NFPA 99]. Quincy, MA: National Fire Protection Association, 1996.)

pressure-sensitive switch, the manifold changeover device. The *operating supply* is the portion of the supply system that normally supplies the piping system. The operating supply consists of a primary supply or a primary and secondary supply.

For larger systems, a reserve supply is added, as shown in Figure 2.3. The reserve supply operates in the event that the operating supply is unable to furnish sufficient gas to the system. The reserve is used for emergencies or when maintenance or repair of the operating supply is needed. An activating switch to indicate when or just before the reserve begins to supply the system must

be connected to the master signal panels. The size of the reserve system depends on the rate of use of the gas.

The reserve may consist of manifolded cylinders. If so, it must either be equipped with a check valve between each cylinder lead and the header or be provided with an activating switch that operates the master signals when the reserve drops to one day's supply. With a cryogenic liquid system, a smaller liquid container may act as a reserve supply. If so, a master signal must indicate when the reserve is reduced to one average day's supply or when the gas pressure available in the reserve unit

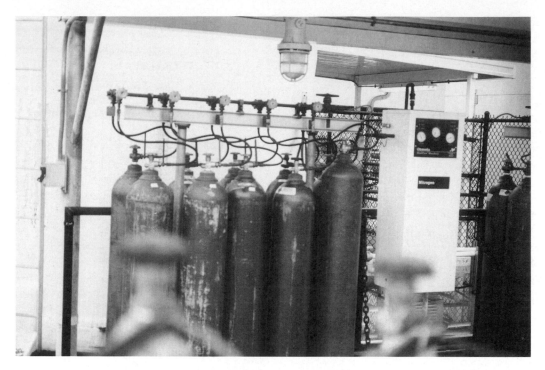

FIGURE 2.2. Cylinder supply system This shows primary and secondary supplies with switching mechanism. Note the header and cylinder leads.

is reduced below the pressure required to function properly.

Check valves between each cylinder lead and the manifold header are not required on the primary and secondary supplies if there is a reserve supply, but a check valve in the primary supply main line upstream of the point of intersection with the secondary or reserve supply is required.

A pressure-reducing (operating) regulator is installed in the main supply line upstream of the pressure relief valve. The pressures at which gases are piped varies with countries. In the United States gases other than nitrogen are normally piped at 345 to 380 kPa (50 to 55 psig). Nitrogen is usually delivered at 1100 kPa (160 psig). NFPA now permits pressures up to 2068 kPa (300 psig) (3). All final line regulators must be duplexed with suitable valving to permit service without completely shutting down the piped gas system.

Oxygen

Oxygen may be stored either as a liquid at low pressures or as a compressed gas in cylinders. A liquid container is usually preferred when large quantities are required. Cylinder supplies are used for small facilities, sections of facilities not piped for oxygen, and auxiliary systems.

Gaseous Supply

Oxygen may be supplied from G or H cylinders that are transported between the distributor and the central supply area or from cylinders that are fixed at the site and refilled by the distributor. A third possible source is oxygen concentrators (see Chapter 3) (11).

Liquid Supply

When large amounts of oxygen are required, it is less expensive and more convenient to store it as a liquid. Most often, liquid oxygen containers are refilled from supply trucks without interruption of service. Alternatively, filled liquid containers may be transported between the supplier and the facility.

Liquid oxygen containers are installed at ground level so they are readily accessible to supply trucks (Fig. 2.4). Liquid oxygen containers should be located where exposure to potential ignition sources is minimal. NFPA standards specify how far the container must be from sidewalks, parked vehicles, and other objects.

To prevent the liquid from evaporating, it must be kept at or below its boiling point ($-297°F$ [$-148°C$]) by keeping it in insulated vessels. Containers vary in size and shape. Containers are constructed similar to thermos bottles with outer and inner metal jackets separated by insulation and a layer of near vacuum to retard heat transfer from the exterior. Each container should have a contents indicator and low liquid level alarm. Gaseous oxygen is drawn off as required and passed through a heater to bring it up to ambient temperature and raise its pressure.

Because liquid oxygen vaporizes at low temper-

atures and a small quantity of liquid will produce a large volume of gas, it is important that these containers be provided with devices to allow some of the gas on top of the liquid to escape if the pressure rises. A minimum vapor space must be maintained.

Although the insulation of such a tank is usually good, a small amount of heat will be absorbed continuously from the surroundings, causing evaporation of the liquefied gas. The amount of this uncontrolled evaporation is normally less than the demand for the piped system. If there is no flow from the container to the pipeline, the pressure in the container will slowly increase until the safety relief valve opens and oxygen is vented to atmosphere. If a liquid system is left standing un-

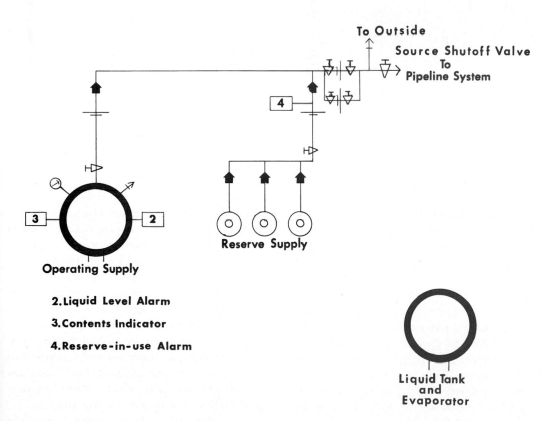

FIGURE 2.3. Bulk supply system. A liquid oxygen container serves as the operating supply with cylinders constituting the reserve supply. The reserve supply may also be a cryogenic liquid oxygen container. Operation of the reserve should activate the reserve-in-use alarm. This is known as a continuous-type system because one pri-

mary source (which is refilled periodically) always supplies the system under normal operating conditions. (Redrawn from a figure in National Fire Protection Association. Standard for Health Care Facilities [NFPA 99]. Quincy, MA: National Fire Protection Association, 1996.)

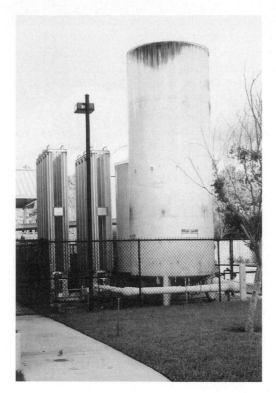

FIGURE 2.4. Liquid oxygen storage tank. Behind the large tank is a smaller liquid oxygen tank. To the left of this are two vaporizers.

used for long periods of time, a significant amount will be lost. The use of liquid containers is economical only when there is a fairly constant demand. Having the proper size container will minimize venting.

Most of the time, the oxygen is kept cold by the latent heat of vaporization as gaseous oxygen is removed and the temperature tends to fall. As the temperature falls, the pressure within the tank also falls. To maintain pressure, liquid oxygen must be removed from the tank and passed through a vaporizer (evaporator, vaporizing column, gasifier), which supplies heat. This consists of a coil, tube, or mesh which is heated by electricity or hot water.

Nitrous Oxide

Most facilities use manifolded cylinders to supply nitrous oxide to the pipeline system. One problem with nitrous oxide cylinders is that the regulator may become so cold that it freezes. Nitrous oxide may also be stored as a liquid at low pressure in insulated vessels similar to those used for oxygen.

Warning signs should be posted around areas where nitrous oxide tanks are located to warn that nitrous oxide is an asphyxiant and that a hypoxic mixture may be produced if there is a leak.

Medical Air

Medical air (air for breathing) is defined by the NFPA as air, regardless of its source, that has no detectable liquid hydrocarbons, less than 25 ppm gaseous hydrocarbons, less than 5 mg/m^3 of particulates of 1 micron size or greater at normal atmospheric pressure and a dew point (the temperature at which water vapor begins to condense when cooled) at 50 psig (345 kPa) of less than 39° F (4°C). (3). A special air system for non-breathing purposes and for gas-powered devices may be provided. The air provided by this system may not meet the requirements for medical air. It is often piped at pressures of up to 175 psig (1210 kPa). The individual use points are separately and manually regulated for individual applications.

Air may be supplied from manifolded cylinders; a proportioning device, which mixes gas from oxygen and nitrogen cylinders; or motor-driven compressors. Air from compressors is usually less clean and dry than that from cylinders but is less expensive if a large volume is required. Low levels of nitric oxide found in ambient air may cause improvement in oxygenation in ventilated patients (12).

The vast majority of piped air systems employ two or more compressors, which operate alternately or simultaneously, depending on demand. A typical system is shown in Figure 2.5. Most components must be duplexed and equipped with upstream and downstream shutoff valves to allow isolation and continued operation of the system in the event of failure of the component.

Each compressor takes in ambient air, compresses it to above the working pressure and supplies it to one or more receivers (accumulators, reservoir tanks, storage receivers, reservoirs, holding tanks, receiver tanks) from which air can be withdrawn as needed. This allows a nonpulsatile

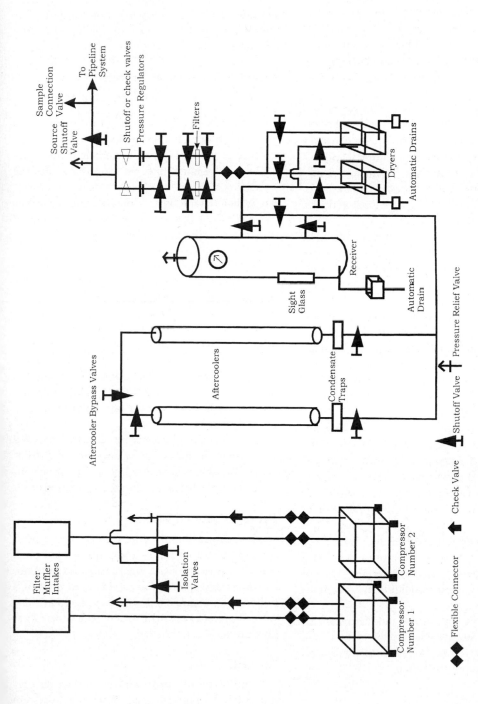

FIGURE 2.5.   Central supply for medical air. The filter/muffler on the inlet side of each compressor removes large particles from air aspirated through the intake. Each compressor is provided with an isolation (shutoff) valve and has a pressure relief valve and a check (one-way) valve in its discharge line. Receivers are sized according to the capacity of the compressors. Final line filters trap particulate, oil, and odors introduced by the system. These must be equipped with a visual indicator showing the status of the filter element life. Special scrubbers may be used to remove this or other pollutants in environments with high concentrations of carbon monoxide. Dryers may be of desiccant or refrigerant type. (Redrawn from a figure in National Fire Protection Association, Standard for Health Care Facilities [NFPA 99]. Quincy, MA: National Fire Protection Association, 1996.)

flow to be delivered to the regulator. It also serves to reduce wear on the compressor. Each compressor must be capable of handling 100% of the estimated peak demand. The receiver must be equipped with a pressure relief valve, automatic drain, sight glass to permit visual checking that the drains are operating properly, and a pressure gauge.

The intake should be in a location where it will take in air that is as free of dirt, fumes, and odors as possible. The location of the intake is usually outside but may be within the building if a source that is equal to or better than outside air is available. The location should not be close to or downwind of vacuum or other exhausts, loading docks, or other sources of polluted air.

Ambient air taken from a location free from auto exhausts or other sources of pollution is normally well within the limits required for compressed air by the *U.S. Pharmacopoeia* and NFPA for medical air (4).

The air at the intake should be checked periodically. Air quality varies from day to day and may exceed the contaminant limits of USP air for unacceptably long periods (4). There are cases in which an intake became improperly located as the environment around the intake changed as a result of changes in the facility (4, 13).

To render air suitable for medical use, its water content is reduced. An aftercooler in which the air is cooled and the condensed moisture removed is usually installed downstream of each compressor. More water may condense in the receiver. Additional water may be removed by running the air through a dryer.

Air downstream of the dryers and upstream of the piping system must be monitored for carbon monoxide and dew point with certain types of compressors and gaseous and liquid hydrocarbons (3).

Valves, pressure regulators, and alarms analogous to those in oxygen supply systems are needed. The reserve may be manifolded cylinders or a separate compressor system.

Nitrogen

Central nitrogen supplies may consist of manifolded high-pressure cylinders or cryogenic liquid containers.

Carbon Dioxide

Carbon dioxide is being piped more frequently because of its use for laparoscopic surgery. The source for piped carbon dioxide is high-pressure cylinders.

Piped Distribution System

There are three general classes of piping:

1) Main lines—pipes connecting the source to risers or branch lines or both.
2) Risers—vertical pipes connecting the main line with branch lines on various levels of the facility.
3) Branch (lateral) lines—the sections of the piping system that service a room or group of rooms on the same level of the facility.

Layouts of piped systems vary considerably. A typical one is shown in Figure 2.6. Pipes are made of copper. Generally oxygen is installed in $\frac{1}{2}$ inch outer diameter (OD) and other gases in $\frac{3}{8}$ inch OD pipes. Identification of the pipes at least every 20 feet and at least once in every room and story traversed by the piping system is required to ensure that personnel installing and maintaining the pipeline are aware of its content. The name and pressure of the gas inside the pipe and its direction of flow must be displayed.

Use of flexible hoses is restricted to exposed areas where the hoses can be inspected and maintained. Flexible hoses cannot penetrate or be concealed in walls, floors, ceilings, or partitions (3).

Pressure Relief Valves

Each central supply system must have a pressure relief valve set at 50% above normal line pressure downstream of the line regulator(s) and upstream of any shutoff valve. This is to prevent a buildup of pressure if a shutoff valve is closed. The valve should close automatically when the excess pressure has been relieved.

Shutoff Valves

Shutoff (on-off, isolating, section) valves permit isolation of specific areas of the piping system in the event of a problem and allow sections to be isolated for maintenance, repair, testing, or expansion without the whole system having to be switched off. Two types of shutoff valves exist: manual and service. Manual shutoff valves must be installed where they are visible and accessible at all times. Service shutoff valves are designed to be used only by authorized personnel. They are in locked cases or have their handles secured and tagged to prevent accidental closing.

Manual shutoff valves are installed in boxes with frangible or removable windows (Fig. 2.7A.). A quarter-turn valve with an indicating handle has become standard (Fig. 2.7B). Each valve should be marked to indicate function, gas, and area controlled and a caution that it should be closed only in an emergency.

Shutoff valves should be located where they will be readily accessible to those who need to use them in an emergency and where access is unlikely to be obstructed. Any person using piped gases should know where shutoff valves are located and exactly what they control. JCAHO has emphasized the importance of properly labeling shutoff valves and informing personnel of the locations of these valves. In the central supply there must be a manually-operated shutoff valve upstream of each regulator and a shutoff or check valve downstream.

A (source) shutoff valve is required at the outlet of the source of supply, upstream of the main line shutoff valve and must be located in the immediate vicinity of the source equipment. This allows the entire source of supply to be isolated.

The main supply line must be equipped with a manual shutoff valve near the entry into the building unless the source shutoff valve is accessible from within the building. It should be at a location well-known and readily accessible to those responsible for maintenance of the system but where any attempt to tamper with it would be noticed.

Each riser must be equipped with a manual shutoff valve adjacent to the connection to the main supply line. Each branch (lateral) line, except those supplying anesthetizing locations and other vital life support and critical areas such as postanesthesia care, intensive care, and coronary care units, must have a service shutoff valve where the lateral branches off the riser. A manual shutoff valve is required immediately outside each vital life sup-

port or critical care area and must be readily accessible in an emergency.

A separate manual shutoff valve is required for each anesthetizing location so that shutting off the supply of gas to one location will not affect other locations. The shutoff valve must be located outside the anesthetizing location so that in an emergency people inside the room can exit and then shut off gas supplies to the room. A facility is not precluded from installing a shutoff valve inside an anesthetizing location, although additional alarms would be required.

Emergency Oxygen Supply Connector

When the central oxygen supply is located outside the building served, a T fitting for connecting a temporary auxiliary source of supply for emergency or maintenance situations is required (3). The inlet must be located on the exterior of the building and must be protected from tampering and unauthorized access. This connection is downstream of the shutoff valve in the main supply line (Fig. 2.6). This connection must be provided with a pressure relief valve.

Alarms
Master Alarm System

A master alarm system monitors the central supply and the pressure in the main line for all medical gas systems. To ensure continuous responsible observation, master signal panels with auditory and visual alarms and pressure gauges must be located in two separate locations and wired in parallel to a single sensor for each condition. One panel should be in the principal working area of the department responsible for maintenance of the system and one or more panels located to ensure continuous surveillance during the working hours of the facility (e.g., telephone switchboard, security office, or other continuously staffed location) (3).

An alarm should signal when a changeover from the primary supply to the secondary bank has occurred, when or just before the reserve supply goes into operation, under certain circumstances when the reserve supply is reduced to one average day's supply, when the pressure in the reserve is below that required to function properly, when the liquid level of a cryogenic supply has

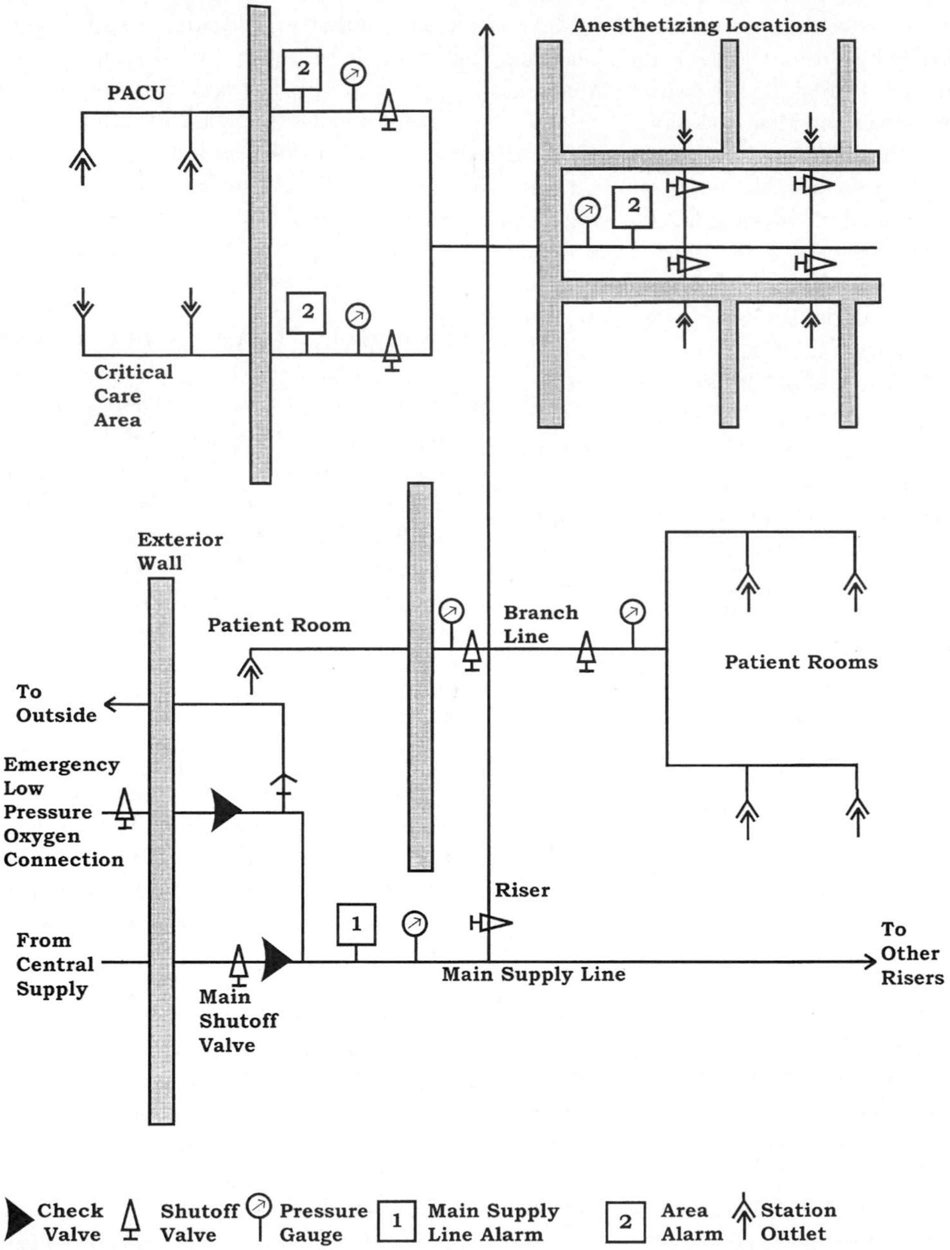

FIGURE 2.6. Typical medical gas piped distribution system. The main line runs on the same level as the central supply and connects it to risers or branch lines or both. In anesthetizing locations, individual room shutoff valves are located downstream of the area alarm. Other locations have a single shutoff valve for the entire area with the area alarm actuator downstream from the shutoff valve. The master alarm is activated by a 20% increase or decrease in the main line pressure. Area alarms must be installed in branch lines leading to intensive care units, postanesthesia care units, and anesthetizing locations to signal if the pressure increases or decreases 20% from normal operating pressure. (Redrawn from a figure in National Fire Protection Association, Standard for Health Care Facilities [NFPA 99]. Quincy, MA: National Fire Protection Association, 1996.)

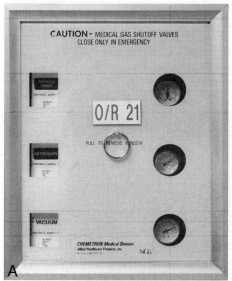

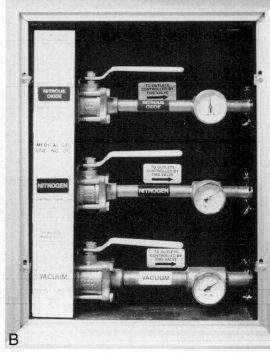

FIGURE 2.7. **A,** Box with shutoff valves. The window can be easily removed by pulling the ring in the center. Note that the operating room controlled by the shutoff valves is identified. **B,** Box with shutoff valves with cover removed. To close a valve, the handle is pulled a quarter turn. Note that the pipe is labeled to show the gases contained. The front cover cannot be installed if a valve is closed.

reached a certain level, and when the pressure in the main line increases or decreases from normal operating pressure. In the medical air system there must be alarms for malfunction of one or more of the compressors or dryers and when the dew point has been exceeded.

Area Alarm Systems

An area alarm system consists of an alarm panel(s) and associated actuating device(s) that provides audible and visual signals for medical gas systems serving a specific area.

Areas of critical life support, such as operating rooms, postanesthesia care units, intensive care units, coronary care units, etc., must have an area (local) alarm system to indicate if the pressure increases or decreases 20% from normal operating pressure. In anesthetizing locations, the alarm will be upstream of the shutoff valves to the individual rooms. In other areas it will be placed downstream of the shutoff valve for the area. Area alarms are sometimes placed in each anesthetizing location.

An appropriately labeled warning signal panel for area alarms must be installed at the nurses' station or other suitable location that will provide responsible surveillance (Fig. 2.8). Many area alarms also sound at the master alarm panel.

General Requirements

Each alarm must be labeled for the gas and area it monitors. Signals should be both audible and visible. Some systems allow the audible signal to be temporarily silenced. The visual signal should continue until the problem is corrected. Each panel should contain a mechanism to test the alarms. Alarms should be designed to function during electric power failure.

Clear, concise instructions should be given to the persons monitoring the alarms to ensure signals are reported promptly to the proper parties.

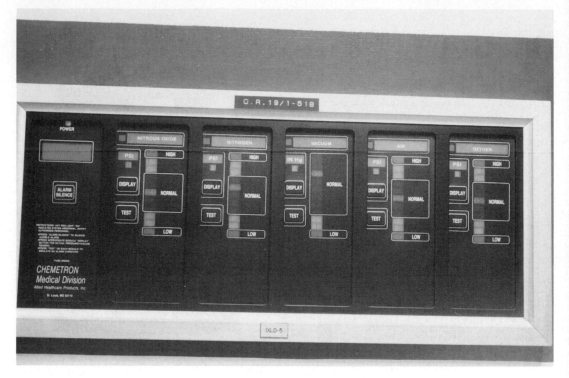

FIGURE 2.8. Area (local) alarm panel. Pressures of gases are monitored and a warning provided if the pressure increases or decreases from the normal operating pressure. A button for testing the alarms is provided. Area alarm systems are provided for anesthetizing locations and other vital life support and critical care areas such as postanesthesia care, intensive care, and coronary care. Note that the panel is labeled for the area being monitored.

Cases have been reported in which a employee did not know what to do when an alarm sounded (10). Activation of the signal should be reported immediately to the department responsible for operation and maintenance of the gas piping system. The action to be taken will depend on the individual arrangements for each facility. These should be recorded in a procedure manual, which is reviewed periodically, and new employees should be given clear instructions regarding actions to be taken.

Pressure Gauges

A pressure gauge must be installed in the main line adjacent to the actuating switch for the main supply line pressure alarm and in each line being monitored at each area alarm panel.

Terminal Units

The terminal unit (station outlet, junctional point, interface, pipeline outlet, end use terminal, service outlet, terminal outlet, outlet point, outlet station, outlet assembly, wall outlet) is the point in a piped gas distribution system at which the user normally makes connections and disconnections. Equipment may be connected to a terminal unit either directly or by means of a flexible hose.

Components
Base Block
The block is the part of a terminal unit that is attached to the pipeline distribution system.
Primary Valve
The primary valve (automatic shutoff valve; terminal unit valve or check valve; terminal valve; self-sealing valve, device, or unit; primary check

valve) opens and allows the gas to flow when the male probe is inserted and closes automatically when the connection is broken. This serves to prevent loss of gas when the nonfixed component is disconnected. Although often called a check valve it is not a unidirectional valve and will permit flow in either direction. The face plate and primary valve are an integral unit in some terminal units.

Secondary Valve

The secondary valve (shutoff valve, terminal stop valve, maintenance valve, automatic service valve, isolating valve, secondary valve, secondary shutoff valve, secondary check valve) is designed so that when the primary valve is removed (e.g., for cleaning or servicing) the flow of gas is shut off. When the primary valve is in place, the secondary valve stays open. The secondary valve is fitted at or near the end of the permanent pipework with hose booms and pendants incorporating hoses.

Gas-Specific Connection Point (Socket Assembly)

The receptor for a noninterchangeable gas-specific connector, which is either part of or attached to the base block, is incorporated into each terminal unit. The connector may be a threaded Diameter Index Safety System (DISS) or a proprietary (manufacturer-specific) quick connector. The corresponding male component of the noninterchangeable connection is attached to the equipment to be used or to a flexible hose leading to the equipment. The female component is called an outlet connector or socket. The male member is called an inlet connector, probe, plug, striker, or jack.

Each DISS or quick connector must be equipped with a backflow check valve to prevent flow of gas from the anesthesia apparatus or other dispensing apparatus into the piping system.

The diameter index safety system (5). The DISS was developed to provide noninterchangeable connections for medical gas lines at pressures of 1380 kPa (200 psig) or less. As shown in Figure 2.9, each DISS connection consists of a body, nipple, and nut combination. There are two concentric and specific bores in the body and two concentric and specific shoulders on the nipple (Fig. 2.10). The small bore (BB) mates with the small shoulder (MM) and the large bore (CC) mates with the large shoulder (NN). To achieve nonin-

terchangeability between different connections, the two diameters on each part vary in opposite directions, so that as one diameter increases, the other decreases. Only properly mated parts will fit together and allow thread engagement. The American Society for Testing and Materials (ASTM) machine standard requires that every anesthesia machine have a DISS fitting for each pipeline inlet (Fig. 2.11) (14).

Quick connectors. Quick connectors (automatic quick couplers valves, quick connects, quick-connect fittings, quick couplers) allow apparatus (e.g., hose, flowmeter) to be connected or disconnected by a single action using one or both hands without the use of tools or undue force. Quick connectors are more convenient than DISS fittings but tend to leak more.

Each quick connector consists of a pair of gas-specific male and female components (Fig. 2.12). A releasable spring mechanism locks the components together. Insertion into an incorrect outlet is prevented by the use of different shapes for mating portions, different spacing of mating portions, or some combination of these. A national standard has not been developed for quick connectors. It is up to each manufacturer to ensure noninterchangeability between connectors for different gases.

Face Plate

The face plate should be permanently marked with the name and/or symbol of the gas it conveys. The identifying color may also be present.

Types

Wall Outlets

Wall outlets (Fig. 2.13) are mechanically simple and well-suited to small rooms where the equipment to be connected will be near the wall. In larger rooms, the hoses to the equipment frequently must be of considerable length and draped across the floor. This leads to problems with tripping, difficulty in moving equipment, wear and tear on the hose, and accumulation of debris along it. More than one set of wall outlets may be advisable for large rooms.

Ceiling-Mounted Hoses

Ceiling-mounted hoses with the terminal unit at the end of the hose (Fig. 2.14) may be used.

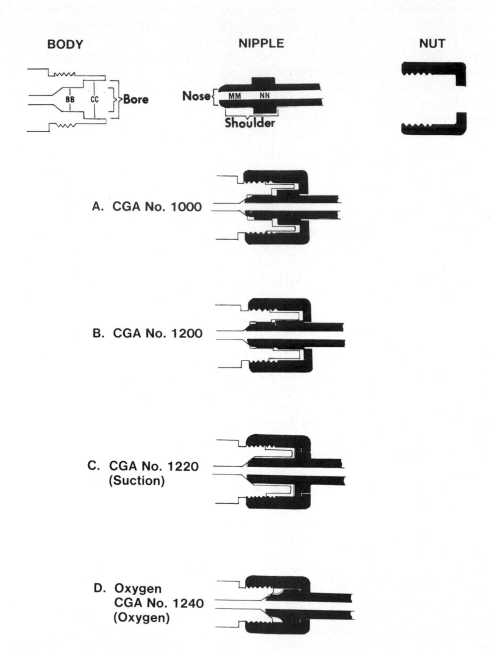

FIGURE 2.9. Diameter Index Safety System (DISS). With increasing Compressed Gas Association (CGA) number, the small shoulder (MM) of the nipple becomes larger and the large diameter becomes smaller. If assembly of a nonmating body and nipple is attempted, either MM will be too large for small bore (BB) or large shoulder (NN) will be too large for large bore (CC). (Redrawn courtesy of the Compressed Gas Association.)

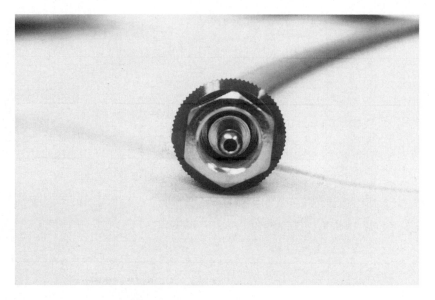

FIGURE 2.10. End of Diameter Index Safety System (DISS) connection. Note the two concentric shoulders on the nipple.

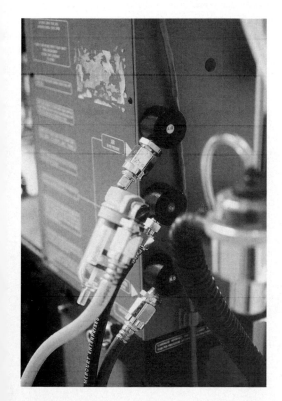

FIGURE 2.11. Pipeline inlets to the anesthesia machine have Diameter Index Safety System (DISS) connections.

Ceiling-Mounted Pendants

A ceiling-mounted pendant with one or more articulated arms (Fig. 2.15) avoids cluttering the floor and can easily be moved to various locations. In addition to terminal units, it may have electric and data management outlets, space for monitors, telephones, intravenous solution mounts, and suction bottles and regulators.

Ceiling Column

Ceiling-mounted columns (Fig. 2.16) can provide the same services as a pendant but are less versatile with respect to positioning (15). They can be made movable by mounting them on tracks. They can also be made retractable so that the column can be lowered for attachment and detachment of lines and then raised to avoid obstruction. They are often positioned at the head and foot ends of the operating room table. Disadvantages include the possibility of people hitting their heads and the difficulty in gaining access to hoses inside the column. Short personnel may have difficulty attaching things to ceiling-mounted columns.

The Nitrogen Piping Terminal Unit

A means of adjusting the pressure at the station outlet is needed because the pressure required for nitrogen-driven tools varies. An adjustable regula-

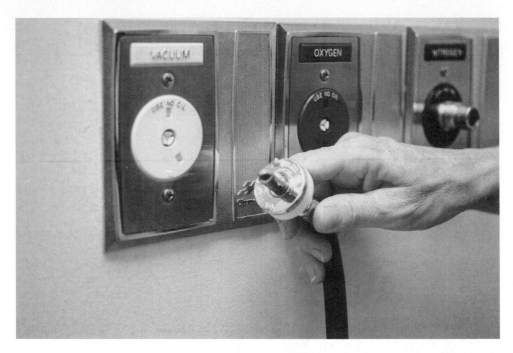

FIGURE 2.12. Quick Connector. The two prominences on the hose connection mate with the two slots on wall outlet to ensure noninterchangeability.

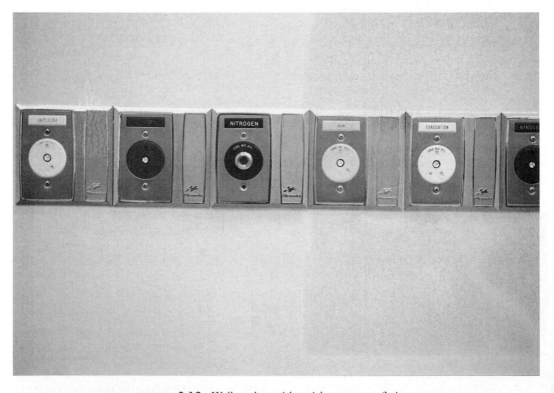

FIGURE 2.13. Wall outlets with quick connector fittings.

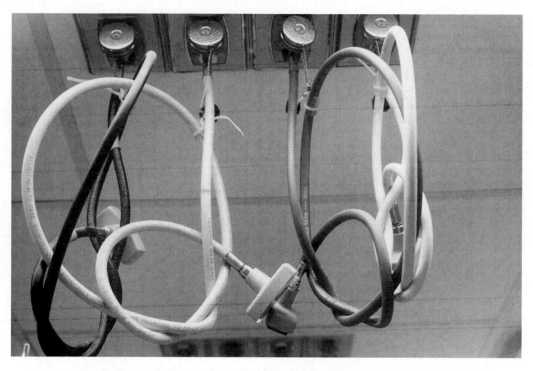

FIGURE **2.14.** Ceiling-mounted hoses. A spring-actuated chain keeps the hose close to the ceiling.

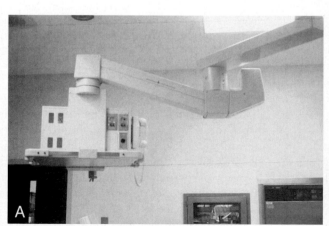

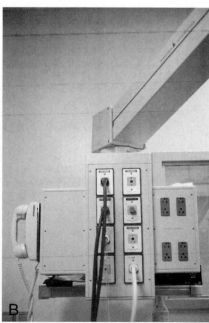

FIGURE **2.15.** Pendant with double-articulated arm. On one side (**A**) is a shelf for equipment and electric and data management system outlets. On the other side (**B**) are terminal units for the piped gases and additional electric outlets. The pendant can be raised or lowered or moved from side to side.

FIGURE **2.16.** Retractable rigid column. Pipeline outlets are on the bottom. Electric outlets and mounts for intravenous solutions are on the sides.

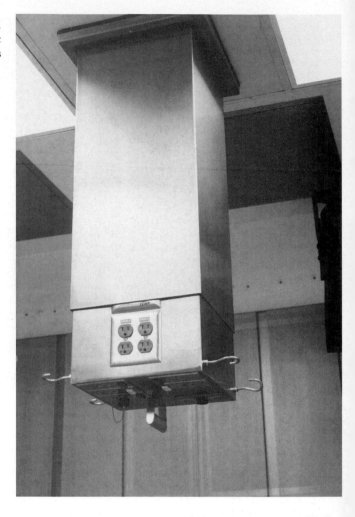

tor of the type described in Chapter 4 is used. Figure 2.17 shows a nitrogen terminal unit built into the wall. Two gauges are present, one indicating the distribution pressure and the other the reduced pressure.

Hoses (8, 16)

Hoses (droplines, hose assemblies, low-pressure hose assemblies, low-pressure flexible connecting assemblies, flexible hose assemblies, pipeline pressure supply hoses, hose pipes) are used to connect anesthesia machines and other apparatus to terminal units. Each end should have a permanently-attached, noninterchangeable connector. The connector that attaches to a terminal unit is called the inlet (supply) connector, and the con-

nector that attaches to equipment such as on an anesthesia machine is the outlet (equipment) connector.

Color coding of the hose and having the name and chemical symbol of the contained gas on each connector are desirable. Most hoses have an imbedded braid in the wall for added strength. Hoses should be kept away from any heat source, especially operating room lights, because contact may cause the hose to rupture (17, 18). Whenever possible, hoses should be kept off the floor.

When an anesthesia machine is moved and a hose must be disconnected, this should be done quickly and preferably without opening the valve of a cylinder on the machine because the cylinder may become depleted if the valve is not closed

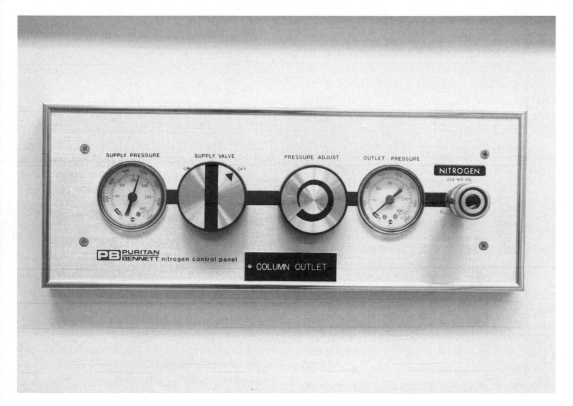

FIGURE 2.17. Termination of nitrogen piping system. Two gauges are present, one showing pipeline and the outlet (reduced) pressure. The reduced pressure can be altered using the regulator. The station outlet is at the right.

after the hose is reconnected. If it is necessary that the hose be disconnected for more than a few seconds, a cylinder should be opened and then closed as soon as the hose is reconnected.

The use of several extension hoses is undesirable. It is better to use one long hose because resistance caused by multiple connections may interfere with flow. One long hose is less likely to leak because most leaks in hoses occur in the connectors or where the connector fits into the hose.

Hoses should be kept in good repair and approach the anesthesia machine at a gentle curve, avoiding acute angulation or stretching. After years of use, hoses can weaken, swell, or crack. Personnel should watch for these problems and have the hoses repaired or replaced.

TESTING OF MEDICAL GAS DISTRIBUTION SYSTEMS (3, 4)

It is essential that medical gas distribution systems be thoroughly tested before being used be-

cause problems are most likely to occur with a new system or one that has been modified or repaired. If a system is brand new, the entire system must be tested. The extent of testing for a new or modified portion of an existing system will depend on how much of the existing system can be isolated and not affected by the work.

There has been controversy over who should carry out the final (commissioning) tests to make sure the piping system complies with regulations. Commercial services that inspect medical gas pipelines and offer certification are available. There are currently no national certification or registration programs for inspectors or testers of medical piped gas systems, so a facility should be careful in the selection of the personnel or companies to perform these tasks. Test procedures and results should be made part of the permanent records of the facility.

There may be local or state requirements for a

permit before a piping system can be installed. The Canadian Standard (9) requires that the pre-operational tests be made by a testing agency experienced in the field and independent of the contractor, gas and equipment suppliers, and the owner. It also requires that a member of the staff of the healthcare facility and a representative of the installer be present to witness testing.

Anesthesia personnel have an obligation to ensure that the system is properly designed and functions correctly so a member of the department should witness the tests performed, especially those for cross-connections. A personal independent check using an oxygen analyzer or other apparatus, such as Raman spectroscopy or mass spectrometer (Chapter 18), is an excellent idea.

Initial Testing

Blow Down

After the pipelines have been installed, but before the installation of terminal units and other components (e.g., pressure-actuating switches for alarms, manifolds, pressure gauges, or pressure relief valves), the line must be blown clear using oil-free dry nitrogen.

Initial Pressure Testing

Before attachment of system components but after installation of the terminal units and before closing of the walls, each section of the piping system must be subjected to a test pressure of 1.5 times the working pressure (minimum 1034 kPa [150 psig]) with oil-free nitrogen with the source valve closed. This pressure is maintained until each joint has been examined for leakage. Any leaks that are found must be corrected.

Standing Pressure Test

After all components of the system have been installed, the entire system is subjected to a 24-hour standing pressure test at 20% above the normal operating line pressure with the source valve closed. This permits testing without damaging system components or opening pressure-relief devices. Leaks, if any, must be located and repaired, and the test must be repeated until no leaks are found.

Piping Purge Test

To remove particulate matter, a heavy intermittent purging must be performed on each outlet until no discoloration on a white cloth held over the outlet is produced.

Test for Cross Connections

Testing for cross-connections (anticonfusion or continuity test) is to ensure that the gas delivered at each terminal unit is that shown on the outlet label and that the proper connecting fittings are present.

One gas system is tested at a time. Each gas is turned off at the source valve, and the pressures reduced to atmospheric. The pipeline being tested is then filled with oil-free nitrogen at its working pressure. Each individual station outlet is checked with appropriate adapters matching outlet labels to ensure that test gas emerges only from the outlets of the medical gas system being tested. Each gas system is tested in turn.

System Verification

After the walls have been closed, the following tests shall be performed with oil-free, dry nitrogen.

Cross-Connection Test

Either of the following tests can be used.

1. All medical gas systems are reduced to atmospheric pressure. All sources of test gas from all medical gas systems, with the exception of the one system to be checked, are disconnected. The system is then pressurized to 345 kPa (50 psig). Each terminal unit of every medical gas system is then checked to determine that test gas is being dispensed only from the outlets of the medical gas system being tested. Each medical gas system is checked in this way.

The pressures of all medical gas system are reduced to atmospheric pressure. The test gas pressure in all medical gas piping system is increased to the following values:

Medical Gas	psig	kPa Gauge
Gas Mixtures	20	140
Nitrogen	30	210
Nitrous Oxide	40	280
Oxygen	50	350
Compressed Air	60	420

Following adjustment of pressures, each station outlet is identified by label and the pressure indicated on the test gauge must be as listed above.

Tests of Values

Valves must be tested to verify proper operation and rooms or areas of control.

Outlet Flow Test

Flow tests must be performed at station outlets using oil-free, dry nitrogen or the gas of the designated system. Oxygen, nitrous oxide, and air outlets must deliver 100 l/min with a pressure drop of no more than 35 kPa (5 psig) at a static pressure of 345 kPa (50 psig). Nitrogen outlets must deliver 140 l/min with a pressure drop of no more than 35 kPa (5 psig) at a static pressure of 1100 kPa (160 psig). Special analyzers that allow quick testing are available (19).

Alarm Testing

Master and area alarm systems must be tested for proper functioning.

Piping Purge Test

To remove particulate matter, purge rates of at least 225 l/min are applied to each outlet until the purge produces no discoloration in a white cloth held over the adapter. Approximately 25% of the zone must be tested at the outlet most remote from the source by flowing 1000 liters of gas through a clean 0.45 micron filter at a minimum flow of 100 l/min. The filter shall accrue no more than 0.1 mg.

Piping Purity Test

Each system must be tested for dew point, methane, and halogenated hydrocarbons at the outlet most remote from the source. Maximum allowable values are given in NFPA 96.

Final Tie-In Test

The final connection between the addition and existing system must be leak-tested at the normal operating pressure with the gas of system designation after connection of any work or extension or addition to an existing piping system.

Operational Pressure Test

Piping systems for gases other than nitrogen must maintain the pressure at 345 + 35 − 0 kPa gauge (50 +5-0 psig) to all terminal units while delivering 100 l/min with a pressure drop of no more than 35 kPa (5 psig) at a static pressure of 345 kPa (50 psig) at terminal units. Piping systems for nitrogen must maintain the pressure at 1100 kPa (160 psig) to all terminal units at a flow of 5.0 standard cubic feet per minute with a pressure drop of no more than 35 kPa (5 psig) at a static pressure of 1100 kPa (160 psig).

Medical Gases Concentrations

Each system must be analyzed for concentrations of gases by volume after purging each system with the gas the system is designed for. Allowable concentrations are given in NFPA 96.

Medical Air Purity Test

The medical air source must be analyzed for dew point, carbon monoxide, carbon dioxide, gaseous hydrocarbons, and halogenated hydrocarbons. Maximum allowable values are given in NFPA 96.

Source Equipment Verification

Source equipment must be tested following installation of pipeline accessories. A pressure test is performed at the highest system operating pressure for 2 hours, with no more than a 10% pressure drop allowed.

All source apparatus, including changeovers, signals, master signal panels, and pressure gauges, must be checked for proper functioning and labeling. In addition, the quality of medical air produced must be checked after a minimum of 24 hours continuous running of the machinery.

Periodic Testing and Preventive Maintenance

A planned preventive maintenance program can stop potentially hazardous conditions and unexpected loss of service, reduce the economic burden of leakage, and reduce repairs performed as emergencies (3, 4, 20). Periodic testing should be performed at least as frequently as recommended by the manufacturer of the pipeline. Maintenance should be scheduled more frequently if required by heavy use or local conditions. The system, as installed, should be examined and the accuracy of existing diagrams verified before maintenance is undertaken. Inspection and testing of piping systems should be performed on a regular basis, and the results recorded in a permanent log. If test buttons are provided at area panels (Fig. 2.8), testing of audible and visual alarm indicators should be performed monthly.

At least annually, all hoses and station outlets in the anesthetizing locations and postanesthesia care units should be checked for wear, damage, and proper function. Terminal units should be checked for ease of insertion and locking of the connectors; ease of unlocking and removal; leakage, wear, and damage; contamination; gas specificity; labeling; flow; and pressure.

Shutoff valves to anesthetizing locations can be checked for tightness and components downstream of the valve for leakage by the following test. An anesthesia machine with a pipeline pressure gauge is connected to the piping system. Cylinder valves on the machines are closed, the zone shutoff valve outside the operating room closed, and gas released until each pipeline pressure gauge reads 280 kPa (40 psig). This pressure is then monitored for 4 hours. It should remain at 280 kPa (40 psig). If the pressure rises, the shutoff valve is not working properly. If the pressure falls, there is a leak in the pipe to the room, the station outlet, or the hose to the anesthesia machine. It is essential that the shutoff valves be reopened after this test has been performed.

Pipeline pressure gauges are included on all new anesthesia machines. These should be checked before administration of anesthesia is begun. If a machine does not have a pipeline pressure gauge, the pressure should be checked on the area pressure gauge (Fig. 2.8).

PLANNED SHUTDOWNS (21)

The process of partially or completely shutting down a medical gas pipeline system is a complex task that involves many risks. The anesthesia department should be actively involved. Careful planning, good communication, and close cooperation will minimize problems and ensure uninterrupted gas service. Following the shutdown,

purity and crossover testing of all outlets involved and immediately adjacent areas should be performed.

PROBLEMS

Many problems in piping systems are the result of a lack of awareness among personnel who have been lulled into believing that the piping system cannot fail and who are not sufficiently familiar with it to make emergency adjustments. Lack of communication between clinical and maintenance departments and commercial suppliers may also be a contributing factor. Finally, lack of adherence to existing codes is responsible for many hazards.

Inadequate Pressure

This is the most frequently reported malfunction (10). Loss of pressure may result in a flow inadequate to power a ventilator but sufficient for other purposes.

Causes

Sources of inadequate pressure include: damage, especially during construction projects unrelated to the piping system (10, 22); fires (23, 24); vehicular accidents; theft of nitrous oxide tanks (10); environmental forces (earthquakes, excessive cold, tornadoes [25], lightning); failure of piped air secondary to compressor failure as a result of an electrical storm (26); depletion of or damage to the central supply (27, 28); human error including closure of a shutoff valve (10, 29, 30); inappropriate adjustment of the main line regulator (31); equipment failures (leaks, closure of a shutoff valve) (32–34); failure of standby supply during routine maintenance (35); regulator malfunction (10, 36, 37); problems with automatic switching gear (36, 38); obstruction of the pipeline (frequently by debris left following installation) (10, 39); failure of a quick coupler to fit into a station outlet or to allow gas to flow (40–43); fracturing of a quick connect (44, 45); plugging of a connector (46); kinking, leak, or obstruction of a hose (17, 18, 22, 47, 48); and detachment of a terminal unit (49). Deliberate tampering is a possibility that should not be overlooked.

Disaster Plan (31, 47)

Because loss of oxygen or air pipeline pressure is not uncommon and the consequences can be severe, each facility should have a plan to deal with it. This section is intended only to provide guidance in the preparation and implementation of a plan because no single plan is feasible for every facility.

One key to effective emergency preparedness planning is flexibility, which is attained by considering all possibilities and developing options for action that are maximally effective under each possibility. It is important that the plan be functional any time of day or night any day of the year. The plan should include conservation of existing supplies and acquisition of additional supplies from other facilities or vendors if necessary. Efforts should be coordinated to determine needs and supplies on hand, and efforts should be coordinated with the department responsible for the piping system to determine how long the loss of piped gas will last.

An effective response must include reliable communication pathways and individual responsibilities that take into account practical circumstances. The details should be discussed and rehearsed in the form of mock disaster drills if an effective response is to be expected during a real emergency. Each individual should be aware of his or her role. Locations of shutoff valves should be known by the staff, so that if the loss of pressure is caused by a leak in one area, the pipeline to that section can be isolated to prevent further loss.

The person discovering a fault in the piped supply should immediately inform the telephone operator who, in turn, should inform the following: the department responsible for maintenance of the system, respiratory therapy, surgery, the postanesthesia care unit, obstetrics, the emergency room, special care units such as intensive care and nursery, the nursing supervisor, and administration. Each department in turn should have carefully established procedures to deal with the emergency. These should be reviewed regularly, revised as necessary, and put in procedure manuals.

There should be no immediate threat to life in the operating rooms because every anesthesia machine should have at least one emergency oxygen cylinder; nevertheless, a prudent course of action would be to use low fresh gas flows and manual ventilation. Elective surgery should be postponed until adequate supplies can be guaranteed. Attention should be focused on the postanesthesia care unit (recovery room). It may be advantageous to move anesthesia machines not in use into the recovery room to supply oxygen until other sources can be obtained. Alternately, patients can be returned to operating rooms. Potential emergency oxygen sources other than compressed cylinders include portable liquid oxygen containers and oxygen concentrators (see Chapter 3). It may be necessary to use manual ventilation for patients on ventilators. Gas-powered ventilators should not be used as these will deplete the contents of a cylinder very quickly.

Emergency Auxiliary Supply

Because of the dangers associated with failure of piped oxygen and air systems, special areas such as intensive care units, recovery rooms, emergency rooms may add an auxiliary oxygen and/or air supply. When an emergency arises, the shutoff valve to the area is closed and the auxiliary source connected to an outlet within the zone not in use or by means of a specially installed T. Outlets within the area can then operate from the auxiliary source.

Leaks

Leaks are also common (10). They may occur anywhere in the piping system. Leaks are expensive and potentially hazardous if oxidizing gases are allowed to accumulate in closed spaces. Leaks of nitrous oxide may pose a health hazard to personnel (see Chapter 12).

Excessive Pressure

Excessive pressure is a relatively common problem (7). High pressures can result in damage to equipment, especially regulators (37, 50), and may cause barotrauma to patients. Few anesthesia machines or ventilators have mechanisms to prevent damage from high pressures. Some ventilators will not operate properly if the line pressure is too high.

As shown in Figure 2.3, a pressure relief valve

in the main supply line is required. However, this can be set improperly or malfunction.

The most common cause of high pressure is failure of a regulator. Ice may form on the vaporizers in a liquid oxygen system in humid atmospheres. This will hamper heat transfer and may result in liquid oxygen passing into the piping system with resultant damage to the regulator and pressure relief valve. Ice formation also has been reported after the addition of liquid oxygen to the main tank (50). Other causes of high pressure include combustion of foreign material in a pipeline (10) and deliberately increasing the pressure setting of the main line regulator in an attempt to compensate for low pressure from the central system (37).

Whenever excessive pipeline pressure occurs, it is best to disconnect apparatus from the pipeline system and use cylinders until the problem is corrected.

Alarm Problems

Failure, absence, or disconnection of an alarm is not uncommon (10, 37). Another problem is that the alarm is not heard or that the person who hears it either does not know the proper course of action or fails to follow it (10, 51).

False alarms are also a common problem. They may result from calibration drift in line pressure sensors (31). Repeated false alarms can cause complacency among personnel, which may have serious consequences if a real emergency occurs.

Cross-Connection of Gases

Although an uncommon event, accidental substitution of one gas for another can have devastating consequences. The most common cross-overs have been between nitrous oxide and oxygen, but various other combinations have also been reported. Pipeline alarms indicate only pressure faults and give no signal if an incorrect gas is present. Because the consequences are most severe when the cross-over results in hypoxia, it is essential that a reliable oxygen analyzer be included as a component of every breathing system (52).

Central Supply

Cases have been reported in which liquid oxygen tanks were filled with nitrogen (53–55) or argon (56). Incorrect tanks have been placed on the central supply manifold (40, 57).

Distribution System

Crossing of pipelines usually occurs during installation, alteration, or repair of a system (58–66). In one case, a fistula was created between two pipes during construction (67).

Flooding of an oxygen line with nitrogen has occurred when nitrogen was used to test for leaks and the shutoff valve to that area did not prevent backflow (23, 68, 69). NFPA now requires that the source gas, rather than nitrogen, be used to test for leaks when connecting new piping to the piping of an existing system. Nitrogen used in the brazing process can enter and contaminate adjacent zones if the shutoff valve leaks.

Terminal Units

There are numerous reports of outlets labeled for one gas that delivered another (70, 71). The wrong outlet connector may be installed (40, 67, 72). A terminal unit may accept an incorrect connector (73–76).

Hoses

Many cases have been reported in which the wrong connector was put on one or more hoses (10, 68, 77–81). Most of these have involved repairs or alterations performed by personnel. Blue hoses turning green have been reported (82). This could result in attachment of an oxygen-specific fitting to one end of a green (previously blue) hose. Whenever a hose is altered or repaired, it should be checked carefully before it is put into service to make certain that the proper connectors are in each end. This is easily performed with extension hoses by inserting one end of the hose into the other.

Peripheral Devices

Numerous cases have been reported in which an air/oxygen mixer or ventilator that used both air and oxygen had a defect such that the gas supplies became interconnected and oxygen flowed into the air pipeline or air flowed into the oxygen piping (36,83–92). The faulty device often was not in use. The level of contamination depends on the difference in supply pressure between the two gases. It is suggested that respiratory equipment be disconnected from the pipeline when not in use.

Contamination of Gases

Particulate

Particulate contamination can be a serious problem, particularly when a new pipeline is opened (50, 67, 93). The NFPA has a number of requirements designed to keep this to a minimum (3). A common source of contamination is air compressors, receivers, or dryers (13, 94). These particles can damage equipment, especially ventilators and blenders, and can cause a significant decrease in flow. Failure of a line pressure sensor owing to foreign material has been reported (31). Particulate matter can be harmful to patients if inhaled.

During installation every effort should be made to keep pipes, fittings, and valves as clean as possible. The majority of particles can be removed by purging, which may require several days, but may never be complete, especially in tall buildings (68).

Gaseous

Inhalation of volatile hydrocarbons can be unpleasant and harmful to patients, may damage equipment, and create a fire hazard. The source of the volatile hydrocarbons may be materials left in the pipes during construction (50, 67) or the inlet to the air compressors (50). In one case, the intake for the air compressor was located at the ambulance entrance and exhaust gases were taken into the piped system (95). In another case, the intake was located in the facility's heating ventilation/air condition–system. The coils of the system were washed with an acidic solution. This resulted in fumes being drawn into the air system (13). In another case, a filter was soaked in cleaning fluid and replaced without allowing it to dry (96). In one reported case, a cleaning solvent was not purged from the hose that connected the delivery truck to maintain the oxygen supply during delivery of liquid oxygen to the main storage tank (97).

In another accident, during the process of switching suppliers, the oxygen supply became contaminated with trichloroethylene, a solvent used to clean pipes and gas tanks, causing the death of several patients (98, 99). The oxygen tank had been cleaned with trichloroethylene and some was left in the tank, which was then filled with oxygen. When this new oxygen source was put online, the volatilized cleaning solvent was inhaled by patients receiving oxygen. In another case, trichloroethylene used to clean a valve was implicated in the death of a child (99). Use of trichloroethylene on-site has been banned by NFPA because controlling and disposing of it can be difficult. Residual trichloroethylene cannot be easily removed and can present a hazard to patients and personnel.

One important lesson to be learned from these accidents is that pipeline odors should always be taken seriously. All medical gases should be odor-free. Any odor originating from a medical gas system must be traced to its source and steps taken to correct the problem. Whenever a pipeline system is breached for any reason, testing of the gases coming from the system should be performed. Gas should be smelled before administering it to patients to ensure that it is odor-free.

Water

Water in an air pipeline can pass through particulate filters and make its way into equipment and patients (13). It can damage equipment such as ventilators and may adversely affect their accuracy (100–102), attack and weaken solder joints (103), cause particulate formation, and provide growth media for bacteria. Water in pipelines that are subjected to low temperatures can freeze and occlude gas flow. A filter with a drain may be used between the station outlet and the equipment (Fig. 2.18).

Bacterial

Piped medical gases are not sterile, and bacterial contamination has been documented (104–106). In some cases, contamination may be mixed, as when a bird became caught in an improperly installed air intake (93). Some manufacturers of devices using piped gases recommend that filters be placed between the station outlet and the equipment (Fig. 2.18), and many incorporate filters in inlets to their apparatus.

Fires

Equipment used with a pipeline system must be clean and free from oil, grease, and particulate

FIGURE 2.18. Filter with drain to remove water, particulate matter, and organisms from medical air. The filter is placed in the hose leading to the anesthesia machine.

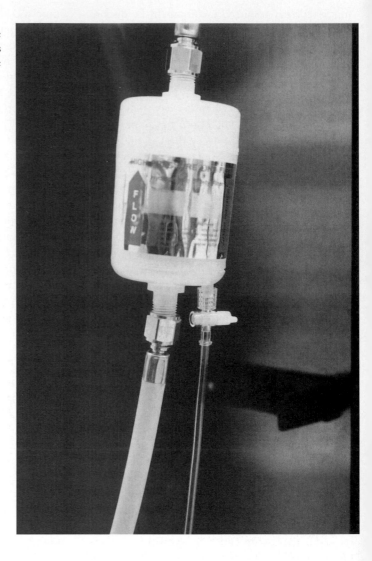

matter to avoid fires. In addition to causing inadequate pressure, a fire may result in hazardous fumes that are inhaled by patients. A hose can rupture and burn if it comes in contact with a light (17, 18).

Depletion of the Reserve Supply

Depletion of the reserve supply caused by failures of connections, pressure imbalances, and leaks has been reported (31, 37).

Theft of Nitrous Oxide Cylinders

Theft of nitrous oxide cylinders from a central supply area for substance-abuse purposes is a recurrent problem (107).

REFERENCES

1. Gjerde GE. Retrograde pressurization of a medical oxygen pipeline system: safety backup or hazard? Crit Care Med 1980;8:219–221.
2. Canadian Standards Association. Nonflammable medical gas piping systems (CSA Z305.1-92). Toronto, Ontario: CSA, 1992.
3. National Fire Protection Association. Standard for health care facilities (NFPA 99). Quincy, MA: National Fire Protection Association, 1996.
4. Klein BR. Health care facilities handbook. 5th ed. Quincy, MA: National Fire Protection Association, 1996.
5. Compressed Gas Association, Inc. Handbook of

compressed gases. 3rd ed. New York, NY: Van Nostrand Reinhold, 1990.

6. International Organization for Standardization. Terminal units for use in medical pipeline systems (ISO 9170:1990(E)). Geneva, Switzerland: ISO, 1990.

7. Canadian Standards Association. Medical gas terminal units (CAN/CSA-Z305.5-M86(R97)). Toronto, Ontario: CSA, 1997.

8. Canadian Standards Association. Low-pressure connecting assemblies for medical gas systems (CSA Z305.2-M88). Toronto, Ontario: CSA, 1988.

9. Canadian Standards Association. Qualification requirements for agencies testing nonflammable medical gas piping systems (CSA Z305.4-M85). Toronto, Ontario: CSA, 1985.

10. Feeley TW, Hedley-Whyte J. Bulk oxygen and nitrous oxide delivery systems: design and dangers. Anesthesiology 1976;44:301–305.

11. Friesen RM. Oxygen concentrators and the practice of anaesthesia. Can J Anaesth 1992;39:R80–R84.

12. Lee KH, Tan PSK, Rico P, et al. Low levels of nitric oxide as contaminant in hospital compressed air: physiological significance? Crit Care Med 1997;25: 1143–1146.

13. Moss E, Nagle T. Medical air systems are complex, usually poorly understood. APSF Newsletter 1996; 11:18–21.

14. American Society for Testing and Materials. Specification for minimum performance and safety requirements for components and systems of anesthesia gas machines (ASTM F1161-88). (Reapproved 1964) West Conshohocken, PA: ASTM, 1988.

15. Wilder RJ, Williams GR. The ceiling-retractable service column. JAMA 1981;246:1403–1404.

16. Low-pressure flexible connecting assemblies (hose assemblies) for use with medical gas systems. Geneva, Switzerland: International Standards Organization, 1989

17. Anderson EF. A potential ignition source in the operating room. Anesth Analg 1976;55:217–218.

18. Anonymous. Unshielded radiant heat sources. Technology for Anesthesia 1985;5:1.

19. Anonymous. Medical gas analyzer tests five outlet types. Biomedical Safety & Standards 1995;15:102.

20. Slack GD. Medical gas and vacuum systems. American Society of Hospital Engineering of the American Hospital Association 1989;3:37–48.

21. Peterson TG. Shutdown of gas supply system need not be danger. Planning minimizes risks. APSF Newsletter 1994;9:32–34.

22. Ewart IA. An unusual cause of gas pipeline failure. Anaesthesia 1990;45:498.

23. Arrowsmith LWM. Medical gas pipelines. Eng Med 1979;8:247–249.

24. Wright CJ, Bostock F. Pipeline hazards—a simple solution. Anaesthesia 1978;33:759.

25. Johnson DL. Central oxygen supply versus mother nature. Respiratory Care 1975;20:1043–1044.

26. Webb RK, Russell WJ, Klepper I, et al. Equipment failure: an analysis of 2000 incident reports. Anaesthesia and Intensive Care 1993;21:673–677.

27. Chi OZ. Another example of hypoxic gas mixture delivery. Anesthesiology 1985;62:543–544.

28. Russell WJ. Oxygen supply at risk. Anaesthesia and Intensive Care 1985;13:216–217.

29. Anonymous. Mystery of turned-off hospital oxygen supply solved by Denver police. Biomedical Safety & Standards 1987;17:18–19.

30. Anonymous. Did accidental O_2 shutdown cause patient death? Biomedical Safety & Standards 1995;25: 105–107.

31. Bancroft ML, du Moulin GC, Hedley-Whyte J. Hazards of hospital bulk oxygen delivery systems. Anesthesiology 1980;52:504–510.

32. Black AE. Extraordinary oxygen pipeline failure. Anaesthesia 1990;45:599.

33. Gibson OB. Another hazardous pipeline isolator valve. Anaesthesia 1979;34:213.

34. MacWhirter GI. An anesthetic pipe line hazard. Anaesthesia 1978;33:639.

35. Francis RN. Failure of nitrous oxide supply to theater pipeline system. Anaesthesia 1990;45:880–882.

36. Carley RH, Houghton IT, Park GR. A near disaster from piped gases. Anaesthesia 1984;39:891–893.

37. Feeley TW, McClelland KJ, Malhotra IV. The hazards of bulk oxygen delivery systems. Lancet 1975; 1:1416–1418.

38. Anonymous. Medical gas delivery manifold could fail. Biomedical Safety & Standards 1996;26:12.

39. Janis KM. Sudden failure of ceiling oxygen connector. Can Anaesth Soc J 1978;25:155.

40. Krenis LJ, Berkowitz DA. Errors in installation of a new gas delivery system found after certification. Anesthesiology 1985;62:677–678.

41. Mather SJ. Put not your trust in: a case of pipeline failure during routine anaesthesia. Anaesthesia 1969; 11:21–22.

42. Craig DB, Culligan J. Sudden interruption of gas flow through a Schrader oxygen couple unit. Can Anaesth Soc J 1980;27:175–177.

43. Chung DC, Hunter DJ, Pavan FJ. The quick-mount pipeline connector: failure of a "fail-safe" device. Can Anaesth Soc J 1986;33:666–668.

44. Anonymous. Puritan-Bennett quick connect valves for medical gases: Canadian medical devices alert warns of possible cracks. Biomedical Safety & Standards 1984;14:52–53.

45. Morrison AB. Puritan-Bennett quick connect valves for medical gases. Medical devices alert. Ottawa: Health and Welfare Canada, April 9, 1984.

46. Anderson B, Chamley D. Wall outlet oxygen failure. Anaesthesia and Intensive Care 1987;15:468–469.

47. Anderson WR, Brock-Utne JG. Oxygen pipeline supply failure: a coping strategy. J Clin Monit 1991;7:39–41.

48. Anonymous. Anesthesia outlet hoses could have gasflow restriction. Biomedical Safety & Standards 1996;26:61.

49. Anonymous: Chemetron (NCG) outlet station adapters. Health Devices 1974;3:124.

50. Eichhorn JH, Bancroft ML, Laasberg LH, et al. Contamination of medical gas and water pipelines in a new hospital building. Anesthesiology 1977;46:286–289.

51. Paul DL. Pipeline failure. Anaesthesia 1989;44:523

52. Shaw SD, Graham IFM, Snowdon SL. Contamination of piped oxygen supplies. Anaesthesia 1991;46:887–888.

53. Sprague DH, Archer GW. Intraoperative hypoxia from an erroneously filled liquid oxygen reservoir. Anesthesiology 1975;42:360–362.

54. Holland R. Foreign correspondence: "wrong gas" disaster in Hong Kong. APSF Newslett 1989;4:26.

55. Bernstein DB, Rosenberg AD. Intraoperative hypoxia from nitrogen tanks with oxygen fittings. Anesth Analg 1997;84:225–227.

56. Smith FP. Multiple deaths from argon contamination of hospital oxygen supply. Journal of Forensic Sciences 1987;32:1098–1102.

57. Anonymous. O_2-N_2O mix-up leads to probe into deaths of two patients. Biomedical Safety & Standards 1981;11:123–124.

58. Anonymous. Medical Gas Systems. Technology for Anesthesia 1982;3:5.

59. Anonymous. Emergency room mixup, deaths linked. American Biomedical News, August 8, 1977, p. 3.

60. Anonymous. Interchanged oxygen and nitrous oxide lines caused death, suit charges. Biomedical Safety & Standards 1980;10:28–29.

61. Anonymous. Undetected crossed air-oxygen lines may have contributed to deaths of 7. Biomedical Safety & Standards 1982;12:41.

62. Anonymous. Cross-connected anesthesia supply lines allegedly result in two deaths: negligence suits filed. Biomedical Safety & Standards 1984;14:15–16.

63. Anonymous. Medical gas/vacuum systems. Technology for Anesthesia 1987;7:1–2.

64. Emmanuel ER, The JL. Dental anaesthetic emergency caused by medical gas pipeline installation error. Aust Dent J 1983;28:79–81.

65. LeBourdais E. Nine deaths linked to cross-contamination: Sudbury General inquest makes hospital history. Dimensions in Health Service 1974;51:10–12.

66. Sato T: Fatal pipeline accidents spur Japanese standards. APSF Newslett 1991;6:14.

67. Tingay MG, Ilsley AH, Willis RJ, et al. Gas identity hazards and major contamination of the medical gas system of a new hospital. Anaesthesia and Intensive Care 1978;6:202–209.

68. Dinnick OP. Medical gases-piping problems. Eng Med 1979;8:243–247.

69. McAleavy JC. Believe your monitors. Anesthesiology 1993;79:409–410.

70. Anonymous. Installation of oxygen system probed in nitrous oxide death suit. Biomedical Safety & Standards 1980;10:41–42.

71. Anonymous. Crossed N_2O & O_2 lines blamed for outpatient surgery death. Biomedical Safety & Standards 1992;22:14.

72. Anonymous. Crossed connections in medical gas systems. Technology for Anesthesia 1984;5:3.

73. Anonymous. Fittings/adapters, pneumatic, quick connect. Technology for Anesthesia 1990;11:11.

74. Scamman, FL. An analysis of the factors leading to crossed gas lines causing profound hypercarbia during general anesthesia. J Clin Anesth 1993;5:439–441.

75. Lane GA. Medical gas outlets—a hazard from interchangeable "quick connect" couplers. Anesthesiology 1980;52:86–87.

76. Anonymous. Misconnection of O_2 line to CO_2 outlet claimed in death. Biomedical Safety & Standards 1991;21:92–93.

77. Anonymous. The Westminster inquiry. Lancet 1977;2:175–176.

78. Anonymous. Anesthesia units. Technology for Anesthesia 1982;3:2.

79. Robinson JS. A continuing saga of piped medical gas supply. Anaesthesia 1979;34:66–70.

80. Neubarth J. Another hazardous gas supply misconnection. Anesth Analg 1995;80:206.

81. Jardine DS. An epidemic of hypoxemia in two intensive care units: cause and human response. Anesthesiology 1992;77:1038–1043.

82. Anonymous. Hoses, compressed gas. Technology for Anesthesia 1986;7:5.

83. Weightman WM, Fenton-May V, Saunders R, et al. Functionally crossed pipelines. An intermittent condition caused by a faulty ventilator. Anaesthesia 1992;47:500–502.

84. Anonymous. Bourns Bear 1 ventilator. Health Devices 1983;12:167–168.

85. Bageant RA, Hoyt JW, Epstein RM. Error in a pipeline gas concentration: an unanticipated consequence of a defective check valve. Anesthesiology 1981;54:166–169.

86. Bedsole SC, Kempf J. More faulty Bear check valves. Respiratory Care 1984;29:1159.

87. Jenner W, George BF. Oxygen-air shunt syndrome strikes again. Respiratory Care 1982;27:604.

88. Shaw A, Richardson W, Railton R. Malfunction of air-mixing valves. Anaesthesia 1985;40:711.

89. Shaw R, Beach W, Metzler M. Medical air contamination with oxygen associated with the Bear 1 and 2 ventilators. Crit Care Med 1988;16:362.

90. Ziecheck HD. Faulty ventilator check valves cause pipeline gas contamination. Respiratory Care 1981; 26:1009–1010.

91. Karmann U, Roth F. Prevention of accidents associated with air-oxygen mixers. Anaesthesia 1982;37: 680–682.

92. Thorp JM, Railton R. Hypoxia due to air in the oxygen pipeline. Anaesthesia 1982;37:683–687.

93. Moss E. Medical gas contamination: an unrecognized patient danger. APSF Newsletter 1994;9:73–76.

94. Bushman JA, Clark PA. Oil mist hazard and piped air supplies. BMJ 1967;3:588–590.

95. RB. Contaminated "medical" air. Respiratory Care 1972;17:125.

96. Lackore LK, Perkins HM. Accidental narcosis, Contamination of compressed air system. JAMA 1970; 211:1846–1847.

97. Gilmour IJ, McComb C, Palahniuk RJ. Contamination of a hospital oxygen supply. Anesth Analg 1990; 71:302–304.

98. Anonymous. Oxygen system contamination probed in patient deaths. Biomedical Safety & Standards 1996;26:57–58.

99 . Moss E. Hospital deaths reportedly due to contaminated O_2. APSF Newsletter 1996;11:13–18.

100. Conely JIM, Railton R, MacKenzie AI. Ventilator problems caused by humidity in the air supplied from simple compressors. Br J Anaesth 1981;53:549–550.

101. McAdams SA, Barnes W. Air compressor failure complicating mechanical ventilation. Respiratory Care 1983;28:1601.

102. Moss E. Dangers seen possible from contaminated medical gases. APSF Newsletter 1993;8:6–7.

103. Anonymous. Soldered medical gas piping. Technology for Anesthesia 1995;16:7.

104. Bjerring P, Oberg B. Bacterial contamination of compressed air for medical use. Anaesthesia 1986;41: 148–150.

105. Bjerring P, Oberg B. Possible role of vacuum systems and compressed air generators in cross-infection in the ICU. Br J Anaesth 1987;59:648–650.

106. Warren RE, Newsom SWB, Matthews JA, et al. Medical grade compressed air. Lancet 1986;1;1438.

107. Stein DW. Anesthetic agent misuse reported. American Society of Anesthesiologists Newsletter, June 1978.

QUESTIONS

1. The normal pipeline pressure for oxygen, nitrous oxide and air in the United States is
   A. 240 to 275 kPa
   B. 275 to 345 kPa
   C. 345 to 380 kPa
   D. 380 to 410 kPa
   E. 410 to 440 kPa.

2. Which of the following gases requires a regulator for use in the operating room?
   A. Oxygen
   B. Nitrous oxide
   C. Air
   D. Nitrogen
   E. All of the above

3. The most frequently reported malfunction of hospital pipeline systems is
   A. Inadequate pressure
   B. Cross connection
   C. Excessive pressure
   D. Alarm dysfunction
   E. Contamination of gases

4. Compressed air is most often supplied by
   A. Proportioning devices
   B. Cylinder banks
   C. Concentrators
   D. Compressors
   E. Liquid containers

5. The Diameter Index Safety System (DISS) is used for devices are pressure of ____ or less
   A. 345 kPa
   B. 690 kPa
   C. 1000 kPa
   D. 1500 kPa
   E. 2000 kPa

Each question below contains four suggested answers of which one or more is correct. Choose the answer:

A If 1, 2, and 3 are correct
B If 1 and 3 are correct
C If 2 and 4 are correct
D If 4 is correct
E If 1, 2, 3, and 4 are correct.

6. The following provide standards for pipeline systems
   1. National Fire Protection Association (NFPA)
   2. Underwriters labs (UL)
   3. Compressed Gas Association (CGA)
   4. Association for the Advancement of Medical Instrumentation (AAMI)

7. Functions of the Joint Commission on Accreditation of Healthcare Organizations (JCAHO) in relation to medical gas pipeline systems include
   1. Inspecting systems
   2. Certifying pipeline installations
   3. Certifying procedures relating to pipeline usage
   4. Ensuring compliance with the various standards that apply to pipeline systems

8. Central gas supplies may be located
   1. Inside in a special room used only for this purpose
   2. Outdoors
   3. In an enclosure
   4. In a nonsterile area of the operating room suite

9. Oxygen may be supplied to the pipeline system by
   1. G and H cylinders
   2. Oxygen concentrators
   3. Bulk liquid systems
   4. C cylinders

10. Vaporization of liquid oxygen in a bulk tank will result in
   1. Loss of oxygen to the atmosphere
   2. Loss of oxygen that may be greater than demand
   3. Significant loss of oxygen even though there is no use
   4. Less loss if the rate of use is low

11. Heat must be supplied to vaporize liquid oxygen because

1. Liquid oxygen will freeze because of the low storage temperature
2. As the temperature falls, the pressure in the tank falls
3. Vaporization causes the pressure to fall
4. The heat of vaporization will cause the temperature to fall

12. NFPA regulations require a shutoff valve
    1. At every lateral branch, adjacent to the connection to the riser
    2. Outside each operating room
    3. Inside each critical care area
    4. At each riser, adjacent to the connection to the main supply line

13. A master alarm system panel should be located
    1. In the office of the person responsible for maintenance of the system
    2. In the operating room
    3. At the switchboard or security office
    4. In critical care areas

14. The diameter index safety system (DISS)
    1. Is used for gases at pressures of 250 psig or less
    2. Is used at all wall outlets
    3. Achieves noninterchangeability by using different screw threads
    4. Is required on all pipeline inlets on anesthesia machines

15. Preuse testing of a pipeline system should include
    1. Pressure testing
    2. Purge testing
    3. Testing for cross connections
    4. Testing for the purity of the gases

16. Quick connectors
    1. Provide noninterchangeable connections at pressures below 200 psig
    2. Allow apparatus to be connected or disconnected by a single action
    3. May require the use of one or both hands
    4. Do not require the use of tools

17. Cross connections of pipelines
    1. Most commonly involve oxygen and nitrogen
    2. May be caused by devices not in use
    3. Can be detected by alarms required by NFPA standards
    4. Are most commonly associated with construction, alterations, or repair

ANSWERS

1. C
2. D
3. A
4. D
5. D
6. B
7. D
8. A
9. A
10. A
11. C
12. C A shutoff valve is required immediately outside each vital life support or critical care area and each anesthetizing location. Lateral branch lines supplying anesthetizing locations and other vital life support and critical care areas do not have a shutoff valve.
13. B
14. D
15. E
16. E
17. C

CHAPTER
3

Oxygen Concentrators

INTRODUCTION

There are circumstances in which obtaining oxygen from cylinders or a pipeline is inconvenient, impossible, or prohibitively expensive. This has resulted in an increased interest in alternative sources of supply, especially oxygen concentrators. There are currently more than 500,000 of these units in use worldwide.

METHOD OF OPERATION
Membrane Filtration

Membrane filtration concentrator uses an oxygen-permeable membrane or lattice to collect oxygen. This type of concentrator will produce 30 to 40% oxygen regardless of flow (1, 2). Membrane filtration will not be discussed further because it is not useful for anesthesia.

Pressure Swing Adsorption

A pressure swing adsorber increases the oxygen concentration by adsorbing nitrogen onto a molecular sieve and allowing oxygen and trace gases, especially argon, to pass through. The result is a gas with between 90 and 96% oxygen (1, 3–8). The argon concentration is usually between 4.3 and 5.5% (8, 9). The product gas from the concentrator is referred to as Oxygen 93% USP or Oxygen 90 (4, 5).

Two international and one United States standards for medical oxygen concentrators have been published (10, 11, 12). Most currently available concentrators use an inorganic silicate, which belongs to a class of crystalline compounds and is known as zeolite, as the molecular sieve. A system of precisely arrayed cavities and pores is located within each zeolite granule. The cavities and pores are uniform in size so that molecules are either readily adsorbed or completely excluded. The molecular size of a gas and its polarity determine whether it is retained by the sieve material. Adsorption efficiency is greatly enhanced if the gas is introduced under pressure.

Air under pressure is passed through a column or bed of molecular sieve. Oxygen (along with argon) passes freely through, while nitrogen, carbon dioxide, carbon monoxide water vapor, and hydrocarbons are trapped. The nitrogen, carbon dioxide, carbon monoxide water vapor, and hydrocarbons are then desorbed (released) by venting the sieve bed to atmosphere, thereby reducing the pressure and the adsorptive force. Regeneration of the sieve bed is then completed by purging with some just-generated product gas.

A continuous output of oxygen-enriched gas is achieved by using two sieve beds in a sequential adsorption-desorption process—the pressure swing adsorption method. As one sieve adsorbs nitrogen under pressure, the other sieve is desorbed and purged to remove nitrogen. The output depends upon the size of the installation.

The molecular sieve has a strong affinity for water, which will displace other molecules. Room humidity does not affect the sieve's adsorbent ability during normal operation. A layer of sieve at the entrance to the bed acts to adsorb humidity. This moisture is returned to the atmosphere during the purge (exhaust) phase. Maintaining this layer through proper purging is critical to long bed life. The beds must be kept sealed from the atmosphere to prevent moisture from migrating into them. Oxygen concentrators can be used under humid conditions if the concentrator has been designed with adequate purges, low dead space, and enough heat to assist desorption of the water (13).

CONCENTRATOR DESIGN

A schematic design for a typical oxygen concentrator is shown in Figure 3.1. Designs vary among manufacturers, and all these components may not be present in a given model.

Inlet Filters and Silencer

Filters at the inlet and outlet of the air compressor trap particles and bacteria, and a muffler reduces the sound level.

Compressor

The compressor receives filtered room air and compresses it to a higher working pressure. The compressor needs to be effectively cooled and often has several fans to promote cooling. Cooling of the compressor is important because, if inefficient, it can lead to a decrease in performance (8).

Heat Exchanger

When a gas is compressed, its temperature increases. A heat exchanger in the form of coiled tubing may be used downstream of the compressor to cool the gas.

Reservoir Canister

In some concentrators, the compressed gas enters a reservoir canister (surge tank), which acts to dampen pulsations generated by the compressor.

Valves

Electrically- or pneumatically-controlled valves direct the flow of gases through the concentrator.

Sieve Beds (Canisters, Columns)

Two beds filled with zeolite allow continuous production of oxygen and regeneration of the sieve.

Product Tank

The product (accumulator) tank functions as a reservoir of product gas. The product tank may also serve as a source of purge gas.

Pressure Regulator

The pressure regulator reduces the pressure of the gas flowing to the outlet to a constant lower value and makes the outlet flow more constant.

Check Valve

A check valve between the pressure regulator and the outlet prevents room air from being

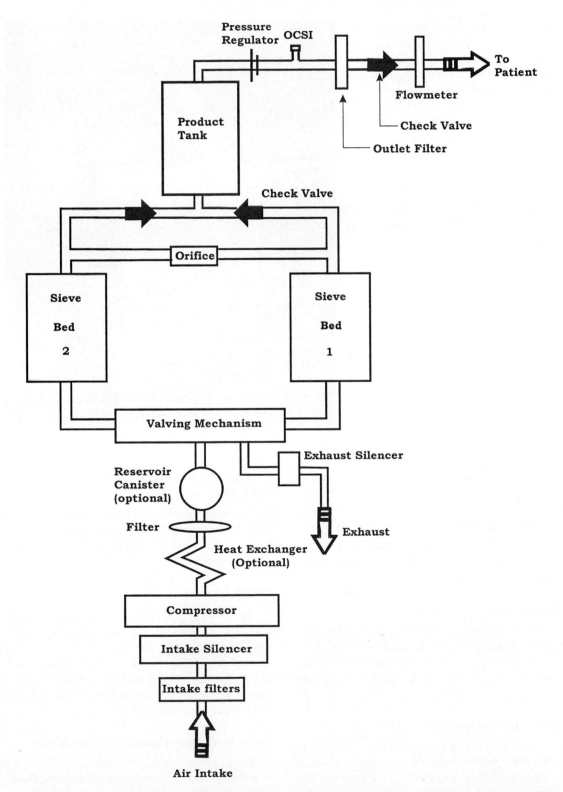

FIGURE **3.1.** Typical Oxygen Concentrator. OCSI = Oxygen-Concentration Status Indicator. See text for details.

FIGURE **3.2.** Oxygen concentrators for domiciliary use. Note flowmeter and oxygen-concentration status indicator on each. (Courtesy of Puritan Bennett, Inc. and Healthdyne Industries)

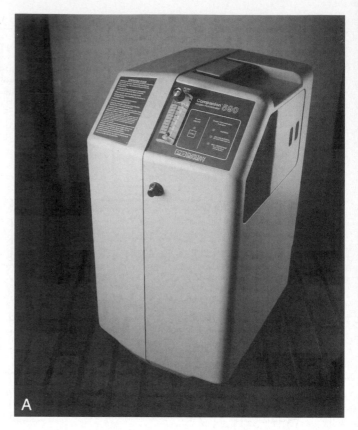

sucked into the sieve beds when the concentrator is turned off.

Outlet Gas Filter

The outlet gas filter is located near the outlet to prevent sieve material, bacteria, and other matter from contaminating the outflow.

Flowmeter

The flowmeter controls the flow of product gas on concentrators for domiciliary use (Fig. 3.2). The flowmeter must be accurate to ± 10% of indicated flow or ± 0.5 l/minute, whichever is greater (10, 11).

Electric Components

Electric components control the cycling of air and purge gases through the sieve beds and other components, including alarms, hour meters, cooling fans, circuit breakers, and oxygen-concentration status indicators.

Oxygen-Concentration Status Indicator

An oxygen-concentration status indicator (OCSI) is required by the United States and international standards to warn of low oxygen in the product gas (10, 11).

OPERATION

Operation of the oxygen concentrator, shown in Figure 3.1, involves admission of air to a molecular sieve bed while the opposite bed is vented and purged with product gas. This cycle is then repeated with the beds reversed. Cycle times vary among manufacturers and depend on the altitude and oxygen output flow rate.

Sieve Bed One Concentrating Cycle

In this phase, valves direct the filtered pressurized air from the air compressor or reservoir canister into sieve bed one where water vapor is attracted and held at the entrance of the bed, and

FIGURE **3.2.** *(continued)*

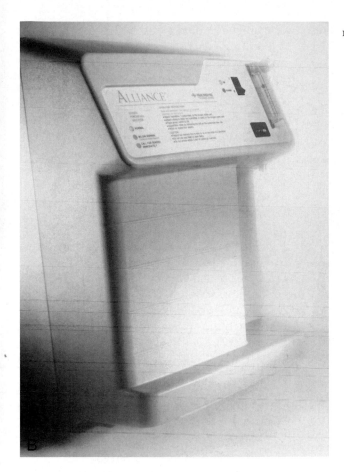

then nitrogen is adsorbed and oxygen-rich gas flows to the product tank. At the same time, the exhaust valve of sieve bed two is opened, causing the gas in the bed to be vented to the atmosphere. This drives water from the sieve bed back into the room. Some oxygen-rich gas passes into sieve bed two as the pressure in the bed exhausts to atmosphere. This removes any nitrogen remaining in the bed and increases the pressure in the bed. This increase in pressure helps ensure immediate oxygen flow from this bed at the beginning of its concentrating cycle.

Sieve Bed Two Concentrating Cycle

In this phase, the cycle reverses itself. Supply air passes into sieve bed two where water vapor is trapped and nitrogen is adsorbed while oxygen-rich gas flows to the product tank. Meanwhile gas is exhausted from sieve bed one to the atmosphere. Some oxygen-rich gas also passes into sieve bed one as the pressure in the sieve bed exhausts to the atmosphere. This cycle duplicates the first concentrating cycle and ensures a relatively constant flow of product gas to the product tank. The apparatus will require 2.5 to 19 minutes to achieve maximum concentration after being turned on (1, 7, 14, 15).

Individual concentrators perform best at particular flow rates, which are dependent upon their size. They have the general characteristic that the concentration process becomes less efficient if the flow rate is increased above the optimum level (1, 5, 7, 14–16). There may be some fluctuation in the concentration related to the cycling between the sieve columns (1, 7).

APPLICATIONS
Domiciliary Use

Oxygen concentrators are widely used to provide oxygen-enriched gas for domestic use (1, 16,

17). These units are compact, lightweight devices and have wheels and a handle for ease in delivery and transport.

Remote Locations

There are locations in the world where oxygen cylinders and liquid oxygen are unavailable or the supply is unreliable or prohibitively expensive (3, 9, 18, 19). Because electricity is almost always available wherever surgery is performed, consideration should be given to the use of oxygen concentrators. Their small size and portability make them a reliable source of oxygen in these circumstances. Combining them with air compressors to power ventilators can provide services similar to those found in more developed areas (18). Use of an oxygen concentrator with a draw-over vaporizer has been described (6).

Oxygen concentrators may also be useful in field hospitals, disaster situations, ambulances, aircraft, and ships at sea.

Hospital Pipeline Systems

Large-scale oxygen concentrator installations have been used to provide oxygen for complete pipeline systems and to supply a pipeline system during deliberate or accidental shutdown (20). In contrast to a domiciliary machine, which has a constant demand, the total flow rate of oxygen for a healthcare facility is quite variable. For this reason, the pipeline system is supplied from a pressurized reservoir of concentrated oxygen that is large enough to cope with the peaks of usage (3, 4, 5). This also provides some protection against temporary failure of electricity. The reservoir is usually supplied by a number of oxygen concentrators connected in parallel so that a fall in pressure in the reservoir can be handled by bringing one or more additional concentrators into use until the pressure is restored.

A reserve supply in the form of a cylinder manifold system, which is permanently connected and operates automatically, must be available in case of a concentrator malfunction or if the oxygen concentration falls below a preset minimum. The system may be set up so that the cylinders are filled with gas from the oxygen concentrator.

Modern anesthesia machines are not adversely affected by the use of oxygen-enriched gas from oxygen concentrators (4). Argon does not alter the flow characteristics of the oxygen (4). However, oxygen monitoring is always advised when using an anesthesia machine.

Other

Oxygen concentrators can be used in situations where for some reasons (e.g., danger of fires) other sources of oxygen cannot be employed.

ADVANTAGES
Cost Savings

An oxygen concentrator can be less expensive than liquid or cylinder oxygen (5, 17, 18, 21, 22). Expense depends on the cost and amount of oxygen usage supplied by other means and the cost of electricity and maintenance. There may be a considerable savings on the labor involved in the delivery and handling of other sources of oxygen. Fortunately the smaller units do not require a high wattage (19).

Filtration of Contaminants

Most airborne contaminants including exhaust hydrocarbons, ethylene oxide, sulfur dioxide, and chemical warfare gases are filtered by the molecular sieve and released back into the air (4).

Non-Interference with Most Gas Monitors

Raman, infrared, galvanic, and paramagnetic gas analyzers (see Chapter 18) are not adversely affected by the presence of argon. Mass spectrometers may need to be reprogrammed for the presence of this gas (4).

Reliability

Most concentrators perform well for long periods of time (18, 21). Concentrators are unaffected significantly by altitude.

Simplicity

Oxygen concentrators provide an increased inspired oxygen concentration without dependence on compressed or liquefied gas and their associated delivery problems.

DISADVANTAGES
Maintenance

Regular servicing is required, particularly for the compressor. It is important that the air intake filters be cleaned at the intervals recommended by the manufacturer.

Backup Supply Needed

Oxygen concentrators can only give an assured supply when either a reserve power supply or a few emergency cylinders of oxygen are available for power cuts.

Less than 100% Oxygen Produced

The maximum attainable oxygen yield for a molecular sieve concentration is approximately 96%. However, in medicine it is rarely essential to use 100% oxygen (23).

HAZARDS

The possible hazards are few, but observing normal electric safety precautions is imperative.

Fires

Oxygen greatly accelerates combustion. Therefore, the concentrator should be kept away from sources of heat, smoking, open flames, or electric equipment that may spark or become heated during operation. Oil and grease should not be allowed to contact the concentrator. Warnings such as "NO SMOKING OR NAKED FLAMES" should be posted in the area where the oxygen concentrator is in use.

Contamination of the Sieve Medium

Water can contaminate the sieve medium. This is not a problem under normal circumstances. However, under extreme circumstances such as high humidity, the oxygen concentration in the product gas will be lowered (24).

Contamination of Intake Air

The air intake must be located where it is not likely to be contaminated by fumes or other atmospheric pollutants (1). These contaminants could cause damage to the sieve medium and lead to premature exhaustion of the molecular sieve (21).

Device Malfunction

Electric or mechanical malfunction may occur and interrupt the flow of oxygen (1). It may be possible for the concentrator to be running but not concentrating oxygen. This has been reported after a liquid caused the intake filter to become nonfunctional (25). Compressor faults can cause cessation of function. Malfunction caused by failure of the valve linking the two sieve beds has also been reported (23). Lastly, cases have been reported where kinked transfer hoses in the units affected the flow of oxygen (26).

Argon Accumulation

Argon is not trapped by the molecular sieve and is concentrated much the same as oxygen (8). Argon can reach concentrations above 5%. The argon may accumulate if Oxygen 93 is added to a circle system used with low fresh gas flows. This has not been found to be a problem if the fresh gas flow is above 0.5 l/minute (9). There are no known patient effects from either long- or short-term exposure to low concentrations of argon (4).

REFERENCES

1. Carter JA, Baskett PJ, Simpson PJ. The "Permox" oxygen concentrator. Anaesthesia 1985;40:560–565.
2. McPherson SP. Respiratory home care equipment. Dubuque, Iowa: Kendall/Hunt Publishing Co., 1988.
3. Ezi-Ashi TI, Papworth DP, Nunn JF. Inhalation anaesthesia in developing countries. Part II: Review of existing apparatus. Anaesthesia 1983;38:736–747.
4. Friesen RM. Oxygen concentrators and the practice of anaesthesia. Can J Anaesth 1992;39:R80–R84.
5. Howell RSC. Oxygen concentrators. Br J Hosp Med 1985;34:221–223.
6. Jarvis DA, Brock-Utne JG. Use of an oxygen concentrator linked to a draw-over vaporizer (anesthesia delivery system for underdeveloped nations). Anesth Analg 1991;72:805–810.
7. Johns DP, Rockford PD, Streeton JA. Evaluation of six oxygen concentrators. Thorax 1985;40:806–810.
8. Lush D. Oxygen concentrators. Anaesthesia 1986;41:83.
9. Dobson M, Peel D, Khallaf N. Field trial of oxygen concentrators in upper Egypt. Lancet 1996;347:1597–1599.
10. Standard specification for oxygen concentrators for domiciliary use. ASTM F1484-93. West Conshohocken, PA: ASTM, 1993.
11. International Standard, Oxygen concentrators for medical use—safety requirements. ISO 8359, 1997. ISO, Geneva, Switzerland
12. International Standard, Oxygen concentrators for use with medical gas pipeline systems, ISO 10083, 1992. ISO, Geneva, Switzerland.

13. Personal Communication, David Peel

14. Easy WR, Douglas GA, Merrifield AJ. A combined oxygen concentrator and compressed air unit. Assessment of a prototype and discussion of its potential applications. Anaesthesia 1988;43:37–41.

15. Harris CE, Simpson PJ. The 'MiniO2' and 'Healthdyne' oxygen concentrators. Their performance and potential application. Anaesthesia 1985;40:1206–1209.

16. Wilson IH, van Heerden PV, Leigh J. Domiciliary oxygen concentrators in anaesthesia: preoxygenation techniques and inspired oxygen concentrations. Br J Anaesth 1990;65:342–345.

17. Stark RD, Bishop JM. New method for oxygen therapy in the home using an oxygen concentrator. BMJ 1973;2:105–106.

18. Fenton PM. The Malawi anaesthetic machine. Anaesthesia 1989;44:498–503.

19. Swan BB. Oxygen concentrators. Can J Anaesth 1987;34:538–539.

20. Robinson JS. An appraisal of piped medical gas systems. Br J Hosp Med 1982;28:160–164.

21. Evans TW, Waterhouse J, Howard P. Clinical experience with the oxygen concentrator. BMJ 1983;287:459–461.

22. Dobson MB. Oxygen concentrators offer cost savings for developing countries. A study based on Papua, New Guinea. Anaesthesia 1991;46:217–219.

23. Petty TL, Block AJ, Cherniak RM, et al. Problems in prescribing and supplying oxygen for Medicare patients. American Review of Respiratory Diseases 1986;134:340–341.

24. Carter MI. Oxygen concentration and water. Anaesthesia 1990;45:68.

25. Solanki T, Neville E. Oxygen concentrator malfunction. Lancet 1990;336:512.

26. Anonymous. Kinked transfer hoses may restrict gas flow in oxygen concentrators. Biomedical Safety & Standards 1996;26:149.

QUESTIONS: Oxygen Concentrators

Select the correct answer

1. In an oxygen concentrator, which of the following is most likely to cause deterioration to the adsorbent medium?
   A. Carbon dioxide
   B. Nitrogen
   C. Hydrocarbons
   D. Water vapor
   E. Carbon monoxide

Each question below contains four suggested answers of which one or more is correct.

Choose the answer:

A if 1, 2, and 3 are correct
B if 1 and 3 are correct
C if 2 and 4 are correct
D if 4 is correct
E if 1, 2, 3 and 4 are correct

2. Which gases can pass through an oxygen concentrator?
   1. Carbon dioxide
   2. Argon
   3. Helium
   4. Oxygen

3. Oxygen from a concentrator is referred to as
   1. USP 96%
   2. Oxygen 90
   3. Oxygen 96
   4. Oxygen USP 93%

4. In an oxygen concentrator
   1. The product gas is used to purge the retained gases from the sieve bed
   2. Aluminum silicates are used to trap specific molecules
   3. Polarity and size determine which molecules are retained by the concentrator medium
   4. Adsorption efficiency is greatly enhanced by the use of subatmospheric pressure

5. Present day applications of oxygen concentrators include
   1. Domiciliary use
   2. Supplying ambulances
   3. Supplying medical gas pipeline systems
   4. Supplying anesthesia machines

6. Advantages of the oxygen concentrator include
   1. Savings associated with purchase, handling, and delivery of gas cylinders
   2. Infrequent maintenance
   3. Contaminants in the air are filtered out of the product gas
   4. Constant oxygen output

7. Hazards associated with using oxygen concentrators include
   1. Argon accumulation
   2. Fires
   3. Unrecognized failure to concentrate
   4. Contamination of the sieve medium

ANSWERS

1. D   5. E
2. C   6. B
3. C   7. E
4. B

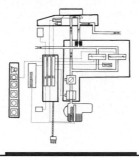

SECTION
II

ANESTHESIA MACHINES
AND BREATHING SYSTEMS

The Anesthesia Machine

ANESTHESIA MACHINES HAVE evolved from simple pneumatic devices to complex computer-based integrated systems with numerous controls, displays, indicators, and alarms. Until recently, the development of anesthesia machines was a slow, relatively unstructured process. In recent years, changes have been occurring at an escalating rate. The prevailing trend is to incorporate and integrate ventilators and vigilance aids such as airway pressure monitors, respirometers, respiratory gas monitors, pulse oximeters, electrocardiograms, and automatic blood pressure monitors into the machine.

MACHINE STANDARDS

In 1979, a standard that defined design, performance, and safety requirements for anesthesia machines was published by the American National Standards Institute (ANSI) (1). Most machines sold since 1979 comply with that standard. In 1988, this standard was superseded by a standard prepared under the auspices of the American Society for Testing and Materials (ASTM) (2). All American anesthesia machine manufacturers have agreed that machines sold after 1988 will comply with that standard.

The anesthesia machine can be conveniently divided into two parts: the electric system and pneumatic system.

THE ELECTRIC SYSTEM

Many components of modern anesthesia machines are powered by electricity supplied through the anesthesia machine. Turning the machine ON enables these devices and overcomes the problem of the operator forgetting to turn individual devices ON. Cellular telephones should not be used near an anesthesia machine because they may interfere with the operation of electronic equipment.

Master Switch

A master switch activates both the pneumatic and electric functions on most anesthesia machines (Figs. 4.1 and 4.2). On some machines, the electric components can be activated without pneumatic power. On most machines, when the switch is in the OFF or STANDBY position only the battery recharger and the convenience electric outlets are active. The master switch can be accidentally turned OFF (3–5).

Power Failure Indicator

Most machines are equipped with a visual or other indicator to alert the anesthesia provider to the loss of power from the facility (Fig. 4.2 and Fig. 4.43).

Backup (Battery) Power

A backup source of power for the occasional outage is necessary because electricity is crucial to the function of the machine.

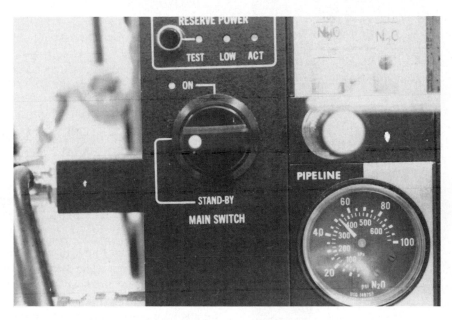

FIGURE 4.1.   Master switch. Turning this to the ON position activates both pneumatic and electric functions of the machine as well as certain alarms and safety fea- tures. Above the switch is a mechanism to check the backup battery power.

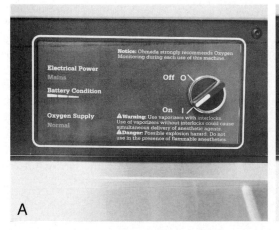 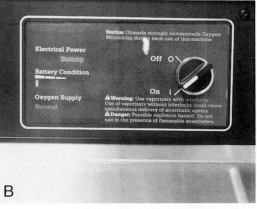

FIGURE 4.2.   **A,** The top indicator shows that the machine is operating on mains power. **B,** The indicator shows that the machine is operating on battery power. The light under the middle indicator shows the charge status of the battery. Note the main ON/OFF Switch to the right and the indicator for oxygen supply pressure below the indicators for electric power.

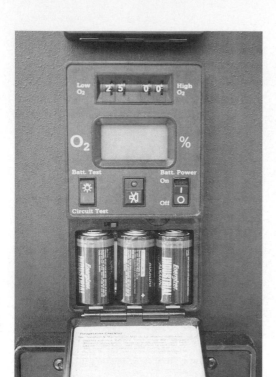

FIGURE 4.3. Some of the monitors, such as this oxygen analyzer, have their own battery backup power. Note the switch that must be turned ON to use battery power.

Equipment-Specific Backup

On some machines, many monitors have their own backup power (Fig. 4.3) These backup systems may need to be turned on individually or may be activated automatically. A disadvantage of this arrangement is that it is necessary to check the battery status of each instrument. The duration of the backup will vary. Some functions may fail before others.

One-Source Backup

Many of the machine components may be backed up with a single power source. The duration will depend on the number of instruments being supported. An advantage of this system is that the status of only one source needs to be checked. Battery life may be extended if manual ventilation is used.

Recharging

Battery recharge times vary. Backup power should be at its highest possible level if the machine is continually connected to power. If a machine is unplugged for an extended period, there may not be a complete charge.

Battery Status Test

Machines with backup systems usually have a means to test their status (Figs. 4.1 and 4.4 and see Fig. 4.43). The anesthesia provider should determine the location of these and include them in the anesthesia machine checkout procedure.

Electric Outlets

Most modern anesthesia machines have convenience electric outlets (Fig. 4.5). The convenience electric outlets are intended to power monitors that may be added to the machine. They are rated for a certain power output. A circuit breaker will be activated if the power requirements exceed that for which the machine was designed. High frequency surgical devices should not be connected to these outlets because this may cause the leakage current to rise above the permitted value. These outlets usually cannot supply electricity in case of a power failure.

Circuit Breakers

There are circuit breakers for both the anesthesia machine and the outlets (Fig. 4.6). Frequently, the maximum electric load is posted. The button will be forced out if this load is exceeded.

Circuit breakers are located in various locations on machines. Anesthesia providers should consult the instruction manual to become familiar with the circuit breaker location on each machine. When a circuit breaker is activated, the electric load should be reduced and the circuit breaker reset by pushing the button.

PNEUMATIC SYSTEM

As shown in Figure 4.7, the pneumatic part of the machine can be conveniently divided into three parts: the high-pressure system, which receives gases at cylinder pressure and lowers the pressure; the intermediate pressure system, which receives gases from the regulators or pipeline sys-

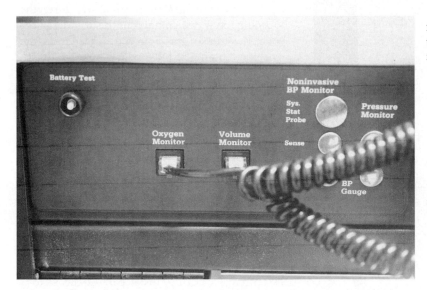

FIGURE **4.4.** Battery test button (at left) on the side of the machine.

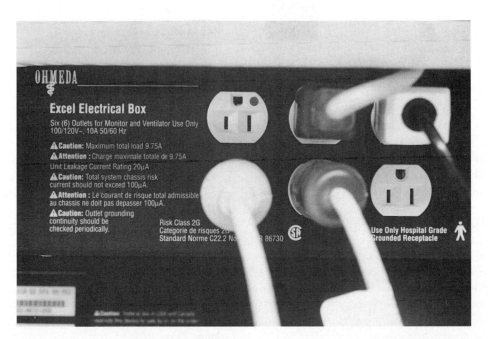

FIGURE **4.5.** Convenience electric outlets on the back of the anesthesia machine. These should be used only for anesthesia monitors and not for general operating room use. Note cautions regarding the total electric load.

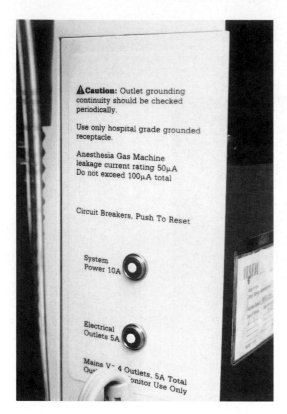

FIGURE 4.6. Circuit Breakers for anesthesia machine itself (above) and electric outlets on the machine (below).

tem and delivers them to the flow control or oxygen flush valves; and the low-pressure system, which takes gases from the flow control valves to the common gas outlet.

The High-Pressure System

The high-pressure system receives gases from a cylinder at a high variable pressure and reduces that pressure to a lower, more constant pressure suitable for use in the machine. It includes the hanger yoke (by which a cylinder is connected to the machine), the cylinder pressure indicator, and the pressure-reducing device.

Hanger Yoke

The functions of the hanger (connecting) yoke (cylinder holder) are to orient and support the cylinder, provide a gas-tight seal, and ensure a unidirectional flow of gas into the machine. It is composed of several parts: the body, which is the principal framework and supporting structure; the retaining screw, which tightens the cylinder in the yoke; the nipple, through which gas enters the machine; the index pins, which prevent attachment of an incorrect cylinder; the washer, which helps to form a seal between the cylinder and the yoke; a filter to remove dirt from the gas in the cylinder; and the check valve assembly, which ensures a unidirectional flow of gas through the yoke. Each yoke assembly must be permanently identified with the name or chemical symbol of the gas it accommodates and should be marked with the color assigned to the gas (2).

Body

The body of the yoke is threaded into the frame of the machine. It provides support for the cylinder(s). On the swinging gate (toggle handle, swivel gate) type, the distal part of the yoke is hinged (Fig. 4.8). The retaining screw is in the middle of this part. When a cylinder is being mounted onto or removed from a yoke, the hinged part can be swung to the side.

Retaining Screw

The retaining screw (clamping device, retaining bar) is threaded into the distal end of the yoke (Fig. 4.8). Tightening the screw presses the outlet of the cylinder valve against the washer and nipple so that a gas-tight seal is achieved. The cylinder is then supported by the retaining screw, the nipple, and the index pins.

The conical point of the retaining screw is shaped to fit the conical depression on the cylinder valve. Its dimensions are specified in the machine standard so that penetration of the safety relief device on the cylinder valve will be prevented.

Nipple

The nipple is the part of the yoke through which the gas enters the machine. It projects from the yoke and fits into the port on the cylinder valve. If the nipple is damaged, it may be impossible to obtain a tight seal with the cylinder valve.

Index Pins

The pins of the Pin Index Safety System are below the nipple (Fig. 4.8). The holes into which the pins are fitted must be of a specific depth. If they extend too far into the body of the yoke, it may be possible to insert an incorrect cylinder into the yoke (6).

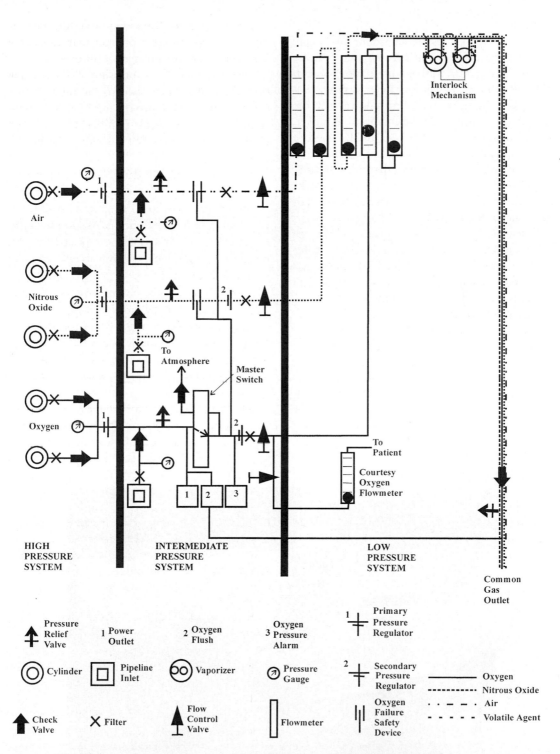

FIGURE 4.7. Diagram of a generic three-gas anesthesia machine. The components and their arrangement may differ somewhat with machines from different manufacturers.

Washer

A washer (gasket) is placed around the nipple (Fig. 4.8) to effect a seal between the cylinder valve and the yoke. A washer is often supplied with each full cylinder. When a cylinder is fitted to a yoke, care should be taken to ensure that the washer is present and in good condition. A broken or curled washer should not be used. An extra washer should be kept in the event a washer becomes damaged. No more than one washer should be used because that may prevent establishment of a tight seal or may nullify the Pin Index Safety System (6).

Filter

The machine standard requires that a filter (100 μm maximum) be installed between the cylinder and reducing device to prevent particulate matter from entering the machine (2).

Check Valve Assembly

The check valve assembly allows gas from a cylinder to enter the machine but prevents gas from exiting the machine when there is no cylinder in the yoke. This allows an empty cylinder to be replaced with a full one without having to turn off the "in-use" cylinder. It also prevents the transfer of gas from one cylinder to another with a lower pressure in a double yoke.

A typical check valve assembly is shown in Figure 4.9. It consists of a plunger that slides away from the side of the greater pressure. When cylinder pressure exceeds the pressure on the machine side, the plunger is pushed to the right and gas passes around it and into the machine. When machine pressure exceeds cylinder pressure, the plunger moves to the left, blocking the flow of gases.

Check valves are not designed to act as permanent seals for empty yokes and may allow a small amount of gas to escape. To minimize such losses, yokes should not be left vacant. As soon as a cylinder is exhausted, it should be replaced by a full one. If a full cylinder is not available, a yoke plug (dummy cylinder block or plug) (Fig. 4.10) should be placed in the empty yoke. A yoke plug is a solid piece of metal or other material that has a conical depression on one side to fit the tip of the retaining screw and a hollowed-out area on the other side to fit over the nipple. When in place, it forms a seal to prevent the escape of gases from the machine. A yoke plug also serves to keep the nipple clean and to prevent damage to the yoke. In the absence of a yoke plug, gas can leak from a yoke through an open flow control valve (7).

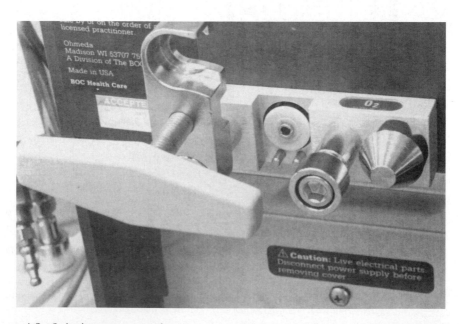

FIGURE **4.8.** Swinging gate type yoke. Note the washer around the nipple and the index pins below.

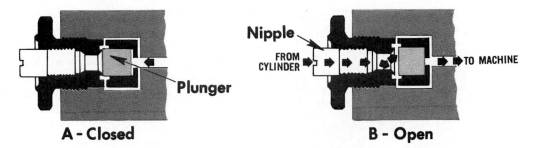

A - Closed   **B - Open**

FIGURE **4.9.** Yoke check valve assembly. This allows gas to enter the machine but does not allow gas to exit the yoke. When the pressure in the machine exceeds that in the cylinder the plunger moves to the left, preventing escape of gas from the machine. When cylinder pressure exceeds machine pressure, the plunger moves to the right and gas flows into the machine. (Adapted with permission from a drawing furnished by Ohmeda, a division of BOC, Inc.)

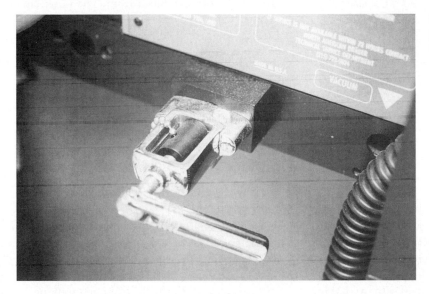

FIGURE **4.10.** Yoke plug in place. Note the chain to the machine.

Manufacturers often chain yoke plugs to the machine (Fig. 4.10).

Only one cylinder should be open at a time to prevent transfilling between paired cylinders as a result of a defective check valve.

Placing a Cylinder in a Yoke

It is important that cylinder valves and yokes not be contaminated with oil or grease. The person placing a cylinder in a yoke should always wash his/her hands beforehand. Before a cylinder is placed, the yoke should be checked to make certain that the two Pin Index Safety System pins are present. A missing pin can allow the safety system to be bypassed (8).

The first step in placing a cylinder in a yoke is to retract the retaining screw as far as possible. With the gate-type yoke, the gate is swung open. The washer is placed over the nipple. The cylinder is then supported with the foot and raised into the yoke (Fig. 4.11). The port of the cylinder valve is slid over the nipple and the index pins engaged in the appropriate holes. The gate is then closed. The retaining screw is tightened so that it contacts the conical depression on the cylinder valve and pushes the valve over the nipple and index pins. It is important to ensure that the cylinder is correctly in place before tightening the retaining screw. Otherwise it may be screwed into the safety

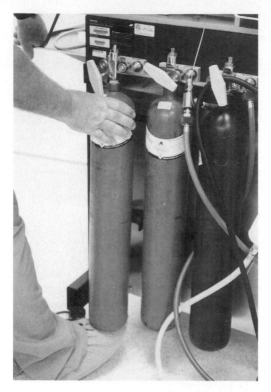

FIGURE **4.11.** Placing cylinder in yoke. The cylinder is supported by the foot and guided into place manually.

relief device on the cylinder (9). The cylinder valve should be opened to make sure that the cylinder is full and that there is no leak (as evidenced by a hissing sound). The cylinder should be returned to the supplier if the valve leaks or is difficult to operate. If a machine is equipped with two E cylinders, only one should be open at a time so that both tanks are not emptied simultaneously.

Cylinder Pressure Indicator (Gauge)

The machine standard requires that each hanger yoke or group of interconnected yokes be provided with a pressure indicator that will display the pressure of cylinder-supplied gas (2). If there is more than one yoke for a gas, one indicator may be provided for each yoke or one indicator may be provided for a group of yokes of the same gas. The indicator may be located near the cylinders or on a panel on the front of the machine (Fig. 4.12).

If the indicator is circular, the lowest pressure indication must be between the 6 o'clock and 9 o'clock positions on a clock face (Fig. 4.12). The scale must be at least 33% more than the maximum filling pressure. These requirements are designed to provide better resolution of the numbers and to facilitate recognition of the empty position on each indicator, which has been a problem in the past (10).

The indicator must be clearly and permanently marked with the name or chemical symbol of the gas it monitors and should be identified by the color assigned to that gas. These indicators are usually of the Bourdon tube (Bourdon spring, elastic element) type, illustrated in Figure 4.13. A hollow metal tube is bent into a curve, sealed, and linked to a clock-like mechanism. The other end is connected to the gas source and soldered into a socket. An increase in pressure of the gas inside the tube causes it to straighten. As the pressure falls, the tube resumes its curved shape. Because the open end is fixed, the sealed end moves. Through the clock-like mechanism these motions are transmitted to the indicator, which moves on a calibrated scale. Gauges are required to be calibrated in kilopascals (kPa), but pounds per square inch (psi) may also be used (Fig. 4.12) (2)

Pressure-Reducing Device (Regulator)

The pressure in a cylinder varies. The anesthesia machine is fitted with pressure-reducing devices (reducing valves, regulators, reducing regulators, reduction valves, regulator valves) to maintain constant flow with changing supply pressure. These reduce the high and variable pressure found in a cylinder to a lower (40 to 48 psig, 272 to 336 kPa) and more constant pressure suitable for use in an anesthesia machine. The machine standard requires reducing devices for each gas supplied to the machine from cylinders (2). Separate yokes for the same gas may be connected to one reducing device.

Physics

Force is defined as a pressure acting against an area. Force can be increased either by increasing the pressure or by increasing the area over which the pressure acts. To illustrate this, consider the simple balance shown in Figure 4.14. A large pressure (Pc) acting on a small area (A1) is balanced

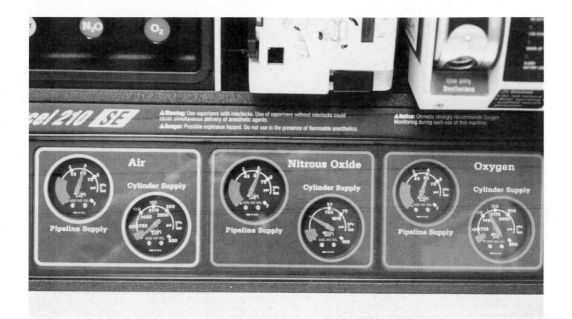

FIGURE 4.12. Cylinder and pipeline pressure indicators. Note that the lowest pressure indication is between the 6 o'clock and 9 o'clock positions on a clock face.

Kpa are indicated in the outside of the dial while psig are on the inside.

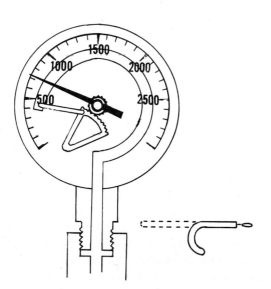

FIGURE 4.13. Bourdon pressure gauge. As gas pressure within the flexible tube increases, the tube tends to straighten. The motion is translated through the gearing mechanism so that the indicator shows a higher pressure. The tail end of the pointer is shorter than the indicating end and blends into the background. The lowest pressure indication is between the 6 o'clock and 9 o'clock positions on a clock face.

by a smaller pressure (Pr) acting on a large area (A2). The force exerted by the higher pressure is:

$$Pc \times A1$$

This is balanced by the force on the right:

$$Pr \times A2$$

Because these forces are equal, it follows that:

$$Pr \times A2 = Pc \times A1$$

Solving for Pr:

$$Pr = A1/A2 \times Pc$$

These same principles apply in a pressure-reducing device. Figure 4.15 shows a cylinder of gas under a high pressure (Pc [inlet pressure]). R is the inside of a reducing device containing gas at reduced pressure (Pr [outlet pressure]). The opening between C and R is occluded by a seat of area A1. A2 is the area of a flexible diaphragm on which Pr acts. The forces are in balance when the stopcock (S) is closed. The seat seals the opening from the cylinder so no gas flows from C into R.

In Figure 4.16, the stopcock is open and gas flows from R, causing the pressure (Pr) to drop.

FIGURE **4.14.** A large pressure acting over a small area is balanced by a smaller pressure acting over a large area. The relative sizes of the arrows represent the magnitudes of the pressures.

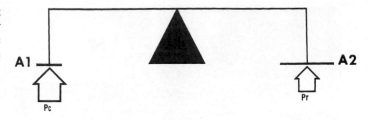

FIGURE **4.15.** The simplified pressure-reducing device is in the closed state (see text for details).

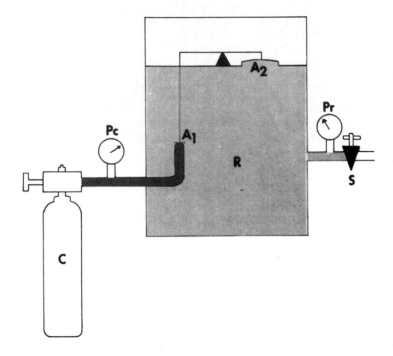

The forces are no longer balanced because Pc × A1 > (Pr × A2). The flexible diaphragm becomes flatter, the balance tips to the right, and the seat no longer occludes the opening from the cylinder so that gas flows from the cylinder into R. As long as the stopcock is open, the forces will be in balance and gas will continue to flow from the cylinder. This is analogous to opening the flow control valve on the anesthesia machine. When the stopcock is closed, gas will continue to flow briefly into R until Pr increases to the point where a balance of forces is restored. The small increase in Pr after the stopcock is closed is called "static increment."

The reducing device shown in Figures 4.15 and 4.16 will yield a constant reduced pressure only if the supplied pressure (Pc) is constant. If Pc decreases, as when the cylinder pressure falls, Pr must

decrease to preserve the balance of forces. With this type of reducing device, the flow indicator would constantly need to be adjusted to compensate for the pressure drop. To remedy this, a main spring (S1) is added (Fig. 4.17). This spring exerts a downward force on the flexible diaphragm. The magnitude of this force depends on an adjustable screw. Now the forces acting to push the diaphragm upward remain at:

$$Pr \times A2$$

Forces acting to push the diaphragm downward are:

$$(Pc \times A1) + F_{s1}$$

where F_{s1} is the force exerted by the spring. If the values for Pc, Pr, A1, and A2 remain un-

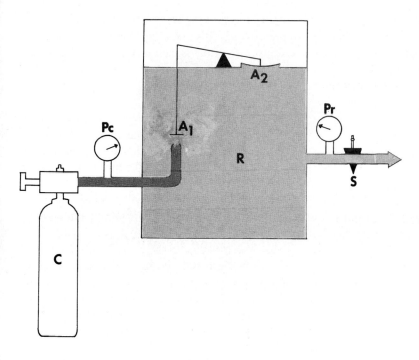

FIGURE **4.16.** The pressure-reducing device with its stopcock (*S*) open. An imbalance of forces is created, allowing gas to pass from the cylinder into the reducing device (see text for details).

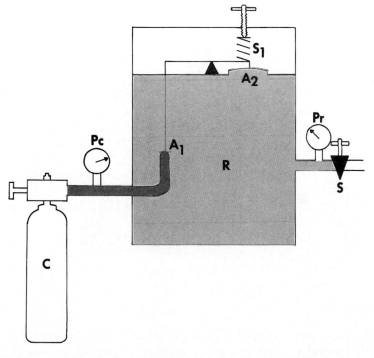

FIGURE **4.17.** A mainspring (*S1*) and adjusting screw have been added to the pressure-reducing device (see text for details).

changed, there would be an imbalance of forces because the force of the main spring would be added to the force of Pc acting on A1. To compensate for this imbalance, A1 may be reduced, A2 may be increased, or both. At equilibrium:

$$(Pc \times A1) + F_{s1} = Pr \times A2$$

Solving this equation for Pr:

$$Pr \times (F_{s1}/A2) + Pc(A1/A2) \qquad (1)$$

The force exerted by Pr acting on the diaphragm, therefore, is opposed by two forces: a constant force from the spring ($F_{s1}/A2$) and a variable force from Pc acting on the seat Pc(A1/A2). If the force exerted by the spring is large in comparison with the force exerted by Pc, large variations in Pc will cause only slight variations in Pr.

The value of Pr will depend on F_{s1}. The tension in the spring can be varied by means of the adjustable screw, and Pr can be varied in this way. For this reason the main spring is sometimes called the adjusting spring. One more addition to the regulator is necessary. A sealing (shutoff) spring (S2) is added in Figure 4.18. This acts to force

the seat against the opening from the cylinder and prevents gas from flowing from C to R when the adjusting spring is completely relaxed and the stopcock open. Equation 1 then becomes:

$$Pr = (F_{s1} - F_{s2})/A2 + Pc(A1/A2) \qquad (2)$$

The value of F_{s2} is considerably smaller than F_{s1} so that $F_{s1} - F_{s2}$ is large compared with Pc, and Pr will remain relatively constant in spite of variations in Pc. There will, however, be some variations in Pr with variations in Pc. A change, ΔPc, in cylinder pressure will produce a change, ΔPr, in the reduced pressure. From Equation 2:

$$\Delta Pr = \Delta Pc(A1/A2)$$

As Pc decreases, Pr also decreases (pressure-proportioned reduction). The magnitude of the change in Pr is governed by the ratio A1:A2.

The reducing device illustrated in Figures 4.15, 4.16, 4.17, and 4.18 is an example of a direct-acting reducing device. The components of a direct-acting reducing device are arranged so that the cylinder pressure tends to open the valve. An indirect-acting reducing device is shown diagram-

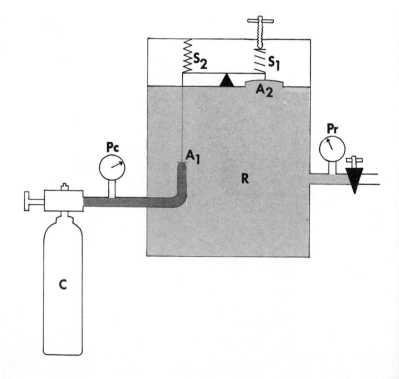

FIGURE **4.18.** A sealing spring has been added to complete the pressure-reducing device (see text for details).

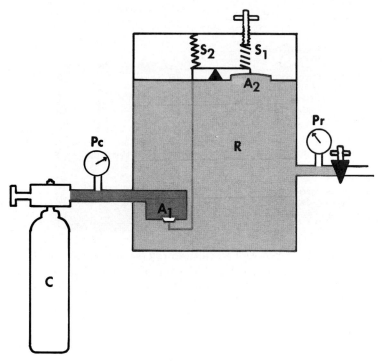

matically in Figure 4.19. In this case, Pc acts to close the valve. Equation 2 then becomes:

$$Pr = (F_{s1} - F_{s2})/A2 - Pc(A1/A2)$$

The variation in Pr with variation in Pc is given by the equation:

$$\Delta Pr = \Delta Pc(A1/A2)$$

As Pc decreases, Pr increases (pressure inversion).

The Modern Reducing Device

The modern reducing device, depicted in Figures 4.20 and 4.21, functions on the same principles as the devices shown in Figures 4.18 and 4.19. Each depends on the balance between high pressure exerted over a small area (the valve seat) and low pressure exerted over a large area (the diaphragm).

A direct-acting reducing device is shown in Figure 4.20. The functioning of a direct-acting reducing device is determined by a balance of forces acting to position the seat (A2). With the valve closed, the force of the sealing spring (S2) pushing the seat up against the nozzle is more than the downward force exerted by the main

spring (S1) and the inlet pressure (Pc) against the seat. No gas flows from the inlet into the reducing device. Pr is 0. The downward force of the main spring (S1) is increased when the valve is opened by tightening the adjusting screw. This force is transmitted along the valve thrust pin to the seat and, in combination with the inlet pressure, overcomes the force of the sealing spring. Gas at reduced pressure (Pr) flows into the space under the diaphragm and exerts an upward force on the diaphragm (Pr $\times$ A2). Gas then flows on to the outlet. The forces are not in balance, but Pr will remain constant because a steady state is soon achieved. Gas will continue to flow until either the cylinder is empty or the gas flow is turned off at a point distal to the reducing device. If it is turned off, gas will continue briefly to flow into the space under the diaphragm. Here, its pressure will increase (static increment) until the force of the reduced gas on the diaphragm (Pr $\times$ A2) plus the force of the sealing spring (S2) balance the force of the cylinder pressure and the main spring (Pc $\times$ A2 + F$_2$), as in Equation 2.

Figure 4.21 illustrates an indirect-acting reducing device. With the valve closed, gas enters

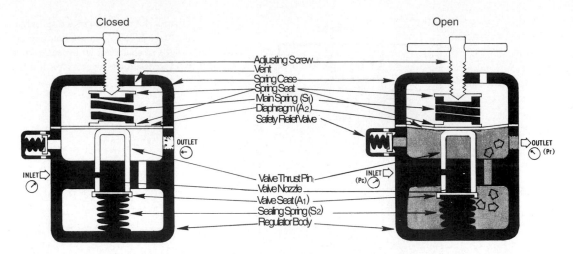

FIGURE 4.20. Direct-acting–reducing device. The *darker shades* are used for gas under high pressure, whereas the *lighter shades* represent gas under reduced pressure. The *arrows* indicate the path of gas flow. The

valve is opened by turning the adjusting screw (see text for details). (Adapted with permission from a drawing furnished by Ohmeda, a division of BOC, Inc.)

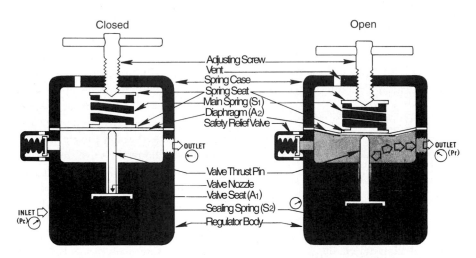

FIGURE 4.21. Indirect-acting–reducing device. The cylinder pressure opposes the opening of the valve. When the adjusting screw is opened, gas flows from the

lower to the upper chamber along the valve thrust pin. (Adapted with permission from a drawing furnished by Ohmeda, a division of BOC, Inc.)

the space surrounding the sealing spring (S2) and the valve seat (A1). Its own pressure (Pc) tends to hold the valve seat against the nozzle. When the adjusting screw is turned so that the main spring exerts a downward force on the diaphragm (F_1), the valve thrust pin moves downward, opening the seat, so that gas at reduced pressure (Pr) expands through the holes for the thrust pin and into the cavity under the diaphragm. When the

gas flow is turned off distal to the reducing device, gas continues to flow briefly into the space under the diaphragm. Here its pressure increases (static increment), pushing the diaphragm upward until the seat closes against the nozzle, stopping further flow.

Reducing devices may be adjustable or preset. An adjustable reducing device has a means for easy user adjustment of the delivery pressure. Tools are required to adjust the delivery pressure with a pre-set reducing device.

Reducing devices used in anesthesia machines are preset at the factory and located under the machine's work surface. One regulator may serve two hanger yokes. The machine standard requires that they be adjusted so that the machine uses only gas from the pipeline when the pipeline inlet pressure is 50 psig (345 kPa) or greater (2). This is to prevent use of gas from a cylinder if the cylinder valve is open while the pipeline supply is in use. This can be accomplished by keeping the pressure from the cylinder pressure-reducing device at a lower level than the pipeline. In addition, when pipeline supplies of gases are being used, cylinder valves should be closed because the machine will always use gas from the source that has the highest pressure. If the pipeline pressure drops below that supplied by the cylinder pressure-reducing device and the cylinder valve is open, some gas will be withdrawn from the cylinder. Eventually, the cylinder will be depleted. In this case, the operator would be unaware that a changeover had occurred until the cylinder became exhausted. Knowing that the pipeline supply has failed allows the operator to make arrangements for additional cylinders to be supplied as those in use are exhausted.

To protect the rest of the machine from excessive pressure, a reducing device must be equipped with a relief valve that opens at not more than four times the normal inlet pressure (2). A defective reducing device may block the flow of gas from a cylinder or cause widely fluctuating flows (11, 12).

Intermediate Pressure System

The intermediate pressure system (Fig. 4.7) receives gases from the regulator or hospital pipeline at pressures of 40 to 55 psig (272 to 375 kPa). It includes the pipeline inlet connections, pipeline pressure indicators, piping, the gas power outlet, the master switch, oxygen pressure failure devices that either interrupt the flow of anesthetic gases or provide an alarm when the oxygen pressure fails, the oxygen flush, additional reducing devices (if so equipped), and the flow control valves.

Pipeline Inlet Connections

The machine standard mandates pipeline inlets for oxygen and nitrous oxide (2). Suction and air inlets are usually available. These inlets are fitted

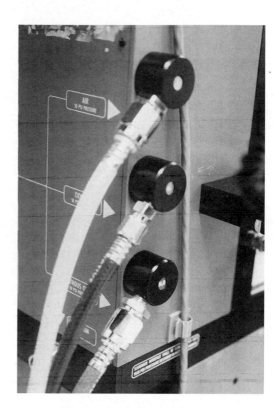

FIGURE 4.22. Pipeline inlets. Note the Diameter Index Safety System connections.

with threaded noninterchangeable Diameter Index Safety System (DISS) fittings (see Chapter 2) (Fig. 4.22). Each inlet must contain a check valve to prevent flow of gas from the machine into the piping system (or to atmosphere if no hose is connected). These check valves function like the hanger yoke check valves. Like hanger yokes, pipeline inlets must have filters with a pore size of 100 micrometers or less. The filter may become clogged, resulting in a decrease in gas flow (13).

Problems have been reported with check valves. In one case it stuck in the closed position, causing obstruction of oxygen flow (14), and there are reports of failure of the valve to prevent reverse flow (15, 16).

Pipeline Pressure Indicators (Gauges)

Indicators to monitor the pressure (Fig. 4.12) of each gas supplied by a pipeline to the machine are required by the machine standard (2). The indicators must meet the same requirements relating to readability as cylinder pressure indicators.

Pipeline pressure indicators are usually found on a panel on the front of the machine and are color coded. On some machines the correct range of pressures is indicated by a green zone. The 1979 and 1988 standards require that the indicator be on the pipeline side of the check valve in the pipeline inlet (Fig. 4.7). On older machines, the indicator may be attached on either the pipeline or machine side of the check valve. If the indicator is on the pipeline side of the check valve, it will monitor pipeline pressure only. If the hose is disconnected or improperly connected, it will read 0 even if a cylinder valve is open (17, 18). If the indicator is on the machine (downstream) side of the check valve, it cannot be depended on to give a true indication of the pipeline supply pressure unless the cylinder valves are closed. If a cylinder valve is open and the pipeline supply fails, there will be no change in the pressure on the indicator until the cylinder is nearly empty (19).

The relationship of the indicator to the check valve is not obvious on inspection of the machine. The user can ascertain the location by disconnecting the pipeline hose and opening the cylinder valve (20). If the reading on the pipeline indicator remains zero, the indicator is on the pipeline side of the check valve. If a reading is obtained, the indicator is connected on the machine side. The indication of an adequate pressure on the pipeline indicator does not guarantee that gas is not being drawn from a cylinder. If, for any reason, the pressure of gas coming from a cylinder through a pressure-reducing device exceeds the pipeline pressure and a cylinder valve is open, gas will be drawn from the cylinder. It follows that cylinders should always remain closed when a pipeline supply is in use.

Pipeline pressure indicators should always be checked before the machine is used. They should register between 45 and 55 psig (310 and 380 kPa). Pipeline pressure indicators should be scanned repeatedly during use.

Piping

Connections between components inside the machine are usually made from metal tubing. Connections must be able to withstand four times the intended service pressure without rupturing. The machine standard specifies that leaks between the pipeline inlet or cylinder pressure-reducing system and the flow control valve not exceed 25 ml per minute at normal service pressure (2). If the pressure-reducing system is included, the maximum allowable leakage is not to exceed 150 ml per minute at maximum inlet pressures.

Cases of cross-connections of piping inside the machine have been reported (21). Although rare, a disconnection in the piping may occur. In one case, a compression fitting had been omitted and replaced by sealant tape. Pressure caused the tube to separate from the connection, causing loss of oxygen (22).

Gas Power Outlet

Most machines are equipped with a connection to supply oxygen or air to a ventilator or jet ventilation system. Most machines currently have a direct connection to the ventilator and do not have a discrete outlet. If provided, the outlet may be fitted with a DISS fitting or quick coupler. The outlet needs to have a check valve so that gas can only flow from the machine. A spring-loaded valve prevents gas from flowing into atmosphere if a hose is not attached.

The reduced pressure issuing from the reducing device may be set just below 50 psig on machines equipped with a power outlet because some ventilators will not function properly at lower pressures. It is possible to operate a ventilator only from pipeline supplies and not from cylinders on some machines.

Master Switch (Pneumatic Component)

One of the characteristics of modern machines is the coordination of all the machine functions under a central control. The master switch (system switch) (Figs. 4.1 and 4.2) is a two- or three-position switch with mutually exclusive positions. The pneumatic portion of the master switch is located in the intermediate pressure system downstream of the inlet from the cylinder and pipeline supplies. Turning on the master switch causes both the pneumatic and electronic functions of the machine to be activated. The oxygen flush is usually independent of this feature. A master switch is shown in Figure 4.23. When the master switch is turned to the OFF or STANDBY position, a port

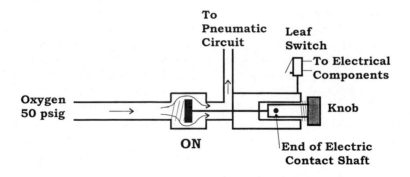

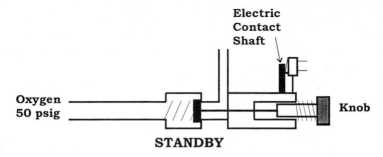

FIGURE 4.23. Master switch, pneumatic component. In the ON position, the knob is depressed. This causes the plunger to move to the left and allows oxygen to flow to the pneumatic circuit. It also allows electricity to flow to components in the machine. In the STANDBY position, oxygen flow to components other than the oxygen flush and the auxiliary oxygen flowmeter is blocked and electricity is not supplied to components of the machine. (Adapted with permission from North American Drager).

is opened to atmosphere and the pressure in the pneumatic system upstream of the switch falls to atmospheric. This causes the oxygen failure safety devices to close, interrupting the flow of anesthetic gases to the common gas outlet.

Cases have been reported in which wear on the master switch caused it to migrate to an intermediate position between OFF and ON. When this occurred, gas supply to the common gas outlet was interrupted (23, 24). Another hazard is that the master switch may be inadvertently turned to the OFF position (3–5).

Oxygen Pressure Failure Devices

One of the most serious mishaps that occurred with early machines was depletion of the oxygen supply (usually from a cylinder) without the user's awareness. The result was delivery of 100% anesthetic gas. Prevention of such an accident has been the object of numerous inventions. Among these have been devices that cut off the supply of gases other than oxygen (oxygen failure safety device) and/or give an audible or visible warning (alarm) when oxygen pressure has fallen to a dangerous level.

Devices

Oxygen failure safety device. The machine standard requires that an anesthesia machine be designed so that whenever the oxygen supply pressure is reduced below normal, the set oxygen concentration at the common gas outlet does not fall below 19% (2). The oxygen failure safety device (oxygen failure safety valve, low-pressure guardian system, oxygen-failure–protection device, pressure sensor shutoff system or valve, fail safe, pressure sensor system, nitrous oxide shutoff valve) shuts off or proportionally decreases and ultimately interrupts the supply of nitrous oxide and other gases if the oxygen supply pressure decreases (25). In some machines, the supply of air is also cut off if the oxygen pressure drops. In the future, the air supply will not be shut off when the oxygen failure safety device is activated.

As shown in Figure 4.7, oxygen failure safety devices are located upstream of the flow control valves. On machines with an ON/OFF switch, turning this to the ON position allows oxygen pressure to reach the oxygen failure safety device, allowing other gases to flow. Turning the switch to the OFF position causes oxygen in the machine to be vented to atmosphere. The resulting decrease in oxygen pressure causes the oxygen failure safety device to interrupt the supply of other gases to their flow control valves.

One such device is shown in Figure 4.24. It is found in certain machines and is similar to an indirect-acting–reducing device with the adjusting spring replaced by oxygen pressure. The opening (B) is connected to the intermediate pressure oxygen system. If oxygen pressure is normal, the diaphragm and stem are pushed downward, allowing anesthetic gas to pass around the seat and on through the machine. Should oxygen pressure drop below 20 to 25 psig (135 to 170 kPa), the combined force of the spring and the pressure of the anesthetic gas in the lower chamber will overcome the downward force from the oxygen and the valve will close, stopping the flow of anesthetic gas. This valve, therefore, is a simple ON/OFF device.

Another such device is shown in Figure 4.25. This is found in Drager machines and is called an oxygen-failure–protection device. When oxygen pressure is normal, the plunger and seal assembly are depressed so that anesthetic gas can flow through the valve. When oxygen pressure is decreased, the spring forces the plunger and seal assembly upward, narrowing the valve opening in proportion to oxygen supply–pressure loss. If oxygen supply–pressure fails completely, the valve closes. This differs from the previous device in that in the event of a partial loss of oxygen pressure, anesthetic gas flow is reduced but is not completely cut off.

Oxygen failure safety devices are present on most anesthesia machines but may not be present on some older machines or may be present for only one gas. To determine if a machine has a properly functioning device, the flows of oxygen and the other gas are turned ON and then the

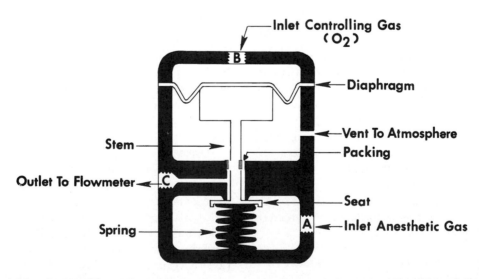

FIGURE 4.24.   Oxygen failure safety valve. When oxygen pressure in the machine is normal, it will push the diaphragm and stem downward, opening the valve. The anesthetic gas then flows in at **A**, around the stem, and out at **C**. When the oxygen pressure falls, the stem moves upward, closing the valve. The middle chamber is vented to atmosphere to prevent mixing of anesthetic gas and oxygen in the event that the diaphragm ruptures or the packing leaks. (Adapted with permission from a drawing furnished by Ohmeda, a division of BOC, Inc.)

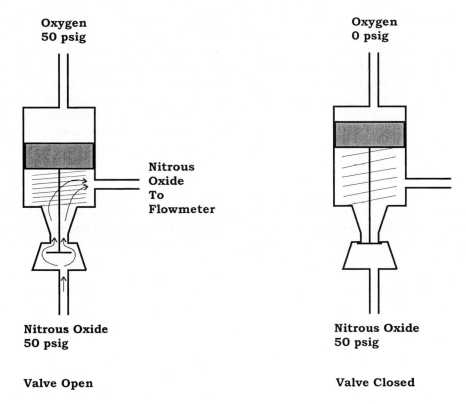

Oxygen
50 psig

Oxygen
0 psig

Nitrous
Oxide
To
Flowmeter

Nitrous Oxide
50 psig

Nitrous Oxide
50 psig

Valve Open

Valve Closed

FIGURE **4.25.**   Drager oxygen-failure–protection device. When oxygen pressure is normal, the plunger and seal assembly are pushed downward, overcoming the upward force of the spring. Anesthetic gas can flow through the valve. When oxygen pressure falls, the spring pushes the plunger upward, so that the valve is closed.

source of oxygen pressure removed. If the oxygen failure safety device is functioning properly, the flow indicator for the other gas will fall to the bottom of the tube. If a machine is lacking such a device for any gas except air, it should be modified or replaced.

A leak in this device has been reported (26, 27). Oxygen was lost through the vent to atmosphere in the center chamber. This resulted in considerable noise but no danger. Cases have been reported in which a tear in the diaphragm resulted in a direct communication between the oxygen and nitrous oxide systems inside the machine (28, 29).

Oxygen supply failure alarm. The machine standard specifies that whenever the oxygen supply pressure falls below a manufacturer-specified threshold (usually 30 psig [205 kPa]), a medium priority alarm shall be enunciated within 5 seconds

(Fig. 4.2 and Fig. 4.43) (2, 30). After the alarm has been activated, it may be silenced for a period not exceeding 120 seconds. The alarm cannot be disabled. If the low pressure condition is corrected, the alarm sound will cease. Some older machines in use may not have such a warning device. Frequently, one can be installed on an existing machine.

ELECTRONIC ALARMS. Some machines use a pressure-operated electric switch to activate the alarm. In Ohmeda machines, the alarm is actuated at pressures around 28 psig (190 kPa). On Drager machines, the threshold is between 30 and 37 psig (207 and 255 kPa) (31).

PNEUMATIC ALARMS. Another alarm mechanism utilizes a pressurized canister that is filled with oxygen when the anesthesia machine is turned ON. When the oxygen pressure falls below a certain value, the alarm directs a stream of oxygen through a whistle. The sound will continue until the reservoir is depleted. It is important to note that the ending of the whistle does not necessarily mean that the low oxygen pressure condition has been corrected. The reservoir is depressurized when the ON/OFF switch is turned to the OFF position.

Limitations

Because both the oxygen failure safety device and alarm depend on pressure and not flow, they have limitations that are not always fully appreciated by the user. If the machine is gas tight, the oxygen system may stay pressurized for weeks without being connected to a source of oxygen. The oxygen failure safety device and alarm do not offer total protection against a hypoxic mixture being delivered because they do not prevent anesthetic gas from flowing if there is no flow of oxygen. The devices aid in preventing hypoxia caused by some problems (disconnected oxygen hose, low oxygen pressure in the pipeline, and depletion of oxygen cylinders) occurring upstream in the machine circuitry. They do not guard against accidents that result from crossovers in the pipeline system or a cylinder containing the wrong gas. Equipment problems (such as leaks) or operator errors (such as a closed or partially closed oxygen flow control valve) that occur downstream are not prevented by these devices. The use of an oxygen analyzer in the breathing system that is turned ON and functioning is essential.

Oxygen Flush Valve

The oxygen flush valve (oxygen bypass, emergency oxygen) receives oxygen from the pipeline inlet or cylinder reducing device and directs a high unmetered flow directly to the common gas outlet (Fig. 4.7). The machine standard requires that the flow be between 35 and 75 liters per minute (2). Flush valves for gases other than oxygen are not permitted. On most anesthesia machines the oxygen flush can be activated regardless of whether the master switch is turned ON or OFF. The standard requires that the oxygen flush be a single-purpose, self-closing device, which is permanently marked to show its function, and designed to minimize accidental activation (2).

An oxygen flush valve is shown in Figure 4.26 and consists of a button and stem connected to a ball. The ball is in contact with the seat. When the button is depressed, the ball is forced away from the seat, allowing the oxygen to flow to the outlet. A spring opposing the ball will close the valve when the button is not depressed. The button is commonly recessed or placed in a collar to prevent accidental activation (Fig. 4.27).

Depending on the particular machine, activation of the oxygen flush may or may not result in other gas flows being shut off. Activation may result in either a positive or negative pressure in the machine circuitry, depending on the design of the inlet of the flush line into the common gas line. This pressure will be transmitted back to other structures in the machine, such as flow indicators and vaporizers, and may change the vaporizer output and the flow indicator readings. The effect of activation will depend on the pressure generated, the presence or absence of check valves in the machine, and the relationship of the oxygen flush valve to other components. The machine standard requires that the connection of the flush valve delivery line to the common gas outlet be designed so that activation does not increase or decrease the pressure at the outlet of a vaporizer by more than 10 kPa or increase the vapor output by more than 20% (2).

Reported hazards associated with the oxygen flush valve include accidental activation (32–35) and internal leakage, which resulted in an oxygen-enriched mixture being delivered (36). There have been reports of flush valves sticking in the ON position (37, 38). There is a report of a flush valve sticking so that it obstructed flow of the gases from the flow indicators (39). Barotrauma and cases of awareness caused by its activation have been reported (35). Activation of the oxygen flush during an inspiration delivered by the anesthesia ventilator will result in delivery of high pressures.

Use of the oxygen flush to ventilate through a catheter inserted percutaneously has been investigated (40). Only machines that delivered the gas at 345 to 380 kPa (50 to 55 psi) were capable of providing effective ventilation.

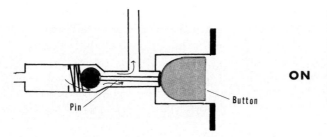

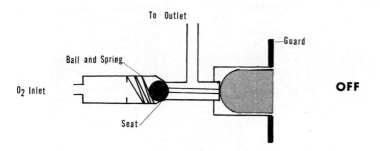

ON

OFF

FIGURE **4.26.** Oxygen flush valve. Depressing the button causes the pin to push the ball away from the seat, allowing oxygen to pass directly to the machine outlet. (Adapted with permission from a diagram furnished by Ohmeda, a division of BOC, Inc.)

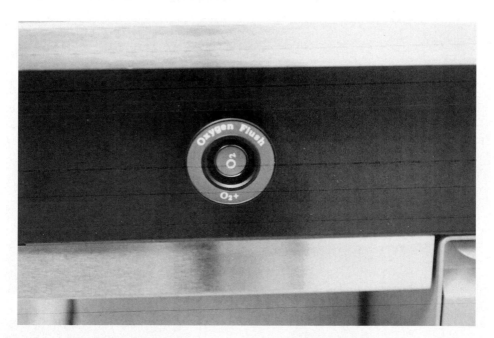

FIGURE **4.27.** Oxygen flush valve. Note the protective ring to prevent accidental activation. O_2+ is a symbol for the oxygen flush valve.

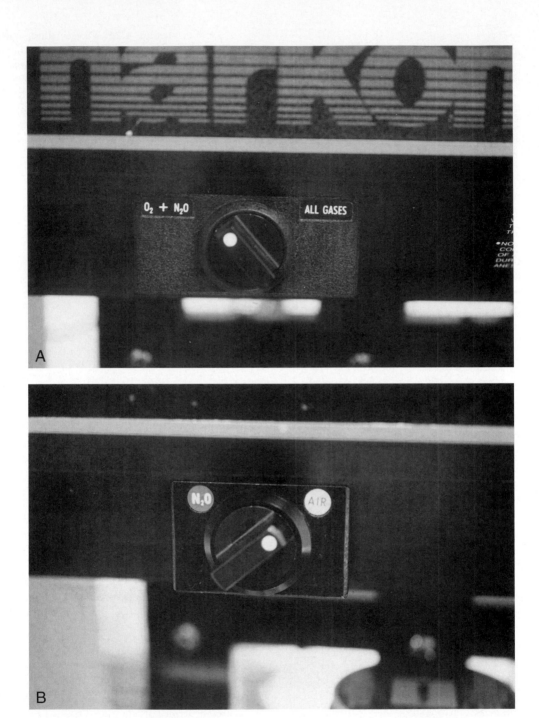

FIGURE 4.28.   Gas Selector Switches **A,** In the N_2O position, only oxygen and nitrous oxide can be used. In the air position, only oxygen and air can be adminis- tered. **B,** This allows selection of either nitrous oxide and oxygen or all gases on the machine.

Gas Selector Switch

Some machines have a gas selector switch with two modes: $O_2 + N_2O$ and ALL GAS (Fig. 4.28 A) or N_2O and air (Fig. 4.28B). In the $O_2 + N_2O$ or N_2O modes, the alarm for the oxygen ratio monitor controller is activated and the minimum oxygen flow is enabled. In the ALL GAS or AIR modes, these are disabled.

Second-Stage–Reducing Device

Some machines have reducing devices just upstream of the nitrous oxide and oxygen flow valves. These receive gas from either the pipeline or the cylinder reducing device and reduce it further to 26 psig (177 kPa) for nitrous oxide and 14 psig (95 kPa) for oxygen. The purpose of this reducing device is to eliminate fluctuations in pressure supplied to the flow indicator caused by fluctuations in pipeline pressure. By reducing the pressures below the normal fluctuation range, the flow will remain constant.

Flow Control Valve

The flow control valve (needle valve, pin valve, fine adjustment valve, flow adjustment control) controls the rate of flow of a gas through its associated flow indicator by manual adjustment of a variable orifice. Most flow control valves have both a control and an ON/OFF function. The ON/OFF function is controlled by the master switch on some machines.

The current standard requires that there be only one flow control valve for each gas (2). It must be adjacent to or identifiable with its flow indicator.

Components

Body. The body of the flow control valve screws into the base of the flow indicator.

Stem and seat. The stem and seat are shown diagrammatically in Figure 4.29. The stem has fine threads so that it moves only a short distance when a complete turn is made. When the valve is closed, the pin at the end of the stem fits onto the seat and no gas can pass through the valve. When the stem is turned outward, an opening between the pin and the seat is created, allowing gas to flow through the valve. The greater the space between the pin and the seat, the greater the volume of gas that can flow. To eliminate any loose-

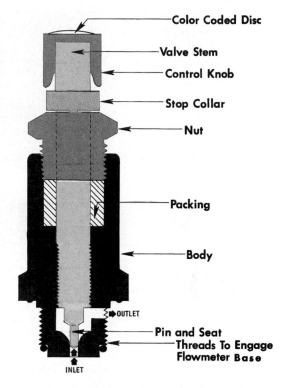

FIGURE 4.29. Flow control valve, shown in the closed position. Turning the stem creates a leak between the pin and seat so that gas flows to the outlet. The stop collar prevents over tightening of the pin in the seat. (Adapted with permission from a drawing furnished by Foregger Co., a division of Puritan Bennett Co., Inc.)

ness in the threads, the valve may be spring-loaded (41). This also minimizes flow fluctuations from lateral or axial pressure applied to the flow control knob. It is advantageous to have stops for the OFF and maximum flow positions. A stop for the OFF position avoids damage to the valve seat. A stop for the maximum flow position prevents the stem from becoming disengaged from the body.

Control knob. The control knob is joined to the stem. It should be large enough that it can be turned easily. If it is a rotary style knob, the oxygen flow control knob must have a fluted profile (Figs. 4.30 and 4.31) and be as large as or larger than that for any other gas, and all other flow control knobs must be round. The oxygen control must look and feel different from the other controls if

FIGURE **4.30.** Flow control valves. Note that the oxygen flow control valve is fluted and larger than the other flow control valve.

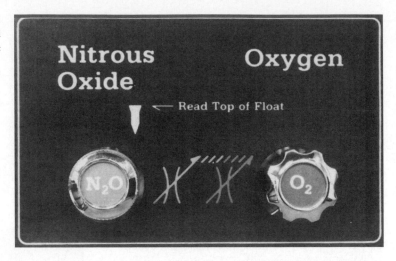

other types of flow adjustment controls are present (2).

The close proximity of the flow control knobs on some machines contributes to the risk of errors. They need to be far enough apart to prevent inadvertent changes in position. Changes in position can also be minimized by a shield, bar, or other protective barrier (Fig. 4.31) and by placing them high above the working surface to lessen the likelihood of contact with objects on that surface.

Knobs are turned counterclockwise to increase flow and clockwise to decrease flow. Flow control knobs should operate smoothly and be easy to adjust, yet resist unintentional changes.

The knob should be turned clockwise only until the flow of gas ceases because further tightening may result in damage to the pin or seat. Some manufacturers provide a stop collar to prevent it from being closed too tightly. However, this can be overridden or changed by overturning. The gas source (cylinder or pipeline) should be closed or disconnected whenever a machine is not being used. The flow control valves should be opened until the gas pressure is bled to zero and then closed.

Before use of the machine is resumed, the flow control valves should be checked to see that they are closed. Sometimes anaesthesia providers develop the habit of leaving the flow control valves open after the gas is bled out. In addition, the flow control valves may be opened when the machine is cleaned or moved by people not in a position to understand the consequences. If the gas supply to an open flow control valve is restored and the associated flow indicator is not observed, the indicator may rise to the top of the tube where its presence may not be noticed by the operator. Even if no harm to the patient results, the sudden rise of the indicator may damage it and impair the accuracy of the flow indicator (42).

Electronic Control of Flow

Conventional flow control valves are not well suited for certain purposes such as servo control. For this reason, anesthesia machines of the future are likely to have electronic flow controls (43). If electronic flow control valves look and feel similar to conventional flow control valves, they must meet the same requirements as conventional valves (2). The oxygen flow control must look and feel different from the flow controls for other gases.

In its simplest form, electronic control of gas flow consists of a motor geared to the control knob of a needle valve. However, modern electronic circuitry and use of computers favor digital systems. These commonly use solenoid valves to control flow by splitting the flow into a number of channels, each controlled by a solenoid valve that is either ON or OFF. An orifice in each channel results in a specific flow rate when the solenoid valve is open. The total flow depends on which channels are open. The solenoid valves are controlled by a computer. Another way solenoids can control flow is to make them pulsed. The volume

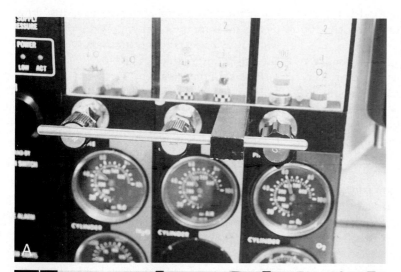

FIGURE 4.31. Flow control knob guards. **A,** The bar serves to protect the knobs from an accidental change.

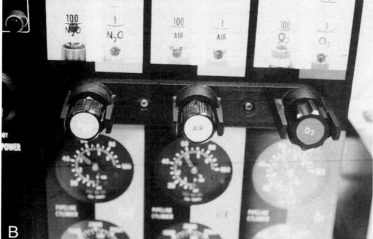

FIGURE 4.31. B, Each knob has guards on either side.

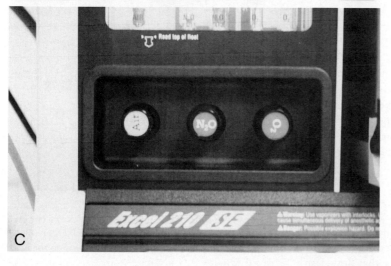

FIGURE 4.31. C, The knobs are recessed. Note the fluted oxygen flow control knobs and ball indicators in A and B.

of gas that passes through the valve depends on how long the valve is open and the frequency of opening.

The type of electronic flow control most likely to be employed is the mass flow controller. This consists of a continuously variable solenoid valve in which the flow is varied by varying the voltage applied to the solenoid. The flow is continually measured, and this information is fed back to the solenoid valve.

Problems with Flow Control Valves

Inadvertent alterations. If the flow control valve knob is loose or worn, it may respond to a light touch or even accidental brushing (44).

Inability to turn control knob. A case has been reported in which the stop pins became locked so that the valve could not be turned ON (45).

Leak through open flow control valve. Flow control valves should be closed when not in use. If there is no yoke plug or cylinder in the yoke or the one-way valve in the pipeline inlet does not work well, gases from the flow indicator manifold can leak to atmosphere (7, 46–49).

Failure to allow adequate gas flow. The stem can break off and block the path of flow (12, 50, 51). The seating into which the stem extends can become detached and obstruct flow (52). Cases have been reported in which the oxygen and nitrous oxide control knobs were linked so that the maximum inspiratory oxygen concentration that could be obtained was less than 100% (53–55).

Low Pressure System

The low-pressure system (Fig. 4.7) is downstream of the flow control valves. Pressure in this section is only slightly above atmospheric. Components found in this section include flow indicators, vaporizer circuit control valves, back pressure safety devices, low-pressure piping, and the common gas outlet. Vaporizers, which are found in the low-pressure system, will be considered in Chapter 5.

Flow Indicators

A flow indicator (flowmeter, flow tube, rotameter) measures and indicates the rate of flow of a gas passing through it. Measurement of the flow of gases is based on the principle that flow past a resistance is proportional to pressure. Most flowmeters measure the drop in pressure that occurs when a gas passes through a resistance and correlate this pressure drop to flow.

Physical Principles

Flow indicators used in anesthesia machines have traditionally been of the variable orifice (variable area, Thorpe tube) type. The tube (Fig. 4.32) is tapered vertically with its smallest diameter at the bottom. It contains an indicator that is free to move up and down inside the tube. When there is no flow of gas, the float rests at the bottom of the tube. As shown in Figure 4.32B, when the flow control valve is opened, gas enters at the bottom and flows up the tube, elevating the indicator. The gas passes through the annular opening between the float and the tube and onto the outlet at the top of the tube. The indicator floats freely in the tube at a position where the downward force on it caused by gravity equals the upward force caused by gas molecules hitting the bottom of the float. As gas flow increases, the number of gas molecules hitting the bottom of the float increases and the float rises. Because the tube is tapered, the size of the annular opening around

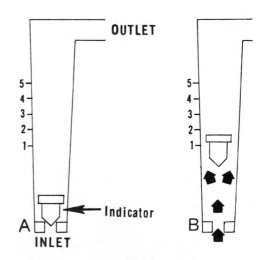

FIGURE 4.32. Variable orifice flow indicator. **A,** No gas flow. **B,** Gas enters at the base and flows through the tube, causing the indicator to rise. The gas passes through the annular opening around the float. The area of this annular space increases with the height of the indicator. Thus the height of the indicator is a measure of gas flow.

the indicator increases with height and more gas flows around the float. When the flow is decreased, gravity causes the indicator to settle to a lower level. A scale marked on or beside the tube shows the gas flow.

The rate of flow through the tube will depend on three factors: the pressure drop across the constriction, the size of the annular opening, and the physical properties of the gas.

Pressure drop across the constriction. As gas flows around the indicator, it encounters frictional resistance between the float and the wall of the tube. The flow also becomes less laminar and more turbulent. There is a resultant loss of energy reflected in a pressure drop. This pressure drop is constant for all positions in the tube and is equal to the weight of the float divided by its cross-sectional area.

Size of the annular opening. The larger the annular opening around the float, the greater the flow of gas. Because the pressure drop across the constriction is always balanced by the weight of the float, the increased or decreased area must be balanced by an increase or decrease in lifting force caused by a change in the gas flow.

In the variable orifice flow indicator, the annular cross-sectional area varies while the pressure drop across the float remains constant for all positions in the tube. For this reason, these flow indicators are often called constant pressure flow indicators. Increasing the flow does not increase the pressure drop but causes the float to rise to a higher position in the tube, thereby providing greater flow area for the gas. The elevation of the float is a measure of the annular area for flow and, therefore, of the flow itself.

Physical characteristics of the gas. When a low flow of gas passes through the Thorpe tube, the annular opening between the float and the wall of the tube will be narrow. As flow increases, the annular opening becomes larger. The physical property that relates gas flow to the pressure difference across the constriction varies with the form of the constriction. With a longer and narrower constriction (low flows), flow is laminar and is a function of the viscosity of the gas (Hagen-Poiseuille equation). Flow is more turbulent and depends on the density of the gas (Graham's law)

when the constriction is shorter and wider (high flows).

Temperature and pressure effects. Flow indicators are calibrated at atmospheric pressure (760 torr) and room temperature (20°C). Temperature and pressure changes will affect both the viscosity and density of a gas and influence the accuracy of the indicated flow rate. Variations in temperature as a rule are slight and do not produce significant changes.

In a hyperbaric chamber, a flow indicator will deliver less gas than indicated by the setting. With decreased barometric pressure (increased altitude), the actual flow rate will be more than that indicated by the flow indicator. The following equation can be used to derive an approximate correction factor for changes in atmospheric pressure (56):

$$F_1 = F_o \times (d_o/d_1)$$

where:

F_1 is the flow at ambient pressure,

F_o is the flow indicated on the scale calibrated at sea level,

d_o is the density of the gas at sea level, and

d_1 is the density of the gas at ambient pressure.

Flow Indicator Blocks

The flow indicator assembly consists of the tube through which the gas flows, the indicator, a stop at the top of the tube, and the scale that indicates the flow. Lights are available on most machines. Each assembly must be clearly and permanently marked with the appropriate color and name or chemical symbol of the gas or gas mixture measured. The flow indicator assembly is usually protected by a plastic shield.

Tube. Flow indicator tubes are usually made of glass. Some tubes have rib guides. These are thickened bars running the length of the tube. Figure 4.33 shows sections at upper and lower parts of the tube. Gas passes between the ball and the inner wall of the tube. Because the tube is tapered, this space increases from below upward. The area occupied by the rib guides varies with the height of the tube.

The flowmeter tube can have either a single or double taper (Fig. 4.34). Single taper tubes have one gradual increase in diameter from the bottom to the top. They are usually used where there are

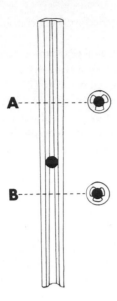

tween the tube and the float. A rotating bobbin
is evidence that gas is flowing and the bobbin is
not stuck. Deviations from the vertical position
will result in the rotor striking the side of the tube.
The reading is taken at the upper rim.

BALL FLOATS. A third type of float is the ball
(Figs. 4.35 and 4.31 A and B and Fig. 4.39). The

FIGURE 4.33. Flow indicator tube with rib guides. This
is used with ball indicators. The triangular thickening
of the inside of the tube keeps the ball centered. The area
through which the gas flows increases with increasing
height in the tube. (Adapted with permission from
Fraser Harlake, Inc.)

different tubes for low and high flows. Dual taper
flowmeter tubes have two different tapers on the
inside of the tube—one corresponding to fine
flows and one for coarse flows.

Float. The float or bobbin is a free-moving device within the tube. The machine standard requires that the point of reference for reading the
float be marked on the flow indicator assembly
(2).

NONROTATING FLOATS. One type of indicator,
the nonrotating float (Fig. 4.35), is designed so
that gas flow keeps it in the center of the tube if
the tube is kept vertical. The reading is taken at
the upper rim.

ROTAMETERS. Rotating floats (Figs. 4.35 and
4.36), have an upper rim whose diameter is larger
than that of the body. Slanted grooves or flutes
are cut into the rim. When gas passes between the
rim and the wall of the tube, it impinges on the
flutes, causing the float to rotate. If the tube is
vertical, the free spinning maintains the float in
the center of the tube. This prevents fluctuations,
reduces wear and tear, assists the passage of small
particles, and reduces errors caused by friction be-

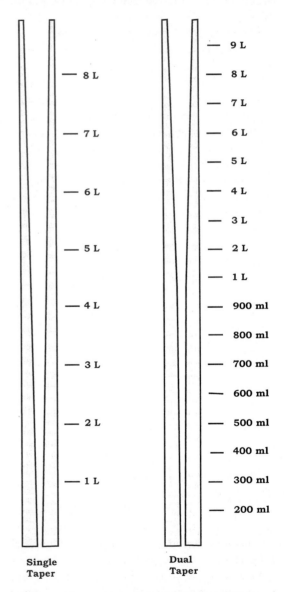

FIGURE 4.34. Single and Dual Taper Flow Indicator
Tubes. With the single taper tube, the opening gradually
increases from the bottom to the top of the tube. With
the dual taper tube the opening size increases more rapidly above 1 l/min.

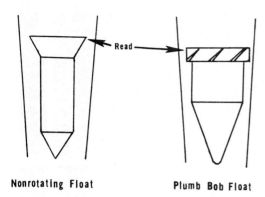

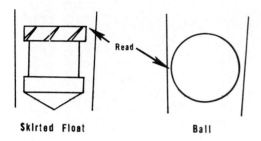

FIGURE **4.35.** Flow indicator indicators. The plumb bob and skirted floats are kept centered in the tube by constant rotation. The reading is taken at the top. The ball indicator is kept centered by rib guides. The reading is taken at the center. The nonrotating float does not rotate and is kept centered by gas flow. (Adapted with permission from Binning R, Hodges EA. Flowmeters. Can they be improved? Anaesthesia 1967;22: 643–646.)

reading is taken at the center of the ball. The ball is kept in the center of the tube by rib guides. The ball may rotate and sometimes has two colors so that the rotation can be easily seen.

It is important to observe the float indicator frequently during use and especially in response to an adjustment of the flow control valve. Erratic movement of the indicator may mean that readings are inaccurate.

Stop. The stop at the top of the flow indicator tube (Fig. 4.37) prevents the float from plugging the outlet, which could lead to damage to the tube (42). It also prevents the indicator from ascending to a point where it cannot be seen. This is important because a flow indicator with the indicator hidden looks much like one that is turned off.

Stops have been known to break off and fall

down into the tube. If the stop descends far enough to rest on the float, it will cause the float to register less flow than is actually occurring.

Scale. The machine standard requires that the flow indicator scale either be marked on the tube (Fig. 4.36 and Fig. 4.39) or be located on the right side of the tube as viewed from the front (2). On some older machines, the scale may be on the left so care must always be taken to read the correct scale.

The standard requires that flow indicators be calibrated in liters per minute (2). For flows up to 1 l/min, the flow may be expressed either in milliliters or in decimal fractions of a liter per minute with a zero before the decimal point. Flow indicator tubes are individually calibrated. The scale, tube, and float should be regarded as an inseparable unit. Should any of the components need replacement, a complete new set must be obtained.

Lights. Flow indicator lights are offered as an option on most modern anesthesia machines. These are useful when the machine is used in a darkened room.

Arrangement of flow indicator tubes. Flow indicator tubes for different gases are grouped side by side. The various gas flows meet at the common manifold (mixing chamber) at the top. Sometimes there are two flow indicators for the same gas—one for low flows and one for high flows. In such a case, the tubes may be arranged either in parallel or in series.

PARALLEL. The parallel arrangement features two complete flow indicator assemblies with a flow control valve for each assembly. The total flow of that gas to the common manifold is the sum of the flows on both flow indicators.

Because accidental use of a low-flow oxygen flow indicator when a high flow was intended is a hazard whenever two oxygen flow control knobs are present, the machine standard (2) requires that only one flow control valve be provided for each gas, so parallel flow indicators are not presently available.

SERIES. With a series (tandem) arrangement (Fig. 4.38), there is one flow control valve for the two flow indicator tubes. Gas from the flow control valve first passes through a tube calibrated up to 1 liter per minute, then passes to a second

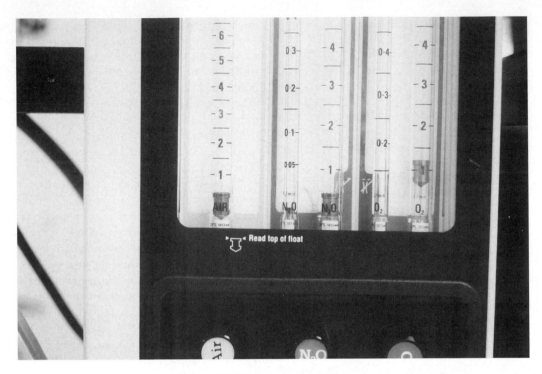

FIGURE 4.36. Skirted float indicators.

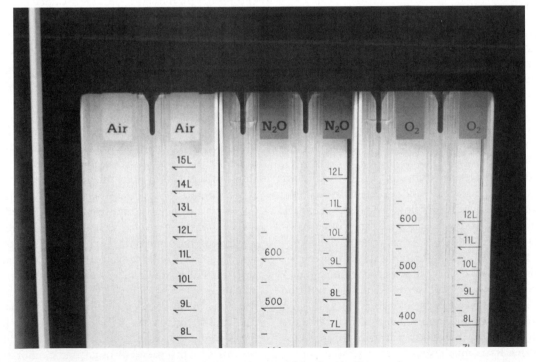

FIGURE 4.37. Stops at the top of the flow indicator tubes.

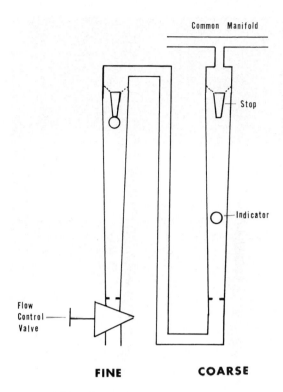

Common Manifold

Stop

Indicator

Flow
Control
Valve

FINE   **COARSE**

FIGURE **4.38.** Flow indicator tubes in series. The total flow is that shown on the higher flow tube, not the sum of the two tubes.

tube that is calibrated for higher flows. The total flow is not the sum of the two tubes but that shown on the higher flow tube. Tandem flow tubes increase accuracy at all flow rates (31).

SEQUENCE OF FLOW INDICATOR TUBES. Flow indicator sequence can be a cause of hypoxia (57). Figure 4.40 shows four different arrangements for oxygen, nitrous oxide, and air flow indicators. Normal gas flow is from bottom to top in each tube and then from left to right at the top. A leak exists in the unused air flow indicator. Potentially dangerous arrangements exist in Figure 4.40A and B because the nitrous oxide flow indicator is located in the downstream position. A substantial portion of oxygen flow passes through the leak while all nitrous oxide is directed to the common gas outlet. Hypoxia from this has been reported (58). Safer configurations that comply with the ASTM standard are shown in Figure 4.40 C and D. By placing the oxygen flow indicator nearest the outlet, a leak upstream from the oxygen results

in loss of nitrous oxide rather than oxygen. Leaks proximal to the oxygen inflow cannot diminish the delivered oxygen concentration, whereas leaks distal to that point result in loss of volume without a qualitative change in the mixture.

Before discovering that the sequence of flow indicators was important in preventing hypoxia, there was no consensus on where the oxygen flow indicator should be in relation to flow indicators for other gases. Thus on older machines, the oxygen flow indicator might be on the right, the left, or the center of the assembly. This was dangerous because users unfamiliar with a particular anesthesia machine might reach for the site where they were used to finding the gas controls and they might turn off the oxygen rather than nitrous oxide because the controls' positions were reversed. To avoid such confusion the ASTM and Canadian standards require that the oxygen flow indicator be placed on the right side of a group of flow indicators as viewed from the front. If a separate vaporizer flow indicator is placed to the right of the oxygen flow indicator, it must be separated by at least 10 cm.

It should be noted that having the oxygen flow indicator on the right is specific to North America and the market supplied by American manufacturers. In many countries the oxygen flow indicator is on the left. This sets the stage for operator error if a user administers anesthesia in a country other than where he or she was trained.

Proper sequence of flow indicators is no guarantee that hypoxia from a broken flow indicator cannot occur. A leak in the oxygen flow indicator tube between the float and the manifold can cause selective loss of oxygen even when the oxygen flow indicator is in the downstream position (59–61).

Safety devices. One of the hazards associated with flow indicators is the possibility that the operator will set the flows so that a hypoxic mixture will be delivered. Various devices have been developed to prevent this.

MANDATORY MINIMUM OXYGEN FLOW. Some anesthesia machines require a minimum (50 to 250 ml/min) flow of oxygen before other gases will flow. This is preset at the factory (sometimes to the customer's specifications). On some machines, the minimum flow may be deleted at the

FIGURE **4.39.** Flowmeters in series. Note that the scales are permanently marked on the tubes.

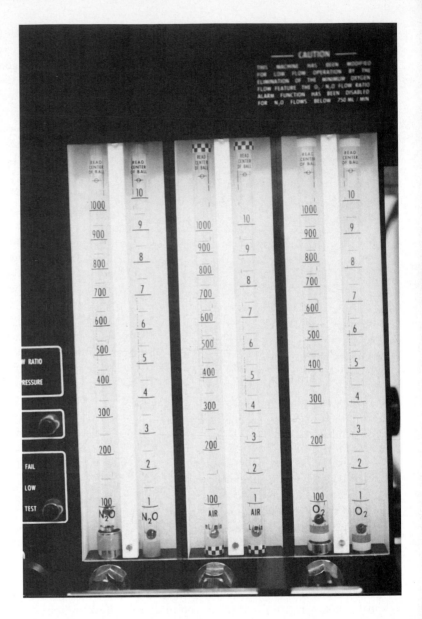

user's request. On some machines, an alarm is activated if the oxygen flow goes below a certain minimum, even if no other gases are being administered.

The minimum flow is activated when the master switch is turned ON. On some machines, it is disabled when air is used. It may be provided by a stop on the oxygen flow control valve or a resistor that permits a small flow to bypass a totally closed oxygen flow control valve (Fig. 4.42) (30, 31).

The minimum oxygen flow does not in itself prevent a hypoxic gas concentration from being delivered. A hypoxic gas mixture can be delivered with only modest anesthetic gas flows. The Julian machine (Dragerwerk) has an oxygen minimum dosing system. For fresh gas flow settings below 1 l/min, the oxygen concentration is automatically increased to a value corresponding to an oxygen flow of 250 ml per minute.

MINIMUM OXYGEN RATIO. Other methods of ensuring that a hypoxic mixture will not be delivered

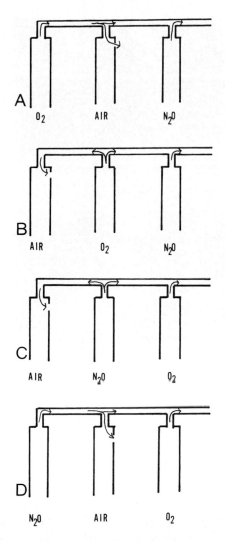

A

O₂   AIR   N₂O

B

AIR   O₂   N₂O

C

AIR   N₂O   O₂

D

N₂O   AIR   O₂

FIGURE 4.40. Flow indicator sequence. **A** and **B**, Potentially dangerous arrangements, with the oxygen flow indicator upstream. If a leak occurs, oxygen will be selectively lost. **C** and **D**, Oxygen is downstream from other gases, which is a safer situation because anesthetic gas rather than oxygen will be lost. *Arrows* represent flows of gases. (Adapted with permission from Eger EI, Hylton RR, Irwin RH, Guadagni N. Anesthetic flow meter sequence—a case for hypoxia. Anesthesiology 1963;24: 396–397.)

are to equip the machine with devices that link flow control valves or with an alarm that is set off if the proportion of oxygen in a mixture is too low.

MINIMUM OXYGEN RATIO DEVICE.

Mechanical Linkage (Ohmeda Link 25 Proportion Limiting Control System). A mechanical linkage involving the nitrous oxide and oxygen flow control valves is shown in Figure 4.41. There is a 14-tooth sprocket on the nitrous oxide flow control valve and a 29-tooth sprocket on the oxygen flow control valve. A pin on the oxygen sprocket engages a pin on the oxygen flow control knob if the flow control valves are adjusted so that a 25% concentration of oxygen is reached. This causes the oxygen and nitrous oxide flow control valves to turn together to maintain a minimum of 25% oxygen. This minimum oxygen ratio device (proportioning system) permits independent control of each gas as long as the percentage of oxygen is above the minimum. The oxygen flow is automatically increased if the operator attempts to increase the nitrous oxide flow beyond that ratio. If the operator attempts to lower the oxygen flow too much, the flow of nitrous oxide is lowered proportionally. It should be noted that these devices only link two gases, nitrous oxide and oxygen. Administration of a third gas such as helium can result in a hypoxic mixture.

Problems have been reported with these devices (53, 54, 62–67).

Pneumatic Linkage. Pneumatic linkage of the oxygen and nitrous oxide flowmeters, which is used on North American Drager Machines, is illustrated in Figure 4.42 (31). A movable horizontal shaft connects the diaphragms of the nitrous oxide and oxygen chambers and the nitrous oxide slave control valve. The slave valve is a ball check valve. Oxygen flow causes a pressure increase in the oxygen chamber, pushing the horizontal shaft to the left. This allows nitrous oxide to flow through the slave control valve. The greater the oxygen flow, the higher the pressure, and the more nitrous oxide will be allowed to flow. This will be independent of the nitrous oxide flow control valve setting unless the setting is less than the maximum allowed by the pressure generated in the oxygen chamber.

If the flow of nitrous oxide is increased beyond 75%, the shaft moves toward the oxygen chamber and the ball check valve restricts the flow of nitrous oxide until it is proportional to the flow of

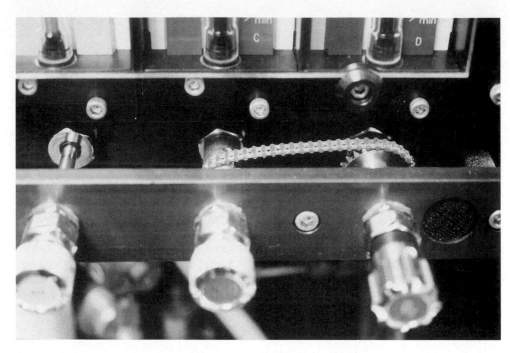

FIGURE 4.41. Mechanically-linked flow control valves. Sprockets are secured to the stems of the oxygen and nitrous oxide flow control valves. A chain linking the sprockets limits the minimum oxygen concentration that can be set. Either nitrous oxide or oxygen flow can be adjusted independently, but the minimum oxygen concentration is maintained. If the nitrous oxide flow is increased beyond the maximum allowed, there is a proportional increase in oxygen flow. If the oxygen flow is lowered, there is a proportional decrease in nitrous oxide flow.

oxygen. The result is that the fresh gas mixture always contains at least 25 (± 3%) oxygen.

Alarms. Alarms are available on some machines to alert the operator when the oxygen:nitrous oxide flow ratio has fallen below a preset value (Fig. 4.43). Such an alarm is often linked to the master switch (if present) so that it is activated whenever the master switch is turned ON (Fig. 4.42). The pressures downstream of the flow control valves are transmitted to diaphragms, which are linked together. If the O_2/N_2O flow ratio is low, the diaphragms move to the right, causing a leaf-spring contact to close and actuate an alarm.

Electronic Flow Measurement

It is likely that the next generation of anesthesia machines will either not be equipped with conven-

FIGURE 4.42. **A**, Oxygen ratio monitor controller and alarm. Flow through Resistor 1 provides the minimum oxygen flow. The nitrous oxide and oxygen flow indicators have resistors downstream from the flow control valves. As gas flows through these resistors, they generate a back pressure that varies in direct proportion to the gas flow. These back pressures are directed to the oxygen and nitrous oxide chambers where they exert force on their respective diaphragms. The diaphragms are connected by a shaft that in turn connects to the proportional valve and the switch to the alarm. Oxygen flow (relative to nitrous oxide flow) generates sufficient back pressure to move the shaft to the left, opening the proportional valve so that nitrous oxide can flow. **B**, If oxygen flow is low (relative to the flow of nitrous oxide), the shaft moves to the right, decreasing the delivery pressure to the proportional valve so that the nitrous oxide flow is lowered. The electronic switch closes and the alarms are activated. (Adapted with permission from drawings furnished by North American Drager, Inc., Telford, Pa.)

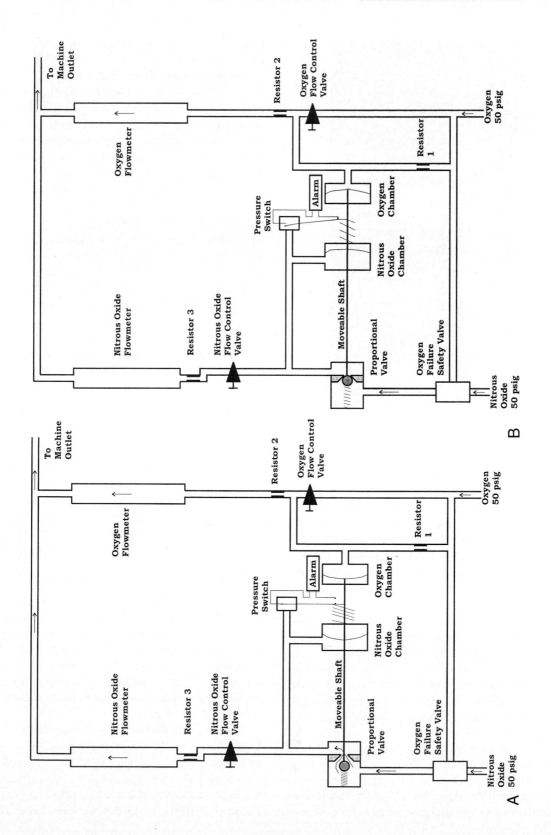

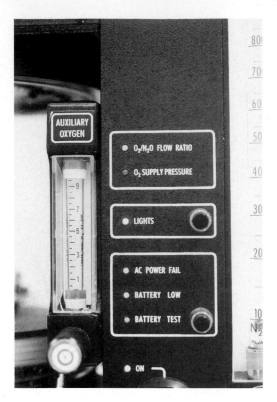

FIGURE 4.43. Auxiliary oxygen flowmeter.

tional flow indicators or will have only small backup ones. Instead, gas flows will be electronically measured and displayed numerically on bar graphs or some other video display as total gas flow and the percentage of each gas (43). This will make such information available for the data management system (see Chapter 25). Electronic measurement of flows will allow servo-control of the inspired gas mixture (43).

Gas flow can be electronically measured in several ways. A signal can be generated by measuring the pressure drop across an orifice, resister, or linear flow element (43). Fluidic flowmeters produce a dynamic instability in the gas flow, which results in oscillations whose frequency is proportional to flow rate (43). Thermister flowmeters may be used. In thermister flowmeters, the tube through which the gas passes is heated and heat sinks cause a temperature gradient along the tube. Thermocouples are attached to either end of the tube. When gas flows along the tube, heat is transferred to the stream, changing the output of the thermo-

couples. The difference in their output is a function of the flow.

Auxiliary Oxygen Flow Indicator

An auxiliary oxygen flow indicator (Fig. 4.43) allows delivery of oxygen to a patient without turning on the main switch. This can be used to supply oxygen directly to patients or can be connected to a resuscitation bag if there is a problem with the anesthesia machine. This can also act as a source of high pressure oxygen for transtracheal jet ventilation (68).

Problems with Flow Indicators

Inaccuracy. Studies of flow indicators in use have shown that the percent of error increases as the flow decreases (69–71). Inaccuracy at low flows is compounded by difficulty reading the low end of flow indicators. There are several causes of inaccuracy.

IMPROPER ASSEMBLY OR CALIBRATION. Routine maintenance by manufacturers may not include flow indicator calibration checks, and a new or recently serviced flow indicator may not be accurate (72).

The flow indicator tube, scale, and indicator are calibrated as a unit. If any parts are broken or damaged, the entire assembly must be replaced. Cases of inaccuracy where indicators or tubes were transposed have been reported (73, 74).

STICKING INDICATOR. Causes of sticking indicators include static electric charges, dirt, and failure to mount the flow tube vertically (43). These rarely cause problems in properly maintained modern equipment.

BACK PRESSURE. Most flow indicators on anesthesia machines are not back-pressure compensated and are affected by increases in pressure transmitted from the breathing system or from use of the oxygen flush valve. These pressure increases cause the float to drop to a lower position so that it reads less than actual flow. The effect of the pressure changes can be reduced by certain devices near the common gas outlet.

Problems with the float. Float damage can result from sudden projection to the top of the tube when a cylinder is opened or a pipeline hose connected with the flow control valve open. Floats can become worn or distorted by handling (75). The stop at the top of the flow indicator tube can became dislodged and rest on top of the float (76, 77).

Indicator unnoticed at top of tube. A tube with the indicator at the top looks much like one with the indicator at the bottom, so this problem can be easily missed.

Blockage of tube outlet. If the stop at the top of the tube is not replaced or breaks off, the float may close the outlet so there is no flow, although the position of the indicator will suggest a flow is present. A leak or rupture of the tube may result.

Reading of wrong flow indicator. An anesthesia care provider will sometimes turn a flow control valve without looking at the flow indicator. If the provider follows up by merely glancing to make sure a float is at an elevation associated with the desired result and does not verify that it is the proper float, the provider may find that he/she has adjusted the wrong gas. Deaths have occurred when an indicator was read beside an adjacent but inappropriate scale. In machines that have parallel flow indicators, the fine control flow indicator may be used in place of the high-flow one and inadequate oxygen given (78).

Changes in float position. Floats should be observed at frequent intervals, particularly soon after the first setting. On some machines, the position of the float may change with a change in supply pressure.

Leaks. A leak in a flow indicator downstream of the indicator but upstream of the common manifold will result in a lower-than-expected concentration of that gas in the fresh gas mixture. A leak can be caused by a crack or chip in the tube or a problem with the connections of the tube (58, 60, 61, 79–83). Obstruction of gas flow downstream may cause the seal at the top of the flow indicator to rupture (84).

A leak may occur if a flow control valve is left open and there is no cylinder or yoke plug in the yoke (7, 46, 48, 85). The indicator at the bottom of the tube will not prevent backflow of gases.

Using the wrong flowmeter. Anesthesia providers are accustomed to a certain flowmeter sequence. When this sequence is altered, there are frequently mistakes that result in an unintended gas being administered (86, 87).

Care of Flow Indicators

Flow indicators should be protected by turning each flow control valve off when cylinder valves are opened or the pipeline hoses are connected to the machine. This prevents a sudden rise of the indicator to the top of the tube, which might damage the indicator or allow it to go unnoticed. In machines with an oxygen failure safety device, the flow indicator for an anesthetic gas or oxygen will register zero when the oxygen pressure is low, even if the flow control valve is open. When the oxygen pressure is restored, there will be a sudden rush of anesthetic gas through the flow indicator, which may cause the indicator to rise abruptly to the top.

Unidirectional (Check) Valve

Positive pressure from the breathing system is transmitted back to the machine when ventilation is controlled or assisted. Use of the oxygen flush valve may also create a positive pressure. Such an increase in pressure can affect the concentration of volatile anesthetic agents issuing from vaporizers on the machine (88). It can also increase leaks and cause inaccurate flow indicator readings. To minimize these problems, a unidirectional (check) valve is present on some machines between the vaporizers and the common gas outlet, upstream of where the oxygen flush flow joins the fresh gas flow. This will lessen the pressure increase, but not prevent it, because gas must still flow from the flow indicators during the time of increased pressure. These check valves are of great importance when checking the machine for leaks. Testing the breathing system for leaks will not detect a leak in a machine equipped with a check valve (89–91).

A hazard has been reported in which a portion of this valve became dislodged and migrated downstream. This caused an obstruction, preventing gas from reaching the common gas outlet (92).

Pressure Relief Device

Some machines have a pressure relief valve near the common gas outlet to prevent high pressure from being transmitted into the machine and to protect the patient from high pressures from the machine. This valve opens to atmosphere and vents gas if a preset pressure is exceeded.

If there is an obstruction in the breathing system or fresh gas delivery hose, this valve may open. If a direct-reading vaporizer with high resistance is placed downstream of such a pressure relief valve, the resistance of the vaporizer may result in a pressure in excess of the opening pressure of the valve, especially when the oxygen flush is activated (93). Such vaporizers must be located between the flow indicators and the common gas outlet.

A pressure relief valve will limit the ability of an anesthesia machine to provide adequate jet ventilation.

Low-Pressure Piping

The low-pressure gas piping has a large number of connections. Components located within this area are subject to breakage and leaks (89). The piping in the machine between the flow control valve and the common gas outlet must not exceed 30 ml per minute at a pressure of 3 kPa (30 cm H_2O) with a vaporizer either in the ON, OFF, or, if possible, in the detached position (2).

Vaporizer Mounting Devices

Vaporizer mounting devices are located in the low pressure system between the flowmeters and the common gas outlet. These devices may allow the vaporizers to be permanently mounted to the anesthesia machine or may allow vaporizers to be changed by the anesthesia provider. Detailed discussion of these devices will be found in Chapter 5.

Common (Fresh) Gas Outlet

The common (fresh) gas outlet receives all the gases and vapors from the machine. Most machine outlets have a 15-mm female slip-joint connection (that will accept a tracheal tube connector), with a coaxial 22-mm male connection. They may also have a load-bearing fitting for secure attachment of accessory apparatus. Because the common gas outlet is a frequent location for a leak or disconnection, the machine standard mandates that it be difficult to accidentally disengage the delivery hose from the outlet (Fig. 4.44) (2). The fresh gas supply tube, which conveys gas to the fresh gas inlet in the breathing system, attaches to the common gas outlet.

THE ANESTHESIA WORKSTATION

A term that will be used frequently in the future is the "anesthesia workstation," which integrates most of the components necessary for anesthesia into one unit (94). The modern anesthesia workstation consists of a gas and vapor delivery system, a breathing system, a ventilator, and a monitoring array. Added to this may be drug delivery systems, a work surface, a data management system, and storage facilities (95).

The movement toward the anesthesia workstation began when manufacturers began making the oxygen analyzer and airway pressure monitor integral parts of the machine so that they were activated when the machine was turned ON. These were followed by other monitors. Finally, central alarm displays and prioritized alarms were developed so that when an alarm sounded there was one place to look to determine which alarm had been activated. Other information such as the suggested checkout procedure is now commonly displayed.

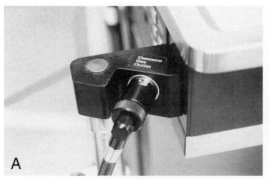
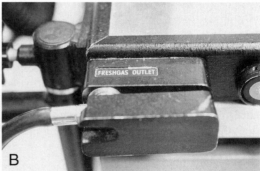

FIGURE 4.44. Common gas outlets with retaining devices.

An advantage of the workstation is that monitoring functions can be integrated. For example, if a blood pressure cuff is on the same arm as the pulse oximeter, inflation of the cuff will not result in the pulse oximeter alarm being activated. Another advantage is that data can be displayed on a single screen so that the user has an overview and can better assimilate the information. Data from different monitors may be analyzed. Potential causes and appropriate responses can be displayed when a problem is sensed. For example, if the problem is a leak or disconnection in the breathing system, the workstation might be able to determine the location of the problem or to advise the user where to look. Finally, the workstation takes up much less space than the anesthesia machine with monitors added onto it.

SERVICING

The Joint Commission on Accreditation of Healthcare Organizations (JCAHO) requires a preventive maintenance procedure for anesthesia machines (96). A frequently asked question is who should service a machine. Because many anesthesiologists are gadgeteers at heart, there may be the temptation to modify the machine or make one's own repairs

Servicing an anesthesia machine requires a detailed knowledge of the components, how they function, and how they fit into the machine. In addition, it is necessary to have the proper replacement parts. It is recommended that the user not perform any services beyond what is suggested in the manual that comes with the machine. Maintenance should not be attempted by hospital maintenance, respiratory therapy, or biomedical personnel who have no particular training with anesthesia machines. Serious hazards have resulted from repairs and alterations made by untrained personnel, and such actions will usually relieve the manufacturer of any responsibility. Some manufacturers will train and certify hospital biomedical personnel to work on machines. Some state laws specify that only certified personnel may work on anesthesia machines.

Manufacturers offer service contracts for maintenance of their machines. With such a contract, a service representative will inspect and perform routine maintenance (including testing, cleaning, lubrication, adjustments, and replacement of damaged parts) on the machine at regular intervals, usually three or four times a year. There is variation in the quality of service. It should not be taken for granted that the work has been performed correctly. Whenever a machine has been serviced, it should be thoroughly checked before use. Service contracts are discussed in more detail in Chapter 26.

Servicing has important medicolegal implications. If a problem occurs with an anesthesia machine and a patient suffers harm, it is important to be able to show that proper servicing was performed. It should be noted, however, that routine servicing does not relieve the user of the responsibility for checking the machine before each use.

Records should be kept on each machine, including problems that occur, service performed, when it was performed, and by whom. Records on equipment are required by the JCAHO and they can be very helpful in the event of legal action.

CHOICE OF ANESTHESIA MACHINE

Only machines that meet all the requirements of the ASTM standard (2) should be considered for purchase. Several things should be considered when choosing an anesthesia machine.

Service

All machines that comply with the ASTM standard should perform well when new. All machines, however, will require servicing. The quality of that service varies among companies and from area to area with the same company. If one company is providing satisfactory service, consider newer models of that company's machines first. If this is not the case, careful shopping is advisable. One way is by inquiring into the experiences of colleagues in the area to determine whether they have long downtimes waiting for repairs, whether servicing is available locally, whether machines for loan are available, and whether service contracts are honored.

Size

Some manufacturers offer compact machines for small operating rooms. A small machine will be easier to move if one needs to be transported outside the operating suite. Larger machines usually offer more drawers and a larger work top.

Special Features and Equipment

Certain machines offer special features that may make them particularly desirable. The ability to add additional equipment is also important. One machine may be more user-friendly than another. Of special note is the MRI-compatible anesthesia machine. This machine has been modified by removing nonessential items and replacing the ferrous metals with nonferromagnetic metals. Aluminum cylinders must be used (97, 98).

REFERENCES

1. American National Standards Institute. Minimum performance and safety requirement for components and systems of continuous flow anesthesia machines for human use (ANSI Z-79. 8). New York: ANSI, 1979.
2. American Society for Testing and Materials. Specification for minimum performance and safety requirements for components and systems of anesthesia gas machines (ASTM F-1161-88). (Reapproved 1994) West Conshohocken, PA: ASTM, 1994.
3. Ng KP, Ho V. Narkomed 4E power failure. Anaesthesia and Intensive Care 1997;25:309.
4. Maurer WG. A disadvantage of similar machine controls. Anesthesiology 1991;75:167–168.
5. Pomykala Z, Schechter H. Design flaw in an anesthesia machine. Anesthesiology 1992;77:399–400.
6. Hogg CE. Pin-indexing failures. Anesthesiology 1973; 38:85–87.
7. McQuillan PJ, Jackson IJB. Potential leaks from anaesthetic machines. Anaesthesia 1987;42:1308–1312.
8. Youatt G, Love J. A funny yoke. Tale of an unscrewed pin. Anaesthesia and Intensive Care 1981;9:79–80.
9. Fox JWC, Fox EJ. Guest discussion. Anesth Analg 1968;51:790–791.
10. Blum LL. Equipment design and human limitations. Anesthesiology 1971;35:101–112.
11. Allberry RAW. Minireg failure. Anaesthesia and Intensive Care 1989;17:234–235.
12. Webb RK, Russell WJ, Klepper I, et al. Equipment failure: an analysis of 2000 incident reports. Anaesthesia and Intensive Care 1993;21:673–677.
13. Okutomi T, Watanabe S, Goto F. Oxygen flow reduction due to dust particle blockage of the oxygen filter. Anesth Analg 1993;76:915–917.
14. Varga DA, Guttery JS, Grundy BL. Intermittent oxygen delivery in an Ohmeda Unitrol anesthesia machine due to a faulty O-ring check valve assembly. Anesth Analg 1987;66:1200–1201.
15. Bamber PA. Possible safety hazard on anaesthetic machines. Anaesthesia 1987;42:782.
16. Heine JF, Adams PM. Another potential failure in an oxygen delivery system. Anesthesiology 1985;63:335–336.
17. Craig DB, Longmuir J. Anaesthetic machine pipeline inlet pressure gauges do not always measure pipeline pressure. Can Anaesth Soc J 1980;27:510–511.
18. Wilson AM. The pressure gauges on the Boyle International anaesthetic machine. Anaesthesia 1982;37:218–219.
19. Dinnick OP. More problems with piped gases. Anaesthesia 1976;31:790–792.
20. Lampotang S. Pipeline pressure gauge location on modern anesthesia machines. J Clin Monit 1994;10:277.
21. Bonsu AK, Stead AL. Accidental cross-connection of oxygen and nitrous oxide in an anaesthetic machine. Anaesthesia 1983;38:767–769.
22. Kua JSW, Tan I. A rare cause of oxygen failure. Anaesthesia 1994;49:650–651.
23. Haynes SR, Best CJ. "On/off" switches on anaesthetic machines. Anaesthesia 1992;47:362.
24. Mandel P. Oxygen supply failure revisited. J Clin Monit 10:405–406.
25. Epstein RM, Rackow H, Lee ASJ, et al. Prevention of accidental breathing of anoxic gas mixtures during anesthesia. Anesthesiology 1962;23:1–4.
26. Jones DE, Watson CB, Goetter C. Oxygen pressure sensor shutoff valve failure in the Ohio "wedge" anesthesia machine. Anesthesiology 1984;61:634–635.
27. Riddle RT. Oxygen pressure sensor shutoff valve failure in the Ohio "wedge" anesthesia machine. In reply. Anesthesiology 1984;61:635–636.
28. Craig DB, Longmuir J. An unusual failure of an oxygen fail-safe device. Can Anaesth Soc J 1971;18:576–577.
29. Puri GD, George MA, Singh H, et al. Awareness under anaesthesia due to a defective gas-loaded regulator. Anaesthesia 1987;42:539–540.
30. Eisenkraft JB. The anesthesia delivery system—part I. Progress in Anesthesiology 1989;3(7):1–7.
31. Cicman JH, Jacoby MI, Skibo VF, et al. Anesthesia systems. Part 1: Operating principles of fundamental components. J Clin Monit 1992;8:295–307.
32. Anderson CE, Rendell-Baker L. Exposed O_2 flush hazard. Anesthesiology 1982;56:328.
33. Cooper CMS. Capnography. Anaesthesia 1987;42:1238–1239.
34. Hanafiah Z, Sellers WFS. Nudging the emergency oxygen. Anaesthesia 1991;46:331.
35. Morris S, Barclay K. Oxygen flush buttons: more critical incidents. Anaesthesia 1993;48:1115–1116.
36. Anonymous. Judge awards $219,000 in oxygen equip-

ment case. Biomedical Safety & Standards 1980;10: 42.

37. Bailey PL. Failed release of an activated oxygen flush valve. Anesthesiology 1983;59:480.

38. Puttick N. Hazard from the oxygen flush control. Anaesthesia 1986;41:222–224.

39. McMahon DJ, Holm R, Batra MS. Yet another machine fault. Anesthesiology 1983;58:586–587.

40. Gaughan SD, Benumof JL, Ozaki GT. Can an anesthesia machine flush valve provide for effective jet ventilation? Anesthesiology 1991;75:A130.

41. Emmett CP, Clutton-Brock TH, Hutton P. The Ohmeda Excel anaesthetic machine. Anaesthesia 1988;43:581–583.

42. Cooper M, Ali D. Oxygen flowmeter dislocation. Anaesthesia and Intensive Care 1989;17:109–110.

43. White DC. Electronic measurement and control of gas flow. Anaesthesia and Intensive Care 1994;22: 409–414.

44. Jenkins IR. A "too close to the door" knob. Anaesth Intensive Care 1991;19:614.

45. Rung GW, Schneider AJL. Oxygen flowmeter failure on the North American Drager Narcomed 2a anesthesia machine. Anesth Analg 1986;65:211–212.

46. Russell WJ, Ward JB. Hypoxia with a third flowmeter tube on the anaesthetic machine. Anaesthesia and Intensive Care 1978;6:355–357.

47. Lenoir RJ, Easy WR. A hazard associated with removal of carbon dioxide cylinders. Anesthesiology 1988;43: 892–893.

48. Williams AR, Hilton PJ. Selective oxygen leak: a potential cause of patient hypoxia. Anaesthesia 1986;41: 1133–1134.

49. Anonymous. Anesthesia units. Technology for Anesthesia 1994;14:7–8.

50. Beudoin MG. Oxygen needle valve obstruction. Anaesthesia and Intensive Care 1988;16:130–131.

51. Khalil SN, Neuman J. Failure of an oxygen flow control valve. Anesthesiology 1990;73:355–356.

52. Fitzpatrick G, Moore KP. Malfunction in a needle valve. Anaesthesia 1988;43:164.

53. Kidd AG, Hall I. Fault with an Ohmeda Excel 210 anaesthetic machine. Anaesthesia 1994;49:83.

54. Lohmann G. Fault with an Ohmeda Excel 410 machine. Anaesthesia 1991;46:695.

55. Davies R. A reply. Anaesthesia 1994;49:83.

56. Camporesi EM. Anesthesia at different environmental pressures. In: Anesthesia equipment. Principles and applications. Ehrenwerth J, Eisenkraft JB, eds. St. Louis: Mosby, 1993: 588–598.

57. Eger EI, Hylton RR, Irwin RH, et al. Anesthetic flowmeter sequence—cause for hypoxia. Anesthesiology 1963;24:396–397.

58. Powell J. Leak from an oxygen flowmeter. Br J Anaesth 1981;53:671.

59. Chung DC, Jing QC, Prins L, et al. Hypoxic gas mixtures delivered by anaesthetic machines equipped with a downstream oxygen flowmeter. Can Anaesth Soc J 1980;27:527–530.

60. Russell WJ. Hypoxia from a selective oxygen leak. Anaesthesia and Intensive Care 1984;12:275–277.

61. McHale S. A critical incident with the Ohmeda Excel 410 machine. Anaesthesia 1991;46:150.

62. Abraham ZA, Basagoitia J. A potentially lethal anesthesia machine failure. Anesthesiology 1987;66: 589–590.

63. Davis TM. Failure of a new system to prevent delivery of hypoxic gas mixture. A reply. Anesthesiology 1981; 54:437.

64. Malone BT. Failure of a new system to prevent delivery of hypoxic gas mixture. Anesthesiology 1981;54: 436–437.

65. Richards C. Failure of a nitrous oxide-oxygen proportioning device. Anesthesiology 1989;71:997–999.

66. Ferguson S, White E. An unusual and dangerous anaesthetic machine failure. Anaesthesia 1997;52: 283–284.

67. Goodyear CM. Failure of nitrous oxide-oxygen proportioning device. Anesthesiology 1990;72:397–398.

68. Good ML. New vaporizer, new FDA check, and a new use (transtracheal jet ventilation) for the anesthesia machine. Orlando, FL: IARS Review Course Lecture, March 1994.

69. Sadove MS, Thomason RD, Thomason CL, et al. An evaluation of flowmeters. Journal of the American Association of Nurse Anesthetists 1976;44:162–165.

70. Waaben J, Stokke DB, Brinklov MM. Accuracy of gas flowmeters determined by the bubble meter method. Br J Anaesth 1978;50:1251–1256.

71. Waaben J, Brinklov MM, Stokke DB. Accuracy of new gas flowmeters. Br J Anaesth 1980;52:97–100.

72. Kelley JM, Gabel RA. The improperly calibrated flowmeter—another hazard. Anesthesiology 1970;33: 467–468.

73. Slater EM. Transposition of rotameter bobbins. Anesthesiology 1974;41:101.

74. Thomas D. Interchangeable rotameter tubes. Anaesthesia and Intensive Care 1983;11:385–386.

75. Hodge EA. Accuracy of anaesthetic gas flowmeters. Br J Anaesth 1979;51:907.

76. Doblar DD, Hinkle JC. Flowmeter malfunction: effect on delivered anesthetic concentration. Anesthesiology 1984;61:220–222.

77. Luich RJ. Flowmeter malfunction: effect on delivered anesthetic concentration: a reply. Anesthesiology 1984;61:222.

78. Rendell-Baker L, Klein OL, Charles P. Hazard of separate low and high flow O$_2$ flowmeters: an interim solution. Anesthesiology 1982;56:155–156.

79. Dudley M, Walsh E. Oxygen loss from rotameter. Br J Anaesth 1986;58:1201–1202.

80. Gupta BL, Varshneya AK. Anaesthetic accident caused by unusual leakage of rotameter. Br J Anaesth 1975;47:805.

81. Hanning CD, Kruchek D, Chunara A. Preferential oxygen leak—an unusual case. Anaesthesia 1987;42:1329–1330.

82. Williams OA. Potential hazard of a cracked rotameter. Anaesthesia 1989;44:523.

83. Wishaw K. Hypoxic gas mixture with Quantiflex Monitored Dial Mixer and induction room safety. Anaesthesia and Intensive Care 1991;19:127.

84. Thompson JB, Fodor IM, Baker AB, et al. Anaesthetic machine hazard from the Select-a-tec block. Anaesthesia 1983;38:175–177.

85. Stoneham MD, Ismail F, Sansome AJ. Leakage of fresh gas from vacant CO$_2$ cylinder yoke. Br J Anaesth 1993;48:730–731.

86. James RH. Rotameter sequence—a variant of "read the label." Anaesthesia 1996;51:87–88.

87. Moon JRA. Rotameter sequence. Anaesthesia 1996;51:508.

88. Hill DW, Lowe HJ. Comparison of concentration of halothane in closed and semiclosed circuits during controlled ventilation. Anesthesiology 1962;23:291–298.

89. Andrews JJ. Understanding your anesthesia machine (ASA Refresher Course No. 272). New Orleans: ASA, 1996.

90. Berner MS. Profound hypercapnia due to disconnection within an anaesthetic machine. Can J Anaesth 1987;34:622–628.

91. Comm G, Rendell-Baker L. Back pressure check valve a hazard. Anesthesiology 1982;56:327–328.

92. Chang J, Larson CE, Bedger RC, et al. An unusual malfunction of an anesthetic machine. Anesthesiology 1980;52:446–447.

93. Kataria B, Price P, Slack M. Delayed filling of the breathing bag due to a portable vaporizer. Anesth Analg 1987;66:1055.

94. Cooper JB. Trends in anaesthesia machine design. Anaesthesia and Intensive Care 1990;18:160.

95. Westhorpe R. The anaesthetic machine and patient safety. Ann Acad Med Singapore 1994;23:592–597.

96. Mahon DJ. A synopsis of current anesthesia machine design. Biomed Instrum Technol 1991;25:190–199.

97. Rao CC, Brandl R, Mashak JN. Modification of Ohmeda® Excel 210 anesthesia machine for use during magnetic resonance imaging. Anesthesiology 1989;71;A364.

98. Rao CC, Krishna G, Emhardt J. Anesthesia machine for use during magnetic resonance imaging. Anesthesiology 1990;73:1054–1055.

QUESTIONS

Each question below contains four suggested answers of which one or more is correct. Choose the answer:

A if 1, 2, and 3 are correct
B if 1 and 3 are correct
C if 2 and 4 are correct
D if 4 is correct
E if 1, 2, 3, and 4 are correct.

1. The high pressure system of the anesthesia machine includes
   1. The oxygen flush valve
   2. Flowmeters
   3. The pipeline inlet
   4. The hanger yokes

2. The pin index safety system
   1. Consists of two pins on the cylinder valve that fit two corresponding holes in the yoke
   2. Is located above the nipple on the yoke
   3. Make it impossible to place an incorrect cylinder in a yoke
   4. Has specific locations for pins and holes for each gas

3. When placing a cylinder in the yoke,
   1. The first step is to fully retract the retaining screw
   2. The washer should be placed on the cylinder valve
   3. The pin-index system components must be mated
   4. The screw is tightened into the cylinder relief valve

4. The pressure regulator
   1. Reduces pipeline pressure to approximately 345 kPa
   2. Supplies a relatively constant outlet pressure while the source pressure is reduced
   3. Will not work properly if gas is being removed from the low pressure side
   4. Can be direct or indirect acting

5. The intermediate pressure system includes:
   1. The pipeline pressure gauge
   2. The flowmeter manifold
   3. The oxygen flush
   4. Vaporizer(s)

6. The oxygen failure safety valve
   1. Will prevent a hypoxic gas mixture from being delivered
   2. Will cut off the flow of oxygen should the nitrous oxide supply fail
   3. Prevents the user from dialing a hypoxic mixture on the flowmeters
   4. May cut off the flow of air should the oxygen supply fail

7. The oxygen supply pressure alarm will
   1. Be activated by a disconnected pipeline hose
   2. Prevent delivery of a hypoxic mixture
   3. Be activated if the pipeline pressure is low
   4. Protect the patient from hypoxia that result from leaks

8. The oxygen flush valve
   1. Will deliver oxygen at between 30 and 60 liters per minute
   2. Can be locked in the ON position
   3. May increase the pressure in vaporizers up to 200 cm H_2O when activated.
   4. Must be protected against accidental activation

9. Which of the following statements about flowmeters are correct?
   1. Parallel flowmeters are used in new anesthesia machines
   2. Flowmeter tubes work on the principle of the variable orifice
   3. The inside of a flow tube containing a ball is smooth
   4. The pressure drop across the indicator is constant for all positions in the tube

10. The rate of flow through a flowmeter tube depends on
    1. The pressure drop across the constriction
    2. The size of the annular opening

3. The physical properties of the gas
4. The length of the tube

11. If a flowmeter tube is broken
   1. Only the tube needs be replaced
   2. The indicator can be used in the new tube if it is a ball
   3. The scale must be replaced if it is integral to the tube
   4. The tube, indicator, and scale must be replaced as a unit

12. Effects of the physical characteristics of the gas passing through the flowmeter include
   1. At low flows, flow is a function of the viscosity of the gas
   2. Viscosity of the gas is more important with a longer and narrower constriction
   3. With high flows, flow depends more on the density of the gas
   4. The density of the gas is more important with a shorter and wider constriction

13. Correct statements concerning the order of flowmeter tubes include
   1. The left tube should be either oxygen or air
   2. A leak in the flowmeter furthermost from the manifold outlet may result in loss of gas from the middle flowmeter
   3. A small leak in the middle flowmeter

will cause loss of gas from the flowmeter next to the manifold
   4. The oxygen flowmeter should be next to the manifold outlet

14. Concerning mandatory minimum oxygen flow
   1. It will prevent delivery of a hypoxic mixture
   2. It cannot be removed
   3. The amount of flow is user adjustable
   4. It is sometimes associated with an alarm

15. Correct statements concerning the minimum oxygen ratio control include
   1. The gases are independently controlled when the oxygen percentage is above the minimum
   2. If the flow of nitrous oxide is increased, the oxygen flow is automatically increased
   3. It can be a mechanical or pneumatic link
   4. It is usually set at 25% nitrous oxide

ANSWERS

1.	D	**9.**	C
2.	D	**10.**	A
3.	B	**11.**	D
4.	C	**12.**	E
5.	B	**13.**	C
6.	D	**14.**	D
7.	B	**15.**	B
8.	D		

CHAPTER
5

Vaporizers (Anesthetic Agent Delivery Devices)

MOST OF THE inhalational anesthetic agents in use today are liquids at atmospheric pressure and room temperature and must be converted into vapors before they can be used. A vapor is the gaseous phase of a substance that is a liquid at room temperature and atmospheric pressure. A vaporizer is an instrument designed to change a liquid anesthetic agent into its vapor and to add a controlled amount of this vapor to the fresh gas flow. As many as three vaporizers are commonly attached to an anesthesia machine.

PHYSICS
Vapor Pressure

Figure 5.1A shows a volatile liquid inside a container closed to atmosphere. Molecules of liquid break away from the surface and enter the space above, forming a vapor. If the container is kept at a constant temperature, a dynamic equilibrium is formed between the liquid and vapor phases so that the number of molecules in the vapor phase remains constant. These molecules bombard the walls of the container, creating a pressure. This is called the "saturated vapor pressure" and is represented by the density of dots above the liquid.

If heat is supplied to the container (Fig. 5.1B), the equilibrium will be shifted so that more molecules enter the vapor phase and the vapor pressure will rise. If heat is taken away from the system (Fig. 5.1C), more molecules will enter the liquid state and the vapor pressure will be lower. It is meaningless, therefore, to talk about vapor pressure of a liquid without specifying the temperature. Vapor pressures of some anesthetic agents at 20°C are shown in Table 5.1. Vapor pressure depends only on the liquid and the temperature. It does not depend on ambient pressure within the range of barometric pressures encountered in anesthesia.

Boiling Point

The boiling point of a liquid is the temperature at which its vapor pressure is equal to the atmospheric pressure. The lower the atmospheric pressure, the lower the boiling point. The boiling points for some anesthetic agents at sea level (760 torr) are shown in Table 5.1.

Concentration of Gases

Two methods are commonly used to express the concentration of a gas or vapor: partial pressure and volumes percent (vol %).

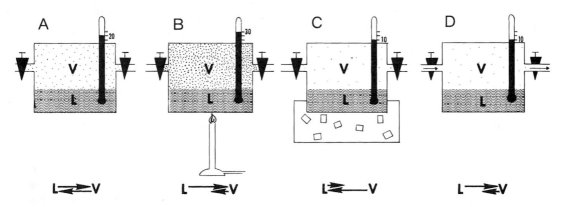

FIGURE 5.1. Vapor pressure changes with varying temperature. **A,** The liquid and vapor are in equilibrium. **B,** The application of heat causes the equilibrium to shift so that more molecules enter the vapor phase, as illustrated by the increased density of dots above the liquid. **C,** Lowering the temperature causes a shift toward the liquid phase and a decrease in vapor pressure. **D,** Passing a carrier gas over the liquid shifts the equilibrium toward the vapor phase. The heat of vaporization is supplied from the remaining liquid. This causes a drop in temperature.

TABLE 5.1. Properties of Common Anesthetic Agents

Agent	Trade Name	Boiling Point (°C, 760 mm Hg)	Vapor Pressure (torr, 20°C)	Density of Liquid (g/ml)	Heat of Vaporization		Specific Heat of Liquid		MAC[a] in O$_2$ (%)
					cal/g	cal/ml	cal/ml	cal/g	
Halothane	Fluothane	50.2	243	1.86 (20°C)	35 (20°C)	65 (20°C)	0.35	0.19	0.75
Enflurane	Ethrane	56.5	175	1.517 (25°C)	42 (25°C)	63 (25°C)			1.68
Isoflurane	Forane	48.5	238	1.496 (25°C)	41 (25°C)	62 (25°C)			1.15
Desflurane	Suprane	22.8	669	1.45 (20°C)					6.4
Sevoflurane	Ultane	58.6	157						2.0

Adapted with permission from Quasha AL, Eger EI, Tinker JH. Determination and applications of MAC. Anesthesiology 1980;53:315–334.
[a] Minimum anesthetic concentration.

Partial Pressure

A mixture of gases in a closed container will exert a pressure on the walls of the container. The part of the total pressure that results from any one gas in the mixture is called the partial pressure of that gas. The total pressure of the mixture is the sum of the partial pressures of the constituent gases. The partial pressure exerted by the vapor of a liquid agent depends only on the temperature of that agent and is unaffected by the total pressure above the liquid. The highest partial pressure that can be exerted by a gas at a given temperature is its vapor pressure.

Volumes Percent

The concentration of a gas in a mixture can also be expressed as its percentage of the total volume. Volumes percent is the number of units of volume of a gas in relationship to a total of 100 units of volume for the total gas mixture. In a mixture of gases, each constituent gas exerts the same proportion of the total pressure as its volume is of the total volume. Volumes percent expresses the relative ratio of gas molecules in a mixture, whereas partial pressure expresses an absolute value.

Partial pressure/Total pressure =
Volumes percent/100

Although gas and vapor concentrations are most commonly expressed in volumes percent, patient uptake and the depth of anesthesia are directly related to partial pressure but only indirectly to volumes percent (1). While a given partial pressure represents the same anesthetic potency under various barometric pressures, this is not the case with volumes percent.

Heat of Vaporization

It takes energy for the molecules in a liquid to break away and enter the gaseous phase. The heat of vaporization of a liquid is the number of calories necessary to convert 1 gm of liquid into a vapor. Heat of vaporization can also be expressed as the number of calories necessary to convert 1 ml of liquid into a vapor (2). The heats of vaporization of the some anesthetic agents are shown in Table 5.1.

Vaporization removes the more energetic molecules so that the remaining molecules have lower kinetic energies. Therefore, the temperature of the liquid decreases as vaporization proceeds. As the temperature falls, a gradient is created so that heat flows from the surroundings to the liquid. The lower the temperature, the greater the gradient and the greater the flow of heat from the surroundings. Eventually, an equilibrium is established so that the heat lost to vaporization is matched by the heat supplied from the surroundings. At this point, the temperature ceases to drop.

In Figure 5.1D, a flow of gas (carrier gas) is passed through the container and carries away with it molecules of vapor. This causes the equilibrium to shift so that more molecules from the liquid enter the vapor phase. Unless some means of supplying heat is available, the liquid will cool. As the temperature drops, so does the vapor pressure of the liquid and fewer molecules will be picked up by the carrier gas so that there is a decrease in concentration in the gas flowing out of the container.

Specific Heat

The specific heat of a substance is the quantity of heat required to raise the temperature of 1 g of the substance 1°C. The higher the specific heat, the more heat required to raise the temperature of a given quantity of that substance. A slightly different definition of specific heat is the amount of heat required to raise the temperature of 1 ml of the substance 1°C (2). Water is the standard with a specific heat of 1 cal/g/°C or 1 cal/ml/°C.

Specific heat is important when considering the amount of heat that must be supplied to a liquid anesthetic to maintain a stable temperature when heat is lost as a result of vaporization. Specific heats for some liquid anesthetic agents are given in Table 5.1.

Specific heat is also important in the choice of material from which a vaporizer is constructed. Temperature changes more gradually for materials with a high specific heat than for those with a low specific heat. Thermal capacity is the product of specific heat and mass and represents the amount of heat stored in the vaporizer body (3). A vaporizer constructed from a substance with a high thermal capacity will change temperature more slowly than one with a low thermal capacity.

Thermal Conductivity

Another consideration in choosing material from which to construct a vaporizer is thermal conductivity. This is a measure of speed with which heat flows through a substance (4). The higher the thermal conductivity, the better the substance conducts heat.

Thermostabilization

Thermostabilization is achieved by constructing vaporizers of metals with high thermal conductivity (copper, bronze) to minimize temperature changes when the vaporizer is in use. In vaporizers containing wicks, it is important that the wicks be in contact with a metal part so heat lost as a result of vaporization can be replaced quickly.

CLASSIFICATION OF VAPORIZERS

The wide variety of available vaporizers makes any single method of classification incomplete. The classification shown in Table 5.2 lists three characteristics that describe most of the important points about each vaporizer.

Methods of Regulating Output Concentrations

The vapor pressures of most anesthetic agents at room temperature are much greater than the partial pressures required to produce anesthesia. To produce clinically useful concentrations, a vaporizer must bring about dilution of the saturated vapor. This can be accomplished in one of two ways.

TABLE **5.2.   Classification of Vaporizers**

Method of regulating output concentration
    Concentration calibrated
    Measured flow
Method of vaporization
    Flow-over
    Bubble through
    Injection
Temperature compensation
    Thermocompensation
    Supplied heat

---

1) The total gas flow from the anesthesia machine goes through the vaporizer and is divided into two parts. Some passes through the vaporizing chamber (the part of the vaporizer containing the liquid anesthetic agent), and the remainder goes through a bypass to the vaporizer outlet. This is known as a concentrated-calibrated vaporizer.

2) A measured amount of gas is supplied to the vaporizer, and all of the gas passes through the vaporizing chamber. It is then diluted by additional flow from the machine. This is known as a measured-flow vaporizer.

Concentration-Calibrated Vaporizers

Concentration-calibrated vaporizers are also called variable bypass, direct-reading, dial-controlled, automatic plenum, percentage-type, and tec-type vaporizers and vaporizer chamber bypass arrangements. The total gas flow from the flowmeters goes through the vaporizer, picks up a predictable amount of vapor, then flows to the common gas outlet. Agent concentration is controlled by a single calibrated knob or dial. This is usually calibrated in volumes percent. Alternatively, the setting may be displayed on a screen.

The machine standard requires that all vaporizers on the anesthesia workstation be concentration-calibrated (5).

Figure 5.2 shows a vaporizer with a variable bypass. In the OFF position, the bypass mechanism (dark squares) occludes the inlet and outlet of the vaporizing chamber. Gas flows through the bypass to the outlet. In the ON position, the incoming gas flow is divided into two portions: one part goes through the bypass and the other flows to the vaporizing chamber, where it picks up vapor of the liquid anesthetic agent. Both gas flows rejoin downstream.

The ratio of bypass gas to gas going to the vaporizing chamber is called the splitting ratio (6, 7) and depends on the ratio of resistances in the two pathways. This in turn depends on the variable (adjustable) orifice. This orifice may be in the inlet to the vaporizing chamber, but in most modern vaporizers it is in the outlet (8). The splitting ratio may also depend on the total flow to the vaporizer.

The composition of the carrier gas affects va-

FIGURE 5.2. Concentration-calibrated vaporizer. **A,** In the OFF position, all the inflowing gas is directed through the bypass. **B,** In the ON position, gas flow is divided between the bypass and the vaporizing chamber. In the MAX position, all of the gas flow allowed by the vaporizer goes to the vaporizing chamber.

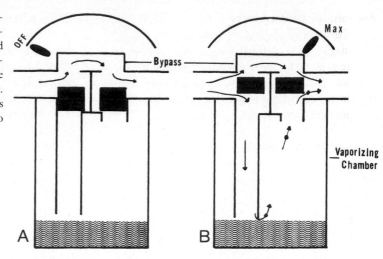

porizer output (vaporizer aberrance) in many concentration-calibrated vaporizers. Most vaporizers are calibrated using oxygen as the carrier gas. Generally, little change in output occurs if air is substituted for oxygen. Addition of nitrous oxide to the carrier gas typically results in both a temporary and a long-lasting effect on vaporizer output. The temporary effect is usually a decrease in vapor concentration. The duration of this effect depends on the gas flow rate and the volume of liquid in the vaporizer. The permanent effect may be an increase or decrease, depending on the construction of the vaporizer (1). With most concentrated-calibrated vaporizers, output decreases as fresh gas flow increases because of incomplete mixing in the vaporizing chamber.

Measured-Flow Vaporizers

Measured-flow vaporizers (kettle-type, flowmetered, and flowmeter-controlled vaporizer systems) use a measured flow of carrier gas, usually oxygen, to pick up anesthetic vapor. These are no longer available for sale. However, there are a great many still in use outside the United States. Each vaporizer system consists of three parts.

Vaporizer

The vaporizer includes the body that holds the liquid. The vaporizer also has a window to view the liquid level, a filler port, and a thermometer to measure the temperature within the vaporizer.

Flowmeter Assembly

The flowmeter may be calibrated either for the flow of gas through the flowmeter or for the vapor flow.

ON-OFF Valve

The ON-OFF valve's function is to isolate the vaporizer. To calculate the vaporizer output one must know the vapor pressure of the agent, the atmospheric pressure, the total flow of gases, the flow to the vaporizer, and the temperature. The formula is

% concentration

= Vaporizer output of anesthetic/Total flow × 100

or

% concentration

$$= \frac{(VF)(V_{pa})}{AP(VF + DF) - (V_{pa})(DF)} \times 100$$

where

DF = diluent flow;
VF = flow to the vaporizer;
V_{pa} = vapor pressure of the liquid anesthetic;
and AP = atmospheric pressure (9).

By using this formula, a vaporizer of this type can be used accurately with a number of different anesthetic agents.

Methods of Vaporization
Flow Over

In a flow-over vaporizer, a stream of carrier gas passes over the surface of the liquid. The efficiency of vaporization can be enhanced by increasing the area of the carrier gas-liquid interface. This can be performed using baffles or spiral tracks to lengthen the pathway of the gas over the liquid. Another method is to employ wicks that have their bases in the liquid. The liquid moves up the wick by capillary action.

Bubble Through

Another means of increasing contact between the carrier gas and the volatile liquid is to bubble the gas through the liquid. There may be a means to break the gas up into small bubbles, further increasing the gas-liquid interface.

Injection

Certain vaporizers control the vapor concentration by injecting a known amount of liquid anesthetic (from a reservoir in the vaporizer or from the bottle of agent) into a known volume of gas (1).

Temperature Compensation

As a liquid is vaporized, energy in the form of heat is lost. As the temperature of the liquid decreases, so does the vapor pressure. Two methods have been employed to maintain a constant vapor output with fluctuations in liquid anesthetic temperature.

Thermocompensation

Most concentration-calibrated vaporizers compensate for changes in vapor pressure with temperature by altering the splitting ratio so that the percentage of the carrier gas that is directed through the vaporizing chamber is changed (7). A thermal element performs this function in mechanical vaporizers. This will be under computer control in electronic vaporizers. Thermocompensation is performed manually by adjusting the flow through the vaporizer in measured-flow vaporizers.

Supplied Heat

An electric heater can be used to supply heat to a vaporizer and maintain it at a constant temperature.

EFFECTS OF ALTERED BAROMETRIC PRESSURE

Most vaporizers are calibrated at standard (sea level) atmospheric pressure. Because they are sometimes used in hyperbaric chambers or at high altitudes where atmospheric pressure is low, it is important to have some knowledge of how vaporizers will perform when the barometric pressure is changed. The American Society for Testing and Materials (ASTM) machine standard requires that the effects of changes in ambient pressure on vaporizer performance be stated in operation manuals (5). Anesthetic agents with low boiling points are more susceptible to the influence of variations in barometric pressure than agents with higher boiling points (7, 10).

Low Atmospheric Pressure
Concentration-Calibrated Vaporizers

A decrease in barometric pressure will affect a concentration-calibrated vaporizer by altering the splitting ratio (7). The high-resistance pathway through the vaporizing chamber offers less resistance under hypobaric conditions, increasing vaporizer output slightly when measured as partial pressure. If concentration is measured as volumes percent, the effect of hypobaric pressure will be greater and can be calculated as follows:

$$c' = c(p/p')$$

where

c' is the output concentration at a different barometric pressure in volumes percent;
c is the vaporizer setting in volumes percent;
p is the barometric pressure for which the vaporizer is calibrated;
and p' is the barometric pressure for which c' is being established (11).

Measured-Flow Vaporizers

With measured-flow vaporizers, the delivered partial pressure increases and volumes percent increases even more if the surrounding pressure is lowered (8). The amount of the increase depends on the barometric pressure and the vapor pressure of the agent (and thus the temperature). The closer the vapor pressure is to the barometric pressure, the greater the effect (8). If nitrous oxide is included in the inspired mixture, the effect of increased partial pressure of the potent agent on anesthetic depth will be at least partially offset by the decreased partial pressure of the nitrous oxide (12).

High Atmospheric Pressures
Concentration-Calibrated Vaporizers

When atmospheric pressure is increased, changes in the density of gases cause more resistance to flow through the vaporizing chamber and a decrease in vaporizer output in both partial pressure and volumes percent (13). At two atmospheres pressure, the concentration in volumes percent is halved (1). The effect on partial pressure is less dramatic.

Measured-Flow Vaporizers

A measured-flow vaporizer will deliver a lower concentration, which is expressed either as partial pressure or volumes percent when atmospheric pressure is increased.

EFFECTS OF INTERMITTENT BACK PRESSURE

When assisted or controlled ventilation is used, the positive pressure generated during inspiration is transmitted from the breathing system back to the machine and the vaporizers. Another source of back pressure is use of the oxygen flush valve. The output from the oxygen flush enters the machine circuitry downstream of the vaporizers, and activating it produces high pressures. This back pressure may either increase (pumping effect) or decrease (pressurizing effect) the output of the vaporizer.

Pumping Effect
Factors

Studies have shown that concentrations delivered by some vaporizers during controlled or assisted ventilation are higher than when the vaporizer was used with free flow to atmosphere (14). This change is most pronounced when there is less agent in the vaporizing chamber, when carrier gas flow is low, when the pressure fluctuations are high and frequent, and when the dial setting is low.

Mechanisms
Concentration-Calibrated Vaporizers

A proposed mechanism for the pumping effect for variable bypass vaporizers is shown in Figure 5.3. Figure 5.3A shows the vaporizer during exhalation. The resistances of the outlets of the bypass and vaporizing chamber determine the flows to each (points 3 and 4 in the figure).

Figure 5.3B shows inspiration. Positive pressure at point C prevents outflow of gases and vapor. The pressure is transmitted to points A and B. This results in compression of gas in the vaporizing chamber and bypass. Because the bypass has a smaller volume than the vaporizing chamber, more gas goes to the vaporizing chamber so that the normal ratio between the flow to the vaporizing chamber and that through the bypass is disturbed. The result is an increased flow to the vaporizing chamber, which then picks up anesthetic vapor.

Figure 5.3C shows the situation just after the beginning of exhalation. The pressure at point C falls rapidly and gas flows from the vaporizing chamber and the bypass to the outlet. Because the bypass has less resistance than the vaporizing chamber outlet, the pressure in the bypass falls more quickly than that in the vaporizing chamber and gas containing vapor flows from the vaporizing chamber into the bypass. The concentration in the vaporizer output is increased because the gas in the bypass (which dilutes the gas from the vaporizing chamber) now carries vapor and the gas flowing from the vaporizing chamber is still saturated.

Measured-Flow Vaporizers

As discussed previously, the gas flow to these vaporizers becomes saturated with vapor and is joined by gas from other flowmeters, which dilutes its concentration. When back pressure is applied, there is a retrograde flow of gas so that the diluted gas mixture is forced back into the vaporizer. Because this gas is not saturated, it will then pick up anesthetic vapor. The result is an increase in output.

Modifications to Minimize the Pumping Effect
Alterations in Concentration-Calibrated Vaporizers

Keeping the vaporizing chamber small or increasing the size of the bypass will decrease the

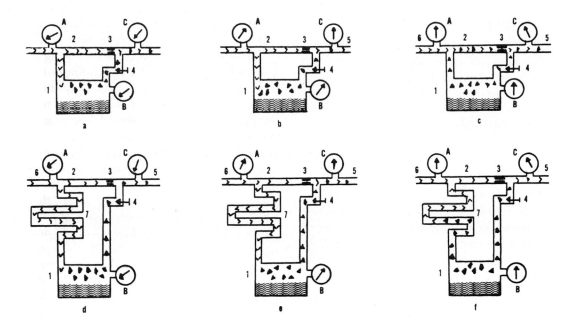

FIGURE 5.3. The pumping effect in a concentration-calibrated vaporizer. See text for details. (Adapted with permission from Hill DW. The design and calibration of vaporizers for volatile anesthetic agents. Br J Anaesth 1968;40:656.)

effects of back pressure because the increase in output in variable bypass vaporizers is related to the relative sizes of the space above the liquid in the vaporizing chamber and the space in the bypass (6). Another method is to employ a long, spiral or large-diameter tube to lead to the vaporizing chamber (Fig. 5.3D, E, and F). The extra gas forced into this tube and subsequently returned to the bypass does not reach the vaporizing chamber. Another method is to exclude wicks from the area where the inlet tube joins the vaporizing chamber. Finally, an overall increase in resistance to gas flow through the vaporizer may be used.

Alterations to the Measured-Flow Vaporizer

Some measured-flow vaporizers have a relief valve at the outlet to limit the pressure. Others have a check valve to prevent backward flow of gas. The outlet tube may be made longer so that unsaturated gas will have to pass farther back before picking up anesthetic vapor. Finally, keeping the vaporizing chamber small will result in less unsaturated gas being forced back into it.

Alterations to the Anesthesia Machine

These devices (pressurizing valve, unidirectional valve, and pressure relief device) were discussed in Chapter 4. A check valve near the machine outlet but upstream of the junction with the oxygen flush offers less protection from the pumping effect than a check valve at the outlet of a vaporizer (15).

The ASTM machine standard (5) requires that the connections of the oxygen flush valve line to the common gas outlet be designed to minimize pressure fluctuations that may produce a pumping effect on vaporizers. It also limits the pressure transmitted to the vaporizers during use of the flush valve to not more than 10 kPa (100 cm H_2O) above normal working pressure when the common gas outlet is open to the atmosphere and limits the change in concentration delivered by a vaporizer to not more than 20% with typical intermittent back pressures. Manufacturers are required to state in catalogs and operations manuals the extent to which back pressure affects a vaporizer's performance.

Pressurizing Effect

Factors

The output of some vaporizers used in conjunction with automatic ventilators has been found to be lower than during free flow to atmosphere (16, 17). The effect is greater with high flows, large pressure fluctuations, and low vaporizer settings.

Mechanism

The explanation for the pressurizing effect is shown in Figure 5.4. Figure 5.4A shows a vaporizer flowing free to atmosphere. The pressure in the vaporizing chamber and the bypass is P. As gas flows to the outlet, the pressure is reduced to R. The number of molecules of anesthetic agent picked up by each milliliter of carrier gas depends on the density of the anesthetic vapor molecules in the vaporizing chamber. This, in turn, depends on the vapor pressure of the agent. The vapor pressure depends solely on the temperature and is not affected by alterations in the atmospheric pressure.

Figure 5.4B shows the situation when an increased pressure (p′) is applied to the vaporizer outlet and transmitted to the vaporizing chamber (p). The increased pressure in the vaporizer will compress the carrier gas so there will be more molecules per milliliter. The number of molecules of anesthetic vapor in the vaporizing chamber will not be increased, however, because this depends on the saturated vapor pressure of the anesthetic and not on the pressure in the container. The net result is a decrease in the concentration of anesthetic in the vaporizing chamber and the vaporizer outlet.

Interplay Between Pressurizing and Pumping Effects

The changes in vaporizer output caused by the pumping effect usually are greater in magnitude than those associated with the pressurizing effect.

FIGURE 5.4. The pressurizing effect. An increase in pressure (p′) causes an increase in pressure (p) inside the vaporizer. The vapor pressure of the volatile anesthetic is unaffected by changes in the total pressure of the gas mixture above it. As a result, the concentration is reduced.

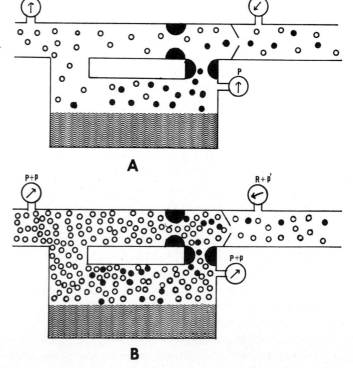

The pressurizing effect is greater with high gas flows and the pumping effect at low flows.

VAPORIZERS AND THE ANESTHESIA MACHINE STANDARD

The 1988 ASTM machine standard (5) contains the following provisions regarding vaporizers:

1) A vaporizer must be capable of accepting a total gas flow of 15 l/min from the anesthesia machine and, in turn, delivering a gas flow with a predictable concentration of vapor.
2) The effects of the conditions of use (including variations in ambient temperature and pressure, back pressure, and input flow rates) on vaporizer performance must be stated in catalogs and operation manuals. The effect of carrier gas composition on vaporizer output should also be supplied.
3) The extent to which temperature and inflow rates influence the vapor concentration must be stated.
4) A system that isolates the vaporizers from each other and prevents gas from passing through the vaporizing chamber of one vaporizer and then through that of another must be provided.
5) Controls must be provided to limit the escape of anesthetic vapor from the vaporizing chamber into the fresh gas so the delivered concentration is less than 0.1% when the vaporizer is turned off.
6) All vaporizer control knobs must turn counterclockwise to increase the concentration.
7) The vaporizer must be equipped with a liquid level indicator visible from the front of the anesthesia machine.
8) The vaporizer must be designed so that it cannot be overfilled when in the normal operating position.
9) The vaporizer must permit maximal calibrated flows of oxygen and nitrous oxide simultaneously in the ON and OFF positions with the vaporizer filled to the maximum safe indicated level without discharging liquid through its outlet when it is mounted and used in accordance with the manufacturer's instructions.
10) Vaporizers unsuitable for use in the breathing system must have noninterchangeable proprietary or 23-mm fittings. The 22-mm and 15-mm fittings cannot be used. The inlet of the vaporizer must be male, the outlet must be female, and the direction of gas flow must be marked when 23-mm fittings are used.
11) Vaporizers suitable for use in the breathing system must have standard 22-mm fittings or screw-threaded, weight-bearing fittings with the inlet female and the outlet male. The inlet and outlet ports must be marked, the direction of gas flow must be indicated by arrows, and the vaporizer must be marked "for use in the breathing system."

SPECIFIC VAPORIZERS
Siemens

This vaporizer is available in a version for halothane, enflurane, and isoflurane.

Classification

Concentration-calibrated, injection, no thermocompensation

Construction

The Siemens vaporizer (Fig. 5.5) is designed to be fitted to the Siemens 900D Ventilator. The ON-OFF valve on the right side has a locking device that must be released before the vaporizer can be turned on. The concentration dial is at the front and above the vaporizing chamber window and liquid level scale. The vaporizing chamber can hold up to 125 ml of liquid agent.

The filling system (Figs. 5.6 and 5.7) consists of an adaptor that fits on a bottle with a collar and fits into the filling receptacle at the back of the vaporizer. Noninterchangeability is accomplished by using different-sized collars to fit different-sized filling ports on the vaporizers. After the collar is fitted into the vaporizer port, a gentle push will open the valve in the filling device and allow agent to enter the vaporizer. The adaptor is self-sealing so it can remain on the bottle when the vaporizer is not being filled.

The vaporizer is diagramed in Figure 5.8. When the ON-OFF valve is in the ON position, gas from the mixing device passes through the

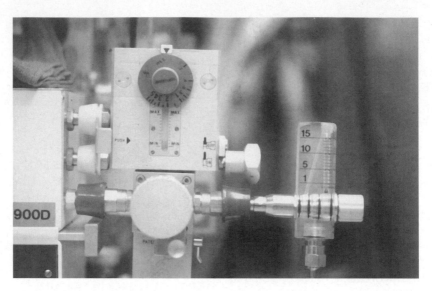

FIGURE 5.5. Siemens vaporizer. The ON-OFF valve with the lock is at the right. In the center is the liquid scale and window, below the concentration dial. The filling mechanism is at the back.

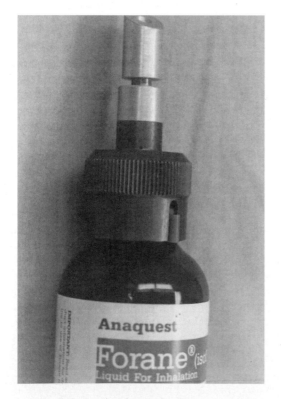

FIGURE 5.6. Bottle adaptor for Siemens vaporizer.

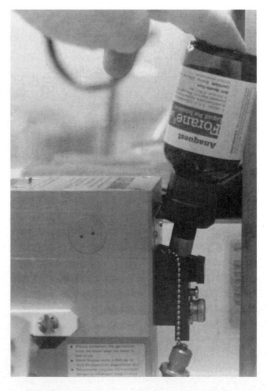

FIGURE 5.7. Filling the Siemens vaporizer. The adaptor is inserted into the filling receptacle. The bottle is pushed downward to allow the liquid to flow.

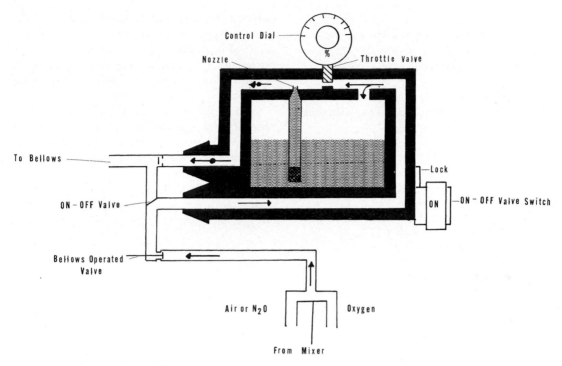

FIGURE 5.8. Diagram of the Siemens vaporizer. (Adapted with permission from a drawing furnished by Siemens.)

vaporizer. The throttle valve, which is adjusted using the concentration dial, causes resistance to gas flow. This results in back pressure that is transmitted to the reservoir, which contains liquid anesthetic. This pressure causes liquid anesthetic to be pushed through the nozzle of the injector into the stream of gas flowing to the bellows. The more the throttle valve constricts the channel, the higher the pressure in the reservoir and the more liquid is pushed through the injector. The liquid quickly vaporizes in this gas stream.

Evaluation

The manufacturer claims an accuracy of ± 10% of set concentration or 0.1 vol %, whichever is greater. The composition of carrier gas affects the output (Fig. 5.9). Output increases with increasing temperature. A 10°C temperature increase causes an increase of 10% of the set value.

Hazards

The vaporizer must not be tipped. A case has been reported in which a malfunctioning valve on the ventilator caused low concentrations to be delivered (18).

Maintenance

The external surface can be cleaned by wiping with a cloth soaked in disinfectant solution. The manufacturer recommends that the halothane vaporizer be drained, the contents discarded, and the vaporizer rinsed monthly with a small amount of halothane or if the vaporizer is out of use for a long time.

The accuracy of the output should be checked periodically using an agent monitor. If none is available, the following test described in the operations manual can be used: the ventilator controls are set at the values marked in green and the inspiratory minute volume is set at 7.5 l/min. The concentration dial is set to 3% for halothane, 3.5% for enflurane, and 3% for isoflurane. The ventilator is set to deliver 35% O_2 and 65% N_2O. If the vaporizer is operating correctly, the liquid level should drop two scale divisions in 18 to 24 minutes.

Tec 3

Tec 3 vaporizers include the Fluotec Mark 3, Enfluratec 3, Fortec 3, and Sevotec III. These vaporizers are no longer being manufactured.

Classification

Concentration-calibrated, flow over with wick, automatic thermocompensation

Construction

The vaporizer is diagramed in Figure 5.10 and shown in Figure 5.11. It consists of a lower va-

porizing chamber and an upper duct and valve system. Control of the delivered concentration is achieved by rotation of the knob at the top. This opens and closes ports and thus regulates the amount of gas passing through the vaporizing chamber.

In the OFF position (Fig. 5.10, Left), gas enters at the inlet, passes through a filter, and then flows to the outlet through two bypass channels. One of these directs a small stream of gas past a bimetallic temperature-sensitive element that is located concentrically within the lower bypass so

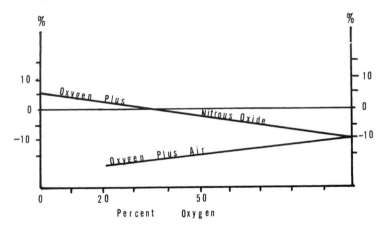

FIGURE **5.9.** Deviation in output with varying gas composition with the Siemens vaporizer. (Adapted with permission from a drawing furnished by Siemens.)

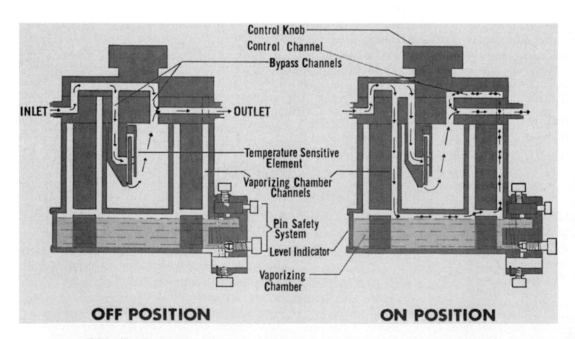

FIGURE **5.10.** Tec 3 vaporizer. The filter at the inlet is not shown. (Adapted with permission from Fraser Harlake.)

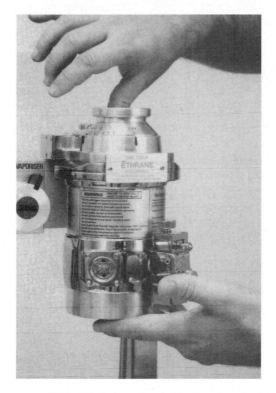

FIGURE 5.11. Enfluratec 3 vaporizer equipped with agent-specific filling device. The locking lever is at the left of the concentration dial. Note the front drain screw and plug chained to the filling device. This vaporizer has a ring that extends the base below the filler block. This allows the vaporizer to be placed upright on a flat surface. The selector valve is to the left of the vaporizer. (Reprinted with permission from Fraser Harlake.)

that its temperature is close to that of the anesthetic agent (19). The inlet and outlet of the vaporizing chamber are closed.

In the ON position (Fig. 5.10, Right), the top bypass channel is closed and the channel to the vaporizing chamber and the control channel (from the vaporizing chamber to the vaporizer outlet) are open. Gas still flows past the temperature-sensitive element in the lower bypass channel. Gas travels down one vaporizing chamber channel, over the liquid, and by the wicks where it becomes saturated with vapor. It then flows out of the chamber through the other lower bypass channel and enters the control channel. The size of the control channel is controlled by the position of the control knob.

The delivered concentration is determined by

resistances to flow past the temperature-sensitive element and in the control channel. Cooling causes increased resistance to flow past the element so that more gas flows through the vaporizing chamber.

The external design of a Tec 3 vaporizer is shown in Figure 5.11. The concentration dial is near the top. To the left of this is a locking lever that must be depressed to turn the vaporizer on. On the Enfluratec 3, this lever must also be depressed to increase the concentration above 5%. At the bottom is a sight window on the left and a filling mechanism on the right.

Evaluation

The manufacturer's performance data are given in Figure 5.12. All are accurate at low dial settings. At higher settings, most put out higher-than-expected concentrations at low flows and lower-than-expected concentrations at high flows.

Studies have shown that these vaporizers are quite accurate (19–27). Most investigations on the effects of carrier gas composition on output show that addition of nitrous oxide results in an initial decrease in output followed by a slow increase to a new value that is less than that seen when the carrier gas is oxygen.

An investigation of the Fluotec 3 showed that in the 0 to 0.5% dial-setting range the output was governed mainly by the position of the concentration dial and was little affected by the fresh gas flow (28). The output was 0 for approximately the first half of the rotation of the dial from OFF to the 0.5% position. In the second half, there was an almost linear increase in output to approximately 0.6% at a dial setting of 0.5%.

A study of Tec 3 vaporizers in clinical service revealed that 17% of Fluotec 3, 3.8% of Isotec 3, and 71% of Enfluratec 3 vaporizers had accuracies of less than 15% (29). Manufacturer's data indicate no effect on output from intermittent back pressure. Studies on the Fluotec 3 have confirmed this finding (19, 21). When Tec 3 vaporizers with no liquid level in the sight glass were set to a dial setting of 1% and a 6 l/min gas flow was passed through the vaporizer, the output concentration was maintained from 55 to 120 minutes because of liquid anesthetic sequestered in the wicks and in the bottom of the vaporizer below the sight indicator (30).

FIGURE **5.12.** Performance of Tec 3 Vaporizers. (Reprinted with permission from graphs furnished by Fraser Harlake.)

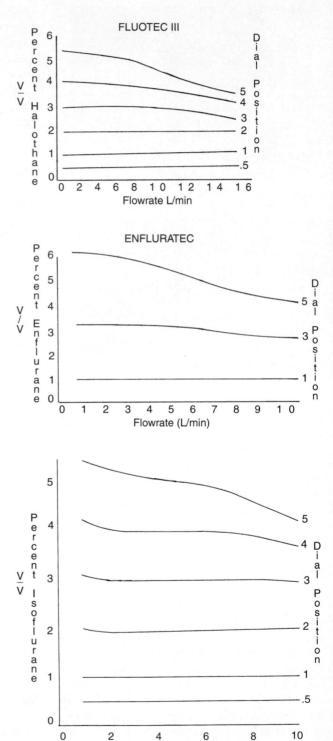

Hazards

The Fluotec 3 has been found to leak small amounts of vapor into the bypass in the OFF position (31, 32). In one case, a Fortec 3 delivered high concentrations, even when turned off (33, 34).

Several cases were reported of a Tec 3 vaporizer on which it was possible to turn the dial beyond the OFF position, resulting in delivery of vapor when none was desired (35–39). The manufacturer redesigned the vaporizer, and there have been no reports of this problem since 1984 (40).

A case was reported in which a damaged gasket in a Fluotec 3 caused a leak that allowed 50% of the fresh gas flow to exit around the top of the vaporizer when the control dial was at a setting other than 0 (41).

Tipping these vaporizers to 90° has no effect on the concentration subsequently delivered (42). However, after inversion to 180° with the dial set at zero or higher, the concentration delivered was much greater than shown on the dial, initially exceeding 12% for all agents. A study of the Fluotec 3 vaporizer filled and securely mounted on a gurney found that movements during normal motion did not cause an increase in delivered concentration (43).

A missing key inside these vaporizers may cause either higher-than-expected (44) or lower-than-expected (45, 46) concentrations.

Reversed flow causes the output to be increased (47, 48).

Maintenance

Yearly return of the vaporizer for maintenance is recommended by the manufacturer.

Tec 4

Tec 4 vaporizers include the Fluotec 4, Enfluratec 4, and the Fortec 4.

Classification

Concentration-calibrated, flow over with wick, automatic thermocompensation

Construction

The Fortec 4 is shown in Figure 5.13. At the top is a control dial. The release button to the left

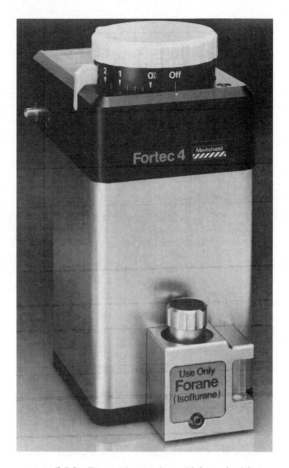

FIGURE 5.13. Fortec 4 vaporizer. (Adapted with permission from Fraser Harlake.)

must be depressed before the vaporizer can be turned on. A locking lever is located to the rear of the control dial. This is connected with the control dial so that the vaporizer cannot be turned on until it is locked on the manifold.

These vaporizers are available with either of two filling mechanisms. One is a screw cap, which is shown in Figure 5.13. Below the cap is a drain plug that extends up into the center of the cap. This plug is unscrewed to drain the vaporizer. The other filling device is a keyed system that has a single port for filling and emptying.

The internal construction of the vaporizer is shown in Figure 5.14. When the vaporizer is in the OFF position, gas from the inlet flows through the bypass and on to the outlet. When the vaporizer is turned on, the inflowing gas is split into

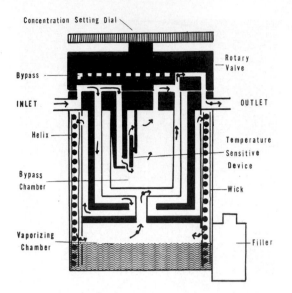

FIGURE 5.14. Diagram of Tec 4 vaporizer in the ON position. (See text for details.) (Adapted with permission from a diagram furnished by Fraser Harlake.)

two streams by the rotary valve attached to the concentration dial. One stream is directed through the vaporizing chamber that surrounds the bypass chamber. After passing through the inner section, the gas flows along the sides of the vaporizer, where two concentric wicks enclose a copper helix. The wicks dip into the liquid and increase contact between the carrier gas and the liquid agent. Gas saturated with vapor leaves the vaporizing chamber and flows past the rotary valve to the outlet. The balance of the fresh gas flow passes through the bypass chamber. Inside this chamber is a temperature-sensitive element that causes more gas to flow into the vaporizing chamber as cooling occurs.

Evaluation

The manufacturer's performance data are given in Figure 5.15. One study showed that delivery was less precise at low and very high flow rates (49). Another study found that at dial settings of 0.25%, the output was decreased by 40% between flows of 0.2 and 1 l/min (50). At dial settings between 0.4 and 0.5%, deviation in output concentration ranged from −5.5% for halothane and isoflurane to +22% for enflurane. Another evalua-

tion found that the vaporizer was accurate in the proximity of an MRI magnet (51).

These vaporizers are calibrated at 21°C. Output tends to rise slightly with elevated ambient temperature, especially with higher dial settings.

Changes in output with alterations in carrier gas composition are normally less than 10% of setting, with output less when nitrous oxide is added to the carrier gas. If helium is used in the carrier gas, the vapor output of the Isotec 4 does not vary by more than 10% except at high flows and high helium concentrations (52).

A surge in output occurs with opening of the vaporizer (53). Peak concentrations up to 3% with a mean of 1.7% have been measured. No serious sequelae were noted but children tended to withdraw from the mask during inhalation inductions.

Hazards

Deviations from the upright position, including tipping up to 180° will not affect the output of the vaporizer but may give a misleading impression of the amount of agent in the vaporizing chamber (42).

Leakage of liquid agent from the drain port caused by inadvertent loosening of the drain plug when the filler cap was removed has been reported (54).

Tec 4 vaporizers with keyed filling systems can be overfilled if the vaporizer is in the ON position and the bottle adaptor is loosened (55). This will result in a large increase in vaporizer output concentration when the vaporizer is turned on.

Reversed gas flow results in an increase in output concentration (48).

Maintenance

Although the manufacturer has recommended that vaporizers for halothane be drained at intervals not exceeding 2 weeks and less frequently for vaporizers for enflurane and isoflurane, studies show that draining every 6 months is probably sufficient (56). The vaporizers should be sent to a service center yearly.

In-house cleaning includes wiping the exterior surface with a damp cloth. No cleaning solution should be allowed to accumulate in the filler, the gas inlet, or around the control dial.

If an incorrect agent is put into the vaporizer,

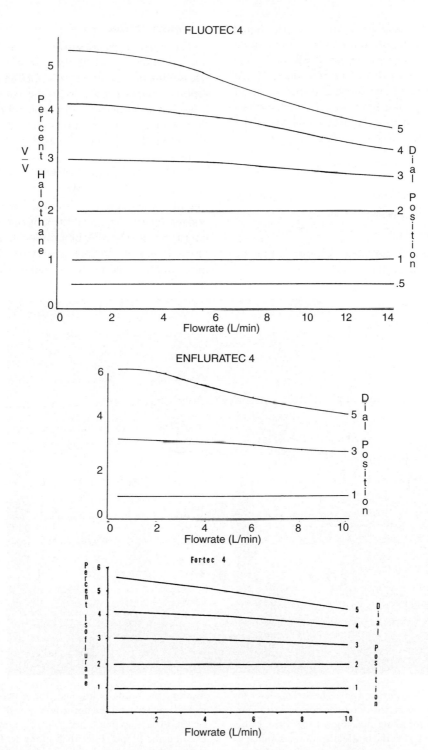

FIGURE 5.15. Performances of Tec 4 vaporizers at various flow rates and vaporizer settings. (Adapted with permission from graphs furnished by Fraser Harlake and Ohmeda, a division of BOC Health Care, Inc.)

the vaporizer should be drained and the liquid discarded. The dial should be set to the highest setting and the vaporizer flushed with a 5 l/min flow until no trace of the agent is detected. At least 2 hours should be allowed for the vaporizer temperature to stabilize before use. The vaporizer must be returned to the manufacturer for service if water or a nonvolatile substance is placed in a vaporizer.

Tec 5

Tec 5 vaporizers include the Isotec 5, Fluotec 5, Enfluratec 5, and Sevotec 5.

Classification

Concentration-calibrated, flow over with wick, automatic thermocompensation

Construction

Tec 5 vaporizers are shown in Figure 5.16. On top is a control dial. At the rear of the dial is a release button that must be pushed in before the vaporizer can be turned on. At the rear is a locking lever that is connected to the control dial so that the vaporizer cannot be turned on until it is locked on the manifold. At the bottom right front of each vaporizer is a sight glass.

Tec 5 vaporizers are available with either of two filling devices. One is a keyed system (Fig. 5.16). The filling-draining port is at the front of the vaporizer on the left near the bottom. A locking lever to secure the filler block is located to the left of the vaporizer. A small lever at the base allows the liquid to be added to or drained from the va-

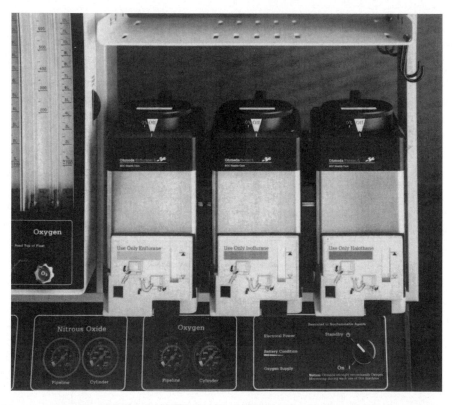

FIGURE 5.16. Tec 5 vaporizers. The locking lever for the filling device is on the lower left side of each vaporizer. The lever for filling-draining is at the base, below the sight glass. To fill, the bottle adaptor is inserted into the port and clamped in place by pulling the locking lever down. The bottle is then lifted up and the filling-draining lever is pulled forward. When filling is completed, the filling-draining lever is returned to the closed position, the bottle is lowered, the clamping lever is pushed upward, and the bottle is removed. Draining of the vaporizer is accomplished using the same levers but lowering the bottle rather than lifting it. Behind each control dial is a locking lever in the locked position. (Reprinted with permission from Ohmeda, a division of BOC Health Care, Inc.)

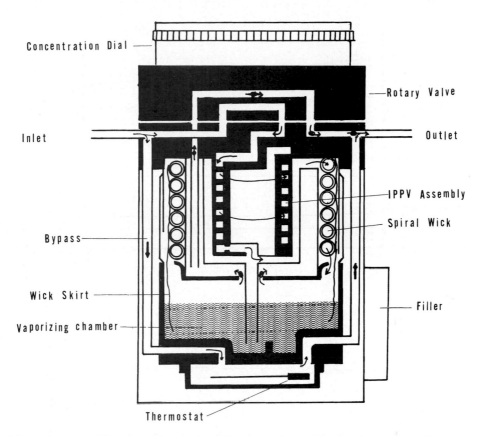

FIGURE 5.17. Diagram of Tec 5 vaporizer in the ON position. (See text for details.) (Adapted with permis- sion from a drawing furnished by Ohmeda, a division of the BOC Health Care, Inc.)

porizer. The other filling device is a screw cap that has a drain plug that can be loosened to drain the vaporizer.

A schematic diagram of a Tec 5 vaporizer is shown in Figure 5.17. The internal baffle system is designed to keep liquid from reaching the outlet if the vaporizer is tipped or inverted.

When the concentration dial is in the zero posi- tion, all incoming gas flows directly to the outlet through the bypass. When the dial is turned past zero, inflowing gas is split into two streams by the rotary valve. One stream is directed to the vaporiz- ing chamber, the other through the bypass.

Gas flowing through the bypass flows down one side of the vaporizer and past the thermostat, a bimetallic strip in the base. As the temperature in the vaporizer decreases, the thermostat allows less gas to flow through the bypass so a greater proportion passes through the vaporizing cham-

ber. From the thermostat, the gas flows up the other side of the vaporizer and joins the gas that has passed through the vaporizing chamber at the vaporizer outlet.

The gas flowing to the vaporizing chamber first passes through the central part of the rotary valve, after which it is directed through the helical inter- mittent positive pressure ventilation assembly and then past a spiral wick, which is designed to give maximum contact between carrier gas and liquid agent. The spiral wick is in contact with the wick skirt, which dips into the liquid agent. Gas with vapor leaves the vaporizing chamber through a channel in the rotary valve and flows to the outlet.

Evaluation

The manufacturer's performance curves are shown in Figure 5.18. Greatest accuracy is at a fresh gas flow of 5 l/min and dial settings less than

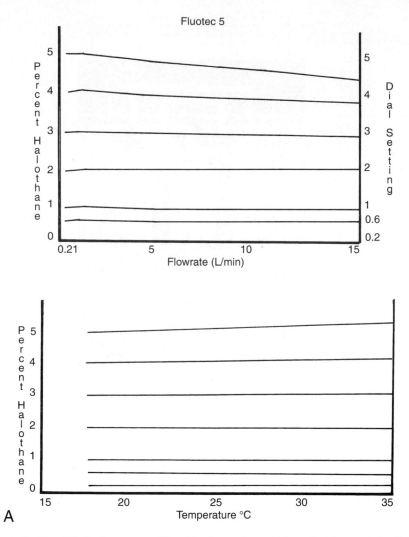

FIGURE 5.18. A, B, C and D, Performances of four Tec 5 vaporizers. (Adapted with permission from drawings furnished by Ohmeda, a division of the BOC Health Care, Inc.)

3%. There is a decrease in output at higher flows and higher dial settings.

The greatest accuracy is between 15° and 35° C. The thermostat does not respond to temperatures below 15° C, and the output will be less than indicated on the dial. The output will be unpredictably high if the temperature is above 35° C.

The Tec 5 is more prone to increases in output concentrations because of the pumping effect than the Tec 4 (57). Carrier gas composition af-

fects the output of the Tec 5 vaporizers. At low flows, the output is less when air or nitrous oxide is used than when oxygen is the carrier gas. At high flows, a small increase in output will occur.

Hazards

If the filling port is accidentally opened while the vaporizer is turned on, there will be a large loss of liquid agent (58). These vaporizers can be overfilled if the bottle adaptor is loose and the

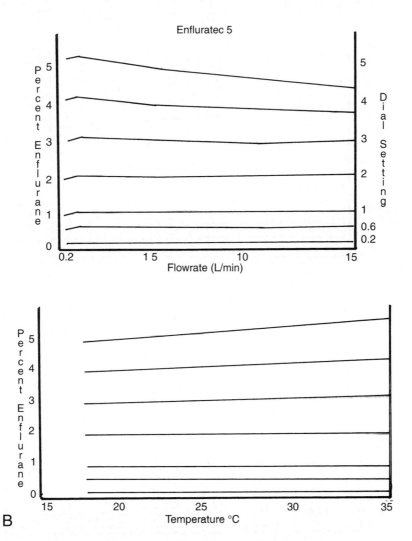

FIGURE **5.18.** *(continued)*

vaporizer is turned to the ON position (59). Reversed flow through the vaporizer results in increased output (48).

Maintenance

It is recommended by the manufacturer that the vaporizer be drained every 2 weeks or when the level is low if the agent contains additives or stabilizing agents. If these are not present, the vaporizer can be drained at less frequent intervals. Every 3 years the vaporizer should be returned to a service center.

The exterior of the vaporizer may be wiped with a damp cloth. No other cleaning or disinfection should be attempted.

Tec 6

Classification

Concentration-calibrated, injection, thermo-compensation by supplied heat

Construction

The Tec 6 vaporizer is shown in Figure 5.19. It is somewhat larger than the Tec 4 and Tec 5 vaporizers.

The concentration dial at the top is calibrated

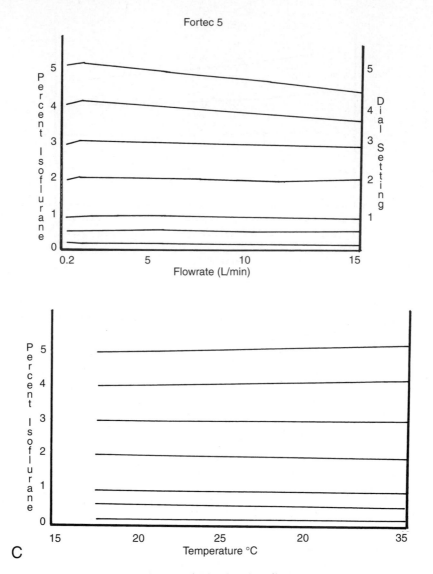

FIGURE **5.18.** *(continued)*

from 1 to 18% in gradations of 1% up to 10% and 2% between 10 and 18%. A dial release is at the back of the dial. This must be depressed to turn the dial from the standby position and to dial concentrations more than 12%. This release cannot be depressed unless the operational light-emitting diode (LED) is illuminated.

The filler port is at the front on the left. Its agent-specific filling system allows only a desflurane bottle to be inserted into it. The power cord attachment and battery case are on the bottom.

A nonrechargeable battery provides power for the alarms and liquid crystal level indicator display during main power failures. The power cord exits at the side. The drain plug is also located at the base of the vaporizer. A draining kit is required to drain the vaporizer.

On the front lower right of the vaporizer is the display panel, which has visual indicators for vaporizer functions (Fig. 5.19). With the exception of the tilt condition, there is a 10-sec delay between detection of a malfunction and alarm ac-

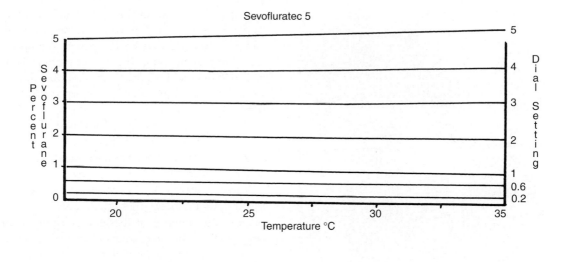

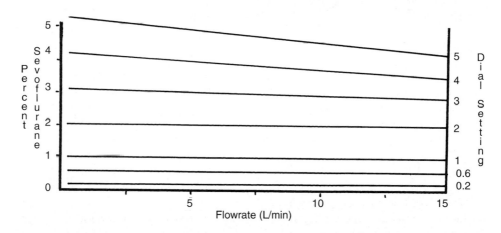

D

FIGURE **5.18.** *(continued)*

tivation. An auditory alarm is mounted behind the upper part of the display panel. A mute button is located above the display panel.

The amber warm-up LED indicates an initial warm-up period after the vaporizer is first connected to the main power. Once warm-up is complete, the green operational LED is illuminated, indicating that the vaporizer has reached its operating temperature and the concentration dial can be turned on. There are no audible signals for these modes except for a short tone that sounds at the transition from warm-up to operational.

The red no-output LED flashes and an auditory alarm of repetitive tones sounds if the vapor-

izer is no longer able to deliver vapor. This can be caused by an agent level less than 20 ml, tilting of the vaporizer, a power failure, or an internal malfunction. Turning the concentration dial to standby will mute this alarm but the red light will illuminate continuously. If the no-output alarm occurs while the concentration dial is in the standby position, it can be silenced by pressing the mute button.

The amber low agent LED accompanied by an audible alarm of repetitive tones flashes if there is less than 50 ml of agent in the vaporizer. This alarm can be muted for 120 seconds.

The amber alarm battery low LED illuminates

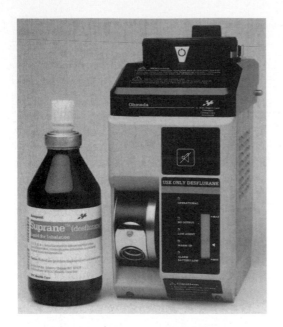

FIGURE 5.19. Tec 6 vaporizer. The filler port is at the bottom left. At the bottom right are the liquid level indicator and the visual signals for monitors of vaporizer function. A bottle of desflurane with the protection cap in place is to the left of the vaporizer. The locking lever behind the control dial is in the unlocked position. (Reprinted with permission from Ohmeda, a division of BOC Health Care, Inc.)

to indicate that a new battery is required. There is no auditory signal for this condition.

The liquid level indicator has a liquid crystal display (LCD) that shows the amount of liquid in the vaporizer between 50 and 425 ml. The LCD is lit whenever the vaporizer is powered. There are 20 bars. A single bar corresponds to a volume of approximately 20 ml. An arrow on the side indicates the 250 ml refill mark. If the level is below this mark, the vaporizer will accept a full bottle (240 ml) of desflurane.

If the vaporizer is tilted more than 10°, the tilt switch is activated. This causes vapor output to cease and activates the red no output LED and auditory alarm.

The electronics go through a self-test when the unit is plugged in. For 2 seconds, the alarm sounds and each LED and LCD illuminates. This self-test can be repeated at any time by pressing the mute button for 4 seconds or more. Once the vaporizer

is plugged in, the power is always on and the sump heaters are operational. Initially, the vaporizer will take 5 to 10 minutes to reach operating temperature. During this time, the concentration dial is locked in the standby position. An internal shutoff valve is closed to prevent flow of vapor from the sump.

The internal construction of this vaporizer is shown in Figure 5.20. It differs from other vaporizers in that none of the fresh gas passes through a vaporizing chamber. In the vaporizer, desflurane is heated to 39°C (102°F), which is well above its boiling point. An external heat source is needed because the potency of desflurane requires that large amounts be vaporized and thermocompensation using the usual mechanical devices is impossible. Power for the heater, alarms, and controls is furnished from a standard electric system. A transformer and AC to DC converter provide a DC power for the vaporizer.

The sump assembly holds the agent and includes the filling port, the drain, the heaters, and the agent level sensor. It has a capacity of 425 ml. Two heaters, which are fitted into the base, heat the agent to 39°C. The temperature is monitored and associated electronics act as a thermostat. There are also two heaters in the upper part of the vaporizer to prevent condensation of agent where the warm vapor meets the cold gas from the common manifold. The current to power the heaters goes back and forth between the sump and the upper part of the vaporizer. This keeps the current requirement to a minimum. The casing of the vaporizer is normally warm to the touch when it is connected to the electric supply.

The level of liquid agent is sensed by a probe and sheath mounted in the sump assembly. These measure the capacitance using the agent as a dielectric. The display is on the front of the vaporizer.

When the proper temperature is attained, the green operational LED illuminates. A signal from the control electronics operates the solenoid interlock, allowing the dial and rotary valve to be turned. When the dial and rotary valve are turned, a signal from the control electronics opens the shutoff valve.

Fresh gas flow enters the vaporizer and encounters a fixed resistor that creates back pressure

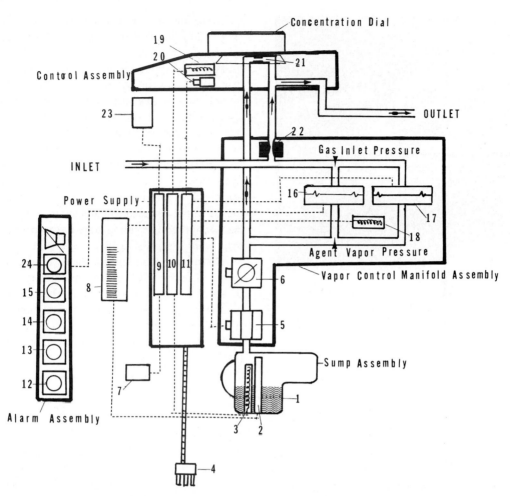

FIGURE 5.20. Diagram of Tec 6 vaporizer. **1**, agent; **2**, level sensor; **3**, sump heaters; **4**, electric mains; **5**, shutoff valve; **6**, agent pressure-regulating valve; **7**, battery for alarms; **8**, liquid crystal display (LCD) level; **9**, alarm electronics; **10**, heater electronics; **11**, control electronics; **12**, alarm battery low light-emitting diode (LED); **13**, warm-up LED; **14**, low agent LED; **15**, no output LED; **16**, pressure transducer; **17**, pressure monitor; **18**, heater in vapor manifold; **19**, heater in valve plate; **20**, solenoid interlock; **21**, variable resistor (controlled by rotary valve); **22**, fixed restrictor; **23**, tilt switch; **24**, operational LED. (See text for details.) (Adapted with permission from a diagram furnished by Ohmeda, a division of BOC Health Care, Inc.)

in the fresh gas portion of the vaporizer. The higher the flow of fresh gas, the higher the back pressure generated. Electromechanical devices operate to maintain the agent vapor pressure at the variable resistor in the rotary valve at the same level as the fresh gas pressure at the fixed restrictor. This pressure balance between the desflurane and the diluent flows compensates for changes in temperature, vapor pressure, or diluent flow rate. The pressures are sensed by a transducer that sends a

signal to the control electronics, which in turn alters the agent pressure at the variable resistor by opening or closing the agent pressure regulating valve to balance the pressures.

With this balance of pressures maintained, the concentration delivered by the vaporizer depends only on the ratio of fresh gas flow through the fixed restrictor and agent vapor flow through the variable resistor, which depends on the setting of the concentration dial. Resistance to desflurane

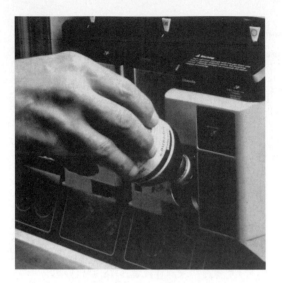

FIGURE **5.21.** Filling Tec 6 vaporizer. The bottle is fitted to the filler port. After it is engaged in the filler port, it is rotated upward. When it reaches the upper stop, agent will enter the vaporizer. (Reprinted with permission from Ohmeda, a division of BOC Health Care, Inc.)

flow decreases and the flow of desflurane increases when the concentration dial is turned to a higher value. With an increase in diluent flow, the electronics will increase the flow in the desflurane limb to maintain the pressure balance. The vapor mixes with fresh gas just before the latter exits the vaporizer.

The Tec 6 filling system is shown in Figures 5.19 and 5.21. Because desflurane boils so close to room temperature, it cannot be poured into a funnel and allowed to drain into the vaporizer. The vaporizer can be filled in use but the fresh gas flow should be less than 8 l/min, the concentration dial should be set at no more than 8%, and the vaporizer should not be subjected to any high back pressure. The vaporizer can be filled while in its warm-up cycle.

The bottle (male component) (Fig. 5.22) has a crimped-on adaptor. This has a spring-loaded valve that opens when the bottle is pushed into the filling port on the vaporizer. The vaporizer (female) component consists of a recessed port on a spindle. The bottle is inserted into this port to a depth at which a spring is activated. The spindle

is then rotated upwards until a stop is encountered (Fig. 5.21). Agent can enter the vaporizer at this point.

To fill the vaporizer, the bottle protection cap is removed and the bottle fitted to the filler port by holding it below and pushing it up against the spring. After the bottle is fully engaged in the port, it is rotated upward (Fig. 5.21). The bottle is held in this position while filling. When the LCD liquid level gauge indicates that the sump is full or when the bottle is empty, the bottle is rotated downward and removed from the vaporizer. The valve on the bottle closes automatically to prevent spillage of agent. The filling port has a spring valve to prevent escape of agent.

There have been few problems reported with this filling system. One study revealed an average of 4.47 cc of residual volume in the bottle after filling the vaporizer. Bottles containing desflurane that did not have the cap replaced, would leak agent, allowing the bottle to empty spontaneously (60).

Evaluation

The manufacturer's data are shown in Figure 5.23. The vaporizer is calibrated for flows from 0.2 to 10 l/min. The output is almost linear at the 3, 7, and 12% settings with slightly lower outputs at flows less than 5 l/min and slightly greater outputs at higher flows. At a dial setting of 18%, the output is higher than setting at flows less than 5 l/min and less at higher flows. The vaporizer is designed to be used at ambient temperatures from 18° to 30°C. Evaluations have found that the output is within 15 % of the dial setting and that tilting the vaporizer did not render it inoperative or dangerous to operate (61, 62).

The Tec 6 vaporizer differs from variable-by-pass vaporizers in its response to changes in barometric pressure. It maintains a constant output concentration in volumes percent but a variable partial pressure with varying barometric pressure. With a decrease in ambient pressure the output in partial pressure at a given setting will be decreased.

Fluctuating back pressure does not affect its output significantly. Carrier gas composition affects vaporizer output (62, 63). Output is highest with pure oxygen, lower with air, and lowest with nitrous oxide in the carrier gas.

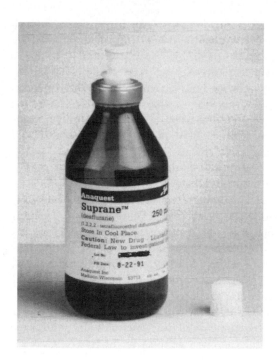

FIGURE **5.22.** Bottle for filling Tec 6 vaporizer. The protection cap has been removed and is at the right. (Reprinted with permission from Ohmeda, a division of BOC Health Care, Inc.)

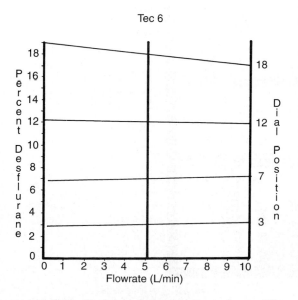

FIGURE **5.23.** Performance of Tec 6 vaporizer, with oxygen as the carrier gas. (Adapted with permission from a graph furnished by Ohmeda, a division of BOC Health Care, Inc).

Electricity consumption by the vaporizer is low (64). The battery must be replaced annually.

Hazards and Precautions

Vapor can leak into the fresh gas flow with the vaporizer turned off. When electricity is supplied to the vaporizer, each LED and all the LCD agent level indicator bars on the front display panel should flash and the auditory alarm should be activated for approximately 1 second. If any of the LEDs or level indicator bars do not illuminate or the audible alarm is not heard, the vaporizer should not be used.

When filling the vaporizer, the bottle must be gripped tightly when it is rotated downward from the upper position to the lower stop position. Otherwise the bottle may be dropped when it is released under pressure at the lower position.

A problem has been reported with the Tec 6 mounted on a North American Drager anesthesia machine (65). A valve piston in the attachment stuck in the depressed position, causing a large leak of fresh gas. Also other vaporizers mounted on the machine could not be turned on. Cases of sparks and smoke around the connection between the main power cord and the socket have been reported (66). This was believed to be the result of a loose plug.

The Tec 6 should be mounted to the far right-hand side on the back bar of the anesthesia machine so the power cord is able to be routed off the side. If mounted on the left or an intermediate position, the power cord may be difficult to route off the machine. A case has been reported where the power cord was draped over the back bar and interfered with the vaporizer interlock mechanism (67).

Maintenance

This vaporizer requires servicing every year at an authorized center. The external surface may be wiped using a cloth slightly dampened with a cleaning agent. No other cleaning or disinfection should be attempted.

Ohio Calibrated Vaporizer

These vaporizers are available in a version for halothane, enflurane, and isoflurane.

Classification

Concentration-calibrated, flow over with wick, automatic thermocompensation

Construction

A schematic view of the Ohio calibrated vaporizer is shown in Figure 5.24. Fresh gases enter the vaporizer and pass through a filter. There are three possible paths for the gases to follow. The first is through the relief valve at the top, which opens when the pressure rises above a set amount.

Most of the gas flows past the temperature-compensating bypass to the outlet. The temperature of the gas leaving the vaporizing chamber is sensed by a bellows. When the vapor is warm, the bellows expands. This increases the size of the opening around the bypass so that more of the incoming gas goes directly to the outlet. When the vapor cools, the bellows contracts and partially closes the bypass. This causes a greater proportion of gas to go through the vaporizing chamber.

The remaining gas flows to the two sets of orifices. Flow through one set is directed to the vaporizer outlet. Flow through the other orifices is directed into the vaporizing chamber. Turning the concentration control dial simultaneously opens one set of orifices while closing the other set and so determines the splitting ratio between gas flowing to the outlet and that going to the vaporizing chamber.

Gas entering the vaporizing chamber flows around a series of wicks where it becomes saturated with vapor. It then leaves the vaporizing chamber, flows around the temperature-sensing bellows and on to the outlet.

The vaporizer is shown in Figure 5.25. There are two sight windows: one with a full and one with an empty indication. The filling port can be either the funnel or keyed block type. The concentration dial is at the top. There are clicks at each increment on the dial. There is a locking button at the top rear that must be depressed before the

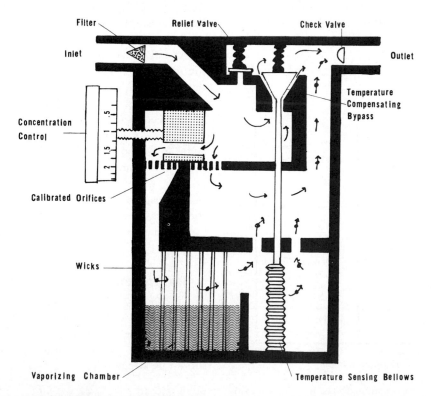

FIGURE 5.24. Schematic drawing of Ohio calibrated vaporizer. For the purpose of illustration, the concentration control dial is shown at the left, although it is actually on top. (Adapted with permission from a drawing furnished by Ohmeda, a division of the BOC Health Care, Inc.)

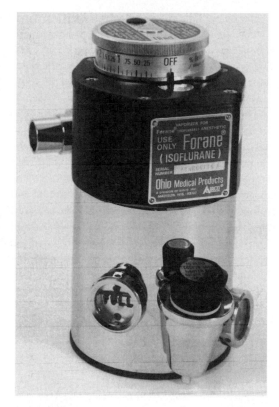

FIGURE **5.25.** Ohio calibrated vaporizer. (Reprinted with permission from Ohmeda, a division of BOC Health Care, Inc.)

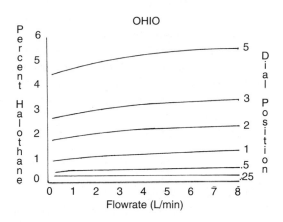

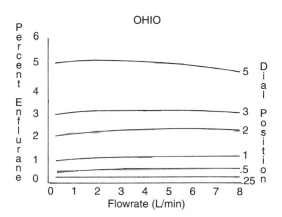

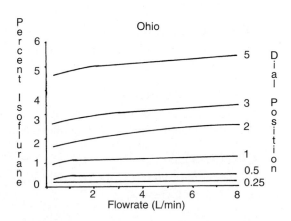

FIGURE **5.26.** Performances of Ohio calibrated vaporizers. **A**, Halothane. **B**, Enflurane. **C**, Isoflurane. (Adapted with permission from Ohmeda, a division of BOC Health Care, Inc.)

dial can be turned on. On the enflurane vaporizer, the dial relocks at the 5% position, and the locking button must again be depressed to dial a concentration more than 5%.

Evaluation

Figure 5.26 shows the manufacturer's data for enflurane, halothane, and isoflurane. The vaporizers are accurate at fresh gas flows from 300 ml to 10 l/min and between 16° and 32°C.

A study of the enflurane and halothane vaporizers at fresh gas flows from 100 to 5000 ml/min found they performed satisfactorily (21). There was a transient but significant increase in output when high flow was suddenly reduced. A transient decrease in output occurred when the flow was increased. Intermittent back pressures affected vaporizer output but mean output was the same as with free flow to atmosphere. Use of the oxygen flush increased the output more than 10% at low fresh gas flows. Another evaluation showed these vaporizers to be reasonably accurate (68).

The manufacturer's literature indicates that the addition of nitrous oxide to the carrier gas will lower the output. Several investigators found this to be true at settings below 3% (21, 22, 24, 26, 69, 70). At settings of 3% and above, the addition of nitrous oxide may increase vapor output slightly (22, 26). Helium in the carrier gas does not cause the output to vary by more than ± 10% (52).

Hazards

When the anesthesia machine is in use and the concentration knob is turned to OFF, a small amount of vapor can diffuse from the vaporizing chamber into the bypass circuit.

These vaporizers can be tilted up to 20° even while in use without effect. If not in use, they can be tilted up to 45° without effect. If tilted more than these amounts, liquid may enter the control head and a higher-than-expected concentration will be delivered when the vaporizer is turned on.

Discoloration of liquid enflurane and isoflurane was noted in early vaporizers of this type (71, 72). This was traced to a reaction between the liquid and plastic wick spacers (73). No evidence of toxicity was found (74, 75).

Reversed gas flow through the vaporizer results in a decreased output (48).

Maintenance

The company recommends that the vaporizer be sent to a service center once a year.

Aladin 2222 Vaporizer

This vaporizer can be used for halothane, enflurane, desflurane, isoflurane, and sevoflurane.

Classification

Concentration-calibrated, flow over, automatic thermocompensation

Construction

The vaporizer has two parts. The electronic control mechanism is in the anesthesia machine itself. The agent is contained in and vaporizes in the cassette.

Electronic Control

This vaporizer is designed to be used with the Datex-Engstrom AS/3 Anesthesia Delivery Unit. The concentration dial is on the anesthesia machine (Fig. 5.27).

Cassette

The cassette is shown in Figure 5.28. It is color-coded according to the agent it is designed to contain and magnetically coded to allow the machine to automatically identify it. There is a temperature sensing mechanism at the rear. The cassettes for desflurane, halothane, enflurane, and isoflurane have keyed fillers. Sevoflurane cassettes may be equipped with either a keyed filler or other (Quik Fill) mechanism. A lock-and-fill wheel on the left locks the keyed filler in place and opens the air vent and liquid filling channel. A handle

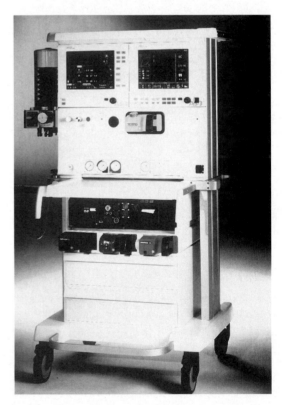

FIGURE 5.27. Aladin Cassette Vaporizer in place. The vaporizer fits into the recess below the screens. The concentration dial is located to the left of the cassette. Unused cassettes are stored below. (Reprinted with permission from Datex-Engstrom, Inc.)

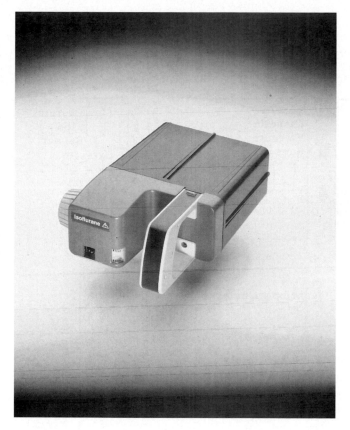

FIGURE **5.28.** Aladin Cassette Vaporizer. The handle is used to transport the vaporizer, which can be held in any position. The wheel on the left is used to lock the filling mechanism in place. The cassette is color-coded according to the agent contained. Note the liquid level indicator to the right of the keyed filler. (Reprinted with permission from Datex-Engstrom, Inc.)

on the front is used to carry the cassette and to insert it into and remove it from the anesthesia machine. The liquid level indicator and the filling port are also located on the front. The cassette holds up to 250 ml of agent when full. When the indicator indicates empty, the cassette contains up to 150 ml.

The cassette is shown diagrammatically in Figure 5.29. Fresh gas enters the vaporizer and is split between the bypass and vaporizing chamber. A check valve in the inlet to the vaporizing chamber protects against back flow of agent into the bypass and prevents liquid from flowing into the bypass when the cassette is handled. The flow control at the outlet of the vaporizing chamber is controlled by the central processing unit in the anesthesia machine. Sensors in the vaporizing chamber outlet and bypass monitor the flows. The electronic control mechanism receives information from the anesthesia gas monitor and the cassette that in-

cludes the anesthetic agent, the temperature and the pressure in the cassette, the flow into the cassette, and the composition of the fresh gas flowing into the vaporizer. This information is used to regulate the amount of gas flowing through the vaporizing chamber to achieve the desired concentration.

The vaporizer is ready for use when the desired cassette is inserted and locked into its slot. To set the concentration, the agent control dial is turned. The setting is displayed on the screen.

To change agents, the cassette is removed and another one inserted. The cassette weighs 2.5 kg. It can be handled and stored in any position.

To fill the cassette, it is first removed from the machine. The keyed filler is screwed firmly on the bottle and inserted into the agent filling port. The filler is locked by turning the lock-and-fill wheel fully clockwise. The bottle is turned upside down. Liquid should then flow into the vaporizer. When

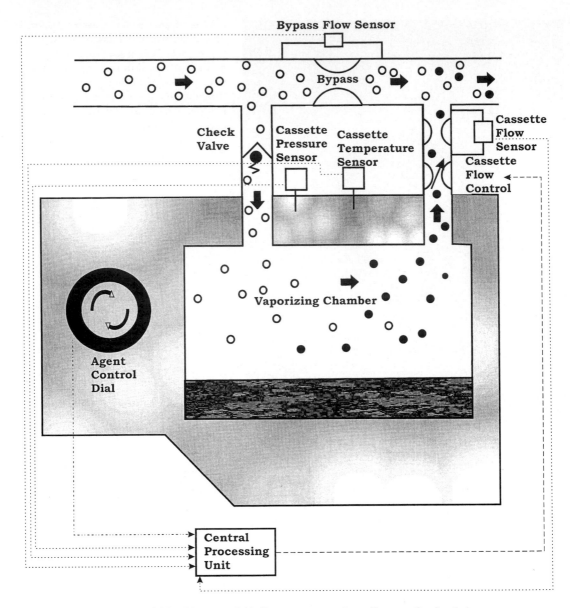

FIGURE **5.29.** Diagram of Aladin cassette vaporizer. (See text for details.)

the vaporizer is filled, the bottle is turned downward and the keyed filler released by turning the lock-and-fill wheel counterclockwise. The filler is then removed from the filling port.

Evaluation

The manufacturer indicates the accuracy for all agents is 10% with fresh gas flows from 200 ml/min to 10 l/min. Figure 5.30 shows variations in output with changes in fresh gas composition. Sevoflurane accuracy in the setting range of 5 to 8% is 20%. If the temperature falls below 20°C or the fresh gas flow is more than 8 l/min, sevoflurane concentrations above 5% may not be produced and messages "insufficient agent" and "decreased flow" will appear on the machine. The delivered

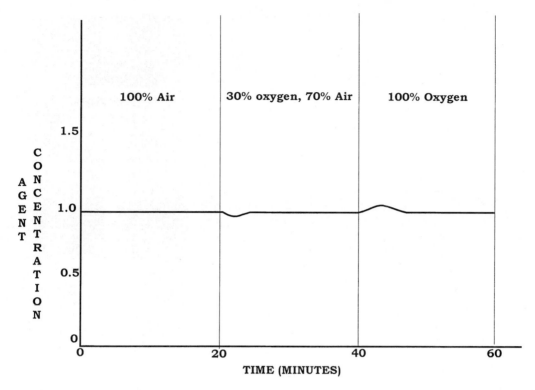

FIGURE 5.30. Output of Aladin Cassette Vaporizer with changes in fresh gas composition. The electronic control unit in the machine makes adjustments for changes in fresh gas composition to maintain a steady output.

concentration will increase with a decrease in ambient pressure. Inaccurate output may temporarily occur if the temperature of liquid agent added to the cassette is considerably colder than the normal operating temperature.

Hazards

There were no reported hazards in the literature at the time of this writing.

Vapor 19.1

The vaporizer is available in a version for halothane, enflurane, isoflurane, and sevoflurane.

Classification

Concentration-calibrated, flow over, automatic thermocompensation.

Construction

The Vapor 19.1 is shown in Figure 5.31. The 0 must be depressed before the concentration dial can be turned. A filling spout, sight glass, and drain are located at the bottom front. The isoflurane Vapor 19.1 has a concentration range from 0.2 to 5.0%; the enflurane, from 0.2 to 5% (or by special model up to 7%); and the halothane from 0.2 to 5% (or 7% by special model).

The Vapor 19.1 is shown schematically in Figure 5.32. In the OFF position, the inlet and outlet of the vaporizing chamber are interconnected and vented to the outside. This prevents anesthetic agent from leaking into the fresh gas. Fresh gas passes directly through the inlet port and ON-OFF switch and to the outlet port without entering the interior of the vaporizer (76).

In the ON position, at dial settings above 0.2%, incoming gases are diverted past the bypass cone to the lower vaporizing section. Part of the fresh gas flows through a pressure compensator that is designed to prevent pressure fluctuations upstream or downstream of the vaporizer from af-

FIGURE **5.31.** Vapor 19.1 vaporizer. (Reprinted with permission from North American Drager.)

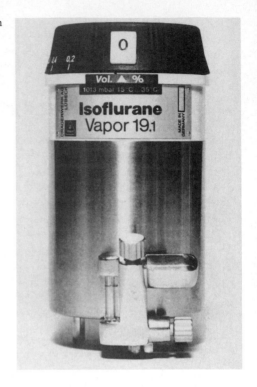

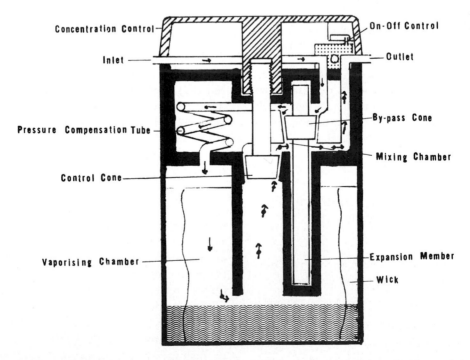

FIGURE **5.32.** Vapor 19.1 vaporizer in the ON position. (See text for details.) (Adapted with permission from a drawing furnished by North American Drager.)

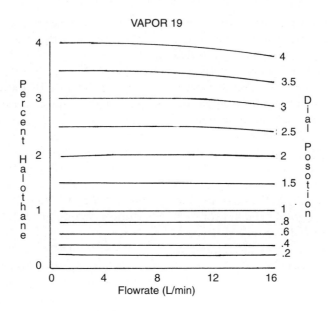

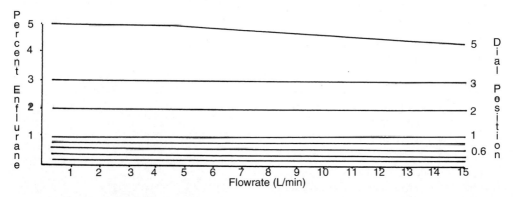

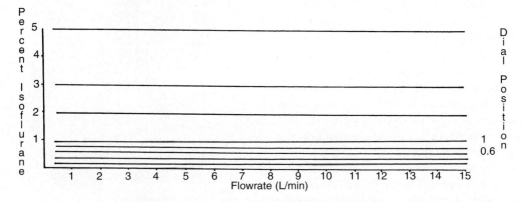

FIGURE 5.33. Output of Vapor 19.1 vaporizers at an ambient temperature of 22°C. (Adapted with permission from graphs furnished by North American Drager.)

fecting the output. Part of the fresh gas then flows to the vaporizing chamber where it becomes saturated. The gas that passes through the vaporizing chamber exits by the control cone, which is controlled by the concentration dial. As the concentration is increased or decreased, the space between the control cone and the cone housing increases or decreases, allowing more or less of the fresh gas/agent mixture to leave the vaporizing chamber (76). The balance is routed past the bypass cone where it mixes with gas from the vaporizing chamber and flows to the vaporizer output. The bypass cone regulates the flow of fresh gas through the bypass and responds to temperature changes. Cooling causes it to direct more gas through the vaporizing chamber (77).

Evaluation

The manufacturer's data for the Vapor 19.1 are shown in Figure 5.33. Output is independent of fresh gas flow in the range of 0.3 to 15 l/min with lower dial settings, but, with high gas flows, total saturation of the gas flowing through the vaporizing chamber is not possible and output falls. An accuracy of 10% can be expected between 10° and 40° C. At temperatures outside this range, the vaporizer will be less accurate.

Investigations of Vapor 19.1 vaporizers for isoflurane, enflurane, and halothane with high and low flows have shown that they perform accurately (21, 49, 50).

The Vapor 19.1 is calibrated using air as the carrier gas. The delivered concentration is 4 to 10% higher than the set concentration when operated on 100% oxygen (21, 78). The concentration is 5 to 10% lower when operated with 30% oxygen and 70% nitrous oxide. Changing from 66% nitrous oxide in oxygen to 100% oxygen results in an increase in output followed by a decrease (27). If helium is in the carrier gas, the output does not vary by more than ± 10% (52).

An investigation of the vaporizer at pressures up to 4 atmospheres showed that output decreased with increasing pressure but remained within 20% of setting (13).

Mounting the vaporizer on a moving trolley does not cause alteration of the output (79).

The Vapor 19.1 with a key filler will not overfill, even when the vaporizer is in the ON position and the bottle adaptor is loosened (55).

Hazards

If a filled Vapor 19.1 is tilted, liquid agent may spill into the control device whether the vaporizer is turned on or off. This can result in either an increase or decrease in delivered concentration. If the vaporizer is tipped more than 45°, it should be flushed with a flow of 10 l/min with the concentration dial on the highest setting for at least 20 minutes. Reverse flow through the vaporizer has no effect on output (48).

Maintenance

The outer part of the vaporizer can be cleaned with a damp cloth soaked with detergent. The manufacturer recommends that the halothane vaporizer be rinsed when the liquid in the sight glass shows discoloration or dirt particles.

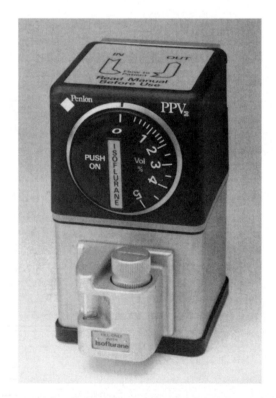

FIGURE **5.34.** PPV Sigma vaporizer with screw cap filler and back entry connections. (Reprinted with permission from Penlon, Ltd.)

The vaporizer should be inspected by trained personnel every 6 months. The vaporizing chamber should be cleaned and the wicks changed every 2 years.

Penlon PPV Sigma

This vaporizer is available in a version for halothane, enflurane, isoflurane, and sevoflurane.

Classification

Concentration-calibrated, flow over, automatic thermocompensation

Construction

The Penlon PPV vaporizer is shown in Figure 5.34. The top of the vaporizer and the bar on the concentration dial are color-coded for the designed agent. The dial is pushed in and rotated to set a concentration. The dial is marked in graduations of 0.2% from 0 to 2% and intervals of 0.5% from 2 to 5%. The filling device can be either a screw cap or keyed filler type. The liquid level indicator has lines for minimum and maximum levels.

A ball rides on top of the liquid meniscus for easy reading. The direction of gas flow through the vaporizer is shown on the top.

The internal construction of the vaporizer is shown in Figure 5.35. Gas enters the vaporizer and is split into two streams, one passing through the bypass and the other passing through the vaporizing chamber. In the zero lock position, the bypass remains open but the vaporizing chamber is completely shut off from gas flow. If the zero lock port is open, gas passes through a spiral tube into the vaporizing chamber that contains a stainless-steel wick. Gas saturated with vapor then exits the vaporizing chamber through the vapor control orifice. The size of this orifice is controlled by the setting of the concentration control dial. Gas saturated with vapor then joins the bypass gas and flows to the outlet.

Temperature compensation is provided by a liquid-filled expansion bellows controlling a variable resistance valve in the bypass. Gas flowing through the bypass passes this variable resistance. As the vaporizing chamber cools, the orifice be-

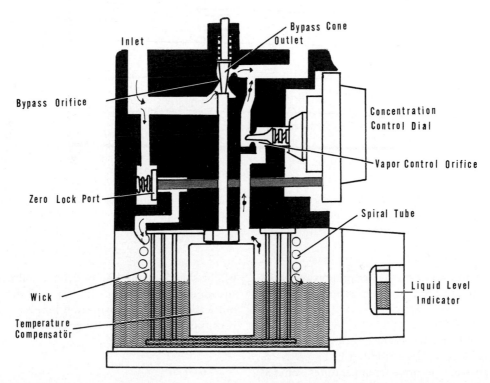

FIGURE 5.35. Diagram of PPV Sigma vaporizer. (See text for details.) (Adapted with permission from a drawing furnished by Penlon, Ltd.)

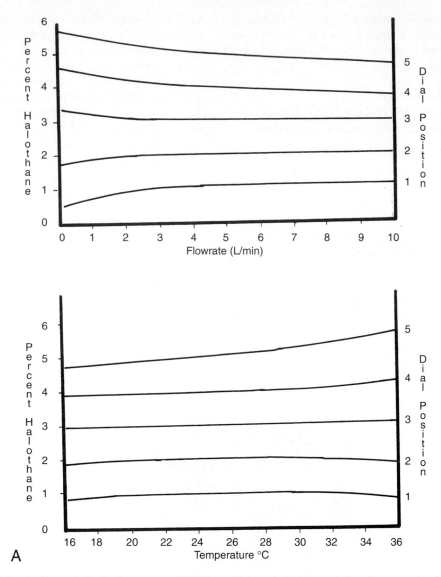

FIGURE 5.36. **A, B**, and **C**, Performances of PPV Sigma vaporizers with oxygen as the carrier gas. (Adapted with permission from graphs furnished by Penlon, Ltd.)

comes smaller so that a greater proportion of gas passes through the vaporizing chamber.

Evaluation

The performance characteristics supplied by the manufacturer are illustrated in Figure 5.36. The vaporizer is accurate at temperatures from 15° to 35° C. Output is increased at higher temperatures. If nitrous oxide is in the carrier gas, output will be slightly higher. Air or helium in the carrier stream causes the output to drop slightly. Intermittent back pressure may result in some increase in output concentration. Reversed gas flow results in increased output (48).

Hazards

If the vaporizer is transported while filled, the control must be in the zero position and at least

2 minutes should elapse with the vaporizer in a secured upright position before use. If the vaporizer has been transported with the control in the open position, it must be flushed with gas at 4 l/min for 2 minutes.

The concentration dial must be in the zero position during filling or draining and the vaporizer must be upright to avoid overfilling. A vaporizer that has been overfilled should be withdrawn from use.

Overfilling can occur if the vaporizer is turned on and the bottle adaptor loosened (80). A high output will then occur when the vaporizer is used.

Maintenance

The vaporizer should be calibrated every 3 to 6 months, with a major overhaul every 5 years. The exterior should be cleaned with a dry cloth. No liquids, including water, should be applied to the surface. The halothane vaporizer should be

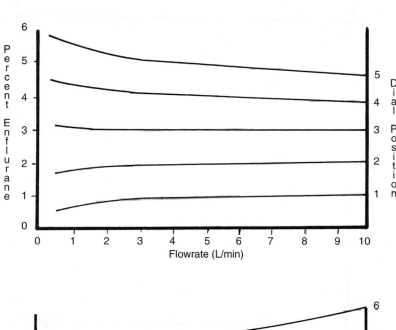

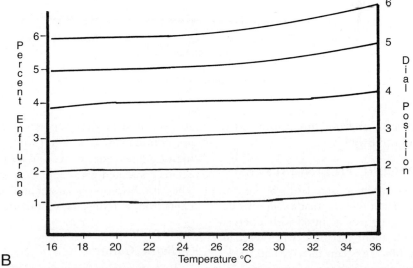

FIGURE 5.36. *(continued)*

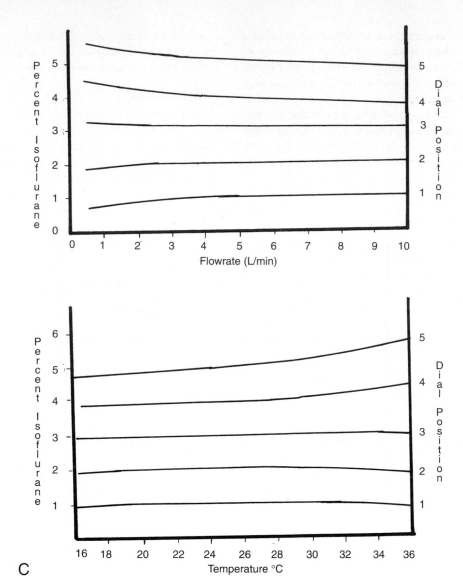

FIGURE **5.36.** *(continued)*

drained periodically and the liquid discarded to prevent buildup of thymol.

AGENT-SPECIFIC FILLING SYSTEMS

The ASTM machine standard (5) recommends, but does not require, that a vaporizer designed for a single agent be fitted with a permanently attached, agent-specific device (keyed or agent-specific filling system, filler system or devices, pin safety system) to prevent accidental filling with the wrong agent. Such a device is avail-

able on most modern vaporizers. In addition to preventing filling a vaporizer with a wrong agent, these systems may reduce the air pollution with agents associated with filling vaporizers (81, 82). They also help prevent water and other contaminants from entering the vaporizing chamber.

Components
Bottle Collar

Each bottle of liquid anesthetic has a special colored collar attached securely at the neck (Fig.

5.37). Each collar has two projections, one thicker than the other, which are designed to mate with corresponding indentations on the bottle adaptor. The colors for the commonly used agents are red for halothane, orange for enflurane, purple for isoflurane, and yellow for sevoflurane. These colors are also used on the bottle labels.

Bottle Adaptor

Bottle adaptors (adaptor tubes or assemblies, tube adaptors, filler tubes) are shown in Figures 5.38 and 5.39. They are color-coded. The adaptor shown in Figure 5.38 has at one end a bottle connector with a screw thread to match the thread on the bottle and a skirt that extends beyond the screw threads and has slots that match the projections on the bottle collar. At the other end is the male adaptor that fits into the vaporizer filler receptacle. A short length of plastic tubing with two inner tubes connects the ends. The tubing allows the bottle to be held higher or lower than the vaporizer.

Figure 5.39 shows a male adaptor (key, probe, tube block, filler plug, male adaptor). It consists of a rectangular piece of plastic with a groove on one side and two holes on another surface. The groove is designed to prevent the probe from

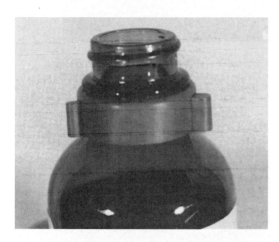

FIGURE 5.37. Bottle collar. The collar is color-coded according to the bottle contents. It has two projections (one thicker than the other), which are designed to mate with corresponding indentations on the bottle adaptor.

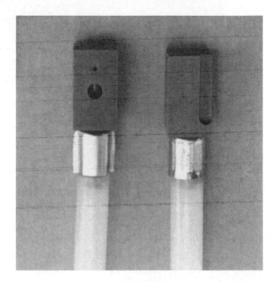

FIGURE 5.39. Male adaptor. The groove corresponds to a projection on the vaporizer filler receptacle. The larger hole is for the anesthetic agent, and the smaller hole is for air.

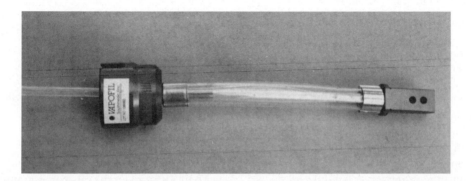

FIGURE 5.38. Bottle adaptor. The bottle connector is at left, and the male adaptor is at the right.

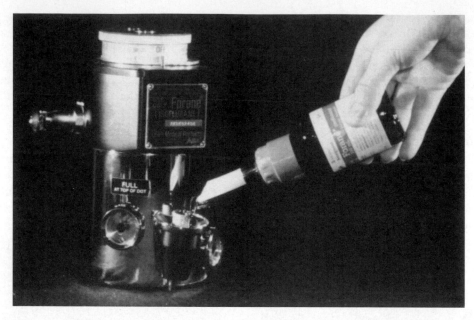

FIGURE 5.40. Bottle adaptor for vaporizers without agent-specific filling devices. It allows filling of a pour- fill vaporizer without excessive spillage. (Reprinted with permission from Southmedic, Inc.)

being placed in an incorrect vaporizer. The larger hole is for the agent to enter or leave the vaporizer, and the smaller hole is for air. There may be a ball valve to facilitate filling.

The adaptor shown in Figure 5.40 is for use with vaporizers without an agent-specific filling system. The bottle connector is the same. The other end has a beveled tip.

A funnel fill can be converted to an agent-specific filling using a commercially available adaptor (Fig. 5.41).

Filler Receptacle (83, 84)

The vaporizer filler receptacle (filler socket or block, vaporizer filler unit, fill and drain system) must permit insertion of only the intended bottle adaptor. There must be a means for tightening the male adaptor to form a seal after insertion. There must also be a means to seal the receptacle when the bottle adaptor is not inserted.

There may be a single port for both filling and draining or two ports (Figs. 5.42 and 5.43). A valve attached to a knob at the top controls the opening into the vaporizer. A ball valve in the air line occludes the air port after the vaporizer is

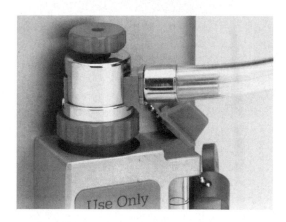

FIGURE 5.41. Adaptor to convert a funnel fill system to an agent-specific keyed filling system. (Reprinted with permission from Sharn Inc.)

filled. This prevents overfilling and flooding of the air line with liquid anesthetic.

Use
Filling

To fill a vaporizer, the cap from the appropriate bottle is removed and the bottle adaptor is screwed to the collar until tight. If the connection is not tight, the vaporizer may be overfilled or a leak may occur. The vaporizer must be turned off before proceeding further. The plug, if present, is removed. The filler block is then inserted with the groove matching that on the vaporizer receptacle. During insertion, the tube should be bent slightly so that the bottle is below the level of the inlet. After the filler block is inserted, the retaining screw is tightened and the fill valve (vent) opened. The bottle is then held higher than the filler receptacle so that liquid enters the vaporizer (Fig. 5.43, top). The air inside the vaporizer, which is displaced by the liquid, moves through the other tube and bubbles through the liquid in the bottle to the air space inside the bottle. Gentle up-and-

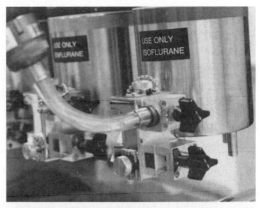

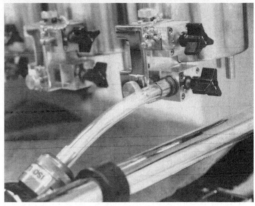

FIGURE **5.43.** Keyed filling device with one front screw and top vent. **Top,** Filling the vaporizer. To fill, the plug is removed, the filler block inserted, and the retaining screw tightened. The vent is opened, and the bottle is tipped upward. **Bottom,** Draining the vaporizer. The filler block is inserted into the drain receptacle, the retaining screw is tightened, and the drain is opened. The bottle is held below the vaporizer.

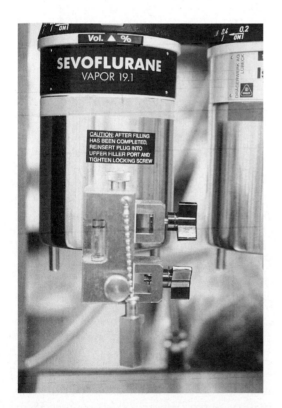

FIGURE **5.42.** Dual-port vaporizer filler receptacle. Note the plug to prevent leaks, the vent at the top, the drain valve at the bottom, and the two retaining screws at the right. A separate vent is not present on all filling receptacles. It must be loosened to fill the vaporizer. The vaporizer will leak if the plug is not reinserted and the screw is not tightened.

down motion may help to clear air bubbles and facilitate filling.

After the desired liquid level in the vaporizer has been reached, the valve on the top is closed, the bottle lowered, and the retaining screw loosened. The bottle adaptor is removed, and the plug, if present, reinserted and tightened in place.

Draining

To drain the vaporizer, the bottle adaptor is first attached to an appropriate bottle. In the dual port filler, the bottom socket is used. The filler plug is removed, the male adaptor inserted, and the retaining screw tightened. The bottle is held below the receptacle (Fig. 5.43, Bottom) and the drain (spool) valve opened. Fluid drains through one tube into the bottle and air moves upward from the bottle through the other tube. After the vaporizer is drained, the drain valve is closed, the retaining screw loosened, and the bottle adaptor removed. The filler plug should be reinserted and the retaining screw tightened.

Storage

Usually the bottle adaptor is removed and replaced with a cap between fillings. If the bottle adaptor is not removed, leakage is minimal (85). However, this may make storage difficult.

Problems With Agent-Specific Filling Devices

Difficulty in Filling

Causes of difficulty in filling include misalignment of the bottle adaptor in the filler receptacle, the adaptor not sealing at the bottle end, a leak in the bottle adaptor, and air bubbles (83).

Lost Bottle Adaptor

It is almost impossible to fill the vaporizer if the filler tube is lost.

Vaporizer Tipping

The filler receptacle on some vaporizers extends below the base of the vaporizer and will prevent the vaporizer from being set upright on a flat surface; therefore, it is necessary to set the vaporizer receptacle at the edge of the surface with the block extending over the edge or to place it on its side. A ring fitted to the base of the vaporizer that extends the base below the projection of the filler block (Fig. 5.11) will allow the vaporizer to be placed upright on a flat surface.

Failure of the Keyed System

One case has been reported in which the bead on the filler receptacle on the vaporizer was too small to prevent incorrect filling (86). In another case the bottle adaptor for one agent fit a bottle for another agent that did not have a collar (87). The bottle adaptor for the other agent will fit if the bottle collar for enflurane or halothane is upside down on the bottle (88–91).

Poor Drainage

Causes of difficulty in draining the vaporizer include the bottle adaptor being wrongly positioned and breakage of one of the inner tubes. Usually a new bottle adaptor will be needed to rectify these problems.

Liquid Leaks

Leakage of liquid can result from failure to tighten the retaining screw, failure to tighten the adaptor on the bottle, blockage of the fluid path inside the vaporizer, or leakage in a valve (83). The filler block can leak from the overfill vent at the beginning or end of the filling cycle. If the fill or drain valve is not closed, liquid can leak (92). Frequent flexing of the tube on the bottle adaptor can result in a leak, usually at the male adaptor (83).

Incomplete Emptying of Bottle

With some filling devices, as much as 27 ml of liquid agent may be left in the bottle after the vaporizer is filled (81, 93, 94). The residual liquid is greater with keyed filling systems than with funnel-fill devices (94).

Overfilling

Some practitioners turn the vaporizer on and loosen the bottle cap to speed filling. One of these maneuvers alone will not cause the vaporizer to overfill but both together will allow this to occur with Penlon PPV (81) and Tec 4 vaporizers (55). Problems in the manufacture of the screw threads of the bottle necks may result in leakage with overfilling (95).

LOCATION
Concentration-Calibrated Vaporizers
Between the Flowmeters and the Common Gas Outlet

Concentration-calibrated vaporizers must be mounted between the flowmeters and the common gas outlet. Vaporizers are mounted to the right of the flowmeter tubes on most machines.

Between the Common Gas Outlet and Breathing System

Locating the vaporizer between the common gas outlet and the breathing system is not recommended for several reasons. It is difficult to secure such a vaporizer properly. This arrangement invites disconnections (96). Some machines have a relief valve near the common gas outlet (see Chapter 4). This vents gas to atmosphere if a certain pressure is exceeded. If a vaporizer is inserted downstream of such a valve, the increased resistance to flow will cause an increase in pressure, especially with use of the oxygen flush. If the opening pressure of the relief valve is exceeded, there will be a decrease in flow (97).

Another potential problem is reversed connection. Because the vaporizers have slip-on connections, it is possible to connect the vaporizer so that the flow of carrier gas is opposite to normal. In most vaporizers this will result in an increase in output (48, 98, 99). With a vaporizer in this location use of the oxygen flush may cause a high concentration to be delivered following the flush (100). Finally, such an installation allows more than one vaporizer to be turned on at a time if they are mounted in a series.

In-System Vaporizers

Currently no vaporizers suitable for use in the breathing system are being manufactured in the United States. A number of these vaporizers are available in other parts of the world. Problems include resistance to flow and unpredictable output.

VAPORIZER MOUNTING SYSTEMS

Permanent Mounting

Permanent mounting means that it requires tools to remove or install a vaporizer on the anes-

thesia machine. If a vaporizer is removed and not replaced, a cap should be placed over the mounting device to prevent leaks (Fig. 5.44).

Advantages of this system are that vaporizers will not be dropped or otherwise abused. Leaks resulting from frequent removal or incorrect installation will be less likely. There are also disadvantages. Machines must have enough mounting locations to accommodate all the vaporizers likely to be needed. Any location that does not have an attached vaporizer will need to be protected to prevent gas leaks.

Detachable Mounting

Detachable mounting systems that allow the vaporizer to be moved by the user are available. The Selectatec system is the most widely used. It consists of a pair of port valves for each vaporizer position on the back bar (Fig. 5.45). A locking lever is on the back of each vaporizer behind the concentration control dial (Figs. 5.16, 5.19, and 5.45). Each vaporizer has a special mounting bracket that fits over the nipples. The weight of the vaporizer and an O-ring around each port valve create a seal between the mounting system and the vaporizer.

Before mounting a vaporizer, the control dial must be in the OFF position and any adjacent vaporizer must be turned off. The locking lever should be in the unlock position. The vaporizer is fitted onto the two port valves. The locking lever is pushed down then turned clockwise to the locked position. To remove a vaporizer, the control dial is turned OFF and the locking lever to

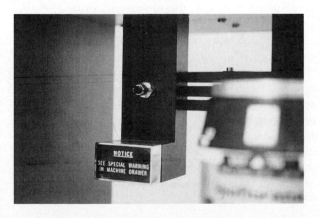

FIGURE 5.44. Mount without vaporizer attached. If a vaporizer is not in place, a special cap needs to be placed over the mounting to prevent leaks.

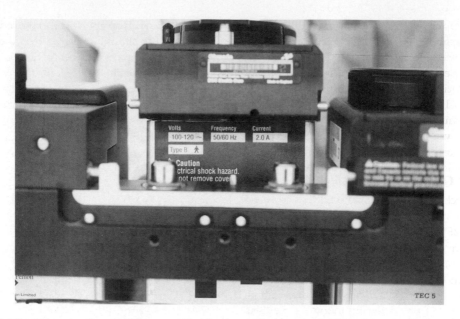

FIGURE **5.45.** Selectatec System. The vaporizer fits over these two valve ports on the back bar. Note the O-ring around each. After the vaporizer is mounted, the locking lever (barely visible at the top) is pushed down and turned to lock the vaporizer in place. When the vaporizer is turned on, the pins on either side are pushed outward. This pushes in pins on the adjacent vaporizers and prevents them from being turned on. The white bar causes interlocking of the outside vaporizers if there is no vaporizer in the center position. Early models of the Modulus II machine did not have this bar.

the unlock position. The vaporizer can then be lifted off the manifold.

When the vaporizer is turned on, two plungers within it open the valve ports in the back bar, connecting the vaporizer into the fresh gas stream. The plungers cause the vaporizer to be isolated from the fresh gas flow when it is turned off. Operation of the dial release also activates two extension rods that prevent operation of any other vaporizer installed on the manifold. On earlier models of the Selectatec system, interlocking was only possible if the vaporizers were mounted side-by-side. Newer versions allow interlocking between vaporizers that are not adjacent.

After a vaporizer has been added to a machine, several checks should be made to ensure proper positioning (101). These include sighting across the tops of the vaporizers to ensure that they are level and at the same height. An attempt should be made to lift each off the manifold without unlocking it. If the vaporizer can be removed, it is improperly positioned. It should be possible to

turn on only one vaporizer at a time. Finally, the anesthesia machine must be checked for leaks with each vaporizer in both the ON and OFF position as described in Chapter 26.

These systems have a number of advantages. The anesthesia machine can have fewer mounting locations. This allows a more compact unit. Vaporizers can be easily removed and replaced even during a case. If malignant hyperthermia is a potential problem, the vaporizers can be removed and the machine decontaminated by continuous flushing. This gives better results than if the vaporizer remains on the machine in the OFF position (102).

Leaks are a common problem in this system (103–109). A common cause is an absent or damaged O-ring (110–115). Another cause is leaving the locking lever in the unlocked position (116). If a Tec 3 vaporizer with a keyed filling system is placed to the left of a Tec 5 vaporizer, neither vaporizer may seat properly and a leak will occur (117).

Partial or complete obstruction to gas flow because of problems with the mounting system has been reported (118–120).

Several cases of failure to delivery anesthetic agent associated with this system have been reported (121–123). In another case a switch malfunction caused fresh gas flow to be directed to the wrong vaporizer (124). This resulted in a delivery of fresh gas with no vapor added.

INTERLOCK DEVICES

Interlock (vaporizer exclusion) systems prevent more than one vaporizer from being turned on at a time (125). The North American Drager interlock system is shown in Figures 5.46 and 5.47. If the screws are not properly adjusted, it may be possible to turn on two vaporizers at the same time (126, 127). Ohmeda interlock systems are shown in Figures 5.45 and 5.48.

Add-on interlock devices are available (128). Their use may require changes in the vaporizer as well as the machine. Failures of interlock devices have been reported (126, 129, 130). Diffusion of agent into the fresh gases is not prevented by an interlock device.

HAZARDS OF VAPORIZERS

Incorrect Agent

Contemporary concentration-calibrated vaporizers are all agent specific. A common hazard involves filling a vaporizer with an agent other than the one for which it was designed (86, 131, 132). One study found that incorrect agent in four of 710 vaporizers (133). None of the affected vaporizers were equipped with agent-specific filling systems.

If an agent of low potency or low volatility is placed in a vaporizer designed for an agent of higher potency or volatility, the output of the vaporizer will be lower (134–139). Conversely, if an agent of high potency or volatility is accidentally used in a vaporizer intended for an agent of low potency or volatility, a dangerously high concentration will be delivered. Filling a conventional vaporizer with desflurane will result is massively high outputs, and a hypoxic mixture will be produced at high settings even with 100% oxygen as the carrier gas (140, 141).

Some anesthetic agent monitors (see Chapter 18) will detect mixtures of agents. Smelling cannot be relied on to tell which agent is in a vaporizer because the smell of a small amount of one agent can completely mask the odor of a less-pungent agent, even if the second agent is present in much higher concentration (142). Anesthesia personnel can detect the presence of a volatile agent but are not able to identify an agent by smell (143).

If a vaporizer is filled with the wrong agent, it must be completely drained and all liquid discarded. Gas should be allowed to flow through it until no agent can be detected in the outflow. Draining cannot be relied on to completely empty a vaporizer (131).

Tipping

If some vaporizers are tipped sufficiently, liquid from the vaporizing chamber may get into the bypass or outlet. If this occurs, a high concentration of agent will be delivered when the vaporizer is again put into use. Vaporizers mounted securely upright on a gurney have been demonstrated to deliver the desired concentration despite motion (144).

Tipping can be prevented by mounting vaporizers securely and handling them with care when they are not mounted. Unless designed to be transported with liquid in the vaporizing chamber, a vaporizer should be drained before being moved.

Should tipping occur, a high flow of gas should be run through the vaporizer with the concentration dial set at a low concentration until the output shows no excessive agent.

Overfilling

If a vaporizer is overfilled, liquid agent may enter the fresh gas line and high concentrations delivered. On most vaporizers the filling port is situated so that overfilling cannot occur. Liquid will pour over the edge of the funnel before the level inside the vaporizer rises to a dangerous level.

Agent-specific filling devices prevent overfilling by connecting the air intake in the bottle to the inside of the vaporizer chamber. Many users of keyed filling devices have found that slightly unscrewing the bottle adaptor can speed the filling process. Turning the concentration dial of the vaporizer on during filling will accomplish the same

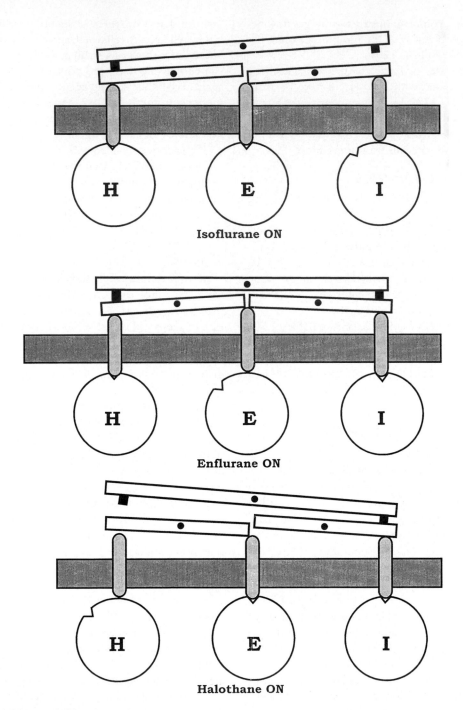

Isoflurane ON

Enflurane ON

Halothane ON

FIGURE 5.46. North American Drager interlock system. When the vaporizer of choice is turned on, a pin is forced into a notch on the concentration control knob of each of the other vaporizers. These vaporizers are then locked in the OFF position. (Adapted with permission from a drawing furnished by North American Drager, Inc, Telford, PA.)

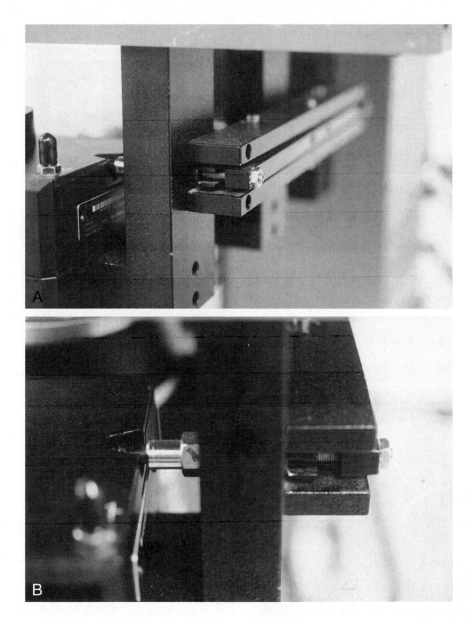

FIGURE 5.47. North American Drager interlock system. **A** shows the adjustment screw at the back. It is connected to the pin (**B**), which interlocks with the concentration control dial of the vaporizer.

end. Such practices should not be allowed because they can result in overfilling (55, 59, 80, 145).

Reversed Flow

Although the machine standard requires that the vaporizer inlet be male and the outlet female, the direction of gas flow be marked, and the inlet and outlet parts labeled (5), it is possible to con-

nect the fresh gas delivery line of the anesthesia machine to the outlet of the vaporizer and the delivery tube to the breathing system to the inlet side of the vaporizer, especially if the vaporizer is free-standing (146). This is easily overlooked. Reversed flow through a vaporizer has been reported after repairs to the selector valve resulted in a plumbing misconnection (148). With most vaporizers, the result of reversed flow will be an increase in output concentration (47, 98, 148).

Concentration Dial in Wrong Position

It is not unusual that previous use of a vaporizer by a colleague or servicing by a technician results in a vaporizer concentration dial's being left on (125, 149–153). For this reason, inspection of vaporizer control dials as well as contents should be part of the preuse checking procedure (see Chapter 26).

The concentration dial may be changed during a case without the operator's knowledge, especially if the vaporizer has the concentration dial at the top. Operating room personnel moving a machine or simply passing by may grab the dial and change the setting.

Leaks

With a leak in a vaporizer, the machine will function normally until the vaporizer is turned on.

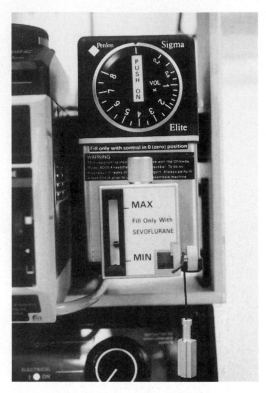

FIGURE **5.49.** Failure to replace the filler plug will result in a leak when the vaporizer is turned on.

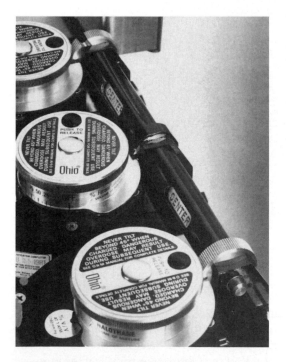

FIGURE **5.48.** Interlock device. The concentration dials on the left and right vaporizers cannot be turned on while the center one is in use. (Reprinted with permission from Ohmeda, a division of BOC Health Care, Inc.)

At that point, fresh gas flow from the machine will be reduced and may contain little or no vapor. The consequences will depend on the size of the leak, its location, and whether there is a check valve at the vaporizer outlet. In addition to affecting fresh gas composition and flow, leaks cause pollution of operating room air.

A common cause of a leak is failure to replace the filler cap or to tighten it adequately. This is usually detected by spillage of liquid anesthetic from the vaporizer when it is turned on (154, 155), but liquid may not be splattered if the level is low (156, 157). A leak will occur if the screw on the fill valve of a keyed filling system is not closed or the plug not replaced and tightened in place (Figs. 5.42 and 5.49) (92, 158). Another cause of a leak is a damaged O-ring around the drain screw shaft (159).

Other locations for leaks include the selector valve (160, 161), mounting mechanism (105, 107, 109, 112, 115–117, 162, 163), interlock device (164), outlet connection (165), and various parts of concentration-calibrated vaporizers (41). The fitting between a vaporizer and its inlet or outlet connection may become loose or broken (96, 166–168).

A leak should be suspected if a vaporizer appears to require filling with unusual frequency or when the odor of an agent can be detected. Splattering of liquid from the filling port may be observed if the cap is not tight. This may not be seen if a keyed filling device is in place and the filling screw is loose. Personnel who fill vaporizers should be instructed to always close filler caps (and screws) tightly. A leak in a vaporizer can be detected when the anesthesia machine is tested before use if the vaporizer is turned on (see Chapter 26).

Vapor Leak Into the Fresh Gas Line

Some vaporizers leak small amounts of vapor into the bypass when turned off (31, 32, 169). Interlock devices will not prevent this problem. A selector valve will not prevent it if there is still a diffusion pathway through the selector valve (32). The amount of such contamination depends on the ambient temperature (and hence the vapor pressure of the liquid) as well as the size and configuration of the internal ports. Although the amounts delivered are usually too small to produce a clinical effect, it might cause a sensitized individual to react to a halogenated agent or trigger an episode of malignant hyperthermia (170). These leaks can be reduced by not turning a vaporizer from the OFF to the 0 setting unless it is to be used.

A vaporizer may deliver vapor when turned off (33, 171). Cases have been reported in which a malfunction prevented a vaporizer from being turned off (172, 173) and in which it was possible to turn the concentration dial past the OFF position (35, 38). In this position, the vaporizer delivered concentrations high enough to produce clinical effects.

Contaminants in the Vaporizing Chamber

It is possible for various substances to be poured into a bottle that should contain anesthetic agent (174). Water and other foreign substances can cause corrosion (Fig. 5.50) and result in excessive carrier gas passing through the vaporizing chamber, causing a greater-than-expected output (175, 176). If these substances are known to have entered the vaporizing chamber,

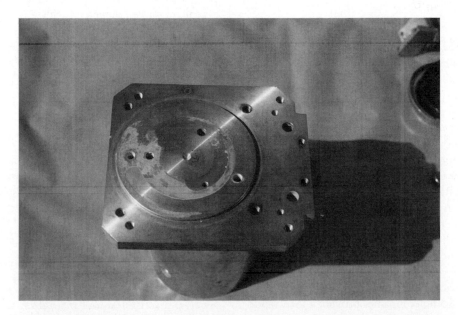

FIGURE 5.50. Corrosion in vaporizer caused by water and other foreign substances.

the manufacturer should be contacted to determine what measures need to be taken.

The output of a halothane vaporizer will be reduced as the concentration of thymol increases (177, 178). A 5% decrease in output will be caused by a 650% increase in thymol concentration.

Physical Damage

Shock, excessive vibration, or mistreatment may lead to malfunction (179, 180). Damage to vaporizers mounted on a machine is significantly less than with those that are disconnected (181). A sufficient number of vaporizers should be purchased so they do not need to be moved around. If a vaporizer must be removed, care should be taken to protect it from physical damage.

Obstruction to Fresh Gas Flow

Problems with mounting systems have caused partial or complete obstruction of the fresh gas flow from the machine (103, 104, 118, 119).

Interlock Malfunction

The interlock system that functions to prevent two vaporizers from being turned on at the same time may malfunction (65, 126, 182). The interlock mechanism should be included with the machine checkout.

PREVENTIVE MAINTENANCE

Vaporizers are precise instruments and require regular, skillful maintenance if they are to remain reliable and precise. Preventive maintenance is not the same as periodic calibration checks or routine use of an agent monitor (183). Preventive maintenance should be carried out by the manufacturer or its certified service agent. If an agent analyzer is in routine use, some manufacturers will lengthen the time between service and recalibration for certain vaporizers.

Because the number of facilities servicing vaporizers is limited, most vaporizers must be sent long distances. It is helpful to have at least one extra agent-specific vaporizer for each agent used so that servicing will result in a minimum of inconvenience. Some companies provide a loan vaporizer during servicing.

REFERENCES

1. White CD. Vaporization and vaporizers. Br J Anaesth 1985;57:658–671.
2. Macintosh R, Mushin WW, Epstein HG. Physics for the anaesthetist. Oxford, UK: Blackwell Scientific, 1963.
3. Eisenkraft JB. Vaporizers and vaporization of volatile anesthetics. Progress in Anesthesiology 1988;2:1–16.
4. Blackwood O, Kelly W. General physics. New York: Wiley, 1955.
5. American Society for Testing and Materials. Standard specification for minimum performance and safety requirements for components and systems of anesthesia gas machines (ASTM F1161-88) (Reapproved 1994). Philadelphia: ASTM, 1994.
6. Jones MJ. Breathing systems and vaporizers. In: Nimmo WS, Smith G, eds. Anaesthesia. Oxford, UK: Blackwell Scientific, 1989.
7. Leigh JM. Variations on a theme: splitting ratio. Anaesthesia 1985;40:70–72.
8. Schreiber P. Effects of barometric pressure on anesthesia equipment. Audio Digest 1975;17(14).
9. Schreiber P. Anesthesia equipment. Performance, classification, and safety. New York: Springer-Verlag, 1972.
10. Camporesi EM. Anesthesia at different environmental pressures. In: Ehrenwerth J, Eisenkraft JB, eds. Anesthesia equipment. Principles and applications. St. Louis, MO: Mosby, 1993.
11. James MFM, White JF. Anesthetic considerations at moderate altitude. Anesth Analg 1984;63:1097–1105.
12. Speer DL. Vaporization of anesthetic agents at high altitude. In: Aldrete JA, Lowe HJ, Virtue RW, eds. Low flow and closed system anesthesia. New York: Grune & Stratton, 1979:235–250.
13. Satterfield JM, Russell GB, Graybeal JM, et al. Anesthetic vaporizers accurately deliver isoflurane in hyperbaric conditions. Anesthesiology 1989;71:A360.
14. Hill DW, Lowe HJ. Comparison of concentration of halothane in closed and semiclosed circuits during controlled ventilation. Anesthesiology 1962;23:291–298.
15. Keet JE, Valentine GW, Riccio JS. An arrangement to prevent pressure effect on the Verni-Trol vaporizer. Anesthesiology 1963;24:734–737.
16. Cole JR. The use of ventilators and vaporizer performance. Br J Anaesth 1966;38:646–651.
17. Heneghan CPH. Vaporizer output and gas driven ventilators. Br J Anaesth 1986;58:932.
18. Slinger PD, Scott WAC, Kliffer AP. Intraoperative

awareness due to malfunction of a Siemens 900B ventilator. Can J Anaesth 1990;37:258–261.

19. Paterson GM, Hulands GH, Nunn JF. Evaluation of a new halothane vaporizer: the Cyprane Fluotec Mark 3. Br J Anaesth 1969;41:109–119.

20. Noble WH. Accuracy of halothane vaporizers in clinical use. Canadian Anaesthetists Society Journal 1970; 17:135–143.

21. Lin C. Assessment of vaporizer performance in low-flow and closed-circuit anesthesia. Anesth Analg 1980;59:359–366.

22. Prins L, Strupat J, Clement J, et al. An evaluation of gas density dependence of anaesthetic vaporizers. Canadian Anaesthetists Society Journal 1980;27: 106–110.

23. Steffey EP, Woliner M, Howland D. Evaluation of an isoflurane vaporizer: the Cyprane Fortec. Anesth Analg 1982;61:457–464.

24. Lin C. Enflurane vaporizer accuracy with nitrous oxide mixtures. Anesth Analg 1979;58:440–441.

25. Palayiwa E, Sanderson MH, Hahn CEW. Effects of carrier gas composition on the output of six anaesthetic vaporizers. Br J Anaesth 1983;55:1025–1038.

26. Stoelting RK, Nawaf K. Enflurane vaporizer accuracy with nitrous oxide mixtures. Anesth Analg 1979;58: 441.

27. Synnott A, Wren WS. Effect of nitrous oxide on the output of three halothane vaporizers. Br J Anaesth 1986;58:1055–1058.

28. Latto IP. Administration of halothane in the 0-0.5% concentration range with the Fluotec Mark 2 and Mark 3 vaporizers. Br J Anaesth 1973;45:563–569.

29. Nielsen J, Pedersen FM, Knudsen F, et al. Accuracy of 94 anaesthetic agent vaporizers in clinical use. Br J Anaesth 1993;71:453–457.

30. Graham SG, Szafranski J, Bland D, et al. The output of an 'empty' Tec 3 vaporizer. Anaesthesia 1995;50: 433–434.

31. Cook TL, Eger EI, Behl RS. Is your vaporizer off? Anesth Analg 1977;56:793–800.

32. Robinson JS, Thompson JM, Barratt RS. Inadvertent contamination of anaesthetic circuits with halothane. Br J Anaesth 1977;49:745–753.

33. Gill RS, Lack JA. Vaporizers—serviced and checked? Anaesthesia 1991;46:695–696.

34. Bridges RT. Vaporizers—serviced and checked? A reply. Anaesthesia 1991;46:696–697.

35. Davies JR. Enfluratec vaporizer. Br J Anaesth 1980; 52:356–357.

36. Davies JR. Broken control on a selectatec vaporizer. Anaesthesia 1987;42:215.

37. Bar ZG. Inadvertent administration of halothane with the Fluotec Mk. 3 vaporizer. Anaesth Intensive Care 1984;12:378.

38. Miller JM, Cascorbi HF. Yet another vaporizer hazard. Anesth Analg 1980;59:805.

39. Novack GD, Ursillo RC. Malfunctioning halothane vaporizer. Anesth Analg 1981;60:121.

40. Smith B. Broken control on Selectatec vaporizer. A reply. Anaesthesia 1987;42:215.

41. Rosenberg M, Solod E, Bourke DL. Gas leak through a Fluotec Mark III vaporizer. Anesth Analg 1979;58: 239–240.

42. Scott DM. Performance of BOC Ohmeda Tec 3 and Tec 4 vaporizers following tipping. Anaesth Intensive Care 1991;19:441–443.

43. Yemen TA, Nelson WW. Are vaporizers in motion safe? Anesth Analg 1992;74:S364.

44. Gill RS, Lack JA. Vaporizers—serviced and checked? Anaesthesia 1991;46:695–696.

45. Duncan JA. Equipment malfunction: possible hazard. Anaesthesia 1986;41:1271.

46. Koga Y, Urushiyama H, Saishu T. A potential defect in an Ohmeda Sevotec III vaporizer. Anesth Analg 1992;74:319.

47. Eisenkraft JB, Bradford C, Silverstein JH. Effect of reversed gas flow through a free-standing isoflurane concentration-calibrated (tec 3) vaporizer. Anesth Analg 1993;76:S91.

48. Eisenkraft JB, Abel M. Effect of gas flow reversal through anesthesia vaporizers. Anesthesiology 1994; 81:A575.

49. Fitzal S, Gilly H, Steinbereithner K. Do modern plenum vaporizers provide accurate anesthetic mixtures irrespective of gas flow? Anesthesiology 1986; 65:A168.

50. Gilly H, Fitzal S, Steinbereithner K. Low flow accuracy of vaporizers: a laboratory comparison between TEC and VAPOR systems. Eur J Anaesthesiol 1987; 4:73–74.

51. Rao CC, Krishna G, Baldwin S, et al. Ohmeda® Fluotec-4 vaporizer output near MRI magnet. Anesthesiology 1990;73:A476.

52. Loeb RG. The output of four modern vaporizers in the presence of helium. Can J Anaesth 1992;39: 888–891.

53. Morrison JE J, McDonald C, Oliver T. A halothane surge phenomenon during paediatric mask induction using the Tec 4 vaporizer in the Ohmeda Modulus II Plus anaesthesia system. Paediatric Anaesthesia 1992;2:111–114.

54. Goldman DB, Mushlin PS. Leakage of anesthetic agent from an Ohmeda Tech IV vaporizer. Anesth Analg 1991;72:567.

55. Palayiwa E, Hahn CEW. Overfill testing of anaesthetic vaporizers. Br J Anaesth 1995;74:100–103.

56. Carter KB, Gray WM, Railton R, et al. Long-term performance of Tec vaporizers. Anaesthesia 1988;43:1042–1046.

57. Loeb R, Santos B. Pumping effect in Ohmeda Tec 5 vaporizers. 1995;11:348.

58. Rajah A, Zideman DA. A problem with the Tec 5 vaporizer. Anaesthesia 1992;97:271–272.

59. Lloyd J. Filling Tec 5 vaporizers. Can J Anaesth 1995;42:839.

60. Uncles DR, Sibell DM, Conway NE. Desflurane and the Tec 6 filler system. Anaesthesia 1994;49:547–548.

61. Joyce TH, Younker D, Pai UT, et al. Clinical evaluation of the accuracy of Tec 6 vaporizer for desflurane. Anesth Analg 1993;76:S174.

62. Weiskopf RB, Sampson D, Moore MA. The desflurane (Tec 6) vaporizer: design, design considerations and performance evaluation. Br J Anaesth 1994;72:474–479.

63. Johnston RV, Andrews J, Deyo DJ, et al. The effects of carrier gas composition on the performance of the Tec 6 desflurane vaporizer. Anesth Analg 1994;79:548–552.

64. Goodman EJ, Cotman FL, Hudson IM, et al. Desflurane vaporizer uses minimal electricity. Anesth Analg 1997;84:S38.

65. Abdi S, Acquadro MA. Technical failure of desflurane vaporizer Tec-6. Anesthesiology 1995;83:226–227.

66. Farmer GM, Zelman V. Tec 6 power cord problem. Anesthesiology 1995;82:1300.

67. Lockey D, Purcell-Jones G. A problem with a desflurane vaporizer. Anaesthesia 1995;50:574.

68. Anonymous. Anesthesia units. Health Devices 1980;10:31–51.

69. Gould DB, Lampert BA, MacKrell TN. Effect of nitrous oxide solubility on vaporizer aberrance. Anesth Analg 1982;61:938–940.

70. Knill R, Prins L, Strupat J, et al. Nitrous oxide and vaporizer outputs: transient or continuous effect? Anesth Analg 1980;59:808–809.

71. Gandolfi AJ, Blitt CD, Weldon S. Discoloration and impurities in isoflurane vaporizer. Anesth Analg 1983;62:366.

72. Wald A. Discoloration of enflurane. Anesth Analg 1981;60:843.

73. Gandolfi AJ, Weldon ST, Blitt CD. Production and characterization of impurities in isoflurane vaporizers. Anesthesiology 1983;59:A159.

74. Blitt CD, Weldon ST, Willians-Van Alstyne SI, et al. Survey of impurities in isoflurane and enflurane vaporizers. Anesth Analg 1984;63:189.

75. Weldon ST, Williams-Van Alstyne SI, Gandolfi AJ, et al. Production and characterization of impurities in isoflurane vaporizers. Anesth Analg 1985;64:634–639.

76. Cicman JH, Skibo VE, Yoder JM. Anesthesia systems. Part II: Operating principles of fundamental components. J Clin Monit 1992;8:295–307.

77. Loeb RG. Anesthesia systems. J Clin Monit 1994;10:68–70.

78. Petty WC. New anesthetic requires new vaporizers for safety. J Clin Monit 1996;12:483.

79. Garden AL, Haberkern CM, Buckon ME, et al. Output from a Drager Vapor 19.1 on a moving trolley. Can J Anaesth 1997;44:227–230.

80. Sinclair A, Van Bergen J. Vaporizer overfilling. Can J Anaesth 1993;40:77–78.

81. Wittmann PH, Wittmann FW, Connor J, et al. A new keyed vaporizer filler. Anaesthesia 1994;49:710–712.

82. Anaesthetic vaporizers—agent-specific filling systems. Geneva: International Standards Organization.

83. Richardson W, Carter KB. Evaluation of keyed fillers on TEC vaporizers. Br J Anaesth 1986;58:353–356.

84. O'Carroll TM, Greenbaum R, Thornton PGN. Agent-specific filling devices. Anaesthesia 1980;35:807–810.

85. Davies JM, Strunin L, Craig DB. Leakage of volatile anaesthetics from agent-specific vapourizer filling devices. Canadian Anaesthetists Society Journal 1982;29:473–476.

86. McBurney R. Letter to the editor. Canadian Anaesthetists Society Journal 1977;24:417–418.

87. Klein SL, Camenzind T. Hazards of bottle adaptors for vaporizers. Anesth Analg 1978;57:596–597.

88. Dickson JJ. Enflurane key filling system. Anaesth Intensive Care 1985;13:331.

89. George TH. Failure of keyed agent-specific filling devices. Anesthesiology 1984;61:228–229.

90. Mar J. A dangerous error in fluothane packaging. Can Med Assoc J 1980;122:990.

91. Riegle EV, Desertspring D. Failure of the agent-specific filling device. Anesthesiology 1990;73:353.

92. Urmey WF, Elliott W, Raemer DB. Vaporizer fill system leak. Anesth Analg 1988;67:711.

93. Wittmann PH, Wittmann FW, Connor T, et al. The "nonempty" empty bottle. Anaesthesia 1992;47:721–722.

94. Uncles DR. A comparison of keyed and non-keyed vaporizer filling modes and volatile agent wastage. Anaesthesia 1993;48:795–798.

95. Anonymous. Safety alert: anesthetic bottle & metal filler incompatibility. Biomedical Safety & Standards 1992;22:37.

96. Capan L, Ramanathan S, Chalon J, et al. A possible hazard with use of the Ohio ethrane vaporizer. Anesth Analg 1980;59:65-68.

97. Kataria B, Price P, Slack M. Delayed filling of the breathing bag due to a portable vaporizer. Anesth Analg 1987;66:1055.

98. Marks WE, Bullard JR. Another hazard of free-standing vaporizers, increased anesthetic concentration with reversed flow of vaporizing gas. Anesthesiology 1976;45:445-446.

99. Rosewarne FA, Duncan IN. Reversed connexions of free-standing vaporizers. Anaesthesia 1990;45:338-339.

100. Kelly DA. Free-standing vaporizers. Another hazard. Anaesthesia 1985;40:661-663.

101. Riddle RT. A potential cause (and cure) of a major gas leak. A reply. Anesthesiology 1985;62:842-843.

102. Ritchie PA, Cheshire MA, Pearce NH. Decontamination of halothane from anaesthetic machines achieved by continuous flushing with oxygen. Br J Anaesth 1988;60:859-863.

103. Childres WF. Malfunction of Ohio Modulus anesthesia machine. Anesthesiology 1982;56:330.

104. Jove F, Milliken RA. Loss of anesthetic gases due to defective safety equipment. Anesth Analg 1983;62:369-370.

105. Jablonski J, Reynolds AC. A potential cause (and cure) of a major gas leak. Anesthesiology 1985;62:842.

106. Pyles ST, Kaplan RF, Munson E. Gas loss from Ohio Modulus vaporizer selector-interlock valve. Anesth Analg 1983;62:1052.

107. Powell JF, Morgan C. Selectatec gas leak. Anaesth Intensive Care 1993;21:892-893.

108. Hartle AJ, Daum REO. Failure of Ohmeda Tec 4 safety interlock. Anaesthesia 1992;47:171.

109. Loughnan TE. Gas leak associated with a Selectatec. Anaesth Intensive Care 1988;16:501.

110. Wraight WJ. Another failure of Selectatec block. Anaesthesia 1990;45:795.

111. James RH. Defective Selectatec O-rings. Anaesthesia 1995;50:184-185.

112. Nott MR, Jacklin F. Missing O-rings and volatile agents. Anaesthesia 1995;50:1001-1002.

113. Tighe SQM, Jones DA. Anaesthetic machine checks during anaesthesia. Anaesthesia 1993;48:88.

114. Pandit JJ, Jakubowski P, Wait CM. Broken O-ring causing hypoventilation. Anaesthesia 1993;48:1114-1115.

115. Berry PD, Ross DG. Missing O-ring causes unrecognized large gas leak. Anaesthesia 1992;47:359.

116. Hung CT, Chieng CF. The Selectatec system: another cause of total leakage. Anaesth Intensive Care 1992;20:532-533.

117. Moore C, Harmon P. More problems with the Selectatec system. Anaesthesia 1993;48:635-636.

118. Riendl J. Hypoxic gas mixture delivery due to malfunctioning inlet port of a Select-a-tec vaporizer manifold. Can J Anaesth 1987;34:431-432.

119. Hogan TS. Selectatec switch malfunction. Anaesthesia 1985;40:66-69.

120. Goddard JM, Abbott TR. Selectatec system: misplaced blood. Anaesthesia 1986;41:439.

121. Duncan JAT. Selectatec switch malfunction. Anaesthesia 1985;40:911-912.

122. Lum ME, Ngan Kee WD, Robinson BJ. Fault in a Selectatec manifold resulting in awareness. Anaesth Intensive Care 1992;20:501-503.

123. Beards SC. Misuse of a Bodok seal. Anaesthesia 1993;48:175-176.

124. Cudmore J, Keogh J. Another Selectatec switch malfunction. Anaesthesia 1990;45:754-756.

125. Petty C. Equipment safety: Vaporizer exclusion or interlock systems. APSF Newslett 1992;7:10.

126. Silvasi DL, Haynes A, Brown ACD. Potentially lethal failure of the vapor exclusion system. Anesthesiology 1989;71:289-291.

127. Viney JP, Gartrell AD. Incorrectly adjusted vaporizer exclusion system. Anesthesiology 1994;81:781.

128. Browne RA, McDonald S. A vapourizer interlocking system. Canadian Anaesthetists Society Journal 1983;30:653-654.

129. Anonymous. Improper setting of anesthesia vaporizer interlock system leads to safety alert. Biomedical Safety & Standards 1990;20:91.

130. Anonymous. Anesthesia unit vaporizers. Technology for Anesthesia 1989;9:4.

131. Karis JH, Menzel DB. Inadvertent change of volatile anesthetics in anesthesia machines. Anesth Analg 1992;61:53-55.

132. Martin ST. Hazards of agent-specific vaporizers: a case report of successful resuscitation after massive isoflurane overdose. Anesthesiology 1992;62:830-883.

133. Popic PM, Jameson LC, Arndt GA. Preliminary results on the incidence of vaporizer contamination in selected U. S. Hospitals. Anesthesiology 1991;75:A902.

134. Deriaz H, Baras E, Duranteau R, et al. Can isoflurane be administered with an halothane vaporizer? Anesthesiology 1989;71:A362.

135. Shih A, Wu W. Potential hazard in using halothane-

specific vaporizers for isoflurane and vice versa. Anesthesiology 1981;55:A115.

136. Eisenkraft JB, Abel M. Performance of a calibrated enflurane vaporizer when filled with sevoflurane. Anesthesiology 1994;81:A572.

137. Sosis M, Braverman B. Determination of the output of mixtures of isoflurane and halothane from a calibrated enflurane vaporizer. Anesthesiology 1991;75: A499.

138. Sosis MB, Braverman B. Determination of the output of an enflurane vaporizer filled with known mixtures of enflurane and halothane. Can J Anaesth 1995;42: A14.

139. Abel M, Eisenkraft JB. Performance of erroneously filled sevoflurane, enflurane and other agent-specific vaporizers. J Clin Monit 1996;12:119–125.

140. Andrews JJ, Johnston RV Jr, Kramer GC. Consequences of misfilling contemporary vaporizers with desflurane. Can J Anaesth 1993;40:71–76.

141. Andrews JJ, Deyo DJ, Johnston RV Jr, et al. Consequences of misfilling isoflurane vaporizers with desflurane. Anesth Analg 1994;78:S7.

142. Paull JD, Sleeman KW. An anaesthetic hazard. Br J Anaesth 1971;3:1202.

143. Roberts SL, Forbes RB, Moyers JR, et al. Can olfaction identify and quantify volatile anesthetics? Anesthesiology 1985;63:A193.

144. Yemen TA, Nelson WW. Are vaporizers in motion safe? Anesth Analg 1992;74:S364.

145. Hardy JF. Vaporizer overfilling. Can J Anaesth 1993; 40:1–2.

146. Anonymous. Death from misconnected vaporizer leads to $750,000 settlement. Biomedical Safety & Standards 1992;22:78.

147. Reference deleted

148. Railton R, Inglis MD. High halothane concentrations from reversed flow in a vaporizer. Anaesthesia 1986;41:672–673.

149. Austin TR. A warning device for the "Fluotec" Mark II and III. Anaesthesia 1971;26:368.

150. Coleshill GG. Safe vaporizers. Can J Anaesth 1988; 35:667–668.

151. Petty C. Equipment safety: Vaporizer exclusion or interlock systems. APSF Newslett 1992;7:10.

152. Williams L, Barton C, McVey JR, et al. A visual warning device for improved safety. Anesth Analg 1986; 65:1364.

153. Ludbrook GL, Webb RK, Fox MA, et al. Problems before induction of anaesthesia: an analysis of 2000 incident reports. Anaesth Intensive Care 1993;21: 593–595.

154. Rajah A, Zideman DA. A problem with the TEC 5 vaporizer. Anaesthesia 1992;47:271–272.

155. Bridges R. A problem with a TEC 5 vaporizer. A reply. Anaesthesia 1992;47:272.

156. Cooper PD. A hazard with a vaporizer. Anaesthesia 1984;39:935.

157. Mullin RA. Letter to the editor. Canadian Anaesthetists Society Journal 1978;25:248–249.

158. Meister GC, Becker KE. Potential fresh gas flow leak through Dräger Vapor 19.1 vaporizer with key-index fill port. Anesthesiology 1993;78:211–212.

159. Anonymous. Anesthesia unit vaporizers. Technology for Anesthesia 1987;7:4.

160. Anonymous. Ohmeda targets June 1 to complete FDA class II recall of vaporizer selector valves. Biomedical Safety & Standards 1985;15:50–51.

161. Loughnan TE. Gas leak associated with a Selectatec. Anaesth Intensive Care 1988;16:501.

162. Anonymous. Anesthesia unit vaporizers. Technology for Anesthesia 1991;12:6–7.

163. Tighe SQM. Defective Selectatex O-rings. Anaesthesia 1995;50:668.

164. Hartle AJ, Daum REO. Failure of Ohmeda Tec 4 safety interlock. Anaesthesia 1992;47:171.

165. Van Besouw JP, Thurlow AC. A hazard of free-standing vaporizers. Anaesthesia 1987;42:671.

166. Anonymous. Anesthesia unit vaporizers. Technology for Anesthesia 1991;12:7.

167. Forrest T, Childs D. An unusual vaporiser leak. Anaesthesia 1992;37:1220–1221.

168. Marsh RHK, Thomas NF. A hazard of the Penlon off-line vaporizer mounting system. Anaesthesia 1986;41:438.

169. Ritchie PA, Cheshire MA, Pearce NH. Decontamination of halothane from anaesthetic machines achieved by continuous flushing with oxygen. Br J Anaesth 1988;60:859–863.

170. Varma RR, Whitsell RC, Iskandarani MM. Halothane hepatitis without halothane: role of inapparent circuit contamination and its prevention. Hepatology 1985;5:1159–1162.

171. Webb RK, Russell WJ, Klepper I, et al. Equipment failure: an analysis of 2000 incident reports. Anaesth Intensive Care 1993;21:673–677.

172. Bahl CP. A cause of inaccuracy in vaporizer delivery. Anaesthesia 1977;32:1037.

173. Lewis JJ, Hicks RG. Malfunction of vaporizers. Anesthesiology 1966;27:324–325.

174. Lippmann M, Foran W, Ginsburg R, et al. Contamination of anesthetic vaporizer contents. Anesthesiology 1993;78:1175–1177.

175. Anonymous. Water in halothane vaporizers. Technology for Anesthesia 1985;5:2–3.

176. Anonymous. Vaporizer, anesthesia, nonheated. Biomedical Safety & Standards 1986;16:18.

177. Gray WM. Dependence of the output of a halothane

vaporizer on thymol concentration. Anaesthesia 1988;43:1047–1049.

178. Rosenberg PH, Alila A. Accumulation of thymol in halothane vaporizers. Anaesthesia 1984;38: 581–583.

179. Anonymous. FDA class I recall of pre-1980 Ohmeda vaporizers "overhalf done": involves testing, possible component replacement. Biomedical Safety & Standards 1985;15:50.

180. Green M, Bugg N, Holt P. Failed inhalational induc-

tion—a faulty vaporizer. Anaesthesia 1995;50: 85–86.

181. Anonymous. Concentration calibrated vaporizers. Technology for Anesthesia 1987;7:2.

182. Anonymous. Improper setting of anesthesia vaporizer interlock system leads to safety alert. Biomedical Safety & Standards 1990;20:91.

183. Huffman LM. Calibrated vaporizers: maintaining clinical performance. J Am Assoc Nurse Anesth 1990; 58:119–120.

QUESTIONS

Each question below contains four suggested answers of which one or more is correct. Choose the answer:

A if 1, 2, and 3 are correct
B if 1 and 3 are correct
C if 2 and 4 are correct
D if 4 is correct
E if 1, 2, 3, and 4 are correct

1. A shift to the vapor phase will be caused by
   1. Heating the vaporizer
   2. Cooling the room
   3. Increasing the flow through the vaporizer
   4. Decreasing atmospheric pressure

2. Which statements concerning boiling point are true?
   1. Boiling point is independent of the atmospheric pressure
   2. Boiling points for commonly used volatile anesthetic agents vary between 48.5 and 58.5° C at 760 torr
   3. Boiling points are determined at normal atmospheric pressure
   4. Atmospheric pressure and the vapor pressure of an agent are equal at the boiling point

3. The concentration of a volatile anesthetic may be expressed as
   1. Volumes percent
   2. The number of units of the vapor in relation to a total of 100 units
   3. The partial pressure
   4. The pressure of the vapor in relationship to the total pressure exerted by all of the gases in the sample

4. Which of the following accurately reflects the heat of vaporization?
   1. It is the amount of heat given off in the process of converting a liquid into a vapor
   2. The temperature of the liquid increases as vaporization proceeds

3. The greater the flow, the higher the temperature of the liquid will become
4. It is expressed as calories per gram

5. Which of the following accurately reflect specific heat?
   1. It is the amount of heat needed to raise the temperature of a substance 1° F
   2. The higher the specific heat, the more heat that is required to raise the temperature of a quantity of a substance
   3. It is the heat required to raise 1 milliliter of a substance 1° F
   4. High specific heat substances are preferred when choosing the material from which to construct a vaporizer

6. Most concentration-calibrated vaporizers
   1. Receive a flow from a dedicated flowmeter
   2. Are calibrated using air as the carrier gas
   3. Have a dial that is turned clockwise to increase the concentration
   4. Are calibrated in volumes percent

7. Methods used by vaporizers to gasify agents include
   1. Bubble through
   2. Flow over
   3. Injection into a vaporizing chamber
   4. Injection into the breathing system

8. Thermal compensation in a vaporizer is accomplished by
   1. Warming the room
   2. Supplying heat to the vaporizer
   3. Using glass in the vaporizing chamber to conduct heat
   4. Altering the flow through the vaporizing chamber

9. Which statements accurately reflect the effects of altered barometric pressure on vaporizer output?
   1. Agents with high boiling points are less susceptible to changes in barometric pressure than those with low boiling points
   2. As atmospheric pressure decreases, the

output measured in partial pressure will increase

3. As atmospheric pressure increases, the output as measured in volumes percent decreases

4. Increases in atmospheric pressure alters the viscosity of agents in vaporizers

10. How do changes in back pressure affect the output of a vaporizer?
    1. The pumping effect will increase vaporizer output
    2. A check valve at the machine outlet is not an effective solution to the pumping effect
    3. The pressurizing effect will decrease vaporizer output
    4. The pumping effect is greater with low fresh gas flows, large pressure fluctuations, and low vaporizer settings

11. Possible locations for the vaporizer on the anesthesia machine include
    1. Between the check valve and the common gas outlet
    2. Between the common gas outlet and the breathing system
    3. Between the oxygen flush and the breathing system
    4. Between the flowmeters and the machine outlet

ANSWERS

1.	B	7.	A
2.	D	8.	C
3.	E	9.	B
4.	D	10.	E
5.	C	11.	D
6.	D		

The Breathing System: General Principles, Common Components, and Classifications

THE BREATHING SYSTEM (breathing or patient circuit, respiratory circuit or system) is a gas pathway in direct connection with the patient, through which gas flows occur at respiratory pressures, and into which a gas mixture of controlled composition may be dispensed (1). The breathing system serves to deliver the gas mixture from the anesthesia machine to the patient, to remove carbon dioxide, to exclude air, and to condition temperature and humidity (2). The breathing system converts a continuous flow from the anesthesia machine to an intermittent flow; facilitates controlled or assisted respiration; and provides for such other functions as gas sampling and airway pressure, flow, and volume measurements (2). In practice, the breathing system is usually regarded as extending from the point of fresh gas inlet to the point at which gas escapes to atmosphere or a scavenging system. Scavenging equipment is not considered part of the breathing system.

GENERAL PRINCIPLES
Resistance (3)
Physics

When gas passes through a tube, the pressure at the outlet will be lower than that at the inlet. The drop in pressure is a measure of the resistance that must be overcome as gas moves through the tube. Resistance varies with the volume of gas passing through per unit of time. Therefore, flow rate must be stated when a specific resistance is mentioned. The nature of the flow is important in determining resistance. There are two types of flow: laminar and turbulent. In clinical practice, flow is usually a mixture of the two.

Laminar Flow

Figure 6.1 A shows a laminar flow of gas through a tube. The flow is smooth and orderly, and particles move parallel to the walls of the tube. Flow is fastest in the center of the tube where there is less friction. When flow is laminar, the Hagen-Poiseuille law applies. This law states that

$$\Delta P = (L \times v \times V)/r^4$$

where r is the radius of the tube, P is the pressure gradient across the tube, v is the viscosity of the gas, and V is the flow rate. Resistance is directly proportional to flow rate with laminar flow.

Turbulent Flow

Figure 6.1B shows a turbulent flow of gas through a tube. The lines of flow are no longer parallel. Eddies, composed of particles moving across or opposite the general direction of flow, are present. The flow rate is the same across the diameter of the tube. For turbulent flow, the factors responsible for the pressure drop along the tube include those described for laminar flow and also gas density, which becomes more important than viscosity.

$$\Delta P = (L \times V^2 \times K)/r^5$$

where K is a constant, including such factors as gravity, friction, gas density, and viscosity. Resistance is proportional to the "square" of the flow rate with turbulent flow. Turbulent flow can be generalized or localized.

Generalized turbulent flow. Generalized turbulent flow results when the flow of gas through a tube exceeds a certain value called "the critical flow rate."

Localized turbulent flow. As seen in Figure 6.1C to F, when gas flow is below the critical flow rate but encounters constrictions, curves, valves, or other irregularities, an area of localized turbulence results. The increase in resistance will depend on the type and number of obstructions encountered. To minimize resistance, gas-conducting pathways should be of minimal length, maximal internal diameter, and without sharp bends or sudden variations in diameter.

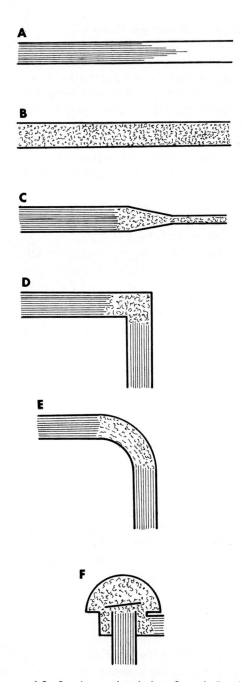

FIGURE 6.1. Laminar and turbulent flow. **A,** Laminar flow; the lines of flow are parallel and flow is slower near the sides of the tube because of friction. **B,** Generalized turbulent flow, which occurs when the critical flow rate is exceeded. Eddies move across or opposite the general direction of flow. **C** to **F,** Localized turbulence, which occurs when there is change in direction or the gas passes through a constriction

Significance of Resistance

Resistance imposes a strain on the patient, especially with ventilatory modes where the patient must do part or all of the respiratory work (e.g., intermittent mandatory ventilation or triggering mechanisms in ventilators). Changes in resistance tend to parallel changes in the work of breathing (4). The tracheal tube is usually the source of more resistance and a more important factor in determining the work of breathing than the breathing system (5). There is lack of agreement about what level of resistance is excessive (6, 7). Anesthesia personnel should be aware of how much resistance components of breathing systems offer and should attempt to employ, wherever possible, components offering the least resistance. For some patients, increased expiratory resistance may be desirable. It is suggested that this be achieved by using devices designed for this purpose.

Rebreathing

Rebreathing means to inhale previously respired gases from which carbon dioxide may have been removed. There is a tendency to associate the word rebreathing with carbon dioxide accumulation. This is unfortunate because, although it is true that rebreathing can result in higher inspired carbon dioxide concentrations than normal, it is possible to have partial or total rebreathing without an increase in carbon dioxide. Total prevention of rebreathing is not always desirable.

Factors Influencing Rebreathing

The amount of rebreathing will depend on the fresh gas flow, the mechanical dead space, and the design of the breathing system.

Fresh Gas Flow

The amount of rebreathing varies inversely with the total fresh gas flow. If the volume of fresh gas supplied per minute is equal to or greater than the patient's minute volume, there will be no rebreathing as long as provision is made for unimpeded expiration to atmosphere or a scavenging system at a point close to the patient's respiratory tract (7). If the total volume of gas supplied per minute is less than the minute volume, some exhaled gases must be rebreathed to make up the required volume (assuming no air dilution).

Mechanical (Apparatus) Dead Space

The mechanical dead space is the space in a breathing system occupied by gases that are rebreathed without any change in composition. The minimum volume of gas that can be rebreathed is equal to the volume of the mechanical dead space. An increase in dead space increases rebreathing. Apparatus dead space may be minimized by separating the inspiratory and expiratory gas streams as close to the patient as possible. The mechanical dead space should be distinguished from the physiologic dead space, which includes

1) anatomic dead space, consisting of the conducting airway of the patient down to the alveoli, and

2) alveolar dead space, which is the volume of alveoli ventilated but not perfused.

The composition of gas in the mechanical dead space will vary according to whether it is occupied by anatomic dead space gas, alveolar gas, or mixed expired gas. Gas exhaled from the anatomic dead space has a composition similar to inspired gas but is saturated with water vapor and warmer. Alveolar gas is saturated with water vapor at body temperature and has less oxygen and more carbon dioxide than inspired gas. The concentration of anesthetic agent in alveolar gas will differ from that in the inspired gas. Mixed expired gas will have a composition intermediate between that of anatomical dead space and alveolar gas.

Design of the Breathing System

In addition to the above factors, the various components of a breathing system may be arranged so that there is more or less rebreathing. This will be discussed more fully under the individual systems.

Backlash

During spontaneous ventilation, breathing tubes tend to collapse on inspiration and bulge on exhalation. This is referred to as "backlash" and may cause some rebreathing.

Effects of Rebreathing

With no rebreathing, the composition of inspired gas is identical to that of the fresh gas delivered by the anesthesia machine. With rebreathing, the inspired gas is composed partly of fresh gas and partly of rebreathed gas.

Retention of Heat and Water

Fresh gas from the anesthesia machine is anhydrous and at room temperature. Exhaled gases are warm and saturated with water. Hence rebreathing reduces heat and water loss from the patient. In most breathing systems, heat is rapidly lost to atmosphere and gas that is reinhaled has a lower temperature and water content than exhaled gas (8).

Alteration of Inspired Gas Tensions

The effects of rebreathing on inspired gas tensions will depend on what parts of the exhaled gases are reinhaled and whether these pass to the alveoli (and so influence gas exchange) or only to the anatomical dead space.

Oxygen. Rebreathing of alveolar gas will cause a decrease in the inspired oxygen tension because of patient uptake of oxygen and the addition of nitrogen, carbon dioxide, and water vapor to the gas.

Inhaled anesthetic agents. Rebreathing of alveolar gas exerts a "cushioning" effect on changes in inspired gas composition with alterations in fresh gas composition. During induction, when alveolar tensions are lower than those in the fresh gas flow, rebreathing of alveolar gas will reduce the inspired tension and prolong induction. During recovery, the alveolar tension exceeds that of the inspired gases and rebreathing slows the elimination of anesthetic agents.

Carbon dioxide. Rebreathing of alveolar gas will cause an increase in inspired carbon dioxide tension unless the gas passes through an absorbent before being rebreathed. Because carbon dioxide is concentrated in the alveolar portion of expired gases, the efficiency with which it is eliminated from a breathing system varies. If the system is designed so that alveolar gas is preferentially eliminated through the adjustable pressure limiting (APL) valve, carbon dioxide retention will be minimal, even with a low fresh gas flow. Breathing systems that do not maintain the separation between fresh gas, dead-space gas, and alveolar gas require high fresh gas flows to eliminate carbon dioxide.

Carbon dioxide retention is generally considered undesirable with spontaneous respiration. Although the patient can compensate by increasing minute volume, a price must be paid in terms of increased work of breathing, and in some cases the compensation may not be adequate. During controlled ventilation, some CO_2 in inhaled gases may be advantageous. Rebreathing will allow normocarbia to be achieved despite hyperventilation (9). Thus hypocarbia is avoided and heat and moisture are retained while the lungs are kept well expanded by large tidal volumes.

Discrepancy Between Inspired and Delivered Volumes

The volume of gas discharged by a ventilator or reservoir bag usually differs from that which enters the patient during inspiration. The volume actually inspired may be less or greater than that delivered.

Causes of Increased Inspired Volume

When an anesthesia ventilator is in use and the fresh gas flow rate is more than the rate at which it is absorbed by the patient or lost through leaks in the breathing system, the fresh gas flow delivered during inspiration is added to the tidal volume delivered by the ventilator (10–12). This augmentation increases with higher fresh gas flows and I:E ratios and lower respiratory rates (10, 13).

Causes of Decreased Inspired Volume

A reduction in tidal volume will result from compression of gases and distention of the components of the breathing system (14, 15). This is referred to as "wasted ventilation" because it results in less volume entering the patient than leaves the ventilator or reservoir bag. Wasted ventilation increases with increases in airway pressure and the volume and distensibility of components of the breathing system (14, 16–19). Proportionally more of the set tidal volume is lost with small patients (14, 20).

Tidal volume is also decreased by leaks in the breathing system. The amount lost will depend on the size and location of the leaks and the pressures during inspiration and expiration. Tidal volumes are most accurately measured between the patient and the breathing system (see Chapter 19). Measuring tidal volume at the end of the expiratory limb will reflect increases caused by fresh gas flow and decreases resulting from leaks but will miss

decreases from compression of gases and distention of components (15).

Discrepancy Between Inspired and Delivered Concentrations

The composition of the gas mixture that exits the machine may be modified by the breathing system so that the mixture the patient inspires differs considerably from that delivered to the system. There are several contributing factors.

Rebreathing

The effect of rebreathing will depend on the volume of the rebreathed gas and its composition. This will depend on the factors discussed previously.

Air Dilution

If the fresh gas supplied per respiration is less than the tidal volume, negative pressure during spontaneous ventilation may cause air dilution if the inspiratory limb is open to atmosphere or there is a leak. The amount of air dilution will depend on the presence of reservoirs in the system, the respiratory pattern, and the total fresh gas flow.

Air dilution makes it difficult to maintain a stable anesthetic state. It causes the concentration of anesthetic in the inspired mixture to fall. This results in a lighter level of anesthesia with stimulation of ventilation. The increased ventilation causes more air dilution. The opposite also is true. Deepening anesthesia depresses ventilation. Depression of respiration decreases air dilution and this causes an increase in the inspired anesthetic agent concentration. This in turn leads to further depression of respiration.

Leaks

When a leak occurs, positive pressure in the system will force gas out of the system. The composition and amount of the gas lost will depend on the location and size of the leak, the pressure in the system, and the compliance and resistance of both the system and the patient.

Uptake of Anesthetic Agent by the Breathing System Components

Uptake of anesthetic agents by rubber, plastics, metal, and carbon dioxide absorbent will produce a lower inspired concentration. Uptake will be directly proportional to the concentration gradient between the gas and the components, the partition coefficient, the surface area, the diffusion coefficient, and the square root of time.

Release of Anesthetic from the System

Elimination of anesthetic agent from the breathing system will depend on the same factors as uptake. The system may function as a low output vaporizer for many hours after a vaporizer has been turned off even if the rubber goods and absorbent are changed (21–23). This can result in inadvertent exposure of a patient to the agent.

COMMON COMPONENTS

Some components are found in only one type of breathing system. These will be discussed under the individual systems. Others are found in more than one system so that their inclusion in a general chapter such as this is appropriate.

Bushings (Mounts)

A bushing serves to modify the internal diameter of a component. Most often it has a cylindrical form and is inserted into and becomes part of a pliable component, such as a reservoir bag or a breathing tube.

Sleeves

A sleeve alters the external diameter of a component.

Connectors and Adaptors

A connector is a fitting intended to join two or more components. An adaptor is a specialized connector that establishes functional continuity between otherwise disparate or incompatible components.

An adaptor or connector may be distinguished by:

1) shape (straight, right-angle or elbow, T, or Y);
2) component(s) to which it is semipermanently attached;
3) added features (with nipple or pop-off) and
4) size and type of fitting at either end (15-mm male, 22-mm female).

All anesthesia systems terminate at the patient connection port, which is the opening at the patient end of the breathing system intended for connection to a tracheal tube connector, face mask, laryngeal mask, or other device connecting to the patient's airway. All face masks have a 22-mm female opening and other devices have a 15-mm male fitting. To facilitate the change from mask to tracheal tube, etc., a component having a 22-mm male fitting with a concentric 15-mm female opening is used at the patient end of the breathing systems. Usually this component is a right-angle connector (Fig. 6.2), also known as an elbow adaptor, elbow joint, elbow connector, mask angle piece, mask adaptor, or mask elbow. Connectors and adaptors can be used to:

1) extend the distance between the patient and the breathing system—this is especially important in patients with head and neck surgery when the presence of the breathing system near the head may make it inaccessible to the anesthesia personnel and interfere with the surgical field
2) change the angle of connection between the patient and the breathing system
3) allow a more flexible and less kinkable connection between the patient and the breathing system
4) increase the dead space

A variety of connectors is available commercially (Fig. 6.2), and many more have been described in the literature. In selecting a connector, several principles should be kept in mind:

1) Resistance increases with sharp curves and rough sidewalls.
2) Connectors add dead space. This may not be of much significance in the adult patient, but any increase in dead space in infants may be excessive.
3) Connectors increase the number of possible locations at which disconnections can take place.

Reservoir Bag

Most breathing systems have a reservoir bag that acts as a counterlung, moving reciprocally with the patient's lungs (2). The reservoir bag is

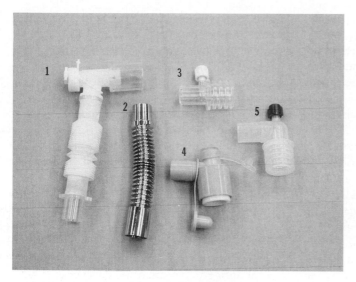

FIGURE **6.2.** Various connectors. **1**, A swivel connector that can be used to insert a flexible fiberscope. A swivel connector has a flexible accordion-type side arm. **2**, A flexible metal connector that can be used between the tracheal tube and the breathing system. A flexible metal connector cannot be used with a mask. **3**, Straight connector with a side gas sampling port. **4**, A right angle connector for insertion of a flexible fiberscope. A right angle connector can accommodate different sized fiberscopes by changing the diaphragm. The large cap is used if no diaphragm is present. **5**, Right-angle connector with gas sampling port.

also known as the respiratory, breathing, or sometimes erroneously, the rebreathing bag. Most bags are composed of rubber or plastic and are ellipsoidal in shape so that they can be grasped easily with one hand. The neck of the bag is the part that connects with the breathing system. The tail is the end opposite from the neck. A hanging loop may be provided near the tail to facilitate drying. The neck of the bag must be a 22-mm female fitting (24, 25).

The bag has the following functions:

1) It allows accumulation of gas during exhalation so a reservoir is available for the next inspiration. This permits rebreathing, allows more economical use of gases, and prevents air dilution.
2) It provides a means whereby ventilation may be assisted or controlled.
3) It can serve through visual and tactile observation as a monitor of a patient's spontaneous respiration (26).
4) It protects the patient from excessive pressure in the breathing system (27–29).

The pressure-volume characteristics of bags become important if there is no way for gases to escape from the system and inflow continues. Adding volume to a bag normally causes a negligible rise in pressure until the nominal capacity is reached. As more volume is added, the pressure

rises rapidly to a peak and then attains a plateau. As the bag distends further, the pressure falls slightly. The peak pressure is of particular interest as this represents the maximal pressure that will develop in a breathing system. The American Society for Testing and Materials (ASTM) standard for reservoir bags (24) requires that for bags of 1.5 liters or smaller the pressure shall be not less than 30 cm H_2O or exceed 50 cm H_2O when the bag is expanded to four times its capacity (24). For bags larger than 1.5 liters, the pressure shall be not less than 35 cm H_2O or exceed 60 cm H_2O when the bag is expanded to four times its size. One study found this pressure was often exceeded, especially if the bag was new and there was a high inflow rate (29).

New bags develop higher pressures when first overinflated than bags that have been overinflated several times or have been prestretched (27, 29). It is good practice to overinflate or stretch a new bag before it is used. This will not limit the ability to produce high airway pressures by squeezing and will increase the margin of safety.

Bags are available in a variety of sizes. The size that should be used will depend on the patient, the breathing system, and the user's preference. A 3-liter bag is traditional for use in adults. A large bag may be difficult to squeeze and will make monitoring of the patient's spontaneous respiration difficult because the excursions will be smaller. A small bag, on the other hand, provides less safety with respect to avoiding high pressures and may not provide a large enough reservoir.

A spare bag should always be kept immediately available. A bag may rupture or become lost while a ventilator is in use.

Breathing Tubes

Large bore, nonrigid breathing (conducting) tubes, which are composed of rubber or plastic and are usually corrugated, are used in most breathing systems to convey gases to and from the patient. Corrugations increase flexibility and help to prevent kinking. Clear plastic tubes are more lightweight (so they cause less drag on the tracheal tube or mask), absorb less halogenated agents, have a lower compliance than rubber tubes, and allow visualization of the interior of the tube.

Smaller diameter tubes are available for use in circle systems designed for pediatric patients. American and International standards require breathing tubes to have 22-mm female fittings at either end (30, 31).

Breathing tubes have two functions. One is to act as a reservoir in certain systems. The second is to provide a flexible, low-resistance, lightweight connection from one part of the system to another. Tubings may also be used to connect the ventilator to the breathing system. Several tubes may be connected in series or extra long tubings can be used if it is desired to have the anesthesia machine at some distance from the patient's head. Special tubings that can be elongated or shortened are available.

Breathing tubes have some distensibility but not enough to prevent excessive pressures from developing (32).

Adjustable Pressure Limiting Valve

The APL valve is a user-adjustable valve that releases gases to atmosphere or a scavenging system and that is intended to provide control of the pressure in the breathing system (1). Other commonly used names for this component include pressure relief valve, venting port, relief valve, overspill valve, pop-off valve, overflow valve, dump valve, blow-off valve, safety relief valve, excess valve, Heidbrink valve, adjustable pressure limiter, excess gas venting valve, spill valve, exhaust valve, expiratory valve, excess gas valve, pressure release valve, and release valve.

Construction

The housing of most APL valves is metal. If the valve is to be used in an magnetic resonance imaging (MRI) environment, it should be constructed from aluminum.

Control Part

The control part serves to control the pressure at which the valve opens. Several types are available.

Spring-Loaded Disc

A commonly used APL valve uses a disc held onto a seat by a spring (Fig. 6.3). A threaded screw cap over the spring allows the pressure exerted by the spring to be varied. When the cap is fully tightened, the disc will prevent any gas from escaping from the system. As the cap is loosened, the tension on the spring is reduced so that the disc can rise.

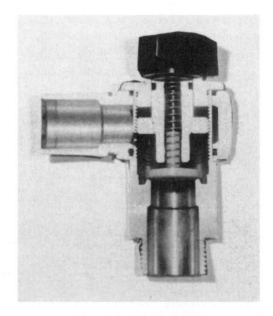

FIGURE 6.3. Adjustable pressure limiting (APL) valve with spring-loaded disc. Gas from the breathing system enters at the base and passes into the gas collecting assembly at left. Turning the control knob varies the tension in the spring and the pressure necessary to lift the disc off its seat. When the cap is fully tightened, the spring is compressed enough to prevent the valve leaflet from lifting at any airway pressure.

When the pressure in the breathing system increases, it exerts an upward force on the disc. When this force exceeds the downward force exerted by the spring, the disc rises and gas flows out of the valve. When the pressure in the system falls, the disc returns to its seat. When the cap is at its maximum upward position, there will be no pressure exerted by the spring. The weight of the disc ensures that the reservoir bag fills before the disc rises.

Stem and Seat

Another control part employed in APL valves is the stem and seat (Fig. 6.4). This is similar to a flow control valve because a threaded stem allows variable contact with a seat. As the valve is opened, the opening at the seat becomes larger and more gas is allowed to escape. A disc or ball that must be moved to open the valve ensures that there will be sufficient pressure in the system to fill the reservoir bag before the valve opens.

Diaphragm

A diaphragm valve is shown in Figure 6.5. It works in a manner similar to the spring-loaded disc valve except that the cap and spring push on a diaphragm rather than a disc. Increased pressure in the breathing system will push the diaphragm off its seat. Increasing or decreasing the tension of the spring controls the amount of gas that will escape through the valve.

If there is negative pressure in the scavenging system, the diaphragm will be pulled onto the seat and gas will not be able to escape from the breathing system. The only quick way to relieve pressure in the breathing system is to disconnect the scavenging system at some point until the source of the negative pressure in the scavenging system has been eliminated.

Control Knob

Most APL valves have a rotary control knob. The ASTM standard requires that valves with ro-

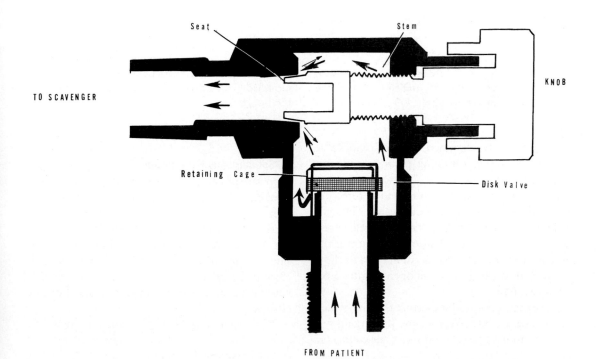

FIGURE 6.4. Adjustable pressure limiting (APL) valve with stem and seat. Rotation of the control knob causes the opening between the stem and seat to change. The disc ensures that the reservoir bag will fill before the valve opens. The disc also prevents transmission of positive pressure or gas from the scavenging system to the breathing system. (Redrawn with permission from North American Drager, Inc.)

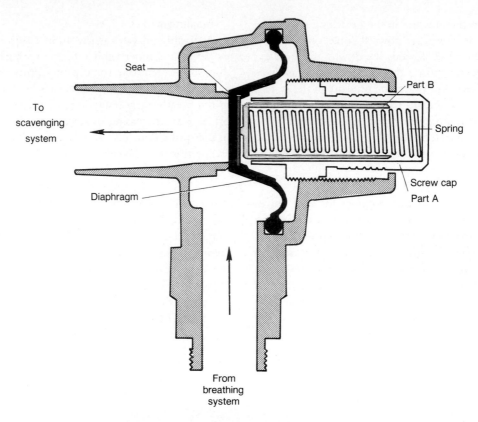

FIGURE 6.5. Adjustable pressure limiting (APL) valve with diaphragm. Turning the control knob (screw cap) varies the tension in the spring and thus controls the amount of gas vented through the valve. Negative pressure in the scavenging systemwill pull the diaphragm onto its seat. (Adapted with permission from a drawing furnished by Ohmeda, a division of BOC Health Care, Inc.)

tating controls be designed so that a clockwise motion increases the limiting pressure and ultimately closes the valve (1). It also requires an arrow or other marking to indicate the direction of movement required to close the valve. The standard recommends that the full range of relief pressure be adjusted by less than one full turn of the control. Some of these valves are marked to show the pressure at which they will open (Figure 6.6).

Exhaust Port

The exhaust port is the aperture through which excess gases are discharged to the scavenging system. It must have a 19- or 30-mm male connector (33).

Collection Device

Almost all APL valves are now fitted with collection devices that collect the gases that are vented and direct them to a scavenging system.

Uses

Spontaneous Respiration

With spontaneous respiration, the APL valve remains closed during inspiration. During exhalation, it opens when its opening pressure is exceeded. Normally, the valve is left fully open during spontaneous ventilation. It should be closed slightly only if the reservoir bag collapses. Partially closing the valve during spontaneous respiration will result in positive end–expiratory pressure (PEEP).

With spontaneous respiration, the anesthesia provider must be constantly aware of the amount of bag inflation. If attention is diverted, the bag may collapse or become overdistended. Negative pressure transmitted from the scavenging system may result in either closure of the valve or evacuation of gases from the system. An obstruction in

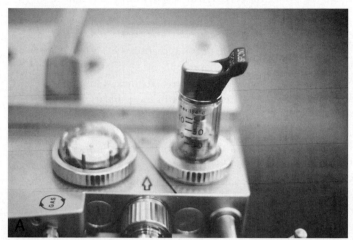

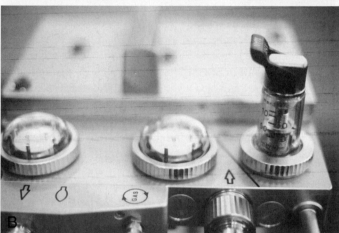

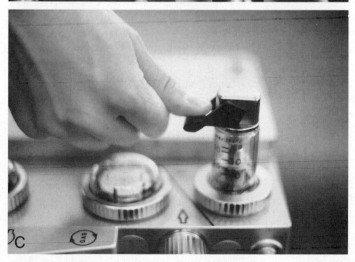

FIGURE **6.6.** Adjustable pressure limiting (APL) valve with spontaneous/manual changeover. **A,** When the lever is in the spontaneous position, the valve is fully open, regardless of the set pressure. **B,** When the lever is placed in the manual position, the knob is rotated to adjust the opening pressure. **C,** In the manual position, the valve can be fully opened by pressing down on the lever. Note the pressure markings.

the scavenging system may result in the bag becoming overdistended.

There is considerable variation in the resistance of APL valves when fully open (34–36) so they should be checked periodically. Fully open APL valves should have a pressure drop between 0.1 and 0.3 kPa (1.0 and 3.0 cm H_2O) at an air flow of 3.0 liters/min and a pressure drop at 30 liters/min of not less than 0.1 kPa (1.0 cm H_2O) and not greater than 0.5 kPa (5.0 cm H_2O) (1).

Manually Controlled or Assisted Ventilation

During manually controlled or assisted ventilation, the valve is usually left partially open. During inspiration, the bag is squeezed and pressure increases until the relief pressure is reached. Before this, the patient receives all of the gas displaced from the bag (less a small amount because of compression of the gases and expansion of the tubes). Once the APL valve opens, the additional volume the patient receives is determined by the relative resistances to flow exerted by the patient and the APL valve. Frequent adjustment of the valve made on the basis of chest movements and exhaled volume measurements may be necessary to achieve the desired level of ventilation and maintain adequate filling of the bag. If compliance falls or resistance increases, the valve must be tightened to maintain the desired tidal volume. The resistance felt during bag compression ("the educated hand") cannot be relied on to ensure adequate ventilation (37, 38). Alternative methods are to close the valve completely and open it periodically to release excess gas or to set the fresh gas flow so that it equals uptake by the patient and the system.

Some APL valves have a lever for spontaneous/manual changeover (Fig. 6.6).

Mechanical Ventilation

When a ventilator is used, gas will be vented from it during expiration. The APL valve should be closed completely. If it is left open, gas will be vented from the system during inspiration. Bag-ventilator selector switches (selector valves) that facilitate the change from manual to automatic ventilation are available and are discussed in Chapter 8. Most of these isolate the APL valve when the selector valve is turned to automatic.

Positive End Expiratory Pressure Valves

On most newer anesthesia machines a PEEP valve is incorporated into the CO_2 absorber assembly (Chapter 8) or ventilator (Chapter 11) (39, 40). For older machines, a disposable PEEP valve can be placed in the exhalation limb for use during manual or artificial ventilation or between the breathing system and the ventilator for use during artificial ventilation. A number of different devices has been used to achieve PEEP (39). A ball PEEP valve must be kept in an upright position. A spring-loaded or magnetic PEEP valve eliminates this need. Electronic PEEP is used on most new anesthesia machines.

Fixed pressure PEEP valves are marked to indicate the amount of PEEP they provide. More than one can be used to obtain an additive effect. Variable pressure ones have a means to adjust the amount of PEEP. Some have a scale that indicates the PEEP at a given setting. If no scale is present, a manometer must be used to measure the pressure.

PEEP valves can be divided into two types: unidirectional and bidirectional (41). A bidirectional valve has a second flow channel with its own one-way valve. It has been recommended that only bidirectional PEEP valves be used (42, 43). Only a bidirectional valve should be used between the breathing system and the ventilator.

When inserting a disposable PEEP valve, it is important that it be placed in the correct position and oriented correctly. The ASTM standard requires that a PEEP valve be marked with an arrow indicating the proper direction of flow or the words "inlet" and "outlet" or both (1). Immediately after placement, the breathing system manometer should be checked to make certain PEEP is being delivered and the patient should be checked for effective ventilation. A unidirectional PEEP valve incorrectly oriented against the flow of gas in the inspiratory or expiratory limb will occlude gas flow (41, 43, 44). Incorrectly orienting a bidirectional PEEP valve in either the inspiratory or expiratory limb will not occlude flow but no PEEP will be applied.

If a PEEP valve is used with a circle breathing system in which the pressure manometer is on the absorber side of the expiratory unidirectional valve, PEEP will not be indicated on the gauge (45, 46). The user must depend on the accuracy of the valve markings to determine the level of PEEP or a second pressure manometer upstream of the PEEP valve used to determine the actual pressures (41).

Use of PEEP in a spontaneously breathing patient will result in increased work of breathing (47, 48). Use of PEEP with a pressure-limited ventilator may result in a substantial decrease in the tidal volume delivered to the patient, unless appropriate adjustments are made to the peak pressure setting on the ventilator.

Filters

Filters (49, 50) have three purposes:

1) Protection of the patient from microorganisms and airborne particulate matter (51).
2) Protection of the anesthesia equipment and the environment from exhaled contaminants.
3) Exchange of heat and moisture when placed between the patient and the breathing system. This will be discussed more fully in Chapter 10.

Filters with more than 99% efficiency in blocking transmission of bacteria and viruses are available (52–59).

Current filters are classified into two groups (60). One group utilizes an extremely compact fiber membrane with small pores but large surface area as a result of pleating. The other group utilizes electrets that are felt-like materials that have been subjected to an electromagnetic field, which gives them a permanent electric polarity (49, 60). The fibers are less dense, hence the pore size is greater.

Hydrophobicity is a characteristic of some filters. Water droplets form on water-repellant fibers and will pass between fibers if pores are large enough. If the pores are sufficiently small, the material is considered to be hydrophobic.

In filters that are not completely hydrophobic, water droplets may move through the filter material, increasing resistance and causing a loss of electrostatic forces. The organism-retaining capability of the filter is seriously diminished by this process, and bacterial contamination of the system can occur (56).

Filters for use in anesthesia are supplied in three forms:

1) attached to the breathing tube of a disposable circle system;
2) attached to a ventilator hose; and
3) as a separate component.

Filters that can be steam sterilized are available, but must be discarded if resistance rises significantly. A filter placed at the patient port may permit disposable breathing systems to be reused. However, the external surface of these systems will not be protected.

Filters that are not completely hydrophobic should not be placed downstream of a humidifier or nebulizer because when wet they may become less efficient. In addition, an increase in resistance, sometimes to a hazardous level, may be seen (61–64).

Obstruction of filters may be caused by exhaled blood, edema fluid, a manufacturing defect, sterilization of a disposable filter, nebulized drugs, and insertion of a unidirectional filter backward (65–67). Aspiration of the filter medium may occur. A hole in a filter can cause a leak (see Fig. 13.6).

Equipment to Administer Bronchodilators

Intraoperative bronchospasm can be a very serious problem. One treatment is topical administration of bronchodilators. Traditionally small volume nebulizers were used to deliver these drugs to patients whose tracheas were intubated, but use of directly-actuated metered dose inhalers (MDIs) has become more common

Apparatus

Manufacturers have adapted MDIs for use with ventilator circuits. An inhaler may be placed inside the barrel of a large syringe (68–71). The inhaler is actuated by pressing the syringe plunger. Most adapters are T-shaped with the injection port on the side (Fig. 6.7). Numerous commercial adapters and homemade devices have been described

FIGURE 6.7. Adaptor for administering bronchodilators using a multidose inhaler. **A**, Side view showing the port into which the inhaler fits. Note the cap that can be fitted over the port when it is not in use. **B**, End view showing hole pointing in one direction. This should point toward the patient unless an upstream spacer is used.

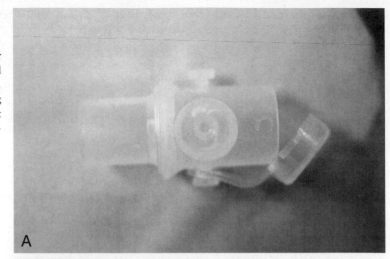

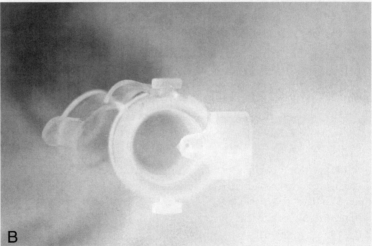

in the literature. (70, 72–79). The gas sampling port or the sampling lumen of a specialized tracheal tube may be used to administer bronchodilators (70, 80). The adapter should be placed close to the patient port (Fig. 6.8). There should not be a filter or HME between the adapter and the patient.

A spacer (aerosol holding chamber, reservoir chamber, auxiliary, or accessory device) (Fig. 6.8) may be placed downstream or upstream of the MDI to slow the flow of aerosol and increase impaction and sedimentation of large particles (81). One study showed that use of rigid spacers resulted in more efficient delivery than collapsible ones (82).

Delivery via a catheter that extends to the tip of the tracheal tube is more efficient (68, 70, 83, 84). However, such administration may cause epithelial lesions in the tracheobronchial tree (85, 86).

Technique of Use

The MDI should be warmed to body temperature and shaken well before administration (87, 88). Bronchodilator discharge is maximal when the canister is upright (68). The hole in the adapter (Fig. 6.7 B) should point toward the patient unless the spacer is upstream. Actuation just after inspiration begins will maximize delivery to the airways (89). If a spacer is used, the MDI

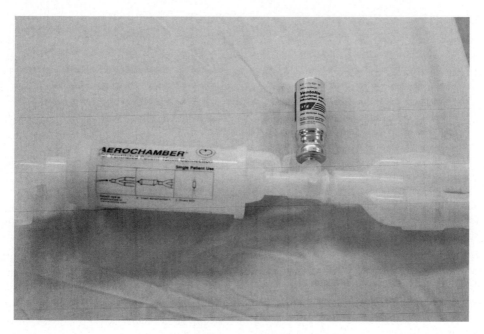

FIGURE 6.8. Multidose inhaler with downstream spacer in place between the breathing system (right) and the patient connection (left).

should be actuated 1 to 2 seconds before inspiration or near end-exhalation, depending on the rate (88).

Airway deposition may be enhanced by a slow, deep inspiration, followed by a pause of 2 to 3 seconds before exhalation (89–91). There should be 30 to 60 seconds between puffs with shaking before each puff (87, 88).

Less humidification is desirable in promoting medication delivery. (82, 87) High humidification causes the aerosol droplets to increase in size, which causes them to rain out. If possible, humidification should be discontinued when MDIs are used.

The optimal number of puffs depends on monitoring of lung function and systemic side effects. Because a high percentage of the medication adheres to the walls of the tube, it usually takes at least twice as many puffs as would be needed in the unintubated patient. A spacer or a extension will reduce the number of puffs that will be needed. However, even with a spacer, as many as 15 puffs may be needed (92). The patient should be monitored for the appearance of beneficial and side effects.

Advantages

Convenience

MDIs are easy to use, take little time to set up, and occupy little space on the anesthesia cart (93).

Efficiency of Drug Administration

Metered dose inhalers are more efficient at delivering medications in intubated patients than nebulizers (94, 95).

Cost

In general, it is less expensive to use MDIs, even with a spacer, than nebulizers (88).

Disadvantages

The main problem with MDIs is that a large amount of drug is lost because of rain out in the breathing system, tracheal tube, and tracheal tube connector.

The size of the tracheal tube influences the amount of the drug that reaches the patient's lungs. There is a decrease in percent reaching the patient as tracheal tube size decreases (82, 84, 89).

Another problem is that the carrier gas may cause erroneous readings by an anesthetic agent analyzer (96).

SIZE AND TYPE OF FITTINGS

The Compressed Gas Association and the ASTM have published standards that specify the size and type of fittings for components in the breathing system (1, 24, 30, 97). Virtually all breathing system components manufactured in the United States in recent years conform to these. The safety provided by standardization of diameters of various connectors can be jeopardized by use of adaptors and adhesive tape.

Any component or accessory of the breathing system that permits only unidirectional flow or any device whose correct function depends on the direction of gas flow through it must be so labeled and marked with an arrow indicating the proper direction of flow or the words "inlet" and "outlet" or both. "Distal" and "proximal" are used to designate the proximity of a component to the patient.

A fitting that is part of a component, such as an absorber, Y piece, or reservoir bag mount, whose purpose is to permit attachment of this component to a reservoir bag, breathing tube, or mask must be male and rigid. Fittings on the breathing tube, mask, and reservoir bag connectors must be female and nonrigid (resilient). All connectors in an adult system are 22 mm. The component that is designed to connect to a tracheal tube connector must have a coaxial 15-mm female fitting at the patient end. The inspiratory and expiratory ports mounted on the absorber and the reservoir bag connector must have male fittings. The exit port for the APL valve has either a 30- or 19-mm male fitting to avoid problems with connections between the breathing and scavenging systems.

CLASSIFICATION OF BREATHING SYSTEMS

A favorite pastime among anesthesia personnel has been the classification of breathing systems. The result has been a hopelessly confused terminology. In an attempt to provide some relief from this confusion, a description of various authors' classifications will be presented. Subsequently, a nomenclature that the present authors believe is more useful will be described.

Classification by Function
Dripps, Echenhoff, and Vandam

With the Dripps, Echenhoff, and Vandam classification, breathing systems are divided into five categories according to the presence or absence of:

1) a reservoir bag;
2) rebreathing;
3) an absorber to remove carbon dioxide; and
4) directional valves (98).

The five systems are insufflation, open, semiopen, semiclosed, and closed. The insufflation system is one in which gases are delivered directly into the patient's airway. There are no valves, reservoir bag, or carbon dioxide absorption.

In the open system, the patient inhales only the mixture delivered by the anesthesia machine. Valves direct each exhaled breath into atmosphere. A reservoir bag may be present. Rebreathing is minimal, and there is no carbon dioxide absorption. This includes systems used with intermittent flow machines and nonrebreathing valves.

In the semiopen system, exhaled gases flow out of the system and also to the inspiratory line of the apparatus to be rebreathed. There is no chemical absorption of carbon dioxide. Rebreathing depends on the fresh gas flow. A reservoir bag and a directional valve are optional.

In the semiclosed system, part of the exhaled gases passes into atmosphere and part mixes with fresh gases and is rebreathed. Chemical absorption of carbon dioxide, directional valves, and a reservoir bag are present.

In the closed system, there is complete rebreathing of expired gas. Carbon dioxide absorption, a reservoir bag, and directional valves are present.

Moyers

The Moyers classification is based on the presence or absence of a reservoir bag and rebreathing (99). An open system has no reservoir or rebreathing. The semiopen system has a reservoir but no rebreathing. The semiclosed system has a reservoir and partial rebreathing, and the closed system has a reservoir and complete rebreathing.

Collins

The Collins classification defines an open system as one in which an anesthetic agent is brought to the patient's respiratory tract with atmospheric air as the diluent (100). The respiratory tract has access to the atmosphere during both inspiration and expiration. There is no reservoir or rebreathing.

A semiopen system is one in which the patient's respiratory system is open to atmosphere during both inspiration and expiration. There is a reservoir that is open to atmosphere, rebreathing is absent, and atmospheric air either carries or dilutes the anesthetic agent.

The semiclosed system is one in which the patient's respiratory system is completely closed to atmosphere on inspiration but open on expiration. A reservoir closed to atmosphere is present. With a closed system, there is no access to atmosphere either during inspiration or expiration. Rebreathing is complete and a reservoir is required.

Adriani

The Adriani classification divides systems into open vaporization, insufflation, semiclosed, and closed (rebreathing) (101). An open system is one employing an open-drop mask. With the insufflation technique, a continuous stream of gas flows to the patient's nasopharynx, oropharynx, or trachea. The semiclosed system is one in which there is complete enclosure of the inspired atmosphere and no air dilution. The closed system permits complete rebreathing.

Conway

With the Conway classification, an open system is one with infinite boundaries and no restriction to fresh gas flow (102). The semiopen system is one partially bounded, with some restriction to fresh gas flow. The closed system is defined as having no provision for gas overflow. The semiclosed system is one allowing for overflow of excess gas. It is divided into semiclosed rebreathing, semiclosed absorption, and semiclosed nonrebreathing systems.

Hall

In the Hall classification, an open system has no reservoir bag or rebreathing (103). The semiopen system also has no reservoir bag but has partial rebreathing. Semiclosed systems have a reservoir bag and partial rebreathing. They are divided into those with and without carbon dioxide absorption. The closed system has complete rebreathing and a reservoir.

McMahon

The McMahon system used rebreathing as the basis for classification of breathing systems into open, semiclosed, and closed (104). An open technique is one in which there is no rebreathing. This includes techniques in which gases are administered at a total flow rate equal to or greater than the respiratory minute volume. Techniques with flows less than the respiratory minute volume would also be considered open if there were no increase in dead space. The semiclosed system would employ some rebreathing. The closed system employs total rebreathing.

Baraka

The Baraka system classified systems according to their mechanism of carbon dioxide elimination (105). Open systems are those that eliminate carbon dioxide by washout and have no reservoir bag. Semiopen systems also wash out carbon dioxide, but have a reservoir bag. Semiclosed systems use carbon dioxide absorption and have a fresh gas flow that exceeds patient uptake. Closed systems also use carbon dioxide absorption and have a fresh gas flow that equals patient uptake.

The International Standards Organization

The International Standards Organization classifies breathing systems as nonrebreathing, partial rebreathing, and complete rebreathing (106). The terms semi-open and semi-closed are deprecated.

Marini, Culver, and Kirk

The Marini, Culver, and Kirk system classifies breathing systems on the basis of carbon dioxide elimination (107). Systems are divided into open, which do not have a reservoir bag, and semiopen, which do have a reservoir bag. Examples of the open variety include the open drop mask, insufflation, and the T piece (Mapleson E). Semiopen systems include the Magill and Lack (Mapleson A), Bain (Mapleson D), Jackson-Rees (Mapleson F), Mera F, and systems with nonrebreathing valves. The carbon dioxide absorption units include the circle system.

Classification by Equipment

Hamilton recognized the shortcomings of the nomenclatures described above and proposed that the terms open, semiopen, etc., be dropped in favor of a description of the equipment and the total fresh gas flow to the system (108). The description of the equipment will be familiar to the reader after reading the next two chapters. The fresh gas flow will determine the amount of rebreathing, if any, that takes place.

REFERENCES

1. American Society for Testing and Materials. Standard specification for minimum performance and safety requirements for anesthesia breathing systems (ASTM F1208–89 (Reapproved 1994). West Conshohocken, PA: ASTM, 1994.
2. Smith TC. Anesthesia breathing systems. In: J Ehrenwerth, JB Eisenkraft, eds. Anesthesia equipment. Principles and applications. St. Louis, MO: Mosby, 1993: 89–113.
3. Martin DG, Kong KL, Lewis GTR. Resistance to airflow in anaesthetic breathing systems. Br J Anaesth 1989;62;456–461.
4. Bolder PM, Healy TEJ, Bolder AR, et al. The extra work of breathing through adult endotracheal tubes. Anesth Analg 1976;65:853–859.
5. Bersten AD, Rutten AJ, Vedig AE, et al. Additional work of breathing imposed by endotracheal tubes, breathing circuits, and intensive care ventilators. Crit Care Med 1989;17:671–677.
6. Davies JM, Hogg MIJ, Rosen M. Upper limits of resistance of apparatus for inhalation analgesia during labour. Br J Anaesth 1974;46:136–144.
7. Hogg MIJ, Davies JM, Mapleson WW, et al. Proposed upper limit of respiratory resistance for inhalation apparatus used in labour. Br J Anaesth 1974;46: 149–152.
8. McMahon J. Rebreathing as a basis for classification of inhalation technics. J Am Assoc Nurse Anesth 1951;19:133–158.
9. Sykes MK. Rebreathing circuits. Br J Anaesth 1968; 40:666–674.
10. Aldrete JA, Castillo RA, Bradley EL. Changes of fresh gas flow affect the tidal volume delivered by anesthesia ventilators. Anesth Analg 1986;65:S4.
11. Ghani GA. Fresh gas flow affects minute volume during mechanical ventilation. Anesth Analg 1984;63: 619.
12. Gravenstein N, Banner MJ, McLaughlin G. Tidal volume changes due to the interaction of anesthesia machine and anesthesia ventilator. Journal of Clinical Monitoring 1987;3:187–190.
13. Scheller MS, Jones BR, Benumof JL. The influence of fresh gas flow and inspiratory/expiratory ratio on tidal volume and arterial CO_2 tension in mechanically ventilated surgical patients. J Cardiothorac Anesth 1989;3:564–567.
14. Cote CJ, Petkau AJ, Ryan JF, et al. Wasted ventilation measured in vitro with eight anesthetic circuits with and without inline humidification. Anesthesiology 1983;59:442–446.
15. Feldman JM, Muller J. Tidal volume measurement errors—the impact of lung compliance and a circuit humidifier. Anesthesiology 1990;73:A469.
16. Aarandia HY, Byles PH. PEEP and the Bain circuit. Canadian Anaesthetists Society Journal 1981;28: 467–470.
17. Elliott WR, Harris AE, Philip JH. Positive end–expiratory pressure: implications for tidal volume changes in anesthesia machine ventilation. Journal of Clinical Monitoring 1989;5:100–104.
18. Elliott WR, Topulos GP. The influence of the mechanics of anesthesia breathing circuits on respiratory monitoring. Biomed Instrum Technol 1990;24: 260–265.
19. Pan PH, van der Aa JJ. Positive end–expiratory pressure and lung compliance: effect on delivered tidal volume. Can J Anaesth 1995;42:831–835.
20. Badgwell JM, Swan J, McDaniel K. Infants are adequately ventilated using volume-limitation and circle systems. Anesthesiology 1994;81:A1324.
21. Dykes MHM, Chir MB, Laasberg LH. Clinical implications of halothane contamination of the anesthetic circle. Anesthesiology 1971;35:648–649.
22. Murray WJ, Fleming P. Patient exposure to residual fluorinated anesthetic agents in anesthesia machine circuits. Anesth Analg 1973;52:23–26.
23. Samulksa HM, Ramaiah S, Noble WH. Unintended exposure to halothane in surgical patients: halothane washout studies. Canadian Anaesthetists Society Journal 1972;19:35–41.
24. American Society for Testing Materials. Standard specification for anesthesia reservoir bags (ASTM F1204–88) (Reapproved 1993). West Conshohocken, PA: ASTM, 1993.
25. International Standards Organization. Anaesthetic reservoir bags (ISO 5362:1986). Geneva, Switzerland: ISO, 1986.

26. Kulkarni PR, Lumb AB, Platt MW, et al. Estimation of tidal volume from the reservoir bag. A laboratory study. Anaesthesia 1992;47:936–938.

27. Parmley JB, Tahir AH, Dascomb HE, et al. Disposable versus reusable rebreathing circuits: advantages, disadvantages, hazards, and bacteriologic studies. Anesth Analg 1972;51:888–894.

28. Johnstone RE, Smith TC. Rebreathing bags as pressure-limiting devices. Anesthesiology 1973;38:192–194.

29. Stone DR, Graves SA. Compliance of pediatric rebreathing bags. Anesthesiology 1980;53:434–435.

30. American Society for Testing Materials. Standard specification for anesthesia breathing tubes (ASTM F1205–88) (Reapproved 1993). West Conshohocken, PA: ASTM, 1993.

31. International Standards Organization. Breathing tubes intended for use with anaesthetic apparatus and ventilators (ISO 5367:1991). Geneva, Switzerland: ISO, 1991.

32. Parmley JB, Tahir AH, Adriani J. Disposable plastic breathing bags and tubes. JAMA 1971;217:1842–1844.

33. American Society for Testing Materials. Specification for anesthetic equipment-scavenging systems for anesthetic gases (ASTM F1343–91). West Conshohocken, PA: ASTM, 1991.

34. Mehta S, Behr G, Chari J, et al. A passive method of disposal of expired anesthetic gases. Br J Anaesth 1977;49:589–593.

35. Morgan BA, Nott MR. Wear in plastic exhaust valves. Anaesthesia 1980;35:717–718.

36. Nott MR, Norman J. Resistance of Heidbrink-type expiratory valves. Br J Anaesth 1978;50:477–480.

37. Robinson RH. Ability to detect changes in compliance and resistance during manual artificial ventilation. Br J Anaesth 1968;40:323–328.

38. Spears RS, Yeh A, Fisher DM, et al. The "educated hand." Can anesthesiologists assess changes in neonatal pulmonary compliance manually? Anesthesiology 1991;75:693–696.

39. Kacmarek RM, Goulet RL. PEEP devices. Anesthesiology Clinics of North America 1987;5:757–776.

40. Cicman JH, Jacoby MI, Skibo VF, et al. Anesthesia systems. Part 1: operating principles of fundamental components. Journal of Clinical Monitoring 1992;8:295–307.

41. Anonymous. Hazard: PEEP valves in anesthesia circuits. Technology for Anesthesia 1983;4(5):1–2.

42. Morse HN. Who is liable when respiratory valve is installed erroneously? Med Elect Prod 1989;(October):32.

43. Lee D. Old equipment PEEP safety cited [Letter to the Editor]. Anesthesia Patient Safety Foundation Newsletter 1990;5:21.

44. Anonymous. Unidirectional PEEP valves and anesthesia. Technology for Anesthesia 1986;6(9):1–2.

45. Mayle LL, Reed SJ, Wyche MQ. Excessive airway pressures occurring concurrently with use of the Fraser Harlake PEEP valve. Anesthesiology Review 1990;17:41–44.

46. Cooper JB. Unidirectional PEEP valves can cause safety hazards. Anesthesia Patient Safety Foundation Newsletter 1990;4:28–29.

47. Banner MJ, Kirby RR. Attention of heavy breathers, vis-a-vis continuous positive airway pressure. Crit Care Med 1994;22:1207–1208.

48. Kacmarek RM, Mang H, Barker N, et al. Effects of disposable or interchangeable positive end–expiratory pressure valves on work of breathing during the application of continuous positive airway pressure. Crit Care Med 1994;22:1219–1226.

49. Hedley RM, Allt-Graham J. Heat and moisture exchangers and breathing filters. Br J Anaesth 1994;73:227–336.

50. Lloyd G, Howells J, Liddle C, et al. Barriers to Hepatitis C transmission within breathing systems: efficacy of a pleated hydrophobic filter. Anesthesia and Intensive Care 1997;25:235–238.

51. Davis R. Soda lime dust. Anesthesia and Intensive Care 1979;7:390.

52. Berry AJ, Nolte FS. An alternative strategy for infection control of anesthesia breathing circuits: a laboratory assessment of the Pall HME filter. Anesth Analg 1991;72:651–655.

53. Fargnoli JM, Arvieux CC, Coppo F, et al. Efficiency and importance of airway filters in reducing microorganisms. Anesth Analg 1992;74:S93.

54. Hedley RM, Allt-Graham J. A comparison of the filtration properties of heat and moisture exchangers. Anaesthesia 1992;47:414–420.

55. Mebius C. Heat and moisture exchangers with bacterial filters: a laboratory evaluation. Acta Anaesthesiol Scand 1992;36:572–576.

56. Hedley RM, Allt-Graham J. A comparison of the filtration properties of heat and moisture exchangers. Anaesthesia 1992;47:414–420.

57. Lee MG, Ford JL, Hunt PB, et al. Bacterial retention properties of heat and moisture exchange filters. Br J Anaesth 1992;69:522–525.

58. Leijten DTM, Rejger VS, Mouton RP. Bacterial contamination and the effect of filters in anaesthetic circuits in a simulated patient model. J Hosp Infect 1992;21:51–60.

59. Vandenbroucke-Grauls CMJE, Teeuw KB, Ballemans K, et al. Bacterial and viral removal efficiency,

heat and moisture exchange properties of four filtration devices. J Hosp Infect 1995;29:45–56.

60. Hogarth I. Anaesthetic machine and breathing system contamination and the efficacy of bacterial-viral filters. Anesthesia and Intensive Care 1996;24: 154–163.

61. Buckley PM. Increase in resistance of in-line breathing filters in humidified air. Br J Anaesth 1984;56: 637–643.

62. Dryden GE, Dryden SR, Brown DG, et al. Performance of bacteria filters. Respiratory Care 1980;25: 1127–1135.

63. Loeser EA. Water-induced resistance in disposable respiratory—circuit bacterial filters. Anesth Analg 1978;57:269–271.

64. Mason J, Tackley R. An acute rise in expiratory resistance due to a blocked ventilator filter. Anaesthesia 1981;36:335.

65. Smith CE, Otworth JR, Kaluszyk P. Bilateral tension pneumothorax due to a defective anesthesia breathing circuit filter. J Clin Anesth 1991;3:229–334.

66. McEwan AI, Dowell L, Karis JH. Bilateral tension pneumothorax caused by a blocked bacterial filter in an anesthesia breathing circuit. Anesth Analg 1993; 76:440–442.

67. Barton RM. Detection of expiratory antibacterial filter occlusion. Anesth Analg 1993;77:197.

68. Dunteman E, Despotis G. A simple method of MDI administration in the intubated patient. Anesth Analg 1992;75:304–305.

69. Jaeger DD. A simpler method of administration of metered dose inhalers during general anesthesia via gas sampling port. Anesth Analg 1993;77:1085.

70. Peterfreund RA, Niven RW, Kacmarek RM. Syringe-actuated meter dose inhalers: a quantitative laboratory evaluation of albuterol delivery through nozzle extensions. Anesth Analg 1994;78:554–558.

71. Wakeling H. Bronchodilator delivery in the operating theatre. Anaesthesia 1996;51:794.

72. Gold MI, Margial E. An anesthetic adapter for all metered dose inhalers. Anesthesiology 1988;68: 964–966.

73. Hess D. How should bronchodilators be administered to patient being mechanically ventilated? Respiratory Care 1991;36:377–394.

74. Koska AJ III, Bjoraker DG. An anesthetic adapter for all metered dose inhalers that is readily available to all. Anesth Analg 1989;69:266–267.

75. Vu H, Kempen PM. Administering metered dose bronchodilators during general anesthesia. Anesthesiology 1996;85:691.

76. Welch WP, Huggins F, Clark RB. Bronchodilator administration through a T-piece during general anesthesia. Anesth Rev 1986;47–48.

77. Bush GL. Aerosol delivery devices for the anesthesia circuit. Anesthesiology 1986;65:240.

78. Duckett JE. A simple device for delivering bronchodilators into the anesthesia circuit. Anesthesiology 1985;62:699–700.

79. Diamond MJ. Delivering bronchodilators into the anesthesia circuit. Anesthesiology 1986;64:531.

80. Newell R, Shulman MS. The administration of bronchodilators into the anesthesia circuit. Anesthesiology 1987;66:716–717.

81. Bishop MJ, Larson RP, Buschman, DL. Metered dose inhaler aerosol characteristics are affected by the endotracheal tube actuator/adapter used. Anesthesiology 1990;73:1263–1265.

82. Garner SS, Wiest DB, Bradley JW, et al. Albuterol delivery by metered-dose inhaler in a mechanically ventilated pediatric lung model. Crit Care Med 1996; 24:870–874.

83. Niven RW, Kacmarek RM, Brain JD, et al. Small bore nozzle extensions to improve the delivery efficiency of drugs from metered dose inhalers: laboratory evaluation. American Review of Respiratory Disease 1993;147:1590–1594.

84. Taylor RH, Lerman J. High-efficiency delivery of salbutamol with a metered-dose inhaler in narrow tracheal tubes and catheters. Anesthesiology 1991;74: 360–363.

85. Spahr-Schopfer IA, Lerman J, Cutz E, et al. Lung lesions induced by metered dose inhaler ventolin: a dose response study in rabbits. Anesth Analg 1993; 76:S414.

86. Spahr-Schopfer IA, Cutz E, Dolovich M. High dose ventolin MDI induces epithelial lesions in the tracheo-bronchial tree in a rabbit mode. Anesth Analg 1993;76:S413.

87. Pierson DJ. Using bronchodilator aerosols effectively during mechanical ventilation. Critical Care Alert 1996;69–72.

88. Kacmarek RM, Hess D. The interface between patient and aerosol generator. Respiratory Care 1991; 36:952–976.

89. Crogan SJ, Bishop MJ. Delivery efficiency of metered dose aerosols given via endotracheal tubes. Anesthesiology 1989;70:1008–1010.

90. O'Doherty MJ, Thomas SHL, Page CJ, et al. Delivery of a nebulized aerosol to a lung model during mechanical ventilation. American Review of Respiratory Disease 1992;146:383–388.

91. Thomas SHL, O'Doherty MJ, Page CJ, et al. Delivery of ultrasonic nebulized aerosols to a lung model during mechanical ventilation. American Review of Respiratory Disease 1993;148:872–877.

92. Manthous CA, Chatila W, Schmidt Gam Hall JB.

Treatment of bronchospasm by metered-dose inhaler albuterol in mechanically ventilated patients. Chest 1995;107:210–213.

93. BS Bishop MJ. Bronchospasm: successful management. ASA Annual Refresher Courses October 19, 1996; New Orleans, No. 123.

94. Fuller HD, Dolovich MB, Posmituck G, et al. Pressurized aerosol versus jet aerosol delivery to mechanically ventilated patients. American Review of Respiratory Disease 1990;141:440–444.

95. Gay PC, Patel HG, Nelson SB, et al. Metered dose inhalers for bronchodilator delivery in intubated, mechanically ventilated patients. Chest 1991;99:66–71.

96. Kharasch ED, Sivarajan M. Aerosol propellant interference with clinical mass spectrometers. Journal of Clinical Monitoring 1991;7:172–174.

97. American Society for Testing and Materials. Standard specification for conical fittings of 15-mm and 22-mm sizes (ASTM F 1054–87) (Reapproved 1994). West Conshohocken, PA: ASTM, 1994.

98. Dripps RD, Echenhoff JE, Vandam LD. Introduction to anesthesia. 3rd ed. Philadelphia, PA: WB Saunders, 1968.

99. Moyers J. A nomenclature for methods of inhalation anesthesia. Anesthesiology 1953;14:609–611.

100. Collins VJ. Principles of anesthesiology. Philadelphia, PA: Lea & Febiger, 1966.

101. Adriani J. The chemistry and physics of anesthesia. Springfield, IL: Charles C Thomas, 1962.

102. Conway CM. Anaesthetic circuits. In: Scurr C, Feldman, S, eds. Foundations of anaesthesia. Philadelphia: FA Davis, 1970:37.

103. Hall J. Wright's veterinary anaesthesia. 6th ed. London: Bailliere, Tindall & Cox, 1966.

104. McMahon J. Rebreathing as a basis for classification of inhalation technics. J Am Assoc Nurse Anesth 1951;19:133–158.

105. Baraka A. Functional classification of anaesthesia circuits. Anesthesia and Intensive Care 1977;5:172–178.

106. International Standards Organization. Anaesthesiology-vocabulary (ISO 4135:1995). Geneva, Switzerland: ISO, 1995.

107. Marini JJ, Culver BH, Kirk W. Flow resistance of exhalation valves and positive end–expiratory pressure devices used in mechanical ventilation. American Review of Respiratory Disease 1984;131:850–854.

108. Hamilton WK. Nomenclature of inhalation anesthetic systems. Anesthesiology 1964;25:3–5.

QUESTIONS

1. Which of the following offers the most resistance?
   A. Nonrebreathing valve
   B. CO_2 canister
   C. Tracheal tube
   D. Y-piece
   E. Breathing tubes

Each question below contains four suggested answers of which one or more is correct. Choose the answer:

A if 1, 2, and 3 are correct
B if 1 and 3 are correct
C if 2 and 4 are correct
D if 4 is correct
E if 1, 2, 3, and 4 are correct.

2. The functions of the breathing system include the following
   1. Conveying oxygen and anesthetic gases to the patient
   2. Delivering positive pressure
   3. Removing waste and anesthetic gases from the patient
   4. Conveying excess gases to the scavenging system

3. Resistance to breathing through a breathing system is influenced by
   1. Laminar flow
   2. Gas flow rate
   3. Turbulent flow
   4. Length of the breathing tubes

4. Rebreathing may be influenced by
   1. Fresh gas flow
   2. Arrangement of components in the breathing system
   3. Mechanical dead space
   4. The size of the reservoir bag

5. Effects of rebreathing include
   1. Reduced loss of heat and water
   2. Reduced inspired oxygen
   3. Less fluctuation in inspired anesthetic agent tensions
   4. Decreased inspired carbon dioxide

6. Factors that cause a discrepancy between the composition of the inspired as mixture and that of the fresh gas include
   1. Rebreathing
   2. Leaks in the breathing system
   3. Uptake of agents by components of the breathing system
   4. Increased fresh gas flow

7. Factors that can cause a discrepancy between the volume of gas discharged from a ventilator or reservoir bag and that inspired by the patient include
   1. Fresh gas flow
   2. Compression of gases in the circuit
   3. Leaks
   4. Distention of breathing system components

8. The reservoir bag
   1. Allows use of lower fresh gas flows
   2. Provides a means for delivering positive pressure
   3. Can serve as a monitor of spontaneous respiration
   4. Can cause excessive pressure if the pressure limiting valve is not open

9. Concerning the peak pressure than can be generated in the breathing system if there is a reservoir bag in place
   1. If the reservoir bag is less than 1.5 liters, the pressure shall not be less than 30 cm H_2O
   2. If the reservoir bag is more than 1.5 liters, the pressure shall not be less than 45 cm H_2O
   3. If a 1.5-liter bag is expanded to four times its normal size, the pressure shall not be more than 50 cm H_2O
   4. If a bag more than 1.5 liters and is expanded to four times its size, the pressure shall not be more than 65 cm H_2O

10. Functions of breathing tubes include
    1. Acting as a reservoir
    2. Protection against excessive pressure
    3. Providing a flexible connection between

the different parts of the breathing
system
4. Expanding during spontaneous
breathing to prevent rebreathing

11. During spontaneous respiration
1. The APL valve should be kept partially
closed
2. Most APL valves open automatically
3. An obstruction in the scavenging
system may result in gas being removed
from the breathing system.
4. Obstruction of the air intake valve in
the scavenging system can result in
positive pressure in the breathing
system.

12. With a PEEP valve in the breathing system
1. An increased exhalation effort is
necessary if the patient is breathing
spontaneously
2. An increase in tidal volume may be seen
with mechanical ventilation
3. The amount of PEEP can be either
fixed or adjustable

4. A spring-loaded PEEP valve must be
kept in the upright position

13. Which of the following connections are
male?
1. Those on the breathing tubes
2. Those on the reservoir bag mount
3. Those on the mask
4. Those on the Y-piece

14. Deposition of bronchodilators in the
patient's tracheobronchial tree is enhanced
by
1. Use of a spacer
2. A low inspiratory flow rate
3. Low humidification
4. An expiratory pause

ANSWERS

1.	C	8.	A
2.	E	9.	B
3.	E	10.	B
4.	A	11.	D
5.	A	12.	B
6.	A	13.	C
7.	E	14.	A

The Mapleson Breathing Systems

THE MAPLESON SYSTEMS are characterized by the absence of valves to direct gases to or from the patient. Because there is no device for absorbing CO_2, the fresh gas flow must wash CO_2 out of the circuit. For this reason, these systems are sometimes called "carbon dioxide washout circuits" or "flow-controlled breathing systems."

These systems were classified by Mapleson into five basic types: A through E (1). A sixth, the Mapleson F system, was added later (2). The classification is shown in Figure 7.1. There are many variations of these systems and only the common ones will be discussed.

Because there is no clear separation of inspired and expired gases, when the inspiratory flow ex-

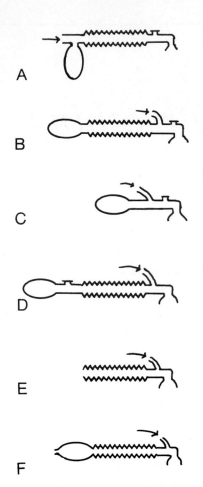

FIGURE 7.1. The Mapleson systems. Components include a reservoir bag, corrugated tubing, adjustable pressure limiting (APL) valve, fresh gas inlet, and patient connection. They lack carbon dioxide absorbers, unidirectional valves, and separate inspiratory and expiratory limbs. (Adapted with permission from Mapleson WW. The elimination of rebreathing in various semiclosed anesthetic systems. Br J Anaesth 1954;26:323–332.)

ceeds the fresh gas flow, rebreathing will occur. The composition of the inspired mixture will depend on how much rebreathing takes place. A large number of studies have been performed to determine the fresh gas flow needed to prevent rebreathing with these systems. These studies have yielded often widely differing results because different criteria have been used to define the onset of rebreathing (3, 4, 5) and because variables such as minute ventilation, respiratory waveform, CO_2

production, patient responsiveness and stimulation, and physiologic dead space may be unpredictable in anesthetized patients. The recommended fresh gas flow may be different using minute volume and weight as predictors (6). Monitoring of end-tidal CO_2 is the best method to determine the optimal fresh gas flow. It should be noted that the arterial CO_2 to end-tidal CO_2 gradient decreases with rebreathing (7).

MAPLESON A SYSTEM
Configurations
Classic Form

The Mapleson A system (Magill attachment or system) is shown in Figure 7.1A. It differs from the other Mapleson systems in that fresh gas does not enter the system near the patient connection but at the other end of the system. A corrugated tubing connects the bag to the adjustable pressure limiting (APL) valve at the patient end of the system.

A sensor for a nondiverting respiratory gas monitor or the sampling site for a diverting monitor (see Chapter 18) may be placed between the APL valve and the corrugated tubing. In adults, it may be placed between the APL valve and the patient. In small patients, this location could result in excessive dead space. It could also be placed between the neck of the bag and its mount, between the bag and the corrugated tubing, or in the fresh gas supply tube, but in these locations the concentration shown on the monitor may differ substantially from the inspired concentration, especially during controlled ventilation.

Lack Modification

The Lack modification of the Mapleson A system (Fig. 7.2) has an added "expiratory" limb, which runs from the patient connection to the APL valve at the machine end of the system (8, 9). This makes it easier to adjust the valve and facilitates scavenging of excess gases. However, it slightly increases the work of breathing (3).

The Lack system is available in both a dual tube (parallel) arrangement and a tube-within-a-tube (coaxial) configuration in which the expiratory limb runs concentrically inside the outer inspiratory limb (10).

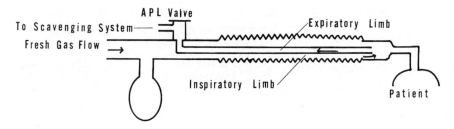

FIGURE 7.2. Lack modification of the Mapleson A system. The coaxial version is shown. APL = adjustable pressure limiting.

Techniques of Use

For spontaneous ventilation, the APL valve is kept in the fully open position. Excess gas exits through it during the latter part of exhalation. For controlled or assisted ventilation, intermittent positive pressure is applied to the bag. The APL valve is tightened so that when the bag is squeezed, sufficient pressure is built up to inflate the lungs. The APL valve opens during inspiration.

Functional Analysis

Spontaneous Respiration

The sequence of events during the respiratory cycle using the Magill system with spontaneous ventilation is shown in Figure 7.3 (11, 12). As the patient exhales (C), first dead-space gas and then alveolar gas flows into the corrugated tubing toward the bag. At the same time, fresh gas flows into the bag. When the bag is full, the pressure in the system rises until the APL valve opens. The first gas vented will be alveolar gas. The remainder of exhalation—containing only alveolar gas—exhausts through the open valve. The continuing inflow of fresh gas reverses the flow of exhaled gases in the corrugated tubing. Some alveolar gas that had bypassed the APL valve now returns and exits through it. If the fresh gas flow is high (A), it will also force the dead-space gas out. If the fresh flow gas is intermediate (D), some dead-space gas will be retained in the system. If the fresh gas flow is low (E), some alveolar gas will be retained.

At the start of inspiration, the first gas inhaled will be from dead space between the patient and the APL valve. The next gas will be either alveolar gas (if the fresh gas flow is low), dead-space gas (if the fresh gas flow is intermediate), or fresh gas (if the fresh gas flow is high) (Fig. 7.3B). Changes in respiratory pattern have little effect on rebreathing (12–14).

With the classic Magill system, investigators have found rebreathing to begin when the fresh gas flow is reduced to 56 to 82 ml/kg per minute (3, 15–21) or 58 to 83% of minute volume (3, 11, 22–25). Fresh gas flows of 51 to 85 mg/kg per minute (3, 15, 20, 26, 27) and 42 to 88% of minute volume (3, 23, 26) have been recommended to avoid rebreathing with the Lack system.

Controlled or Assisted Ventilation

The pattern of gas flow changes during controlled or assisted ventilation (Fig. 7.4). During exhalation (A), the pressure in the system will remain low and no gas will escape through the APL valve, unless the bag becomes distended. All exhaled gases, both dead space and alveolar, remain in the corrugated tubing, with alveolar gas nearest the patient. If the tidal volume is large, some alveolar gas may enter the bag (28).

At the start of inspiration (Fig. 7.4B), exhaled gases in the tubing flow to the patient. Because alveolar gases occupy the space nearest the patient, they will be inhaled first. As the pressure in the system rises, the APL valve opens so that gas exits through the APL valve and flows to the patient. When all the exhaled gas has been driven from the tube, fresh gas fills the tubing (C). Some fresh gas enters the patient and some is vented through the valve. Thus, during controlled ventilation, there is considerable rebreathing of alveolar gases and venting of fresh gas. The composition of the

FIGURE 7.3. Magill system with spontaneous ventilation. (See text for details.) (Adapted with permission from Kain ML, Nunn JF. Fresh gas economies of the Magill circuit. Anesthesiology 1968;29:964–974.)

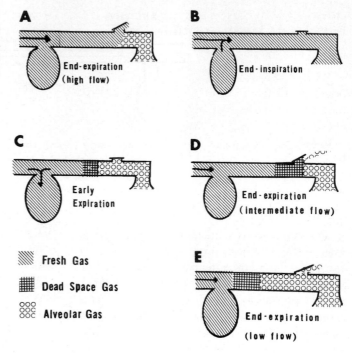

inspired gas mixture depends on the respiratory pattern (28, 29). The system becomes more efficient as the expiratory phase is prolonged. Most investigators believe that the Mapleson A is an illogical system to use for controlled ventilation.

During assisted ventilation, the Mapleson A system is somewhat less efficient than with spontaneous ventilation but more efficient than with controlled ventilation (30).

Hazards

A mechanical ventilator that vents excess gases should not be used with this system because the entire system then becomes dead space. The ventilators found on most anesthesia machines in the United States are unsuitable.

A case has been reported in which a Lack circuit was incorrectly manufactured so that the inner expiratory tube that should have been connected to the APL valve was connected to the reservoir bag (31). This converted the entire tubing into dead space.

Misassembly of the Lack system so that the fresh gas inlet was mounted adjacent to the APL valve rather than the reservoir bag has been reported (32). This would result in a substantial in-

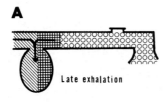

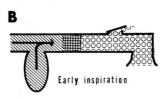

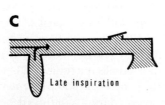

FIGURE 7.4. Magill system with controlled ventilation. (See text for details.)

crease in dead space. This problem has reportedly been corrected (33).

Tests of the Mapleson A Systems

The Mapleson A system is tested for leaks by occluding the patient end of the system, closing the APL valve, and pressurizing the system. Opening the APL valve will confirm proper functioning of that component. In addition, the user or a patient should breathe through the system.

The coaxial Lack system requires additional testing to confirm the integrity of the inner tube. One method is to attach a tracheal tube to the inner tubing at the patient end of the system (34). Blowing down the tube with the APL valve closed will produce movement of the bag if there is leakage between the two limbs. Another method is to occlude both limbs at the patient connection with the APL valve open, then squeeze the bag (35). If there is a leak in the inner limb, gas will escape through the APL valve and the bag will collapse.

MAPLESON B SYSTEM

The Mapleson B system is shown in Figure 7.1B. The fresh gas inlet and APL valve are both located near the patient port. The reservoir bag is at the distal end of the system, separated from the fresh gas inlet by corrugated tubing.

Techniques of Use

To use the Mapleson B system with spontaneous respiration, the APL valve is opened completely. Excess gas is vented through the valve during exhalation.

Assisted or controlled ventilation is accomplished by tightening the APL valve sufficiently to allow the lungs to be inflated. Excess gases are vented during inspiration.

Functional Analysis
Spontaneous Respiration

As the patient exhales, dead-space gas will pass down the corrugated tubing, along with fresh gas. At the end of exhalation, the tubing near the patient will be filled with fresh gas and some alveolar gas. When the bag reaches full capacity, the APL valve opens and fresh gas and alveolar gas will exit from the system. When the patient begins to inspire, the APL valve closes and the patient inhales

fresh gas and gas from the tubing. No gas will be inhaled from the bag if the volume of the tubing exceeds the tidal volume.

The amount of rebreathing will depend on the fresh gas flow. The fresh gas flow must be equal to peak inspiratory flow (normally 20 to 25 l/min) to avoid rebreathing (36). A fresh gas flow more than double minute volume has been recommended (1, 36), but flows as low as 0.8 to 1.2 times minute volume may be sufficient (28).

Controlled or Assisted Ventilation

The behavior of the Mapleson B system during controlled or assisted ventilation is similar to that of the Mapleson A, but it is slightly more efficient because fresh gas accumulates at the patient end of the tubing during the expiratory pause (28, 36). This system has variable performance during controlled ventilation because the composition of inspired gas is greatly influenced by the ventilatory pattern (28). A fresh gas flow of 2 to 2.5 times minute volume has been recommended (28, 36, 37).

MAPLESON C SYSTEM

The Mapleson C system is identical to the Mapleson B system except that the corrugated tubing is omitted (Fig. 7.1C).

Techniques of Use

Use of this system is similar to that described for the Mapleson B system.

Functional Analysis

The Mapleson C system behaves similarly to the Mapleson B system. With spontaneous ventilation, the Mapleson C system is almost as efficient as the Mapleson A when the expiratory pause is minimal but the Mapleson C system becomes less efficient as the expiratory pause increases (12, 38). A fresh gas flow of 2 times minute volume has been recommended. During controlled ventilation, a fresh gas flow of 2 to 2.5 times minute volume is recommended (28, 39).

MAPLESON D SYSTEM

The Mapleson D, E, and F systems all have a T piece near the patient and function similarly. The T piece is a three-way tubular connector with a patient connection port, a fresh gas port, and a port for connection to corrugated tubing. The Mapleson D system is popular because scavenging of excess gases is relatively easy and it is the most efficient of the Mapleson systems during controlled ventilation.

Configuration

Classic Form

The Mapleson D system is shown in Figures 7.1D and 7.5. A length of tubing connects the T piece at the patient end to the APL valve and the reservoir bag adjacent to it. The length of the tubing determines the distance the user can be from the patient but has minimal effects on ventilation (40).

The sensor or sampling site for a respiratory gas monitor may be placed between the bag and its mount, between the corrugated tubing and the T piece, or between the corrugated tubing and the APL valve. In adults, it may be placed between the T piece and the patient.

Bain Modification

The fresh gas supply tube runs coaxially inside the corrugated tubing in the Bain modification (41). The outer tubing of most commercially available versions of the Bain system is narrower than conventional corrugated tubing (28).

The Bain modification is available with a metal head with channels drilled into it (Fig. 7.6). This provides a fixed position for the reservoir bag and APL valve. Some heads also have a pressure manometer.

Positive end–expiratory pressure (PEEP) devices have been used with the Mapleson D system. A bidirectional PEEP valve may be placed between the corrugated tubing and the APL valve (42). This permits PEEP to be administered during manual or mechanical ventilation. However, some PEEP valves will close when a negative pressure is applied so spontaneous breathing is impossible with such a valve in the system. The PEEP valve may be placed in the hose leading to the anesthesia ventilator. In this location, it will be effective only during mechanical ventilation. A unidirectional PEEP valve can be used at the bag attachment site using special connectors and unidirectional valves (43). Such an arrangement allows application of PEEP during spontaneous or mechanical but not manual ventilation (42, 44, 45).

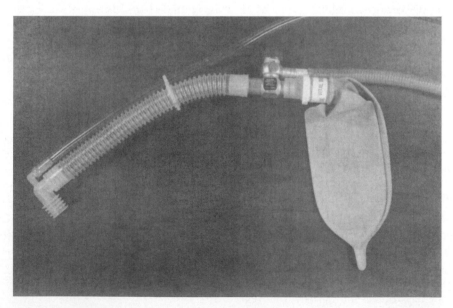

FIGURE 7.5. Mapleson D system. A tube leading to the scavenging system is attached to the adjustable pressure limiting (APL) valve.

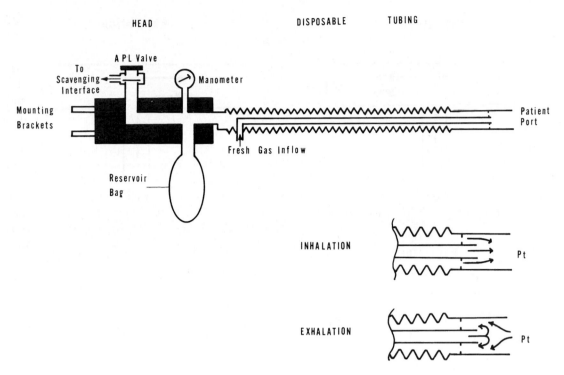

HEAD   DISPOSABLE   TUBING

FIGURE 7.6. Bain modification of the Mapleson D system. The fresh gas supply tube is inside the corrugated tubing. APL = adjustable pressure limiting.

Techniques of Use

For spontaneous respiration, the APL valve is left completely open and excess gases are vented during expiration. Manually controlled or assisted ventilation is performed by partially closing the APL valve and squeezing the bag. Excess gases are vented during inspiration. Mechanically controlled ventilation is achieved by connecting the hose of an anesthesia ventilator in place of the reservoir bag and closing the APL valve. Excess gases are vented through the ventilator.

Functional Analysis

Spontaneous Breathing

During exhalation (Fig. 7.7), exhaled gases mix with fresh gases and move through the corrugated tube toward the bag. After the bag has filled, gas exits via the APL valve. During the expiratory pause, fresh gas flows down the corrugated tubing, pushing exhaled gases in front of it.

During inspiration, the patient will inhale gas from the fresh gas inlet and the corrugated tubing. If the fresh gas flow is high, all the gas drawn from the corrugated tube will be fresh gas. If the fresh gas flow is low, some exhaled gas containing CO_2 will be inhaled. The ventilatory pattern will help to determine the amount of rebreathing (46). Factors that tend to decrease rebreathing include a high inspiratory:expiratory time ratio, a slow rise in inspiratory flow rate, a low flow rate during the last part of exhalation, and a long expiratory pause, with the expiratory pause having the most effect (12, 13, 38, 47–49).

As gas containing CO_2 is inhaled, the end-tidal CO_2 will rise. If the patient's spontaneous respiration then increases, the end-tidal CO_2 will fall while inspired CO_2 will increase (50). Provided rebreathing is not extreme, a normal end-tidal CO_2 can be achieved but only at the cost of increased work on the part of the patient. The end-tidal CO_2 tends to reach a plateau. At that point, no matter how hard the patient works, the end-

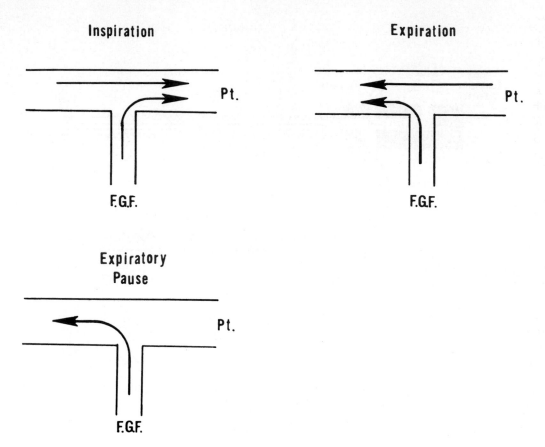

FIGURE 7.7. Functioning of the Mapleson D system. (See text for details.) Pt = patient; F.G.F. = fresh gas flow.

tidal CO_2 cannot be lowered further (51). If the patient's respiration is depressed, end-tidal CO_2 will rise further (50).

End-tidal CO_2 depends on both the ratio of minute volume and fresh gas flow and their absolute values (50, 52). If expired volume is greater than fresh gas flow, end-tidal CO_2 will be determined mainly by fresh gas flow. If fresh gas flow is greater than minute volume, end-tidal CO_2 will be determined mainly by minute volume. Recommendations for fresh gas flows based on body weight vary from 100 to 300 ml/kg per minute (15, 16, 21, 26, 27, 31, 53, 54). Most studies have recommended that the fresh gas flow be 1.5 to 3.0 times the minute volume (2, 16, 24, 26, 55–60), although others have held that a fresh gas flow approximately equal to total ventilation is adequate (61). In terms of body surface area,

fresh gas flows of 4000 to 4700 ml/m^2 per minute have been recommended (54, 62).

Controlled Ventilation

During exhalation, gases flow from the patient down the corrugated tubing. At the same time, fresh gas enters the tubing. During the expiratory pause, the fresh gas flow continues and pushes exhaled gases down the tubing.

During inspiration, fresh gas and gas from the corrugated tubing enter the patient. If the fresh gas flow is low, some exhaled gases may be inhaled. Prolonging the inspiratory time, increasing the respiratory rate, or adding an inspiratory plateau will increase rebreathing (48, 63, 64). Rebreathing can be decreased by allowing a long expiratory pause so that fresh gas can flush exhaled gases from the tubing.

When the fresh gas flow is high, there is little rebreathing and the end-tidal CO_2 is determined mainly by minute ventilation (65). Tidal volume, the volume of the expiratory limb, and expiratory resistance also affect it (63). When minute volume substantially exceeds the fresh gas flow, the fresh gas flow is the main factor controlling carbon dioxide elimination. The higher the fresh gas flow, the lower the end-tidal CO_2.

A series of curves can be constructed by combining fresh gas flow, minute volume, and arterial CO_2 levels (Fig. 7.8). An infinite number of combinations of fresh gas flow and minute volume can be used to produce a given $PaCO_2$. High fresh gas flows and low minute volumes or high minute volumes and low fresh gas flows or combinations in between can be used. In Figure 7.8, at the left, with a high fresh gas flow, the circuit is a nonrebreathing one and end-tidal CO_2 depends only on ventilation. Such high flows are uneconomical and associated with loss of heat and humidity. End-tidal CO_2 depends on minute volume, which is difficult to adjust accurately, especially in small patients (51). On the right is the region of hyperventilation and partial rebreathing. End-tidal CO_2 is regulated by adjusting the fresh gas flow. Lowering fresh gas flows (and increased rebreathing) is associated with higher humidity, less heat loss, and greater economy of fresh gases. Hyperventilation can be used without inducing hypocarbia. In-

dividual differences in dead space:tidal volume are minimized at high levels of minute volume (51). For these reasons, it is advantageous in most cases to aim for the right side of the graph. Exceptions might be patients with stiff lungs, poor cardiac performance, or hypovolemia.

Formulas to predict fresh gas flow requirements have been based on body weight (51, 66–72), minute volume (51, 73), and body surface area (74).

With assisted ventilation, the efficiency of the Mapleson D system is intermediate between that for spontaneous and controlled ventilation (30, 75) so slightly higher fresh gas flows should be used.

Hazards of the Bain System

Special hazards are associated with the Bain system. It should not be used with an intermittent-flow machine unless the machine is set for continuous flow (76, 77). The entire exhalation limb becomes dead space if the inner tube becomes detached from its connections at either end or develops a leak at the machine end (78–82, 83) or the fresh gas supply tube becomes kinked or twisted (84–86). Incorrect assembly, including adding standard tubing, can also cause this (87, 88).

An incident of improper assembly has been reported in which the large bore tubing was connected to the common gas outlet of the anesthesia

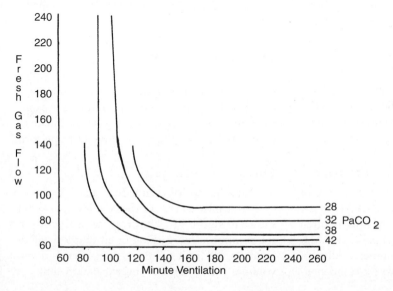

FIGURE **7.8.** Mapleson D system used with controlled ventilation. Each isopleth represents a constant level of $PaCO_2$. Note that essentially the same $PaCO_2$ is achieved for fresh gas flows from 100 to 240 ml/kg/min. (Adapted with permission from Froese AB. Anesthesia circuits for children [ASA Refresher Course]. Park Ridge, IL: ASA, 1978.)

machine and the small bore tube was attached to the APL valve (89). High inflation pressures were needed for ventilation.

A conventional wide-bore tubing may be attached to the system in departments that use a Bain and other circuits such as the Mapleson A (90, 91).

In some Bain systems the inner tubing is smaller and longer, causing an increase in flow resistance that may be excessive (92).

Testing Before Use

The Mapleson D System is tested for leaks by occluding the patient end, closing the APL valve, and pressurizing the system. The APL valve is then opened. The bag should deflate easily if the valve and scavenging system are working properly. In addition, either the user or a patient should breathe through the system to detect obstructions.

The Bain modification of the Mapleson D requires special testing to confirm the integrity of the inner tubing. This can be performed by setting a low flow of oxygen on a flowmeter and occluding the inner tube (with a finger or the barrel of a small syringe) at the patient end while observing the flowmeter indicator. If the inner tube is intact and correctly connected, the indicator will fall (82, 93–95). The integrity of the inner tube can also be confirmed by activating the oxygen flush and observing the bag (96). A Venturi effect caused by the high flow at the patient end will create a negative pressure in the outer exhalation tubing, and this will cause the bag to deflate. If the inner tube is not intact, this maneuver will cause the bag to inflate slightly. However, this test would not expose a system in which the inner tube is omitted or does not extend to the patient port or one that has holes at the patient end of the inner tube (97–99).

Continuous Positive Airway Pressure

During one-lung ventilation, application of continuous positive airway pressure (CPAP) to the up (nondependent, nonventilated) lung is often used to enhance oxygenation. A modified Mapleson D system attached to the lumen leading to that lung is often used. This allows the nondependent lung to be ventilated with intermittent positive pressure when desired.

A number of configurations have been described (100–111). One is shown in Figure 7.9. A source of gas is connected to the system. The APL valve is set so that the desired pressure, which is read from the manometer, is maintained. A PEEP valve may be added to function as a high-pressure relief device (112).

MAPLESON E (T PIECE) SYSTEM

Use of the Mapleson E system for anesthesia has decreased because of difficulties in scavenging excess gases, but it is still commonly used to administer oxygen or humidified gas to intubated patients breathing spontaneously.

The Mapleson E system is shown in Figure 7.1E. A length of tubing may be attached to the T piece to form a reservoir. The expiratory port may be enclosed in a chamber from which excess gases are evacuated.

The sensor or sampling site for the respiratory gas monitor may be placed between the expiratory port and the expiratory tubing. In larger patients, it may be placed between the T piece and the patient, but this should be avoided in small patients because it increases dead space.

Numerous modifications of the original T piece have been made. Many have the fresh gas inlet extending inside the body of the T piece toward the patient connection to minimize dead space. A pressure-limiting device may be added to the system.

Techniques of Use

For spontaneous ventilation, the expiratory limb is left open. Controlled ventilation can be performed by intermittently occluding the expiratory limb and letting the fresh gas flow inflate the lungs. Assisted respiration is difficult to perform.

Functional Analysis

The sequence of events during the respiratory cycle is similar to that of the Mapleson D system shown in Figure 7.7. The presence or absence and the amount of rebreathing or air dilution will depend on the fresh gas flow, the patient's minute volume, the volume of the exhalation limb, the

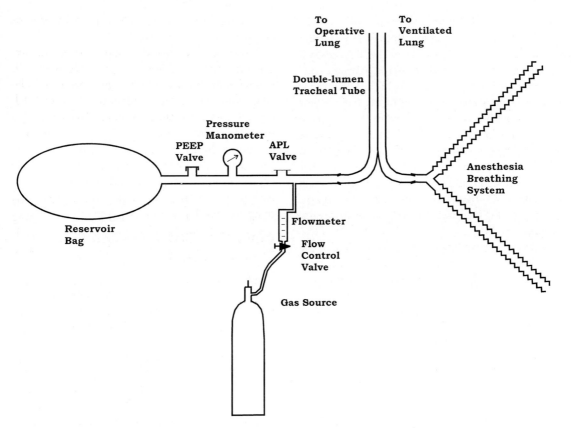

FIGURE 7.9. System for continuous positive airway pressure (CPAP). (See text for details.) APL = adjustable pressure limiting; PEEP = positive end–expiratory pressure.

type of ventilation (spontaneous or controlled), and the respiratory pattern.

Rebreathing

With spontaneous ventilation, if there is no exhalation limb, no rebreathing can occur. If there is an expiratory limb, the fresh gas flow needed to prevent rebreathing will be the same as for the Mapleson D system. During controlled ventilation, there can be no rebreathing because only fresh gas will inflate the lungs.

Air Dilution

No air dilution can occur during controlled ventilation. During spontaneous ventilation, air dilution cannot occur if the volume of the tubing is greater than the patient's tidal volume. If there is no expiratory limb or the volume of the limb is less than the patient's tidal volume, air dilution

can be prevented by providing a fresh gas flow that exceeds the peak inspiratory flow rate (normally 3 to 5 times the minute volume). A fresh gas flow of 2 × minute volume and a reservoir volume 33% of the tidal volume will prevent air dilution (113).

Hazard of Barotrauma with the T Piece System

Controlling ventilation by intermittently occluding the expiratory limb may lead to overinflation and barotrauma (114). This is particularly a danger with this system because of the following: the user does not have the "feel" of inflation that he or she has with a system containing a bag, the pressure-buffering effect of the bag is absent, and there is no APL valve. To overcome this potential hazard, it has been recommended that a pressure-limiting device be placed in the system (115, 116).

MAPLESON F SYSTEM

The Mapleson F (Jackson-Rees or Rees system or Jackson-Rees modification of the T piece) system has a bag with a mechanism for venting excess gases on the tubing (Fig. 7.1F) (117). The mechanism is often a hole in the tail of the bag. It may be fitted with a device to prevent the bag from collapsing while at the same time allowing excess gases to escape. Alternately, the hole may be in the side of the bag so the user can place his or her finger over it. An anesthesia ventilator may be used in place of the bag (118). An adjustable pop-off valve may be included to provide overpressure protection (119).

Scavenging can be performed by enclosing the bag in a plastic chamber from which waste gases are suctioned (120) or by attaching various devices to the relief mechanism in the bag.

Techniques of Use

For spontaneous respiration, the relief mechanism is left fully open. For assisted or controlled respiration, the relief mechanism is occluded sufficiently to distend the bag. Respiration can then be controlled or assisted by squeezing the bag. Alternately, the hole in the bag can be occluded by the user's finger during inspiration. For mechanical ventilation, the bag is replaced by the hose from a ventilator.

Functional Analysis

The Mapleson F system functions much like the Mapleson D system. The flows required to prevent rebreathing during spontaneous and controlled respiration are the same as those required with the Mapleson D system. Two studies found higher carbon dioxide levels with manually than with mechanically-controlled ventilation (121, 122).

PEEP does not affect end-tidal carbon dioxide during controlled ventilation but causes an increase during spontaneous breathing when fresh gas flow is less than three × minute volume (123). PEEP should not be applied using an underwater seal (124).

Hazards

The hazards of the Mapleson F system are the same as those described for the Mapleson E system. Excessive pressure is less likely to develop because there is a bag in the system.

None of the above-described systems is ideal for every situation. Some systems are better for spontaneous breathing and others are more efficient with controlled ventilation. When comparing the systems during spontaneous ventilation, the relative order of merit is A, D, F, E (with an expiratory limb), C, and B. During controlled ventilation, the order becomes D, F, E (with an expiratory limb), B, C, and A. A number of combination systems have been introduced in an attempt to develop a universal system.

COMBINATION SYSTEMS
Humphrey ADE System
Description

The ADE system can be used in different configurations (125). In the A configuration, it is similar to the Lack variation of the Mapleson A system. In the D configuration, it resembles the Bain modification of the Mapleson D system. It also allows the APL valve to be bypassed in the D configuration so that it resembles the Mapleson E system.

The system is shown in Figure 7.10. It is available in coaxial and noncoaxial versions. It has two levers whose positions determine the functioning of the system. A self-locking mechanism prevents accidental displacement of either lever from its selected position. In the coaxial version, the expiratory tubing runs concentrically inside the inspiratory limb. In the noncoaxial version, the two tubes are held together by a metal bridge at the machine end.

The inspiratory limb consists of a fresh gas inlet, a reservoir bag with a lever, and a length of corrugated tubing that runs to the patient connection port. When the lever is vertical, gases can flow in and out of the bag. When the lever is horizontal, gas flow into the bag is blocked, making the inspiratory limb a simple tube.

The expiratory limb consists of a length of tubing running from the patient connection, an APL valve, a valve bypass outlet, and a lever that directs the flow of gases through either the APL valve or valve bypass outlet. When the lever is vertical, the gases pass through the APL valve. When it is hori-

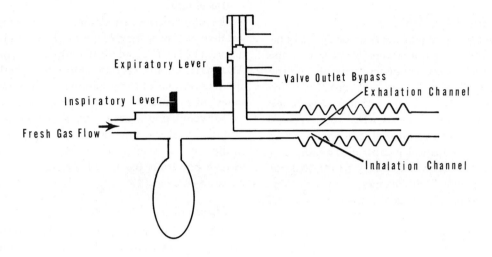

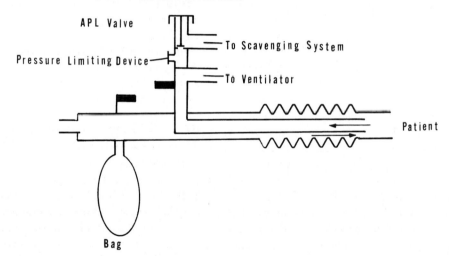

FIGURE **7.10.** Humphrey ADE system. The dual-lever coaxial version is shown. APL = adjustable pressure limiting.

zontal, the APL valve is isolated and gases flow through the valve-bypass outlet. Both outlets have 30-mm external diameters for attachment of scavenging devices. The valve-bypass outlet also has a 22-mm internal diameter for attachment of a hose leading to a ventilator or reservoir bag. A pressure-limiting device may be fitted near the APL valve (18).

A single-lever Humphrey ADE system has been developed (18). It is also available in coaxial and parallel forms. The lever controls a single rotating cylinder that passes through the inspiratory and expiratory limbs. When the lever is upright, the reservoir bag and APL valve are in circuit and the valve bypass outlet is excluded. When the lever is turned down, the bag and APL valve are excluded from the system and the valve bypass outlet is connected into the system.

Techniques of Use

To use the system in the A mode (for spontaneous ventilation), both levers (or the lever in the single-lever version) are placed vertically and the APL valve is left open (Fig. 7.10, top). The ventilator hose can be left connected and ready for use because it will be excluded when the levers are vertical. If manual ventilation is desired, the bag is squeezed and the leak is controlled by adjusting the APL valve. However, this system should not be used very long in this manner, because the Mapleson A system is inefficient with controlled ventilation.

To use the system in the D/E mode (for controlled ventilation), both levers are moved to the horizontal position (Fig. 7.10, bottom). For the single-lever version, the lever is turned downward. If mechanical ventilation is desired, the hose from a ventilator is attached to the valve-bypass outlet. Excess gases are scavenged through the ventilator. The APL valve does not need to be closed because it is bypassed.

To use manual ventilation in the D/E mode, a length of flexible tubing with a bag is attached to the valve bypass outlet. The bag is squeezed to ventilate the patient. Excess gases are eliminated by rotating the expiratory lever between vertical and horizontal with the APL valve fully open. Scavenging is easily accomplished (126).

To use spontaneous ventilation in the D/E mode, the expiratory lever is placed horizontal and the valve-bypass outlet is connected to the scavenging system.

Functional Analysis

A Mode

When placed in the A mode, the system functions like the Lack modification of the Mapleson A. Mean fresh gas flows ranging from 46 to 56 ml/kg per minute have been found to prevent rebreathing (17, 125, 127). If the APL valve is excluded by placing the expiratory lever horizontally, dead-space gas can escape without hindrance at the beginning of expiration so the system is less efficient and fresh gas flows need to be increased up to 33% (125). The ADE system in the A mode

with controlled ventilation is more efficient than the Magill (128) (but still inefficient).

D or E mode

For spontaneous ventilation, 33% of the fresh gas flow necessary for a Mapleson F system is required (125). The only difference between the ADE system in the D configuration and the Bain are the positions of the inspiratory and expiratory tubes. Most studies have found that when controlled ventilation is used with the system in the D mode, fresh gas flow requirements are similar to those of the Mapleson D (126, 129, 130), although one study has found the Bain system to be more efficient (131).

Hazards

With the dual-lever system, incorrect positioning or accidental displacement of the expiratory lever from a vertical to a horizontal position or obstruction of the expiratory port in the A mode may result in a dangerous rise in pressure (132, 133).

If a ventilator is used and the sensor for the low airway pressure monitor is in the inspiratory limb, the alarm may fail to provide a warning if there is a disconnection (134).

RESPIRATORY GAS MONITORING AND THE MAPLESON SYSTEMS

All the Mapleson systems except the A have the fresh gas inlet near the patient connection port. This may make it difficult to get a reliable sample of exhaled gases. One study examined four sampling sites (Fig. 7.11): at the junction of the breathing system and elbow connector, at the corner of the elbow connector, 2 cm distal in the elbow connector, and in the tracheal tube connector (135). It was found that if sampling were carried out at the two sites closest to the patient, values were accurate. Significant errors were noted when samples were taken from the corner of the elbow connector but only if a high fresh gas flow was used. Significant errors were noted when sampling was performed at the junction of the breathing system and elbow connector even if low fresh gas flows were used. A cannula that projects into the airway can be used to improve sampling (136).

In another study involving infants and children, sampling at the junction of the tracheal tube

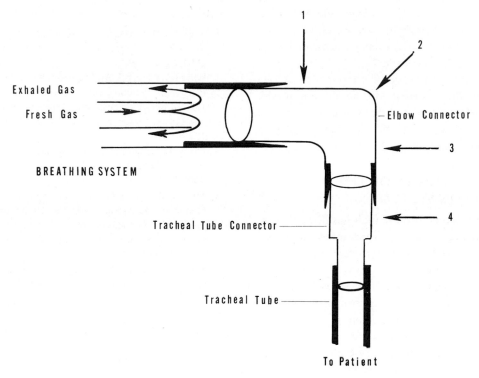

FIGURE 7.11. Respiratory gas sampling with a Mapleson system. Accurate values for expiratory concentrations can be obtained by sampling at sites 3 and 4. Sampling at site 2 will yield accurate values only if the fresh gas flow is not high. Sampling at site 1 will yield inaccurate values even at low fresh gas flows. (Adapted with permission from Gravenstein N, Lampotang S, Beneken JEW. Factors influencing capnography in the Bain circuit. J Clin Monit 1985;1:6–10.)

and breathing system resulted in falsely low end-tidal CO_2 values in patients weighing less than 8 kg (64). The accuracy of measurements can be improved by inserting a small heat and moisture exchanger between the breathing system and the tracheal tube connector (137). However, use of a device at this site will result in an increase in dead space (138) and may result in excessive resistance so that spontaneous respiration cannot be used (139).

ADVANTAGES OF THE MAPLESON SYSTEMS

1) The equipment is simple, inexpensive, and rugged. With the exception of the APL valve, there are no moving parts. The components are easy to disassemble and can be disinfected or sterilized in a variety of ways.

2) The systems provide a buffering effect so that variations in minute volume affect end-tidal CO_2 less than in a circle system.
3) Rebreathing will result in retention of heat and moisture. In coaxial systems (Lack, Bain, Humphrey ADE), the inspiratory limb is heated by the warm exhaled gas in the coaxial expiratory tubing.
4) Resistance is usually within the recommended ranges at flows likely to be experienced in normal clinical practice (140–143). A commonly held view is that the work of breathing during spontaneous ventilation is significantly less with these systems than with the circle system. However, studies indicate this is not always the case (144–147). The work of breathing will be increased if the APL valve is not oriented properly (145).

5) These systems are lightweight and not bulky. They are not likely to cause excessive drag on the mask or tracheal tube, facial distortion, or accidental extubation.

6) They are easy to position conveniently. A long Mapleson D system with an aluminum APL valve may be used to ventilate a patient undergoing magnetic resonance imaging (MRI) (148).

DISADVANTAGES OF THE MAPLESON SYSTEMS

1) These systems require high gas flows that result in higher costs, increased atmospheric pollution, and difficulties in assessment of spontaneous ventilation.

2) The optimal fresh gas flow may be difficult to determine. It is necessary to change the flow when changing from spontaneous to controlled ventilation or vice versa.

3) Anything that causes the fresh gas flow to be lowered presents a hazard because dangerous rebreathing may occur. This has been reported with emptying of a nitrous oxide tank (149), loss of gas through a loose vaporizer filler cap (150, 151), and a leak in a humidification device (152).

4) An increase in dead space will occur if any components (such as a respiratory gas monitor or heat and moisture exchanger [HME]) is placed between the fresh gas inlet and the patient connection port. This can result in dangerous rebreathing (138).

5) In the Mapleson A, B, and C systems, the APL valve is located close to the patient where it may be inaccessible to the user. In addition, scavenging is awkward. This disadvantage can be overcome by using the Lack modification of the Mapleson A.

6) The Mapleson E and F systems are difficult to scavenge, and air dilution can occur with the Mapleson E system.

7) Mapleson systems are not suitable for patients with malignant hyperthermia because it may not be possible to increase the fresh gas flow enough to remove the increased carbon dioxide load (153).

REFERENCES

1. Mapleson WW. The elimination of rebreathing in various semiclosed anaesthetic systems. Br J Anaesth 1954;26:323–332.

2. Willis BA, Pender JWM, Mapleson WW. Rebreathing in a T-piece: volunteer and theoretical studies of the Jackson-Rees modification of Ayre's T-piece during spontaneous respiration. Br J Anaesth 1975;47:1239–1246.

3. Ooi R, Lack A, Soni N, et al. The parallel Lack anaesthetic breathing system. Anaesthesia 1993;48:409–414.

4. Miller DM, Palm A. Comparison in spontaneous ventilation of the Maxima with the Humphrey ADE breathing system and between four methods for detecting rebreathing. Anaesthesia and Intensive Care 1995;23:296–301.

5. Barrie JR, Beatty PCW. Rebreathing and semiclosed anaesthetic breathing systems. Anaesthesia 1992;48:86–87.

6. Soni N, Ooi R. Fresh gas flow requirements during spontaneous ventilation: fresh gas flow to total ventilation ratio or ml kg^{-1} min^{-1}? Br J Anaesth 1993;71:796–799.

7. Bowie JR, Knox P, Downs JB, et al. Rebreathing improves accuracy of ventilatory monitoring. Journal of Clinical Monitoring 1995;11:354–357.

8. Lack JA. Pollution control by co-axial circuits. Anaesthesia 1976;31:561–562.

9. Lack JA. Theatre pollution control. Anaesthesia 1976;31:259–262.

10. Robinson DA, Lack JA. The Lack parallel breathing system. Anaesthesia 1985;40:1236–1237.

11. Kain ML, Nunn JF. Fresh gas economies of the Magill circuit. Anesthesiology 1968;29:964–974.

12. Cook LB. Respiratory pattern and rebreathing in the Mapleson A, C and D breathing systems with spontaneous ventilation. A theory. Anaesthesia 1996;51:371–385.

13. Jonsson LO, Zetterstrom H. Influence of the respiratory flow pattern on rebreathing in Mapleson A and D circuits. Acta Anaesthesiol Scand 1987;31:174–178.

14. Cook LB. The importance of the expiratory pause. Comparison of the Mapleson A, C and D breathing system using a lung model. Anaesthesia 1996;51:453–460.

15. Humphrey D. The Lack, Magill and Bain anaesthetic breathing systems: a direct comparison in spontaneously-breathing anesthetized adults. J R Soc Med 1982;75:513–524.

16. Alexander JP. Clinical comparison of the Bain and Magill Anaesthetic systems during spontaneous respiration. Br J Anaesth 1982;54:1031–1036.

17. Dixon J, Charabarti MK, Morgan M. An assessment of the Humphrey ADE anaesthetic system in the Mapleson A mode during spontaneous ventilation. Anaesthesia 1984;39:593–596.

18. Humphrey D, Brock-Utne JG, Downing JW. Single lever Humphrey A.D.E. low flow universal anaesthetic breathing system. Canadian Anaesthetists Society Journal 1986;33:698–709.

19. Millar SW, Barnes PK, Soni N. Comparison of the Magill and Lack anaesthetic breathing systems in anaesthetized patients. Br J Anaesth 1987;59:930P.

20. Millar SW, Barnes PK, Soni N, et al. Comparison of the Magill and Lack anaesthetic breathing systems in anaesthetized patients. Br J Anaesth 1989;62:153–158.

21. Ungerer MJ. A comparison between the Bain and Magill anaesthetic systems during spontaneous breathing. Canadian Anaesthetists Society Journal 1978;25:122–124.

22. Soni N, Ooi R, Pattison J. Rebreathing in the Magill breathing system. Br J Anaesth 1992;69:215P–216P.

23. Ooi R, Pattison J, Soni N. Parallel Lack breathing system: fresh gas flow requirements during spontaneous ventilation. Br J Anaesth 1992;69:216P.

24. Chan ASH, Bruce WE, Soni N. A comparison of anaesthetic breathing systems during spontaneous ventilation. An in-vitro study using a lung model. Anaesthesia 1989;44:194–199.

25. Miller DM, Couper JL. Comparison of the fresh gas flow requirements and resistance of the preferential flow system with those of the Magill system. Br J Anaesth 1983;55:569–574.

26. Jonsson LO, Zetterstrom H. Fresh gas flow in coaxial Mapleson A and D circuits during spontaneous breathing. Acta Anaesthesiol Scand 1986;30:588–593.

27. Jonsson IO, Johansson SLG, Zetterstrom H. Rebreathing and ventilatory response to different fresh gas flows in the Bain and Lack systems. Acta Anaesthesiol Scand 1987;31:179–186.

28. Conway CM. Anaesthetic breathing systems. Br J Anaesth 1985;57:649–657.

29. Tyler CKG, Barnes PK, Rafferty MP. Controlled ventilation with a Mapleson A (Magill) breathing system: reassessment using a lung model. Br J Anaesth 1989;62:462–466.

30. Joshi S, Walker A, Rice CP, et al. In vitro performance of three semiclosed anesthetic breathing systems during assisted ventilation. Anesthesiology 1995;83:A472.

31. Muir J, Davidson-Lamb R. Apparatus failure; cause for concern. Br J Anaesth 1980;52:705–706.

32. Jones PL. Hazard: single-use parallel Lack breathing system. Anaesthesia 1991;46:316–317.

33. Williams SK. Hazard: single-use parallel Lack breathing system. A reply. Anaesthesia 1991;46:317.

34. Furst B, Laffey DA. An alternative test for the Lack system. Anaesthesia 1984;39:834.

35. Martin LVH, McKeown DW. An alternative test for the Lack system. Anaesthesia 1985;40:80–81.

36. Sykes MK. Rebreathing circuits. Br J Anaesth 1968;40:666–674.

37. Christensen KN, Thomsen A, Hansen OL, et al. Flow requirements in the Hafnia modification of the Mapleson circuits during spontaneous respiration. Acta Anaesthesiol Scand 1978;22:27–32.

38. Cook LB. The importance of the expiratory pause. Comparison of the Mapleson A, C and D breathing system using a lung model. Anaesthesia 1996;51:453–460.

39. Christensen KN. The flow requirement in a nonpolluting Mapleson C circuit. Acta Anaesthesiol Scand 1976;20:307–312.

40. Jackson E, Tan S, Yarwood G, et al. Increasing the length of the expiratory limb of the Ayre's T-piece: implications for remote mechanical ventilation in infants and young children. Br J Anaesth 1994;73:154–156.

41. Bain JA, Spoerel WE. A streamlined anaesthetic system. Canadian Anaesthetists Society Journal 1972;19:426–435.

42. Arandia HY, Byles PH. PEEP and the Bain circuit. Canadian Anaesthetists Society Journal 1981;28:467–470.

43. Erceg GW. PEEP for the Bain breathing circuit. Anesthesiology 1979;50:542–543.

44. Arandia HY. Bain PEEP. Anesthesiology 1980;52:193–194.

45. Erceg GW. Bain PEEP. A reply. Anesthesiology 1980;52:194.

46. Byrick RJ, Janssen EG. Respiratory waveform and rebreathing in T-piece circuits: a comparison of enflurane and halothane waveforms. Anesthesiology 1980;53:371–378.

47. Dorrington KL, Lehane JR. Minimum fresh gas flow requirements of anaesthetic breathing systems during spontaneous ventilation: a graphical approach. Anaesthesia 1987;42:732–737.

48. Gabrielsen J, van den Berg JT, Dirksen H, et al. Effect of inspiration-expiration ratio on rebreathing with the Mapleson D system (Bain's modification; coaxial system). Acta Anaesthesiol Scand 1980;24:336–338.

49. Stenqvist O, Sonander H. Rebreathing characteristics of the Bain circuit. An experimental and theoretical study. Br J Anaesth 1984;56:303–310.

50. Spoerel WE. Rebreathing and end-tidal CO_2 during spontaneous breathing with the Bain circuit. Canadian Anaesthetists Society Journal 1983;30: 148–154.

51. Froese AB. Anesthesia circuits for children (ASA Refresher Course). Park Ridge, IL: ASA, 1978.

52. Goodwin K. Letter to the editor. Canadian Anaesthetists Society Journal 1976;23:675.

53. Spoerel WE, Aitkieh RR, Bain JA. Spontaneous respiration with the Bain breathing circuit. Canadian Anaesthetists Society Journal 1978;25:30–35.

54. Soliman MG, Laberge R. The use of the Bain circuit in spontaneously breathing paediatric patients. Canadian Anaesthetists Society Journal 1978;25: 276–281.

55. Nott MR, Walters FJM, Norman J. The Lack and Bain systems in spontaneous respiration. Anaesthesia and Intensive Care 1982;10:333–339.

56. Dean SE, Keenan RL. Spontaneous breathing with a T-piece circuit. Anesthesiology 1982;56:449–452.

57. Conway CM, Seeley HF, Barnes PK. Spontaneous ventilation with the Bain anaesthetic system. Br J Anaesth 1977;49:1245–1249.

58. Lindahl SGE, Charlton AJ, Hatch DJ. Accuracy of prediction of fresh gas flow requirements during spontaneous breathing with the T-piece. Eur J Anaesthiol 1984;1:269–274.

59. Lindahl SGE, Charlton AJ, Hatch DJ. Ventilatory responses to rebreathing and carbon dioxide inhalation during anaesthesia in children. Br J Anaesth 1985;57:1188–1196.

60. Miller DM. Early detection of "rebreathing" in afferent and efferent reservoir breathing systems using capnography. Br J Anaesth 1990;64:251–255.

61. Meakin G, Coates AL. An evaluation of rebreathing with the Bain system during anaesthesia with spontaneous ventilation. Br J Anaesth 1983;55:487–495.

62. Rayburn RL. Pediatric anaesthesia circuits. (ASA Refresher Course). Park Ridge, IL: ASA, 1981.

63. Lovich MA, Simon BA, Venegas JG, et al. A mass balance model for the Mapleson D anaesthesia breathing system. Can J Anaesth 40:554–567.

64. Badgwell JM, Heavner JE, May WS, et al. End-tidal PCO_2 monitoring in infants and children ventilated with either a partial-rebreathing or a non-rebreathing circuit. Anesthesiology 1987;56:405–410.

65. Bain JA, Spoerel WE. Flow requirements for a modified Mapleson D system during controlled ventilation. Canadian Anaesthetists Society Journal 1973; 20:629–636.

66. Bain JA, Spoerel WE. Prediction of arterial carbon dioxide tension during controlled ventilation with a modified Mapleson D system. Canadian Anaesthetists Society Journal 1975;22:34–38.

67. Bain JA, Spoerel WE. Carbon dioxide output and elimination in children under anaesthesia. Canadian Anaesthetists Society Journal 1977;24:533–539.

68. Chu YK, Rah KH, Boyan CP. Is the Bain breathing circuit the future anaesthesia system? An evaluation. Anesth Analg 1977;56:84–87.

69. Henville JD, Adams AP. The Bain anaesthetic system: an assessment during controlled ventilation. Anaesthesia 1976;31:247–256.

70. Kneeshaw JD, Harvey P, Thomas TA. A method for producing normocarbia during general anaesthesia for caesarean section. Anaesthesia. 1984;39: 922–925.

71. Rose DK, Froese AB. The regulation of $PaCO_2$ during controlled ventilation of children with a T-piece. Canadian Anaesthetists Society Journal 1979;26: 104–113.

72. Savva D. Controlled ventilation with the Bain coaxial system. A rationalisation of gender-related minute volume requirements and carbon dioxide replacement therapy. Anaesthesia 1993;48:1072–1074.

73. Badgwell JM, Wolf AR, McEvedy BAB, et al. Fresh gas formulae do not accurately predict end-tidal PCO_2 in paediatric patients. Can J Anaesth 1988;35: 581–586.

74. Rayburn RL, Graves SA. A new concept in controlled ventilation of children with the Bain anesthetic circuit. Anesthesiology 1978;48:250–253.

75. Shah NK, Bedford RF. Conservation of anesthetic gases using the Bain circuit. Anesthesiology 1987;67: A212.

76. Padfield A, Perks ER. Misuse of coaxial circuits. Anaesthesia 1978;33:77–78.

77. Sugg BR. Misuse of coaxial circuits. A reply. Anaesthesia 1978;33:78.

78. Breen M. Letter to the editor. Canadian Anaesthetists Society Journal 1975;22:247.

79. Hannallah R, Rosales JK. A hazard connected with reuse of the Bain's circuit: a case report. Canadian Anaesthetists Society Journal 1974;21:511–513.

80. Wildsmith JAW, Grubb DJ. Defective and misused co-axial circuits. Anaesthesia 1977;32:293.

81. Williams AR, Hasselt GV. Adequacy of preoperative safety checks of the Bain breathing system. Br J Anaesth 1992;68:637.

82. Jackson IJB. Tests for co-axial systems. Anaesthesia 1988;43:1060–1061.

83. Bell CT, Ball AJ. An unusual communication? Anaesthesia 1994;49:830.

84. Goresky GV. Bain circuit delivery tube obstructions. Can J Anaesth 1990;37:385.

85. Inglis MS. Torsion of the inner tube. Br J Anaesth 1980;52:705.

86. Mansell WH. Bain circuit: the hazard of the hidden tube. Canadian Anaesthetists Society Journal 1976; 23:227.

87. Paterson JG, Vanhooydonk V. A hazard associated with improper connection of the Bain breathing circuit. Canadian Anaesthetists Society Journal 1975; 22:373–377.

88. Robinson DN. Hazardous modification of Bain breathing attachment. Can J Anaesth 1992;39: 515–516.

89. Pfitzner J. Apparatus misconnection: Mapleson D systems and scavenging. Anaesthesia and Intensive Care 1981;9:396–397.

90. Boyd CH. Another hazard of coaxial circuits. Anaesthesia 1977;32:675.

91. Robinson DN. Hazardous modification of Bain breathing attachment. Can J Anaesth 1992;39: 515–516.

92. Sinclair A, Van Bergen J. Flow resistance of coaxial breathing systems: investigation of a circuit disconnect. Can J Anaesth 1992;39:90–94.

93. Foex P, Crampton-Smith A. A test for coaxial circuits. Anaesthesia 1977;32:294.

94. Ghani GA. Safety check for the Bain circuit. Canadian Anaesthetists Society Journal 1984;31:487.

95. Jackson IJB. Tests for co-axial systems. Anaesthesia 1988;43:1060–1061.

96. Pethick SL. Correspondence. Canadian Anaesthetists Society Journal 1975;22:115.

97. Beauprie IG, Clark AG, Keith IC, et al. Pre-use testing of coaxial circuits: the perils of Pethick. Can J Anaesth 1990;37:S103.

98. Peterson WC. Bain circuit. Canadian Anaesthetists Society Journal 1978;25:532.

99. Robinson S, Fisher DM. Safety check for the CPRAM circuit. Anesthesiology 1983;59:488–489.

100. Baraka A, Sibai AN, Muallem M, et al. CPAP oxygenation during one-lung ventilation using an underwater seal assembly. Anesthesiology 1986;65:102–103.

101. Brown DL, Davis RF. A simple device for oxygen insufflation with continuous positive airway pressure during one-lung ventilation. Anesthesiology 1984; 61:481–482.

102. Benumof JL, Gaughan S, Ozaki GT. Operative lung constant positive airway pressure with the Univent blocker tube. Anesth Analg 1992;74:406–410.

103. Cook CE, Wilson R. Dangers of using an improvised underwater seal for CPAP oxygenation during one-lung ventilation. Anesthesiology 1987;66:707–708.

104. Hughes SA, Benumof JL. Operative lung continuous positive pressure to minimize FIO_2 one-lung ventilation. Anesth Analg 1990;71:92–95.

105. Galloway DW, Howler BMR. A simple CPAP system during one-lung anaesthesia. Anaesthesia 1988;43: 708–709.

106. Hannenberg AA, Satwicz PR, Dienes RS, et al. A device for applying CPAP to the nonventilated upper lung during one-lung ventilation. II. Anesthesiology 1984;60:254–255.

107. Lyons TE. A simplified method of CPAP delivery to the nonventilated lung during unilateral pulmonary ventilation. Anesthesiology 1984;61:216–217.

108. Shah JB, Skerman JH, Till WJ, et al. Improving the efficacy of a CPAP system during one-lung anesthesia. Anesth Analg 1988;67:715–716.

109. Slinger P, Triolet W, Chang M. CPAP circuit for nonventilated lung during thoracic surgery. Can J Anaesth 1987;34:654–655.

110. Scheller MS, Varvel JR. CPAP oxygenation during one-lung ventilation using a Bain circuit. Anesthesiology 1987;66:708–709.

111. Thiagarajah S, Job C, Rao A. A device for applying CPAP to the nonventilated upper lung during one–lung ventilation. I. Anesthesiology 1984;60: 253–254.

112. Hensley FA, Martin F, Skeehan TM. High pressure pop-off safety device when using the Bain circuit for CPAP oxygenation during one-lung ventilation. Anesthesiology 1987;67:863.

113. Naunton A. The minimum reservoir capacity necessary to avoid air-dilution. Br J Anaesth 1985;57: 803–806.

114. Arens JF. A hazard in the use of an Ayre T-Piece. Anesth Analg 1971;50:943–946.

115. Inkster JS. Kinked breathing systems. Anaesthesia 1990;45:173.

116. Ramanathan S, Chalon J, Turndorf H. A safety valve for the pediatric Rees system. Anesth Analg 1976;53: 741–743.

117. Rees GJ. Anaesthesia in the newborn. BMJ 1950;2: 1419–1422.

118. Hatch DJ, Yates AP, Lindahl SGE. Flow requirements and rebreathing during mechanically controlled ventilation in a T-piece (Mapleson E) system. Br J Anaesth 1987;59:1533–1540.

119. Anonymous. Mislocated pop-off valve can produce airway overpressure in manual resuscitator breathing circuits. Health Devices 1996;25:212–214.

120. Chan MSH, Kong AS. T-piece scavenging—the double bag system. Anaesthesia 1993;48:647.

121. Akkineni S, Patel KP, Bennett EJ, et al. Fresh gas flow to limit $PaCO_2$ in T and circle systems without CO_2 absorption. Anesthesiology Review 1977;4: 33–37.

122. Kuwabara S, McCaughey TJ. Artificial ventilation in infants and young children using a new ventilator

with the T-piece. Canadian Anaesthetists Society Journal 1966;13:576–584.

123. Dobbinson TL, Fawcett ER, Bolton DPG. The effects of positive end–expiratory pressure on rebreathing and gas dilution in the Ayre's T-piece system—laboratory study. Anaesthesia and Intensive Care 1978;6:19–25.

124. Lawrence JC. PEEP and the Ayre's T-piece system. Anaesthesia and Intensive Care 1978;6:359.

125. Humphrey D. A new anaesthetic breathing system combining Mapleson A, D, and E principles. A simple apparatus for low flow universal use without carbon dioxide absorption. Anaesthesia 1983;38:361–372.

126. Humphrey D. Eliminating pollution in paediatric and adult anaesthesia. Anaesthesia 1992;47:640–641.

127. Shulman MS, Brodsky JB. The A.D.E. system—a new anesthetic breathing system. Anesth Analg 1984; 63:273.

128. Humphrey D, Brock-Utne JG. Manual ventilation with the Humphrey ADE system. Can J Anaesth 1987;34:S128–S129.

129. Humphrey D, Brock-Utne JG, Downing JW. Single lever Humphrey A.D.E. low flow universal anaesthesia breathing system. Part II: comparison with Bain system in anaesthetized adults during controlled ventilation. Canadian Anaesthetists Society Journal 1986;33:710–718.

130. Criswell J, McKenzie S, Day S, et al. The Bain, ADE, and enclosed Magill breathing systems. A comparative study during controlled ventilation. Anaesthesia 1990;45:113–117.

131. Shah NK, Loughlin CJ, Bedford RF. Comparison of the Bain and the ADE systems during controlled ventilation in adults. Br J Anaesth 1989;62:150–152.

132. Taylor MB. A suggestion. Anaesthesia 1983;38:906.

133. Newton N, Cundy JM. The ultimate goal? Anaesthesia 1983;38:906–907.

134. Murphy PJ, Rabey PG. The Humphrey ADE breathing system and ventilator alarms. Anaesthesia 1991; 46:1000.

135. Gravenstein N, Lampotang S, Beneken JEW. Factors influencing capnography in the Bain circuit. Journal of Clinical Monitoring 1985;1:6–10.

136. Ball AJ. Paediatric capnography. Anaesthesia 1995; 50:833–834.

137. Brock-Utne JC, Humphrey D. Multipurpose anaesthetic breathing systems—the ultimate goal. Acta Anaesthesiol Scand Suppl 1985;80:67.

138. Fox LM. Equipment dead space in paediatric breathing systems. Anaesthesia 1992;47:1101–1102.

139. Goddard JM, Bennett HR. Filters and Ayre's T-piece. Anaesthesia 1996;51:605.

140. Martin DG, Kong KL, Lewis GTR. Resistance to airflow in anaesthetic breathing systems. Br J Anaesth 1989;62:456–461.

141. Ooi R, Pattison J, Soni N. The additional work of breathing imposed by Mapleson A systems. Anaesthesia 1993;48:599–603.

142. Sinclair A, Ban Bergen J. Flow resistance of coaxial breathing systems: investigation of a circuit disconnect. Can J Anaesth 1992;39:90–94.

143. Blumgart CH, Hargrave SA. Modified parallel 'Lack' breathing system for use in dental anaesthesia. Anaesthesia 1992;47:993–995.

144. Conterato JP, Lindahl GE, Meyer DM, et al. Assessment of spontaneous ventilation in anesthetized children with use of a pediatric circle or a Jackson-Rees system. Anesth Analg 1989;69:484–490.

145. Gravenstein N, Gallagher RC. External flow-resistive, circuit-related work of breathing: Bain vs circle. Anesthesiology 1985;63:A183.

146. Kay B, Beatty PCW, Healy TEJ, et al. Change in the work of breathing imposed by five anesthetic breathing systems. Br J Anaesth 1983;55:1239–1247.

147. Rasch DK, Bunegin L, Ledbetter, et al. Comparison of circle absorber and Jackson-Rees systems for paediatric anaesthesia. Can J Anaesth 1988;35:25–30.

148. Boutros A, Pavlicek W. Anesthesia for magnetic resonance imaging. Anesth Analg 1987;66:367.

149. Dunn AJ. Empty tanks and Bain circuits. Canadian Anaesthetists Society Journal 1978;25:337.

150. Mullin RA. Letter to the editor. Canadian Anaesthetists Society Journal 1978;25:248–249.

151. Mullin RA. Bain circuit (a reply). Canadian Anaesthetists Society Journal 1979;26:239.

152. Nimocks JA, Modell JH, Perry PA. Carbon dioxide retention using a humidified "nonrebreathing" system. Anesth Analg 1975;54:271–273.

153. Rogers KH, Rose DK, Byrick RJ. Severe hypercarbia with a Bain breathing circuit during malignant hyperthermia reaction. Can J Anaesth 1987;34:652–653.

QUESTIONS

1. In which of the following is the fresh gas port most distant from the patient connection port?
   A. Mapleson A
   B. Mapleson B
   C. Mapleson C
   D. Mapleson D
   E. Mapleson E

2. Which of the following is most efficient during spontaneous ventilation?
   A. Mapleson A
   B. Mapleson B
   C. Mapleson C
   D. Mapleson D
   E. Mapleson E

3. Which of the following systems lacks a reservoir bag?
   A. Mapleson A
   B. Mapleson B
   C. Mapleson C
   D. Mapleson D
   E. Mapleson E

4. Which of the following is the most efficient during controlled ventilation?
   A. Mapleson A
   B. Mapleson B
   C. Mapleson C
   D. Mapleson D
   E. Mapleson E

5. Advantages of the Mapleson systems include all of the following except
   A. Buffering effect on end-tidal CO_2
   B. Simple, inexpensive equipment
   C. Useful in treating malignant hyperthermia
   D. Light weight
   E. Ease of disassembly

ANSWERS

1. A
2. A
3. E
4. D
5. C

CHAPTER
8

The Circle System

I. Components
  A. Carbon Dioxide Absorber
    1. Canisters
      a. Construction
      b. Size
      c. Pattern and Direction of Flow
    2. Housing
    3. Baffles
    4. Side Tube
    5. Bypass
  B. Carbon Dioxide Absorption
    1. Absorbents
      a. Soda Lime
        (1). Composition
        (2). Chemistry
        (3). Shape and Size of Granules
        (4). Hardness
      b. Barium Hydroxide Lime
        (1). Composition
        (2). Chemistry
        (3). Size and Shape
        (4). Hardness
    2. Absorbents and Anesthetic Agents
    3. Indicators
    4. Contents
      a. Granular Space
      b. Air Space
        (1). Void Space
        (2). Pore Space
    5. Storage and Handling of Absorbents
    6. Changing the Absorbent
      a. Carbon Dioxide in the Inspiratory Gas
      b. Indicator Color Change
      c. Heat in the Canister
  C. Unidirectional Valves
  D. Inspiratory and Expiratory Ports
  E. Y-piece
  F. Fresh Gas Inlet
  G. Adjustable Pressure Limiting Valve

  H. Pressure Gauge (Manometer)
  I. Breathing Tubes
  J. Reservoir Bag
  K. Bag/Ventilator Selector Switch
    1. Without Adjustable Pressure Limiting Valve
    2. With Adjustable Pressure Limiting Valve
    3. With Ventilator Interconnect
  L. Respiratory Gas Monitor Sensor or Connector
  M. Sensor or Connector for Airway Pressure Monitor
  N. Optional Equipment
    1. Positive End–Expiratory Pressure Valve
    2. Filters
    3. Heated Humidifier
    4. Respirometer

II. Arrangement of Components
  A. Objectives
  B. Consideration of Individual Components
    1. Fresh Gas Inlet
    2. Reservoir Bag
    3. Unidirectional Valves
    4. Adjustable Pressure Limiting Valve
    5. Filters
    6. Respiratory Gas Monitor Sensor or Connector
      a. Mainstream Devices
        (1). Oxygen Monitor
        (2). Mainstream CO_2 Monitor
      b. Sidestream Devices
    7. Respirometer
    8. Sensor or Connector for Airway Pressure Monitor
    9. Positive End–Expiratory Pressure Valve
    10. Pressure Manometer

III. Resistance and Work or Breathing in the Circle System

IV. Dead Space of the Circle System

V. Heat and Humidity

THE CIRCLE SYSTEM is so named because gases flow in a circular pathway through separate inspiratory and expiratory channels. The system prevents rebreathing of carbon dioxide by absorption but allows rebreathing of other exhaled gases. A United States standard and an international standard for breathing systems with particular emphasis on circle systems have been published (1, 2).

COMPONENTS

A typical circle absorption system is diagrammed in Figure 8.1. It contains a number of components.

Carbon Dioxide Absorber

The absorber is a heavy, bulky component that is usually attached to the anesthesia machine but may be a separate unit. An absorber assembly has an absorber and may include two ports for connection to breathing tubes, a fresh gas inlet, inspiratory and expiratory unidirectional valves, an adjustable pressure limiting (APL) valve, and a bag mount. Disposable absorbers and absorber assemblies are available.

Canisters

Construction

The canisters (carbon dioxide absorbent containers, chambers, units, or cartridges), which hold the absorbent, make up the main part of the absorber. The side walls are usually constructed of a transparent material. A screen at the bottom of each canister holds the absorbent in place. Modern absorbers use two canisters in apposition (Fig. 8.2). With fresh absorbent in both chambers, carbon dioxide is absorbed mostly in the upstream chamber. As that absorbent becomes exhausted, carbon dioxide will enter the downstream chamber where absorption will continue. Disposable canisters are available. They eliminate the need

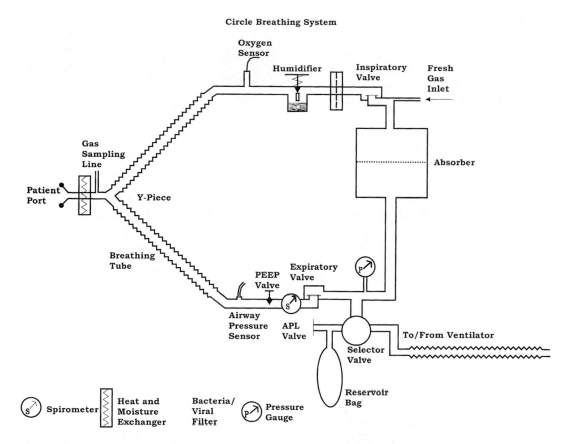

FIGURE 8.1. A commonly used arrangement of the circle system. Not all these components may be present in a given system. For example, a heat and moisture exchanger and a humidifier would not be used at the same time. APL = adjustable pressure limiting; PEEP = positive end–expiratory pressure.

for emptying and refilling but can be a source of obstruction if a label or wrap is not removed or an excessive number of holes are occluded (3, 4).

Size

Canisters of varying capacity have been used. Advantages of large canisters include better utilization of absorbent and longer intervals between absorbent changes. Use of a canister with a large cross-sectional area results in lower flows through it so that resistance and absorbent dust migration are reduced.

Pattern and Direction of Flow

The pattern of absorption within a correctly packed canister is shown in Figure 8.3. It makes no difference whether the gases enter at the top or bottom. The first absorption occurs at the inlet and along the sides. The tendency of gases to travel along the periphery of the canister is known as the wall effect.

Flow through the canister is pulsatile. The direction of flow during the respiratory cycle will depend on the location of other components of the circle system. In the configuration shown in Figure 8.1, with the reservoir bag upstream of the absorber and the fresh gas inlet downstream, gases upstream of the absorber move through it during inspiration. During the expiratory pause, fresh gases from the anesthesia machine will push gases retrograde through the absorber.

Housing

The head and base of the absorber are usually constructed of metal. Gaskets at the bottom and top fit against the interposed canisters. The housing (canister support) and canisters are tightened together by raising the base of the housing so that the upper canister seals against the upper gasket. Lowering the base creates a gap between the rim of the upper canister and the upper gasket.

Two methods have been employed to raise and lower the base. One uses a screw or wing nut. This often does not turn freely and is difficult to operate. Most of the newer absorbers have a lever-actuated cam (Fig. 8.4). The lever may be accidentally displaced (5, 6). To prevent this, a lever that points toward the front of the absorber can often be altered to face upward and toward the side (Fig. 8.4) or toward the rear of the absorber, making it less susceptible to inadvertent displacement.

There are spaces at the top and bottom of the absorber for incoming gases to disperse before passing through the absorbent or for outgoing

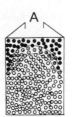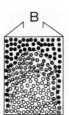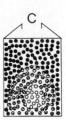

FIGURE 8.3. Pattern of carbon dioxide absorption in a canister. Darkened circles represent exhausted absorbent. It makes no difference whether the gases enter at the top or bottom of the absorber. **A,** After limited use; absorption has occurred primarily at the inlet and to a lesser extent along the sides. **B,** After extensive use; the granules at the inlet and along the sides are exhausted. **C,** Carbon dioxide is filtering through the canister; in the distal third of the canister a spot remains where the granules are still capable of absorbing carbon dioxide. (Adapted with permission from Adriani J, Rovenstein EA. Experimental studies on carbon dioxide absorbers for anesthesia. Anesthesiology 1941;2:10.)

gases to collect before passing on through the circle. This promotes even distribution of flow through the absorber (7). In the base, this space allows dust and condensed water to accumulate (Figs. 8.2 and 8.4). This helps to prevent caking in the bottom layers of absorbent. Some bases have a means of draining water from the bottom. Care should be taken that this water does not contact skin because it will be highly alkaline.

Baffles

Baffles, annular rings that serve to direct gas flow toward the central part of the canister, are frequently placed at the top and bottom of the absorber. Baffles increase the path of travel for gases along the sides and help to compensate for the reduced resistance to flow along the walls of the canister (7).

Side Tube

A tube external to the canisters conducts gases either to or from the bottom of the absorber (Fig. 8.2). The main flow of gases passing through the absorber will be in the opposite direction to that of gases passing through the side tube.

Bypass

An absorber may be equipped with a bypass (cutout control, rebreathing valve, bypass channel

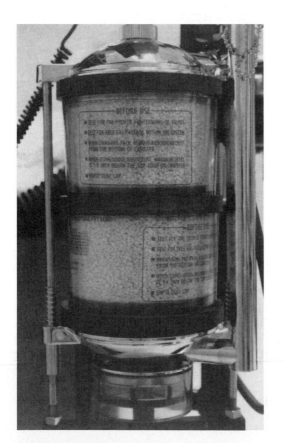

FIGURE 8.2. Absorber with two canisters, a dust/moisture trap at the bottom and a side tube at the right.

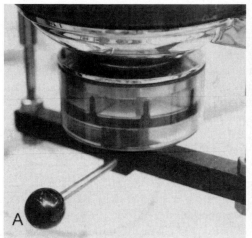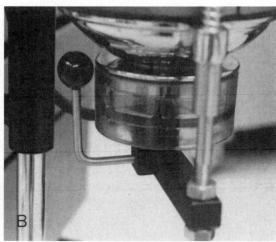

FIGURE 8.4.   The lever connects to a geared arrangement at the base of the absorber and is used to lower or raise the bottom. **A,** The lever projects straight out, making it susceptible to accidental displacement. **B,** The lever is bent to prevent accidental displacement. Note the dust and moisture trap at the bottom of the absorber.

or control) controlled by a manually operated valve. Bypasses are no longer available in the United States but are used in other countries. A complete bypass diverts all of the gases entering the absorber to the outlet without passing through the absorbent (8). A partial bypass allows a portion of the incoming gas to bypass the absorbent. A complete bypass allows the absorbent to be changed during a case, whereas a partial bypass does not because there would be a loss of integrity of the circuit (9).

A hazard with a bypass is that if it is in the bypass position and the fresh gas flow is low, carbon dioxide accumulation can occur. On one absorber, the bypass is located on the side of the absorber opposite from where the operator normally stands or sits and is not easily seen (Fig. 8.5).

Carbon Dioxide Absorption

Absorbents

Carbon dioxide absorption (neutralization) employs the general principle of a base neutralizing an acid. The acid is carbonic acid formed by the reaction of carbon dioxide with water. The base is the hydroxide of an alkali or alkaline earth metal. The end products of the reaction are water and a carbonate.

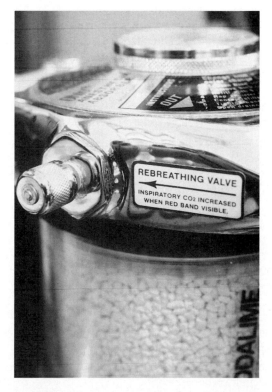

FIGURE 8.5. Partial bypass at side of the absorber. This is located on the opposite side of the absorber from where the user normally stands and is easily overlooked.

There are two absorbents in common use today: soda lime and barium hydroxide lime (baralyme).

Soda Lime

Composition. The composition of soda lime has varied over the years. Most soda lime used today is the "wet" or "high-moisture" variety. By weight it is 4% sodium hydroxide, 1% potassium hydroxide, 14 to 19% water, and enough calcium hydroxide to make 100%. Small amounts of silica and kieselguhr are added to give hardness (and thus minimize the formation of dust), and indicators are added to allow assessment of absorption capacity.

Water is present as a thin film on the granule surface (10). Moisture is essential because the reactions take place between ions that exist only in the presence of water. Absorbents with low moisture exhaust rapidly. On the other hand, those with high moisture have a slower rate of absorption, stickiness, and increased resistance (11). The humidity of the gas does not affect the capacity of soda lime to absorb carbon dioxide (12). Absorption is as effective when the gases are dry as when they are humidified, provided the soda lime has a high moisture content. Soda lime in absorbers may dry in routine clinical use (13).

Chemistry. To initiate the chemical reaction, carbon dioxide must first react with the water on the surface of the granule to form carbonic acid:

$$CO_2 + H_2O \rightleftharpoons H_2CO_3$$

This is a weak acid and is incompletely dissociated into its ions:

$$H_2CO_3 \rightleftharpoons H^+ + HCO_3^-$$
$$\downarrow$$
$$H^+ + CO_3^{-2}$$

Sodium hydroxide and calcium hydroxide are likewise dissociated into their ions:

$$NaOH \rightleftharpoons OH^- + Na^+$$
$$Ca(OH)_2 \rightleftharpoons 2OH^- + Ca^{2+}$$

The sodium and calcium ions combine with the carbonate ions, forming sodium carbonate and calcium carbonate:

$$2NaOH + 2H_2CO_3 + Ca(OH)_2 \rightleftharpoons$$
$$CaCO_3 + Na_2CO_3 + 4H_2O$$

Water is formed from the hydrogen and hydroxyl ions. 100 grams of soda lime can absorb approximately 26 liters of carbon dioxide.

Heat is liberated at the rate of 13,700 calories/mole of water produced (or CO_2 absorbed). This heat does not affect absorption efficiency (14). It can be detected by warmth of the canister. Failure of the canister to become warm to external touch may be a sign that absorption is not taking place.

A phenomenon known as "peaking" or "regeneration" is seen with soda lime. The soda lime appears to be reactivated with rest. The amount of regeneration depends on the length of the period of rest (15). After a number of such periods of efficient absorption with intervening periods of rest, terminal exhaustion occurs. There is general agreement that with modern "wet" soda lime the absorption capacity regenerated with rest is slight and affords no appreciable increase in the overall life of the absorbent (16, 17).

Regeneration does have some importance when indicators are used. Soda lime that shows an exhausted color, if allowed to rest, will often reveal a reversal of color. The absorption capacity of that soda lime will be low and the exhausted color will reappear after only a brief exposure to carbon dioxide.

Shape and Size of Granules. Soda lime is supplied in granules that have irregular surfaces to provide maximum area for absorption. The size of the granules is important. Small granules provide greater surface area and decrease channeling, the passage of gas occurring preferentially along low-resistance pathways and bypassing the bulk of the absorbent (18, 19). However, they cause more resistance and caking (18–21). Studies show that a blend of larger and smaller granules will minimize resistance with little sacrifice in absorption efficiency (22).

Granule size is measured by mesh number. A 4-mesh strainer has four openings per inch whereas one of 8 mesh has eight openings per inch. Soda lime granules graded 4 mesh will pass through the 4-mesh strainer but not through a strainer with smaller holes. In other words, the higher the mesh number, the smaller the particles. Soda lime used in anesthesia today consists of granules in the range of 4 to 8 mesh (10).

Hardness. Soda lime granules fragment easily, producing dust (fines). There may be variations in the dust content of different brands of absorbent (23). Excessive powder produces channeling, resistance to flow, and caking. Dust may be blown through the system to the patient or may cause system components to malfunction (24–26). To prevent this, small amounts of silica are added to increase hardness (10). Silica tends to clog the pores of the soda lime and reduce its efficiency, a drawback overcome by the addition of kieselguhr (27). Some manufacturers coat the outside of the granules with a film to which dust particles adhere.

Hardness is tested by placing a weighed amount of absorbent in a pan with steel ball bearings and agitating it. The soda lime is then sifted onto an 8-mesh screen. The percentage of the original sample remaining on the screen is the hardness number, which should be more than 75 (10).

Barium Hydroxide Lime

Composition. Baralyme is a mixture of approximately 20% barium hydroxide and 80% calcium hydroxide. It may also contain some potassium hydroxide and an indicator (27). Barium hydroxide is the more active component, acting much as sodium hydroxide in soda lime. Moisture is incorporated into the structure of the barium hydroxide as an octahydrate: $Ba(OH)_2 \cdot 8H_2O$. Some moisture is also present on the surface. Compared with soda lime, the water content is less variable and less likely to be lost through evaporation. Water will be lost, however, if barium hydroxide lime is heated over 100°C.

Chemistry. The reactions between barium hydroxide lime and carbon dioxide are as follows:

$$Ba(OH)_2 \cdot 8H_2O + CO_2 \rightarrow BaCO_3 + 9H_2O$$
$$9H_2O + 9CO_2 \rightarrow 9H_2CO_3$$
$$9H_2CO_3 + 9Ca(OH)_2 \rightarrow 9CaCO_3 + 18H_2O$$
$$2KOH + H_2CO_3 \rightarrow K_2CO_3 + 2H_2O$$
$$Ca(OH)_2 + K_2CO_3 \rightarrow CaCO_3 + 2KOH$$

Heat and water formation vary little from soda lime under identical conditions (28). There is some regeneration with barium hydroxide lime (17).

Size and Shape. Baralyme is supplied in granular form (4 to 8 mesh) similar to soda lime. In the past it was supplied in the form of pellets, which had shorter lives than granules.

Hardness. It is not necessary to add a hardening agent to baralyme because the water of crystallization imparts sufficient hardness to prevent dust formation (17, 20).

Absorbents and Anesthetic Agents

Sevoflurane, isoflurane, enflurane, desflurane, and halothane are all degraded by absorbents to some extent (13, 29–32). The most extensive degradation occurs with sevoflurane. The following increase the concentration of the major degradation product of sevoflurane (compound A):

1) low fresh gas flows;
2) use of baralyme rather than soda lime;
3) higher concentrations of sevoflurane;
4) higher absorbent temperatures; and
5) drying of the absorbent (33–43).

The significance of this degradation has not yet been determined.

Absorbents can remove volatile anesthetic agents by adsorption or solution (30, 31, 44–47). This can result in slower inductions and exposure of subsequent patients to volatile agents. Dry absorbent removes more agent than wet (13, 30, 45, 46, 48).

High concentrations of carbon monoxide (CO) have been reported when volatile agents were administered using absorbers that have not been used for at least 24 hours (49, 50). Levels of carbon monoxide are higher with the following:

1) use of baralyme rather than soda lime,
2) higher temperatures in the absorber,
3) dry absorbent,
4) high anesthetic concentrations, and
5) increased length of time (49, 51).

Highest levels have been seen with desflurane followed by enflurane then isoflurane. The amounts seen with halothane and sevoflurane are small.

Of all these factors, drying of the absorbent appears to be the most important. It is important to ensure that standard absorbents containing the full complement of water are used and that prolonged dry gas flushing of the absorbent is avoided

(52). Adding water to the absorbent will reduce CO formation (53).

Respiratory gas monitors in current use cannot detect CO directly. However, a compound produced when desflurane or isoflurane interacts with absorbent to produce CO may be read erroneously as enflurane by a mass spectrometer (54).

Indicators

An indicator is an acid or base whose color depends on pH and that is added to the absorbent to signify when exhaustion has occurred. The indicator does not affect absorption. Some of the commonly used indicators and their colors are shown in Table 8.1. Confusion may result because one indicator is white when fresh whereas another is white when exhausted. Ethyl violet is most commonly employed because the color change is vivid and of high contrast (55). Ethyl violet undergoes deactivation even if stored in the dark (56). Deactivation is accelerated in the presence of light, especially high-intensity light.

Contents

Granular Space

The granular space is occupied by solid absorbent.

Air Space

The air space occupies 48 to 55% of the volume of the canister (17). It is divided into the void space and the pore space.

Void space. The void (intergranular or interstitial) space is between the granules. Void space varies with the size of the granules and how tightly they are packed. The smaller the granules and the closer they fit together, the smaller the void space.

TABLE **8.1. Indicators for Absorbents**

Indicator	Color When Fresh	Color When Exhausted
Phenolphthalein	white	pink
Ethyl violet	white	purple
Clayton yellow	red	yellow
Ethyl orange	orange	yellow
Mimosa Z	red	white

The void space of soda lime is 40 to 47% of its volume (17). For barium hydroxide lime, it is 45%.

Pore space. The pore (intragranular) space is within the pores of the granules. The pore volume for fresh absorbent is 8% of the total volume. As absorption proceeds, the pore space decreases (10).

Storage and Handling of Absorbents

Absorbents are supplied in several types of containers: resealable packages, pails, cans, cartons, and disposable prefilled containers. Once opened, containers should be resealed as soon as possible to prevent reaction of the absorbent with carbon dioxide in the air, deactivation of the indicator, and moisture loss. High temperatures will have no effect on absorbents if the containers are sealed, but any temperature below freezing is harmful because the moisture will expand and cause fragmentation of the granules.

Absorbents should always be handled gently to avoid fragmentation and dust formation. All personnel involved in the handling of absorbents should be periodically warned that absorbent dust is irritating to the eyes and respiratory tract and that absorbents are caustic to the skin, particularly when damp. When a canister is emptied, care should be taken to remove dust particles along the rubber surfaces as they will cause the seals to warp, making it difficult to achieve a tight fit. Screens should be cleaned to reduce resistance to gas flow.

Filling of the canister should always be performed with care. The canister should be held over a suitable container to avoid getting particles on the floor. The absorbent should be poured slowly into the canister while the canister is rotated, stopping occasionally to tap the sides to settle the granules (57). The canister should be filled completely but not overfilled. A small space should be left at the top to promote even flow of gases through the canister. The upper layer of the absorbent should be level.

With disposable, prefilled containers, it is important to remove the top and bottom labels or plastic wrap, if present, before insertion. If this is not done, gas cannot flow through the container (3).

Changing the Absorbent

Several methods have been used to determine when the absorbent should be changed.

Carbon Dioxide in the Inspiratory Gas

The appearance of carbon dioxide in the inspiratory gas is the most reliable method to detect absorbent exhaustion.

Indicator Color Change

Confidence should not be placed in indicator color change because this does not reliably demonstrate CO_2 breakthrough (58). The following should be kept in mind when using a color indicator:

1) When the exhausted color shows strongly, the absorbent is at or near the point of exhaustion. When little or no color change shows, active absorbent may be present but the amount is indeterminate and may be quite small.
2) When a canister is rested, the color may revert back to its preexhaustion color even when the absorbent is sufficiently exhausted to be of no value clinically. Upon reuse, the indicator color will rapidly return to its exhausted state. The rested canister, therefore, can give a false impression of its usefulness.
3) When channeling occurs, the absorbent along the channels will become exhausted and carbon dioxide will filter through the canister. If the channeling occurs at other sites than the sides of the canister, the color change along the channels may not be visible (59).
4) Use of absorbent without indicators has been reported (60, 61).
5) Ethyl violet undergoes deactivation even if it is stored in the dark (56). Light, especially ultraviolet, accelerates this process.

Heat in the Canister

The reaction of carbon dioxide with absorbent produces heat, and changes in absorbent temperature occur earlier than changes in the color of the indicator. Periodically checking the temperature of the canisters is useful (62). Some heat production should be apparent unless high fresh gas flows are used. Studies suggest that when the temperature of the downstream canister exceeds that of the upstream chamber, the absorbent in the upstream canister should be changed (63).

To change the absorbent, the base of the absorber housing is lowered and the canisters removed. The absorbent in the upstream canister is discarded, and the canister is filled with fresh absorbent. Care should be taken when placing the last of the absorbent into the canister. If excessive dust is present, the remaining absorbent should be discarded and filling completed from a new container (64). The canisters are then reversed in position so that the canister that was downstream is placed in the upstream position.

Unidirectional Valves

Two unidirectional (flutter, one-way, check, directional, dome, flap, nonreturn, inspiratory, and expiratory) valves are used in each circle system to ensure that gases flow toward the patient in one breathing tube and away in the other. They are usually part of the absorber assembly. The 22-mm male connector next to the inspiratory unidirectional valve is called the inspiratory port, and that next to the expiratory unidirectional valve is called the expiratory port. The American Society for Testing and Materials (ASTM) standard requires that the direction of intended gas flow be permanently marked on the valve housing or near its associated hose terminal with either a directional arrow or with the marking "inspiration" or "expiration" so that it is visible to the user (1).

A typical unidirectional valve is shown diagrammatically in Figure 8.6. A light, thin disc (leaflet or poppet) seats horizontally on an annular seat. The disc has a slightly larger diameter than the circular knife edge it sits on. A cage or guide mechanism (retainer) (such as projections from the seat and dome) may be present to prevent the disc from becoming dislodged laterally or vertically (Fig. 8.7). The disc must be hydrophobic so that condensate does not cause it to stick to the knife edge and increase the resistance to opening. The top of the valve is covered by a removable clear plastic dome so that the disc can be seen. Gas enters at the bottom and flows through the center of the valve, raising the disc from its seat. The gas then passes under the dome and on through the breathing system. Reversing the gas flow will cause the disc to contact the seat, stopping further retrograde flow. Unidirectional valves are positional and must be vertical for the disc to seat properly. The inspiratory valve opens

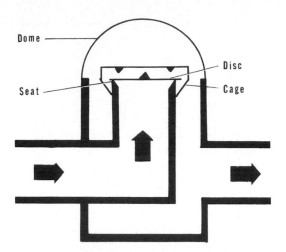

FIGURE 8.6. Unidirectional valve in closed position. Gas flowing into the valve raises the disc from its seat, then passes through the valve. Reversing the gas flow causes the disc to contact its seat, stopping further retrograde flow. The guide (cage) prevents lateral or vertical displacement of the disc. The transparent dome allows observation of disc movement.

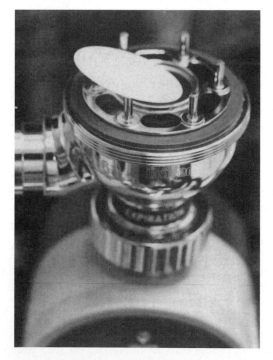

FIGURE 8.7. Unidirectional valve with dome removed. The disc is displaced from its seat. The projections on the seat prevent lateral displacement of the disc.

on inspiration and closes on expiration, preventing backflow of exhaled gas in the inspiratory tubing. The expiratory valve works in reciprocal fashion.

As can be seen in Figure 6.1F, turbulence results from gas flow through a unidirectional valve. Although this was a significant problem with older valves, modern valves have light discs and present only slight resistance.

Incompetence of one or both unidirectional valves is not uncommon (65). The disc may adhere to the dome unless a guard is present. Moisture may cause the disc to stick (66). Electrostatic charges may cause the disc to be attracted to the top of the valve (67). An unsecured cage may allow the disc to move laterally (68). The disc may catch on a pin of a cage (67). Foreign material such as absorbent granules may hold the valve open (68). Because an open valve offers less resistance to flow than one that must open, the flow of gas will be primarily through the incompetent side, resulting in rebreathing.

A unidirectional valve may jam, obstructing gas flow (69, 70). In one reported case, the disc was lost during cleaning and not recovered (71). It was later found out of sight below the seat, where it had moved into such a position that it covered the opening to the bag mount and functioned as a one-way valve. Gas could flow into the system, but not back out again.

Inspiratory and Expiratory Ports

The inspiratory port of the circle system is the opening through which gases pass during inspiration. The expiratory port is the opening through which gases pass during expiration. These are traditionally mounted on the absorber. The ASTM standard requires that each port be a 22-mm conical male fitting (1).

Y-piece

The Y-piece (Y-piece connector, Y-connector, Y-yoke, Y-adaptor, three-way breathing system connector) is a three-way tubular connector with two 22-mm male ports for connection to the breathing tubes and a 15-mm female patient connection port. The patient connection port may have a coaxial 22-mm male fitting to allow direct connection between the Y-piece and face mask.

In most disposable systems, the Y-piece and breathing tubes are permanently attached. The Y-piece may be designed so that the patient port swivels. A septum may be placed in the Y-piece to decrease the dead space.

Y-pieces on some disposable systems may become detached from the breathing tubes (72), and many leak, especially those with swivel joints (73).

Fresh Gas Inlet

The fresh gas inlet is usually incorporated with other components near the absorber. It is often connected to the common gas outlet on the anesthesia machine by a flexible rubber tubing—the fresh gas supply tube (delivery hose). The ASTM standard requires that the fresh gas inlet port, or nipple, have an inside diameter of at least 4.0 mm and that the fresh gas delivery tube have an inside diameter of at least 6.4 mm (1).

Adjustable Pressure Limiting Valve

APL valves were discussed in Chapter 6. The valve should be fully open during spontaneous breathing. The valve will open after the bag has become distended during expiration or the expiratory pause. When manually-assisted or controlled ventilation is used, the APL valve should be closed enough that the desired inspiratory pressure can be achieved. When this pressure is attained, the valve opens and excess gas is vented. Some modern APL valves have two positions: manual and spontaneous (Figure 6.6). In the spontaneous mode, the valve is fully open. In the manual position, the valve can be adjusted.

Pressure Gauge (Manometer)

Most circle systems have a pressure gauge attached to the absorber. The ASTM Standard requires that they be marked in units of kPa and/or cm water (1).

The gauge is usually the diaphragm type shown in Figure 8.8. Changes in pressure in the breathing system are transmitted to the space between two diaphragms, causing them to move inward or outward. Movements of one diaphragm are transmitted to the pointer, which moves over a calibrated scale.

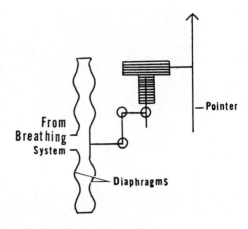

FIGURE **8.8.** Diaphragm-activated pressure gauge. Two thin metal diaphragms are sealed together, with a space between them. This space is connected to the breathing system. Variations in pressure in the breathing system are transmitted to the diaphragms, which bulge outward or inward. A series of levers is activated, moving the pointer, which records the pressure.

Breathing Tubes

Two breathing tubings carry gases to and from the patient. Each tube connects to a port on the absorber assembly at one end and the Y-piece at the other. The length of the tubes does not affect the amount of dead space or rebreathing. Longer tubes allows the anesthesia machine and other equipment to be located farther from the patient's head (74).

A coaxial circle is available. As shown in Figure 8.9, the tubings attach to a conventional valved absorber assembly. The inner tube is connected to the inspiratory port and the outer tube to the expiratory port. Gases flow through the corrugated inner tube to the patient and exhaled gases flow to the absorber via the outer corrugated tube. The inspired gas is warmed in the process. Advantages of this system include its light weight, compactness, and increased inspired heat and humidity.

Reservoir Bag

Reservoir bags were discussed in Chapter 6. The bag is usually attached to the 22-mm male bag port (bag mount or extension). It may also be placed at the end of a length of corrugated tubing leading from the bag mount, providing

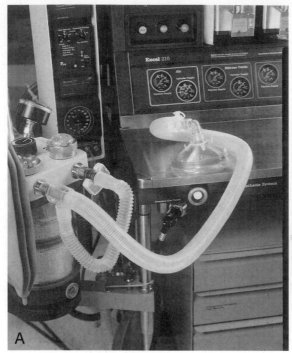

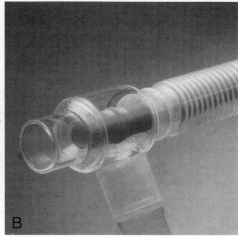

FIGURE **8.9.** Universal F system. **A,** Gases pass through the inspiratory unidirectional valve into the inner tube of the coaxial tubing and on to the patient. Exhaled gases flow to the expiratory unidirectional valve via the outer corrugated tube. **B,** Patient end of the system. (Reprinted with permission from King Systems Corporation.)

some freedom of movement for the anesthesia care provider (55). A case has been reported in which the bag mount broke off, preventing use of the system (75).

Bag/Ventilator Selector Switch

A bag/ventilator selector switch (switch valve, mode selector valve, selector valve, bag-ventilator switch valve, switching valve, switchover valve, manual/automatic selector valve, ventilator valve assembly) provides a convenient method to shift rapidly between manual or spontaneous respiration and automatic ventilation without removing the bag or the ventilator hose from its mount. On some modern anesthesia machines, turning the selector switch to the ventilator position causes the ventilator to be turned ON.

As shown in Figure 8.10, the selector switch is essentially a three-way stopcock. One port connects to the breathing system. The second is attached to the bag mount. The third attaches to the ventilator hose. The handle or knob used to select the position indicates the position in which the switch is set (Fig. 8.11). There are two types of selector switches (Fig. 8.10).

Without Adjustable Pressure Limiting Valve

The selector switch without an APL valve (Fig. 8.10A and B) is found on some older anesthesia machines. Operation of the selector switch does not affect the APL valve. It is necessary to close the valve when switching from bag to ventilator. Failure to close the valve in the ventilator mode may result in inadequate ventilation.

Breathing System

APL Valve

To Ventilator

Bag

A   B   C

FIGURE 8.10.   Bag/ventilator selector switch. **A** and **B**, Older type. In **A**, the switch is set for manual or spontaneous ventilation. The bag is connected to the breathing system. **B** shows the switch set for automatic ventilation; the adjustable pressure limiting (APL) valve is still connected to the system and must be closed. **C**, Newer type. The APL valve is on the bag side of the valve. When the switch is set for automatic ventilation, the APL valve is excluded from the system so it is not necessary to close it.

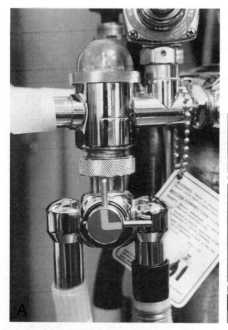

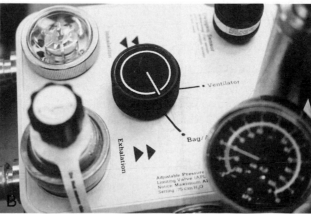

FIGURE 8.11.   Bag/ventilator selector switches. **A**, Older style. The adjustable pressure limiting (APL) valve is not excluded from the breathing system when the valve is set for ventilator use. The position of the handle indicates whether the valve is set for manual or automatic ventilation. **B**, Newer style. When the switch is in the ventilator position, the APL valve is excluded from the circuit.

With Adjustable Pressure Limiting Valve

The selector switch with an APL valve (Fig. 8.10C) is the only type allowed by the ASTM standard (1) and is on newer anesthesia machines. The APL valve is located near the bag mount. When the switch is in the ventilator position, the APL valve is isolated along with the reservoir bag so it does not need to be closed. Switching to the bag mode causes the APL valve to be connected to the breathing system.

A hazard with one of these valves has been reported. A missing retainer ring allowed the valve handle to be positioned so that gas escaped toward the ventilator when the bag was squeezed (76).

With Ventilator Interconnect

On some new anesthesia machines the bag/ventilator selector switch is linked with the ventilator actuating switch so the ventilator is turned on when the switch is placed in the ventilator position.

Respiratory Gas Monitor Sensor or Connector

Respiratory gas monitor sensors are discussed in Chapter 18. Both mainstream and sidestream devices can be used with the circle system but care must be taken when selecting the best position within the system.

Sensor or Connector for Airway Pressure Monitor

Airway pressure monitors are discussed in Chapter 19. The sensor can be inserted into the circle system using a T-shaped adaptor or it may be incorporated into the absorber assembly.

Optional Equipment

Positive End–Expiratory Pressure Valves

Positive end–expiratory pressure (PEEP) valves are discussed in Chapter 6. They are integral parts of some absorber assemblies. One can also be added to a circle system. If the PEEP valve is a separate component, it usually has a fixed pressure. It is essential that such a valve be placed in the expiratory limb and that it be oriented cor-

rectly. Placing a unidirectional PEEP valve backward will occlude gas flow. If a bidirectional PEEP valve is placed backward, gas flow will not be occluded but PEEP will not be produced. PEEP valves that are an integral part of the absorber assembly are usually of the variable pressure type. The amount of PEEP is dialed on the valve and read on the manometer (Fig. 8.12). A hazard with this device is that if it is not returned to zero at the end of a case, the next user may not notice this. Some of the newer PEEP valves have a method to indicate when they are turned on (Fig. 8.13).

Filters

One of the disadvantages of the circle system is that it is difficult to clean and/or sterilize certain components, particularly the absorber, ventilator, and unidirectional valves. Filters may been used to avoid transmission of pathogens. These were discussed in Chapter 6.

Heated Humidifier

A heated humidifier can be placed in the inspiratory limb of the circle system. These will be discussed in Chapter 10.

Respirometer

A respirometer to measure ventilatory volumes is commonly used in the circle system. These are discussed in Chapter 19.

ARRANGEMENT OF COMPONENTS

The relative placement of components comprising the circle system influences its function. Figure 8.1 illustrates a common arrangement.

Objectives

1) Maximum inclusion of fresh and dead-space gases in the inspired mixture and maximum venting of alveolar gas should be one objective (77, 78). Fresh gas should be preferentially included in the inspired mixture so that the inspired concentrations approach those in the fresh gas. This will result in faster inductions and emergences. The lower the fresh gas flow, the more important this objective becomes because one of the effects of using lower fresh gas flows is that changes in concentration in

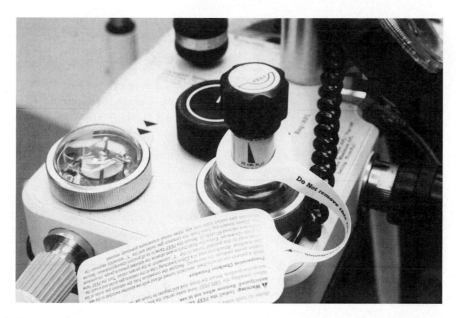

FIGURE 8.12. Positive end–expiratory pressure (PEEP) valve built into absorber assembly. The amount of PEEP is dialed by turning the knob and is read on the manometer. A hazard with this valve is that it may be left on and a subsequent user may be unaware of this. Another hazard is that it may be accidentally altered.

the fresh gas flow are reflected more slowly in inspired concentrations.

Faster induction and emergence will also be aided by selective venting of alveolar gases. During induction, it is advantageous if alveolar gases containing low concentrations of anesthetic agents (rather than fresh or dead-space gases containing higher concentrations) be eliminated through the APL valve. During emergence, the opposite is true.

2) Minimal consumption of absorbent should be a goal (79). For efficient absorbent use, the gas vented through the APL valve should have the highest possible concentration of carbon dioxide. This will occur when

A) exhaled gas does not pass through the absorber before being vented,

B) exhaled gas is diluted as little as possible before venting, and

C) the vented gas is that exhaled late in exhalation, as the first gas exhaled is that from the dead space and contains a low concentration of carbon dioxide.

As fresh gas flow is reduced, more exhaled gas must pass through the absorbent, so this objective becomes less important. When using a closed system, the arrangement of components should have no effect on the utilization of absorbent because all exhaled gases will pass through the absorber.

3) Accurate readings from a respirometer placed in the system are important (80–82). If the fresh gas inlet is positioned so that the fresh gas continuously flows through the respirometer, measured ventilatory volumes will not be accurate.

4) Meaningful pressures on a manometer or transmitted by the sensor for an airway pressure monitor should be a goal.

5) Maximal humidification of inspired gases is always desirable.

6) Minimal dead space is desirable.

7) Low resistance is beneficial.

8) Pull on the tracheal tube or mask should be avoided. Components should be so arranged that they do not create difficulties during use. Tubings and wires should not become tangled.

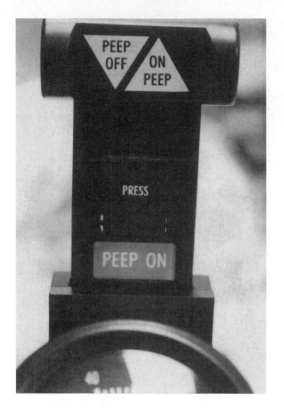

FIGURE 8.13. Positive end-expiratory pressure (PEEP) ON/OFF indicator. The handle must be raised before the PEEP can be dialed. This alerts the user that the PEEP is being applied.

There is no single arrangement of components that will meet all of the above objectives. Objectives may conflict in some cases. For example, venting carbon dioxide upstream of the absorber will conserve absorbent but will tend to reduce inspired humidity because the amount of heat and humidity produced are directly proportional to the volume of carbon dioxide entering the canister. In certain clinical situations, particular objectives need to be given priority. For example, in pediatric patients, dead space and humidification are more significant than in adults.

Consideration of Individual Components

Fresh Gas Inlet

Figure 8.14 shows possible locations of the fresh gas inlet. It is most commonly placed upstream of the inspiratory unidirectional valve and

downstream of the absorber (position A). In this position, during exhalation and the expiratory pause, fresh gas will flow into the absorber and then components between the expiratory unidirectional valve and the absorber. At low fresh gas flows, no gas vented through the APL valve will have passed through the absorber. With higher flows, some gas that has been in the absorber may be vented. At very high flows, some fresh gas may be vented.

Placing the fresh gas inlet just upstream of the absorber (position B) would result in less inclusion of fresh gas in the inspired mixture. Fresh gas would be vented because of the proximity to the APL valve. Anesthetic agent in the fresh gas would be retained in the absorbent, resulting in slower inductions (83). Placement in this position will improve humidification of inspired gases (84–86) but will result in more drying of the absorbent. Another problem is that absorbent dust could be blown into the inspiratory limb when the oxygen flush is activated.

Placing the fresh gas inlet upstream of the bag and the APL valve (position E) would have all the disadvantages of position B and would result in more venting of fresh gas and dilution of exhaled gas before it is vented.

Placing the fresh gas inlet upstream of the expiratory unidirectional valve (position D) has all the disadvantages of positions B and E. In addition, during inspiration, the fresh gas flow would force exhaled gases containing carbon dioxide back toward the patient.

Position C, downstream of the inspiratory unidirectional valve, was originally advocated to reduce dead space by sweeping exhaled gases out of the Y-piece during exhalation (79). However, if the unidirectional valves are competent, there will be only slight retrograde flow at the Y-piece. With an incompetent valve, even a high inflow cannot prevent rebreathing of exhaled gases (79). With the inflow in position C, during exhalation, fresh gas would join exhaled gases and escape though the APL valve without reaching the patient. This would result in poor economy of fresh gas (87) and inefficient use of absorbent because fresh gas would dilute the concentration of carbon dioxide in the gas vented through the APL valve. Another

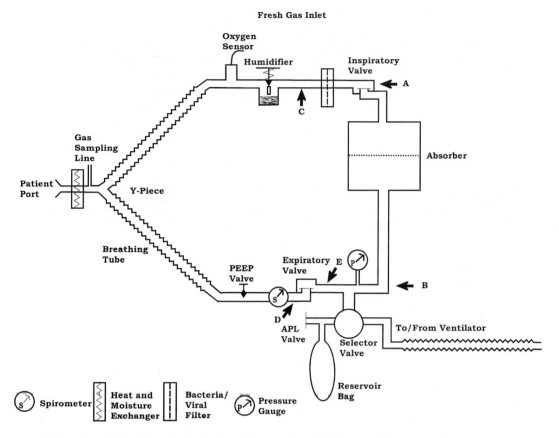

FIGURE 8.14. Possible locations for the fresh gas inlet. (See text for details.) APL = adjustable pressure limit- ing; PEEP = positive end–expiratory pressure; S = spirometer.

disadvantage of position C is that a respirometer placed on the exhalation side of the circuit will not record volumes accurately unless the fresh gas flow is turned off (80–82, 88).

Another disadvantage of position C is that if the oxygen flush were used and if there were an obstruction upstream, the patient could be exposed to a sudden rapid increase in pressure (89). With the fresh gas inlet in other positions, the increase in pressure would be slower because gas could exit through the APL valve and the pressure increase would be buffered by the bag. Use of position C would cause changes in the fresh gas composition to appear more rapidly in the inspired gases. If the Y-piece has a septum, placement of the fresh gas inlet in this position will wash out dead space under a mask.

Reservoir Bag

Figure 8.15 shows possible locations for the reservoir bag. It is most commonly placed between the expiratory unidirectional valve and the absorber (position A). A disadvantage of placing the bag upstream of the absorber is that a sudden increase in pressure from squeezing the bag may force dust from the absorber into the inspiratory tubing (90).

During spontaneous respiration, absorbent use is equally efficient if the bag is downstream (position D) or upstream (position A or E) of the absorber (79). With manually controlled or assisted ventilation, more efficient use occurs with the bag upstream of the absorber. If the bag were in position D, exhaled gases would pass through the absorber to the bag during exhalation. Squeezing

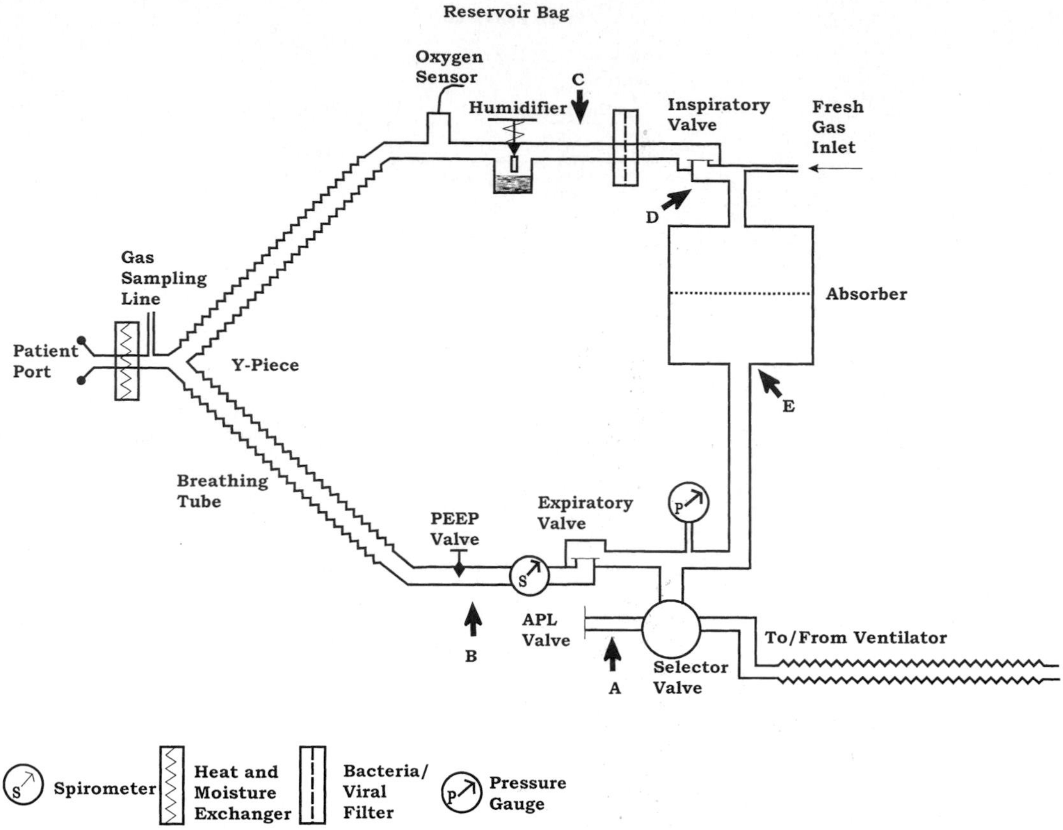

FIGURE 8.15. Possible locations for the reservoir bag. (See text for details.) APL = adjustable pressure limit ing; PEEP = positive end–expiratory pressure; S = spirometer.

the bag during inhalation would cause the gases to reverse flow and pass retrograde through the absorber to be vented through the APL valve. This would result in inefficient absorbent use because gases cleared of carbon dioxide would be vented. When a mechanical ventilator is used, the APL valve is closed and excess gases are vented through the ventilator so the position of the bag will determine which gas is vented. If the bag is placed in position D during mechanical ventilation, exhaled gases must pass through the absorber before being vented. If the bag is placed between the patient and either of the unidirectional valves (position B or C), it would form a reservoir for exhaled gases that would then be rebreathed.

Another possible position for the bag is position E, at the bottom of the absorber. A disadvantage is that absorbent dust may collect in this area,

and a hard squeeze of the bag could force this dust into the inspiratory limb (25).

Unidirectional Valves

Two locations have been used for the unidirectional valves: in the Y-piece and attached to the absorber. Valved Y-pieces are no longer available commercially and are not permitted by the ASTM standard (1).

Placing the valves in the Y-piece offers the advantage of eliminating backflow of exhaled gases into the inspiratory tubing. However, under normal circumstances, backflow into this tubing is insignificant. With controlled ventilation, placing the valves in the Y-piece results in more efficient absorbent use (79).

Disadvantages of placing the valves in the Y-piece include the fact that they are bulky and difficult to see and have a higher resistance than unidirectional valves at the absorber (77). Serious accidents have occurred when a valved Y-piece was placed in a circle system containing absorber-mounted valves (91–94). If this error occurs, there is a 50% chance that the valves in the Y-piece will be opposed to those on the absorber and there will be no gas flow through the breathing system. If the unidirectional valves are mounted in the Y-piece they may be mounted backwards and make the sequence of other components incorrect. For these reasons, it is recommended that they not be used.

Adjustable Pressure Limiting Valve

Figure 8.16 shows possible locations for the APL valve. It is most commonly located downstream of the expiratory unidirectional valve and upstream of the absorber (Position A), permanently mounted near the absorber. In this position fresh gas will be vented only if the fresh gas flow is high (95).

During manually controlled or assisted ventilation, overflow of excess gases occurs during inspiration. Considerable venting of fresh gas and gas that has passed through the absorber will occur with the APL valve between the fresh gas inlet and the patient at position B, C, or D (77, 79). If the valve were located at position E, upstream of the expiratory unidirectional valve, absorbent use would be inefficient because all gas in the reservoir bag would have to pass through the absorber before being vented.

Locating the APL valve at the reservoir bag with an extender hose between the bag and the bag mount has been suggested (96). This would

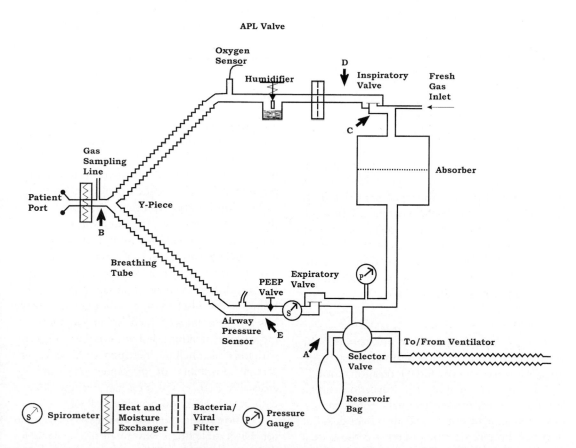

FIGURE 8.16. Possible locations for the adjustable pressure limiting (APL) valve. (See text for details.) PEEP = positive end–expiratory pressure; S = spirometer.

allow fresh gas that travels retrograde through the absorber during exhalation more space in which to collect.

During automatic ventilation the APL valve is closed or isolated, so its location is of no significance.

During spontaneous respiration, the most efficient use of absorbent will occur with the APL valve on the Y-piece (position B) (77, 79). This is because overflow occurs in the latter part of expiration during spontaneous respiration. Gas exhaled during the first part of expiration is dead-space gas with a low concentration of carbon dioxide. Because the APL valve is not open, this gas passes by it. When the bag is filled, the pressure in the system rises and the APL valve opens. Because this opening occurs during the latter part of exhalation, the gas vented through the APL valve is mainly alveolar gas (with a high carbon dioxide content). No such discrimination is possible when the APL valve is distant from the patient (77). However, if the APL valve is at the Y-piece, the added weight (especially when scavenging apparatus is added) may increase the incidence of disconnections. Transfer tubing to the scavenging interface may become entangled with other objects. The valve will be difficult to adjust during head and neck surgery. Finally, placing the valve at position B will cause a decrease in inspired heat and humidity (97). During spontaneous ventilation, absorbent use is inefficient if the APL valve is downstream of the absorber (positions C and D) because vented gas would have passed through the absorber. If the APL valve is placed at position C, fresh gas will be vented. If the APL valve were in position D, exhaled gases would move retrograde in the inspiratory tubing during exhalation, causing an increase in dead space.

Filters

Figure 8.17 shows possible positions within the circle system for a filter. Most disposable systems do not allow placement of a filter at position A or B.

Position A is between the inhalation tubing and the Y-piece. A filter here will protect the patient from contamination and absorbent dust but does not protect the components of the system or the operating room environment from contamination from the patient. If the filter is heavy or bulky, placing it in this position may be awkward. A filter should not be placed in this location if a humidifier is located upstream.

Position B is between the Y-piece and the exhalation tubing. In this position, the components of the system and operating room will be protected. Water, mucus, or edema fluid can collect in the filter in this position, causing an increase in resistance or obstruction to gas flow (98, 99). The bulk and weight of a filter may make it unsuitable for this location.

Position C is between the inspiratory tubing and the inspiratory unidirectional valve. The size or weight of the filter is not a problem in this position. If a humidifier is used, it should be downstream of the filter. A filter in this position will protect the patient from contamination from the absorber and its attached parts but not the inhalation tubing. The filter will catch absorbent dust (90). It will not protect the circle system components or the operating room air from contamination from the patient. Use of a filter in this position has been shown not to reduce the incidence of pneumonia after inhalation anesthesia (100).

Position D is between the exhalation tubing and the expiratory unidirectional valve. In this position, the filter will protect the components of the system from contamination. Because the filter is on the expiratory side, obstruction from fluid is possible, although less likely than with position B.

Position E is between the Y-piece and the patient. In this position, the filter will protect the patient from the equipment and the equipment from the patient. It will also act as a heat and moisture exchanger (101). This suggests a strategy for infection control in anesthesia (102). Using a new filter between the patient and the breathing system with each patient would permit reuse of the breathing system. Potential problems with this site include increased dead space, increased possibility of disconnections, and increased resistance. The filter may become clogged with blood, secretions, or edema fluid.

Position F is in the hose leading to the ventilator. Disposable hoses with filters are available for this purpose. This will protect the patient from the ventilator and the ventilator from the patient

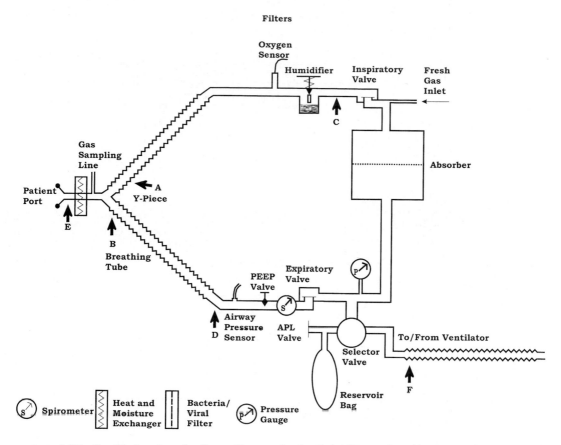

FIGURE 8.17. Possible locations for filters. (See text for details.) APL = adjustable pressure limiting; PEEP = positive end–expiratory pressure; S = spirometer.

but will not offer protection for other components.

Respiratory Gas Monitor Sensor or Connector

Mainstream Devices

Oxygen monitor. Figure 8.18 shows possible locations for an oxygen monitor sensor. It may be fitted into the dome of a unidirectional valve, the top of the absorber, or a T-shaped adapter. The sensor should be placed so that the tip points downward to prevent water from accumulating on the membrane. Most disposable systems do not permit the sensor to be placed at position F or G and between the tubing and the Y-piece.

Positions A, F, and H are on the inspiratory side, whereas positions C, E, G, and I are on the exhalation side. Placing the sensor on the expira-

tory side will usually expose it to more humidity, but with most sensors this is not a problem. If low fresh gas flows are used, the reading on the expiratory side will be lower than on the inspiratory side, but the inspired-expired difference is only 4% to 6% even with a closed system (103).

It has been advocated that the oxygen analyzer be placed near the Y-piece (position G, F, or B) so that it will alarm in the event of a disconnection between the breathing system and the tracheal tube. However, an oxygen analyzer should not be relied on as a disconnect alarm. Although this is the most common site for disconnections, they occur in other locations. Furthermore, with a high fresh gas flow, the oxygen concentration may not fall sufficiently for the alarm to sound. Placing the sensor near the patient in position B, F, or G may make it difficult to maintain in an upright posi-

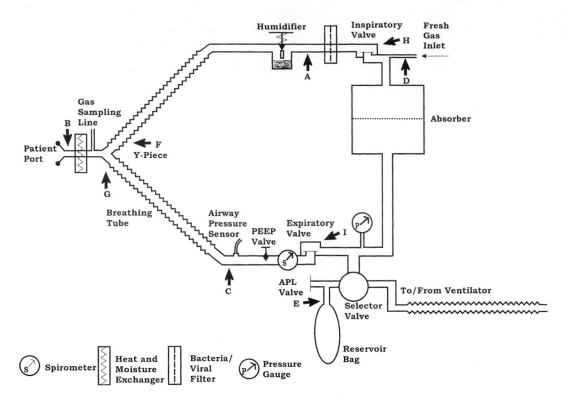

FIGURE 8.18. Possible locations for oxygen monitor sensor. (See text for details.) APL = adjustable pressure limiting; PEEP = positive end–expiratory pressure; S = spirometer.

tion. In addition, the cable to the monitor may become entangled with other tubings or stretched, resulting in a pull on the Y-piece. Placing it in position B, between the Y-piece and the patient, will increase dead space.

Position D is in the fresh gas line. This position is not recommended because the monitor will indicate only the concentration of oxygen in the gas mixture delivered to the breathing system and not in that inspired by the patient.

Mainstream CO₂ monitor. To obtain satisfactory exhaled values, a mainstream CO_2 sensor must be placed as close as possible to the patient, between the patient and the breathing system (position B in Fig. 8.18).

Sidestream Devices

Gases can be aspirated from an adaptor in the breathing system or from a port in a component such as an elbow adaptor. To obtain satisfactory samples of inhaled and exhaled gases, the site should be close to the patient.

Respirometer

Figure 8.19 shows possible locations for a respirometer in the circle system. Some have special adaptors for attaching them securely at particular locations.

A respirometer is usually placed on the expiratory side, on either side of the expiratory unidirectional valve (positions A and B). During spontaneous respiration, the volumes recorded will be accurate. During controlled respiration, a spirometer in this location will overread inspired volumes because of expansion of the breathing tubes and compression of gases (81, 82). If the spirometer

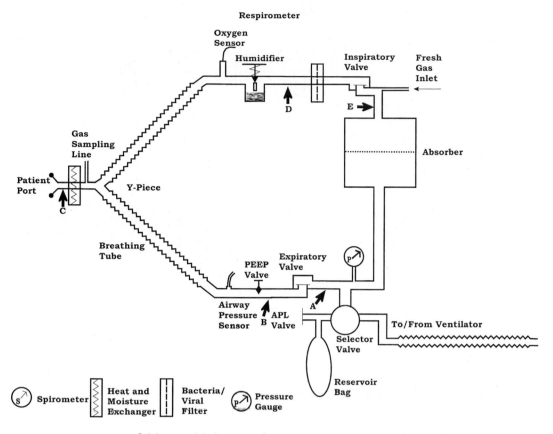

FIGURE **8.19.** Possible locations for a respirometer. (See text for details.)

can detect reverse flow, a malfunctioning unidirectional valve may be detected.

A spirometer placed between the patient and the Y-piece (position C) will record accurately with both spontaneous and controlled ventilation if it can read bidirectional flow. Sidestream spirometers must be placed in this position. Problems such as a leaking tracheal tube cuff can be detected by measuring inhaled and exhaled volumes. However, some respirometers are too bulky to place in this position and the increase in dead space may be significant. Use of this position may result in increased risk of damage to the spirometer, disconnections, and kinking of the tracheal tube. Condensation, mucus, edema, and secretions can cause problems with the respirometer in this position.

If the spirometer is placed on the inspiratory side (position D), it will overread volumes during controlled or assisted ventilation because of expansion of the tubings and leaks between the spirometer and the patient.

A spirometer should not be located downstream of the absorber (position E) because the absorption of carbon dioxide will decrease the volume of gas measured.

Sensor or Connector for Airway Pressure Monitor

Possible positions for the sensor or connector for an airway pressure monitor are shown in Figure 8.20. Placing the sensor in Position C, between the patient and the breathing system, will ensure that the pressure measured is close to that of the patient's airway. The more distant the site is from the patient, the less accurately it reflects airway pressure (104, 105). Breathing system resistance, leaks, obstructions, and other mechanical

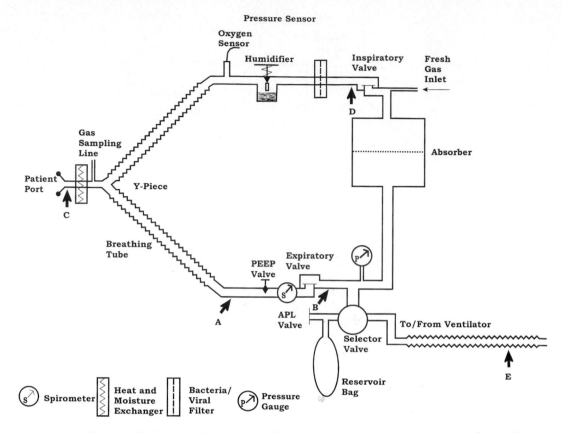

FIGURE **8.20.** Possible locations for the sensor for an airway pressure monitor. (See text for details.)

factors may result in a measured pressure that differs substantially from the pressure in the patient's airway (106). Problems with this site include increased dead space, disconnections, tracheal tube kinking, contamination, and water buildup in the pilot line. It is necessary to connect the pilot line for every case.

T-adaptors must be used for positions A and D. Placing the sensor on the expiratory side (positions A and B) has an advantage over the inspiratory side (position D). If there is obstruction to flow in the inspiratory limb and the sensor for airway pressures is located upstream of the obstruction, the low pressure near the patient will not be sensed. If the sensor is located downstream from the obstruction or on the expiratory side, the low pressure will be detected. Position E, in the ventilator itself, was used in the past but is now not recommended. Certain circumstances

may cause sufficient back pressure to develop to inhibit the minimum pressure alarm (106, 107). Also placement in the ventilator may result in failure to detect an incorrectly set bag/ventilator selector valve.

Positive End–Expiratory Pressure Valve

The PEEP valve must be placed in the expiratory side of the breathing system. A disposable PEEP valve should be placed between the expiratory breathing tube and the expiratory unidirectional valve (position B in Fig. 8.21). Built-in PEEP valves are usually situated downstream of the expiratory unidirectional valve and upstream of the absorber (position A in Fig. 8.21). A bidirectional PEEP valve may be inserted between the anesthesia ventilator and breathing system (position C in Fig 8.21).

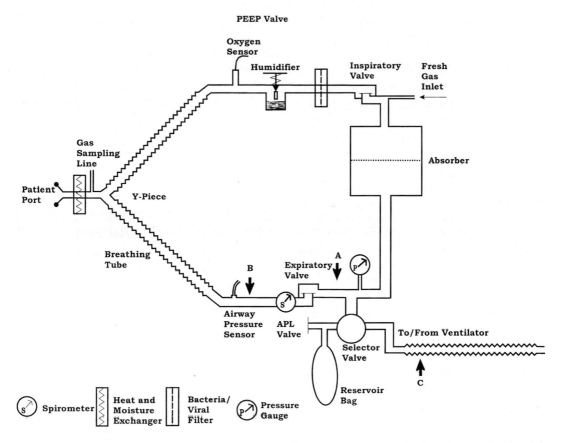

FIGURE 8.21. Possible locations for a positive end–expiratory pressure (PEEP) valve. (See text for details.)

Pressure Manometer

To measure PEEP accurately, the pressure manometer must be on the same side (patient or absorber) of the expiratory unidirectional valve as the PEEP valve (108). On most older absorber assemblies the manometer is on the absorber side. If a PEEP valve is added to the expiratory limb on the patient side of the unidirectional valve, PEEP will not register on the manometer gauge. Most newer absorber assemblies have a built-in PEEP valve located on the absorber side of the unidirectional valve with the pressure manometer in close proximity.

RESISTANCE AND WORK OF BREATHING IN THE CIRCLE SYSTEM

In the past, one of the objections to using a circle system with small children was that it had a high resistance. However, investigations have shown that the resistance or work of breathing with the circle system is not significantly greater than with other breathing systems and may be less (109, 110–114). Use of coaxial tubings increases resistance (109).

DEAD SPACE OF THE CIRCLE SYSTEM

In the circle system, dead space extends from the patient port of the Y-piece to the partition. Use of a Y-piece with a septum will decrease dead space. When exhalation or inhalation starts, the gases in the breathing tubes move in the opposite direction from their usual flow until stopped by closure of one of the unidirectional valves. This is referred to as "backlash" and causes a slight increase in dead space. If the unidirectional valves are competent, however, backlash will be clinically insignificant.

HEAT AND HUMIDITY

In the circle system, moisture is available from exhaled gases, the absorbent, and water liberated from the neutralization of carbon dioxide. Most inspired humidity is supplied by the absorbent (115). The amount derived from the neutralization of carbon dioxide is negligible.

Gases in the inspiratory limb of a circle system are near room temperature (116, 117). Even with low fresh gas flows, gases reach the Y-piece only 1° to 3°C above ambient temperature (118). The humidity of a standard adult circle system using a fresh gas flow of 5 l/min is shown in Figure 8.22. The initial inspired humidity was 30%. This rose to 61% in 90 minutes, stabilizing at this level. These values may be altered by the following factors:

1. Higher humidity results when lower fresh gas flows are used (97, 118–121).
2. A decrease in the patient's carbon dioxide output will cause a decrease in the initial and final humidity (116).
3. Increasing ventilation will increase the inspired humidity (102, 116).
4. Prior use of the system will result in an initially higher humidity that stabilizes in the same period of time at the same final humidity (116).
5. An increase in humidity of inspired gas occurs when the fresh gas inlet is upstream of the absorber (86, 97, 122).

6. Wetting the inspiratory tubing (123, 124) or using a humidifier will increase humidity.
7. Heating the canister (122) or the breathing tubes (125, 126) will increase the inspired temperature and humidity.
8. Use of smaller canisters will result in higher heat and humidity (97).
9. Use of coaxial tubings (97, 127–129) and the use of the heat of reaction to vaporize water (128, 130, 131) will increase inspired heat and humidity.

RELATIONSHIP BETWEEN INSPIRED AND DELIVERED CONCENTRATIONS

In a system with no rebreathing, the concentrations of gases and vapors in the inspired mixture will be close to those in fresh gas. With rebreathing, however, the concentrations in the inspired mixture may differ considerably from those in the fresh gas.

Nitrogen

The importance of nitrogen lies in the fact that it hinders the establishment of high concentrations of nitrous oxide and may cause low inspired oxygen concentrations (132). Before any fresh gas is delivered, the concentration of nitrogen in the breathing system is approximately 80%. Nitrogen enters the system from exhaled gases and leaves through the APL valve or ventilator and leaks. Using high fresh gas flows for a few minutes to eliminate most of the nitrogen in the system and

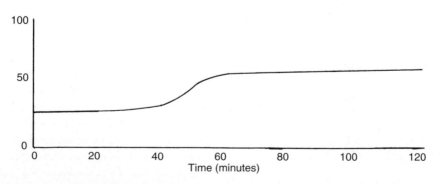

FIGURE 8.22. Humidity changes in the circle system. Fresh gas flow 5000 ml/min; CO_2 inflow 200 ml/min; respiratory rate 12/min; and tidal volume 500 ml. (Adapted with permission from Chalon J, Kao ZI, Dolorico VN, et al. Humidity output of the circle absorber system. Anesthesiology 1973;38:462.)

much of that in the patient is called "denitrogenation." Different methods have been described, with varying flows and times. A fresh gas flow of 10 l/min for 1 minute followed by 5 l/min for 6 minutes after intubation will wash out most nitrogen in the system (133).

After denitrogenation, nitrogen elimination by the patient will proceed at a slower rate. In a closed system, the nitrogen concentration will gradually rise. Provided denitrogenation has been carried out, even if all the body's nitrogen is exhaled, the concentration in the breathing system should not increase to more than 18% in the average adult (133–138).

Carbon Dioxide
With Absorbent

The inspired carbon dioxide concentration should be near zero unless there is failure of one or both unidirectional valves (139, 140), exhausted absorbent, or the absorber is in the bypass position. If one of these conditions exists, a high fresh gas flow will limit the increase in inspired carbon dioxide concentration.

Without Absorbent

A number of studies using the circle system without absorbent have been published (141–150). The arterial carbon dioxide level achieved will depend on the fresh gas flow, the arrangement of circle system components, and ventilation. Advantages of not using absorbent include the ability to achieve the desired level of arterial carbon dioxide with hyperventilation, lack of danger of inhaling absorbent dust, lack of dependence on absorbent to eliminate CO_2, and low resistance. Disadvantages include the need for uneconomical high flows and lower heat and humidity.

Oxygen

The concentration of oxygen in the inspired mixture is affected by the rate of uptake by the patient, uptake and elimination of other gases by the patient, arrangement of the components of the circle, ventilation, fresh gas flow, volume of the system, and the concentration of oxygen in the fresh gas. Use of a reliable oxygen analyzer in the breathing system should be mandatory because so many of these factors are unpredictable and uncontrollable.

Anesthetic Agent

The following influence the concentration of anesthetic agent in the inspired mixture: uptake by the patient, uptake by components of the system, arrangement of system components, uptake and elimination of other gases by the patient, volume of the system, concentration in the fresh gas flow, and fresh gas flow (151). It is not possible to predict the concentration accurately unless a high fresh gas flow is used. The greatest variation occurs during induction, when anesthetic uptake is high and nitrogen excretion by the patient dilutes the gases in the circuit. For this reason, most authors recommend that anesthesia be begun with high fresh gas flows. Several devices are now available to measure the inspired anesthetic agent concentration (see Chapter 18). When malignant hyperthermia is suspected, increasing the fresh gas flow is the most important measure that will aid in the washout of anesthetic agents from the patient. Use of a charcoal filter in the inspiratory limb or changing the anesthesia machine and breathing system are of no clinical advantage (152).

USE OF CIRCLE SYSTEM WITH LOW FRESH GAS FLOWS
Definitions

Low-flow anesthesia has been variously defined as an inhalation technique in which a circle system with absorbent is used with a fresh gas inflow of:

1) less than the patient's alveolar minute volume,
2) 1 l/min or less (153),
3) less than 1.5 l/min (154)
4) 3 l/min or less (155),
5) 0.5 to 2 l/min (118), and
6) less than 4 l/min (156)
7) 500 ml/min (157),
8) 500–100 ml/min (158), or
9) 0.5 to 1 l/min (159).

Closed system anesthesia is a form of low-flow anesthesia in which the fresh gas flow equals uptake of anesthetic gases and oxygen by the patient and system. There is complete rebreathing of exhaled gases after absorption of carbon dioxide and no gas is vented through the APL valve.

Equipment

Anesthesia Machine

A standard anesthesia machine can be used but it must have flowmeters that will provide low flows.

Circle System

A standard circle system with the absorber filled with active absorbent is used. If the absorber has a bypass, this should be removed or the absorber replaced with one that does not have a bypass. The system must have low leakage. Requirements include intubation with a cuffed tube or a tight mask fit.

Vaporizers

Anesthetic agent can be added to the circle in two ways.

Direct Injection into the Expiratory Limb

If direct injection is used, care must be taken that only small amounts are injected at a time and that the syringe containing the liquid agent is not confused with those containing agents for intravenous injection (160–164). Another problem is that the liquid agent may cause deterioration of components in the system (165).

Calibrated Vaporizers

Vaporizers capable of delivering high concentrations are required for low-flow anesthesia (160). Settings may need to be as high as 5% for halothane and isoflurane and 7% for enflurane (166). Some vaporizers cannot deliver high concentrations, and some are not accurate at low fresh gas flows (167).

Ventilator

A ventilator whose bellows rises during exhalation will result in easier detection of disconnections and large leaks than one whose bellows descends (168, 169). If a ventilator whose bellows descends during exhalation is used, leaks may lead to entrainment of driving gas or air.

Respiratory Gas Monitor Sensor or Connector

Continuous measurement of oxygen concentrations should be mandatory. Monitoring of other gases is helpful. Lower flows can be used with mainstream analyzers, but with aspirating types, the fresh gas flow must be increased to compensate for the gases removed by the monitor unless the gases are returned to the breathing system (170).

Techniques (171, 172)

Induction

Induction using low fresh gas flows can be accomplished by injecting measured amounts of liquid anesthetic directly into the expiratory limb of the circuit. Problems associated with this include the following:

1) Large body stores of nitrogen will be released into the breathing system and will dilute concentrations of other gases.
2) If nitrous oxide is being used, it will take a prolonged period of time to establish concentrations high enough to have a clinical effect.
3) Rapidly changing uptake of nitrous oxide and volatile agent as well as high oxygen consumption during this period mean that the anesthesia provider will have to make frequent injections and adjustments at a time when he or she is likely to be busy with other tasks.

More commonly, induction is accomplished using high flows to allow denitrogenation, establishment of anesthetic agent concentrations, and provide oxygen well in excess of consumption. After gas exchange has stabilized, low flows are used.

Maintenance

During maintenance, nitrous oxide and oxygen flows and vaporizer settings should be adjusted to maintain a satisfactory oxygen concentration and the desired level of anesthesia. If closed system anesthesia is used, a constant circuit volume is achieved by one of the following methods (166, 173).

Constant Reservoir Bag Size

If the bag decreases in size, the fresh gas flow rate is increased. If the bag increases in size, the flow must be decreased.

Ventilator with Ascending (Upright or Standing) Bellows

Constant volume can be achieved by adjusting the fresh gas flow so that the bellows is below the top of its housing at the end of exhalation. It is important that no negative pressure be transmitted to the bellows from the scavenging system because this could cause the bellows to be held aloft in the presence of inadequate fresh gas flow (174).

Ventilator with Descending (Inverted or Hanging) Bellows

The fresh gas flow should be adjusted so that the bellows just reaches the bottom of its housing at the end of exhalation.

If a rapid change in any component of the inspired mixture is desired, the fresh gas flow should be increased. If, for any reason, the integrity of the circle is broken, high flows with desired inspired concentrations should be used for several minutes before returning to low flows. If closed system anesthesia is used, it is recommended that high flows be used for 1 to 2 minutes at least once an hour to eliminate gases such as nitrogen and carbon monoxide that accumulate in the system.

Emergence

Recovery from anesthesia will be slow when low flows are used. High flows are usually needed at least briefly to clear nitrous oxide. Coasting, in which anesthetic administration is stopped toward the end of the operation and the circuit is maintained closed with enough oxygen flow to maintain a constant end-tidal volume of the ventilator or reservoir bag, can be used (175). A charcoal filter placed in the inspiratory limb will cause a rapid decrease in volatile agent concentration (176–178).

Advantages (179)

Economy

Significant savings can be achieved with lower flows of nitrous oxide and oxygen but the greatest savings occurs with the potent volatile agents. These savings are partly offset by increased absorbent usage, but this is small (188–190). There will be a savings in energy if an active scavenging system is used because the amount of excess gases and vapors that must be removed from the operating room is reduced.

Decreased Operating Room Pollution

Pollution of the operating room with trace gases is discussed in Chapter 12. With lower flows, there will be less anesthetic agent put into the operating room. One study showed that the concentrations inhaled by operating room personnel were within the OSHA limits without scavenging with nitrous oxide flows of 300 ml/min (191). However, use of low-flow techniques does not eliminate the need for scavenging because high flows are still necessary at times. Because a less volatile agent is used, vaporizers have to be filled less frequently so exposure of personnel to anesthetic vapors during filling is decreased.

Reduced Environmental Pollution

Fluorocarbons and nitrous oxide attack the earth's ozone layer, and nitrous oxide contributes to the greenhouse effect (192–196). With low flows, the ecologic dangers are reduced.

Estimation of Anesthetic Agent Uptake and Oxygen Consumption

In a closed system without significant leaks, fresh gas flow is matched by the patient's uptake of oxygen and anesthetic agents (197, 198). Changes in volume may be attributed to changes in uptake of oxygen or nitrous oxide because the volume contributed by the potent inhalational agents is not significant.

Buffering of Changes in Inspired Concentrations

The lower the fresh gas flow, the longer it takes for a change in concentration in the fresh gas flow to cause a comparable change in the inspired concentration.

Conservation of Heat and Humidity

With lower gas flows, inspired humidity will be increased (97, 118–120, 199). The incidence of shivering is lowered (200).

Less Danger of Barotrauma

High pressures in the breathing system take longer to develop with lower flows.

Disadvantages

More Attention Required

With closed system anesthesia, fresh gas flow into the system must be kept in balance with uptake. This could lead to insufficient attention to other aspects of the patient's care.

Inability to Alter Quickly Inspired Concentrations

This inability is a significant disadvantage only if the user insists on using low flows at all times. The user of low flows should accept that higher flows should be used when it is necessary to change inspired concentrations rapidly.

Danger of Hypercarbia

Hypercarbia resulting from exhausted absorbent, incompetent unidirectional valves, or the absorber being left in the bypass position will be greater when low flows are used.

Greater Knowledge Required

Use of low-flow anesthesia requires knowledge of uptake. However, it is arguable whether the need to acquire this knowledge is a disadvantage.

Accumulation of Undesirable Gases in the System

The accumulation of undesirable gases is probably only a problem with closed circuit anesthesia because low flows provide a continuous flush of the system. With closed system anesthesia, flushing with high fresh gas flows once an hour will decrease the concentration of most of these substances. Alternately, a diverting gas monitor can be used to remove small amounts of gas (154). To date, there have been no reported cases of significant patient harm from breathing any of these substances.

Carbon Monoxide

Carbon monoxide from the breakdown of hemoglobin can accumulate in the closed circle system (201). However, the levels reported are unlikely to cause clinically significant effects. One study found that carboxyhemoglobin concentrations decreased during closed circuit anesthesia (160). Although the levels reported with normal patients should be innocuous, patients with severe hemolytic anemia, high COHb levels and/or a reduced total hemoglobin may be at some risk (202).

Acetone, Methane, Hydrogen, and Ethanol

Hydrogen, methane, and acetone accumulate during closed system anesthesia (136, 203–207).

However, dangerous levels are reached only after hours of closed system anesthesia (208). The common intoxicant ethanol can also accumulate. Flushing with high flows will decrease the concentrations of methane and hydrogen but will not significantly affect the concentration of ethanol or acetone (136). Methane can disturb infrared analyzers (205, 207) (see Chapter 18). High concentrations of acetone can cause nausea, vomiting, and stupor in the postoperative patient (206).

Metabolites of Anesthetic Agents

One study showed that low concentrations of two volatile metabolites of halothane and a metabolic decomposition product—which has been shown to be mutagenic in one study (209) but not in another (210)—could be found in exhaled gases of patients anesthetized with halothane using a circle system but not a system without absorbent (32). However, the levels found were well below those demonstrated to be toxic in laboratory animals (211).

The safety of using sevoflurane with low flows is still under investigation. At the time of writing, the Food and Drug Administration (FDA) was still recommending that sevoflurane not be used with fresh gas flows of less than 2 l/min.

Argon

If oxygen is supplied from an oxygen concentrator (see Chapter 3), there will be an accumulation of argon (212). Raman gas analyzers (see Chapter 18) add a small amount of argon during its calibration cycle (213). If the gas exhausted from the monitor is returned to the breathing system, argon levels will increase.

Nitrogen

Even with initial denitrogenation, nitrogen will accumulate in the closed breathing circuit (133, 134, 136, 160). If oxygen is being supplied by an oxygen concentrator (see Chapter 3), malfunction of one of the concentrator modules can cause nitrogen to appear in the product gas (212). Infrared and Raman monitors (see Chapter 18) add air to the sample gas after the sample is analyzed (154, 213). If the gas exhausted is returned to the breathing system, nitrogen accumulation will be more than expected.

Other

Acrylic monomer is exhaled when joint prostheses are surgically cemented (214). During this period, the system should be vented to prevent rebreathing of this chemical.

Uncertainty About Inspired Concentrations

One of the effects of rebreathing is that the inspired concentrations cannot be predicted accurately. However, absolute or near-absolute knowledge of inspired concentration of anesthetic agents is not necessary for safe conduct of anesthesia because patients' responses to drugs vary widely.

USE OF CIRCLE SYSTEM FOR PEDIATRIC ANESTHESIA

It was once believed that small patients required special breathing circuits and ventilators (215). However, recent evidence indicates that circle systems can be used even in small infants (113, 215, 216).

In the past, special pediatric circle systems with small absorbers were used. These are no longer available commercially. What is referred to as a pediatric circle system is usually a standard absorber assembly with short, small-diameter tubings and a small bag attached (186, 217). This allows rapid and easy changeover from an adult to a pediatric system. However, the work of breathing in spontaneous-breathing pediatric patients with the pediatric circle system is greater than with the Jackson-Rees (218). The circle system can be used with low flows with pediatric patients (219–223).

USE OF THE CIRCLE SYSTEM TO DELIVER OXYGEN

In some institutions supplemental oxygen may be delivered to patients by attaching the oxygen tubing to a mask or nasal prongs to the Y-piece of a circle system. Studies show that this method is less accurate than use of a distinct flowmeter or the common gas outlet as a source of oxygen (224). Another disadvantage is that this may lead to drying of the absorbent (225). If the Y-piece is the only available source, it is important that the APL valve be completely closed.

ADVANTAGES OF CIRCLE SYSTEM

1. Low fresh gas flows can be used with the physiologic, economic, and environmental advantages of rebreathing.

2. $PaCO_2$ depends only on ventilation, not fresh gas flow.
3. Normocarbia can be achieved when a malignant hyperthermia syndrome develops.
4. The lengths of the tubings can be varied so that the machine can be placed away from the patient to allow optimal surgical exposure in head and neck surgery (74).

DISADVANTAGES OF CIRCLE SYSTEM

1. It is composed of many parts that can be arranged incorrectly or may malfunction. It also has a large number of connections, all of which can become disconnected and leak.
2. Some components are difficult to clean.
3. The system is bulky and not easily moved.
4. Minute volume must be limited to avoid profound hypocarbia.
5. The compliance of the circle system is high compared to other systems. This may make consistent ventilation more difficult with the circle system than with the Mapleson D or F systems (226).

REFERENCES

1. American Society for Testing and Materials. Standard specification for minimum performance and safety requirements for anesthesia breathing systems (ASTM F1208–89 [Reapproved 1994]). West Conshohocken, PA: ASTM, 1994.
2. International Standards Organization. Inhalational anaesthesia systems – Part 2: Anaesthetic circle breathing systems (ISO 8835-2:1993). Geneva, Switzerland: ISO, 1993.
3. Anonymous. Sodasorb prePak CO_2 absorption cartridges. Health Devices 1988;17:35–36.
4. Anonymous. Anesthesia unit carbon dioxide absorbents. Technology for Anesthesia 1992;12:4.
5. Anonymous. North American Drager Narkomed 2A carbon dioxide absorbers. Health Devices 1986;15:178–179.
6. Anonymous. Anesthesia machine owners alerted to potential breathing circuit leak. Biomedical Safety & Standards 1989;19:122.
7. Elam JO. The design of circle absorbers. Anesthesiology 1958;19:99–100.
8. Neufeld PD, Johnson DL. Results of the Canadian Anaesthetists' Society opinion survey on anesthetic equipment. Canadian Anaesthetists Society Journal 1983;30:469–473.

9. Tarbrett DG, de Jersey I. Equipment hazard alert. Anaesthesia and Intensive Care 1986;14:208.

10. Adriani J. Disposal of carbon dioxide from devices used for inhalational anesthesia. Anesthesiology 1960;21:742–758.

11. Brown ES, Bakamjian V, Seniff AM. Performance of absorbents: effect of moisture. Anesthesiology 1959; 20:613–617.

12. Miles G, Adriani J. Carbon dioxide absorption. Anesth Analg 1959;38:293–300.

13. Strum DP, Johnson BH, Eger EI II. Stability of sevo flurane in soda lime. Anesthesiology 1987;67: 779–781.

14. Adriani J, Rovenstine EA. Experimental studies on carbon dioxide absorbers for anesthesia. Anesthesiology 1941;2:1–19.

15. Foregger R. The regeneration of soda lime following absorption of carbon dioxide. Anesthesiology 1948; 9:15–20.

16. Jorgensen B, Jorgensen S. The 600 gram CO_2 absorption canister: an experimental study. Acta Anaesthesiol Scand 1977;21:437–444.

17. Sato T. New aspects of carbon dioxide absorption in anesthetic circuits. Med J Osaka Univ 1971;22: 173–206.

18. Bracken A, Sanderson DM. Some observations on anaesthetic soda lime. Br J Anaesth 1955;27: 422–427.

19. Lund I, Lund O, Erikson H. Model experiments on absorption efficiency of soda lime. Br J Anaesth 1957; 29:17–20.

20. Adriani J, Batten DH. The efficiency of mixtures of barium and calcium hydroxides in the absorption of carbon dioxide in rebreathing appliances. Anesthesiology 1942;3:1–10.

21. Hunt HK. Resistance in respiratory valves and canisters. Anesthesiology 1955;16:190–205.

22. Adriani J. The removal of carbon dioxide from rebreathing appliances. Journal of Aviation Medicine 1941;12:304–309.

23. Maycock E. Soda lime dust. Anaesthesia and Intensive Care 1980;8:217.

24. Davis R. Soda lime dust. Anaesthesia and Intensive Care 1979;7:390.

25. Lauria JI. Soda-lime dust contamination of breathing circuits. Anesthesiology 1975;42:628–629.

26. Williams N. A leaky circuit. Anaesthesia 1996;51: 406–407.

27. Hale DE. The rise and fall of soda lime. Anesth Analg 1967;46:648–655.

28. Adriani J. Rebreathing in anesthesia. South Med J 1942;35:798–804.

29. Eger EI II. Stability of I-653 in soda lime. Anesth Analg 1987;66:983–985.

30. Eger EI, Strum DP. The absorption and degradation of isoflurane and I-653 by dry soda lime at various temperatures. Anesth Analg 1987;66:1312–1315.

31. Liu J, Laster MJ, Eger EI II, et al. Absorption and degradation of sevoflurane and isoflurane in a conventional anesthetic circuit. Anesth Analg 1991;72: 785–789.

32. Sharp JH, Trudell JR, Cohen EN. Volatile metabolites and decomposition products of halothane in man. Anesthesiology 1979;50:2–8.

33. Frink EJ, Malan TP, Morgan SE, et al. Quantification of the degradation products of sevoflurane in two CO_2 absorbants during low-flow anesthesia in surgical patients. Anesthesiology 1992;77:1064–1069.

34. Bito H, Ikeda K. Effect of total flow rate on the concentration of degradation products generated by reaction between sevoflurane and soda lime. Br J Anaesth 1995;74:667–669.

35. Bito H, Ikeda K. Long-duration, low-flow sevoflurane anesthesia using two carbon dioxide absorbents. Quantification of degradation products in the circuit. Anesthesiology 1994;81:340–345.

36. Strum DP, Johnson BH, Eger EI II. Stability of sevoflurane in soda lime Anesthesiology 1987;67: 779–781.

37. Inhibition of volatile sevoflurane degradation product formation in an anesthesia circuit by a reduction in soda lime temperature. Anesthesiology 1994;81: 238–244.

38. Munday IT, Ward PM, Foden ND, et al. Sevoflurane degradation by soda lime in a circle breathing system. Anaesthesia 1996;51:622–626.

39. Liu J, Laster MJ, Eger EI II, et al. Absorption and degradation of sevoflurane and isoflurane in a conventional anesthetic circuit. Anesth Analg 1991;72: 785–789.

40. Fang ZX, Kandel L, Laster MJ, et al. Factors affecting production of Compound A from the interaction of sevoflurane with Baralyme and soda lime. Anesth Analg 1996;82:775–781.

41. Frink EJ, Green WB, Brown EA, et al. Compound A concentrations during sevoflurane anesthesia in children. Anesthesiology 1996;84:566–571.

42. Fang ZX, Eger EI II. Factors affecting the concentration of Compound A resulting from the degradation of sevoflurane by soda lime and Baralyme in a standard anesthetic circuit. Anesth Analg 1995;81: 564–568.

43. Wong DT, Lerman J. Factors affecting the rate of disappearance of sevoflurane in Baralyme. Can J Anaesth 1992;39:366–369.

44. Grodin WK, Epstein MAF, Epstein RA. Enflurane and isoflurane adsorption by soda lime. Anesthesiology 1981;55:A124.

45. Grodin WK, Epstein RA. Halothane adsorption complicating the use of soda-lime to humidify anaesthetic gases. Br J Anaesth 1982;54:555–559.

46. Grodin WK, Epstein MAF, Epstein RA. Mechanisms of halothane adsorption by dry soda-lime. Br J Anaesth 1982;54:561–565.

47. Tanifuji Y, Takagi K, Kobayashi K, et al. The interaction between sevoflurane and soda lime or baralyme. Anesth Analg 1989;68:S285.

48. Grodin WK, Epstein MAF, Epstein RA. Soda lime adsorption of isoflurane and enflurane. Anesthesiology 1985;62:60–64.

49. Fang ZX, Eger EI II, Laster MJ, et al. Carbon monoxide production from degradation of desflurane, enflurane, isoflurane, halothane and sevoflurane by soda lime and Baralyme. Anesth Analg 1995;80:1187–1193.

50. Woehick MJ, Dunning M III, Gandhi S, et al. Indirect detection of intraoperative carbon monoxide exposure by mass spectrometry during isoflurane anesthesia. Anesthesiology 1995;83:213–217.

51. Harrison N, Knowles AC, Welchew EA. Carbon monoxide within circle systems. Anaesthesia 1996;51:1037–1040.

52. Fang ZX, Eger EI. Source of toxic CO explained: -CHF$_2$ anesthetic + dry absorbent. Anesthesia Patient Safety Foundation Newsletter 1994;9:26–30.

53. Baxter PJ, Kharasch ED. Rehydration of desiccated baralyme prevents carbon monoxide formation from desflurane in an anesthesia machine. Anesthesiology 1997;86:1061–1065.

54. Eisenkraft JB. Complications of anesthesia delivery systems. ASA Annual Refresher Courses, No. 255, 1996.

55. Smith TC. Anesthesia breathing systems. In: Ehrenwerth J, Eisenkraft JB, eds. Anesthesia equipment, principles and applications. St. Louis: Mosby, 1993.

56. Andrews JJ, Johnston RV, Bee DE, et al. Photodeactivation of ethyl violet: a potential hazard of Sodasorb. Anesthesiology 1990;72:59–64.

57. Elam JO. Channeling and overpacking in carbon dioxide absorbers. Anesthesiology 1958;19:403–404.

58. Lamb KSR, Cummings GC, Asbury AJ. Comparison of three commercially available preparations of soda-lime. Br J Anaesth 1988;60:329P–330P.

59. Bell, GT. Problems with soda lime. Anaesthesia 1994;49:550.

60. Detmer MD, Chandra P, Cohen PJ. Occurrence of hypercarbia due to an unusual failure of anesthetic equipment. Anesthesiology 1980;52:278–279.

61. Liley A. Problems with soda lime. Anaesthesia 1994;49:550.

62. James MFM. Problems with soda lime. Anaesthesia 1994;49:1101–1102.

63. Tsuchiya M, Ueda W. Heat generation as an index of exhaustion of soda lime. Anesth Analg 1989;68:683–687.

64. Anonymous. Soda lime in anaesthesia. Australian Therapeutic Device Bulletin 1990;90(2):3.

65. Kim J, Kovac AL, Mathewson HS. A method for detection of incompetent unidirectional dome valves. Anesth Analg 1985;64:745–747.

66. Nunn BJ, Rosewarne FA. Expiratory valve failure. Anaesthesia and Intensive Care 1990;18:273–274.

67. Schreiber P. Anaesthesia Equipment. Performance, classification, and safety. New York: Springer-Verlag, 1974.

68. Rosewarne F, Wells D. Three cases of valve incompetence in a circle system. Anaesthesia and Intensive Care 1988;16:376–377.

69. Amir M. Caught by a cage. Anaesthesia and Intensive Care 1992;20:389–390.

70. Thompson AR, Gordon NH. One-way valve malfunction in a circle system. Anaesthesia 1995;50:920–921.

71. Dean HN, Parsons DE, Raphaely RC. Case report: bilateral tension pneumothorax from mechanical failure of anesthesia machine due to misplaced expiratory valve. Anesth Analg 1971;50:195–198.

72. Cottrell JE, Bernhard W, Turndorf H. Hazards of disposable rebreathing circuits. Anesth Analg 1976;55:743–744.

73. Wang JS, Hung WT, Lin CY. Leakage of disposable breathing circuits. J Clin Anesth 1992;4:111–115.

74. Boyd GL, Funderberg BJ, Vasconez LO, et al. Long-distance anesthesia. Anesth Analg 1992;74:477.

75. Stevenson PH, McLeskey CH. Breakage of a reservoir bag mount, an unusual anesthesia machine failure. Anesthesiology 1980;53:270–271.

76. Warren PR, Gintautas J. Problems with Dupaco ventilator valve assembly. Anesthesiology 1980;53:524–525.

77. Eger EI, Ethans CT. The effects of inflow, over-flow and valve placement on economy of the circle system. Anesthesiology 1968;29:93–100.

78. Zbinden AM, Feigenwinter P, Hutmacher M. Fresh gas utilization of eight circle systems. Br J Anaesth 1991;67:492–499.

79. Brown ES, Seniff AM, Elam JO. Carbon dioxide elimination in semiclosed systems. Anesthesiology 1964;25:31–36.

80. Briere C, Patoine JG, Audet R. Inaccurate ventimetry by fresh gas inlet position. Canadian Anaesthetists Society Journal 1974;21:117–119.

81. Campbell DI. Volumeter attachment on Boyle circle absorber. Br J Anaesth 1971;43:206–207.

82. Purnell RJ. The position of the Wright anemometer in the circle absorber system. Br J Anaesth 1968;40:917–918.

83. Grodin WK, Epstein RA. Halothane adsorption by soda lime. Anesthesiology 1979;51:S317.

84. Berry FA, Hughes-Davies DI. Methods of increasing the humidity and temperature of the inspired gases in the infant circle system. Anesthesiology 1972;37:456–462.

85. Shanks CA, Sara CA. Estimation of inspiratory-limb humidity in the circle system. Anesthesiology 1974;40:99–100.

86. Weeks DB. Higher humidity, an additional benefit of a disposable anesthesia circle. Anesthesiology 1975;43:375–377.

87. Harper M, Eger EI. A comparison of the efficiency of three anesthesia circle systems. Anesth Analg 1976;55:724–729.

88. Campbell DI. Change of gas inflow siting on Boyle MK3 absorbers. Anaesthesia 1971;26:104.

89. Russell WJ, Drew SE. A potential hazard with an inspiratory valve of a circle system. Anaesthesia and Intensive Care 1977;5:269–271.

90. Amaranath L, Boutros AR. Circle absorber and soda lime contamination. Anesth Analg 1980;59:711–712.

91. Dogu TS, Davis HS. Hazards of inadvertently opposed valves. Anesthesiology 1970;33:122–123.

92. LeBourdais E. Doctors say connector units are dangerous. Dimensions in Heath Service 1976;(Feb):10–11.

93. Rendell-Baker L. Another close call with crossed valves. Anesthesiology 1969;31:194–195.

94. White CW. Hazards of the valved Y-piece. Anesthesiology 1970;32:567.

95. Varma YS, Puri GD. Location of the adjustable pressure limiting valve. Anaesthesia 1986;41:773–774.

96. Puri GD, Varma YS. A new site for the adjustable pressure limiting valve on a circle absorber. Anaesthesia 1985;40:889–891.

97. Bengtson JP, Bengtson A, Stenqvist O. The circle system as a humidifier. Br J Anaesth 1989;63:453–457.

98. Kopman AF. Obstruction of bacterial filters by edema fluid. Anesthesiology 1976;44:169–170.

99. Mason J, Tackley R. An acute rise in expiratory resistance due to a blocked ventilator filter. Anaesthesia 1981;36:335.

100. Garibaldi RA, Britt MR, Webster C, et al. Failure of bacterial filters to reduce the incidence of pneumonia after inhalation anesthesia. Anesthesiology 1981;54:364–368.

101. Chalon J, Markham JP, Ali MM, et al. The Pall Ulti-por breathing circuit filter—an efficient heat and moisture exchanger. Anesth Analg 1984;63:566–570.

102. Berry AJ, Nolte FS. An alternative strategy for infection control of anesthesia breathing circuits: a laboratory assessment of the Pall HME filter. Anesth Analg 1991;72:651–655.

103. MacKrell TN. Intravenous anesthesia plus nitrous oxide in a closed system. In: Aldrete JA, Lowe HJ, Virtue RW, eds. Low flows and closed system anesthesia. New York: Grune & Stratton, 1979:99–101.

104. Elliott WR, Topulas GP. The influence of the mechanics of anesthesia breathing circuits on respiratory monitoring. Biomed Instrum Technol 1990;24:260–265.

105. Sola A, Farina D, Rodriguez S, et al. Lack of relationship between the true airway pressure and the pressure displayed with an infant ventilator. Crit Care Med 1992;20:778–781.

106. Sinclair A, VanBergen J. Flow resistance of coaxial breathing systems: investigation of a circuit disconnect. Can J Anaesth 1992;39:90–94.

107. McEwen JA, Small CF, Jenkins LC. Detection of interruptions in the breathing gas of ventilated anaesthetized patients. Can J Anaesth 1997;35:549–561.

108. Mayle LL, Reed SJ, Wyche MQ. Excessive airway pressures occurring concurrently with use of the Fraser Harlake PEEP valve. Anesthesiology Review 1990;17:41–44.

109. Shandro J. A coaxial circle circuit: comparison with conventional circle and Bain circuit. Canadian Anaesthetists Society Journal 1982;29:121–125.

110. Conterato JP, Lindahl GE, Meyer DM, et al. Assessment of spontaneous ventilation in anesthetized children with use of a pediatric circle or a Jackson-Rees system. Anesth Analg 1989;69:484–490.

111. Gravenstein N, Gallagher RC. External flow-resistive, circuit-related work of breathing: Bain vs circle. Anesthesiology 1985;63:A183.

112. Kay B, Beatty PCW, Healy TEJ, et al. Change in the work of breathing imposed by five anaesthetic breathing systems. Br J Anaesth 1983;55:1239–1246.

113. Rasch DK, Bunegin L, Ledbetter J, et al. Comparison of circle absorber and Jackson-Rees systems for paediatric anaesthesia. Can J Anaesth 1988;35:25–30.

114. Shandro J. Resistance to gas flow in the "new" anaesthesia circuits: a comparative study. Canadian Anaesthetists Society Journal 1982;29:387–390.

115. Dery R, Pelletier J, Jacques A, et al. Humidity in anaesthesiology II. Evolution of heat and moisture in the large carbon dioxide absorbers. Canadian Anaesthetists Society Journal 1967;14:205–219.

116. Chalon J, Kao ZL, Dolorico VN, et al. Humidity output of the circle absorber system. Anesthesiology 1973;38:458–465.

117. Dery R, Pelletier J, Jacques A, et al. Humidity in anaesthesiology. Heat and moisture patterns in the respiratory tract during anaesthesia with the semi-closed system. Canadian Anaesthetists Society Journal 1967; 14:287–298.

118. Aldrete JA, Cubillos P, Sherrill D. Humidity and temperature changes during low flow and closed system anaesthesia. Acta Anaesthesiol Scand 1981;25: 312–314.

119. Aldrete JA. Closed circuit anesthesia prevents moderate hypothermia occurring in patients having extremity surgery. Circular 1987;4:3–4.

120. Kleeman PP, Jantzen FP, Erdmann W. Fresh gas flow effects on airway climate: a controlled clinical study. Circular 1988;5:11.

121. Henriksson BA, Sundling J, Hellman A. The effects of a heat and moisture exchanger on humidity in a low-flow anaesthesia system. Anaesthesia 1997;52: 144–149.

122. Berry FA, Ball CG, Blankenbaker WL. Humidification of anesthetic systems for prolonged procedures. Anesth Analg 1975;54:50–54.

123. Chase HF, Kilmore MA, Trotta R. Respiratory water loss via anesthesia systems; mask breathing. Anesthesiology 1961;22:205–209.

124. Shanks CA, Sara CA. Airway heat and humidity during endotracheal intubation. 4: connotations of delivered water vapour content. Anaesthesia and Intensive Care 1974;2:212–220.

125. Kadim MY, Lockwood GG, Chakrabarti MK, et al. A low-flow to-and-fro system. Laboratory study of mixing of anaesthetic and driving gases during mechanical ventilation. Anaesthesia 1991;46:948–951.

126. Kleeman PP, Schickel BK, Jantzen J-PAH. Heated breathing tubes affect humidity output of circle absorber systems. J Clin Anesth 1993;5:463–467.

127. Chalon J, Patel C, Ramanathan S, et al. Humidification of the circle absorber system. Anesthesiology 1978;48:142–146.

128. Chalon J, Goldman C, Amirdivani M, et al. Humidification in a modified circle system. Anesth Analg 1979;58:216–220.

129. Ramanathan S, Chalon J, Turndorf H. Compact well-humidified breathing circuit for the circle system. Anesthesiology 1976;44:238–242.

130. Chalon J, Ramanathan S. Water vaporizer heated by the reaction of neutralization of carbon dioxide. Anesthesiology 1974;41:400–404.

131. Paspa P, Tang CK, Dwarkmanath R, et al. A percolator vaporizer heated by reaction of neutralization of lime by carbon dioxide. Anesth Analg 1981;60: 146–149.

132. Conway CM. Gaseous homeostasis and the circle system. Validation of a model. Br J Anaesth 1986;58: 337–344.

133. Bengtson JP, Sonander H, Stenqvist O. Gaseous homeostasis during low-flow anaesthesia. Acta Anaesthesiol Scand 1988;32:516–521.

134. Barton F, Nunn JF. Totally closed circuit nitrous oxide/oxygen anaesthesia. Br J Anaesth 1975;47: 350–357.

135. Anonymous. Action required on scavenging systems. Br J Anaesth 1976;48:397.

136. Morita S, Latta W, Hambro K, et al. Accumulation of methane, acetone, and nitrogen in the inspired gas during closed-circuit anesthesia. Anesth Analg 1985; 64:343–347.

137. Philip JH. Nitrogen build-up in a closed circuit. Journal of Clinical Monitoring 1991;7:89.

138. Luttropp H, Rydgren G, Thomasson R, et al. A minimal-flow system for xenon anesthesia. Anesthesiology 1991;75:896–902.

139. Kerr JH, Evers JL. Carbon dioxide accumulation: valve leaks and inadequate absorption. Canadian Anaesthetists Society Journal 1958;5:154–160.

140. Schultz EA, Buckley JJ, Oswald AJ, et al. Profound acidosis in an anesthetized human: report of a case. Anesthesiology 1960;21:285–291.

141. Schoonbee CG, Conway CM. Factors affecting carbon dioxide homeostasis during controlled ventilation with circle systems. Br J Anaesth 1981;53: 471–477.

142. Akkineni S, Patel KP, Bennett EJ, et al. Fresh gas flow to limit PaCO$_2$ in T and circle systems without CO$_2$ absorption. Anesthesiology Review 1977;4: 33–37.

143. deSilva AJC. Normocapnic ventilation using the circle system. Canadian Anaesthetists Society Journal 1976;23:657–666.

144. Gibb DB, Prior G, Pollard B. Methods of conserving carbon dioxide in artificially ventilated patients. A clinical investigation. Anaesthesia and Intensive Care 1977;5:122–127.

145. Harris PHP, Kerr JH, Edmonds-Seal J. Artificial ventilation using a circle circuit without an absorber. Anaesthesia 1975;30:269–270.

146. Keenan RL, Boyan CP. How rebreathing anaesthetic systems control PaCO$_2$ studies with a mechanical and mathematical model. Canadian Anaesthetists Society Journal 1978;25:117–121.

147. Ladegaard-Pedersen HJ. A circle system without carbon dioxide absorption. Acta Anaesthesiol Scand 1978;22:281–286.

148. Patel K, Bennett EJ, Grundy EM, et al. Relation of $PaCO_2$ to fresh gas flow in a circle system. Anesth Analg 1976;55:706–708.

149. Scholfield EJ, Williams NE. Prediction of arterial carbon dioxide tension using a circle system without carbon dioxide absorption. Br J Anaesth 1974;46: 442–445.

150. Snowdon SL, Powell DL, Fadl ET, et al. The circle system without absorber. Anaesthesia 1975;30: 323–332.

151. Conway CM. Gaseous homeostasis and the circle system. Factors influencing anaesthetic gas exchange. Br J Anaesth 1986;58:1167–1180.

152. Reber A, Schumacher P, Urwyler A. Effects of three different types of management on the elimination kinetics of volatile anaesthetics. Implications for malignant hyperthermia treatment. Anaesthesia 1993;48: 862–865.

153. Stone SB, Greene NM. Low-flow anesthesia. Current Review in Clinical Anesthesia 1981;1:114.

154. Bengtson JP, Bengtsson J, Bengtsson A, et al. Sampled gas need not be returned during low-flow anesthesia. Journal of Clinical Monitoring 1993;9: 330–334.

155. Spence AA, Alison RH, Wishart HY. Low flow and closed systems for the administration of inhalation anaesthesia. Br J Anaesth 1981;53:69S–73S.

156. Cotter SM, Petros AJ, Barber ND, et al. Cost of low flow anaesthesia. Br J Anaesth 1991;66:408P–409P.

157. Lee DJH, Robinson DL, Soni N. Efficiency of a circle system for short surgical cases: comparison of desflurane with isoflurane. Br J Anaesth 1996;76:780–782.

158. Baker AB. Low flow and closed circuits. Anaesthesia and Intensive Care 1994;22:341–342.

159. Baxter AD. Low and minimal flow inhalational anaesthesia. Can J Anaesth 1997;44:643–653.

160. Lowe HJ, Ernst EA. The quantitative practice of anesthesia. Use of closed circuit. Baltimore, MD: Williams & Wilkins, 1981.

161. Boulogne P, Demontoux MH, Colin D, et al. Isoflurane requirements during low and high flow anesthesia. Circular 1988;5:10–11.

162. Dennison PH. Coaxial tubing for conventional anesthetic systems. Anaesthesia 1984;39:841.

163. O'Callaghan AC, Hawes DW, Ross JAS, et al. Uptake of isoflurane during clinical anaesthesia. Servo-control of liquid anaesthetic injection into a closed-circuit breathing system. Br J Anaesth 1983;55: 1061–1064.

164. El-Attar AM. Guided isoflurane injection in a totally closed circuit. Anaesthesia 1991;46:1059–1063.

165. Ferderbar PJ, Kettler RE, Jablonski J, et al. A cause of breathing system leak during closed circuit anesthesia. Anesthesiology 1986;65:661–663.

166. Ernst EA. A clinical approach to closed circuit anesthesia. Circular 1985;2:5–7.

167. Lin C. Assessment of vaporizer performance in low-flow and closed-circuit anesthesia. Anesth Analg 1980;59:359–366.

168. Graham DH. Advantages of standing bellows ventilators and low-flow techniques. Anesthesiology 1983; 58:486.

169. Lin CY, Mostert JW, Benson DW. Closed circle systems. A new direction in the practice of anesthesia. Acta Anaesthesiol Scand 1980;24:354–361.

170. Huffman LM, Riddle RT. Mass spectrometer and/or capnograph use during low-flow closed circuit anesthesia administration. Anesthesiology 1987;66: 439–440.

171. Baker AB. Back to basics—a simplified non-mathematical approach to low flow techniques in anaesthesia. Anaesthesia and Intensive Care 1994;22: 394–395.

172. Dale O, Stenqvist O. Low-flow anesthesia: available today—a routine tomorrow. Survey of Anesthesia 1992;36:334–336.

173. Lowe HJ. The anesthetic continuum. In: Aldrete JA, Lowe HJ, Virtue RW, eds. Low flow and closed system anesthesia. New York: Grune & Stratton, 1979: 11–37.

174. Blackstock D. Advantages of standing bellows ventilators and low-flow techniques. Anesthesiology 1984;60:167.

175. El-Attar AM. Closed-circuit coasting from high flow isoflurane anesthesia. Journal of Clinical Monitoring 1992;8:182–183.

176. Baumgarten RK. Simple charcoal filter for closed circuit anesthesia. Anesthesiology 1985;63:125.

177. Ernst EA. Use of charcoal to rapidly decrease depth of anesthesia while maintaining a closed circuit. Anesthesiology 1982;57:343.

178. Jan-Peter AH, Jantzen DEAA. More on black and white granules in the closed circuit. Anesthesiology 1988;69:437–438.

179. Baum JA, Aitkenhead AR. Low-flow anaesthesia. Anaesthesia 1995;50(Suppl):37–44.

180. Aldrete JA, Hendricks PL. Differences in costs: how much can we save? Anesthesiology 1986;64: 656–657.

181. Bengtson JP, Sonander H, Stenqvist O. Comparison of costs of different anaesthetic techniques. Acta Anaesthesiol Scand 1988;32:33–35.

182. Christensen KN, Thomsen A, Jorgensen S, et al. Analysis of costs of anaesthetic breathing systems. Br J Anaesth 1987;59:389–390.

183. Cotter SM, Petros AJ, Dore CJ, et al. Low-flow anaesthesia. Anaesthesia 1991;46:1009–1012.

184. Matjasko J. Economic impact of low-flow anesthesia. Anesthesiology 1987;67:863–864.

185. Pedersen FM, Nielsen J, Ibsen M, et al. Low-flow isoflurane-nitrous oxide anaesthesia offers substantial economic advantages over high- and medium-flow isoflurane-nitrous oxide anaesthesia. Acta Anaesthiol Scand 1993;37:509–512.

186. Perkins R, Meakin G. Economies of low-flow anaesthesia in children. Anaesthesia 1996;51:1089–1092.

187. Logan M. Breathing systems: effect of fresh gas flow rate on enflurane consumption. Br J Anaesth 1994; 73:775–778.

188. Virtue RW, Aldrete JA. Costs of delivery of anesthetic gases reexamined. II. Anesthesiology 1981;55:711.

189. Spain JA. Cost of delivery of anesthetic gases reexamined. III. Anesthesiology 1981;55:711–712.

190. Patel A, Milliken RA. Costs of delivery of anesthetic gases re-examined. I. Anesthesiology 1981;55:710.

191. Virtue RW, Escobar A, Modell J. Nitrous oxide levels in operating room air with various gas flows. Canadian Anaesthetists Society Journal 1979;26: 313–318.

192. Logan M, Farmer JG. Anaesthesia and the ozone layer. Br J Anaesth 1989;63:645–647.

193. Sherman SJ, Cullen BF. Nitrous oxide and the greenhouse effect. Anesthesiology 1988;68:816–817.

194. Westhorpe R, Blutstein H. Anaesthetic agents and the ozone layer. Anaesthesia and Intensive Care 1990;18:102–109.

195. Brown AC, Canosa-Mas CE, Parr AD, et al. Tropospheric lifetimes of halogenated anaesthetics. Nature 1989;341:635–637.

196. Dale O. Inhalational anesthetics and the global environment. Acta Anaesthiol Scand 1992;35:40–41.

197. Cohen AT, Beatty PCW, Kay B, et al. Measurement of oxygen uptake: a method for use during nitrous oxide in oxygen anaesthesia. Eur J Anaesthiol 1984; 1:63–75.

198. Bengtson JP, Bengtsson A, Stenqvist O. Predictable nitrous oxide uptake enables simple oxygen uptake monitoring during low flow anaesthesia. Anaesthesia 1994;49:29–31.

199. Kleeman PP. Humidity of anaesthetic gases with respect to low flow anaesthesia. Anaesthesia and Intensive Care 1994;22:396–408.

200. Panah M, Rosenblatt M, Kahn P, et al. Incidence of shivering in patients undergoing ambulatory gynecological laparoscopy increases by fresh gas flow rate and surgical time. Anesth Analg 1997;84:S18.

201. Rolly G, Versichelen L, Vermeulen H. CO concentrations during closed circuit anesthesia conditions. Anesth Analg 1993;76:S353.

202. Spiess W. To what degree should we be concerned about carbon monoxide accumulation in closed circuit anesthesia? Circular 1984;1:8.

203. Morita S. Inspired gas contamination by non-anesthetic gases during closed circuit anesthesia. Circular 1985;2:24–25.

204. Rolly G, Versichelen L. Methane accumulation during closed circuit anesthesia. Anesth Analg 1992;74: S253.

205. Tolly G, Versichelen LF, Mortier E. Methane accumulation during closed-circuit anesthesia. Anesth Analg 1994;79:545–547.

206. Straub JM, Hausdorfer J. Accumulation of acetone in blood during long-term anaesthesia with closed systems. Br J Anaesth 1993;70:363–364.

207. Versichelen L, Rolly G, Vermeulen H. Accumulation of foreign gases during closed-system anaesthesia. Br J Anaesth 1996;76:668–672.

208. Baumgarten RK, Reynolds WJ. Much ado about nothing: Trace gaseous metabolites in the closed circuit. Anesth Analg 1985;64:1029–1030.

209. Garro AJ, Phillips RA. Mutagenicity of the halogenated olefin, 2-bromo-2-chloro-1,1-difluoro-ethylene, a presumed metabolite of the inhalation anesthetic, halothane. Environ Health Perspect 1977;21: 65–69.

210. Waskell L. Lack of mutagenicity of two possible metabolites of halothane. Anesthesiology 1979;50: 9–12.

211. Eger EI. Dragons and other scientific hazards (Editorial). Anesthesiology 1979;50:1.

212. Parker CJR, Snowdon SL. Predicted and measured oxygen concentrations in the circle system using low fresh gas flows with oxygen supplied by an oxygen concentratior. Br J Anaesth 1988;61:397–402.

213. Stevens WC, Nash JA, Burney R. A source of nitrogen in the breathing circuit during closed system anesthesia. Anesthesiology 1996;85:1492–1493.

214. Philip JH. Closed circuit anesthesia. In: Ehrenwerth J, Eisenkraft JB, eds. Anesthesia equipment, principles and applications. St. Louis, MO: Mosby, 1993

215. Badgwell JM, Swan J, Foster AC. Volume-controlled ventilation is made possible in infants by using compliant breathing circuits with large compression volume. Anesth Analg 1996;82:719–723.

216. Conteraro JP, Lindahl SGE, Meyer DM, et al. Assessment of spontaneous ventilation in children with use of a paediatric circle or a Jackson-Rees system. Anesth Analg 1989;69:484–490.

217. Berry FA. Clinical pharmacology of inhalational anesthetics, muscle relaxants, vasoactive agents, and narcotics, and techniques of general anesthesia. In: Berry FA, ed. Anesthetic management of difficult and routine pediatric patients. 2nd ed. New York: Churchill Livingstone, 1990:83–84.

218. Nakae Y, Miyabe M, Sonoda H, et al. Comparison of the Jackson-Rees circuit, the pediatric circle and the MERA F breathing system for pediatric anesthesia. Anesth Analg 1996;83:488–492.

219. Aldrete JA. . . . and the frog turned into a prince: closed circuit in pediatric anesthesia. Circular 1985; 2:13.

220. Aldrete JA. Closed circuit and the pediatric patient. Circular 1988;5:12–13.

221. da Silva JMC, Tubino PJ, Vieira ZEG, et al. Closed circuit anesthesia in infants and children. Anesth Analg 1984;63:765–769.

222. Pappas ALS, Santos E, Sukhani R, et al. Low flow closed circuit anesthesia in pediatrics—its safety and applicability. Circular 1988;5:13.

223. Pappas AS, Santos E, Sukhani R, et al. Applicability and safety of low flow closed circuit anesthesia in pediatrics. Anesthesiology 1988;69:A783.

224. Henderson CL, Rosen HD, Arney KL. Oxygen flow through nasal cannulae. Can J Anaesth 1996;43: 636–639.

225. Woehlick HJ, Dunning MB III, Connolly L. Reduction in the incidence of carbon monoxide exposures during inhalation anesthesia in humans. Anesthesiology 1996;85:A1017.

226. Hillier SC, McNiece WL. Pediatric anesthesia and equipment. In: Ehrenwerth J, Eisenkraft JB, eds. Anesthesia equipment, principles and applications, esthesia systems and equipment. St. Louis, MO: Mosby, 1993.

QUESTIONS

1. Concerning degradation of sevoflurane by absorbent
   A. It is degraded more by baralyme than soda lime
   B. More degradation occurs at lower temperatures
   C. More degradation occurs with lower concentrations
   D. Drying of the absorbent decreases degradation
   E. Low fresh gas flows decrease degradation

2. The most common location for the fresh gas inlet in the circle system is
   A. Just upstream of the inspiratory unidirectional valve
   B. Between the pressure manometer and the absorber
   C. Between the inspiratory unidirectional valve and the Y-piece
   D. Between the spirometer and the expiratory unidirectional valve
   E. Between the inspiratory unidirectional valve and the PEEP valve

3. The most common location for the reservoir bag is
   A. Just upstream of the inspiratory unidirectional valve
   B. Between the inspiratory unidirectional valve and the absorber
   C. Between the inspiratory unidirectional valve and the Y-piece
   D. Between the exhalational unidirectional valve and the absorber
   E. Between the Y-piece and the spirometer

4. The best location for the fresh gas inlet to the circle breathing system is
   A. Upstream of the inspiratory valve
   B. Between the pressure manometer and the absorber
   C. Between the inspiratory unidirectional valve and the Y-piece
   D. Between the spirometer and the expiratory unidirectional valve
   E. Between the inspiratory unidirectional valve and the PEEP valve

5. The best position for the reservoir bag is
   A. Upstream of the inspiratory valve
   B. Between the pressure manometer and the absorber
   C. Between the inspiratory unidirectional valve and the Y-piece
   D. Between the PEEP valve and the pressure manometer
   E. Between the Y-piece and the spirometer

Each question below contains four suggested answers of which one or more is correct.
Choose the answer:

A if 1, 2, and 3 are correct
B if 1 and 3 are correct
C if 2 and 4 are correct
D if 4 is correct
E if 1, 2, 3, and 4 are correct.

6. Which statements correctly reflect the flow through a CO_2 absorber?
   1. Flow is continuous
   2. It makes no difference if the flow is from bottom to top or from top to bottom
   3. Larger canisters do not allow more CO_2 absorption
   4. Absorption takes place first at the inlet and along the sides of the cannister

7. Baffles in the absorber
   1. Increase resistance
   2. Separate the absorbent into different compartments
   3. Increase the path of travel for gases in the absorber
   4. Act as a buffer for dust and water generated in the cannister

8. A partial absorber bypass
   1. Allows the absorbent to rest and regenerate
   2. Increases the inspired CO_2
   3. Allows the absorbent to be changed during an anesthetic
   4. Can be especially dangerous if actuated used during low flow anesthesia

9. Regarding carbon dioxide absorption
   1. The general principle is that of a base neutralizing an acid
   2. Carbonic acid is formed
   3. An alkaline earth metal is commonly used as the base
   4. The sodalime presently in use is of the dry type

10. Which statements correctly reflect the importance of size and shape of granules in soda lime?
    1. Small granules provide a greater surface area for absorption
    2. Small granules cause more resistance and caking
    3. Granule size used today range in size between 4 to 8 mesh
    4. Small granules decrease channeling

11. Concerning the hardness of soda lime granules
    1. If the granule is too hard, its absorptive properties will be decreased
    2. If the granule is too soft, it will fragment easily and produce dust
    3. Kieselghur is added to granules to increase the absorptive properties
    4. Dust will increase resistance and channeling

12. The absorbent in the canister should be changed when
    1. CO_2 appears in the inhaled gases
    2. There is no heat production with low fresh gas flows
    3. Heat is generated in the downstream canister
    4. Color change is seen in the downstream canister

13. Concerning the storage and handling of carbon dioxide absorbents
    1. They should not be stored at high temperatures
    2. Absorbent dust can be an irritant to the eyes, respiratory tract, and skin
    3. When filling the canister with absorbent, a small space should be left at the top
    4. Absorbent dust will cause the seals to warp

14. Which of the following are objectives in the arrangement of components of the circle breathing system?
    1. Maximal humidification of inspired gases
    2. Minimal resistance
    3. Minimal consumption of carbon dioxide absorbents
    4. Maximal inclusion of dead space gases in the inspired mixture

15. Disadvantages of placing the unidirectional valve in the Y-piece include
    1. The valves are bulky
    2. The dead space is increased
    3. The Y-piece could be used in a system that had absorber-mounted valves, and complete obstruction could occur
    4. Absorbent use is increased

16. Which position(s) of the APL valve in the circle system would cause inefficient use of the carbon dioxide absorbent during controlled ventilation?
    1. Just upstream of the inspiratory valve
    2. Between the inspiratory unidirectional valve and the Y-piece
    3. At the Y-piece
    4. Between the exhalation unidirectional valve and the absorber

17. If a bacterial filter is located on the inspiratory side of a circle system downstream of the inspiratory valve
    1. The patient will be protected from bacterial contamination by the anesthesia machine and components of the breathing system
    2. It will catch absorbent dust
    3. If a humidifiers is used, it should be attached downstream of this filter
    4. Use of a filter in this position has not been shown to reduce the incidence of pneumonia after anesthesia

18. Sources of naturally occurring humidity in the circle breathing system include
    1. Neutralization of carbon dioxide
    2. Water content of the absorbent granules
    3. Exhaled gases
    4. The fresh gas flow

19. Which techniques are used during the emergence of anesthesia with low fresh gas flows?
    1. Turn off all anesthetics and allow the patient to awaken slowly
    2. Use a charcoal filter to remove volatile agents
    3. Use high fresh gas flows to wash out anesthetics
    4. Activate the absorber bypass in order to increase CO_2

20. Humidity in the circle system is increased by
    1. Low fresh gas flows
    2. A decrease of carbon dioxide output from the patient
    3. Increased minute ventilation
    4. Cooling the canister

21. Inspired CO_2 using a circle breathing system may be caused by
    1. Not activating the bypass mechanism
    2. Failure of one or both unidirectional valves
    3. High fresh gas flow into the system
    4. Exhausted absorbent

22. What equipment is essential for performing low flow anesthesia with a circle breathing system?
    1. Oxygen analyzer
    2. Anesthetic agent analyzer
    3. Vaporizers with accuracy in the high range of the scale
    4. A ventilator with a bellows that descends on exhalation

23. Which gases may accumulate in the circle breathing system during closed circle anesthesia?
    1. Carbon monoxide
    2. Acetone
    3. Toxic metabolites of anesthetic agents
    4. Hydrogen

24. At which location(s) in the circle system will a spirometer overread the inspired volume?
    1. Just upstream of the inspiratory unidirectional valve

    2. Between the pressure manometer and the absorber
    3. Between the inspiratory unidirectional valve and the Y-piece
    4. Between the Y-piece and the expiratory unidirectional valve

25. Concerning unidirectional valves
    1. Movement of the disc does not assure competence
    2. The disc can obstruct gas flow through the valve
    3. Electrostatic charges can cause the disc to be attracted to the top of the valve
    4. Unidirectional valves are not positional and can be operated in a number of positions

26. What are some of the advantages of low flow anesthesia?
    1. Less danger of barotrauma
    2. Buffering of changes in inspired concentrations
    3. Conservation of heat and humidity
    4. Elimination of the need for scavenging

27. Which of the following are commonly found in soda lime?
    1. Sodium hydroxide
    2. Potassium hydroxide
    3. Calcium hydroxide
    4. Silica

ANSWERS

1.	A	15.	B
2.	A	16.	A
3.	D	17.	E
4.	A	18.	A
5.	D	19.	A
6.	C	20.	B
7.	B	21.	C
8.	C	22.	B
9.	A	23.	E
10.	E	24.	E
11.	E	25.	A
12.	E	26.	A
13.	C	27.	E
14.	A		

Manual Resuscitators

INTRODUCTION

Breathing systems using nonrebreathing valves have largely disappeared from anesthesia practice. However, these valves are still used in small portable manual resuscitators, which are used for patient transport and emergency situations. They can also be used to administer anesthesia. A manual resuscitator may be adapted for manual ventilation during magnetic resonance imaging (MRI) (1).

Manual resuscitators are known by many different terms, including: bag ventilators; bag-assist devices; bag-type resuscitators; bag-valve devices, units, or resuscitators; bag-valve-mask units, resuscitators, or ventilators; emergency manual ventilators; hand ventilators; hand-operated bag resuscitators; manual ventilators; hand-operated emergency ventilators; hand- or operator- powered resuscitators; handbag resuscitators; manual bag ventilators; manually-operated resuscitators; manual pulmonary resuscitators; respiratory bags; resuscitator or resuscitation bags; self-inflating manual resuscitators; self-inflating respirator bags or resuscitators; ventilator bags; and self-inflating bag-valve devices. United States, Canadian, and international standards for resuscitators have been published (2–4).

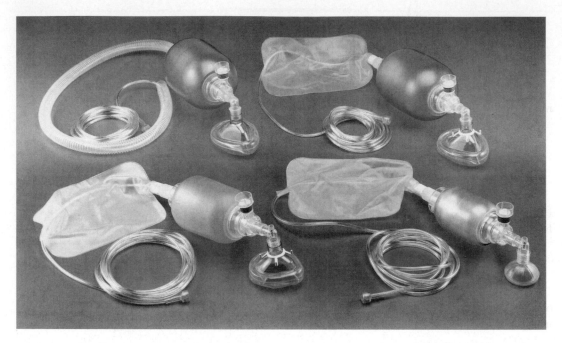

FIGURE 9.1. Manual Resuscitators. The resuscitator at the bottom right is for pediatric patients. The resuscitator at the top left has an open reservoir. The others have closed reservoirs. Each has a pressure-limiting device that can be overridden by placing a finger on top. (Courtesy of Rusch Inc.)

These devices are frequently supplied in three sizes: adult, child, and infant (Fig. 9.1). The United States standard classifies devices delivering a tidal volume of 600 ml and over as adult resuscitators and notes that resuscitators designed to deliver a tidal volume of 20 to 50 ml are usually suitable for neonatal use (2). Disposable manual resuscitators that avoid the inconvenience and hazards associated with reprocessing and sterilizing of reusable resuscitators are available and in common use.

COMPONENTS

Some typical manual resuscitators are shown in Figures 9.1 and 9.2. It has a compressible self-expanding bag, a bag refill valve, and a nonrebreathing valve. The two valves are combined in some units. Optional components include a pressure-limiting device, oxygen enrichment device, positive end–expiratory pressure (PEEP) valve, and mechanism for scavenging anesthetic gases.

Self-Expanding Bag

The self-expanding bag (ventilating or ventilation bag, self-inflating bag, compressible unit,

compressible reservoir) is constructed so that it is inflated in its resting state. The self-expanding bag may be cylindrical or football shaped. Some bags collapse like an accordion for storage. During expiration, the bag expands. If the volume of oxygen from the delivery source is inadequate to fill the bag, the difference is made up by intake of air. The rate at which the bag reinflates will determine the maximum respiratory rate.

Nonrebreathing Valve

The nonrebreathing valve is sometimes referred to as the directional control valve, exhalation valve, expiratory valve, inflating valve, inhalation-exhalation valve, inflating-exhalation valve, inspiratory-expiratory valve, nonreturn valve, patient valve, routing valve, or one-way inflating valve.

Body

Most nonrebreathing valves are T-shaped. The expiratory port is the opening through which exhaled gases pass to the atmosphere. A PEEP valve may be connected at this point (5). The expiratory

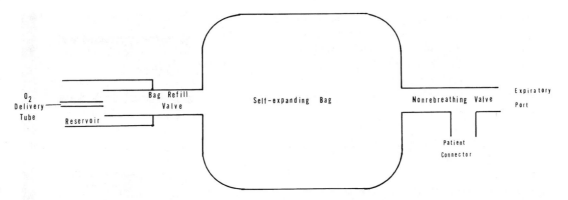

FIGURE **9.2.** Components of a manual resuscitator. The nonrebreathing valve directs the gas from the bag to the patient during inspiration. During expiration, the nonrebreathing valve directs exhaled gases from the pa- tient to atmosphere through the expiratory port and the bag refill valve opens to allow the bag to fill. An open reservoir is attached to the bag refill valve.

port may have a tapered 19- or 30-mm connector for attachment of the transfer tube of a scavenging system. The American Society for Testing and Materials (ASTM) standard (2) requires that such a connector have ridges in its internal lumen so that it cannot accept a 22-mm male connector.

The patient connector is the part that connects to a tracheal tube, face mask, laryngeal mask, or other device that connects to the patient's airway. It has 15-mm female and 22-mm male coaxial fittings. The patient connector may be designed to swivel.

The inspiratory port is the opening through which gas enters the valve from the bag. It may be permanently attached to the bag. During inspiration, the nonrebreathing valve directs gas from the bag to the patient connection port. At the same time, the expiratory port is blocked. As exhalation begins, the expiratory port opens and the patient exhales to atmosphere. Simultaneously, gas flow from the bag is blocked. The valve may have a means to prevent air intake so that the spontaneously breathing patient will inhale only from the bag. It is preferable that the housing be constructed so that operation of the mechanism can be observed by the operator.

Unidirectional Valves

A nonrebreathing valve usually contains at least two unidirectional valves (moving mechanisms, active parts). One ensures unidirectional flow

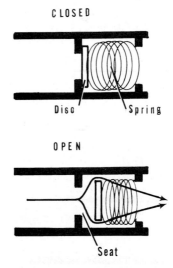

FIGURE **9.3.** Spring-disc unidirectional valve. In the closed position, the spring holds the disc against the seat. When the pressure to the left of the disc increases above the pressure of the spring, the disc is forced away from the seat. When the pressure to the left of the disc drops, the valve closes.

from the bag to the patient, another from the patient to atmosphere.

Spring-Disc Valve

A spring-disc valve is shown in Figure 9.3. A spring holds the disc against a seat. When the pressure on the disc is great enough to overcome the force of the spring, the valve opens. As the pressure drops, the spring causes the disc to move to the left. Some unidirectional valves have a ball in place of the disc. The ball or disc may be held in place by gravity rather than a spring. An example of a spring-disc nonrebreathing valve is shown in Figure 9.7.

Flap Valve

The flap (leaf) valve has a rigid or flexible flap that moves. The flap may be fixed at the center or the edge (Figs. 9.4 and 9.5).

Fishmouth Valve

The fishmouth (duckbill) valve is so named because it opens and closes like a fish's mouth (Fig. 9.6). As the pressure upstream of the valve increases, it opens at the slit in the center. An increase in pressure downstream pushes the leaflets together, closing the valve.

Diaphragm Valve

A diaphragm valve has a flexible diaphragm attached at the side. When pressure is applied to one side of the diaphragm, the central part moves, which causes the gas path to be opened or occluded (Fig. 9.8).

Mushroom Valve

A mushroom valve is a hollow balloon-like device that occludes an opening when inflated (Fig. 9.9).

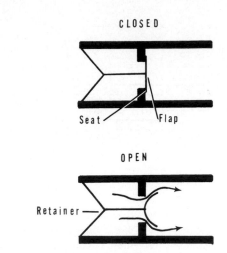

FIGURE 9.5. Center-mounted flap unidirectional valve. The flap valve is secured by a tab at the center. The tab is secured by a retainer, which is part of the valve body.

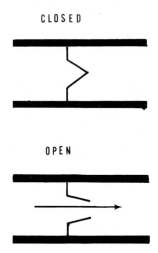

FIGURE 9.6. Fishmouth unidirectional valve. As pressure to the left increases, the leaflets open, allowing gas to flow through the valve. An increase in pressure to the right pushes the leaflets together, closing the valve, and preventing backflow of gas.

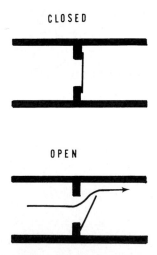

FIGURE 9.4. Edge-mounted flap unidirectional valve. Increased pressure upstream of the flap pushes the flap away from the seat, opening the valve. When the pressure downstream of the flap increases above the pressure upstream, the flap is forced back against the seat, blocking the flow of gas.

Figure 9.7 shows a valve with a spring disc. In the resting position, the spring holds the disc away from the expiratory port and against the inspiratory port so that a spontaneously breathing patient may inhale room air through the exhalation port. A guide pin keeps the disc centered. When the bag is compressed, the disc is pushed across the

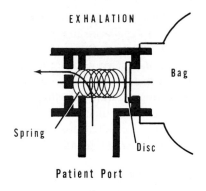

EXHALATION

Bag

Spring

Disc

Patient Port

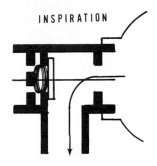

INSPIRATION

FIGURE 9.7. Spring-disc nonrebreathing valve. The disc is held on the seat by the spring. When the bag is squeezed, the disc moves to the left, closing the expiratory port. At the end of inspiration, the spring forces the disc to the right, so that the patient exhales to atmosphere and not into the bag. A guide pin keeps the disc in the center. A spontaneously breathing patient can inhale room air unless a valve is placed over the expiratory port to prevent air entrainment.

valve, connecting the inspiratory port with the patient port and at the same time occluding the expiratory port. When the bag is released, the disc moves back toward the bag and exhaled gases pass out through the expiratory port. If the patient is breathing spontaneously, the disc will not close the exhalation port and air will be inhaled.

Figure 9.8 shows a diaphragm-flap valve. The diaphragm is attached at its periphery. When the bag is squeezed, the diaphragm is pushed to the left and occludes the expiratory port. Flap valves at the side of the diaphragm open, allowing the gas from the bag to flow to the patient. When inhalation ends, the diaphragm returns to its resting position, and the flap valves close so the pa-

tient can exhale through the expiratory port. A spontaneously breathing patient may inhale room air through the exhalation port.

The valve illustrated in Figure 9.9 combines one mushroom and two flap valves. The inside of the mushroom is connected to a pressure channel. During inspiration, the mushroom is inflated against the seat, preventing flow of gas through the expiratory port, and the inhalational flap opens. During expiration, the inhalational flap prevents flow back into the bag. The mushroom collapses and opens the exhalation channel. A flap valve over the expiratory port prevents the inhalation of room air during spontaneous ventilation.

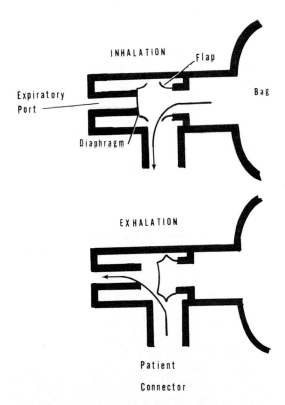

INHALATION

Flap

Bag

Expiratory
Port

Diaphragm

EXHALATION

Patient

Connector

FIGURE 9.8. Diaphragm-flap nonrebreathing valve. During inspiration when the bag is squeezed, the pressure to the right increases and the diaphragm is pushed to the left, closing the exhalation channel. At the same time, the flaps at the edge of the diaphragm open, allowing gas from the bag to flow to the patient connector. When inspiration ends, the diaphragm moves away from the exhalation channel and the flaps close, blocking the inspiratory port.

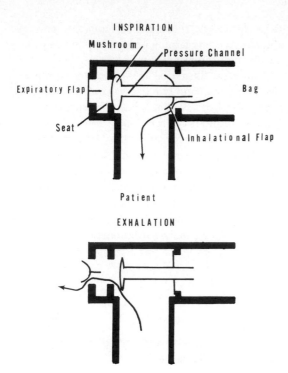

FIGURE **9.9.** Diaphragm-flap nonrebreathing valve. This valve has one diaphragm and two flap valves. During inspiration the diaphragm is inflated and blocks the expiratory channel, preventing flow of gas to atmosphere. At the same time, the inhalation flap valve opens so that gas flows to the patient. At the end of inspiration, the diaphragm collapses, opening the exhalation channel. The inhalational flap valve prevents flow of gas back into the bag. The expiratory flap opens during exhalation. It prevents room air from being inspired during spontaneous ventilation.

The valve diagrammed in Figure 9.10 and pictured disassembled in Figure 9.11 has one fishmouth and two flap valves. The fishmouth and two circular flap valves are combined into one piece, with the flap valves surrounding the central fishmouth. Outside the main body of the valve is another circular flap valve. During inspiration, the fishmouth opens and the circular flap valve closes the exhalation ports. The outside flap valve prevents room air from entering the valve during spontaneous respiration. During expiration, the fishmouth section closes. The circular flap valve attached to it is lifted off the expiratory apertures, allowing exhaled gas to escape.

Figure 9.12 shows a nonrebreathing valve that incorporates two flap valves. During inspiration, the center-mounted flap valve moves to the right. The peripheral flap valve covers the exhalation ports. During exhalation, the flap valves move to the left, preventing gas from entering the bag and the exhalation ports are uncovered. The peripheral flap valve prevents inhalation of room air in the spontaneously breathing patient.

Bag Refill Valve

The bag refill (inlet) valve is a one-way valve that is opened by negative pressure inside the bag. When the bag is squeezed, the valve closes to prevent flow of gas back through the inlet. A simple flap valve (Figs. 9.4 and 9.5) is most commonly used. A spring disc (Fig. 9.3) may also be used.

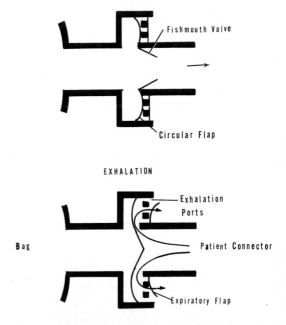

FIGURE **9.10.** Fishmouth-flap nonrebreathing valve. The circular flap and fishmouth valves are attached with the diaphragm around the periphery. When the bag is squeezed, the diaphragm is seated against the exhalation ports and the fishmouth portion of the valve opens. During expiration, the fishmouth closes and the flap falls away from the exhalation channel. A second flap valve over the exhalation ports prevents air from being inspired during spontaneous respiration.

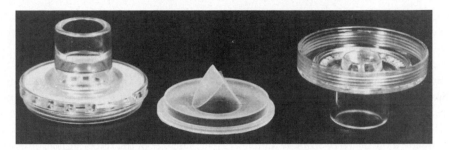

FIGURE **9.11.** Components of the fishmouth-flap nonrebreathing valve. At the left is the patient connection with the expiratory flap. In the center is the fish-mouth with its concentric flap. The right piece is the part of the housing closest to the bag.

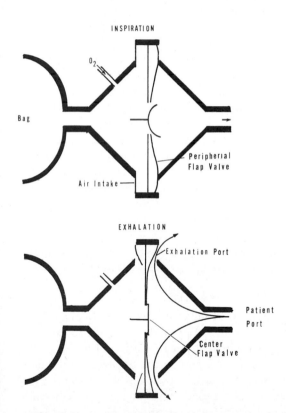

FIGURE **9.12.** Nonrebreathing valve with two flap valves. During inspiration, the center-mounted flap valve opens and the peripheral flap closes over the exhalation ports. During exhalation, the central flap valve closes and the peripheral flap falls away from the exhalation ports. This valve has an oxygen inlet and two bag refill valves, which open if the oxygen flow is not sufficient to prevent a negative pressure from developing in the space to the left.

This valve is usually located at the opposite end of the bag from the nonrebreathing valve (Fig. 9.2) but may be at the same end and may be combined with the nonrebreathing valve.

Pressure-Limiting Device

The pressure-limiting device is also called the pressure relief device, valve, or system; overpressure-limiting system; overpressure valve; pop-off valve; and pressure-limiting system. The ASTM standard (2) requires a pressure-limiting system with an opening pressure of 4.5 kPa (45 cm H_2O) with the option of an override for infant and child resuscitators. For adult resuscitators, the standard requires that there be an override mechanism if there is a device that limits the pressure to below 6 kPa (60 cm H_2O). If the override mechanism can be locked, it must be designed so that the operating mode (i.e., on or off) is readily apparent to the user. The standard recommends that if a resuscitator is equipped with a pressure-limiting device, there be an audible or visible warning to the operator when the pressure-limiting device is operating. It also requires that with a pressure-limiting device set at a fixed pressure, the pressure at which the device is activated must be marked on the resuscitator.

A variety of devices have been used. One is a spring-loaded disc with the tension on the spring adjusted so that it opens at the desired pressure. Another is a magnetic device with the force of the magnet adjusted to open at the desired pressure. Some systems provide a small hole. The maximum pressure depends on the size of the hole and how firmly the bag is compressed (6). Another resuscitator employs a double-bag design. An inner bag with elastic recoil properties similar to most resuscitation bags is contained within a thin outer bag. As pressure within the bags builds up, holes in the inner bag allow gas to enter the outer bag, causing it to balloon.

Many resuscitators with a pressure-limiting mechanism provide a means to override it. Often all that is required is to place a finger over the device. However, even such a simple action may be difficult when ventilating a patient, especially if a mask is being used. Another problem is that an override mechanism may cause confusion.

Means to create a higher inflation pressure is especially important in a resuscitator designed for infants. The first few breaths in neonatal resuscitation may require pressures as high as 5 to 7 kPa (50 to 70 cm H_2O), and the pressure needed to overcome the resistance to flow in a narrow tracheal tube and to expand the stiff lungs of a premature infant may exceed 3 to 4 kPa (30 to 40 cm H_2O) (7).

Oxygen Enrichment Device
Delivery of Oxygen Near the Bag Refill Valve

Attachment of a tubing from an oxygen flowmeter near the bag refill valve is a simple means of increasing the concentration of oxygen in the bag. The oxygen does not enter the bag directly. The increase in oxygen concentration is limited because air will still be drawn into the bag. The delivered oxygen concentration can be increased by increasing the oxygen flow but this is of limited value because most flowmeters do not deliver over 15 l/min. The higher the minute volume and the greater the I:E ratio, the lower the delivered oxygen concentration.

Delivery of Oxygen Directly Into the Bag

Delivery of oxygen directly into the bag will result in high delivered oxygen concentrations without making the resuscitator cumbersome. If the oxygen flow is less than the filling rate of the bag, the bag refill valve will open and admit air. However, provision must be made for venting excess oxygen to minimize the danger of the nonrebreathing valve locking in the inspiratory position.

Reservoir

Some units have a reservoir (accumulator) into which oxygen flows when the bag is not filling. It may be a tube or a bag. When the bag refill valve opens, oxygen from the reservoir enters the bag. The size of the reservoir may limit the oxygen concentration delivered. If the volume of the reservoir is less than that of the bag, the inflowing oxygen may not be sufficient to make up the difference and room air will be drawn in. On the other hand, a large reservoir makes a resuscitator more cumbersome.

Open Reservoir

Open reservoirs are shown in Figures 9.1 and 9.13. A piece of corrugated tubing or other material open to atmosphere at its distal end is placed like a sleeve around the bag refill valve. When the bag is not filling, oxygen flows into the reservoir. If the flow is high, oxygen will flow into atmosphere at the open end of the reservoir.

Closed Reservoir

Closed reservoirs are shown in Figures 9.1 and 9.14. It has two valves: an overflow valve that vents excess gases and an air intake valve that draws in ambient air if there is insufficient oxygen flow. A bag provides a visual indication that the reservoir is receiving sufficient oxygen flow. A deflated reservoir bag means there is a problem with the oxygen supply or a hole in the bag.

Demand Valve

A demand valve connecting a compressed gas source to the self-expanding bag will consistently provide a high inspired oxygen concentration (8). A negative pressure in the bag triggers the flow of oxygen, which stops at a preset pressure. A demand valve provides warning of problems with supplemental oxygen. Should the demand valve become stuck or the oxygen supply depleted, the bag will not refill.

Positive End–Expiratory Pressure Device

A PEEP valve is available on some resuscitators and can be added to the expiratory port on others (5, 9).

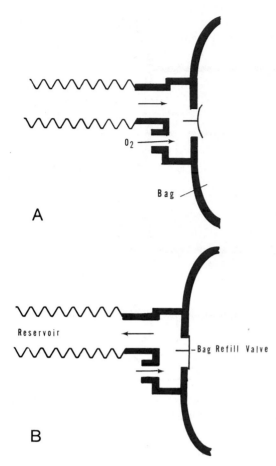

A

B

FIGURE 9.13. Open reservoir. **A**, The bag is filling. Oxygen from the delivery tubing as well as that in the reservoir flows into the bag. If the volume entering the bag exceeds that in the reservoir and flowing through the delivery tubing, room air will make up the difference. The size of the reservoir is, therefore, important. **B**, The bag refill valve is closed. Oxygen from the delivery tubing flows into the reservoir. Some oxygen will be lost if the flow is high because the reservoir is open to atmosphere.

Scavenging Mechanism

A means for scavenging expired gases (see Chapter 12) can be mounted on the expiratory port of some resuscitators.

FUNCTIONAL ANALYSIS
Minute Volume

The minute volume will be determined by the tidal volume and respiratory rate. These will be determined by the performance of the resuscitator and also the operator. The volume delivered when the bag is compressed will vary with the size of the user's hand and whether one or two hands are used (10–20). Tidal volume may be increased by compressing the bag against a solid surface such as a thigh or the operating room table. Another method is to compress the bag between the open palm and body (21).The respiratory rate may be limited by how fast the bag reexpands, which depends on the construction of the bag and the size of the refill valve inlet. The maximum compression rate may be reduced at low temperatures (11, 22, 23) and with the use of certain oxygen input adapters (23).

Delivered Oxygen Concentration

The ASTM standard (2) states that a resuscitator for use with adults shall be capable, when an oxygen source is available, of delivering an inspired oxygen concentration of at least 40% when connected to an oxygen source supplying not more than 15 l/min and at least 85% with an attachment made available by the manufacturer.

The delivered oxygen concentration is limited by size of the reservoir and the oxygen flow. If the volume of the reservoir is greater than the volume of the bag and the oxygen flow is greater than the minute volume, the delivered oxygen concentration may approach 100%. If the tidal volume is greater than the reservoir volume plus the volume of oxygen delivered during inspiration, then air will be drawn into the unit and reduce the percentage of oxygen delivered (24).

Controlled Ventilation

The oxygen concentrations delivered during controlled ventilation have been investigated under a variety of conditions with and without enrichment devices (8, 22, 23, 25–33). It is recommended that only the most recent evaluations be considered because modifications to these devices are made frequently.

The delivered oxygen concentration will be determined by the minute volume; the size of the reservoir, if present; the oxygen flow; and the technique of bag squeezing and release. If bag filling is allowed to proceed at its most rapid rate, all the oxygen in the reservoir may be exhausted

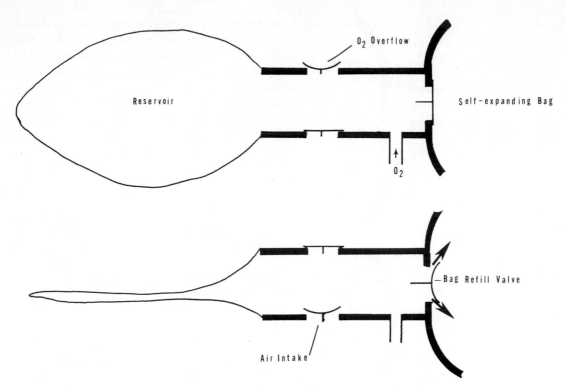

FIGURE 9.14.   Closed reservoir. **Top**, The reservoir is full and the pressure increases. Oxygen flows through the overflow valve. **Bottom**, The resuscitator bag is fill-ing. Air enters through the intake valve because there is insufficient gas in the reservoir.

and air drawn in. If bag filling is manually re-tarded, the delivered oxygen concentration will be higher (8, 34). Manually restricting bag refill may be useful when low oxygen flows must be used or when a reservoir is small or not present, but it limits the respiratory rate and thus the minute vol-ume that can be achieved. Furthermore, this ma-neuver may cause the nonrebreathing valve to jam in the inspiratory position (22).

Activation of the pressure-limiting device may cause the delivered oxygen concentration to be decreased (7, 32).

Spontaneous Ventilation

With spontaneous ventilation, inspired gas may come from the exhalation port as well as the bag. The portion coming from the bag may vary from 0 to 97% (23, 24).

Rebreathing

If the nonrebreathing valve is competent, mix-ing of inhaled and exhaled gases should not occur. If the valve is incompetent, back leak will allow exhaled gases to pass back into the resuscitator and be reinhaled by the patient.

USE

A bag size appropriate for the patient should be selected. For adults, an oxygen flow of 10 to 15 l/min is most commonly used. For children and infants, lower flows are recommended.

If anesthetic gases are to be administered, the transfer tube from a scavenging system should be attached to the expiratory port. A manual resusci-tator can be adapted for manual ventilation during MRI by inserting an extension tube long enough to cover the distance between the patient and the person squeezing the bag between the nonrebreathing valve and the bag (1).

HAZARDS
High Airway Pressure

High airway pressure is a hazard only if the patient is intubated. It is very difficult to achieve a dangerously high pressure using a mask.

Sticking of the Nonrebreathing Valve in the Inspiratory Position

If the nonrebreathing valve sticks (valve lockup) in the inspiratory position, the patient will be attempting to exhale against a closed outlet and continued inflow can cause a continuous and dangerous increase in pressure in a short period of time. A variety of conditions can cause this, including cessation of manual ventilation for observation of spontaneous respiratory efforts, manually restricting bag refill, contamination of the valve with foreign material, a squeeze or bump on the bag, the patient coughing, improper assembly, attachment of an oxygen inlet nipple without vent holes directly to the resuscitator, and kinking of the reservoir tail (25, 35–47). In several cases, a sliding ball separated into two halves and one half wedged in the expiratory outlet (48–50). The expiratory flap valve may fail to open (51).

High Oxygen Inflow

The ASTM resuscitator standard (2) requires that the valve not jam at an input flow of up to 30 l/min. Infant resuscitators are more prone to obstruction with high flows because the bag is so small.

Use of a Demand Valve

Manual activation of a demand valve while the patient is exhaling can cause dangerously high pressures (8).

Failure of the Pressure-Limiting Device

Studies show that pressure-limiting devices often malfunction, opening well above an acceptable pressure (32, 52, 53).

Excessive Resistance

Resuscitators with high resistance predispose the patient to airway pressure elevations and barotrauma during conditions of high expiratory flows (54).

Rebreathing

Rebreathing of exhaled gases can occur if the valve is not competent or is improperly assembled (40, 55, 56).

Hypoventilation

A defective nonrebreathing valve may have forward leak where part of the tidal volume expelled from the bag during inspiration escapes through the expiratory port (55, 57, 58). Obstruction of the part of the valve that closes the expiratory port can cause unwanted venting. Unrecognized venting through the pressure relief device may result in hypoventilation (59, 60).

Squeezing the bag may require considerable physical effort. During extended use, performance may deteriorate as the operator becomes fatigued. Operators with small hands may have difficulty delivering adequate tidal volumes. Adequate tidal volumes are frequently not delivered when a mask is used unless two persons participate, one holding the mask and one squeezing the bag (14). Squeezing the bag using one hand instead of two tends to lower the delivered volume (10, 18).

Because resuscitators are used away from the hospital, it is possible that they will be subjected to low temperatures. In this situation the maximum cycling rate is often greatly reduced and the units may become inoperable or incapable of delivering satisfactory ventilation (22, 23, 42, 44, 61).

Cases have been reported in which it was possible to connect the patient connector into the bag (55, 62), the tracheal tube to a part of the resuscitator other than the patient connector (22), and the expiratory port to the mask (63). In all these cases when the bag was squeezed, the contents were exhausted to atmosphere. The bag can become detached from the nonrebreathing valve (64).

If a resuscitator with an oxygen reservoir bag does not have an auxiliary air intake valve or unobstructed air intake port, it can become nonfunctional if there is not enough oxygen flow to inflate the compressible bag.

If the pressure-relief device is incorrectly set it may open at low pressures, causing hypoventilation (65, 66).

Decreased tidal volume may be seen with increased resistance or decreased compliance (10, 18, 67).

Delivery of Low Oxygen Concentrations

Delivery of low oxygen concentrations may be the result of insufficient oxygen flow, detachment of the oxygen tubing, or problems with the oxygen enrichment device. The reservoir may be too small for the tidal volume. Incorrect assembly of a nonrebreathing valve can result in ambient air rather than gas from the bag being inhaled (68).

During spontaneous ventilation, the patient may inhale room air from the expiratory port as well as oxygen-enriched gas from the bag. Studies have shown that percentage of minute volume coming through the bag varies from 0 to 97% (23, 24).

Low temperatures may result in low inspired oxygen concentrations being delivered (61). With some resuscitators, a high oxygen concentration may not be delivered during spontaneous breathing (29).

High Resistance

Some nonrebreathing valves offer high resistance to flow, so that high negative pressures must be generated during spontaneous ventilation (24, 54). Imposed work of breathing may be quite high. It has been recommended that patients not be allowed to spontaneously breathe through manual resuscitators (29).

Contamination

These devices frequently become contaminated because they are often used on patients who have respiratory infections (69, 70). Oxygen flowing through the valve may aerosolize bacteria and spread them into the surrounding air. For these reasons and because these devices are somewhat difficult to clean, disposable units have become popular.

Inhalation of Foreign Substances

Part of the inside of the bag may break off (71). Parts of the resuscitator may break off and be inhaled (72–74).

ADVANTAGES

1) The equipment is compact, lightweight, and mobile, allowing it to be placed throughout the healthcare facility and to be used outside.
2) The equipment is inexpensive yet rugged.
3) The equipment is simple with a small number of parts. Disassembly and reassembly are usually easy to perform.
4) Dead space and rebreathing are minimal if the valve functions properly. Resistance is generally low.
5) It is possible to administer close to 100% oxygen with most resuscitators with proper attention to the oxygen enrichment device, oxygen flow, and technique of ventilation.
6) In emergency situations in which a connection to a gas source is not readily available, the resuscitator can be used with room air until such a source becomes available.
7) The operator has some feel for pressures and volumes delivered. Barotrauma is less likely with these devices than with gas-powered resuscitators, which do not allow the operator to sense when the patient's lungs are fully inflated.

DISADVANTAGES

1) Some of the valves are noisy and stick, particularly when wet.
2) There may be considerable loss of heat and humidity from the patient with prolonged use. Consideration should be given to using a heat and moisture exchanger with prolonged transport.
3) The feel of the bag is different from that in other breathing systems. The user's hand must be reeducated.
4) The valve must be located at the patient's head. Its bulk may be troublesome and its weight may cause the tracheal tube to kink or be displaced downward.

REFERENCES

1. Taylor WF, Pangburn PD, Paschall A. Manual ventilation during magnetic resonance imaging. Respiratory Care 1991;36:1207–1210.

2. American Society for Testing and Materials. Standard specification for minimum performance and safety requirements for resuscitators intended for use with humans (F 920–93). West Conshohocken, PA: ASTM, 1993.
3. Canadian Standards Association. Resuscitators intended for use with humans (Z8382–94) Rexdale, Ontario, Canada: CSA, 1994.
4. International Organization for Standardization. Resuscitators intended for use with humans (ISO 8382). Geneva: ISO, 1988.
5. Perel A, Eimerl D, Grossberg M. A PEEP device for a manual bag ventilator. Anesth Analg 1976;52:745.
6. Anonymous. Manually operated infant resuscitators. Health Devices 1973;2:240–248.
7. Breivik H. A safe multipurpose pediatric ventilation bag. Crit Care Med 1976;4:32–39.
8. Campbell TP, Stewart RD, Kaplan RM, et al. Oxygen enrichment of bag-valve-mask units during positive-pressure ventilation: a comparison of various techniques. Ann Emerg Med 1988;17:232–235.
9. Anonymous. A simple PEEP system for the Laerdal resuscitation bag. Respiratory Therapy 1981;12:120.
10. Hess D, Goff G. The effects of two-hand versus one-hand ventilation on volumes delivered bag-valve ventilation at various resistances and compliances. Respiratory Care 1987;32:1025–1028.
11. Kissoon N, Nykanen D, Tiffin N, et al. Evaluation of performance characteristics of disposable bag-valve resuscitators. Crit Care Med 1991;19:102–107.
12. Law GD. Effects of hand size on Ve, Vt, and FIO_2 during manual resuscitation. Respiratory Care 1982;27:1236–1237.
13. Tiffin NH, Kissoon N, Clarke G, et al. An evaluation of eight disposable and two nondisposable adult resuscitators. Can J Respir Ther 1989;25:13–19.
14. Jesudian MCS, Harrison RR, Keenan RL, et al. Bag-valve-mask ventilation; two rescuers are better than one: preliminary report. Crit Care Med 1985;13:122–123.
15. Elling R, Politis J. An evaluation of emergency medical technicians' ability to use manual ventilation devices. Ann Emerg Med 1983;12:765–768.
16. Augustine JA, Seidel DR, McCabe JB. Ventilation performance using a self-inflating anesthesia bag: effect of operator characteristics. Am J Emerg Med 1987;5:267–270.
17. Hess D, Goff G, Johnson K. The effect of hand size, resuscitator brand, and use of two hands on volumes delivered during adult bag-valve ventilation. Respiratory Care 1989;34:805–809.
18. Hess D, Simmons M, Blaukovitch S, et al. An evaluation of the effects of fatigue, impedance, and use of two hands on volumes delivered during bag-valve ventilation. Respiratory Care 1993;38:271–275.
19. Hess D, Baran C. Ventilatory volumes using mouth-to-mouth, mouth-to-mask, and bag-valve-mask techniques. Am J Emerg Med 1985;3:292–296.
20. Hess D, Spahr C. An evaluation of volumes delivered by selected adult disposable resuscitators: the effects of hand size, number of hands used, and use of disposable medical gloves. Resp Care 1990;35:800–805.
21. Thomas AN, Dang PT, Hyatt J, et al. A new technique for two-hand bag valve mask ventilation. BMJ 1993;70:397–398.
22. Anonymous. Manual resuscitators. Health Devices 1979;8:133–146.
23. LeBouef LL. 1980 Assessment of eight adult manual resuscitators. Respiratory Care 1980;25:1136–1142.
24. Mills PJ, Baptiste J, Preston J, et al. Manual resuscitators and spontaneous ventilation—an evaluation. Crit Care Med 1991;19:1425–1431.
25. Anonymous. Manually operated resuscitators. Health Devices 1974;3:164–176.
26. Barnes TA, Watson ME. Oxygen delivery performance of old and new designs of the Laerdal, Vitalograph and AMBU adult manual resuscitators. Respiratory Care 1983;28:1121–1128.
27. Barnes TA, Watson ME. Oxygen delivery performance of four adult resuscitation bags. Respiratory Care 1982;27:139–146.
28. Barnes TA, Potash R. Evaluation of five adult disposable operator-powered resuscitators. Respiratory Care 1989;34:254–261.
29. Hess D, Hirsch C, Marquis-D'Amico C, et al. Imposed work and oxygen delivery during spontaneous breathing with adult disposable manual ventilators. Anesthesiology 1994;81:1256–1263.
30. Fitzmaurice MW, Barnes TA. Fractional delivered oxygen concentrations of resuscitation bags. Respiratory Care 1981;26:581–583.
31. Fitzmaurice MW, Barnes TA. Oxygen delivery performance of three adult resuscitation bags. Respiratory Care 1980;25:928–933.
32. Finer NN, Barrington KJ, Al-Fadley F, et al. Limitations of self-inflating resuscitators. Pediatrics 1986;77:417–420.
33. Eaton JM. Adult manual resuscitators. Br J Hosp Med 1984;31:67–70.
34. Priano LL, Ham J. A simple method to increase the FIO_2 of resuscitator bags. Crit Care Med 1978;6:48–49.
35. Anonymous. Silicone resuscitators may have partial blockade. Biomedical Safety & Standards 1993;23:172.
36. Anonymous. Manual reusable pulmonary resuscitators. Technology for Anesthesia 1994;14, 8:5–6.

37. Tucker J, Hanson CW, Chen L. Pneumothorax reexacerbated by a self-inflating bag-valve device. Anesthesiology 1992;76:1067–1068.

38. Dolan PF, Shapiro S, Steinbach RB. Valve misassembly—manually operated resuscitation bag. Anesth Analg 1981;60:66–67.

39. Hunter WAH, Duthie RA. Malfunction of a Laerdal resuscitation valve. Anaesthesia 1991;46:505–506.

40. Klick JM, Bushnell LS, Bancroft ML. Barotrauma, a potential hazard of manual resuscitators. Anesthesiology 1978;49:363–365.

41. Kelly MP. Ventilation equipment. BMJ 1968;2:176.

42. Anonymous. Manually operated resuscitators. Health Devices 1971;1:13–17.

43. Anonymous. New component designed for resuscitator valve sticking problem. Biomedical Safety & Standards 1991;21:123.

44. Carden E, Hughes T. An evaluation of manually operated self-inflating resuscitation bags. Anesth Analg 1975;54:133–138.

45. Hillman K, Albin M. Pulmonary barotrauma during cardiopulmonary resuscitation. Crit Care Med 1986;14:606–609.

46. Newton NI, Adams AP. Excessive airway pressure during anaesthesia. Anaesthesia 1978;33:689–699.

47. Ho Am-H, Shragge W, Tittley JG, et al. Exhalation obstruction due to Laerdal valve misassembly. Crit Care Med 1996;24:362–364.

48. Anonymous. Ohio Hope II resuscitators. Health Devices 1981;10:199.

49. Anonymous. Resuscitator ball valve alert extended: germicidal solutions may crack new component. Biomedical Safety & Standards 1988;18:43.

50. Jumper A, Desai S, Liu P, et al. Pulmonary barotrauma resulting from a faulty Hope II resuscitation bag. Anesthesiology 1983;58:572–574.

51. Myers DP, de Leon-Casasola OA, Bacon DR, et al. Bilateral pneumothoraces from a malfunctioning resuscitation valve. J Clin Anesth 1993;5:433–435.

52. Kissoon N, Connors R, Tiffin N, et al. An evaluation of the physical and functional characteristics of resuscitators for use in pediatrics. Crit Care Med 1992;20:292–296.

53. Barnes TA, McGarry WP. Evaluation of ten disposable manual resuscitators. Respiratory Care 1990;35:960.

54. Hess D, Simmons M. An evaluation of the resistance to flow through the patient valves of twelve adult manual resuscitators. Respiratory Care 1992;37:432–438.

55. Munford BJ, Wishaw KJ. Critical incidents with nonrebreathing valves. Anaesthesia and Intensive Care 1990;18:560–563.

56. Day CJE, Nolan JP. A rebreathing non-rebreathing valve. Anaesthesia 1994;49:456.

57. Anonymous. Valve component on resuscitation kits may leak. Biomedical Safety & Standards 1989;19:35–36.

58. Anonymous. Pulmonary resuscitators. Health Devices 1989;18:333–352.

59. Hirschman AM, Kravath RE. Venting vs ventilating. A danger of manual resuscitation. Chest 1982;82:369–370.

60. Kain ZN, Berde CB, Benjamin PK, et al. Performance of pediatric resuscitation bags assessed with an infant lung simulator. Anesthesiology 1992;77:A509.

61. Barnes TA, Stockwell DL. Evaluation of ten manual resuscitators across an operational temperature range of −18°C to 50°C. Respiratory Care 1991;36:161–172.

62. Oliver JJ, Pope R. Potential hazard, with silicone resuscitators. Anaesthesia 1984;39:933–934.

63. Anonymous. Mismating of Laerdal exhalation diverters and intertech masks. Technology for Anesthesia 1988;8:1–2.

64. Anonymous. Inspiron disposable adult manual pulmonary resuscitators. Technology for Anesthesia 1987;8:2–3.

65. Freeman G, Hannallah M. Severe hypoventilation resulting from improper use of a disposable manual resuscitator. J Clin Anesth 1995;7:267.

66. Kain ZN, Berde CB, Benjamin PK, et al. Performance of pediatric resuscitation bags assessed with an infant lung simulator. Anesth Analg 1993;77:261–264.

67. Johannigman JA, Branson RD, Davis K, et al. Techniques of emergency ventilation: a model to evaluate tidal volume, airway pressure, and gastric insufflation. J Trauma 1991;31:93–98.

68. Cramond T, Mead P. Non-rebreathing valve assembly. Anaesthesia and Intensive Care 1986;14:465.

69. Thompson AC, Wilder BJ, Powner DJ. Bedside resuscitation bags: A source of bacterial contamination. Infection Control 1985;6:231–232.

70. Hartstein AI, Rashad AL, Liebler JM, et al. Multiple intensive care unit outbreak of *Acinetobacter colcoaceticus* subspecies *anitratus* respiratory infection and colonization associated with contaminated, reusable ventilator circuits and resuscitation bags. Am J Med 1988;85:624–631.

71. Anonymous. Resuscitators, pulmonary manual reusable. Technology for Anesthesia 1991;12:9.

72. Anonymous. Resuscitators, pulmonary manual. Technology for Anesthesia 1985;7:11.

73. Anonymous. Nonrebreathing valves. Biomedical Safety & Standards 1986;16:19.

74. Pauca AL, Jenkins TE. Airway obstruction by breakdown of a nonrebreathing valve: how foolproof? Anesth Analg 1981;60:529–531.

QUESTIONS

1. What minimum tidal volume should resuscitators be capable of delivering to be considered useable for adults?
   A. 250 to 300 ml
   B. 300 to 400 ml
   C. 400 to 500 ml
   D. 500 to 600 ml
   E. 600 ml or more

Each question below contains four suggested answers of which one or more is correct. Choose the answer:

A if 1, 2, and 3 are correct
B if 1 and 3 are correct
C if 2 and 4 are correct
D if 4 is correct
E if 1, 2, 3, and 4 are correct.

2. The amount of oxygen that will be delivered from a resuscitation bag will be increased by
   1. Increasing the oxygen flow
   2. Low minute volume
   3. Addition of a reservoir to the inlet
   4. A smaller I:E ratio

3. Problems with delivering oxygen directly into the resuscitation bag include
   1. Difficulty attaining high oxygen levels
   2. Inspiratory valve locking in the inspiratory position
   3. Inability to deliver adequate tidal volume because the flowmeter can only deliver up to 15 l/min
   4. Excess pressure

4. Characteristics of an open reservoir include
   1. Oxygen flows into the reservoir during exhalation
   2. If the tidal volume is high, air will be added to inspiration
   3. Oxygen enters the bag from the source during exhalation
   4. Ambient air can make up deficiencies in oxygen during inhalation

5. Characteristics of the closed reservoir include

   1. A valve to let in ambient air during the patient's inspiration
   2. A valve to vent excess oxygen
   3. A valve to provide warning of excess oxygen pressure
   4. Presence of a bag

6. Minimum oxygen concentrations required by the ASTM standard include
   1. 40% with an oxygen delivery of up to 15 l/min
   2. 100% if the reservoir is smaller than the tidal volume
   3. 85% with the addition of a reservoir
   4. 90% if the reservoir is larger than the tidal volume

7. Benefits of manually restricting refill of the resuscitation bag include
   1. A lower flow of oxygen may be used
   2. A reservoir may not be needed to deliver high oxygen concentrations
   3. Higher oxygen concentration will be delivered
   4. Higher minute volume can be achieved

8. Situations that can result in high airway pressure include
   1. Nonrebreathing valve stuck in expiratory position
   2. High oxygen inflow
   3. Use of a demand valve during inhalation
   4. Kinking of the reservoir tail

9. Causes of hypoventilation when using a manual resuscitator include
   1. Incomplete closure of the expiratory port
   2. Low temperature
   3. Venting through the pressure relief device
   4. No auxiliary air intake

10. The ASTM standard on resuscitators includes the following provisions concerning pressure-limiting devices
    1. For adults, an opening pressure of 50 cm H_2O

2. For infant and child resuscitators, an opening pressure of 45 cm H_2O

3. Optional override for infant and child resuscitators

4. In adults, if the override mechanism can be locked, it must be designed so that the operating mode is readily apparent to the user

11. Hazards associated with use of a manual resuscitator include
    1. Barotrauma

2. Inhalation of foreign substances
3. Delivery of low oxygen concentrations
4. Hyperventilation

ANSWERS

1.	E	7.	A
2.	E	8.	C
3.	C	9.	E
4.	A	10.	E
5.	C	11.	A
6.	B		

CHAPTER
10

Humidification Methods

I. General Considerations
  A. Terminology
    1. Absolute Humidity
    2. Humidity at Saturation
    3. Relative Humidity
    4. Water Vapor Pressure
  B. Interrelationships
II. Considerations for Anesthesia
  A. Normal Mechanics of Humidification
  B. Effects of Anesthesia
  C. Effects of Inhaling Dry Gases
    1. Damage to the Respiratory Tract
    2. Loss of Body Heat
III. Sources of Humidity
  A. Carbon Dioxide Absorbent
  B. Exhaled Gases
  C. Moistening Breathing Tubes and Reservoir Bag
  D. Low Flow Techniques
  E. Heat and Moisture Exchanger
    1. Description
      a. Hydrophobic Membrane
      b. Composite Hygroscopic
    2. Indications and Contraindications for Use
    3. Factors Affecting Moisture Output
      a. Heat and Moisture Exchanger Type
      b. Initial Humidity
      c. Inspiratory and Expiratory Flows
      d. Continuity of the System
    4. Use
    5. Advantages
    6. Disadvantages
    7. Hazards
      a. Excessive Resistance
      b. Airway Obstruction
      c. Inefficient Filtration
      d. Aspiration of Particles
      e. Rebreathing
      f. Interference with Monitoring

    g. Leaks and Disconnections
  F. Heated Breathing Tubes
  G. Humidifiers
    1. Unheated
    2. Heated
      a. Description
        (1). Humidification Chamber
        (2). Heat Source
        (3). Delivery Tube
        (4). Temperature Monitor(s)
        (5). Thermostats
          (a). Servo-Controlled Units
          (b). Nonservo-Controlled Units
        (6). Controls
        (7). Alarms
      b. Action
      c. Standard Requirements
      d. Use
      e. Advantages
      f. Disadvantages
      g. Hazards
        (1). Infection
        (2). Breathing System Problems
        (3). Tracheal Lavage or Aspiration of Water
        (4). Overhydration
        (5). Thermal Injury
        (6). Underhydration
        (7). Increased Work of Breathing
        (8). Pharyngeal Complaints
        (9). Interference with Monitoring
        (10). Alteration of Anesthetic Agents
  H. Nebulizers
    1. Description
    2. Use
    3. Hazards
    4. Advantages
    5. Disadvantages

SOME HUMIDIFICATION IS considered beneficial during anesthesia to avoid the effects of inspiring dry gases. This chapter discusses various methods and equipment for humidifying inspired gases.

GENERAL CONSIDERATIONS
Terminology

Humidity is a general term used to describe the amount of water vapor in a gas. It may be expressed several ways.

Absolute Humidity

Absolute humidity is the mass of water vapor present in a volume of gas. It is commonly expressed in milligrams of water per liter of gas.

Humidity at Saturation

The amount of water vapor that a gas can hold at any given temperature is limited. The maximum that can be carried in a volume of gas is the humidity at saturation. This will vary with the temperature. Table 10.1 shows the absolute humidity of saturated gas at various temperatures. It is 44 mg H_2O/liter at a body temperature of 37°C.

Relative Humidity

Relative humidity, or percent saturation, is the amount of water vapor at a particular temperature expressed as a percentage of the amount that would be held if the gas were saturated.

Water Vapor Pressure

Humidity may also be expressed as the pressure exerted by water vapor in a gas mixture.

Interrelationships

The amount of water that can be held as vapor depends on the ambient temperature. The warmer the temperature, the more water vapor a gas can hold.

If a gas saturated with water vapor is heated, its capacity to hold moisture increases and it becomes unsaturated (has less than 100% relative humidity). Its absolute humidity remains unchanged. Gas that is 100% saturated at room temperature and warmed to body temperature without additional humidity will be approximately 40% saturated (1). This gas will absorb water by evapora-

TABLE 10.1. **Water Vapor Pressure and Absolute Humidity in Moisture-Saturated Gas**

Temperature °C	mg H_2O/liter	mm Hg
0	4.84	4.58
1	5.19	4.93
2	5.56	5.29
3	5.95	5.69
4	6.36	6.10
5	6.80	6.54
6	7.26	7.01
7	7.75	7.51
8	8.27	8.05
9	8.81	8.61
10	9.40	9.21
11	10.01	9.84
12	10.66	10.52
13	11.33	11.23
14	12.07	11.99
15	12.82	12.79
16	13.62	13.63
17	14.47	14.53
18	15.35	15.48
19	16.30	16.48
20	17.28	17.54
21	18.33	18.65
22	19.41	19.83
23	20.57	21.07
24	21.76	22.38
25	23.04	23.76
26	24.35	25.21
27	25.75	26.74
28	27.19	28.35
29	28.74	30.04
30	30.32	31.82
31	32.01	33.70
32	33.79	35.66
33	35.59	37.73
34	37.54	39.90
35	39.57	42.18
36	41.53	44.56
37	43.85	47.07
38	46.16	49.69
39	48.58	52.44
40	51.03	55.32
41	53.66	58.34
42	56.40	61.50

tion from the wet surface of the respiratory tract mucosa until it becomes saturated.

If gas saturated with water vapor is cooled, it will condense (rain out) the amount of water vapor it held at the original temperature less the amount it can hold at the lower temperature. The absolute humidity will fall but relative humidity will remain 100%.

If inspired gas is to have a relative humidity of 100% at body temperature, it must be maintained at body temperature after leaving the humidifier or heated above body temperature at the humidifier and allowed to cool as it flows to the patient. This will result in condensation (rain out) in the breathing system.

The specific heats of gases are low. As a consequence, they quickly assume the temperature of the surrounding environment. Inhaled gases quickly approach body temperature and gases in corrugated tubes rapidly approach room temperature.

The heat of vaporization of water is relatively high. Evaporation of water, therefore, requires considerably more heat than warming of gases. Likewise, condensation of water yields more heat than cooling of gases.

CONSIDERATIONS FOR ANESTHESIA
Normal Mechanics of Humidification

In its passage to the alveoli, inspired gas is brought to body temperature (either by heating or cooling) and 100% relative humidity (either by evaporation or condensation). In the unintubated patient, the upper respiratory tract (especially the nose) functions as the principle heat and moisture exchanger (HME).

Effects of Anesthesia

Water is intentionally removed from medical gases—piped or from cylinders—to prevent corrosion and condensation in regulators and valves. Gases emerging from the anesthesia machine are dry and at room temperature. The breathing system may add some humidity to the inspired gases.

Tracheal intubation or use of an laryngeal mask airway (LMA) bypasses the upper airway, modifying the pattern of heat and moisture exchange, so that the tracheobronchial mucosa must assume

more of the burden of heating and humidifying gases.

Effects of Inhaling Dry Gases
Damage to the Respiratory Tract

As the respiratory mucosa dries and its temperature drops, secretions thicken, ciliary function is reduced, surfactant activity is impaired, and the mucosa becomes more susceptible to injury. If secretions are not cleared, atelectasis or obstruction of the airway can result. Thickened plugs may provide loci for infection. There may be a fall in functional residual capacity and compliance and a rise in the alveolar-arterial oxygen difference (2, 3). Dry gases can cause bronchoconstriction, further compromising respiratory function. Dry gases may increase the incidence of respiratory complications associated with inhalation induction with isoflurane (4–6).

The duration of exposure should be considered. It is unlikely that a brief exposure of the tracheobronchial tree to dry inspired gases will result in damage, but the likelihood of a significant effect rises as exposure time increases.

In humans during normal breathing, the temperature in the upper trachea is between 30 and 33°C, with a relative humidity of approximately 95%, providing a water content of 30 ml/l (7). There is no agreement as to the minimum humidity necessary to prevent pathologic changes. Recommendations in terms of absolute humidity have ranged from 12 to 44 mg water/liter (8–18). It has been suggested that the optimal level is core temperature and 100% relative humidity (1).

Loss of Body Heat

Body temperature is lowered as the airways bring the inspired gas into thermal equilibrium and saturate it with water. Use of a humidification device can decrease the heat loss that occurs during anesthesia and may provide heat input (19–28).

The importance of humidification in anesthesia remains uncertain. It is of greatest benefit in pediatric patients, patients at increased risk for developing pulmonary complications, and in procedures of long duration. Several studies have shown a decrease in postoperative pulmonary complications when gases are humidified (19, 29–31) but one study showed no difference (32). The benefits of increased humidity must be weighed against its hazards and cost.

SOURCES OF HUMIDITY
Carbon Dioxide Absorbent

The reaction of absorbent with carbon dioxide liberates water (see Chapter 8). Water is also contained in the absorbent granules.

Exhaled Gases

In systems that allow rebreathing, the humidity and temperature of inspired gases depend on the relative proportions of fresh gases and expired gases inhaled. This will depend on the system and the fresh gas flow. As the fresh gas flow is increased, the temperature and humidity of inspired gases are reduced.

Previous use of a system can increase the initial inspired humidity caused by water condensed in parts of the system that are not changed between cases (33).

Moistening Breathing Tubes and Reservoir Bag

Rinsing the inside of the breathing tubes and reservoir bag with water before use increases the inspired humidity (34).

Low Flow Techniques

Using low fresh gas flows with a circle breathing system will conserve moisture (see Chapter 8).

Heat and Moisture Exchangers

An HME conserves some of the exhaled water and heat and returns them to the inspired gases. Many also perform bacterial/viral filtration and prevent inhalation of small particles. An HME is also called a condenser humidifier, Swedish nose, artificial nose, nose humidifier, passive humidifier, regenerative humidifier, moisture exchanger, and vapor condenser. It is called a heat and moisture exchanging filter (HMEF) when combined with a filter.

Description

Most HMEs are disposable devices with the exchanging medium enclosed in a plastic housing (27, 35, 36). Typical ones are shown in Figure 10.1. The size and configuration vary. Each has a 15-mm female connection port at its proximal (patient) end and a 22-mm male port at the other end. The patient port may also have a concentric 22-mm male fitting (Fig. 10.1C and D). There may be a port to attach the gas sampling line for a respiratory gas monitor (Fig 10.1B and D).

The dead space of HMEs varies. Pediatric and neonatal HMEs with less dead space than adult models are available (37–39).

A variety of materials have been used for the exchange medium (40). HMEs having more than one type of element are available. Most modern HMEs are one of two types, as shown in Table 10.2

Hydrophobic Membrane

These have a hydrophobic membrane with small pores. The surface area of the membrane must be high to achieve high gas flows with low resistance. This is accomplished by pleating the membrane.

A pleated hydrophobic membrane provides moderate moisture output. A temperature gradient in the element is caused by the low thermal conductivity of the hydrophobic material and the large surface area. Temperatures 15 to 20°C less than ambient may be attained (27). Performance of these HMEs may be impaired with high ambient temperatures (7, 41).

These are efficient bacterial and viral filters (35, 42–45). A pleated hydrophobic filter will consistently prevent the passage of the hepatitis C virus while a hygroscopic filter may be ineffective (46). The hydrophobicity and small pores allow the passage of water vapor but not liquid water at usual ventilation pressures (35, 47). Hydrophobic membrane HMEs are associated with small increases in resistance even after use (20, 27, 48). Resistance is not increased by nebulization of medications (45).

Composite Hygroscopic

Hygroscopic HMEs contain a wool, foam, or paper-like material coated with moisture-retaining chemicals (27, 35). The medium may be impregnated with a bactericide (49). Composite hygroscopic filters consist of a hygroscopic layer plus a layer of thin, non-woven fiber membrane that has been subjected to an electric field to increase

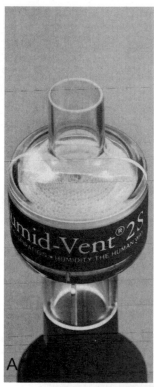
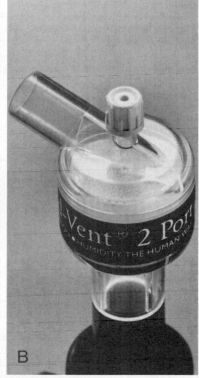
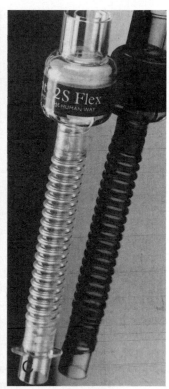
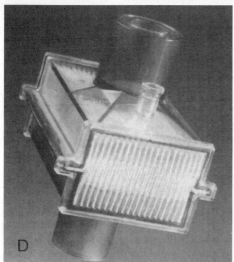
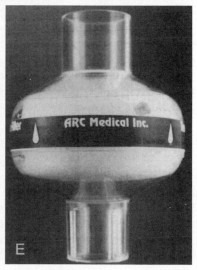

FIGURE 10.1. Heat and moisture exchangers (HMEs). **A** and **E,** Straight variety. **B,** Right-angle HME with port for aspiration of respiratory gases on the breathing system side. **C,** The flexible tube attached to the HME extends the distance between the patient and the breathing system and allows the angle between the breathing system and the patient to be altered. Be-

cause this HME has significant dead space, it should be used only with high tidal volumes and controlled ventilation with monitoring of inspired and expired CO_2. **D,** Hydrophobic HME with respiratory gas aspiration port. (Pictures C, D, and E reprinted with permission from Gibeck Respiration, Pall Biomedical Products Corp., and ARC Medical Inc.)

TABLE 10.2. **Comparison of Hydrophobic and Hygroscopic Heat and Moisture Exchangers**

	Hygroscopic	Hydrophobic
Heat and moisture exchanging efficiency	Good	Fair
Effect of increased tidal volume on heat and moisture exchange	Slight decrease	Significant decrease
Filtration efficiency when dry	Good (86 to > 99%)	Greater than 99%
Filtration efficiency when wet	Poor	Greater than 99%
Resistance when dry	Low	Low
Resistance when wet	Increased	Low
Effect of nebulized medications	Increased resistance	Little effect

its polarity. This improves filtration efficiency and hydrophobicity.

A number of studies have shown that hygroscopic HMEs are more efficient at moisture and temperature conservation than hydrophobic ones (7, 40, 50–58). These devices show variable efficiency as filters. Reported bacterial and viral removal efficiencies are between 86 and 99.9% (45, 59, 60). Although the material in the composite filters is hydrophobic, the large pore size allows the ingress of fluids into and passage through the filter material. They will lose their airborne filtration efficiency if they become wet, and microorganisms held by the filter medium will be washed through the device. The resistance of a composite hygroscopic HME increases more than that of a hydrophobic one with use (54, 61). Resistance is increased by nebulization of medications (45).

Indications and Contraindications for Use

HMEs are most useful during short-term ventilation in patients who are adequately hydrated. HMEs may be especially useful during transport of an intubated patient because this is rarely for more than a few hours and transport ventilators frequently have no means for humidifying inspired gases.

An HME may be used in a patient with a tracheostomy in place (62). An HME can be used as an oxygen therapy device in the intubated patient (63). Oxygen tubing is connected to the gas sampling port. An HMEF should be used in a patient with a known infectious disease.

The American Association of Respiratory Care has listed some contraindications for the use of HMEs during mechanical ventilation (64). These include:

1. Patients with thick, copious, or bloody secretions
2. Patients with an expired tidal volume less than 70% of delivered tidal volume (e.g., bronchopleurocutaneous fistula or leaking or absent tracheal tube cuff)
3. Patients with body temperatures less than 32°C

HMEs may be contraindicated in patients with spontaneous minute volumes greater than 10 l/min. An HME should be removed from the patient circuit during aerosol treatment. An HME will increase the work of breathing during weaning from respiratory support or pressure support ventilation so it may be beneficial to remove it (65).

Factors Affecting Moisture Output

Heat and Moisture Exchanger Type

As noted above, composite hygroscopic HMEs have better heat and moisture exchanging properties than hydrophobic ones.

Initial Humidity

Increasing the humidity of the gas entering the HME will increase the humidity in its output (66, 67).

Inspiratory and Expiratory Flows

The faster gas passes through the HME, the less time there is to absorb or deposit moisture so an increased tidal volume will cause the humidity of the inspired gas to fall (18, 40, 49, 54, 58, 68,

69). The output of hydrophobic HMEs is more affected by tidal volume than that of hygroscopic ones (50, 56).

Continuity of the System

A leak around the tracheal tube or between the tracheal tube and the HME will result in a decrease in inspired humidity (37, 49, 70).

Use

The HME selected should be of an appropriate size for the patient's tidal volume. Dead space is especially important in small patients. If a small HME is used in large patients, there will not be enough surface area to absorb the moisture and the HME will become inefficient (71). Connecting more than one HME in series will improve performance (9, 72). Care must be taken that the units are pushed firmly together and the increase in dead space is not excessive.

The greatest inspired relative humidity occurs with the HME positioned next to the tracheal tube or LMA (73). The relative humidity declines as the space between the tracheal tube and HME increases.

An HME can be used with any breathing system. With the Mapleson systems, dead space can be reduced by utilizing the gas sampling port as the fresh gas inlet (74). A port for airway pressure monitoring should be between the patient and the HME so that the low pressure alarm is activated if there is a disconnection between the patient and the HME (75–77).

An HME may be used as the sole source of humidity or may be combined with another source such as an unheated humidifier (78). HMEs should not be used with a heated humidifier. Some HMEs can be moistened before use to increase efficiency (79). Hygroscopic unit should not be moistened because this reduces their filtering efficiency.

During prolonged use, regular tracheobronchial suctioning, preceded by instillation of small volumes of normal saline should be carried out (27, 36). However, instillation of saline with a closed suction system may cause a significant increase in resistance with a hygroscopic HME (80).

If a nebulizer or metered dose inhaler is used to deliver medication, it should be inserted between the HME and the tracheal tube (81).

HMEs should be inspected and replaced if contaminated with secretions.

Advantages

HMEs are inexpensive, easy to use, small, lightweight, reliable, simple in design, and silent in operation. They have low compliance and resistance when dry. Disposable ones require no cleaning or sterilization. Disposable HMEs do not require water, an external source of energy, temperature monitors, or alarms. There is no danger of overhydration, hyperthermia, burns of the skin or respiratory tract, or electric shock. They eliminate condensation of water. The workload on nursing and respiratory personnel is lessened (82).

HMEs act as a barrier to large particles, and some are efficient bacterial and viral filters (20, 44, 83–85). HMEs may reduce the incidence of nosocomial pneumonia and contamination of the breathing system (42, 48, 86). Their use may increase the correlation between esophageal and core temperatures (87).

Disadvantages

The main disadvantage of HMEs is the limited humidity these devices can deliver. Their contribution to temperature preservation is not significant (73). Active heating and humidification are more effective than an HME in retaining body heat (88, 89).

Placing an HME between the breathing system and the patient increases dead space. This may necessitate an increase in tidal volume and can lead to dangerous rebreathing (90).

Hazards

Excessive Resistance

Use of an HME increases resistance to respiration although the work of breathing associated with them is not a major component of total work (91). In some cases, the increased resistance may make it necessary to use controlled rather than spontaneous ventilation (92). Resistance may increase with use (38, 42, 45, 80, 86, 91, 93–103). Heavy viscous secretions can greatly increase resistance (102, 104, 105).

Use of nebulized medication increases the resistance of hygroscopic (but not hydrophobic)

HMEs (35, 45). Use of a hygroscopic HME and a closed suction system may increase resistance significantly (80). HMEs should not be used in conjunction with a heated humidifier because this can cause a dangerous increase in resistance (106, 107).

High resistance may result in sufficient back pressure to prevent the low pressure airway pressure alarm from being activated if there is a disconnection between the patient and the HME (75–77).

It is important to observe the HME frequently for plugging. The spontaneously breathing patient should be observed for signs of increased work of breathing. If the peak pressure increases during controlled ventilation, it should be measured with and without the HME in place.

Airway Obstruction

An HME can become obstructed because of fluids, blood (108), secretions, a manufacturing defect (109–111), or nebulized drugs (112–116). The weight of an HME may cause the tracheal tube to kink. If HMEs are used for long-term ventilation, occlusion of the tracheal tube from secretions may occur, especially if a hydrophobic membrane type is used and instillation of normal saline is not consistently performed before suctioning (41, 53, 117–120).

Inefficient Filtration

Liquid will break through composite hygroscopic HMEs, and this may be associated with contamination of the breathing system (35, 47).

Aspiration of Particles

Some HMEs contain materials that may be released in the form of particles and then inhaled by the patient (9, 121–123).

Rebreathing

The dead space of the HME may cause excessive rebreathing, especially with small tidal volumes. Special low volume devices are available for pediatrics.

Interference with Monitoring

If the gas sampling line is connected on the machine side of an HME, end-tidal carbon dioxide values may be significantly lower, especially in spontaneously breathing patients (101–124). Tidal volume measurements may also be affected.

Leaks and Disconnections

Adding an additional component to a breathing system increases the potential for disconnection. In addition, the HME can come apart and cause a leak (108, 125).

Heated Breathing Tubes

Heating the breathing tubes will result in an increase in inspired humidity during low flow anesthesia (126).

Humidifiers

A humidifier (vaporizer or vaporizing humidifier) is an instrument that passes a stream of gas over water or across wicks dipped in water (pass-over or blow-by) or through water (bubble or cascade).

Unheated

Most unheated humidifiers are disposable bubble-through devices that are used to increase the humidity of oxygen supplied to patients via a face mask or nasal cannulae. Unheated humidifiers cannot deliver more than approximately 9 mg H_2O/liter.

Heated

Heated humidifiers incorporate a device that warms the water in the humidifier. Some also heat the delivery tube.

Description

Humidification chamber. The humidification chamber is the part from which water is immediately derived for humidification of inspired gases. It may be disposable or reusable. Clear plastic chambers have the advantage of allowing a quick visual check of the water level. Some humidifiers have an integral or remote reservoir that supplies liquid water to the humidification chamber (Fig. 10.2)

Heat source. Heat may be supplied by heated rods immersed in the water or a plate at the bottom of the humidification chamber (Fig. 10.3).

Delivery tube. The delivery tube conveys humidified gas from the humidifier outlet. If it is not heated, the gas will cool and lose some of its moisture as it travels to the patient. This water will collect in the inspiratory tubing. Water traps must be used to prevent water from entering the patient's lungs.

Methods of heating the delivery tube have included an electric wire inside the tube (Fig. 10.3)

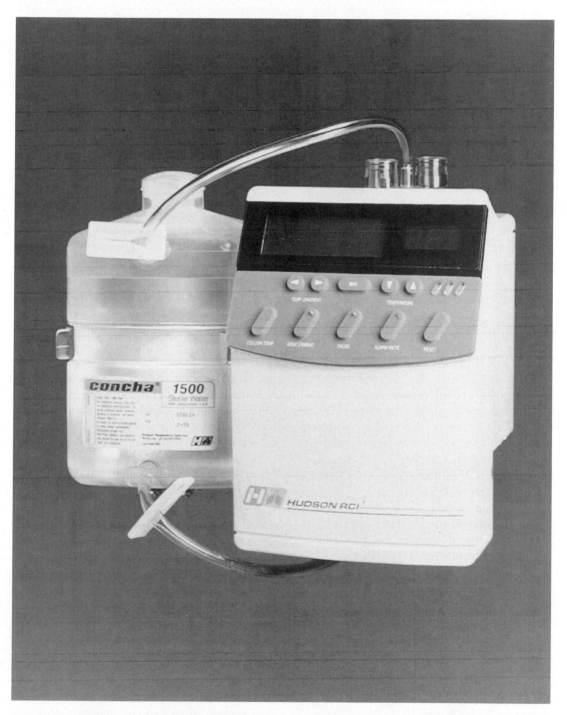

FIGURE 10.2.   Heated humidifier with separate water reservoir. (Reprinted with permission from Hudson RCI.)

FIGURE 10.3. Heated humidifier. Heat is supplied from a heated plate below the humidification chamber. Note the probe for monitoring the temperature of gas leaving the humidification chamber. A heating wire is inside the delivery tube. (Reprinted with permission from Marquest Medical Products, Inc.)

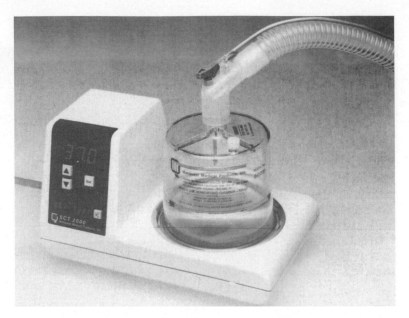

(127, 128), heating tape, orthopedic cast padding or an air or water jacket around the tube (129–132), and placing it inside the expiratory limb (133–135).

The heating wire has the advantage of still allowing visualization of the tube (Fig. 10.3). It should extend as close to the patient connection as possible. Disposable wires in preassembled disposable breathing systems are available. A reusable wire must be inserted manually into the delivery tube using a draw wire (136).

An advantage of heated delivery tubes is that there is no rainout of moisture. However, they may deliver a low relative humidity (16, 137, 138).

Temperature monitor(s). Most heated humidifiers have a means to measure the delivered gas temperature (the temperature of the gas at the patient end of the breathing system). In systems using a heated wire, there is usually a second probe to measure the temperature at the humidifier outlet. A low temperature alarm may be the means of detecting lack of ventilation (139). There may be temperature sensors in the water reservoir or in contact with the heater plate to activate alarms and shut off heater power.

Thermostats

SERVO-CONTROLLED UNITS. A servo-controlled unit regulates power to the heating element in response to the temperature sensed by a probe near the patient connection or the humidifier outlet (140–142). Usually there are two thermostats so that if one fails, the other will cut off the power before a dangerous temperature is reached.

NONSERVO-CONTROLLED UNITS. A nonservo-controlled unit provides power to the heating element according to the setting of a control, irrespective of the delivery temperature. A nonservo-controlled unit may include a servo-controlled circuit but this maintains heat rather than delivery temperature (140, 142).

Controls. Most humidifiers allow selection of different temperatures at the end of the delivery tube or the humidification chamber outlet. Some allow less than 100% relative humidity to be delivered (143). Some models generate saturated vapor only at a preset temperature (3).

Alarms. Alarms may warn when the following occurs: the temperature at the patient end of the circuit deviates from the set temperature by a fixed amount, the temperature probe is not in place, the heater wire is not connected, the water level in the humidification chamber is low, or the airway temperature probe does not sense an increase in temperature within a certain time after activation

Action

Some humidifiers heat the gas to a temperature exceeding the desired patient airway temperature (superheating) so that the cooling that occurs as it flows to the patient will result in the desired temperature at the patient connection. In other units, temperature increases as it passes through the delivery tube so that gas with less than 100% relative humidity is delivered.

The temperature will drop as it flows to the patient with any humidifier in which the delivery tube is not heated. The magnitude of the drop depends on many factors, including the ambient temperature; gas flow; and the length, diameter, and thermal mass of the breathing system. Cooling can be reduced by shortening or insulating the delivery tube and using higher inspiratory flows (144). If the gas is saturated at the humidifier outlet, the temperature drop will cause condensation of water vapor (rainout) to occur.

Standard Requirements

An international standard on humidifiers has been published (145). It contains the following provisions:

1. All humidifiers must be capable of producing an output of at least 10 mg H_2O/l. Those intended for use with patients whose supraglottic airways have been bypassed must be capable of producing an output of at least 33 mg H_2O/l.
2. The average temperature at the delivery tube outlet shall not fluctuate by more than 2°C from the set temperature after a state of thermal equilibrium has been established following a change in gas flow or set temperature. If the measured gas temperature differs from the set temperature by more than the range specified by the manufacturer, a medium priority (caution) alarm must be generated.
3. The volume of liquid exiting the humidifier shall not exceed 1 ml/min or 20 ml/hr for humidifiers intended for use with neonates or 5 ml/min or 20 ml/hr for all other humidifiers.
4. If the humidifier is heated, the gas temperature at the delivery tube outlet shall not exceed 41°C or the gas temperature at the humidifier outlet shall be indicated continuously and the temperature measuring device shall activate a medium priority alarm when the temperature exceeds 41°C. The humidifier shall interrupt heating when the measured gas temperature exceeds 41°C.
5. The accessible surface temperature of the delivery tube must not exceed 44°C within 25 cm of the patient connection port.
6. When the humidifier is tilted 20° from its normal operating position, there shall be no spillage of water into the breathing system.
7. All calibrated controls and indicators shall be accurate to within 5% of their full-scale value, except for temperature displays and controls. The measured gas temperature shall be accurate to ± 2°C.

The American Society for Testing and Materials (ASTM) standard for breathing systems requires a flow-direction sensitive humidifier to be marked with an arrow indicating the proper directional flow and/or the words "inlet" and "outlet" (146).

Use

In the circle system, a heated humidifier is placed in the inspiratory limb downstream of the unidirectional valve. Care should be taken to be certain that it is in the inspiratory and not the expiratory limb (147, 148). If a filter is used, it should be upstream of the humidifier to prevent it from becoming clogged.

In Mapleson systems, the humidifier is usually placed in the fresh gas supply tube (132, 149–152). Using a large-diameter tubing and placing the humidifier near the end of the tube will decrease condensation (150). The delivery tube temperature probe may be placed between the fresh gas supply tube and the T piece or between the T piece and the patient (150).

The humidifier should be lower than the patient to avoid the risk of water running down the tube into the patient. Clear tubing should be used so this water can be seen. The condensate should be drained periodically or a water trap inserted in the dependent part of the tubing to prevent blockage or aspiration. If high fresh gas flows are used, it may be necessary to combine two humidifiers in series to obtain adequate humidification (153). The heater wire in a delivery tube should not be bunched but strung evenly along the length of the tube. The delivery tube should not rest on other surfaces or be covered with sheets, blankets, or other materials. A boom arm or tube tree may be used to support it (154).

Advantages

Most heated humidifiers are capable of delivering saturated gas at body temperature or above, even with high flow rates.

Disadvantages

Humidifiers are bulky and somewhat complex. Humidifiers are more costly than HMEs. Their use involves high maintenance costs, electric hazards, and increased workload (control of temperature, refilling of the reservoir, drainage of condensate, cleaning and sterilization after use). Compared to both water and forced-air warming blankets, the heated humidifier offers relatively little protection against heat loss during anesthesia (155).

Hazards

Infection. Bacterial growth can occur in water stored in a reservoir or the condensate in the delivery tube. Bacterial contamination is especially a problem with cascade humidifiers (156, 157).

Breathing system problems. Reported breathing system problems include sticking valves, leaks, disconnections, incorrect connections, obstruction of the fresh gas line or inspiratory limb, noise, and clogging of filters and HMEs (150, 158–165). If the humidifier is placed in the fresh gas line, a sudden obstruction may result in water splashing back into the anesthesia machine (166). A leak may occur as a result of the heating wire being caught between the Y-piece and the tube (167).

Melting of the delivery tubing may occur, resulting in an obstruction or leak (136, 162, 168–174). Fires have been reported (140, 175, 176). Charring of the breathing system may result in fumes entering the patient's lungs (136). Overheating of breathing circuits with melting may be caused by defects in or damage to the heated wire; bunching of the heated-wire coils within the breathing system; electric incompatibility between the heated-wire breathing circuit and the humidifier; operating the device outside the specified range of flows or minute volumes; or covering the delivery tube with sheets, blankets, or other materials (154, 169, 172, 173, 177). Problems may occur if circuits from a supplier other than the humidifier manufacturer are used. Even when electric connectors for heated-wire circuits are physically compatible, they may not be electrically interchangeable (154).

Obstruction of the inspiratory limb by the heating coils of a humidifier has been reported (178).

Adding a humidifier may change the breathing system volume and compliance significantly (179). This can complicate delivery of small tidal volumes.

Tracheal lavage or aspiration of water. Overfilling, misassembly, or malfunction can cause water to enter the breathing system (180–183). There is also danger of liquid water entering the tracheal tube and drowning the patient or causing a burn of the respiratory tract. These risks can be decreased by configuring the breathing system so that it does not allow condensate to drain into the patient, installing a water trap in the dependent portion of the tube, draining condensate frequently, and placing the humidifier and tubes below the patient.

Overhydration. Use of a humidifier can produce a positive water balance and even overhydration. Undesirable heat gain may occur. Although most anesthetics are of sufficiently short duration that this is not a significant problem, it can be a problem with infants.

Thermal Injury. Delivery of excessively heated gases can cause hyperthermia or damage to the tissues lining the tracheobronchial tree (174, 184–188). Burns to the skin have been reported from heated oxygen administered nasally (189) and to the nares and face during delivery of continuous positive airway pressure (142). Overheating of inspired gas may be caused by omitting, misplacing, dislodging, or not fully inserting the airway temperature probe (140, 189–191).

A humidifier may overheat if turned on with a low gas flow through it (140, 188). A temporary increase in inspired gas temperature may occur following a period of interrupted flow or an increase in flow rate (192).

Skin contact with heated breathing circuits may cause burns (193–196). Care must be taken not to allow the tubing containing a heated wire to contact the skin.

Underhydration. Failure to deliver adequate humidity can lead to impaction of secretions and tracheal tube obstruction. The delivered humidity may fall with high flows (137, 153) so that it may be necessary to use two humidifiers in series to obtain adequate humidification. Heating the delivery tube may result in less than 100% relative humidity being delivered (16, 197).

Increased work of breathing. A bubble humidifier may present an unacceptable inspiratory load during spontaneous breathing (198).

Pharyngeal complaints. Heated humidification may increase the incidence of postoperative pharyngeal complaints when used with an LMA or tracheal tube (199, 200).

Interference with monitoring. A humidifier may add enough resistance to prevent activation of a low airway pressure alarm if the sensor is upstream of the humidifier (76). High humidity can cause problems with sidestream (aspirating) respiratory gas monitors (201). Inserting a filter between the sampling line and the sensing port in the breathing system may help.

Alteration of anesthetic agents. Halothane may be altered by passage through a humidifier whose heating element is in direct contact with the gas at a temperature of 68°C (202).

Nebulizers

Description

A nebulizer (aerosol generator, atomizer, nebulizing humidifier) emits water in the form of an aerosol mist (water vapor plus particulate water). The most commonly used nebulizers are the pneumatic (gas driven, jet, high pressure, compressed gas) and ultrasonic. Both can be heated. In addition to providing humidification, nebulizers may be used to deliver drugs to the breathing system (203).

In a pneumatic nebulizer, a jet of high-pressure gas encounters the liquid, inducing shearing forces and breaking the water up into fine particles. An ultrasonic nebulizer produces a fine mist by subjecting the liquid to a high-frequency resonator. The frequency of oscillation determines the size of the droplets. There is no need for a driving gas. Ultrasonic nebulizers create a denser mist than pneumatic nebulizers (141).

Use

Because a high flow of gas must be used with a pneumatic nebulizer, it should be placed in the fresh gas line (204). An ultrasonic nebulizer can be used in the fresh gas line or the inspiratory limb (31).

Hazards

Nebulized drugs may cause obstruction of an HME or filter in the breathing system (112, 205). Overhydration can occur. If the droplets are not warmed, hypothermia may result. Transmission of infection can occur, because microorganisms can be suspended in the water droplets (206)

Advantages

Nebulizers can deliver gases saturated with water without heat and, if desired, can produce gases carrying more water.

Disadvantages

Nebulizers are somewhat costly. Pneumatic nebulizers require high gas flows. Ultrasonic nebulizers require a source of electricity and may present electric hazards. There may be considerable water deposition in the tubings, requiring frequent draining and increasing the danger of water draining into the patient or blocking the tubing.

REFERENCES

1. Williams R, Rankin N, Smith T, et al. Relationship between the humidity and temperature of inspired gas and the function of the airway mucosa. Crit Care Med 1996;24:1920–1929.
2. Rashad K, Wilson K, Hurt HH Jr, et al. Effect of humidification of anesthetic gases on static compliance. Anesth Analg 1967;46:127–133.
3. Shelly MP, Lloyd GM, Park GR. A review of the mechanisms and methods of humidification of inspired gases. Intensive Care Med 1988;14:1–9.
4. Van Heerden PV, Wilson IH, Marshall FPF, et al. Effect of humidification on inhalation induction with isoflurane. Br J Anaesth 1990;64:235–237.
5. van Heerden PV, Bukofzer M, Edge KR, et al. Rapid inhalational induction of anaesthesia with isoflurane or halothane in humidified oxygen. Can J Anaesth 1992;39:242–246.
6. Cregg N, Wall C, Green D, et al. Humidification reduces coughing and breath-holding during inhalation induction with isoflurane in children. Can J Anaesth 1996;43:1090–1094.
7. Martin C, Papazian L, Perrin G, et al. Preservation of humidity and heat of respiratory gases in patients with a minute ventilation greater than 10 L/min. Crit Care Med 1994;22:1871–1876.
8. Dery R, Pelletier J, Jacques A, et al. Humidity in anesthesiology. Heat and moisture patterns in the respira-

tory tract during anaesthesia with the semi-closed system. Canadian Anaesthetists Society Journal 1967; 14:287–298.

9. Anonymous. Heat and moisture exchangers. Health Devices 1983;12:155–167.

10. Chamney AR. Humidification requirements and techniques. Including a review of the performance of equipment in current use. Anaesthesia 1969;24: 602–617.

11. Chalon J, Loew DAY, Malebranche J. Effects of dry anesthetic gases on tracheobronchial ciliated epithelium. Anesthesiology 1972;37:338–343.

12. Forbes AR. Humidification and mucus flow in the intubated trachea. Br J Anaesth 1973;45:874–878.

13. Noguchi H, Takumi Y, Aochi O. A study of humidification in tracheostomized dogs. Br J Anaesth 1973; 45:844–848.

14. Tsuda T, Noguchi H, Takkumi Y, et al. Optimum humidification of air administered to a tracheostomy in dogs. Scanning electron microscopy and surfactant studies. Br J Anaesth 1977;49:965–977.

15. Weeks DB. Humidification during anesthesia. N Y State J Med 1975;75:1216–1218.

16. Miyao H, Hirokawa T, Miyasaka K, et al. Relative humidity, not absolute humidity, is of great importance when using a humidifier with a heating wire. Crit Care Med 1992;20:674–679.

17. Chatburn RL, Primiano FP. A rational basis for humidity therapy. Respiratory Care 1987;32:249–254.

18. Mebius C. A comparative evaluation of disposable humidifiers. Acta Anaesthesiol Scand 1983;27: 403–409.

19. Chalon J, Patel C, Ali M, et al. Humidity and the anesthetized patient. Anesthesiology 1979;50: 195–198.

20. Chalon J, Markham JP, Ali MM, et al. The Pall ultipore breathing circuit filter—an efficient heat and moisture exchanger. Anesth Analg 1984;63: 566–570.

21. Haslam KR, Nielsen CH. Do passive heat and moisture exchangers keep the patient warm? Anesthesiology 1986;64:379–381.

22. Morton GH, Flewellen EH. Prevention of intraoperative hypothermia in geriatric patients. Anesth Analg 1989;68:S204.

23. Pflug AE, Aasheim GM, Foster C, et al. Prevention of post-anaesthesia shivering. Canadian Anaesthetists Society Journal 1978;25:41–47.

24. Stone DR, Downs JB, Paul WL, et al. Adult body temperature and heated humidification of anesthetic gases during general anesthesia. Anesth Analg 1981; 60:736–741.

25. Tausk HC, Miller R, Roberts RB. Maintenance of body temperature by heated humidification. Anesth Analg 1976;55:719–723.

26. Wallace CT, Baker JD, Brown CS. Heated humidification for infants during anesthesia. Anesthesiology 1978;48:80.

27. Hedley RM, Allt-Graham J. Heat and moisture exchangers and breathing filters. Br J Anaesth 1994;73: 227–236.

28. Kulkarni P, Webster J, Carli F. Body heat transfer during hip surgery using active core warming. Can J Anaesth 1995;42:571–576.

29. Fonkalsrud EW, Calmes S, Barcliff LT, et al. Reduction of operative heat loss and pulmonary secretions in neonates by use of heated and humidified anesthetic gases. J Thorac Cardiovasc Surg 1980;80: 718–723.

30. Gawley TH, Dundee JW. Attempts to reduce respiratory complications following upper abdominal operations. Br J Anaesth 1981;53:1073–1078.

31. Stevens HL, Kennedy RL. The ultrasonic approach to humidification of anesthesia gases. Journal of Asthma Research 1968;5:325–333.

32. Knudsen J, Lomholt N, Wisborg K. Postoperative pulmonary complications using dry and humidified anaesthetic gases. Br J Anaesth 1973;45:363–368.

33. Chalon J. Low humidity and damage to tracheal mucosa. Bull N Y Acad Med 1980;56:314–322.

34. Chase HF, Trotta R, Kilmore MA. Simple methods for humidifying nonrebreathing anesthesia gas systems. Anesth Analg 1962;41:249–256.

35. Hedley RM, Allt-Graham J. A comparison of the filtration properties of heat and moisture exchangers. Anaesthesia 1992;47:414–420.

36. Linden BM. Heat and moisture exchanging bacterial filters. Evaluating humidification efficacy for mechanically ventilated patients. British Journal of Intensive Care 1993;3:330–337.

37. Gedeon A, Mebius C, Palmer K. Neonatal hygroscopic condenser humidifier. Crit Care Med 1987; 15:51–54.

38. Wilkinson KA, Cranston A, Hatch DJ, et al. Assessment of a hygroscopic heat and moisture exchanger for paediatric use. Anaesthesia 1991;46:296–299.

39. Roustan JP, Kienlen J, Aubas P, et al. Comparison of hydrophobic heat and moisture exchangers with heated humidifier during prolonged mechanical ventilation. Intensive Care Medicine 1992;18:97–100.

40. Branson RD, Hurst JM. Laboratory evaluation of moisture output of seven airway heat and moisture exchangers. Respiratory Care 1987;32:741–745.

41. Roustan JP, Kienlen J, Aubas P, et al. Comparison of hydrophobic heat and moisture exchangers with

heated humidifier during prolonged mechanical ventilation. Intensive Care Medicine 1992;18:97–100.

42. Berry AJ, Nolte FS. An alternative strategy for infection control of anesthesia breathing circuits: a laboratory assessment of the Pall HME filter. Anesth Analg 1991;72:651–655.

43. Lee MG, Ford JL, Hunt PB, et al. Bacterial retention properties of heat and moisture exchange filters. Br J Anaesth 1992;69:522–525.

44. Leitjen DTM, Rejger VS, Mouton RP. Bacterial contamination and the effect of filters in anaesthetic circuits in a simulated patient mode. J Hosp Infect 1992;21:51–60.

45. Vandenbroucke-Grauls CMJE, Teeuw KB, Ballemans K, et al. Bacterial and viral removal efficiency, heat and moisture exchange properties of four filtration devices. J Hosp Infect 1995;29:45–56.

46. Lloyd G, Howells J, Liddle C, et al. Barriers to Hepatitis C transmission within breathing systems: efficacy of a pleated hydrophobic filter. Anaesthesia and Intensive Care 1997;25:235–238.

47. Lee MG, Ford JL, Hunt PB, et al. Bacterial retention properties of heat and moisture exchange filters. Br J Anaesth 1992;69:522–525.

48. Gallagher J, Strangeways JEM, Allt-Graham J. Contamination control in long-term ventilation. A clinical study using a heat-and-moisture-exchanger filter. Anaesthesia 1987;42:476–481.

49. Anonymous. Evaluation report: heat and moisture exchangers. J Med Eng Technol 1987;11:117–127.

50. Cigada M, Elena A, Solca M, et al. The efficiency of twelve heat and moisture exchangers: an in vitro evaluation. Intensive Care World 1990;7:98–101.

51. Jackson C, Webb AR. An evaluation of the heat and moisture exchange performance of four ventilator circuit filters. Intensive Care Medicine 1992;18:264–268.

52. Sottiaus T, Mignolet G, Damas P, et al. Comparative evaluation of three heat and moisture exchangers during short-term postoperative mechanical ventilation. Chest 1993;104:220–224.

53. Villafane MC, Cinnella G, Lofaso F, et al. Gradual reduction of endotracheal tube diameter during mechanical ventilation via different humidification devices. Anesthesiology 1996;85:1341–1349.

54. Eckerbom B, Lindholm C-E. Performance evaluation of six heat and moisture exchangers according to the Draft International Standard (ISO/DIS 9360). Acta Anaesthesiol Scand 1990;34:404–409.

55. Bickler PE, Sessler DI. Efficiency of airway heat and moisture exchangers in anesthetized humans. Anesth Analg 1990;71:415–418.

56. Mebius C. Heat and moisture exchangers with bacterial filters: a laboratory evaluation. Acta Anaesthesiol Scand 1992;36:572–576.

57. Martin C, Papazian L, Perrin G, et al. Performance evaluation of three vaporizing humidifiers and two heat and moisture exchangers in patients with minute ventilation > 10 L/min. Chest 1992;102:1347–1350.

58. Mebius C. A comparative evaluation of disposable humidifiers. Acta Anaesthesiol Scand 1983;27:403–409.

59. Linden BM. Heat and moisture exchanging bacterial filters. Evaluating humidification efficacy for mechanically ventilated patients. British Journal of Intensive Care 1993;3:330–337.

60. Holton J, Webb AR. An evaluation of the microbial retention performance of three ventilator-circuit filters. Intensive Care Medicine 1994;20:233–237

61. Quinn AC, Newman PJ, Allt-Graham J, et al. In vivo assessment of the work of breathing through dry and wet heat and moisture exchanging devices. Br J Anaesth 1994;72(Supp 11):A17.

62. Myer CM III, McDonald JS, Hubbell RN, et al. Study of humidification potential of a heat and moisture exchanger in tracheotomized dogs. Ann Otol Rhinol Laryngol 1988;97:322–325.

63. Chui PT, Poon M. Using the Pall HME filter as an oxygen therapy device in recovery room. Anaesthesia and Intensive Care 1996;24:514.

64. Branson RD, Campbell RS, Chatburn RL, et al. AARC clinical practice guideline. Humidification during mechanical ventilation. Respiratory Care 1992;37:887–890.

65. Pelosi P, Solca M, Ravagnan I, et al. Effects of heat and moisture exchangers on minute ventilation, ventilatory drive, and work of breathing during pressure-support ventilation in acute respiratory failure. Crit Care Med 1996;24:1184–1188.

66. Usuda Y, Suzukawa M, Yamaguchi O, et al. Increased moisture output from heat and moisture exchangers combined with an unheated humidifier. Crit Care Med 1989;17:S35.

67. Shanks CA. Clinical anesthesia and multiple-gauze condenser humidifier. Br J Anaesth 1974;46:773–777.

68. Hay R, Miller WC. Efficacy of a new hygroscopic condenser humidifier. Crit Care Med 1982;10:49–51.

69. Ogino M, Kopotic R, Mannino FL. Moisture-conserving efficiency of condenser humidifiers. Anaesthesia 1985;40:990–995.

70. Tilling, SE, Hayes B. Heat and moisture exchangers in artificial ventilation. Br J Anaesth 1987;59:1181–1188.

71. Gedeon A, Mebius C. The hygroscopic condenser humidifier. A new device for general use in anaesthesia and intensive care. Anaesthesia 1979;34:1043–1047.

72. Shanks CA, Sara CA. A reappraisal of the multiple gauze heat and moisture exchanger. Anaesthesia and Intensive Care 1973;1:428–432.

73. Nebbia S, Bissonnette B. Efficiency of passive airway humidification as a function of the dead space between hygroscopic filter and endotracheal tube. Can J Anaesth 1993;40:A25.

74. Jerwood DC, Jones SEF. HME filter and Ayre's piece. Anaesthesia 1995;50:915–916.

75. Milligan KA. Disablement of a ventilator disconnect alarm by a heat and moisture exchanger. Anaesthesia 1992;47:279.

76. Slee TA, Pavlin EG. Failure of low pressure alarm associated with the use of a humidifier. Anesthesiology 1988;69:791–793.

77. Milligan KA. Disablement of a ventilator disconnect alarm by a heat and moisture exchanger. Anaesthesia 1992;47:279.

78. Suzukawa M, Usuda Y, Numata K. The effects on sputum characteristics of combining an unheated humidifier with a heat-moisture exchanging filter. Respiratory Care 1989;34:976–984.

79. Duncan A. Use of disposable condenser humidifiers in children. Anaesthesia and Intensive Care 1985;13:330–337.

80. Martinez FJ, Pietchel S, Wise C, et al. Increased resistance of hygroscopic condenser humidifiers when using a closed circuit suction system. Crit Care Med 1994;22:1668–1673.

81. Leigh JM, White MG. A new condenser humidifier. Anaesthesia 1984;39:492–493.

82. Tenaillon A, Cholley GM, Boiteau R, et al. Heat and moisture exchanging bacterial filter versus heated humidifier in long-term mechanical ventilation. Care of the Critically Ill. 1991;7:56–61.

83. Shelly M, Bethune DW, Latimer RD. A comparison of five heat and moisture exchangers. Anaesthesia 1986;41:527–532.

84. Bygdeman S, von Euler C, Nystrom B. Moisture exchangers do not prevent patient contamination of ventilators. A microbiological study. Acta Anaesthesiol Scand 1984;28:591–594.

85. Luttropp HH, Berntman L. Bacterial filters protect anaesthetic equipment in a low-flow system. Anaesthesia 1993;48:520–523.

86. Branson RD, Davis K Jr, Campbell RS, et al. Humidification in the intensive care unit. Prospective study of a new protocol utilizing heated humidification and a hygroscopic condenser humidifier. Chest 1993;104:1800–1805.

87. Siegel MN, Gravenstein N. Passive warming of airway gases (artificial nose) improves accuracy of esophageal temperature monitoring. Journal of Clinical Monitoring 1990;6:89–92.

88. Bissonnette B, Sessler DI, LaFlamme P. Passive and active inspired gas humidification in infants and children. Anesthesiology 1989;71:350–354.

89. Bissonnette B, Sessler DI. Passive or active inspired gas humidification increases thermal steady-state temperatures in anesthetized infants. Anesthesiology 1989;71:350–354.

90. Mason DG, Edmondson L, McHugh P. Humidifier-induced hypercarbia. Anaesthesia 1987;42:672–673.

91. Johnson PA, Raper RF, Fisher MM. The impact of heat and moisture exchanging humidifiers on work of breathing. Anaesthesia and Intensive Care 1995;23:697–701.

92. Goddard JM, Bennett HR. Filters and Ayre's T-piece. Anaesthesia 1996;51:605.

93. Buckley PM. Increase in resistance of in-line breathing filters in humidified air. Br J Anaesth 1984;56:637–642.

94. Chung R, Soni NC. Work of ventilating heat and moisture exchangers. Br J Anaesth 1991;67:647P–648P.

95. Jones BR, Ozaki GT, Benumof JL, et al. Airway resistance caused by a pediatric heat and moisture exchanger. Anesthesiology 1988;69:A786.

96. Ploysongsang Y, Branson R, Rashkin MC, et al. Pressure flow characteristics of commonly used heat-moisture exchangers. American Review of Respiratory Disease 1988;138:675–678.

97. Ploysongsang Y, Branson RD, Rashkin MC, et al. Effect of flow rate and duration of use on the pressure drop across six artificial noses. Respiratory Care 1989;34:902–907.

98. Rodes WD, Banner MJ, Gravenstein N. Variations in imposed work of breathing with heat and moisture exchangers. Anesth Analg 1991;72:S226.

99. Steward DJ. A disposable condenser humidifier for use during anaesthesia. Canadian Anaesthetists Society Journal 1976;23:191–195.

100. Manthous CA, Schmidt GA. Resistive pressure of a condenser humidifier in mechanically ventilated patients. Crit Care Med 1994;22:1792–1795.

101. Costigan SN, Snowdon SL. Breathing system filters can affect the performance of anaesthetic monitors. Anaesthesia 1993;48:1015–1016.

102. Chiaranda M, Verona L, Pinamonti O, et al. Use of heat and moisture exchanging (HME) filters in mechanically ventilated ICU patients: influence on airway flow-resistance. Intensive Care Medicine 1993;19:462–466.

103. Ploysongsang Y, Branson R, Rashkin MC, et al. Pressure flow characteristics of commonly used heat-moisture exchangers. American Review of Respiratory Disease 1988;138:675–678.

104. Kong KL, Rainbow C, Ford DB. Heat and moisture exchanging bacterial filters. Anesthesia 1988;43:254.

105. Branson RD. Artificial noses: the unanswered questions. Respiratory Care 1989;34:969–971.

106. Barnes SD, Normoyle DA. Failure of ventilation in an infant due to increased resistance of a disposable heat and moisture exchanger. Anesth Analg 1996;83:193.

107. Warmington A, Peck D. HME plus heated humidifier danger. Anaesthesia and Intensive Care 1995;23:125.

108. Prasad KK, Chen L. Complications related to the use of a heat and moisture exchanger. Anesthesiology 1990;72:958.

109. Anonymous. Breathing system components—Gibeck humidifiers. Anaesthesia 1991;46:612.

110. Anonymous. Heat & moisture exchangers block breathing circuit airway. Biomedical Safety & Standards 1996;28:43.

111. Prados W. A dangerous defect in a heat and moisture exchanger. Anesthesiology 1989;71:804.

112. Anonymous. Heat/moisture exchange humidifiers. Technology for Anesthesia 1991;11(8):5.

113. Reference deleted.

114. Martin C, Perrin G, Gevaudan MJ, et al. Heat and moisture exchangers and vaporising humidifiers in the intensive care unit. Chest 1990;97:144–149.

115. Anonymous. Hazard notice. Anaesthesia 1994;49:563.

116. Stacey MRW, Asai T, Wilkes A, et al. Obstruction of a breathing system filter. Can J Anaesth 1996;43:1276.

117. Cohen IL, Weinberg PF, Fein IA, et al. Endotracheal tube occlusion associated with the use of heat and moisture exchangers in the intensive care unit. Crit Care Med 1988;16:277–279.

118. Misset B, Escudier B, Rivara D, et al. Heat and moisture exchanger vs heated humidifier during long-term mechanical ventilation. A prospective randomized study. Chest 1991;100:160–163.

119. Martin C, Perrin G, Gevaudan M-J, et al. Heat and moisture exchangers and vaporizing humidifiers in the intensive care unit. Chest 1990;97:144–149.

120. Turner DAB, Wright EM. Efficiency of heat and moisture exchangers. Anaesthesia 1987;42:1117–1118.

121. Anonymous. Humidifiers, heat/moisture exchange. Technology for Anesthesia 1985;6(3):8.

122. James PD, Gothard JWW. Possible hazard from the inserts of condenser humidifiers. Anaesthesia 1984;39:70.

123. Casta A, Houck CS. Acute intraoperative endotracheal tube obstruction associated with a heat and moisture exchanger in an infant. Anesth Analg 1997;84:939–940.

124. Hardman JG, Curran J, Mahajan RP. End-tidal carbon dioxide measurement and breathing system filters. Anaesthesia 1997;52:646–648.

125. Bengtsson M, Johnson A. Failure of a heat and moisture exchanger as a cause of disconnection during anaesthesia. Acta Anaesthesiol Scand 1989;33:522–523.

126. Kleemann PP, Schickel BK, Jantzen J-PAH. Heated breathing tubes affect humidity output of circle absorber systems. J Clin Anesth 1993;5:463–467.

127. Baker JD, Wallace CT, Brown CS. Maintenance of body temperature in infants during surgery. Anesthesiol Rev 1977;4:21–25.

128. Shanks CA, Gibbs JM. A comparison of two heated water-bath humidifiers. Anaesthesia and Intensive Care 1975;3:41–47.

129. Berry FA, Hughes-Davies DI, Difazio CA. A system for minimizing respiratory heat loss in infants during operation. Anesth Analg 1973;52:170–175.

130. Epstein RA. Humidification during positive pressure ventilation of infants. Anesthesiology 1971;35:532–536.

131. Mizutani AR, Ozaki G, Rusk R. Insulated circuit hose improves heated humidifier performance in anesthesia ventilation circuits. Anesth Analg 1991;72:566–567.

132. Racz GB. Humidification in a semiopen system for infant anesthesia. Anesth Analg 1971;50:995–1002.

133. Ramanathan S, Chalon J, Turndorf H. A compact, well-humidified breathing circuit for the circle system. Anesthesiology 1976;44:238–242.

134. Chalon J, Patel C, Ramanathan S, et al. Humidification of the circle absorber system. Anesthesiology 1978;48:142–146.

135. Branson RD, Davis K Jr, Porembka DT. Reassessment of humidification supplied by the circle system using ISO 9360: conventional vs a co-axial circuit. Anesthesiology 1995;83:A401.

136. Anonymous. Heated wires can melt disposable breathing circuits. Technology for Anesthesia 1989;9(11):2–3.

137. Gilmour IJ, Boyle MJ, Rozenberg A, et al. The effect of heated wire circuits on humidification of inspired gases. Anesth Analg 1994;79:160–164.

138. Wilkes AR. Low relative humidity delivered by a humidifier with a heating wire. Crit Care Med 1993;21:948.

139. Russell WJ, Webb RK, van der Walt JH, et al. Problems with ventilation: an analysis of 2000 incident reports. Anaesthesia and Intensive Care 1993;21:617–620.

140. Anonymous. Heated humidifiers. Technology for Anesthesia 1987;8(3):1–5.

141. Anonymous. Heated humidifiers. Health Devices 1987;16:223–250.

142. Anonymous. An overview of heated humidifiers. Technology for Anesthesia 1994;15(6):1–5.

143. Cook RI, Potter SS, Woods DD, et al. Evaluating the human engineering of microprocessor-controlled operating room devices. Journal of Clinical Monitoring 1991;7:217–226.

144. Anonymous. Heated humidifiers. Health Devices 1980;9:167–180.

145. International Organization for Standards. Humidifiers for medical use—Part 1: General requirements for humidification systems (ISO 8185-1). Geneva: ISO, 1997.

146. American Society for Testing and Materials Standard specifications for minimum performance and safety requirements for anesthesia breathing systems (ASTM F1208–89, Reapproved 1994). West Conshohocken, PA: ASTM, 1994.

147. Hawkins C, Ross A. Unexplained humidifier failure. Anaesthesia and Intensive Care 1994;22:739–740.

148. Spencer M. Unexplained humidifier failure. Anaesthesia and Intensive Care 1994;22:740.

149. Garg GP. Humidification of the Rees-Ayre T-piece system for neonates. Anesth Analg 1973;52:207–209.

150. Hannallah RS, McGill WA. A practical way of using heated humidifiers with pediatric T- piece systems. Anesthesiology 1983;59:156–157.

151. Kovac AL, Filardi JP, Goto H. Water trap for fresh gas flow line of Bain or CPRAM circuit. Can J Anaesth 1987;34:102–103.

152. Weeks DB. Provision of endogenous and exogenous humidity for the Bain breathing circuit. Canadian Anaesthetists Society Journal 1976;23:185–190.

153. Harrison DA, Breen DP, Harris ND, et al. The performance of two intensive care humidifiers at high gas flows. Anaesthesia 1993;48:902–905.

154. Burlington DB. FDA safety alert. Hazards of heated-wire breathing circuits. Rockville, MD: Food and Drug Administration, July 14, 1993.

155. Hynson JM, Sessler DI. Intraoperative warming therapies: a comparison of three devices. J Clin Anesth 1992;4:194–199.

156. Rhame FS, Streifel A, McComb C, et al. Bubbling humidifiers produce microaerosols which can carry bacteria. Infect Control 1986;7:403–407.

157. Goularte TA, Manning M, Craven DE. Bacterial colonization in humidifying cascade reservoirs after 24 and 48 hours of continuous mechanical ventilation. Infect Control 1987;8:200–203.

158. Anonymous. Humidifiers, heat/moisture exchange. Technology for Anesthesia 1985;6(2):7.

159. Bancroft ML. Problems with humidifiers. In: Rendell-Baker L, ed. Problems with anesthetic and respiratory therapy equipment. Int Anesthesiol Clin 1982;20(3):93–102.

160. McNulty S, Barringer L, Browder J. Carbon dioxide retention associated with a humidifier defect. Can J Anaesth 1987;34:519–521.

161. Nimocks JA, Modell JH, Perry PA. Carbon dioxide retention using a humidified "nonrebreathing" system. Anesth Analg 1975;54:271–273.

162. Patil AR. Melting of anesthesia circuit by humidifier. Another cause of "ventilator disconnect." Anesthesia Progress 1989;36:63–65.

163. Shroff PK, Skerman JH. Humidifier malfunction—a cause of anesthesia circuit occlusion. Anesth Analg 1988;67:710–711.

164. Shampaine EL, Helfaer M. A modest proposal for improved humidifier design. Anesth Analg 1991;72:130–131.

165. Wang J, Hung W, Lin C. Leakage of disposable breathing circuits. J Clin Anesth 1992;4:111–115.

166. Amirdivani M, Siegel D, Chalon J, et al. A heated water humidifier with a rotating wick. Anesth Analg 1979;58:244–246.

167. Warmington A, Peck D. Another complication of heated hose humidification. Anaesthesia and Intensive Care 1994;22:740–741.

168. Wong DHW. Melted delivery hose—a complication of a heated humidifier. Can J Anaesth 1988;35:183–186.

169. Wood D, Boyd M, Campbell C. Insulation of heated wire circuits. Anesth Analg 1992;74:471.

170. Sprague DH, Maccioli GA. Disposable circuit tubing melted by heated humidifier. Anesth Analg 1986;65:1247.

171. Anonymous. Anesthesia breathing circuits. Technology for Anesthesia 12(2):8.

172. Wood D, Boyd M, Campbell C. Insulation of heated wire circuits. Anesth Analg 1992;74:471–472.

173. Anonymous. Incompatibility of disposable heated-wire breathing circuits and heated-wire humidifiers. Technology for Anesthesia 1993;14(2):4–5.

174. Webb RK, Russell WJ, Klepper I, et al. Equipment failure: an analysis of 2000 incident reports. Anaesthesia and Intensive Care 1993;21:673–677.

175. Anonymous. "Potential fire hazard" from nebulizers reported. Biomedical Safety & Standards 1988;18:58.

176. Anonymous. Breathing circuit heating component could short and cause fire. Biomedical Safety & Standards 1990;20:67–68.

177. Anonymous. Anesthesia breathing circuits may overheat & melt tubing. Biomedical Safety & Standards 1994;24:85.

178. Beards SC, Payne T. An unexpected complication of heated hose humidification. Anaesthesia and Intensive Care 1994;22:232.

179. Cote CJ, Petkau AJ, Ryan JF, et al. Wasted ventilation measured in vitro with eight anesthetic circuits with and without inline humidification. Anesthesiology 1983;59:442–446.

180. Poulton TJ. Humidification hazard. Chest 1984;85:583–584.

181. Poplak TM, Leiman BC, Braude BM. A hazardous humidifier misconnexion. Anaesthesia 1984;39:937.

182. Railton R, Shaw A. Filling humidifiers. Avoiding a hazard. Anaesthesia 1982;37:105–106.

183. Ward CF, Reisner LS, Zlott LS. Murphy's law and humidification. Anesth Analg 1983;62:457–461.

184. Kirch TJ, DeKornfeld TJ. An unexpected complication (hyperthemia) while using the Emerson postoperative ventilator. Anesthesiology 1967;28:1106–1107.

185. Klein EF, Graves SA. "Hot pot" tracheitis. Chest 1974;65:225–226.

186. Spurring PW, Shenolikar BK. Hazards in anaesthetic equipment. Br J Anaesth 1978;50:641–644.

187. Sims NM, Geoffrion CA, Welch JP, et al. Respiratory tract burns caused by heated humidification of anesthetic gases in intubated, mechanically ventilated dogs—a light microscopic study. Anesthesiology 1986;65:A490.

188. Anonymous. Safety action bulletin. Heated humidifiers when used with lung ventilators: risk of excessive temperatures. Anaesthesia 1992;47:547.

189. Anonymous. Heated humidifiers can burn infants during CPAP. Health Devices 1987;16:404–406.

190. Anonymous. Heated humidifiers can burn infants during CPAP. Technology for Anesthesia 1988;8:7–9.

191. Anonymous. Safety action bulletin. Anaesthesia 1992;47:547.

192. Smith HS, Allen R. Another hazard of heated water humidifiers. Anaesthesia 1986;41:215–216.

193. Anonymous. Possible burn injury from heated breathing circuit. Biomedical Safety & Standards 1991;21:147.

194. Anonymous. Possible burn from heated breathing circuit. Biomedical Safety & Standards 1991;21:147.

195. Whiteley SM. A hazard of heated humidifiers. Anaesthesia 1992;47:909.

196. Wilkes AR. Resistance to gas flow heat and moisture exchangers. Anaesthesia 1992;47:1095–1096.

197. Levy H, Simpson SQ, Duval D. Hazards of humidifiers with heated wires. Crit Care Med 1993;21:477–478.

198. Oh TE, Lin ES, Bhatt S. Resistance of humidifiers, and inspiratory work imposed by a ventilator-humidifier circuit. Br J Anaesth 1991;66:258–263.

199. O'Neill BL, Foley EP, Chang A. Effects of humidification of inspired gases with the laryngeal mask airway. Anesthesiology 1994;81:A52.

200. Rose K, Cohen MM. Sore throat and hoarse voice in postoperative patients. Anesth Analg 1994;78:S367.

201. Sprung J, Cheng EY. Modification to an anesthesia breathing circuit to prolong monitoring of gases during the use of humidifiers. Anesth Analg 1991;72:264–265.

202. Karis JH. Alteration of halothane in heated humidifiers. Anesth Analg 1980;59:518.

203. Weeks DB. Micronebulizer for anesthesia circuits. Anesth Analg 1981;60:537–538.

204. Fortin G, Blanc VF. Miniature ventilators with interrupted non-rebreathing circle systems and other anaesthetic circuits. Canadian Anaesthetists Society Journal 1970;17:613–623.

205. Barton RM. Detection of expiratory antibacterial filter occlusion. Anesth Analg 1993;77:197.

206. Craven DE, Goularte TA, Make BS. Contaminated condensate in mechanical ventilator circuits. A risk factor for nosocomial pneumonia. American Review of Respiratory Disease 1984;129:625–628.

QUESTIONS

1. Which is not an effect of inhaling dry gases?
   A. Drying of the mucosa
   B. Decreased compliance
   C. Development of loci for infection
   D. Impairment of surfactant activity
   E. Decreased alveolar-arterial oxygen difference

2. Where should a heated humidifier be located in the circle system?
   A. Between the exhalation tubing and the carbon dioxide absorber
   B. Between the Y-piece and tracheal tube
   C. Between the inspiratory tubing and the Y-piece
   D. Between the absorber and the inspiratory tubing
   E. Between the Y-piece and the mask

3. If a bacterial filter is used in a circle system that has a heated humidifier, where should the filter be placed?
   A. Between the Y-piece and the tracheal tube
   B. Between the Y-piece and the inhalational tubing
   C. Between the inhalational tubing and the humidifier
   D. Between the inhalational unidirectional valve and the humidifier
   E. Between the Y-piece and the exhalation tubing

Each question below contains four suggested answers of which one or more is correct. Choose the answer:

A if 1, 2, and 3 are correct
B if 1 and 3 are correct
C if 2 and 4 are correct
D if 4 is correct
E if 1, 2, 3, and 4 are correct

4. Which of the following statements about humidity and ambient conditions are true?
   1. If a gas saturated with water is heated it can hold more water
   2. Gas that is 100% saturated at room temperature and warmed to body temperature will be approximately 60% saturated
   3. If a gas saturated with water is heated, the absolute humidity remains the same
   4. If a gas saturated with water is heated, the relative humidity increases

5. A result of the low specific heat of gases is
   1. Inhaled gas will quickly assume body temperature
   2. Water will condense in the exhalation side of a circle system
   3. Gas in breathing tubes will quickly assume room temperature
   4. Gas has a tendency to change temperature slowly

6. Heat and moisture are normally lost during anesthesia because
   1. Dry gases are supplied from the anesthesia machine
   2. The breathing system does not supply humidity
   3. Tracheal intubation bypasses normal humidification mechanisms
   4. The tracheal tube does not act to conserve heat or moisture

7. Physiologic effects of lowered body temperature seen in the postoperative period include
   1. Shivering
   2. Decreased metabolism
   3. Increased cardiac output
   4. Lowered oxygen demand

8. Sources of humidity in the breathing system include
   1. Carbon dioxide absorbent
   2. Exhaled water from a previous patient
   3. Rebreathing of previously exhaled gases
   4. Fresh gas

9. Advantages of a hydrophobic HME over a composite hygroscopic HME include
   1. Better filtration
   2. Less resistance
   3. Nebulized drugs have little effect on resistance
   4. Better humidification

10. Use of a heated breathing tube with a heated humidifier will result in
    1. A higher temperature at the Y-piece
    2. Rainout in the delivery tube
    3. Drying of secretions
    4. A delivered relative humidity of 100%

11. Hazards of heated humidifiers include
    1. Sticking valves
    2. Overhydration
    3. Alteration of anesthetic agents
    4. Obstruction of sidestream gas monitors

12. Advantages of HMEs include
    1. Fluctuating temperatures and humidities
    2. Decease in dead space
    3. Low compliance
    4. Decreased resistance to breathing

13. Contraindications to HME use include
    1. Bloody secretions
    2. Patient temperature less than 35°C
    3. Bronchopleurocutaneous fistula
    4. Patient with tracheotomy

14. When using an HME, the inspired humidity can be increased by
    1. Use of an uncuffed tube
    2. Increasing the minute volume
    3. Lowering the humidity of gas entering the HME
    4. Use of a hygroscopic rather than a hydrophobic HME

ANSWERS

1.	E	8.	A
2.	D	9.	A
3.	D	10.	B
4.	B	11.	E
5.	A	12.	B
6.	B	13.	B
7.	B	14.	D

CHAPTER
11

Anesthesia Ventilators

G. Ohmeda 7900 Series Ventilator
  1. Description
  2. Alarms
  3. Special Features
  4. Internal Construction
  5. Control of Ventilation
    a. Volume Control Mode
    b. Pressure Control Mode
  6. Hazards
H. Anodyne™ CC Anesthesia Workstation Ventilator
  1. Description
  2. Alarms
  3. Special Features
  4. Internal Construction
  5. Spontaneous Respiration
    a. Manual Ventilation
    b. Automatic Ventilation
  6. Control of Ventilation
  7. Hazards
V. General Hazards
  A. Hypoventilation
    1. Ventilator Dysfunction
      a. Cycling Failure
      b. Inadequate Design
      c. Driving Gas Leak
      d. Loss of Breathing System Gas
    2. Incorrect Settings
    3. Ventilator Turned Off
    4. Obstruction to Flow
    5. Addition of Positive End–Expiratory Pressure
  B. Hyperventilation
  C. Hyperoxia
  D. Excessive Airway Pressure
  E. Negative Pressure During Expiration
  F. Alarm Failure
VI. Advantages
VII. Disadvantages

MOST PATIENTS GIVEN general anesthesia are administered muscle relaxants. As a result, control of ventilation is required. A ventilator (breathing machine) is an automatic device designed to provide or augment the patient's ventilation. Presently most anesthesia machines come with an attached or built-in ventilator.

RELATIONSHIP OF THE VENTILATOR TO THE BREATHING SYSTEM

A ventilator replaces the reservoir bag in the breathing system. It may be connected to the breathing system using a hose that is attached at the bag mount or the bag/ventilator selector valve. Newer anesthesia ventilators are connected to the breathing system without a hose. During automatic ventilation, the adjustable pressure limiting (APL) valve in the breathing system must be closed or isolated. Most selector valves when turned for automatic ventilation isolate the APL valve from the rest of the system. With these, it is not necessary to close the APL valve when the ventilator is used.

Most anesthesia ventilators have a "bellows in a box" (bag in a bottle or double circuit) design (Fig. 11.1). With this arrangement, the bellows is housed in a chamber and the inside of the bellows is connected to the breathing system. The bellows acts as an interface between the breathing system and the ventilator driving gas, just as the reservoir bag acts as an interface between the breathing system and the anesthesia provider's hand. It separates breathing system gases from driving gas. The pressure of the anesthesia provider's hand is replaced by the pressure of driving gas.

During inspiration, driving gas (oxygen and/or air) is delivered into the space between the bellows and its housing. This causes pressure to be exerted on the bellows, causing it to be compressed. At the same time, the spill valve (which vents excess gases to the scavenging system) and exhaust valve (which vents driving gas to atmosphere) are closed. The compression of the bellows causes gas to flow into the breathing system.

During expiration the bellows reexpands as breathing system gases flow into it. Driving gas is vented to atmosphere through the exhaust valve. After the bellows is fully expanded, excess gases from the breathing system are vented to the scavenging system through the spill valve. Thus, during mechanically controlled or assisted ventilation, excess gases are vented during expiration, which is in contrast to manually-assisted or -controlled ventilation when they are vented during inspiration.

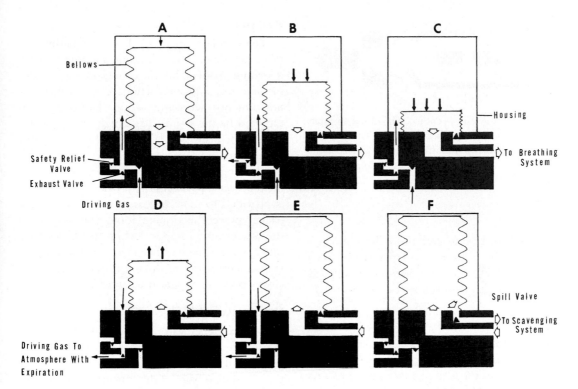

FIGURE 11.1.   Functioning of the bellows-in-box ventilator. **A**, Beginning of inspiration. Driving gas begins to be delivered into the space between the bellows and its housing. The exhaust valve (which connects the driving gas pathway with atmosphere) is closed. The spill valve (which vents excess breathing system gases to the scavenging system) is also closed. **B**, Middle of inspiration. As driving gas continues to flow into the space around the bellows, its pressure increases, exerting a force that causes the bellows to be compressed. This pushes the gas inside the bellows toward breathing system. The exhaust and spill valves remain closed. If the pressure of the driving gas exceeds the opening pressure of the safety-relief valve, the valve will open and vent driving gas to atmosphere. **C**, End of inspiration. The bellows is fully compressed. The exhaust and spill valves remain closed. **D**, Beginning of expiration. Breathing system (exhaled and fresh) gases flow into the bellows, which begins to expand. The expanding bellows displaces driving gas from the interior of the housing. The exhaust valve opens and driving gas flows through it to atmosphere. The spill valve remains closed. **E**, Middle of expiration. The bellows is nearly fully expanded. Driving gas continues to flow to atmosphere. The spill valve remains closed. **F**, End of expiration. Continued flow of gas into the bellows after it is fully expanded creates a positive pressure that causes the spill valve at the base of the bellows to open. Breathing system gases are vented through the spill valve into the scavenging system.

As noted in Chapter 6, the tidal volume exiting the ventilator may differ substantially from that which flows through the patient connection port. Newer ventilators have mechanisms to compensate for changes in fresh gas flow (fresh gas decoupling) and changes in compliance.

COMPONENTS

A standard for ventilators intended for use during anesthesia that sets down basic performance and safety requirements for components has been published by the American Society for Testing and Materials (ASTM) (1).

Driving Gas Supply

The driving gas supply is also called the "power gas supply." Most currently available anesthesia ventilators are pneumatically powered, most often by oxygen. The ventilator standard specifies that the ventilator shall continue to function within

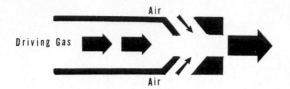

FIGURE 11.2. Injector (Venturi). Gas flows through the constricted area at a high velocity. The pressure around it drops below atmospheric levels and air is entrained. The net result is an increase in total gas flow leaving the outlet of the injector.

the manufacturer's specifications throughout a range of supply pressures of 380 kPa (55 psig) +20% and -25%. Most ventilators are supplied with DISS oxygen connections (see Chapter 2).

Injector

Some ventilators use a device called an injector (Venturi mechanism) to increase the flow of driving gas. An injector is shown in Figure 11.2. As the gas flow meets a restriction, its lateral pressure drops (Bernoulli principle). Air will be entrained when the lateral pressure drops below atmospheric. The end result is an increase in the total gas flow leaving the outlet of the injector but no increase in consumption of driving gas.

Controls

The ventilator controls regulate the flow, volume, timing, and pressure of the driving gas that compresses the bellows. This is done through the pneumatic circuitry (Fig. 11.1). Ventilator controls may be pneumatic or electronic.

Pneumatic

Pneumatic control uses pressure changes to initiate changes in the respiratory cycle.

Electronic

Newer ventilators have a wider variety of controls and alarms than older ones. Such complexity requires use of electronic controls. This type of ventilator requires electric power and a source of driving gas. If there is an electric power failure, it must be operated on batteries.

Alarms

The ventilator standard (1) groups alarms into three categories: high, medium, and low priority, depending on whether the condition requires immediate action, prompt action, or operator awareness but not necessarily action. The only alarm required by the standard is a high-priority alarm for loss of main power supply. The alarm must have a duration of at least 2 minutes, and a means of silencing it following disconnection from the main power supply must be provided. If an alarm is provided to indicate loss of main power with backup power functioning, it must be assigned to the low-priority category. Most ventilators have other alarms. These will be mentioned when individual ventilators are discussed. (See section on airway pressure alarms in Chapter 19.)

Safety-Relief Valve

A safety-relief valve (pressure-limiting valve, maximum limited pressure mechanism, driving gas pressure relief valve) is built into a ventilator to limit the pressure of the driving gas in the bellows. On some ventilators, it is preset (usually 65 to 80 cm H_2O); on others, the pressure is adjustable. The appropriate relief pressure is difficult to define. Patients with high airway resistance or low compliance may require peak pressures well in excess of 60 cm H_2O, whereas those pressures may cause serious injuries with other patients. An adjustable safety-relief valve carries the hazard of operator error, whereas a factory-adjusted valve will prevent use of high peak pressures during artificial ventilation.

There are two types of safety-relief valves (2): The first is a spring-loaded valve assembly. When the pressure exceeds the closing force of the spring, the disc lifts and excess pressure is vented to atmosphere. The lungs are held inflated at the set pressure until the cycling mechanism terminates the inspiratory phase. The second type has a diaphragm and two electric contacts suspended by rigid metal strips. With this type, once the pressure-limiting device is activated, the inspiratory phase time is terminated.

Bellows Assembly

The bellows assembly may be attached to the rest of the ventilator or separate from it.

Bellows

The bellows (concertina bellows) is an accordion-like device that is attached at the top or bottom of the bellows assembly. There are two types of bellows that are distinguished by their motion during exhalation: ascending (standing, upright) and descending (hanging, inverted). Ventilators with descending bellows were common until the mid-1980s. Since then, most new ventilators have ascending bellows.

With an ascending bellows, the bellows is attached at the base of the assembly and is compressed downward during inspiration. During exhalation, the bellows expands upward. These ventilators impose a slight resistance at the end of exhalation, at which time the pressure in the bellows rises enough (2 to 4 cm H_2O) to open the spill valve. Tidal volume may be regulated by adjusting the inspiratory time and flow or by a plate that limits upward excursion of the bellows.

With a descending bellows (Fig. 11.5), the bellows is attached at its top and is compressed upward during inspiration. Inside, the dependent portion of the bellows is a weight that facilitates reexpansion downward during exhalation. As the weight descends, negative pressure develops in the bellows and breathing system. Tidal volume is controlled by limiting the excursion of the bellows on filling. One method is to use a chain inside the bellows. When the control at the top of the bellows is turned, the length of the chain is altered. Another means is to have an adjustable plate that contacts the lower end of the bellows and limits its excursion.

An important difference between the two types of bellows is that when there is a disconnection or major leak, the ascending bellows will usually collapse unless this is prevented by the scavenger system (3). However, the ventilator may continue to deliver small tidal volumes (4). When a disconnection occurs with a descending bellows ventilator, the ventilator will continue its up-and-down movement, drawing in room air during its descent and discharging it during the upward movement. Gas flow during the upward movement may generate sufficient pressure that the low airway pressure alarm is not activated (5).

Housing

The bellows is surrounded by a clear plastic cylinder that allows the bellows's movement to be observed. A scale on the side of the housing provides a rough approximation of the tidal volume being delivered. The housing is also called the canister or bellows chamber or cylinder.

Exhaust Valve

The exhaust valve (exhalation valve, patient system relief valve, ventilator relief valve, compressed gas exhaust) communicates with the inside of the bellows housing. It is closed during inspiration. During exhalation, it opens to allow driving gas inside the housing to be exhausted to atmosphere.

Spill Valve

Because the APL valve in the breathing system is closed or isolated during ventilator operation, each ventilator must contain a spill valve (vent valve, dump valve, overflow valve, expired gas outlet, expiratory valve or port, safety dump valve, pop-off valve, relief valve, flapper valve, pressure relief valve, overspill valve, gas evacuation outlet valve, exhaust gas valve, gas evacuation or evacuator valve; expiratory pressure relief valve) for venting excess gases into the scavenging system. It is usually located within the bellows. During inspiration, this valve closes. During expiration, it remains closed until the bellows is fully expanded. Then it opens to vent excess breathing system gases.

The spill valve has a minimum opening pressure of 2 to 4 cm H_2O with an ascending bellows design (6, 7). This enables the bellows to fill during exhalation. This amount of positive end–expiratory pressure (PEEP) is applied to the breathing system. The scavenging transfer means connects the exhalation port of the spill valve to the scavenging system interface. The transfer mean's connections must be 19 or 30 mm.

Ventilator Hose Connection

The ventilator standard requires that the fitting for the tubing that connects the ventilator to the breathing system be a standard 22-mm male conical fitting. A filter may be used on the tubing to lessen the transmission of organisms.

CONTROL OF PARAMETERS OF VENTILATION

Tidal Volume

Most anesthesia ventilators are designed so that tidal volume is set directly. On others, tidal volume is determined indirectly by setting minute volume and respiratory rate. With time-cycled ventilators, tidal volume is set indirectly by varying the inspiratory time and flow. The tidal volume control may be separate from other controls and part of the bellows assembly.

Minute Volume

Minute volume may be set directly or indirectly as the product of tidal volume and respiratory rate. The ventilator standard requires that delivered volumes of the ventilator be indicated to the operator and be accurate to 15%.

Frequency

Frequency may be controlled directly or indirectly. Indirect control is achieved by varying the inspiratory time and expiratory pause. The ventilator standard requires that calibrated devices controlling frequency be accurate to within one breath per minute or 10% of the set value, whichever is smaller.

I:E Ratio

The I:E ratio can be varied directly on some ventilators; on others, it is determined indirectly by the settings of other controls, and on still others it is fixed. It is essential that there be sufficient inspiratory time for the desired tidal volume to be delivered and sufficient expiratory time to allow full expiration. Insufficient inspiratory time may be indicated by a bellows that does not make a full excursion or a respirometer that indicates a less-than-expected tidal volume. Insufficient expiratory time may be indicated by a bellows that does not expand fully.

Inspiratory Flow Rate

On some anesthesia ventilators, the inspiratory flow rate can be set directly. On others, it is determined indirectly by setting the minute volume, respiratory rate, and I:E ratio. If the inspiratory flow rate is too low to provide the set tidal volume, the bellows will not complete its excursion. If the flow is set at a faster rate than is needed to provide the tidal volume, there will be an inspiratory pause time. An excessively high peak inspiratory pressure may result from setting the inspiratory flow rate too high (8).

Maximum Working Pressure

The maximum working pressure control (pressure limit controller or inspiratory pressure limit) limits the pressure that can be attained during the inspiratory phase when the ventilator is functioning normally. It may limit the tidal volume.

SPECIFIC VENTILATORS

Datex-Engstrom AS/3 Anesthesia Delivery Unit (ADU) Ventilator

Description

This ventilator is an integrated part of the Datex-Engstrom Anesthesia AS/3 Delivery Unit (Fig. 11.3). The bellows assembly that is located

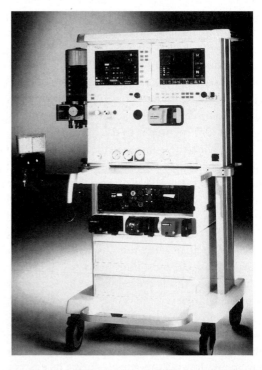

FIGURE 11.3. Datex-Engstrom AS/3 Anesthesia Delivery Unit (ADU) Ventilator. The ON/OFF control is on the ventilator. To the right of this is the adjustable pressure limiting (APL) valve. (Reprinted with permission from Datex-Engstrom.)

to the left of the control unit is similar to other standing bellows. Air or oxygen can be used as the driving gas. If the supply of one of these is interrupted, the ventilator automatically switches to the other.

The AUTO/MAN switch is located below the bellows. It has two settings: AUTO for ventilator function and MANUAL/SPONTANEOUS for when the ventilator is not in use. This also acts to direct the circuit gases to the bag or bellows as appropriate. The APL valve is excluded from the circuit in the AUTO mode but is included in the MANUAL/SPONTANEOUS mode. The APL valve may be located on the ventilator or in the circuit.

There are two screens: one for patient data and one for anesthesia delivery data. Ventilator controls keys are next to the lower right side of the anesthesia delivery data screen. When a parameter is selected, it is adjusted by rotating the handwheel just below the screen. Pushing the wheel confirms the displayed value. Pressing the ventilator key to the right of the PEEP key or depressing the wheel causes menus from which the ventilator parameters can be accessed and altered to be displayed.

Tidal volume can be set from 20 to 1400 ml. Respiratory rate can be set from two to 60 breaths per minute (bpm). Available inspiratory to expiratory ratios are 1:4.5, 1:3, 1:2.5, 1:2, 1:1.5, 1:1, and 2:1.

Inspiratory pause can be set from 0 to 60% of the inspiratory time in 5% increments. PEEP can be set OFF or from 5 to 30 cm H_2O. In the OFF position, there is 2 to 4 cm H_2O PEEP, which results from the weight of the overflow (spill) valve. A sigh of 1.5 times tidal volume every 100 breaths can be set if desired.

Alarms

Alarms are accessed through the alarm set-up key to the upper right of the screen and set using the wheel below the screen. The high pressure and low pressure alarms are adjustable. There are nonadjustable alarms for subatmospheric pressure, sustained pressure, and high PEEP (defaulted at 10 cm H_2O for manual ventilation). There are additional alarms relating to the vaporizer and other components.

Special Features

In the AUTO mode, there is an adjustable maximum pressure release. There is an overpressure release valve at the fresh gas outlet that is set at 80 cm H_2O. This machine has battery back-up for the entire machine and the ventilator for 30 minutes. There is a battery charge indicator. A red alarm message indicates "battery empty go to manual" when approximately 30 seconds remain in the battery. There is an automatic full-check procedure, which can be bypassed in an emergency. Automatic and manual leak tests are available. The compliance of the system, the compression volume of gases, and the leakage are measured. The fresh gas flow is measured continuously. The bellows excursion will vary as the fresh gas flow is altered. Gas usage is displayed on newer models. During spontaneous breathing, subatmospheric pressure is limited to -3 cm H_2O.

Internal Construction

A diagram of the bellows block is shown in Figure 11.4A. During inspiration, the control unit directs driving gas into the block. The bellows canister is pressurized, driving the bellows downward. At the same time, the pressure in the overflow (spill) valve housing increases, pushing downward on the rubber membrane and metal lid in the overflow valve. This closes the valve, preventing gas from inside the bellows from being lost to atmosphere. At the end of the inspiratory phase, the pressure in the outer canister returns to zero.

Figure 11.4B depicts the ventilator during late expiration. Exhaled gases cause the bellows to return to its uppermost position. The pressure in the overflow valve housing returns to zero, allowing the rubber membrane and metal lid to rise from the seat so that excess gas can escape to the scavenging system.

Control of Ventilation

This ventilator allows volume-controlled, pressure-controlled, and synchronized–intermittent-mandatory ventilation (SIMV).

Volume-Controlled Ventilation

The ventilator is time cycled in the volume control mode. Parameters settings (tidal volume, respiratory rate, I:E ratio, PEEP, inspiratory pause,

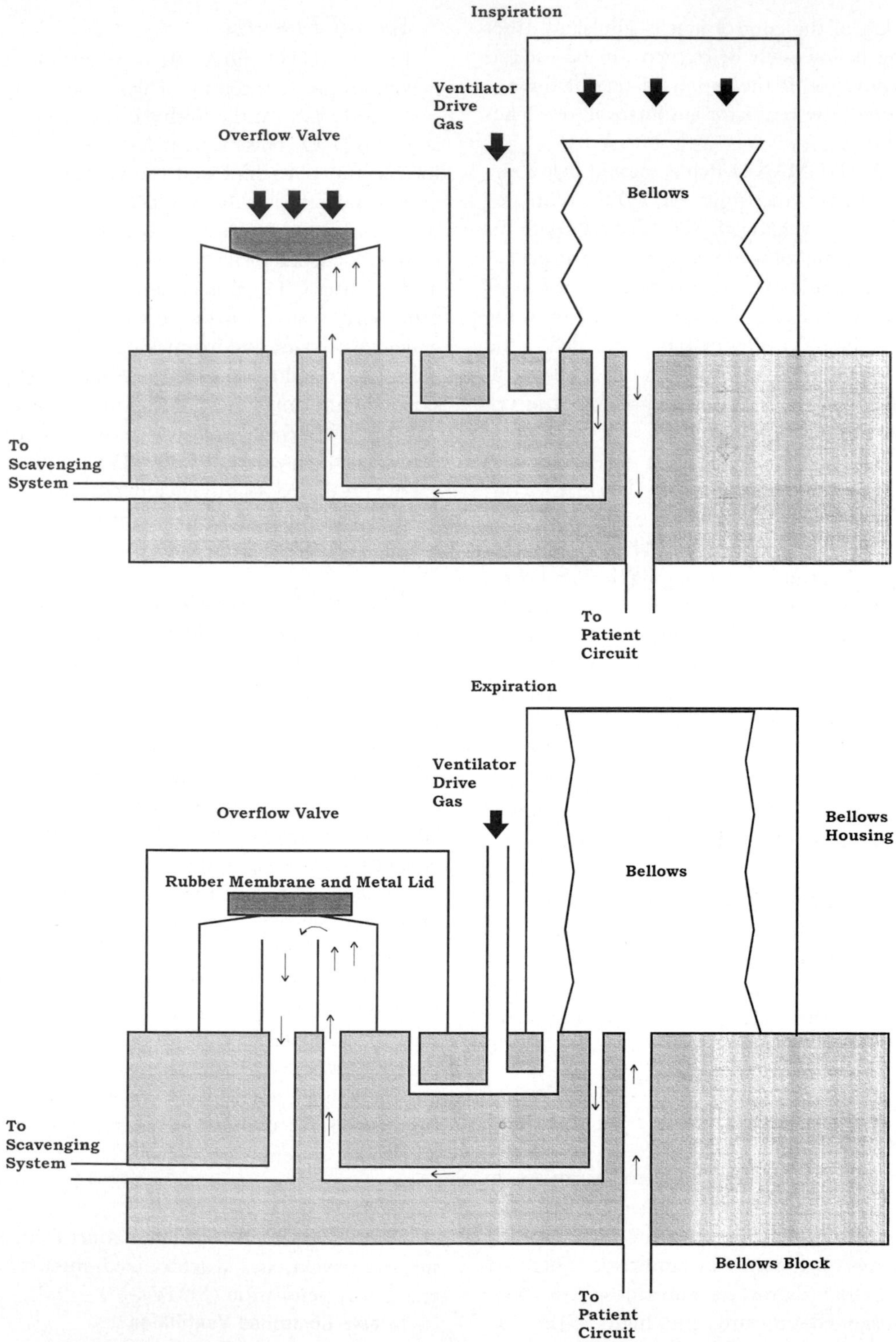

FIGURE 11.4. Datex Ventilator. **Top**, Inspiration. **Bottom**, Expiration.

and sigh) are adjusted by the operator. Volume and rate can be preset, based on patient weight. Changes in parameters are made over a period of four respiratory cycles to avoid sudden changes in patient ventilation. The ventilator automatically switches to exhalation if the maximum pressure is reached.

Pressure-Controlled Ventilation

With pressure-controlled ventilation, the operator sets the pressure above measured PEEP and the inspiratory rise time. Tidal volume and inspiratory time are determined by the rise time and the set pressure.

Synchronized–Intermittent-Mandatory Ventilation

With SIMV, the operator adjusts the trigger sensitivity, the trigger window, and the I:E ratio so spontaneous breaths can trigger volume-controlled inspirations delivered by the ventilator. Spontaneous and mandatory breaths are synchronized by allowing a minimum expiratory time of 0.5 seconds.

Drager AV Anesthesia Ventilator

Description

The Drager AV ventilator is shown in Figure 11.5. The controls are usually incorporated into the anesthesia machine. The ON/OFF switch is at the left. The dial at the middle is the frequency (respiratory rate) control. The frequency gauge is to its left. The ventilatory rate can be set at 6 to 18 or 10 to 30 bpm. Higher rates may be obtained with settings beyond the maximum calibration mark on the dial. The flow control valve and gauge are to the right. The gauge is divided into three sections labeled "low" (green), "medium" (yellow), and "high" (orange). The bellows assembly is to the left of the controls. It has a chrome-plated dome. A volume scale is on the side of the housing. The bellows may be hanging or upright. A plate limits the bellows ascent or descent. The position of the plate is controlled by turning a knob immediately below the bellows assembly. A self-locking mechanism prevents inadvertent movement of the knob. The tidal volume can be set between 250 and 1750 ml. A pediatric bellows is available for smaller tidal volumes.

Alarms

The alarms for low, subatmospheric, continuing, and high airway pressures are located to the left of the flowmeters on the anesthesia machine.

Special Features

The maximum pressure is limited to 60 cm H_2O when the inspiratory flow is in the low area; 90 cm H_2O in the medium area; and 120 cm H_2O in the high area. When the limit is reached, inflation pressure is held constant for the preset time before exhalation begins.

Internal Construction

A diagram of the ventilator is shown in Figure 11.6. When the ON/OFF switch is in the ON position, driving gas is supplied to two adjustable pressure regulators: the frequency regulator and the flow regulator. The frequency regulator, whose setting is determined by the frequency control, adjusts the input pressure to the pneumatic timer. A pilot line connects the timer to the manifold (ON/OFF) valve. This valve, which consists of a piston operating against a spring, opens and closes with a frequency determined by the timer. The ratio of open time to closed time is always 1:2. The flow pressure regulator controls the pressure of driving gas delivered to the manifold valve. The pressure adjusted at this regulator is displayed on the flow control gauge on the front of the machine.

During inspiration, driving gas flows through the open manifold valve to the injector and into the bellows housing. This causes the bellows to be compressed. The chamber relief (exhaust) valve, which is parallel to the injector and consists of a piston operating against a spring, is held closed. Changing the setting of the flow regulator results in alteration of both flow rate into the housing and the maximum pressure in it. A pilot line connects the housing with the spill valve. This valve will be closed as long as the pressure in the housing is greater than the pressure in the breathing system.

After all the gas contained in the bellows has been discharged into the ventilator hose, the pressure in the housing rises until it reaches a value that causes the injector to cut off the flow of driving gas to the bellows housing and discharge it to atmosphere through the intake opening of the injector. After a time determined by the setting of the

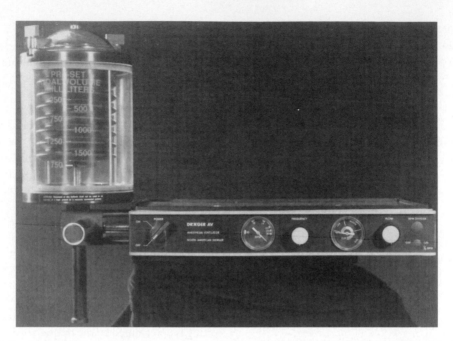

FIGURE 11.5. Drager AV ventilator. This model has a hanging bellows. The controls and gauges are on the front of the anesthesia machine, below the shelf. The alarms, not shown here, are to the left of the flowmeters on the anesthesia machine. (Reprinted with permission from North American Drager.)

FIGURE 11.6. Internal construction of the Drager AV ventilator. **1**, driving gas; **2**, ON/OFF switch; **3**, flow regulator and control; **4**, flow gauge; **5**, manifold (ON/OFF) valve; **6**, frequency regulator and control; **7**, frequency gauge; **8**, timer valve; **9**, chamber relief (exhaust) valve; **10**, injector; **11**, tidal volume control; **12**, tidal volume adjustment plate; **13**, bellows; **14**, bellows housing; **15**, spill valve; **16**, to scavenging system; **17**, to breathing system; **18**, spill valve open at end expiration. (Adapted with permission from a diagram furnished by North American Drager.)

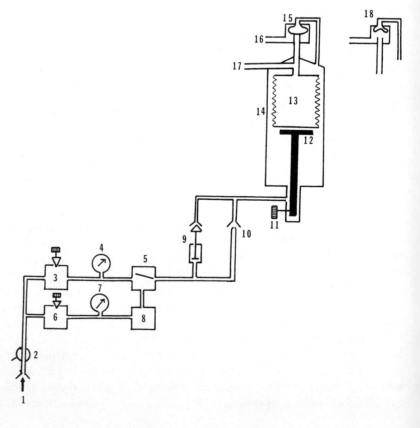

frequency control, the timer closes the manifold valve and the flow of gas to the injector stops. The pressure on the chamber relief valve falls and it opens so that driving gas flows from the bellows housing to atmosphere. Exhaled gases flow through the ventilator hose into the bellows, which re-expands. During this time, the pressure in the housing remains higher than the pressure in the breathing system so that the spill valve remains closed. When the bellows is fully expanded, the spill valve opens and excess gases are vented to the scavenging system.

After a time determined by the frequency control setting, the manifold valve is again opened by the timer and another inspiration begins.

Control of Ventilation

The ventilator is volume preset and time cycled. Tidal volume is adjusted by altering the position of the plate in the bellows assembly. The inspiratory flow rate can affect tidal volume. If the flow rate is set too low, it may not provide the full tidal volume in the allotted time. Minute volume is the product of tidal volume and respiratory rate. The I:E ratio is fixed at 1:2, and the unit has

a fixed inspiratory phase time. An increase in tidal volume will result in a lengthening of inspiratory flow time and a shortening of the inspiratory pause. An increase in frequency will result in shortening of the inspiratory pause time.

Hazards

Air or oxygen must be provided as driving gas at a pressure between 280 and 420 kPa (40 and 60 psig). A supply pressure below 280 kPa but higher than 140 kPa will reduce the maximum minute volume obtainable but will not affect the functioning of the ventilator. The use of air as a driving gas will reduce the frequency by approximately 10% from the setting of the frequency gauge.

Drager AV-E Anesthesia Ventilator

The Drager AV-E ventilator is supplied with several North American Drager machines. It is not available as a free-standing unit.

Description

The ventilator is shown in Figure 11.7. The controls are built into a shelf above the anesthesia

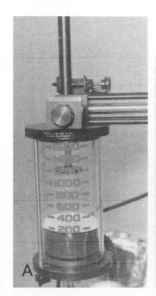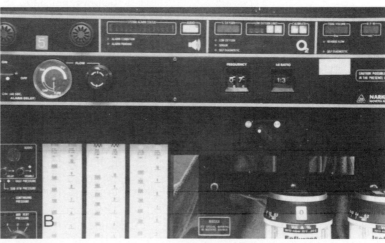

FIGURE 11.7. Drager AV-E ventilator. **A**, Bellows assembly with upright bellows. Turning the knob at the top alters the position of the footplate and so limits the tidal volume. **B**, Ventilator controls and gauges. Note

that the ON/OFF switch has two ON positions. Placing this switch in the 6 o'clock position results in a 60-second delay in the low airway pressure alarm.

machine. The ON/OFF switch is to the left. On some models, this switch has two ON positions: at the 6 and 12 o'clock locations. In the 12 o'clock position, there is a 15 second delay before the low airway pressure alarm is activated. Placing it in the 6 o'clock position increases the time until the alarm is activated to 60 seconds. This allows use of respiratory rates of less than 4/min.

The flow control valve and gauge are to the right of the ON/OFF valve. The gauge has three sections that are labeled "low" (green), "medium" (yellow), and "high" (orange). The frequency (rate) control and I:E ratio are set by adjusting the thumb switches at the right. The respiratory rate can be set from 1 to 99 bpm, and I:E ratio can be set from 1:1 to 1:4.5 in 0.5 increments.

The bellows assembly is shown in Figure 11.7. The bellows may be upright or hanging. A pediatric bellows is available. A volume scale is marked on the side of the bellows housing. Control of tidal volume is by means of a knob with a locking bar immediately above or below the bellows assembly. The locking bar is depressed, and the desired tidal volume is set by rotating the knob. The tidal volume can be set from 250 to 1750 ml for the hanging bellows and 200 to 1600 ml for the upright bellows. Smaller volumes are available with use of the pediatric bellows. A plate inside the bellows housing limits the expansion of the bellows. The pediatric bellows attachment incorporates a fine flow control valve downstream of the regular flow control valve. The fine flow control valve can be used to fine tune the inspiratory flow but cannot increase the inspiratory flow beyond that set on the ventilator.

A pressure limit control is available as an add-on accessory. This provides a means to limit the peak inspiratory pressure to a preselected value, which can be as low as 15 cm H_2O. When the preselected inspiratory pressure is reached, a valve opens and bleeds off some of the driving gas into the atmosphere for the remainder of the inspiratory phase time. On newer models, turning the bag/ventilator selection switch to automatic ventilation turns on the ventilator.

Alarms

There are alarms for low, subatmospheric, high, and continuing airway pressures and a PEEP advisory and an excessive PEEP caution.

Internal Construction

The internal construction of the Drager AV-E ventilator is shown in Figure 11.8. The Drager AV-E ventilator utilizes electric power for the timing circuits and control of the solenoid valve. The primary electric supply is a 120-V alternating current. The secondary supply is a 5-V direct current battery. The ventilator utilizes oxygen or air to drive the pneumatic section.

When the ON/OFF switch is in the ON position, electric power is supplied to the control module and gas is supplied to the pneumatic portion of the ventilator. The gas switch supplies pressure to a transducer, which acts as an electronic ON/OFF switch. A solenoid valve, which is controlled by the electronic circuits, delivers a pressure signal to the pneumatic control valve that opens and closes with a frequency determined by the settings of the frequency and I:E ratio controls. Driving gas passes through the flow regulator and to the control valve. The flow is controlled by the flow regulator, is adjusted using the control knob, and is indicated on the flow gauge.

During inspiration, the solenoid valve opens the control valve and driving gas flows into the injector where it entrains ambient air and flows into the bellows housing, compressing the bellows. This in turn forces the gas contained into the breathing system. While gas is flowing to the bellows housing, the relief (exhaust) valve is closed. The increased pressure within the housing closes the spill valve.

Exhalation begins when the solenoid valve causes the control valve to close, terminating driving gas flow. The exhaust valve opens and driving gas from the housing exits the bellows chamber and is vented to atmosphere through a muffler. Exhaled gases flow into the bellows, causing it to expand until it is stopped by the footplate. The spill valve remains closed until the bellows is fully expanded. Further gas inflow causes the pressure inside the bellows to increase until the spill valve opens and excess gases are vented into the scavenging system.

Control of Ventilation

The ventilator is time cycled. Tidal volume is dialed directly, and minute volume is the product of tidal volume and respiratory rate. An increase in flow rate with no change in tidal volume will

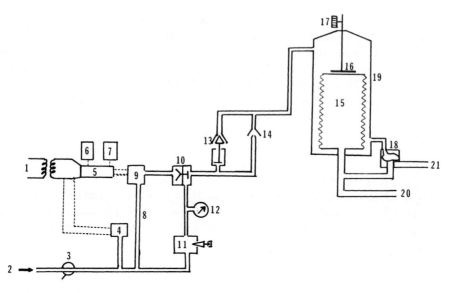

FIGURE 11.8.   Internal construction of a Drager AV-E ventilator. **1**, electric power supply; **2**, driving gas; **3**, ON/OFF switch; **4**, transducer; **5**, electronic control module; **6**, I:E phase time ratio control; **7**, frequency control; **8**, pilot pressure line; **9**, solenoid valve; **10**, control valve; **11**, flow regulator; **12**, flow gauge; **13**, ventilator relief (exhaust) valve; **14**, injector; **15**, bellows; **16**, tidal volume adjustment plate; **17**, tidal volume adjustment control knob; **18**, spill valve; **19**, bellows housing; **20**, to breathing system; **21**, to scavenging system. (Adapted with permission from a drawing furnished by North American Drager.)

result in an increase in the inspiratory pause time. An increase in the I:E ratio will result in a lengthening of the inspiratory pause time and a decrease in the expiratory phase time but will not affect the respiratory rate. If the flow rate is set too low, the full tidal volume may not be delivered. Studies indicate that the Drager AV-E anesthesia ventilator may be suitable for high- frequency ventilation (9).

Hazards

A case has been described in which the muffler placed over the driving gas exhaust became saturated with water and obstructed the flow from the bellows chamber during expiration (10). This prevented exhalation, and high airway pressures resulted as gas continued to flow into the ventilator. In another reported case, malfunction of the control valve resulted in the ventilator becoming stuck in the inspiratory mode (11). High airway pressures resulted as closure of the spill valve prevented venting of excess gas. There has been a report of the exhaust valve becoming incompetent, resulting in hypoventilation (12).

In other reported cases, the pilot line connecting the bellows chamber to the spill valve became kinked during inspiration so the valve could not close (13, 14). This caused an increase in pressure in the breathing system. If the line became occluded during expiration, hypoventilation would result because the spill valve would not close.

Prolongation of the inspiratory phase as a result of insufficient lubrication of parts has been reported (15).Ventilatory irregularities have been reported because of improper seating of the bellows on its mount (16).

If the frequency control wheel is left between settings, the ventilator may not cycle (17). A brief cessation of cycling may occur when the I:E ratio or frequency setting is changed abruptly (18). At the highest settings of the inspiratory flow rate, the peak pressure may exceed the minimum pressure threshold for the low pressure alarm (19).

Divan (Digital Ventilator for Anaesthesia)

The DIVAN is supplied on certain anesthesia machines made by Dragerwerk in Germany. It will be on certain North America Drager machines.

Description

The front of the anesthesia machine is shown in Figure 11.9. The ventilator control panel is situated at the front below the desktop. The breathing system is to the left. The APL valve (Fig. 11.10) has two positions: manual (MAN) and spontaneous (SPONT). The absorber has a single chamber. Gas flow is from bottom to top. Airway pressure, inspired oxygen concentration, expired tidal volume, and CO_2 and anesthetic agent concentrations along with various patient data are displayed on the screen above the counter space. The alarm silence button is to the right of this screen. Pressing it silences alarms for 2 minutes. Above it are two bar indicators that show the alarm status even when the alarms have been silenced. To the right of the system screen are five keys that are used to control the content of the screen. Beside the screen on the right-hand side is an unmarked touch-sensitive keypad. The function of these keys depends on the software and is indicated on the screen itself.

The ventilator control panel is shown in Figure 11.10. A display window is in the center. Keys for testing, SIMV, and the master switch are to the right. The manual/spontaneous (MAN/SPONT) and intermittent positive pressure ventilation (IPPV) buttons are at the left.

The set value for the maximum pressure during IPPV and SIMV is displayed above the button marked P_{max}. Depressing this button causes the set value to appear on the right and left sides of the lower part of the display box. The units of value are also displayed. Turning the rotary control to the right of the dialogue box will change the value shown on the right. This value can be confirmed by depressing the control. The new value is then displayed above the P_{max} button. If the control is not turned for 10 seconds, the previous setting is retained. Buttons for tidal volume and respiratory frequency for IPPV are to the right of the P_{max} button. Maximum tidal volume is 1.4 liters. An indication of the relative piston movement is shown above these three buttons. I:E ratio is accessed by the key marked Ti:Te. The relation of the inspiratory pause to inspiratory time can be altered using the button marked Tip:Ti.

To the right of this is the PEEP button. The final key, fimv, is used to set ventilation frequency in the SIMV mode. Each of these parameters is adjusted in the same manner as P_{max}.

Alarms

Alarm limits depend on the ventilatory mode and the patient. There are different sets of limits for adults and neonates and for MANUAL/SPONTANEOUS, SIMV with a respiratory frequency of less than six, SIMV at frequencies greater than six, and IPPV. If an alarm limit is exceeded or not attained, the alarm limits menu is displayed and the value is highlighted. Alarmed parameters include tidal volume, inspiratory anesthetic agent concentration, airway pressure, apnea flow, apnea pressure, and apnea carbon dioxide. Related alarms are combined to minimize unnecessary alarms. A message that indi-

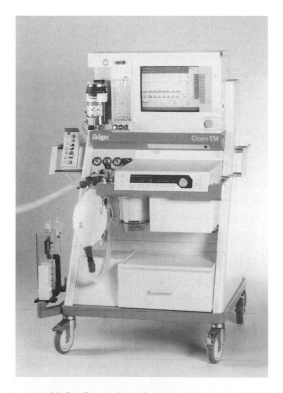

FIGURE 11.9. Cicero Anesthesia machine with DIVAN ventilator. The control panel for the ventilator is just below the counter top. The system screen is above the counter top. The reservoir bag is at the end of a piece of corrugated tubing. The breathing system is to the left of the ventilator control module. (Reprinted with permission from Dragerwerk, Lubeck, Germany.)

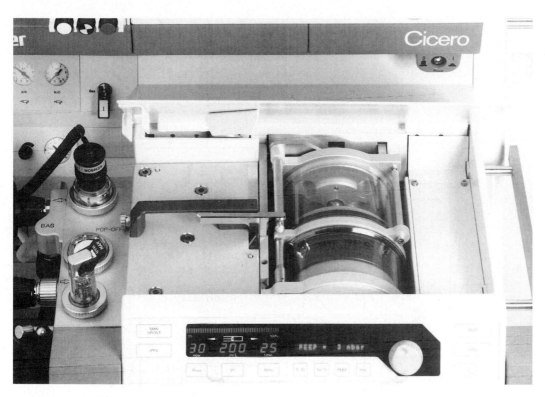

FIGURE 11.10.   Control module for divan ventilator. The piston cylinder unit is behind it to the right. The breathing system is to the left. Note that the adjustable pressure limiting (APL) valve is in the manual position.

cates the computer analysis of the problem will appear.

Special Features

In case of air failure, the system automatically switches over to the O_2 supply. In case of O_2 failure, the system switches over to the air supply and an alarm is sounded. The supply of N_2O is disabled. An uninterruptible power supply is available as an option. This can supply the anesthesia machine with electric power for approximately 1 hour.

A microprocessor supervises all ventilator functions. In case of malfunction, the electric power is shut off and valves of the breathing system are set in the MAN/SPONT mode. A leakage test can be performed automatically. The compliance of the breathing system and ventilator is measured during the self-test or when the leakage test is performed manually. Decreases in tidal volume because of compliance are then corrected for auto-

matically. A safety pressure relief valve limits pressure in the breathing system to 80 mbar. Tidal volumes as low as 20 ml are possible. The only modification needed for pediatrics is to use smaller breathing tubes.

Internal Construction

The internal construction is shown in Figure 11.11. V1 is the fresh gas decoupling valve. V2 is the surplus gas valve. Gas is aspirated from near the patient port, analyzed, and returned to the circuit downstream of the expiratory valve. A respirometer and PEEP valve are located in the expiratory limb. The piston cylinder unit, which generates the inspiratory flow, consists of an outer cylinder and a piston that is powered by a motor-gear unit. The piston is directed and sealed by two membranes. Between the two membranes is an air pressure of 160 mbar to ensure horizontal movement and low friction load on the piston. With volume-controlled IPPV or SIMV, the piston

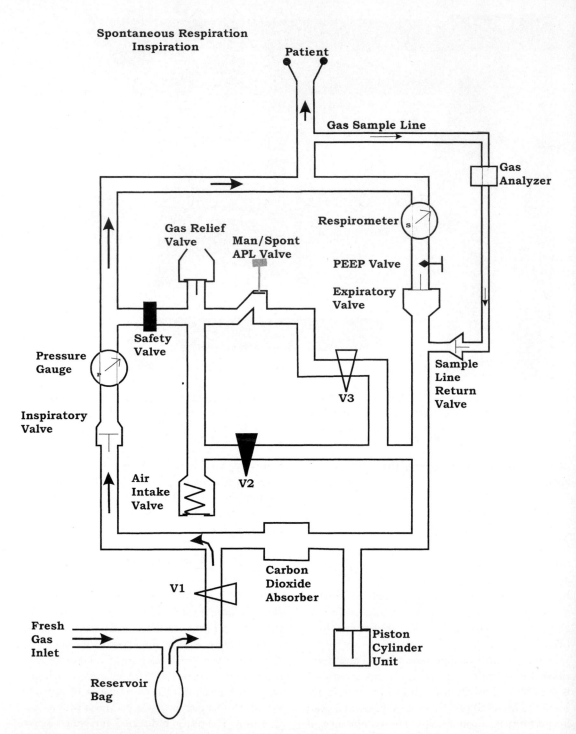

FIGURE 11.11. Divan ventilator during spontaneous inspiration. V1 is the fresh gas decoupling valve. V2 is the surplus gas valve. The air intake valve will open if the fresh gas is not sufficient to supply the gas taken up by the patient.

stops during plateau time in the end position. When the maximum airway pressure is reached in volume-controlled or pressure-controlled ventilation, inspiratory flow will be reduced so that the pressure is kept at a constant level.

Ventilatory Modes

Spontaneous Respiration

For spontaneous respiration, the MAN/ SPONT button is pressed and the APL valve is set to SPONT. Valves V1 and V3 are open while V2 is closed. The piston is held in its end position. When the patient inhales (Fig. 11.11), the inspiratory valve opens, the expiratory valve closes and gas flows from the reservoir bag. With exhalation (Fig. 11.12), the expiratory valve opens and the inspiratory valve closes. Exhaled gases pass through the absorber and into the bag. During late exhalation, the pressure rises and excess gas flows through V3 and the gas relief valve to the scavenging system.

Manual Ventilation

For manual ventilation (Fig. 11.13), the MAN/SPONT button is pressed and the APL valve is set to manual. The pressure during inspiration will be limited by the setting of the APL valve. When the pressure limit is reached, excess gas will flow through V3 and the APL valve to the scavenging system through the gas relief valve. During expiration, exhaled gases flow through the absorber into the reservoir bag.

Mechanical Ventilation

When mechanical ventilation is selected, the MAN/SPONT APL valve is closed. The bag functions as a reservoir for fresh gas. During inspiration (Fig. 11.14), valves V1, V2, and V3 are closed. The inspiratory valve opens, and the expiratory valve closes. Movement of the piston produces flow through the inspiratory valve to the patient port. Fresh gas continues to enter the reservoir bag but does not affect the tidal volume.

When exhalation begins, the expiratory valve opens, allowing exhaled gases to flow to the absorber and to the reservoir bag through V1, which is open. Valves V2 and V3 remain closed. Fresh gas flowing into the system mixes with some of the exhaled gases in the piston cylinder unit.

Mid-exhalation is depicted in Figure 11.15. The piston moves backward, allowing the cylinder

housing to fill with gases. Some gases from the reservoir bag will flow back through the absorber into the cylinder. Some fresh gas will go to the piston unit and some will enter the reservoir bag.

During the later part of exhalation (Fig. 11.16), the piston attains its maximum excursion. If the fresh gas flow is greater than the uptake by the patient and losses through leaks, V2 opens and gases are vented to the scavenging system through the gas relief valve.

Control of Ventilation

Spontaneous Respiration

For spontaneous respiration, the MAN/ SPONT button is pressed. The APL valve is set to SPONT. It is now open, regardless of the set pressure limit.

Manual Ventilation

For manual ventilation the MAN/SPONT button is pressed. The APL valve is set to MAN. Airway pressure is limited by rotating the lever on the APL valve.

Mechanical Ventilation

For mechanical ventilation, the IPPV button is pressed. The system screen and the IPPV alarm limits are activated. The parameters should be adjusted according to the clinical situation. Inspiratory flow will be influenced by tidal volume, Tip: Ti, and Ti:Te. The maximum pressure (P_{max}) should be set 5 to 10 mbar above peak pressure.

Volume constant. During volume-controlled ventilation, the inspiratory pattern is determined by time and volume variables, while airway pressure serves as a safety limit. If the set P_{max} is reached, the ventilator will adjust flow to maintain a constant pressure until the end of inspiration. If P_{max} is exceeded by more than 5 mbr, inspiration is stopped and exhalation begins. This could occur if the patient coughs or bucks. Tidal volume is limited to 1.4 l and minute volume to 25 l/min. The maximum flow is 75 l/min.

Synchronized–intermittent mandatory ventilation. SIMV is set by pressing the button to the right of the screen. PEEP cannot be used in this mode. A dialogue box is displayed and SIMV confirmed by pressing the handwheel. SIMV limits are adjusted and confirmed in the usual manner. If the ventilatory rate is less than 6 per minute, special alarm limits become active. If the fre-

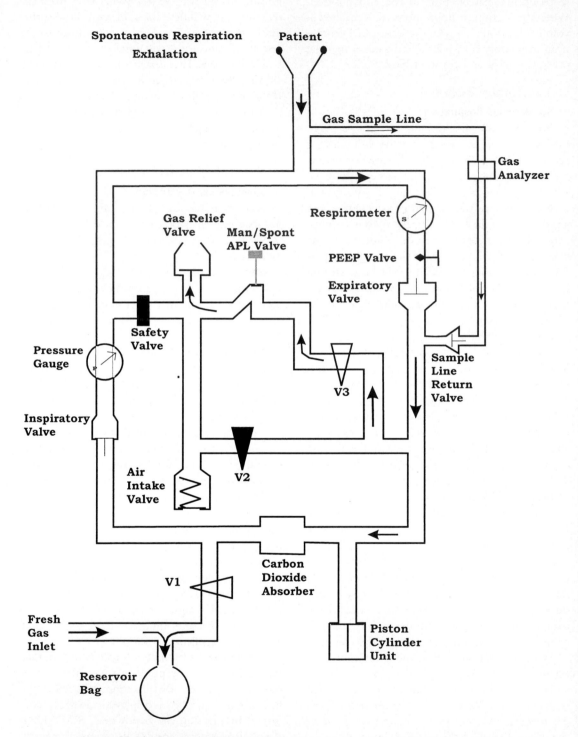

FIGURE 11.12. Divan ventilator during spontaneous exhalation. (See text for details.)

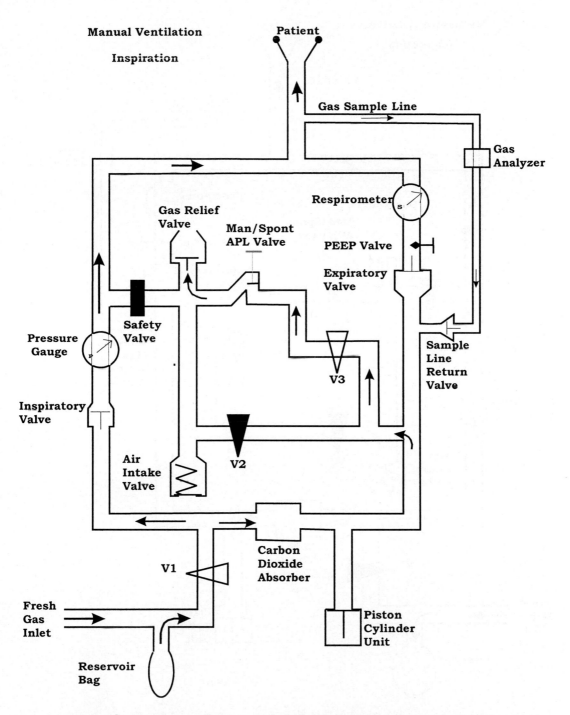

FIGURE 11.13. Divan ventilator, manual ventilation, inspiration. (See text for details.)

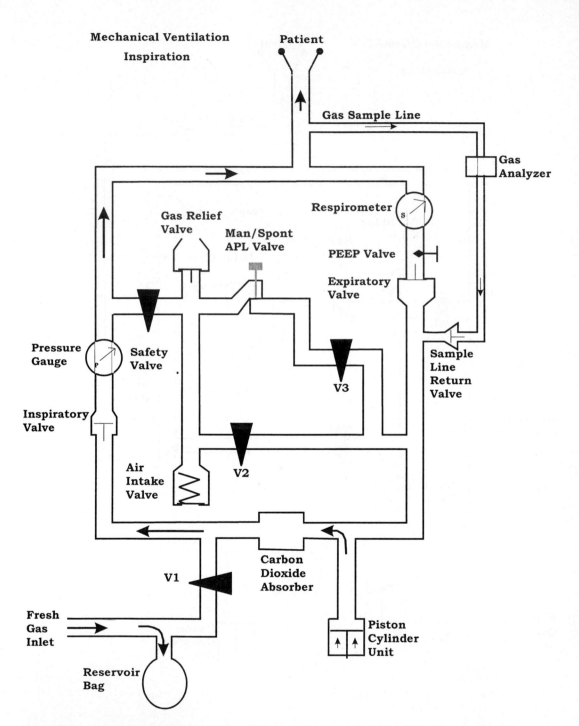

FIGURE 11.14. Divan ventilator, mechanical ventilation, inspiration. V1, the fresh gas decoupling valve, closes so that the fresh gas flow does not affect the inspired tidal volume.

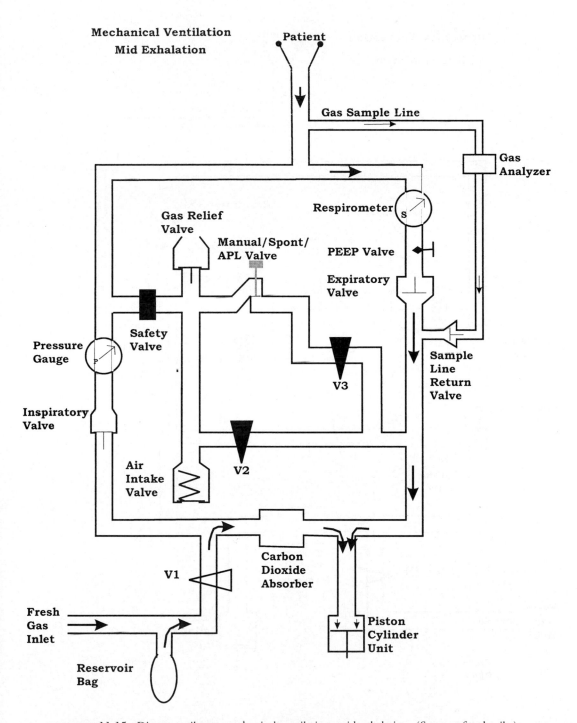

FIGURE 11.15. Divan ventilator, mechanical ventilation, mid exhalation. (See text for details.)

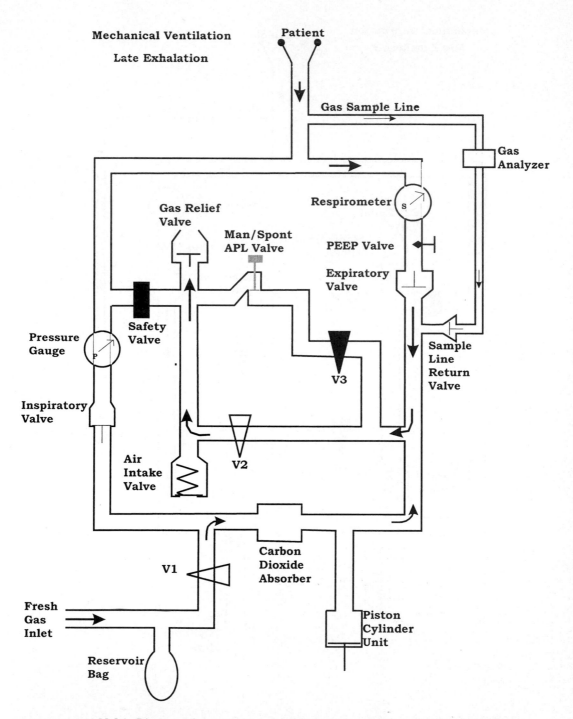

Mechanical Ventilation

Late Exhalation

FIGURE 11.16. Divan ventilator, mechanical ventilation, late exhalation. (See text for details.)

quency is greater than 6 per minute, the preceding IPPV alarm limits are in effect. To prevent the mechanical mandatory ventilation stroke from being applied during expiration, a special trigger ensures that the stroke is synchronized with spontaneous breathing.

Pressure Constant Ventilation The inspiratory pattern is determined first by inspiratory flow during pressure constant ventilation. When P_{max} is reached, inspiratory flow is reduced. The rest of the tidal volume will be delivered at constant pressure. Inspiratory flow will stop when inspiratory time has expired or the tidal volume is reached. Tidal volume is limited to 1.4 liters.

Hazards

At the time of writing, no hazards had been reported in the literature.

Ohmeda 7000 Anesthesia Ventilator

Description

The Ohmeda 7000 ventilator is shown with adult and pediatric bellows assemblies in Figure 11.17. It consists of two parts: the bellows assembly and the control module. They may be attached to each other with either the bellows assembly mounted on top or separate and connected by flexible hoses. The bellows assembly may be mounted behind a carbon dioxide absorber assembly. The bellows is the standing variety. The clear plastic housing has a volume scale marked on the front. Parts of the bellows assembly can be steam autoclaved.

The control module (Fig. 11.18) contains the controls, monitoring, and alarm functions. An abbreviated preoperative checklist, which can be pulled out, is just below the front of the control module. The power and sigh controls have toggle switches, while the manual cycle has a push button. In addition, there are three circular control dials. The power switch turns the AC electric power ON or OFF.

The minute volume can be set from 2 to 30 l/min with the adult bellows assembly and 2 to 12 l/min with the pediatric bellows assembly. The respiratory rate can be set from 6 to 40 bpm. The I:E ratio can be set from 1.1 to 1.3 for minute volumes from 2 to 15.5 l/min. Above this range, the actual I:E ratio may be less than the dial setting.

When the sigh is turned on, 150% of the set tidal volume to a maximum of 1600 ml is delivered every 64 breaths. The manual control allows the operator to initiate an inspiration manually.

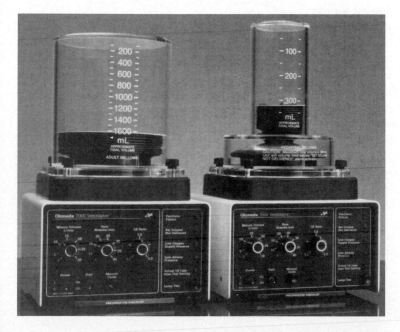

FIGURE 11.17. Ohmeda 7000 ventilators. The stand-alone ventilator is shown with adult (left) and pediatric (right) bellows. (Reprinted with permission from Ohmeda, a division of BOC Health Care, Inc.)

FIGURE 11.18. Control module of the Ohmeda 7000 ventilator.

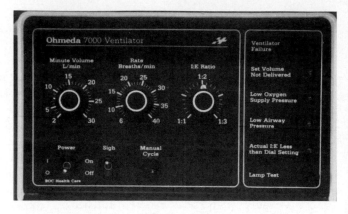

The cycle can be activated only during the expiratory phase.

Alarms

The alarms are arranged vertically to the right of the control panel. Six of the alarms (ventilator failure, set volume not delivered, low drive gas (oxygen) supply pressure, low airway pressure, actual I:E less than dial setting, and power failure) are visible and audible. The seventh, power failure, is audible only. There is a lamp test located below the alarms.

Special Features

The maximal tidal volume is 1500 ml for the adult bellows and 300 ml for the pediatric bellows. Inspiratory flow is limited to a maximum of 62 l/min. Pressure in the bellows housing is limited to 65 cm H_2O. When this pressure is sensed, some of the driving gas is vented and the ventilator will stop cycling. The vent failure alarm will be activated and the ventilator must be turned off. There are batteries in the monitors to continue operation during a power failure.

Internal Construction

The internal construction of this ventilator is shown in Figure 11.19. Driving gas (oxygen) at 345 kPa (50 psig) enters the ventilator and passes through a filter en route to the pressure regulator. Here the pressure is reduced to 273 kPa (38 psig) at a flow of 24 l/min. From here, the gas flows to five solenoid flow control valves in parallel.

During inspiration, the electronically-con-trolled solenoid valves direct gas flow through orifices calibrated for flows of 2, 4, 8, 16, and 32 l/min. The range of flow is from 4 to 62 l/min in steps of 2 l/min. By opening and closing selected solenoid valves, the volume of oxygen corresponding to the set tidal volume and flow rate is delivered. The exhaust valve closes during inspiration so that the flow from the selected valves is delivered into the space between the housing and the bellows. This compresses the bellows. The tidal volume delivered is determined by the driving gas volume entering the bellows housing. The bellows does not fully descend except when delivering the maximum tidal volume (20).

At the end of inspiration, the solenoid valves close and the exhaust valve opens. Gas from the breathing system enters the bellows. As the bellows expands, driving gas from the housing is discharged through the exhaust valve to atmosphere. When the bellows is fully expanded, the spill valve opens and vents excess gas to the scavenging system. The opening pressure of the spill valve is approximately 2.5 cm H_2O.

The pressure of the driving gas upstream of the pressure regulator is monitored. If a pressure of less than 280 kPa (40 psig) is sensed, the low supply pressure switch sends a signal to the control circuitry and the low oxygen supply pressure alarm is actuated. Pressure in the breathing system is also monitored. If a pressure of at least 6 cm H_2O is not sensed after three consecutive cycles, a signal is sent to the control circuitry and the low airway pressure alarm is activated.

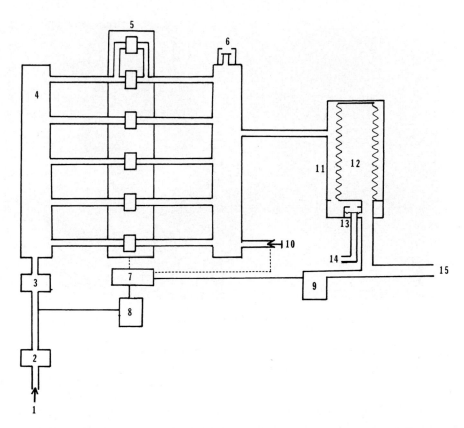

FIGURE 11.19. Internal construction of Ohmeda 7000 ventilator. **1**, driving gas; **2**, filter; **3**, pressure regulator; **4**, regulated gas supply; **5**, solenoid flow valves; **6**, safety-relief valve; **7**, control circuitry; **8**, low supply pressure switch; **9**, pressure switch; **10**, exhaust valve; **11**, bellows housing; **12**, bellows; **13**, spill valve; **14**, to scavenging system; **15**, to breathing system.

Control of Ventilation

The three controls (minute volume, respiratory rate, and I:E ratio) are not interactive. If minute volume is increased and the ventilatory rate is held constant, the tidal volume will increase. If the rate is increased and the minute volume is held constant, the tidal volume will decrease. Changes in the I:E ratio have no effect on tidal volume, minute volume, or frequency.

Hazards

The ventilator is designed to be powered by oxygen only. Use of any other gas will cause inaccurate operation and may damage the ventilator. Low driving gas pressure will cause the ventilator to deliver less than the set minute volume. Very sick patients with low compliance may not be effectively ventilated with this ventilator because the pressure is limited to 65 cm water. The sigh control may inadvertently be left in the ON position (15).

Ohmeda 7800 Series Anesthesia Ventilators

The Ohmeda 7800 may be a stand-alone ventilator or a component of certain Ohmeda machines. On the 7810 and 7850 ventilators, the control module and bellows assembly are separate from each other; the control module is above the flowmeters on the machine and the bellows assembly is mounted on the absorber arm (Fig. 11.20) or to the left of the machine. With the 7850, the ventilator's liquid crystal screen is blank unless one of the controls is altered or pressed. If

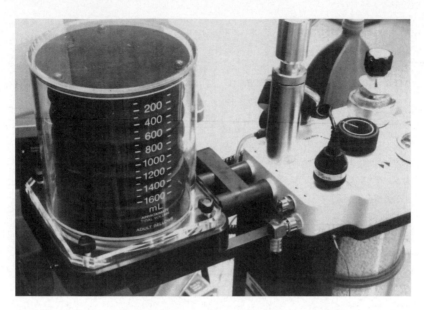

FIGURE 11.20. Ohmeda 7800 ventilator mounted on absorber assembly.

the display pod is not functional, certain information will be displayed on the ventilator screen.

Description

The bellows assembly is the same as that found on the 7000 ventilators. The front panels of the 7800 and 7850 ventilators are shown in Figures 11.21 and 11.22. The screen has a liquid crystal display that provides numeric readouts for tidal volume, respiratory rate, minute volume, and inspired oxygen concentration. Below these are control and alarm messages. The ON/OFF control is a toggle switch. The tidal volume, respiratory rate, inspiratory flow, and inspiratory pressure limits have circular knobs while the inspiratory pause is a push button. Adjusting or merely touching one of the circular control knobs results in that control's setting being displayed. A light above the inspiratory pause button is illuminated when the inspiratory pause is being used.

Tidal volume can be set from 50 to 1500 ml. Respiratory rate can be set from 2 to 100 bpm. Inspiratory flow rate can be set from 10 to 100 l/min.

The inspiratory pressure limit can be set from 20 to 100 cm H_2O. Both the maximum inspiratory pressure and sustained pressure alarm limits are set using this dial. For inspiratory pressure limits from 20 to 60 cm H_2O, the ventilator sets the

sustained pressure limit at 50% the inspiratory pressure limit. Any inspiratory pressure limit setting higher than 60 cm H_2O results in a sustained pressure limit of 30 cm H_2O. The maximum inspiratory pressure limit is active during mechanical and manual ventilation. If the pressure exceeds the set limit, the control circuitry terminates the inspiration, switches to exhalation, and produces an alarm.

An inspiratory pause that is 25% of the set inspiratory time can be added to the inspiratory cycle by pushing the inspiratory pause button located above the alarm limit settings. The expiratory time is decreased automatically to maintain the same ventilatory frequency. The I:E ratio is displayed when the inspiratory pause button is pressed.

The mechanical ventilation ON/OFF switch and the alarm silence button are to the left of the controls. Pressing the alarm silence button will silence some alarms for 30 seconds and some permanently. If this button is pressed while the ventilator is not being used, the apnea and low minute volume alarms are canceled. If, however, another breath is sensed, these alarms will again be activated.

Alarms

Above the alarm silence button are red and yellow light-emitting diodes (LEDs). When an alarm

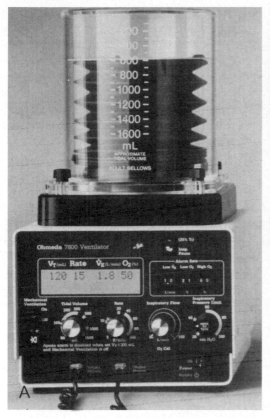

FIGURE 11.21.   Ohmeda 7800 ventilators. The model on the right has an autoclavable bellows assembly. (Reprinted with permission from Ohmeda, a division of BOC Health Care, Inc.)

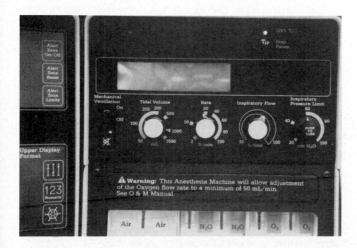

FIGURE 11.22. Control module of the Ohmeda 7850 ventilator. Courtesy of Ohmeda, a division of BOC Health Care, Inc.

condition occurs, a message will appear on the screen, a tone will sound, and an LED will flash. The red LED light indicates that immediate operator response is required. The yellow LED light signals the need for prompt operator response or awareness. If the alarm silence is activated, the LED is lighted continuously to remind the user that the alarm condition still exists.

The alarm set points for low and high oxygen concentrations and low tidal volume are set with a series of pushwheels to the right of the screen. To increase or decrease a value, the user pushes the button above or beneath the value that is to be changed. The low oxygen concentration cannot be set below 18%. If the value is set below this level, a "limit set error" message is displayed. There is a similar message if the high alarm limit is set equal to or below the low limit. The high oxygen alarm limit can be disabled by setting the value to zero.

Alarms

Alarms for the 7800 ventilator include apnea; high, low, sustained, and subatmospheric airway pressure; reverse flow; high and low oxygen concentration; low minute volume; open drive circuit; low battery; incorrect control combinations; oxygen sensor calibration needed; power failure; high and low supply pressure; and ventilator or monitoring malfunction. The sensing port for airway pressure is located immediately downstream of the unidirectional inspiratory valve in the circle system (21, 22).

Special Features

If the inspiratory pressure limit is reached, the ventilator terminates the inspiratory phase. The ventilator displays a reminder if the inspired pressure is set above 60 cm H_2O, even if the ventilator is not turned on. There is a battery to continue ventilator operation for 20 minutes during a power failure.

Internal Construction

The internal parts of the ventilator control module are shown diagrammatically in Figure 11.23. When the ventilator is turned on, the gas inlet solenoid is energized, allowing the gas inlet valve to open and supplying driving gas to the primary regulator. The output of the primary regulator is monitored by the high-pressure transducer. If the driving gas pressure is greater than or equal to 210 kPa (30 psig), the microprocessor will not allow ventilation and an error message is displayed. The primary regulator connects directly to the pneumatic manifold. The driving gas flow is controlled by a flow control valve inside the pneumatic manifold. The flow control valve varies the size of an orifice in proportion to the current supplied to it. The amount of current supplied to the flow control and the time it is applied are determined by the microprocessor and is based on the control settings.

Just before inspiration begins, the exhaust valve is supplied with pressure from the secondary regulator through the exhalation solenoid, closing the valve. This valve remains closed during the inspiratory phase when driving gas is being delivered into the bellows housing. It opens at the end of the inspiratory phase to provide an outlet for the driving gas that is displaced from the bellows housing during expiration. After the inspiratory phase time is ended, the flow control valve is deenergized and is returned to the closed position by its internal spring. Simultaneously, the exhalation solenoid is deenergized. This allows the exhaust valve to open. Driving gas flows to atmosphere through the exhaust port. When the expiratory phase time is completed, the cycle is repeated by energizing the exhalation solenoid (closing the exhaust valve) and opening the flow control valve to begin the next inspiratory cycle. If the patient breathes spontaneously while connected to the ventilator, the air inlet valve in the pneumatic manifold will open.

Control of Ventilation

The tidal volume, respiratory rate and inspiratory flow controls are not interactive. The I:E ratio will be changed whenever any of these is altered or when the inspiratory pause is activated. The I:E ratio can be varied from 1:0.5 to 1:999. The 7800 ventilator has been found to be suitable for use in a high frequency mode (9).

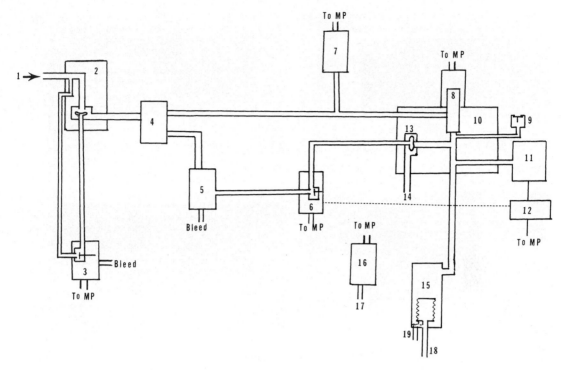

FIGURE 11.23.   Ohmeda 7800 ventilator. **1**, driving gas; **2**, gas inlet valve; **3**, gas inlet solenoid valve; **4**, primary regulator; **5**, secondary regulator; **6**, exhalation solenoid valve; **7**, high-pressure transducer; **8**, flow control valve; **9**, air inlet valve; **10**, pneumatic manifold; **11**, high-pressure safety switch; **12**, relay; **13**, exhaust valve; **14**, exhaust port for driving gas; **15**, bellows assembly; **16**, low-pressure transducer; **17**, to breathing system for pressure monitoring; **18**, to breathing system; **19**, to scavenging system; MP, microprocessor. Bleed used to reduce the pressure in a component.

Hazards

Electromagnetic interference or power line disturbances may cause the ventilator to stop cycling, the monitoring functions to cease, or unintelligible messages to be displayed (23). If any of these problems occurs, manual ventilation should be instituted and the ON/OFF switch should be turned off for approximately 5 seconds.

Ohmeda 7900 Series Ventilator

Description

The 7900 ventilator is an integral part of certain Ohmeda anesthesia machines. The bellows assembly is separate and is the same as that supplied with the 7000 and 7800 series ventilators. The bellows is steam autoclavable and latex free. PEEP is set electronically.

The front panel (Fig. 11.24) has the controls for the ventilator functions and a display screen. The ON/OFF switch is to the left and is identified by a bellows icon. Above the ON/OFF switch is a switch to silence the alarms. On the right side is a button to disable the apnea and volume monitor alarms. Below this is a menu access switch. Below the menu switch is an adjustment knob. The adjustable knob is used to change set values, to select menus, and to change the values on menus. Pushing the knob confirms the selections and keeps them in memory.

The screen is the integral contrast enhancement (ICE) type. It displays alarm messages, alarm status, ventilatory values, and waveforms when the ventilator is used. The displayed waves will be volume against time or pressure against time, depending on the ventilatory mode being

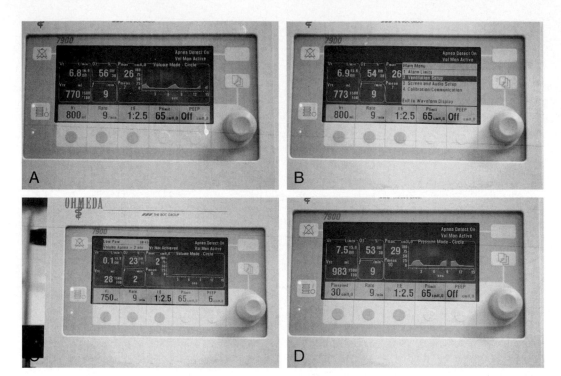

FIGURE 11.24.   **A,** Front of Ohmeda 7900 ventilator control module in volume mode. At bottom left is the ON/OFF switch (with the bellows icon). Above this is the alarm silence switch. To the right is the apnea alarm ON/OFF and volume monitor ON/Standby switch. Below this is the menu switch and the adjustment knob. Below the screen are selection switches with the setting for each parameter displayed just above each. High and low alarm limits are shown to the right of the tidal volume, minute volume, and oxygen concentration displays. Note that the displayed waveform shows time against volume. Above this is the APNEA DETECT ON, VOL MON ACTIVE message. **B,** 7900 ventilator with main menu displayed. **C,** 7900 ventilator with alarm messages. Note the Low Paw, Volume Apnea and V_T Not Achieved messages. **D,** 7900 ventilator in pressure mode. Note that the inspired pressure rather than the tidal volume is set. The delivered tidal volume is still displayed. The waveform displayed is pressure against time. The ventilator maintains the set inspired pressure plus set PEEP through the end of the inspiratory phase time.

used. The mode is shown above the waveform. The status of the apnea alarm and the volume monitor setting are displayed above this. Inspired oxygen concentration; exhaled tidal and minute volumes; respiratory rate; and peak, mean, and plateau airway pressures are indicated on the left side of the screen. Alarm limits are displayed to the right of some values.

Below the screen are a series of selection switches that are related to values on the screen. The number in the yellow background indicates the setting of the parameter. When a selection switch is pressed, the setting can be adjusted by turning the adjustment knob on the right. Pressing the selection switch or the knob confirms the value and causes the ventilator to make the necessary adjustments.

Tidal volume can be set from 20 to 1500 ml. The range for respiratory rate is 4 to 100 bpm. The I:E ratio can be adjusted from 1:8 to 2:1. The airway pressure limit can be set from 12 to 100 cm H_2O. The range for PEEP is from 4 to 30 cm H_2O. The airway pressure during inspiration can be set from 5 to 60 cm H_2O for pressure control ventilation. To the upper right of the screen is an Apnea Detect ON/OFF and volume monitor STANDBY/ACTIVE switch. The Apnea Detect is automatically turned on if a breath is detected.

Menus (Fig. 11.24B) are accessed by pressing the button above the adjustment knob. Menus are used for settings that are changed less frequently. The ventilation menu is used to set the ventilatory mode, inspiratory pause, breathing system, and correction factors to be used if the fresh gas includes helium. The calibration/communication menu is used to calibrate the oxygen sensor or zero the flow sensors. Adjustments to communicate with various monitors are also made with this menu. The alarm limits menu is used to adjust the limits for oxygen concentration, minute volume, and tidal volume. The screen and audio menu allows adjustment of screen brightness and alarm volume. It also permits the alarm limits and units of measure to be displayed or hidden.

Alarms

Alarm limits are displayed on the screen next to the parameters with which they are associated. They are accessed from the alarm limits menu. The alarm value to be altered is selected, then set and confirmed using the handwheel.

There are alarms for high and low oxygen concentrations; high, low, sustained and subatmospheric airway pressures; volume apnea; high and low exhaled minute and tidal volumes; reverse flow; set breath not supplied; empty bellows; incorrect control settings; incorrect flow sensor connections; oxygen sensor calibration needed; low supply pressure to the ventilator; high drive pressure to the bellows; low oxygen supply pressure; ventilator or monitoring malfunctions; electric power failure; and low battery. The sensing port for airway pressure is in the inspiratory limb. The low-airway pressure is set for 4 cm H_2O above baseline pressure. Alarm messages are displayed at the top of the screen (Fig. 11.24C). Alarms can be silenced for 120 seconds using the alarm silence button to the upper left of the screen.

Special Features

Battery backup permits approximately 30 minutes of mechanical ventilation and operation of monitors during a power failure. During some malfunctions, the ventilator automatically changes modes. The backup volume mode supplies the set tidal volume. However, it cannot adjust the ventilator output to supply the set breath. The minimum monitoring mode shows patient data, but does not permit mechanical ventilation.

Internal Construction

The 7900 ventilator consists of a pneumatic engine, a transducer section, a computer control system with a user interface, and displays. The pneumatic engine uses compressed gas to control the flow and pressure of the gases delivered to the bellows assembly. Sensors in the breathing system measure flow, pressure, and oxygen concentration. The ventilator monitors its own function through its built-in software. Should malfunction occur, the affected sections are shut down and the operator is alerted.

Control of Ventilation

When the ventilator is activated, the previous control settings are in effect. These may need to be altered. To do this, the button below the parameter to be changed is pushed. The box around the display window for that parameter flashes on and off. The parameter setting is altered using the adjustment knob. The knob is pushed to confirm the value. If the setting is not confirmed in 8 seconds, the setting remains unchanged. Once a change in a parameter is confirmed, it usually takes several breaths for the ventilator to adjust for the new setting. The 7900 ventilator offers a choice of pressure- or volume-controlled ventilation. This choice is accessed through the ventilation menu. PEEP is available in both modes.

Volume Control Mode

During volume control ventilation (Fig. 11.24A), the tidal volume is selected and the ventilator is programmed to deliver that volume. A constant flow is delivered during inspiration. The displayed waveform is volume versus time. The set and the actual tidal volumes are compared and there is automatic adjustment for fresh gas flow (fresh gas decoupling), small leaks, changing compliance, and compression losses in the ventilator bellows and absorber. This is accomplished using flow sensors in both the inspiratory and exhalation sides of the circle system. These are discussed in Chapter 19.

Pressure Control Mode

In the pressure control mode (Fig. 11.24D), the inspiratory pressure is set by the operator. During inspiration, the ventilator delivers the required flow, high initially, to generate this pressure plus the set PEEP, then delivers sufficient flow to maintain this pressure for the duration of the inspiratory phase time. The waveform portion of the screen displays a pressure against time curve.

Hazards

At this writing, there were no published hazards.

Anodyne™ CC Anesthesia Workstation Ventilator

Description

This ventilator is an integral part of the Anodyne™ CC Anesthesia Workstation (Fig. 11.25). The heated aluminum patient module (block), which contains the valves, CO_2 absorber, ventilator bellows, and housing, and various other built-in components is at the front left of the machine (Fig. 11.26). The module is attached using an electric retraction system. When in place, all the electronic and pneumatic connections are secured. Air (primary) or oxygen (secondary) can be used as the driving gas for the ventilator. Failure of the piped air supply will result in automatic switch over to piped oxygen. If this is unavailable, the machine will switch to oxygen from cylinders. If this is unavailable, ambient air will be used.

The main (ON/OFF) button at the top left of the machine controls the electric and pneumatic power. To the right of the ON/OFF control are four buttons for selecting the gases to be administered. They are labeled "O2 only," "O2/AIR," "O2/N2O" and "All gases." Above each button is an indicator that changes from black to white when the button below is pressed.

Below these is a screen on which menus, measured data, alarm settings, alarm messages, and graphics of airway pressure and expiratory flow are displayed. Ventilator parameters and alarm settings can be adjusted using this screen. Ventilator settings are on the control panel that is at the left

front of the anesthesia machine, above the patient module (Fig. 11.27). The panel is divided into several sections. Near the center is a dial that allows selection of the ventilatory mode. The choices include "standby," "manual/spontaneous ventilation," "CMV (continuous mechanical ventilation) child," and "CMV adult."

To the left of the dial are touch keys for inspiratory and expiratory pause. These are available in the CMV modes. When the key for inspiratory pause is pressed, the adjacent LED starts blinking and a 5-second inspiratory pause is added to the cycle. Pressing the key a second time cancels the pause. Pressing the expiratory pause key will add a pause of up to 30 seconds after expiration. This is canceled by pressing the key a second time.

A Rotary Mouse dial is located in the upper right quadrant of the control panel. The dial is used to select and change parameters. Turning the dial moves the cursor on the screen. Once the cursor is positioned on the desired field, the dial is depressed to enter that field. The parameter can then be adjusted by turning the dial clockwise to increase the value or counterclockwise to decrease it. Once the desired value is displayed, the dial is depressed to confirm the setting and return to the cursor function.

In the left lower quadrant are three touch keys marked "menu," "graphics," and "option." Pressing the menu key opens the window for general settings on the screen. Pressing the graphics key opens a window for adjustment of graphics. The parameters in these menus can be changed using the Rotary Mouse dial. The option key is used to switch the driving gas.

Below the Rotary Mouse dial are four "hot keys" that allow quick adjustment of certain ventilator parameters (tidal volume, respiratory rate, I:E ratio, and PEEP) in the controlled mechanical ventilation modes. Pressing one of these keys opens a window on the screen and allows that parameter to be changed by depressing the Rotary Mouse dial and then rotating it. The dial is depressed again to confirm the setting. Tidal volume can be varied from 50 to 400 ml in the pediatric mode and 300 to 1400 ml in the adult mode. The respiratory rate can be varied from 20 to 60 bpm in the pediatric mode and 4 to 30 bpm in the adult mode. Possible I:E ratios are 3:1, 2:1, 1:1,

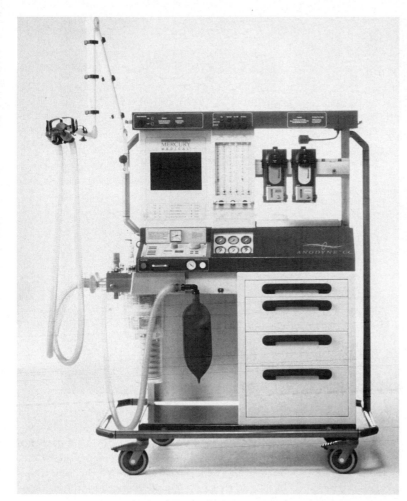

FIGURE 11.25. Anodyne™ CC Workstation. Note the CO_2 canister and ventilator assembly with descending bellow extending below the patient module. The main ON/OFF button is at the top left. The gas selector buttons are to the right of the main switch, above the flowmeters. Above each button is a light that is illuminated when the button is pressed. Below the screen is a panel displaying the status of the electric and pneumatic supplies. Below this is the ventilatory control panel. (Reprinted with permission from Mercury Medical.)

1:2, and 1:3 and 1:4. The end inspiratory plateau can be set to OFF or 20 or 30% of inspiratory time. The maximum inspiratory pressure limit can be set from 10 to 80 cm H_2O.

Default settings in the adult mode include a tidal volume of 500 ml, a respiratory rate of 10 bpm, and an I:E ratio of 1:2. Plateau, sigh, and PEEP are off. In the pediatric mode, the default tidal volume is 200 ml, the respiratory rate 20 bpm, and the I:E ratio 1:2. Plateau, sigh, and PEEP are off. A sigh that is delivered once every 100 breaths and is equivalent to 1.5 times the set tidal volume can be set during controlled mechanical ventilation.

In the lower midportion of the control panel are the touch keys for alarms. Pressing the Limits key opens a window on the screen on which alarm settings can be altered. Alarms are accessed and set in a similar manner to other functions using the Rotary Mouse dial. Alarm volume is adjusted in the menu window. There is also a key for a 2-minute silencing of alarms.

Alarms

The alarms shown on the screen vary with the mode of ventilation. In the MANUAL/SPONTANEOUS mode, there are alarms for high and low airway pressures; minimum tidal and minute volumes; minimum and maximum respiratory rate; and maximum and minimum oxygen concentrations. For mechanical ventilation there are alarms for minimum tidal and minute volumes;

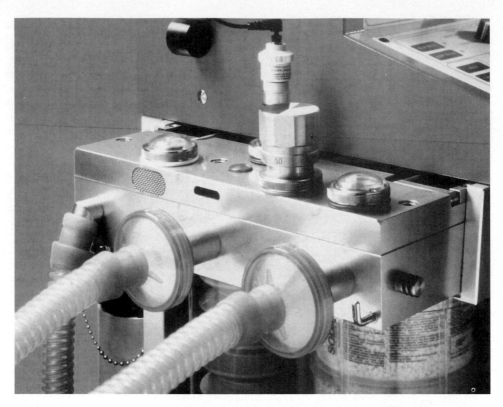

FIGURE 11.26.   Anodyne™ CC Workstation Patient Module. Anodyne™ CC workstation with connections for (from left to right) the bag tubing, the inspiratory tubing, and the expiratory tubing. At the top of the module are (from left to right) the subatmospheric pressure relief valve, the pressure relief (safety pop-off) valve, the adjustable pressure limiting (APL) valve, and the expiratory unidirectional valve dome. The top of the APL valve is marked with pressures. Behind the red pressure relief valve is the inspiratory unidirectional valve with the oxygen sensor connection in its dome. The oxygen sensor calibration adapter is on the side of the machine above the patient module. At the front is the block over which the Y-piece is placed for the leak and compliance tests during the setup procedure. (Reprinted with permission from Mercury Medical.)

low and high airway pressures; and minimum and maximum oxygen concentrations. Alarm messages along with suggestions for operator action are displayed in a window in the lower right section of the screen. The message field will turn to yellow to highlight the message.

Special Features

During automatic ventilation, the tidal volume is unaffected by changes in fresh gas flow (fresh gas decoupling). It is also unaffected by changes in compliance. In order to accomplish this, the system compliance is measured during the sensor test portion of the setup procedure. The patient block is heated to 36°C (97°F). This prevents con-densation of moisture and minimizes dehydration and cooling of inspired gases.

In the event of power failure, a battery will power the ventilator and monitoring for 30 minutes. If an optional second battery is present, this time is doubled. Power from the battery is not used to heat the patient module.

An ambient air intake (subatmospheric pressure relief) valve will admit air to the system when there is subatmospheric pressure in the patient module. A safety pop-off valve for fast pressure relief in case of an emergency is located next to the APL valve (Figure 11.26).

A Mapleson breathing system can be used by selecting a certain setting in one of the MANUAL/

SPONTANEOUS windows. Absorber pre-paks can be changed during use. Ambient air is drawn into the system through the subatmospheric pressure relief valve so that ventilation is not affected.

Internal Construction

The internal construction of the system is shown in Figures 11.28 through 11.34. The fresh gas decoupling valve controls the flow of fresh gas from the anesthesia machine. When it is closed, all the fresh gas flows into the reservoir bag. When it is open, fresh gas can flow into the rest of the system and gas can flow from the system into the reservoir bag. The expiratory control valve is a pneumatically-powered, microprocessor-controlled diaphragm valve. During continuous mechanical ventilation, it closes during inspiration, preventing gases from flowing through the absorber or to the APL valve.

The oxygen flush has two connections to the breathing system. When it is activated, 30 l/min of oxygen will flow through the larger connection through the fresh gas decoupling valve or into the reservoir bag. An oxygen flow of 10 l/min will be delivered downstream of the fresh gas decoupling valve and connection to the ventilator.

Expired volume is measured in the expiratory limb using a hot-wire anemometer. During controlled ventilation, the delivered tidal volume is measured using an internal flow sensor and is independent of the expired volume measurement. Airway pressure is measured in the inspiratory limb.

Spontaneous Respiration

During spontaneous respiration, the ventilator bellows remains fully expanded. During inspiration (Fig. 11.28), gases flow from the reservoir bag. If the bag empties, the subatmospheric pressure relief valve opens and air is drawn into the system. During expiration (Fig. 11.29), exhaled gases pass through the CO_2 absorber and mix with fresh gas in the reservoir bag. Excess gases are vented to the scavenging system through the APL valve.

Manual Ventilation

With manual ventilation, the ventilator bellows stays fully expanded. During inspiration (Fig. 11.30), the reservoir bag is squeezed, so that gases

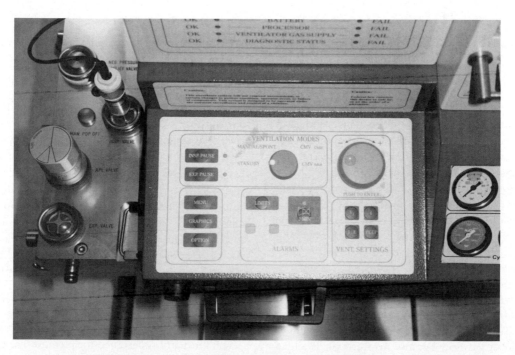

FIGURE 11.27. Anodyne™ CC Workstation Control Panel. (See text for details.)

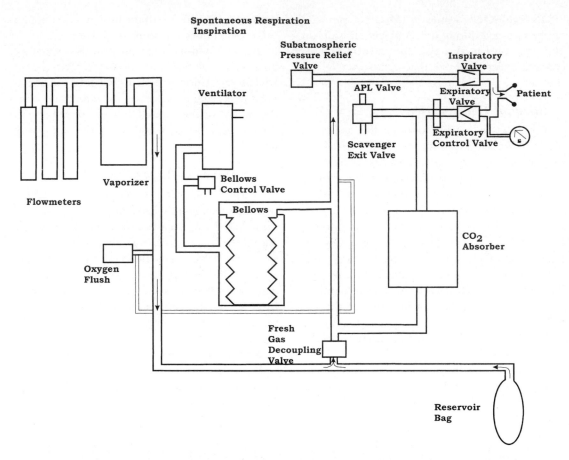

FIGURE 11.28. Anodyne™ CC Workstation: Spontaneous Respiration, Inspiration. Fresh gas from the anesthesia machine and gases from the reservoir bag flow through the inspiratory valve to the patient. If the bag empties, the subatmospheric pressure relief valve will open and admit room air into the system.

flow out of it. These include fresh gases and gases that passed through the CO_2 absorber during the previous exhalation. During the latter part of inspiration, some gas may be vented through the partly open APL valve. During expiration (Fig. 11.31), the inspiratory valve closes. Fresh gas flows into the reservoir bag. Exhaled gas from the patient passes through the CO_2 absorber and mixes with fresh gas in the reservoir bag.

Automatic Ventilation

During inspiration with mechanical ventilation (Fig. 11.32), the fresh gas decoupling valve is closed so all the fresh gas flows into the reservoir bag. The delivered tidal volume is independent of the fresh gas flow because no fresh gas is added to the ventilator's flow. The APL valve is excluded from the breathing system by the closed expiratory control valve. Compression of the bellows by the driving gas causes gases to flow to the patient port.

During expiration (Fig. 11.33), the fresh gas decoupling valve opens. The gas stored in the reservoir bag is drawn into the breathing system by the negative pressure caused by the descending bellows. After the bellows has filled (Fig. 11.34), the pressure in the breathing system increases. When it reaches approximately 2 cm H_2O, the APL valve opens and excess gases pass through it to the scavenging system.

Control of Ventilation

The ventilator is designed for pressure-limited, volume-constant, time-cycled ventilation in patients down to 3.5 kg.

Hazards

At the time of this writing, this ventilator has not been used to any great extent in the United States and no hazards have been reported.

GENERAL HAZARDS
Hypoventilation
Ventilator Dysfunction

Most anesthesia ventilators perform reliably for long periods of time. Nevertheless, one can occasionally fail to perform properly. Some problems may be insidious and result in less-than-total failure. Accuracy of any of the controls on a ventilator can result in inadequate ventilation. Malfunction may not be readily apparent. A false sense of security may be generated by the constant noise the ventilator makes.

Cycling Failure

Causes of cycling failure include disconnection from or failure of the power source and an internal mechanical dysfunction (24–26). Intermediate frequency settings have been associated with cycling failure (17).

Inadequate Design

Some anesthesia ventilators are not capable of delivering adequate volumes to patients with high airway resistance and/or poor compliance (27, 28).

Driving Gas Leak

If the bellows housing is not tightly secured, driving gas can leak, causing a reduction in the tidal volume (29, 30). The housing may hit ceiling columns or other objects as the ventilator is moved. Operating room personnel may attempt to move a ventilator by grabbing the housing.

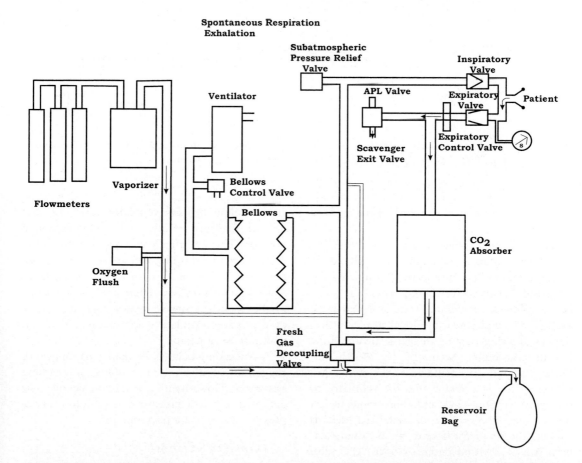

FIGURE 11.29.   Anodyne™ CC Workstation: Spontaneous Respiration, Exhalation. Gases exhaled by the patient flow through the absorber and join fresh gases flowing into the reservoir bag. At the end of exhalation, excess gases flow through the adjustable pressure limiting (APL) valve to the scavenging system.

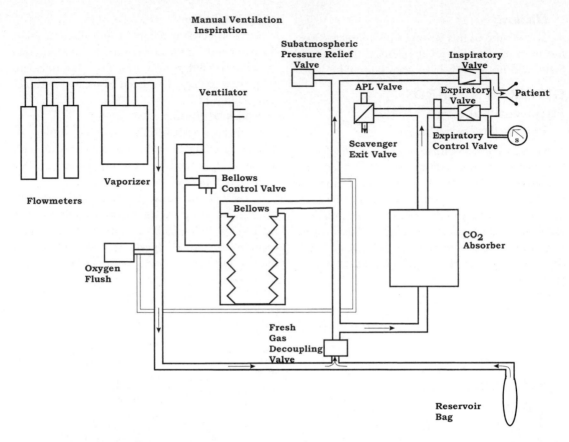

FIGURE 11.30. Anodyne™ CC Workstation: Manual Ventilation, Inspiration. When the bag is squeezed, gases from it and fresh gases flow through the inspiratory valve to the patient.

These maneuvers may loosen the housing or cause it to break.

Loss of Breathing System Gas

Most anesthesia ventilators are volume or time cycled and have no means of compensating for loss of gas in the breathing system. This can be an insidious problem. A ventilator may cycle but fail to occlude the exit port of the spill valve, thereby blowing part or all of the tidal volume into the scavenging system (12, 13, 24, 31, 32). Other reported sites of leaks are the spirometer box (33), the pole connecting the ventilator to the ventilator hose (34), and connections within the ventilator (35). The operator may fail to connect the ventilator hose to the breathing system. A leak, disconnection, or open APL valve in the breathing system can cause loss of gas.

If there is loss of breathing system gas and an ascending bellows ventilator is in use, the bellows may not return to its fully expanded position. This will usually be obvious (36). However, with the introduction of scavenging systems, the bellows may remain expanded if there is a disconnection (3). There may be a change in the sound of the ventilator, although some of the newer ventilators are so quiet that this may not be apparent.

A descending bellows ventilator may appear to function normally in the face of loss of breathing system gas. Upward movement of the bellows may generate sufficient pressure to fool a low airway pressure alarm and a respirometer.

Incorrect Settings

In a crowded anesthetizing area, ventilator switches or dials may be inadvertently changed as personnel move around (37). An operator may fail to adjust respiratory rate and volumes with a new case. For ventilators that provide a control for setting the peak inspiratory pressure, setting that pressure too low may result in an inadequate tidal volume being delivered.

Ventilator Turned Off

There are times during administration of anesthesia when the ventilator must be turned off, such as during radiologic procedures during which movement would compromise the quality of the picture. The operator may forget to turn it back on. Some ON/OFF ventilator switches can be placed in an intermediate position. The poten-

tial exists for reverting to the OFF position with only a slight impact (38).

Obstruction to Flow

As is pointed out in Chapter 13, occlusion of gas flow to the patient can occur in a variety of sites and because of a variety of mechanisms. One is failure to change the position of the bag-ventilator selector valve when converting to automatic ventilation. If the valve is left in the bag position, the ventilator will operate against a dead end. With obstruction to flow, the excursion of the bellows will be reduced but not totally eliminated. The pressure shown on the breathing system pressure gauge will vary, de-

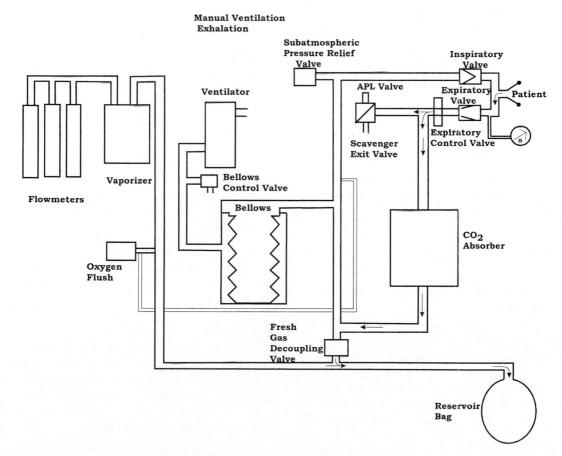

FIGURE 11.31.   Anodyne™ CC Workstation: Manual Ventilation, Exhalation. Exhaled gases from the patient pass through the absorber and join fresh gas flowing into the reservoir bag. When the pressure set on the adjustable pressure limiting (APL) valve is exceeded, excess gases will pass through it to the scavenging system.

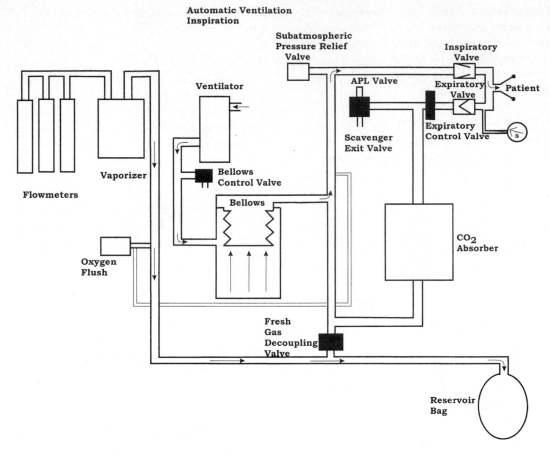

FIGURE 11.32. Anodyne™ CC Workstation: Automatic Ventilation, Inspiration. The fresh gas decoupling valve is closed so all the fresh gas flows into the reservoir bag. The bellows is compressed so that gas flows through the inspiratory valve to the patient.

pending on the locations of the obstruction and the gauge.

Addition of Positive End–Expiratory Pressure

Addition of PEEP may decrease the tidal volume delivered by some ventilators. The effect is more pronounced with low tidal volumes. If the lung compliance is low, there is less effect than if it were high. If PEEP is used, the tidal volume needs to be measured and may need to be increased to maintain the same minute volume (39, 40).

Hyperventilation

With a hole in the bellows or a loose connection between the bellows and its base assembly, driving gas from the housing can enter the bellows, causing an unexpectedly high tidal volume (41–43). This can be accentuated by a high inspiratory flow rate (24).

Hyperoxia

A hole or tear in the bellows with oxygen as the driving gas can result in an increase in the inspired oxygen concentration and a lower-than-expected anesthetic depth (42, 44–49).

Excessive Airway Pressure

Excessive airway pressure can develop rapidly, especially if high fresh gas flows are being used. Quick action may be required to prevent injury to the patient. Because the spill valve is closed during inspiration and the APL valve in the breathing system is closed or isolated, activating the oxygen flush during the inspiratory phase can result in barotrauma (6). A hole in the bellows or a loose connection between the bellows and its base may allow driving gas to enter the bellows, resulting in a higher-than-expected pressure during inspiration. If the spill valve becomes stuck in the closed position, the pressure in the breathing system will continue to rise as fresh gas flows into the system (13, 50–52). Excessive suction applied to the scavenging attachment can hold the spill valve closed (30, 53).

In one reported case, a muffler designed to silence the exhaust of driving gas from the ventilator became saturated with water and prevented gas from exiting from the bellows housing (10). Malfunction of a control valve can result in the ventilator becoming stuck in the inspiratory position (54).

A properly set pressure relief valve on a ventilator should reduce the risk of barotrauma but will not eliminate it (30). Some ventilators have adjustable high-pressure alarms. On others, the alarms are preset. Such an alarm may give warning of a problem in time to prevent harm to the patient. If a ventilator does not have a high-pressure alarm, it is suggested that this be added to the breathing system.

When there is high airway pressure while a ventilator is in use, a disconnection at the tracheal tube should be made immediately and manual

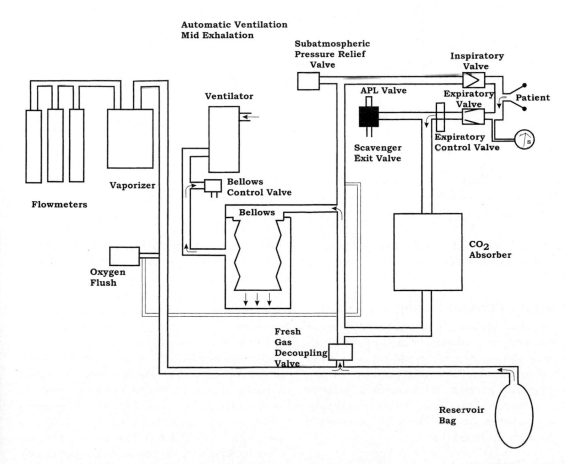

FIGURE 11.33. Anodyne™ CC Workstation: Automatic Ventilation, Mid Exhalation. The bellows expands, drawing in fresh gas and gas from the reservoir bag. Gas exhaled by the patient passes toward the absorber.

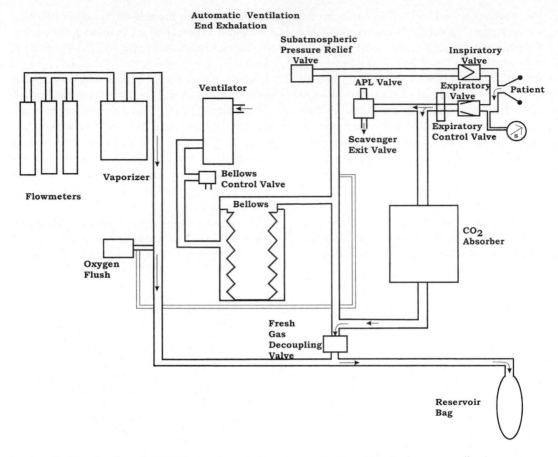

FIGURE 11.34. Anodyne™ CC Workstation: Automatic Ventilation, End Exhalation. The adjustable pres-sure limiting (APL) valve opens, allowing excess gases to flow into the scavenging system.

ventilation instituted. Taking time to find the source of the problem may place the patient at risk.

Negative Pressure During Expiration

Negative pressure is considered undesirable under most circumstances because of adverse effects on pulmonary function and increased risk of air embolism. Ventilators with weighted hanging bellows can generate subatmospheric pressure during the early part of expiration if expiratory flow is not impeded (24). This will be accentuated if the fresh gas flow is low.

Alarm Failure

Low airway pressure alarms that do not depend on the bellows's collapsing may fail to alarm if

there is failure of the cycling mechanism (55) or a negative pressure is transmitted from the scavenging system to the bellows housing (56). Although low-pressure alarms have significantly advanced patient safety, they can fail (57, 58).

When the low airway pressure alarm threshold is adjustable, it should be set just below the peak inspiratory pressure. Cases have been reported in which resistance (from tracheal tube connectors, Y pieces, bacterial filters, and other components or from the patient port of the breathing system being pressed against the patient or a pillow) coupled with high inspiratory flow rates created sufficient back pressure to generate a false-positive signal at the sensing site when the threshold was set too low.

Use of a PEEP valve in the breathing system

may cause a low-pressure alarm not to be activated if the PEEP valve raises the pressure above the alarm threshold.

ADVANTAGES

1. Use of a ventilator allows anesthesia personnel to devote time and energy to other tasks and eliminates the fatigue resulting from squeezing a bag (59).
2. A ventilator produces more regular ventilation with respect to rate, rhythm, and tidal volume than manual ventilation.
3. Compared with critical care ventilators, anesthesia ventilators are relatively simple in design and have fewer controls.
4. Some anesthesia ventilators can be used to administer high-frequency ventilation (9). Most patients, including children, can be ventilated in a satisfactory manner using these devices, provided the adequacy of ventilation is continuously monitored.

DISADVANTAGES

1. Probably the greatest disadvantage to the use of ventilators is the loss of contact between the anesthesia provider and the patient. The feel of the bag can reveal such things as disconnections, changes in resistance or compliance, continuous positive pressure, and spontaneous respiratory movements. With mechanical ventilation, these may go undetected for a considerable period of time.
2. A ventilator may induce a false sense of security in the user if it continues to make the appropriate sounds even when it malfunctions.
3. Some ventilators are large and cumbersome.
4. Some older ventilators lack proper monitoring and alarm capabilities.
5. Most anesthesia ventilators do not include the newer modes of ventilation (60). Some cannot develop high enough inspiratory pressure, flow, or PEEP to ventilate certain patients adequately (27, 28). It may be necessary to take a critical care ventilator into the operating room to provide adequate ventilation for critically ill patients (61).

6. Components subject to contamination may not be easy to remove or clean.
7. Disinfection and sterilizing procedures may take considerable time and effort.
8. Some ventilators are not user-friendly. There is room for improvement in the design and grouping of controls.
9. Some ventilators are disturbingly noisy.
10. Some ventilators require relatively high flows of driving or fresh gas (62). Oxygen consumption increases with increased minute volume, and, with some ventilators, oxygen consumption increases with an increased I:E ratio.

REFERENCES

1. American Society for Testing and Materials. Standard specification for ventilators intended for use during anesthesia (ASTM F1101–90) (Reapproved 1996). West Conshohocken, PA: ASTM, 1996.
2. Dupuis YG. Ventilators, theory and clinical application. St. Louis, MO: CV Mosby, 1986.
3. Blackstock D. Advantages of standing bellows ventilators and low-flow techniques. Anesthesiology 1984; 60:167.
4. Gravenstein JS, Nederstigt JA. Monitoring for disconnection: ventilators with bellows rising on expiration can deliver tidal volumes after disconnection. Journal of Clinical Monitoring 1990;6:207–210.
5. Sinclair A, Van Bergen J. Flow resistance of coaxial breathing systems: investigation of a circuit disconnect. Can J Anaesth 1992;39:90–94.
6. Andrews JJ. Understanding anesthesia ventilators (ASA Refresher Course No. 242). Park Ridge, IL: ASA, 1990.
7. Eisenkraft JB. The anesthesia delivery system. Part II. Prog Anesth 1989;3:1–12.
8. Grogono AW, Travis JT. Anesthesia ventilators. In: J Ehrenwerth, JB Eisenkraft, eds. Anesthesia equipment. Principles and applications. St. Louis, MO: Mosby, 1993:140–171.
9. Tessler MJ, Ruiz-Neto PP, Finlayson R, et al. Can anesthesia ventilators provide high-frequency ventilation? Anesth Analg 1994;79:563–566.
10. Roth S, Tweedie E, Sommer RM. Excessive airway pressure due to a malfunctioning anesthesia ventilator. Anesthesiology 1986;65:532–534.
11. Sprung J, Samaan F, Hensler T, et al. Excessive airway pressure due to ventilator control valve malfunction during anesthesia for open heart surgery. Anesthesiology 1990;73:1035–1038.

12. Sommer RM, Bhalla GS, Jackson JM, et al. Hypoventilation caused by ventilator valve rupture. Anesth Analg 1988;67:999–1001.

13. Eisenkraft JB. Potential for barotrauma or hypoventilation with the Drager AV-E ventilator. J Clin Anesth 1989;1:452–456.

14. Chaney MA. Delivery of excessive airway pressure to a patient by the anesthesia machine. Anesth Analg 1993;76:1166–1167.

15. Anonymous. Anesthesia unit ventilators. Technology for Anesthesia 1990;11(2):6.

16. Johnstone R, Graf D. Bellows failure with Drager anesthesia ventilator. Anesth Analg 1993;76:685–686.

17. Sosis MB. Drager ventilator failure on changing the respiratory rate setting. Anesth Analg 1993;76:453–454.

18. Ananthanarayan C, Fisher JA. Drager ventilator failure. Anesth Analg 1993;77:638.

19. Picard UM, Hancock DE, Pinchak AC. Pressure transients in anesthesia ventilators—failure of disconnect alarm system. Anesthesiology 1987;67:A189.

20. Elliott WR, Topulos GP. The influence of the mechanics of anesthesia breathing circuits on respiratory monitoring. Biomed Instrum Technol 1990;24:260–265.

21. Beahan PG. A hazardous sigh. Anaesthesia and Intensive Care 1989;17:515.

22. Raphael DT. An algorithmic response for the breathing system low-pressure alarm condition. Progress in Anesthesiology 1997;11:219–244.

23. Anonymous. Anesthesia unit ventilators. Technology for Anesthesia 1992;13:8–9.

24. Wyant GM, Craig DB, Pietak SP, et al. A panel discussion: safety in the operating room. Canadian Anaesthetists Society Journal 1984;31:287–301.

25. Sarnquist FH, Demas K. The silent ventilator. Anesth Analg 1982;61:713–714.

26. Gruneberg A. Ventilator hazard identified and rectified. BMJ 1984;288:1763.

27. Marks JD, Schapera A, Kraemer RW, et al. Pressure and flow limitations of anesthesia ventilators. Anesthesiology 1989;71:403–408.

28. Pinchak AC, Hancock DE, Shepard LS. Limitations of anesthesia ventilators in severe lung injury. Anesthesiology 1986;65:A149.

29. Lee K. Leak of driving gas from Air-Shields ventilator. Canadian Anaesthetists Society Journal 1986;33:263–264.

30. Feeley TW, Bancroft ML. Problems with mechanical ventilators. In: Rendell-Baker L, ed. Problems with anesthetic and respiratory therapy equipment. Int Anes Clin 1982;20(3):83–93.

31. Choi JJ, Guida J, Wu W. Hypoventilatory hazard of an anesthetic scavenging device. Anesthesiology 1986;65:126–127.

32. Khalil SN, Gholston TK, Binderman J, et al. Flapper valve malfunction in an Ohio closed scavenging system. Anesth Analg 1987;66:1334–1336.

33. Judkins KC, Sage M. Routine servicing of the Cape-Wane ventilator. Anaesthesia 1983;38:1102.

34. Rolbin S. An unusual cause of ventilator leak. Canadian Anaesthetists Society Journal 1977;24:522–524.

35. Anonymous. Valves, positive end expiratory pressure. Technology for Anesthesia 1991;11(7):7.

36. Graham DH. Advantages of standing bellows ventilators and low-flow techniques. Anesthesiology 1983;58:486.

37. Wald A, Neidzwski TJ. Front panel cover for Frazer Harlake ventilator. Anesth Analg 1983;62:619–620.

38. Ciobanu M, Meyer JA. Ventilator hazard revealed. Anesthesiology 1980;52:186–187.

39. Pan PH, van der Aa JJ. Positive end-expiratory pressure: effect on delivered tidal volume. J Clin Anesth 1995;7:443–444.

40. Pan PH, van der Aa JJ. Positive end-expiratory pressure and lung compliance: effect on delivered tidal volume. Can J Anaesth 1995;42:831–835.

41. Waterman PW, Pautler S, Smith RB. Accidental ventilator-induced hyperventilation. Anesthesiology 1978;48:141.

42. Rigg D, Joseph M. Split ventilator bellows. Anaesthesia and Intensive Care 1985;13:213.

43. Harris TL, Podraza A, Salem MR, et al. Effects of bellows leaks on anesthesia ventilator function. Journal of Clinical Monitoring 1991;7:120–121.

44. Baraka A, Muallem M. Awareness during anaesthesia due to a ventilator malfunction. Anaesthesia 1979;34:678–679.

45. Longmuir J, Craig DB. Inadvertent increase in inspired oxygen concentration due to defect in ventilator bellows. Canadian Anaesthetists Society Journal 1976;23:327–329.

46. Love JB. Missassembly of a Campbell ventilator causing leakage of the driving gas to a patient. Anaesthesia and Intensive Care 1980;8:376–377.

47. Marsland AR, Solomos J. Ventilator malfunction detected by O_2 analyser. Anaesthesia and Intensive Care 1981;9:395.

48. Ripp CH, Chapin JW. A bellow's leak in an Ohio anesthesia ventilator. Anesth Analg 1985;64:942.

49. Webb RK, Russell WJ, Klepper I, et al. Equipment failure: an analysis of 2000 incident reports. Anaesthesia and Intensive Care 1993;21:673–677.

50. Anonymous. Wrongful death suit dismissal over-

turned. American Medical News, November 13, 1981: 19.

51. Henzig D. Insidious PEEP from a defective ventilator gas evacuation outlet valve. Anesthesiology 1982;57: 251–252.

52. Hilton PJ, Clement JA. Surgical emphysema resulting from a ventilator malfunction. Anaesthesia 1983;38: 342–345.

53. Anonymous. Pre-use testing prevents "helpful" reconnection of anesthesia components. Technology for Anesthesia 1987;8(1):1–2.

54. Murray AW, Easton JC. Another problem with an expiratory valve. Anaesthesia 1988;43:891–892.

55. Sarnquist FH, Demas K. The silent ventilator. Anesth Analg 1982;61:713–714.

56. Heard SO, Munson ES. Ventilator alarm nonfunction associated with a scavenging system for waste gases. Anesth Analg 1983;62:230–232.

57. Mazza N, Wald A. Failure of battery-operated alarms. Anesthesiology 1980;53:246–248.

58. Lahay WD. Defective pressure/flow alarm. Canadian Anaesthetists Society Journal 1982;29:404–405.

59. Amaranath L, Boutros AR. Circle absorber and soda lime contamination. Anesth Analg 1980;59:711–712.

60. Del Valle RM, Hecker RB. A review of ventilatory modalities used in the intensive care unit. American Journal of Anesthesiology 1995;22:23–30.

61. Bishop MJ. Bronchospasm: managing and avoiding a potential anesthetic disaster. ASA Refresher Courses 1993:272.

62. Raessler KL, Kretzman WE, Gravenstein N. Oxygen consumption by anesthesia ventilators. Anesthesiology 1988;69:A271.

QUESTIONS

Each question below contains four suggested answers of which one or more is correct. Choose the answer:

A. if 1, 2, and 3 are correct
B. if 1 and 3 are correct
C. if 2 and 4 are correct
D. if 4 is correct
E. if 1, 2, 3, and 4 are correct.

1. A hole or tear in the bellows may result in
   1. Hyperventilation
   2. Hyperoxia
   3. Barotrauma
   4. Patient awareness

2. Excessive airway pressure may be caused by
   1. Excessive negative pressure in the scavenging system
   2. A hole in the bellows housing
   3. A stuck spill valve
   4. Ascension of the bellows

3. The low airway pressure alarm limit should be set
   1. Low enough to prevent nuisance alarms
   2. Lower if there is increased resistance to gas flow
   3. Lower when PEEP is used
   4. Just below the peak pressure during inspiration

4. Functions controlled by the pneumatic circuitry include
   1. Flow of the inspired gas
   2. Inspiratory-to-expiratory ratio
   3. Volume of inspired gas
   4. Flow rate of the respiratory gas

5. Required alarm(s) for an anesthesia ventilator include
   1. Loss of airway pressure
   2. Minute volume less than the alarm set point
   3. High airway pressure
   4. Loss of main power supply

6. Characteristics of a pressure-limiting valve include
   1. It limits the pressure of the driving gas in the bellows assembly
   2. It may be preset at the factory
   3. It may be a spring-loaded valve assembly
   4. Preset pressure is usually 80 to 90 cm H_2O

7. Characteristics of ascending and descending bellows ventilators include
   1. Negative pressure is generated during exhalation with the descending bellows version
   2. A footplate is used to limit excursion on the ascending bellows ventilator
   3. A weight in the bellows facilitates exhalation with the descending bellows version
   4. It is easier to detect disconnections with the descending bellows

8. Possible mechanisms for hypoventilation when a ventilator is in use include
   1. Loose bellows housing
   2. Decreased compliance
   3. The rate control being between settings
   4. Closure of the spill valve

ANSWERS

1.	E	5.	D
2.	B	6.	A
3.	D	7.	B
4.	A	8.	A

Controlling Trace Gas Levels

INTRODUCTION

In the past the usual practice was to discharge excess anesthetic gases and vapors directly into room air. As a consequence, operating room personnel were exposed to low concentrations of these drugs. For many decades there was little thought about any detrimental effects that might result from such exposure. In recent times, questions have been raised about the possible hazards from exposure to trace amounts of anesthetic gases and vapors (1). (Through the remainder of this chapter anesthetic gases and vapors will be referred to as *gases*, because most vapors behave as gases.)

A trace level of an anesthetic gas is far below that needed for clinical anesthesia or that can be detected by smell (2). Trace gas levels are usually expressed in parts per million (ppm), which is volume/volume (100% of a gas is 1,000,000 ppm; 1% is 10,000 ppm).

Reported trace gas concentrations vary greatly, depending on the fresh gas flow in use, the ventilation system, the length of time that anesthesia has been administered, the measurement site, and other variables. The degree of pollution may be particularly high in hospitals devoted to pediatric surgery (3, 4). This is probably related to use of mask inductions and uncuffed tracheal tubes (5).

METHODS OF STUDY (6)

Despite many studies and much discussion, opinions differ on whether a problem exists and what levels should be allowed in the working environment. To interpret the data it is first necessary to understand how they were gathered. Four basic methods of study have been used. All have major limitations and disadvantages.

Animal Investigations

In these studies, laboratory animals are exposed to varying levels of gases for varying periods of time and studied to determine effects. These studies should be interpreted warily. Large numbers of animals need to be studied to achieve statistical significance (7). In animals diet affects tumor susceptibility and stress affects reproduction (7). Toxicity usually depends on both exposure time and concentration, and it is difficult to correlate exposure time in animals with that in humans, because the lifespans are so different. Finally, variations in drug effects among species create uncertainty about the relevance of these findings to humans.

Human Volunteer Studies

Human volunteers have been used to study the effects of trace gases on skilled performance, immune responses, and drug metabolism.

Epidemiological Studies of Exposed Humans

A number of epidemiological studies of exposed personnel have been made. All have serious flaws. Most were retrospective and used questionnaires sent through the mail. They suffer from low response rates, inappropriate control groups, poor recollections and biases on the part of the respondents, poor wording, failure to include significant points in the questionnaires, and misinterpretations because of differences in education and experience on the part of the respondents (7–11). Interpretation of the data is hampered by a lack of agreement as to what level of significance to accept (7, 12). Finally, the studies have not been designed to test the cause-and-effect relationship between trace gases and problems in exposed personnel. Some show increased risk for specific groups but not for other equally exposed groups (13). Others have shown problems in groups with and without exposure to trace gases, suggesting that the risk may be related to some other factor. Finally, many of the studies were performed before scavenging and other methods to control trace gas levels were implemented. Prospective studies are needed to determine whether there is a relationship between current levels of occupational exposure to anesthetic gases and adverse outcomes.

Mortality Studies

Studies on the causes of death and the age at which death occurred among anesthesiologists have provided interesting data, despite some questions about the appropriateness of the control group and rather small numbers.

PROBLEMS
Spontaneous Abortions
Epidemiological Studies

Epidemiological studies from several countries have shown higher rates of spontaneous abortion in operating room and dental operatory personnel than women in different environments (14–24).

Other studies have failed to find significant increases in spontaneous abortions in exposed personnel (25–31). One study found that the frequency of miscarriages among nurses working in intensive care units was approximately equal to that of nurses in the operating room, suggesting that psychic and/or physical stress may be the causative factors (20).

If anesthetic gases caused spontaneous abortions, a higher rate of miscarriage would be expected in those with greatest exposure. Statistics show that the incidence of miscarriage among operating room staff is higher in the United States than in the United Kingdom, despite the fact that routine use of carbon dioxide absorption and low flow rates plus air-conditioning in the United States probably result in lower average atmospheric contamination than in the United Kingdom where high flow rates are more common and air-conditioning less common.

In summary, while most of the epidemiological studies on spontaneous abortions are flawed and subject to reporting bias, there are data to support the contention that there is a slightly increased risk of spontaneous abortions among women exposed to trace anesthetics (32).

Animal Studies

Isoflurane

Investigations have found no evidence of increased spontaneous abortion in mice exposed to up to 10,500 ppm isoflurane (33, 34).

Enflurane

Several investigations failed to show any toxic effects to fetuses in animals exposed to concentrations as high as 16,500 ppm (34–37).

Halothane

Investigations have shown no lethal effects to embryos from exposures of up to 8000 ppm (34, 38, 39).

Nitrous Oxide

One study found that prolonged exposure to 1000 ppm nitrous oxide caused fetal death and resorption, but no effect was seen when 500 ppm was used (40). A later study found that the threshold for fetal death was higher (between 1000 and 5000 ppm) with intermittent exposure (41).

Mixtures

Investigations using mixtures of halothane and nitrous oxide found no effect with concentrations as high as 1,600 ppm halothane plus 100,000 ppm nitrous oxide (39). Nitrous oxide 500,000

ppm plus isoflurane 3500 ppm had no effect on spontaneous abortions (42).

In summary, with the possible exception of nitrous oxide, animal studies indicate that if a threshold concentration of inhalation anesthetics causing increased spontaneous abortions exists, it is 10 to 100 or even 1000 times that commonly found in operating rooms. A finding of some interest in one study (39) was that animals stressed by experimental handling had dramatically higher fetal losses.

Spontaneous Abortion in Spouses

Although several studies have shown an increased spontaneous abortion rate in wives of exposed males (16, 21, 43, 44), results from the majority of studies suggest there is no increase (11, 14, 18, 31).

One study found no changes in sperm concentration or morphology in male anesthesiologists working in hospitals with scavenging equipment (45). Studies have failed to show any adverse effect on reproductive processes of male animals exposed to up to 5000 ppm enflurane (34, 46) or 10 ppm halothane plus 500 ppm nitrous oxide (47).

Infertility

Epidemiological Studies

Studies have found higher-than-expected rates of involuntary infertility among exposed personnel (17, 21, 48). One study found no effect from paternal exposure (18), and no changes in sperm count or morphology have been found in male anesthesiologists working in scavenged operating rooms (45).

Animal Studies

Isoflurane

Exposure of female mice to up to 4000 ppm isoflurane had no effect on fertility (33). Exposure of male mice to 10,000 ppm caused no increase in percentage of abnormal spermatozoa (49). No effect on fertility was seen in flies exposed to 160,000 ppm.

Enflurane

No effect on fertility in male or female mice was found from exposure to up to 5000 ppm (35,

46). One study did find an increase in abnormal spermatozoa in mice exposed to 12,000 ppm (49). No effect on fertility was seen in male or female flies exposed to as high as 160,000 ppm (50).

Halothane

Studies show no effect on male fertility with exposure of up to 160,000 ppm halothane (50–52). Exposure of male mice to 8000 ppm halothane caused no increase in percentage of abnormal spermatozoa (49). In studies on female fertility, one found a decrease in fertility in rats exposed to 3000, but not 1000 ppm halothane (51). Other studies found no effect from exposure to 14,000 ppm in rats (52) or 160,000 ppm in flies (50).

Nitrous Oxide

No changes in male fertility and no sperm abnormalities were found in mice after exposure to up to 800,000 ppm (49, 53). However, prolonged exposure of male rats to 200,000 ppm resulted in abnormalities in spermatogenic cells (54). One study found that male rats mated after exposure to 5,000 ppm nitrous oxide produced significantly smaller liters (55). This was reversible with time. Exposure to up to 800,000 ppm caused no changes in fertility in male or female flies (50).

Mixtures

Decreased fertility was seen in female rats exposed to halothane 10 ppm plus nitrous oxide 500 ppm before mating (47). Male rats exposed to these concentrations showed greater frequency of chromosomal aberrations in spermatogenic cells, but the aberrations were probably too infrequent to cause decreased fertility (50).

Birth Defects

Epidemiological Studies

Several studies in humans have found an increase in congenital abnormalities in children of exposed personnel (14, 16, 17, 21, 25, 28, 30, 44, 56, 22). Interpretations of the data have been questioned (7, 12, 13, 56, 57), and several investigators have found no increase in birth defects among the offspring of exposed parents (11, 18–20, 27, 31, 23). No increase in chromosomal abnormalities in exposed nurses or changes in sperm morphology in male anesthesiologists working in operating rooms have been found (45, 58).

Animal Studies

Isoflurane

Exposures to concentrations up to 10,500 failed to cause any significant teratogenic effect (42, 34).

Enflurane

Studies have found no teratogenic effects of exposure to up to 16,500 ppm (34, 35, 59). However, one study found changes in spermatozoa after exposure to 12,000 ppm (49).

Halothane

Several investigations have found exposure of pregnant rats to concentrations of halothane of up to 8000 ppm produced no effects that could be expected to result in permanent abnormalities or decreased survival (34, 37–39, 60, 61). Chronic exposure of rats to 10 and 12.5 ppm of halothane in utero has been shown to produce later deficits in learning (62, 63). However, the interpretation of these data have been questioned (13).

Nitrous Oxide

Studies have shown no gross abnormalities in animals exposed to up to 750,000 ppm (34, 40, 53, 64).

Mixtures

No major teratogenic effects were seen with exposure to halothane 10 ppm and nitrous oxide 500 ppm (47). Decreases in fetal weight and slight developmental retardation have been found with exposure to mixtures as high as 100,000 ppm nitrous oxide and 1600 ppm halothane, but this was unaccompanied by evidence of gross abnormalities (39, 47).

In summary, studies of laboratory animals show that concentrations of inhalation agents that produce gross malformations are well above those found in even unscavenged operating rooms. The question of learning deficits, however, deserves more study.

Impairment of Skilled Performance

Operating room personnel are subjected to many stimuli that require precise, rapid, and complicated responses. Because the patient's survival depends on the alertness and performance of the professional team, anything that interferes with its ability to perceive changes and react quickly and appropriately may cause harm to a patient.

Studies that have tested operating room personnel exposed to trace gases have failed to demonstrate decreased performance in exposed personnel (65–69).

Although a few early studies found exposure of volunteers to trace concentrations of nitrous oxide, halothane, or enflurane caused significant decreases in performance (70–72) efforts to duplicate these results have failed (73–77). These studies found that the concentrations needed to decrease performance were hundreds of times greater than the average levels found in unscavenged operating rooms. In another study, neuropsychological symptoms and tiredness were reported more by individuals in operating rooms that were less scavenged (78).

In laboratory tests, exposure of adult rats to 10 ppm halothane failed to affect learning (79).

Cancer

Epidemiological Studies

A large study found no increase in cancer in exposed males but indicated that females in the operating room were at higher risk for cancer than nonexposed females (14). The significance of these data has been questioned (12, 13). Similar results have been reported for female dental operatory assistants (16). Two studies of dentists have shown that the incidence of cancer is not significantly different among those exposed and those not exposed to trace concentrations of anesthetics (16, 44). A review of combined data from six studies found an increased cancer risk among women but not men (32).

Mortality Studies

There is no increased death rate from cancer in male anesthesiologists (80–84). The death rate from cancer among female anesthesiologists is high compared with male anesthesiologists and control groups (82), but the numbers are too small to permit any strong conclusions. Also, new therapeutic modalities have resulted in higher cancer cure rates, so the incidence of cancer cannot be inferred using only mortality data.

Animal Studies

Halothane

Studies have found no evidence of increased carcinogenicity in animals exposed to up to 5000 ppm halothane (85, 86).

Enflurane

Mice exposed to up to 10,000 ppm enflurane have been found to have no increased risk of neoplasms (86, 87).

Isoflurane

One study found hepatic neoplasms in mice exposed during gestation and early life to 1000 to 5000 ppm isoflurane (88), but the validity of this study has been questioned and it appears that the increased incidence of tumors may have been the result of other factors. In later studies, no evidence of increased carcinogenicity could be found in animals exposed to up to 6000 ppm isoflurane (86, 89)

Nitrous Oxide

No evidence of increased carcinogenicity in mice has been found with exposure to up to 800,000 ppm (86, 90).

Mixtures

No increase in neoplasms has been found in rats exposed to 10 ppm halothane plus 500 ppm nitrous oxide (91).

Mutagenicity Testing

Testing for carcinogenicity requires large numbers of animals and a great expenditure of money and effort. A more rapid and inexpensive method is to look for an increase in mutagens in a bacterial system exposed to an inhalational anesthetic. One of the mechanisms by which environmental agents are thought to produce cancer involves mutation of DNA (92, 93). Because the DNA of all organisms is chemically similar, a study of mutagenic effects in a simpler organism may predict carcinogenicity in humans.

Cytogenetic methods are used increasingly for monitoring exposure to potential mutagens in the environment. Examination of sister chromatid exchanges in peripheral lymphocytes has been used to study anesthetic agents.

Although mutagenicity tests have predictive value in detecting carcinogens, lack of mutagenicity does not exclude the possibility that an agent may be carcinogenic to chronically exposed personnel. Furthermore, there is the possibility that an anesthetic agent could increase the carcinogenic effect of other chemical and physical factors.

Human Studies

One study found increased mutagenic activity in the urine of anesthesiologists (94), but another study found no difference in mutagenic activity in the urine of individuals working in scavenged and unscavenged operating rooms (95). Also, the urine of individuals collected before and after beginning training in anesthesia had similar mutagenic activity.

Most studies of sister chromatic exchanges in personnel exposed to trace gases have shown no evidence of a mutagenic effect (96–100), but some studies in unscavenged rooms did find an increase (101, 102).

Animal Studies

Halothane. Several studies have found halothane and its metabolites not mutagenic (92, 103–107). Others have found it and/or its metabolites weakly mutagenic (108–112).

Enflurane. Several investigations (103, 113, 114) were unable to demonstrate mutagenic effects from enflurane.

Isoflurane. Several investigations (103, 105, 114) have found isoflurane not to be mutagenic.

Nitrous oxide. Investigations (103, 115) have found nitrous oxide not mutagenic.

Mixtures. One investigation found that halothane plus nitrous oxide did not increase mutagenesis (106). Another found that nitrous oxide had no effect on the mutagenicity of halothane (108). The same study found no mutagenicity with mixtures of nitrous oxide and enflurane or isoflurane.

Liver Disease

Epidemiological Studies

Studies have found that operating room personnel have higher-than-expected rates of hepatic disease (6, 14, 116). Interpretation of these data has been questioned (12). Similar results have been reported in male dentists (16, 44) and female chair-side assistants (16). Analysis of the data suggests that there is an increased risk of developing liver disease, especially among men (32).

Anesthesia personnel working in unscavenged operating rooms have been found to have normal levels of hepatic enzymes (117).

Recurrent hepatitis on exposure to halothane has been demonstrated in a few individuals (118–121), and exposure to trace anesthetic agents enhances hepatic metabolism of some drugs (122, 123). The relevance of these facts to the effects of trace concentrations is not clear.

Mortality Studies

No increase in the death rate as a result of liver disease among anesthesiologists has been found (82).

Animal Studies

Exposure to halothane in concentrations as low as 20 ppm may be associated with mild toxic effects to the liver in rats (124–126). No evidence of such effects have been found from enflurane (124, 126) or isoflurane (124).

Renal Disease

Epidemiological Studies

The ASA National Study found that male and female operating room nurses and technicians and female anesthesiologists had a higher risk of kidney disease than did comparable groups outside the operating room (14). These differences were not found in male anesthesiologists. These results have been questioned (12). Another study failed to find any increase in kidney disease in male anesthesiologists (6). An early study in exposed dentists showed no increase in renal disease (43), but a later study showed an increase in both exposed dentists and female chair-side assistants (16). An analysis of several studies found an increased risk of renal disease only among women (56).

Mortality Studies

No increase in deaths caused by renal disease among anesthesiologists has been found (82).

Hematological Studies

Several studies have shown that inhalation of nitrous oxide inactivates vitamin B_{12} which may lead to impaired synthesis of DNA in the bone marrow (127). Changes can occur in patients exposed to nitrous oxide over prolonged periods, after multiple short-term exposures, and in the period immediately after operation.

Epidemiological Studies

In one study a higher-than-expected rate of leukemia was found in female anesthesiologists, but the small database makes any valid conclusions difficult (14). Other studies have found no significant alterations in hematological function in exposed individuals (117, 128–130). However, three of 20 dentists exposed to concentrations of nitrous oxide higher than those normally found in operating rooms showed abnormalities in their bone marrows (131). Two had abnormalities in their peripheral blood.

Animal Studies

Halothane

No hematological effects were found from exposure of mice to 500 ppm halothane (85).

Enflurane

Exposure to 3000 ppm enflurane had no effect on hematopoiesis in mice (132).

Nitrous Oxide

Exposure to 10,000 ppm nitrous oxide caused no changes in hematopoiesis in rats (133).

Mixtures

Cytogenetic damage to bone marrow was found in rats exposed to 10 ppm halothane plus 500 ppm nitrous oxide (46).

Neurological Symptoms

A nonspecific polyneuropathy following chronic exposure to nitrous oxide has been described (134, 135). Two studies found an increase in neurological symptoms (numbness, tingling, and/or muscle weakness) in dentists and female chair-side assistants exposed to anesthetic gases (16, 136). Another study showed no difference in neurological symptoms or signs, sensory perception, or nerve conduction between dentists using nitrous oxide extensively and those using it sparingly or not at all (137).

In animals, high levels of nitrous oxide have not been shown to cause neuromuscular or neurological abnormalities (137.)

Alterations in Immune Response

Several studies have found that work in operating rooms does not change the immunologic profile of individuals (138–141). However, a study of individuals working in unscavenged rooms with trace gas concentrations several times the recommended levels had changes that reversed when the individuals were removed from that environment (142).

Cardiac Disease

Studies have shown a greater-than-expected frequency of hypertension and dysrhythmias (6, 143), and there is one case report of atrial fibrillation secondary to halothane exposure (144). However, mortality studies give no evidence that anesthesiologists have a higher-than-expected risk of dying from heart disease (80–83).

Miscellaneous

Various studies have reported higher-than-expected incidences of bone and joint disease (6), ulcers (6, 143), ulcerative colitis (143), gallbladder disease (6), migraine (143) and headache and fatigue (145) in exposed personnel. Case reports of exposed personnel who developed asthmatic symptoms (146), laryngitis (147), ophthalmic hypersensitivity (148), conjunctivitis (149), exacerbation of myasthenia gravis (150), and skin eruptions (151, 152) have been published. Mortality statistics show a high incidence of suicide among anesthesiologists (80, 82).

Summary

The evidence that trace anesthetic gases are harmful is at present suggestive rather than conclusive. The hazard, if it exists, is not great and is more properly regarded as disquieting than alarming. Researchers who have systematically examined the published data feel that adverse reproductive problems in women such as spontaneous abortion and fetal injury were the only health effects for which there is reasonably convincing evidence (9). While it is somewhat reassuring to note that studies have shown that anesthesiologists have a mortality rate less than that expected for physicians or the general population (81–83), reproductive problems are not reflected in mortality data and high cure rates may be responsible for the low mortality. One study showed an increased rate of early retirement as a result of permanent ill health and a high rate of deaths while working among anesthesia personnel (153).

A cause-and-effect relationship between occupational exposure and the problems described has not been established. If there is an increased risk, it may be related to other factors such as mental and physical stress; strenuous physical demands; disturbed night rest; need for constant alertness; long and inconvenient working hours often interfering with domestic life; irregular routine; exposure to transmissible infections, solvents, propellants, cleaning substances, lasers, methylmethacrylate, radiation, or ultraviolet light; preexisting health and reproductive problems; hormonal or dietary disturbances; the physical or emotional makeup of those who choose to work in operating rooms; socioeconomic factors; or some other as yet undefined factor. Proof that trace amounts of anesthetic gases contribute to the increased risk must await demonstration that measures to reduce their levels also reduce the risk.

While reducing trace gas levels appears to be of little benefit to the patient (other than perhaps resulting in a healthier person administering the anesthesia), definite hazards to the patient have been created by the introduction of scavenging equipment (see "Hazards of Scavenging Equipment," in this chapter). Use of scavenging equipment and/or changing work practices also may be inconvenient or awkward for anesthesia personnel.

The authors of this text believe that the most prudent approach is to take action to reduce the levels of trace anesthetics to the lowest level consistent with reasonable cost, risk to the patient, and inconvenience.

The Committee on Occupational Health of Operating Room Personnel suggests that through some formal process, health care institutions bring to the attention of operating and recovery room personnel pertinent information on the claimed risks of excess anesthetic gases and ways by which these risks can be minimized (154). A sample letter is available (155).

CONTROL MEASURES

Complete elimination of all anesthetic molecules from the ambient atmosphere is impossible. The goal should be to reduce concentrations to the lowest level consistent with a reasonable expenditure of effort and money. To achieve this, attention must be focused on four areas: scavenging, leaks, work techniques, and the room ventilation system. If pollution is to be controlled, attention must be paid to all of these areas. Even with scavenging systems in place, exposure to nitrous oxide can be as high as 12 times the NIOSH recommended limit, and in dental operations, more than 40 times the recommended limit (1).

Scavenging Systems

Scavenging is defined as the collection of excess gases from equipment used in administering anesthesia or exhaled by the patient and removal of these gases to an appropriate place of discharge outside the working environment. Scavenging systems are also called evacuation systems, waste anesthetic gas disposal systems, and excess anesthetic gas-scavenging systems. The flowmeters on the anesthesia machine are usually set to deliver more gases than the patient can take up. In the absence of scavenging, these gases will flow into the operating room air. Installation of an efficient scavenging system is the most important step in reducing trace gas levels, lowering ambient concentrations by up to 90% (156–165).

A scavenging system consists of five basic parts (Fig. 12.1): a gas-collecting assembly, which captures gases at the site of emission; a transfer means, which conveys them to the interface; the interface, which provides positive (and sometimes negative) pressure relief and may provide reservoir capacity; the gas-disposal tubing, which conducts the gases from the interface to the gas-disposal assembly; and the gas-disposal assembly, which conveys them to a point where they can be discharged safely. Frequently, some or all of these components are combined.

A U.S. standard (166) and an international standard (167) for scavenging systems have been published (166). The international standard differs from the U.S. standard in that some fittings are male rather than female and vice versa.

Gas-Collecting Assembly

The gas-collecting assembly (scavenger adapter; gas-capturing assembly, device, or valve;

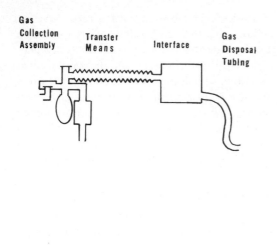

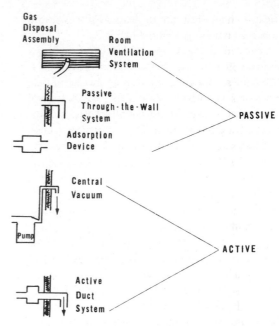

FIGURE 12.1. Complete scavenging system. The gas-collecting assembly may be an integral part of the breathing system, ventilator, or extracorporeal pump oxygenator. The interface may be an integral part of the gas-collecting assembly or some other portion of the scavenging system.

scavenging trap or valve; collecting or collection valve; scavenging exhale valve; evacuator; antipollution valve; ducted expiratory valve; collecting system exhaust valve; scavenging trap) collects excess gases from their sources and delivers them to the transfer means. It may attach to, or be an integral part of, a source. Frequently the outlets of two or more sources are joined together.

The ASTM standard and international standards specify that the outlet connection must be a 30-mm male fitting. In the past, 19-mm fittings were permitted, but their use is being phased out. The size is important because it should not be possible to connect components of the breathing system to the outlet. Some early assemblies had a 22-mm fitting and cases of misconnection with breathing system hoses occurred (168, 169).

Breathing Systems

Systems containing an adjustable pressure-limiting valve. Systems with an adjustable pressure-limiting (APL) valve include the circle system and the Mapleson A, B, C, and D systems. The APL valve can be fitted with a shroud (Fig. 12.2). With the circle and Mapleson D systems and the Lack

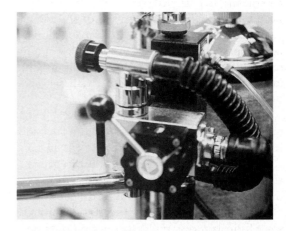

FIGURE 12.2. Gas-collecting assembly attached to an adjustable pressure-limiting (APL) valve.

variant of the Mapleson A system, the weight of the assembly can be supported by the anesthesia machine and the transfer means can be quite short. Smaller and lighter APL valves with gas-collecting assemblies are available for the Mapleson A, B, and C systems. APL valves sometimes have a mechanism built into them that will prevent positive or negative pressure from the scavenging system from being transmitted to the breathing system (169a).

T-piece systems without an APL valve. Numerous devices for removing gases from the bag have been described (170–189). Other methods use a container attached to suction (190, 191). The waste gases are discharged into the container and a disposal system removes them before they can enter the room. Other methods attach the gas-collecting assembly between the bag and its attachment to the tubing (193–196).

Resuscitation Equipment

A nonrebreathing valve with a scavenging adapter is commercially available. It is fairly simple to devise a means to attach transfer means to the exhalation port of some existing nonrebreathing valves without affecting valve function.

Masks or Nasal Cannulae

It is common practice in some institutions to administer nitrous oxide to patients through a nasal cannula or face mask for sedation. Placing a tent or hood around the patient's head and attaching a suction source can reduce the ambient concentrations of gases (197–199).

A double mask consisting of an inner smaller mask separated from an outer larger mask by a space connected to a scavenging device will reduce exposure to anesthetic gases (200, 201).

Ventilators

Most anesthesia ventilators are now equipped with gas-collecting assemblies, and most also come with an interface and gas-disposal assembly.

For a ventilator with a gas-collecting assembly, it is useful to attach the assembly outlet to a Y that joins the effluent from the APL valve in the breathing system (see Fig. 12.7). With some ventilators, it is necessary to have a unidirectional valve between the ventilator and the Y to prevent flow of gases back into the ventilator and the operating room air when the ventilator is not in use.

With some older ventilators, the exhaust includes not only the excess breathing system gases but also the driving gas for the ventilator, so that a disposal system with high flows is required. Thus a scavenging system that functions efficiently with spontaneously breathing patients may fail to do so when used with some automatic ventilators (202).

Extracorporeal Pump Oxygenators

The outlet port of an extracorporeal pump oxygenator is a potential source of anesthetic pollution (203). Gas-collecting assemblies for these are available. It is important to provide an effective interface with these devices because significant positive or negative pressure alterations at the outflow port can markedly alter function (204).

Respiratory Gas Monitors

Some respiratory gas monitors that withdraw a sample of gas from the breathing system expel this sample into the room. This constitutes a source of contamination that is often ignored (205–207). Many monitors are now designed so that the aspirated sample travels either back to the breathing system or to a scavenging system (Fig. 12.3)(208).

Cryosurgical Units

Many cryosurgical units use nitrous oxide. These can contribute to operating room contami-

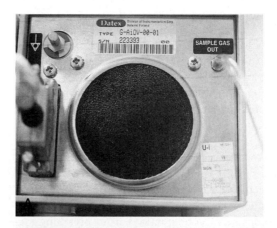

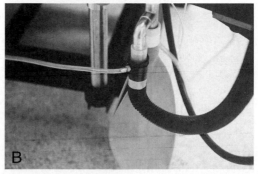

FIGURE 12.3. **A,** Gas sampling monitor with sample gas outlet. **B,** Connection of transfer tubing near the interface.

nation (209). These units should be fitted with scavengers or carbon dioxide should be used instead of nitrous oxide (210).

Leak Sites

When there is a definite leak site (as when a face mask or laryngeal mask is used or a vaporizer is filled), close (local) scavenging of contaminated air through a separate scavenging device or a low negative pressure hood can be used to lower ambient concentrations (211–214).

Transfer Means

The transfer means (exhaust tubing, hose, and transfer system) conveys gas from the collecting assembly to the interface when the interface is not an integral part of the gas-collecting assembly.

It is most commonly a length of tubing with a connector at either end. The inlet and outlet fittings should be either 30- or 19-mm. It should be as short as possible (this is facilitated by mounting the interface on the anesthesia machine) and of large enough diameter to carry a high flow of gas without a significant increase in pressure. It should be resistant to kinking. If the transfer means is not kink-resistant, a pressure relief valve can be added to the collector to prevent pressure increases that could result from occlusion of the tubing between the collector and the interface. If it must run along the floor it should be designed to prevent occlusion (154). It should be easily seen and easy to disconnect from the gas-collecting assembly in the event of malfunction or occlusion of the scavenging system. To discourage misconnections it is desirable that it be different (by color and/or configuration) from breathing system tubing.

Interface

The interface (balancing valve or device, pressure balancing valve or device, interface system or block, intermediate site, safety block, air break receiver, receiver unit, air break, receiving system, interface valve, and scavenging valve) serves to prevent pressure increases or decreases in the scavenging system from being transmitted to the breathing system, ventilator, or extracorporeal oxygenator. The American standard requires that the interface limit pressures immediately downstream

of the gas-collecting assembly to between -0.5 and $+10$ cm H_2O during normal operating conditions and up to $+15$ cm H_2O with obstruction of the scavenging system for scavenging from a breathing system or ventilator (154). In the proposed international standard these limits are -0.5 cm H_2O and $+3.5$ cm H_2O. For scavenging from an extracorporeal oxygenator, the recommended limits are -0.25 to 0 cm H_2O (154).

The inlet should have a 30- or 19-mm male connection. The size of the outlet connection is optional, but should be different from breathing system connections and from the inlet connection if the device is sensitive to the direction of flow (154).

The interface may be part of the gas-collecting assembly in a breathing system, incorporated into a ventilator, or a separate device. It should be situated as close to the gas-collecting assembly as possible, preferably on the anesthesia machine, and where it can be readily observed and reached by anesthesia personnel.

There are three basic elements to an interface: positive pressure relief, negative pressure relief, and reservoir capacity. Irrespective of what type of disposal system is used, positive pressure relief must be provided to protect the equipment and patient if occlusion of the scavenging system occurs. If an active disposal system is used, negative pressure relief is needed to limit subatmospheric pressure. A reservoir is necessary to match the intermittent flow from the gas-collecting assembly to the continuous flow of the disposal system. A device that gives an audible signal may be fitted to the interface to indicate operation of the positive or negative pressure relief device. A flow indicator may be provided to monitor flow from the interface to the gas-disposal assembly (Fig. 12.5).

The reservoir may be a rigid container, wide tubing, a bag, or a combination of these. A distensible bag allows monitoring of the scavenging system. It should only be used with active disposal systems and should be of a different color from, and situated away from, the reservoir bag in the breathing system.

Interfaces can be divided into two types: open and closed, depending on the means to provide positive and negative pressure relief.

Open Interface (215–217)

An open interface (air break receiver unit) is open to atmosphere (allowing positive and negative pressure relief) and contains no valves. It should be used only with an active disposal system.

Because the discharge of waste gases is usually intermittent and flow through an active disposal assembly is continuous, a reservoir is needed to hold the surges of gas that enter the interface at an inflow greater than the disposal system flow until the disposal system removes them. The reservoir allows the flow rate in the disposal system to be kept just above the average, rather than at the peak flow rate of gases from the gas-collecting assembly.

It is important that the reservoir have adequate capacity, especially if a ventilator in which the driving gas mixes with waste gases is used or if high tidal volumes or high nitrous oxide flows are used (218). If a large amount of turbulence occurs, leakage into the atmosphere can occur before the volume of excess gas entering the interface equals the reservoir volume (215).

The safety afforded by an open system depends on the patency of the vents to atmosphere so it is good to have redundancy in case some are accidentally blocked (219, 220). Regular checking and cleaning of the vents are also necessary.

With an open interface, it is important that the inlet for waste gases, the disposal system connection, and the opening to atmosphere be arranged so that waste gases are removed preferentially before room air is entrained.

T-piece (221). An example of a simple type of open interface, known as a T tube, is shown in Figure 12.4A. One limb of the T attaches to the transfer means with the side limb leading to the active disposal system. The third limb of the T is fitted with a piece of tubing that serves as a reservoir. Surges of gases flowing out of the transfer means flow partly into the disposal system and partly into the reservoir tubing. They can then be removed from the reservoir by the disposal system.

As long as the free end of the reservoir remains open to atmosphere there is no danger that significant negative or positive pressure will be applied

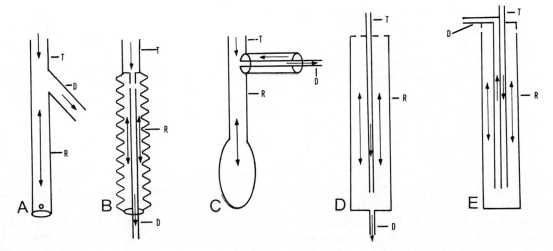

FIGURE 12.4. Open interfaces. **A,** T-tube interface. Note the escape-inlet hole near the free end of the reservoir tubing. **B,** Tube-within-a-tube interface. **C,** Tube-within-a-tube interface with distensible bag for monitoring efficiency of scavenging. **D,** Tube-within-a-tube with the escape holes at top. **E,** Two parallel tubes are inside the canister, which acts as a reservoir. Gases from the breathing system travel down in one and are removed by suction applied to the other tube. The relief ports provide positive and negative pressure relief. *T,* transfer means; *R,* reservoir; *D,* active disposal system. (Partly redrawn from a drawing furnished by Boehringer Laboratories, Inc.)

to the breathing system. It is important that a guard be placed at the free end to prevent occlusion or that holes be provided near the end (see Fig. 12.4A) so that an opening to atmosphere is still present if the end of the tubing is occluded.

Tube-within-a-tube. A second type of open interface, known as the tube-within-a-tube (or coaxial), is shown in Figure 12.4B. It consists of two coaxial tubes. The proximal end of the inner tube is open to the outer tube and the distal end is connected to the active disposal device. The outer tube is connected to the transfer means proximally and the distal end is open to atmosphere. A variation of this is shown in Figure 12.4C. A distensible bag has been added so that the adequacy of scavenging can be monitored.

Another variation of this type of open interface is shown in Figure 12.4D. Anesthetic gases from the transfer means enter at the top and are conducted to the base where they are dispersed by wire mesh. The mesh acts as a silencer, reducing the hiss generated by flow into the disposal tubing (222). Suction is applied to the base, and this serves to remove the gases. Gases are stored in the reservoir between exhalations. The holes at the top are open to atmosphere.

A commonly used open interface is shown in Figures 12.4E and Figure 12.5. Gases from the transfer tubing enter at the top and travel to the base in a tube. A parallel tube is connected at the top to the active disposal system. The space around both tubes acts as a reservoir. Holes at the top are open to atmosphere.

The open interface is simple but is fraught with the danger of polluting the atmosphere should the reservoir not have sufficient volume to contain the boluses of waste gases. Turbulence will increase with the size of the reservoir, which contains air contaminated with anesthetic gases (215). Turbulence is greatest when gases from the breathing system flow against the disposal system flow and least when flow is in the same direction. In addition, anesthesia staff may forget to turn on the suction to evacuate gases.

Closed Interfaces

In a closed interface the connection(s) with the atmosphere are through valve(s). A positive pressure relief valve is always required to allow release of gases into the room if there is obstruction of the

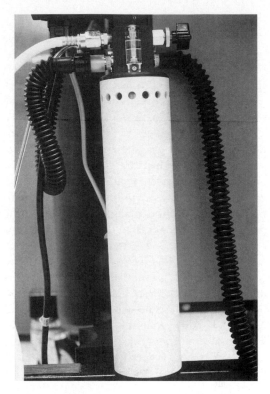

FIGURE 12.5. Open interface. The open ports in the reservoir provide positive and negative pressure relief. The adjustable needle valve regulates the suction flow. The flowmeter indicates whether or not the suction flow is within the range recommended by the manufacturer. The float should be between the two lines on the flowmeter. There are connections for transfer tubing on either side. Inside the canister one tube conducts waste gases to the bottom. Another tube conducts gases from the bottom of the canister to suction (see Fig. 12.3E)

scavenging system downstream of the interface. If an active disposal system is to be used, a negative pressure relief valve (dumping valve, pop-in valve, inlet relief valve) is necessary to allow entrainment of air when the pressure falls below atmospheric.

A reservoir is not required with a closed interface and should not be used unless an active disposal system is used, in which case a distensible bag is useful for monitoring the functioning of the scavenging system.

Positive pressure relief only. A closed interface with only positive pressure relief should be used only with passive disposal systems. An example is

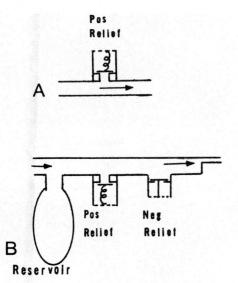

FIGURE 12.6. Closed interfaces. **A,** Without reservoir or negative relief device; for use with passive disposal systems only. **B,** With reservoir bag and negative pressure relief valve; for use with either a passive or active disposal system. If an active disposal system is used, the bag will be collapsed, except during periods of high flow from the gas collection assembly, and inadequate outflow will be indicated by bag distention.

shown in Figure 12.6A. The positive pressure relief valve remains closed unless there is a problem downstream of the interface. The device may be spring loaded or work by gravity.

Positive and negative pressure relief. If an active disposal system is used, a negative pressure relief valve must be present. Subatmospheric pressures greater than -0.5 H_2O water can raise or lower the opening pressure of some APL valves (223).

Examples of this type of closed interface are shown in Figures 12.6B and Figure 12.7. When a passive disposal system is used, the negative pressure relief will remain closed at all times. If an active disposal system is used, it should close during high peak flow rates from the gas-collecting assembly and open when the gas-disposal assembly flow is greater than the flow of gases from the gas-collecting assembly.

The rate of flow into the gas-disposal assembly should be adjusted to the optimal level by observing the bag (if present) and the positive and negative relief valves. In an optimally adjusted system,

the bag should expand and deflate and never become overextended or completely deflated (224, 225, 226). If the bag is continually collapsed or the negative pressure relief valve opens frequently, the flow should be lowered. If the bag becomes distended or the positive pressure relief valve opens frequently, flow should be increased.

A closed interface can be used with any type of disposal system but valves add to the complexity. They must be designed so that they do not stick or leak. Interfaces with two negative pressure relief valves are available and add a margin of safety.

Gas-Disposal Assembly Tubing

The gas-disposal assembly tubing (receiving hose, disposal tubing) connects the interface to the disposal assembly (see Fig. 12.1). It should be different in size and appearance from the breathing system hoses to avoid misconnections. It should be resistant to collapse and free of leaks. With a passive gas-disposal assembly it is important that the hose be as short and wide as practical to minimize resistance.

Ideally, the gas-disposal tubing should be run overhead to minimize the risk of occlusion and to avoid the dangers of personnel tripping over it or other apparatus becoming entangled in it. Should the disposal point be a significant distance from the anesthesia machine or the tubing obstruct personnel or equipment movement, it may be hidden in a false ceiling (185). If the tubing must be run across the floor, it should be routed where it is least likely to be stepped on or have equipment rolled onto it. If it must pass a doorway, it should follow the door frame.

Gas-Disposal Assembly

The gas-disposal assembly (elimination system or route, disposal-exhaust route, disposal system) contains the components used to remove waste gases from the anesthetizing location. The gases must be vented at a point that is isolated from personnel and any air intakes.

Disposal assemblies are of two types: active, in which a flow-inducing device moves the gases, and passive, in which the pressure is raised above atmospheric by the patient exhaling, manual squeezing of the reservoir bag, or a ventilator. With an active system there will be a negative pressure in the gas

FIGURE 12.7. Closed interface. There are three inlet ports to accommodate evacuation from an adjustable pressure-limiting (APL) valve and ventilator joined by a Y connection (**A**) and from another gas collection assembly (**B**). An adjustment knob for a needle valve to regulate suction flow is at top left (**C**). To the left is the suction tubing attachment. The reservoir bag (**D**) allows monitoring of the scavenging efficiency and permits adjustment of suction flow to the minimum necessary. **E** is a test button and **F** is the positive pressure relief. The negative pressure relief is below this. If a passive disposal system is used, the reservoir bag is removed and the mount capped. The needle valve is closed and a tubing is attached from **B** to the gas disposal system. (Courtesy of Ohmeda, a division of BOC Health Care, Inc.)

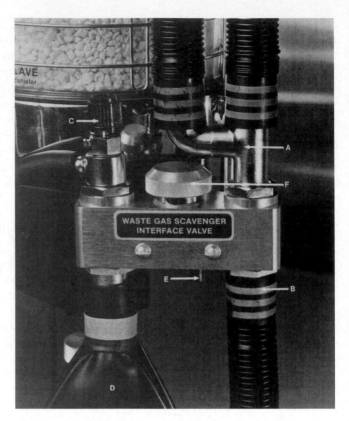

disposal tubing. With a passive system, the pressure will be positive.

Active systems are usually more effective in keeping pollution levels low, because most leaks will be inward (157, 227, 228). They have the advantage that small-bore gas-disposal tubing can be used and excessive resistance is not a problem. They also aid room air exchange. They are, however, expensive in terms of energy costs. They are not automatic and must be turned on and off. If they are not turned on, air pollution will occur; if they are not turned off, there will be needless waste of energy. Active systems are more complex than passive ones. Their use requires that the interface have negative pressure relief.

Passive systems are simpler, but may not be as effective in lowering trace gas levels, because the positive pressure encourages outward leaks. They are less expensive to operate than active systems.

Passive Systems

Room ventilation system (162, 185, 229, 230). Ventilation systems used in operating rooms are of two types: nonrecirculating (one-pass, single pass, 100% fresh air) and recirculating. In the proposed international standard the room ventilation system is classified as an active disposal system, because a powered device is used for removal. It has also been called assisted-passive (231).

A nonrecirculating system takes in exterior air and processes it by filtering and adjusting the humidity and temperature. The processed air is circulated through the room then all of it is exhausted to atmosphere. This type of ventilation system can be used for waste gas disposal by securing the disposal tubing to a convenient exhaust grill. Air flowing into the ventilation system will remove the gases from the room.

Concern for economy has lead to increased use of systems that recirculate air. With a recirculating system, a small amount of air is taken in from the atmosphere. Most of the gases exhausted from the room are shunted back into the intake and recirculated, while a volume of circulated air equal to the fresh air is exhausted. With this type of system waste gases must be vented beyond the point of recirculation.

The hospital engineer should know which type of ventilation system is present. If not, absence of recirculation can be determined by sampling the room air inlet to see if it is free of trace gases after they have been released in another room.

An important consideration in using the room ventilation system for waste gas disposal is the increase in negative pressure downstream in the exhaust duct, away from the grille. If the waste gases are introduced at the exhaust grille, the negative pressure is usually low and its effect negligible (219). If waste gases are introduced at a distance downstream in the duct (as they must be with a recirculating system), negative pressure relief must be provided in the interface.

Using the room ventilation system is economical because an existing structure is used and no expenditure of energy is necessary. It is automatic, so there is no need to turn anything on or off or make adjustments.

In many operating rooms, the exhaust grilles are not located close to the anesthesia machine. Tubing should not lie on the floor because this increases the risk of occlusion. In some cases, the disposal tubing can be extended to a wall- or ceiling-mounted connection that leads to a pipe in the wall (162). The pipe connects to the exhaust duct, preferably near the exhaust grille to avoid excessive negative pressure.

Piping direct to atmosphere (227, 232). Piping direct to the atmosphere is also known as a direct duct or vent, specialized duct system, direct disposal line, and through-the-wall system. With this system, excess gases are vented through the wall, window, ceiling, or floor to the outside, using only the slight pressure of the gases leaving the gas-collecting assembly to provide the flow. To prevent cross-flow between rooms, each room should have its own duct.

The inlet to the system in each room should be close to the anesthesia machine. There should be a means to cap the opening to the duct when it is not connected to the gas-disposal tubing. The duct should be constructed of a material resistant to anesthetic gases and should be relatively short and of large diameter if excessive back pressure is to be avoided. This type of system is not suitable for an operating room far from an outside wall (219). A unidirectional valve may be placed in the duct to prevent outside air from entering the operating room and to minimize the effects of wind pressure on the disposal system (233). The duct should be inclined so that water will not accumulate.

The discharge point on the outside should be selected so that it is away from wind pressures, ignition hazards, windows, and the inlets for the ventilation system. It may be advantageous to attach a short T piece as a terminal (234). The open end(s) should point downward to minimize the entry of water and dirt and be fitted with netting to prevent insects, rodents, and foreign matter from entering the pipe.

Such a disposal assembly is easy to use, but requires a special installation. In redesigning an existing operating room or designing a new room, construction of a separate scavenging system should be considered. If the operating rooms are not near the outside of the building, this type of disposal assembly may not be practical.

Problems that can occur with this system include both positive and negative pressure caused by wind currents, obstruction from ice buildup (235), and accumulation of foreign matter at the outlet. There needs to be a means to determine the patency of the system. It is important to do trace gas monitoring under conditions of use with this system, to make sure a flow-inducing device is not needed.

Adsorption device (160, 236–244). An adsorption device removes some or all excess anesthetic agents by adsorbing them or converting them to harmless substances. Canisters of varying shape and capacity filled with activated charcoal have been used as waste gas disposal assemblies. The effectiveness of individual canisters and various brands of charcoal vary widely (236, 237). Some can be regenerated by autoclaving (245). Different volatile agents are adsorbed with varying efficiency. The efficiency of adsorption also depends on the rate of flow through the canister (246). Moisture may reduce the efficacy of adsorption (247).

Charcoal canisters have the advantages of being simple and portable and not requiring expensive installation or maintenance. An additional advantage is that halogenated anesthetic vapors are not released to the ozone layer (246).

They also have a number of disadvantages. At present, there is no adsorption device for removal of nitrous oxide. They are fairly expensive and effective for only relatively short periods of time. They must be replaced regularly and pose problems of storage and disposal. Determination that the adsorber is saturated requires continuous monitoring or weighing of the adsorber. Finally, a large canister may impose significant resistance (236).

It is recommended that use of these devices be limited to situations in which nitrous oxide is not being employed and no other means of eliminating waste gases is available.

Active Systems

Piped vacuum (185, 221, 248). The central vacuum system is a popular method for gas disposal because no new equipment or installation is required. The system should be capable of providing high volume (30 l/min) flow, but only slight negative pressure is needed. There should be a means to allow the user to control the suction flow (see Figs. 12.5 and 12.7). This will conserve energy, cut down the wear and tear on the central pumps, and reduce the noise level in the room. For some units, this is done by observing the bag and the positive and negative pressure relief valves. Others have a means to allow the user to adjust the flow to that recommended by the manufacturer (see Fig. 12.5). A restrictive orifice may be placed in the suction nipple to limit the flow (249).

There are a number of problems associated with use of a central piped vacuum system for scavenging.

INADEQUATE NUMBER OF OUTLETS Many operating rooms have only two suction outlets. This is barely enough for some surgical procedures, let alone anesthesia requirements. Ideally, anesthesia personnel should have two suction outlets available, one for suctioning the airway and one for scavenging waste gases.

If there are not enough outlets, a Y may be inserted into the suction line to create two lines. Unfortunately, this may reduce the flow so that it is inadequate for either purpose.

Some anesthesia providers use a single suction line for scavenging and patient suctioning. The suction line remains attached to the interface most of the time and is detached when needed for patient suctioning. If the flow of anesthesia gases is not turned off, there will be escape of anesthetic gases into the room air.

INCONVENIENT OUTLETS If a suction outlet is not near the anesthesia machine, long tubings must reach across the floor, with the dangers of occlusion, tripping of personnel, and entanglement with other apparatus.

OVERLOAD OF THE SYSTEM Because scavenging requires high flows, it is possible to overload the central vacuum system if too many devices are in use at once. Overcoming this problem may require a major renovation of the system. The drain can be reduced if anesthesia personnel will adjust the flow down to that necessary to prevent spillage of gases into room air and turn off the suction after use.

DAMAGE TO THE SUCTION PUMP Wear and tear on the suction pump can be expected to increase if the central vacuum system is used for disposal of waste gases. Widespread use of central vacuum systems for disposal of anesthetic gases and the paucity of reports of problems suggest that this is not a great problem.

PERSONNEL EXPOSURE If the exhaust from the central vacuum pump goes to an area frequented by personnel or is situated near an air intake, open window, or door, use of the system for gas disposal will result in additional exposure of personnel to waste gases. It may be necessary to relocate the pump exhaust.

INCONVENIENCE To conserve energy, the suction system should be turned on just before anesthesia is begun and turned off at the termination of a procedure. For further energy conservation, the anesthesia provider should regulate the suction flow according to the volume of waste gases. These extra duties may be neglected and there will be either wasted energy or operating room pollution.

Active duct system (219, 227, 250–252). The other type of active disposal assembly is a dedicated duct system that leads to the outside and employs flow-inducing devices (fans, pumps, blowers, etc.) that can move large volumes of gas at low pressures. Each operating room is supplied with a duct, two or three of which are connected together to a common duct that leads outside. The flow-inducing device is located in the common duct and provides movement of gases at a low negative pressure. Balancing dampers should be provided to prevent pressure imbalances from developing between the operating rooms that are connected to the system (223, 252). The negative pressure ensures that cross-contamination between operating rooms will not occur and prevents atmospheric conditions from affecting the outflow from the system. It has been recommended that two flow-inducing devices be provided and arranged so that if one fails the second one will run. It is recommended that there be a means to indicate to the user that the scavenging system is operational. The outlet to atmosphere must be away from windows and ventilation intakes. A means to adjust the flow may be incorporated into the common duct.

A station inlet for excess anesthetic gases may be installed in an operating room. It should not be interchangeable with other systems, including the medical-surgical vacuum system. The piping system for such a system is covered in NFPA 96 (252). Labeling is required on the network and at least once in or above each room and story traversed by the piping.

The advantages of this system are that resistance is not a problem and wind currents do not affect the system.

Disadvantages include those of any active system: added complexity and the need for negative pressure relief and reservoir capacity in the interface. It requires a special installation, which should be considered during renovation or when a new operating room is being designed. Installing such a system is fairly expensive. The flow-inducing device means added energy consumption and requires regular maintenance.

Work Practices (9, 253–256)

A number of work practices allow anesthetic gases to enter room air. Most of this pollution can be prevented. Trace gas monitoring can be used to demonstrate to personnel the techniques needed to avoid pollution.

Adherence to the following practices will significantly reduce contamination. Most can be followed without compromising safety and some of them are beneficial to the patient. However, adherence to them should not distract from the comfort and safety of the patient. For example, in pediatric anesthesia, leakage of anesthetic agents around uncuffed tracheal tubes may be needed to avoid trauma to the trachea and holding the mask tightly against the face may be frightening to a child.

Checking before Use

Before starting an anesthetic, secure connection and lack of occlusion of all components of the scavenging system should be verified. If an active gas disposal assembly is to be used, the flow should be turned on.

Nitrous oxide should be turned on only momentarily during preuse checkout of equipment. All other tests should be conducted using oxygen.

Using Scavenging Equipment

Failure to use available scavenging equipment correctly is commonplace (257, 258). In some cases, the reasons relate to equipment design and difficulty in scavenging in specific circumstances. Commonly, however, lack of concern is the problem.

Proper Mask Fit

Obtaining a good mask fit requires skill but is critical to maintain low levels of anesthetic gases in the room, especially during assisted or controlled ventilation, when higher pressures will magnify the leak between the patient and the mask. Anesthesia by face mask causes the highest levels of pollution (213, 259). Lower levels are found with the laryngeal mask airway (259, 260). Most investigators have found it difficult to keep trace anesthetic levels within safe limits unless the face mask was strapped extremely tightly (261, 262).

Reduction of high levels of anesthetic gases associated with poor mask fit can be reduced by placing an active scavenging device near the mask (184, 214, 263) or using a double mask (264, 265).

Prevention of Flow from the Breathing System into Room Air

Nitrous oxide or a vaporizer should not be turned on until the mask is fitted to the patient's face or the patient is intubated and connected to the breathing system. Nitrous oxide and vaporizers should be turned off when not in use. Turning the gas flow off, but leaving the vaporizer on, may also be a good practice (266).

Disconnections can be prevented by making certain that all connections are tight before use. An airway pressure monitor (see Chapter 19, "Airway Pressure, Volume, and Flow Measurements") will aid in early detection of disconnections. Nonessential disconnections for activities such as taping the tracheal tube or positioning the patient should be kept to a minimum. If it is necessary to make a disconnection, release of anesthetic gases into the room can be minimized if the reservoir bag is first emptied (gradually rather than violently dumping it) into the scavenging system and all flowmeters turned off. Alternately, the patient port can be occluded and the APL valve opened so that the gases will enter the scavenging system (267–269). If a ventilator (which has its own spill valve) is being used, the APL valve need not be opened. Keeping the mask pointed floorward next to the patient's head will result in slightly lower levels (268).

Washout of Anesthetic Gases at the End of a Case

At the end of a case, 100% oxygen should be administered before extubation or removal of the face mask, to flush most of the anesthetic gases into the scavenging system.

Prevention of Liquid Agent Spillage

It is easy to spill liquid agent when filling a vaporizer, so care should be exercised. Use of a pin-indexed vaporizer (see Chapter 5, "Vaporizers") will reduce spillage. Close scavenging will reduce contamination associated with filling and draining of vaporizers (213).

The connections for filling and draining a vaporizer must be kept tight. If one or the other is loose agent may escape (270).

Keeping Keyed Filler on the Bottle

There is less loss of agent if the keyed filler remains on the bottle after a vaporizer is filled (271). However, this may present storage problems.

Avoidance of Certain Techniques

Insufflation techniques in which an anesthetic mixture is introduced into the patient's respiratory system on inhalation are still used for laryngoscopy and bronchoscopy (272, 273). High flow rates are required to avoid dilution with room air and result in a cloud of anesthetic gases escaping into the room air.

Proper Use of Tracheal Tubes

Cuffed tracheal tubes should always be used in adults and the cuff inflated until there is no leak. Only small leaks should be permitted around uncuffed tubes in pediatric patients. Reduction of contamination with an uncuffed tube can be achieved by placing a suction catheter in the mouth (274, 275) and using a throat pack (276).

Disconnection of Nitrous Oxide Sources

Nitrous oxide and oxygen pipeline hoses leading to the machine should be disconnected at the end of the operating schedule. The disconnection should be made as close to the terminal unit as possible and not at the back of the anesthesia machine, so that if there is a leak in the hose, no gases will escape to room air while the hose is disconnected. This will result in lower levels of nitrous oxide in the operating room and will conserve gases.

When cylinders are used, the cylinder valve should be closed at the end of the operating schedule. Gas remaining in the machine should be "bled out" and evacuated through the scavenging system.

Use of Low Fresh Gas Flows (277–279)

Use of low fresh gas flows will reduce the volume of anesthetic gases added to the room by reducing the pollution resulting from disconnections in the breathing system and from inefficient scavenging. It also allows use of low removal flows with active disposal assemblies, resulting in energy conservation and reduced wear and tear on the disposal device. Use of low flows does not make scavenging unnecessary, because high flows must still be used at times.

Use of Intravenous Agents and Regional Anesthesia

Use of an intravenous induction technique significantly reduces trace gas exposure (280).

Keeping Scavenging Hoses off the Floor

Scavenging hoses on the floor can be obstructed by equipment rolling over it, reducing scavenging.

Action by Post-Anesthesia Care Unit Personnel

Post-anesthesia personnel should breathe off to the side or well above the patient's head (256).

Leakage Control (9, 171, 253, 255, 256, 281–283)

Leakage of gases from equipment may account for 2.5 to 87% of total contamination (284). Some leakage is unavoidable, but it should be minimized. Control of leakage may require replacement of equipment that cannot be made gas tight.

Most anesthesia machines are under contract to undergo servicing at regular intervals. Unfortunately, this servicing does not always identify or correct all leak points. In addition, leakage in some equipment develops fairly frequently so that quarterly servicing is not sufficient. In-house monitoring and maintenance are necessary to minimize leakage.

Initially, elimination of significant leakage will take a fair amount of time and effort, but following this, anesthesia equipment can usually be maintained in an acceptable state with a minimum of effort. It is recommended that one individual supervise leakage control.

Pressure Terminology

Some literature on scavenging has referred to all equipment upstream of the flow control valves as the high-pressure system and all equipment between the flow control valves and the patient plus the scavenging equipment as the low-pressure system (255, 285, 286). However, older terminology established by the National Fire Protection Association defines high pressure as more than 200 psig.

In this book, the high-pressure system refers to those components that contain gas whose pressure is normally above 50 psig (340 kPa). This includes the components between the cylinder and the regulator. The intermediate-pressure system includes components normally subjected to a pressure of approximately 50 psig. This includes the hospital pipeline pipes and hoses and the components of the machine between the regulators or pipeline inlets and the flow control valves. The low-pressure system consists of components downstream of the flow control valves to the patient, plus the scavenging system. Pressures in this system vary, but seldom exceed 40 cm H_2O.

Identification of Leak Sites

Once it has been determined that significant leakage exists, there are several techniques for locating the leak sites. A continuous infrared nitrous oxide analyzer can be used. The equipment under test is pressurized with nitrous oxide and the sampling probe directed at suspected leak sites. The meter reading indicates the presence or absence of leakage. This will identify most leaks. An exception would be leakage in a vaporizer. Use of an infrared analyzer may be the only way to find leakage in complicated pieces of equipment such as ventilators.

Leak sites can be identified by application of a solution of 50% liquid soap and 50% water or a commercial leak test solution to a piece of equipment under pressure. Leakage will be revealed by bubbling.

Leakage can be assessed by testing the capacity of the equipment to sustain pressurization. The total leak rate for a system is determined, after which a component of the system is excluded and the leak rate redetermined. The difference is the leak rate for that piece of equipment.

High-Pressure System

To test for leakage in the high-pressure system, the pipeline hoses should be disconnected and the flow control valves closed. The valve on a nitrous oxide cylinder should be opened fully, the pressure recorded, and the cylinder valve closed. The pressure should be recorded again 1 hour later. If little or no pressure drop has occurred, there is no significant leakage. If it falls, the high-pressure system is not tight. The test should be repeated with the other nitrous oxide cylinder if there is a double yoke.

If significant leakage is found, the most common site is the yoke, and application of a leak test solution will demonstrate a poor seal. Tightening the cylinder in its yoke will often seal off the leak. Other easily correctable causes include double, absent, or deformed washers. If found, these should be replaced. If fixing these problems does not cause the pressure to hold, the leak is inside the machine and must be corrected by the manufacturer's service representative.

Because leakage in this area does not occur often, checking every 2 to 4 months and after a cylinder has been changed should be sufficient (175, 253, 255).

Intermediate-Pressure System

Leakage in intermediate-pressure system components can be determined by measuring the nitrous oxide concentrations in the operating room when no anesthesia is being administered (255). The survey should be begun at least 1 hour after administration of anesthesia has been discontinued. If a recirculating air-conditioning system is in use, a longer period may be required. The early morning is an excellent time to perform this test.

Flow control valves should be closed, pipeline hoses connected, and cylinder valves closed. Any of the area sampling and monitoring methods (dosimetry, grab samples in bags or cartridges, or infrared [IR] analysis) can be used. Room air should be sampled from the anesthesia breathing zone (4 to 5 feet above the floor within 3 feet of the front of the anesthesia machine) and the room air intake and outlet. Nitrous oxide concentrations should be less than 5 ppm (8, 204). If a higher level is found, the pipeline hoses should be disconnected and the measurements repeated. If a high level is still present, this indicates a leak in the nitrous oxide pipe leading into the room or the station outlet and should be reported to the hospital engineer. If the level falls, this indicates a leak in the pipeline hose or the anesthesia machine.

Common problems with pipeline hoses include worn or broken connections, loose connections (especially quick-connects), deformed compression fittings, and holes. These should be corrected or the hoses replaced. Leaks inside the anesthesia machine require correction by a service representative.

Once leakage is corrected, it is suggested that testing of the intermediate pressure system be performed every 2 to 4 months (171, 204, 253, 255).

Low-Pressure System

The low-pressure portion of the system develops leaks more frequently than other parts. The preuse test for leaks in the breathing system (described in Chapter 26, "Equipment Checking and Maintenance") is sufficient for the safe conduct of anesthesia yet can miss leaks that emit large amounts of anesthetic gases into room air.

One way to quantify leakage in most of the low-pressure system is shown in Figure 12.8. The breathing system is assembled as for clinical use. Components that are normally used should be present in their usual positions. The patient port is occluded. The bag is removed and the bag mount occluded. This is necessary because the bag's compliance makes it hard to quantitate low leak rates. The bag should be tested separately for leaks by pressurization. A vaporizer on the anesthesia machine should be turned on. The APL valve should be fully open and the scavenging system occluded upstream of the interface. The oxygen flow control valve is now opened sufficiently to establish and maintain a steady pressure of 30 cm H_2O on the pressure gauge in the breathing system. The flow on the oxygen flowmeter is the leak rate and should be less than 1000 ml/min (287). Leakage of 1000 ml/minute of nitrous oxide would result in a mean concentration of only 30 ppm in a 4000 cubic foot room with 15 air changes per hour (223). The leakage test should be repeated with other vaporizers on the machine turned on.

If the leak rate exceeds 1000 ml/min, the APL valve should be closed and the leak rate redetermined. The difference is the leak rate in the scavenging system. The remaining leakage can be divided into that associated with the machine and that associated with the breathing system by attaching a sphygmomanometer bulb to the common gas outlet of the anesthesia machine and determining the oxygen flow necessary to achieve and maintain a pressure of 30 cm H_2O (22 mm Hg). This is the portion of the low-pressure leak-

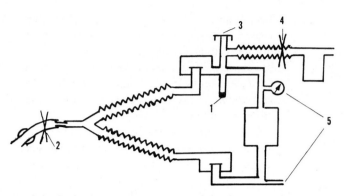

FIGURE 12.8. Test for quantifying low-pressure leakage. *1*, The reservoir bag is removed and the bag mount is occluded. *2*, The patient port is occluded. *3*, The adjustable pressure-limiting (APL) valve is opened fully. *4*, The transfer means is occluded just upstream of the interface. *5*, Oxygen flow is turned on and adjusted to maintain a pressure of 30 cm H_2O on pressure gauge in breathing system.

age associated with the machine. The machine leakage can be further divided by turning off the vaporizer and redetermining the leak rate.

Problems in the scavenging system may be as simple as a crack in a tubing (especially where it becomes kinked) or a poor connection.

The breathing system is the most common location of significant low-pressure leakage, and the most common site in the breathing system is the absorber. Common causes include defective gaskets or seals, improper closure, inadequate tightening, and open or leaking drain cocks. Absorbent on the gaskets can prevent a tight seal. Many of these problems are easily corrected. Complicated repairs should be done by the manufacturer's representative.

Domes over unidirectional valves may become cracked or loose and should be replaced or tightened. Fittings for oxygen analyzer sensors that leak should be replaced.

The above test does not check for leakage in the ventilator. The ventilator and the low-pressure system can be tested using an IR nitrous oxide analyzer. The anesthesia machine and breathing system are set up as for clinical use. The patient port outlet is occluded and the bag-ventilator selector switch is put in the bag mode. The APL valve is closed. Using the flowmeters, the breathing system is pressurized to 30 cm H_2O with a 50% mixture of nitrous oxide and oxygen. The machine and breathing system are scanned for nitrous oxide leakage. The selector valve is then put in the ventilator mode and the flowmeters set to deliver 2 l/min oxygen and 2 l/min nitrous oxide. The ventilator is turned on and set to a tidal volume such that a peak pressure of 30 cm H_2O is

reached, with an I:E ratio of 0.5 at a rate of 10 to 20 breaths per minute. The scavenger system is activated. The machine, ventilator, breathing system, and scavenging system are scanned. Readings should not be greater than 25 ppm nitrous oxide.

How often the low-pressure system should be tested for leakage is controversial. Suggested intervals vary from daily (204, 253), to every other week (255) to monthly (171). It should be repeated with new equipment and when the absorbent is changed.

Room Ventilation System (284, 288–290)

The room ventilation system serves as an important adjunct to trace gas control by diluting and removing anesthetic gases resulting from leaks, errors in technique, and scavenging system malfunctions. The American Society of Heating, Refrigerating and Air-Conditioning Engineers recommends 25 air changes per hour for recirculating systems and 15 air changes for nonrecirculating systems (256).

Recirculating systems are less effective in removing trace gases than nonrecirculating systems. A downward displacement ventilation system is more effective than a turbulent flow system (158, 287).

The anesthesia machine should be placed as close to the exhaust grille as possible. This will ensure maximum removal of gases by the ventilation system and make it easy to use the ventilation system as the gas-disposal assembly. This should be taken into consideration when constructing a new operating room or renovating an older one.

HAZARDS OF SCAVENGING EQUIPMENT

Misassembly

Misconnections involving the scavenging system are not uncommon (291). Most scavenging components have 19- or 30-mm connections rather than the 15- and 22-mm sizes found in breathing systems. This will not completely prevent misconnections because there may be another apparatus in the room that will accept 19- or 30-mm connections (284). The safety potential provided by 19- and 30-mm connectors can be bypassed by using cheater adapters or tape for making connections.

Connection of a circle system hose to the outlet of the APL valve has been reported (168, 169, 292, 293). Measures to prevent this include turning the exhaust port of the gas-collecting assembly so it points in the opposite direction from the breathing system ports, use of transfer and gas-disposal hoses of different colors and/or configurations from breathing system hoses, and using either 19- or 30-mm connections in the scavenging system.

Pressure Alterations in the Breathing System

The scavenging system extends the breathing system all the way to the disposal point. When a scavenging system malfunctions or is misused, positive or negative pressure can be transmitted to the breathing system, with potential harm to the patient.

Measures to prevent these untoward incidents include employing a collapse-proof material in all disposal lines, making the transfer means easy to disconnect, using scavenging tubing that has a distinctive appearance, incorporation of positive and negative pressure relief mechanisms in the interface (and regular checking of these for proper functioning), and use of airway pressure monitors (see Chapter 19, "Airway Pressure, Volume, and Flow Measurements").

Positive Pressure

Positive pressure in the scavenging system can result from occlusion of the gas disposal assembly, transfer tubing, or gas-disposal assembly by a wheel of an anesthesia machine (169, 294, 295), ice (235), insects, water, or other foreign matter. Another cause is defective components (296). Misassembly of the connection to the exhaust grille (297), and failure to include an opening between the inner and outer tubes of a tube-within-a-tube interface (298) have been reported.

These malfunctions may not result in a pressure buildup if a positive pressure relief mechanism is incorporated into the interface. However, the positive pressure relief mechanism may be incorrectly assembled, may not open at a low pressure, or may be blocked (299). Obstruction or misconnection of the transfer means may occur (300–304). Because these problems are on the patient side of the interface, disconnection of the transfer means from the gas-collecting assembly may be necessary to prevent a dangerous increase in pressure. In one reported case, kinking of the transfer means caused back pressure to develop in the gas jacket of an extracorporeal oxygenator. This resulted in gas being forced into the blood (305).

Application of subatmospheric pressure to some APL valves can result in a buildup of positive pressure in the breathing system (298, 306). In one reported case, subatmospheric pressure in the scavenging system drew a ventilator relief valve diaphragm to its seat and closed the valve, resulting in a buildup of pressure in the system (307).

Negative Pressure

In systems with an active disposal assembly, there is the danger that subambient pressure will be applied to the breathing system. Monitoring expired volumes (but not airway pressure) may fail to detect a disconnection in the breathing system because the scavenging system may draw a considerable flow of room air through the expiratory pathway (308, 309).

Gas can be evacuated from the breathing system if the APL valve in the breathing system allows gas to be drawn through it at a pressure less than that needed to open the negative pressure valve on the interface (310, 311). This can be overcome by partially closing the APL valve (312), increasing the fresh gas flow, or lowering the flow in the gas disposal assembly.

A malfunction of the negative pressure relief

mechanism may occur. In one case, the valve disc became stuck in the closed position (313). In other cases, the valve was covered by a plastic bag so that air could not be entrained (314, 315). In still another case, the opening to atmosphere of an open interface was taped over (299). Blockage of the opening to atmosphere as a result of dust and other material has been reported (316). Another problem is using an interface for a passive system (which has no means to prevent development of a subatmospheric pressure) in an active scavenging system (301). With some scavenging systems that use a central vacuum system a restrictive orifice is incorporated into the vacuum hose fitting to limit the evacuation of gas, regardless of the pressure applied by the central vacuum source (249). Should this orifice be omitted or become damaged, full vacuum would be applied to the interface and the capacity of the negative pressure relief mechanism could be exceeded.

Means to prevent these problems include provision of one or more negative relief mechanisms in the interface with an active disposal system (317), adjustment of gas disposal assembly flow to the minimum necessary, and protection of the openings to atmosphere from accidental occlusion.

Loss of Means of Monitoring

Use of a scavenging system may mask the strong odor of an inhalation anesthetic, delaying recognition of an overdose (300, 318). Increasing use of agent monitoring should largely eliminate this problem.

Adding a gas-collecting assembly to an APL valve has the effect of silencing it, thereby removing one means of monitoring a patient's ventilation. The sounds emitted by a mechanical ventilator can be altered when scavenging lines are attached.

Ventilator Function Disruption

A case has been reported in which negative pressure from the scavenging interface prevented the bellows of a ventilator from collapsing when a disconnection in the breathing system occurred (319). The low airway pressure alarm in the ventilator was not activated.

Noise Pollution

The gas scavenging system can be a significant cause of noise in anesthetizing locations (320). This can have significant physiological and psychological effects.

MONITORING TRACE GASES
Rationale

Air monitoring is the best indicator of the success of a waste gas control program. It reflects how well leaks and errors in technique are being controlled plus the efficiency of the scavenging and room ventilation systems and documents that low trace levels are being maintained. Many anesthetic departments do not have their working areas monitored for anesthetic pollution in the belief that scavenging devices have solved the problem (321).

Monitoring is necessary because a scavenging system that appears adequate in design may perform inefficiently in use. Sites of gas leakage are diverse, frequently obscure and sometimes inaccessible (286). Even relatively large leaks may be inaudible. Nitrous oxide is odorless and the threshold for smelling potent agents such as halothane varies from 5 to 300 ppm (322, 323). Without monitoring, operating room personnel may be unaware that atmospheric contamination is at unacceptable levels. A properly conducted monitoring program provides a constructive method of reminding anesthesia personnel to avoid careless work habits. Another advantage of monitoring is that it can detect problems with delivery of gases to equipment (324).

Although such a program will increase a health care facility's operating expense, it will help to reduce the institution's liability to claims by employees alleging overexposure to waste gases. Also, correction of leakage in nitrous oxide lines will result in a savings to the facility.

In-House Versus Commercial
Laboratory (286)

The monitoring program should be directed by an interested and qualified person, preferably from the anesthesia department. Samples may be analyzed by either hospital-based personnel or outside commercial laboratories. Use of outside laboratories avoids the cost of purchasing, operating, maintaining, and calibrating a gas analyzer. The responsibility for record keeping is shared. The chief disadvantage is the delay in reporting results. The precise circumstances of sampling are likely to have been forgotten and the effect of corrective measures cannot be immediately assessed. In addition, analysis of a large number of samples is expensive.

Advantages of in-house analysis include a virtually unlimited number of analyses at modest cost and immediate on-site reporting. Leaks can be found quickly and the effectiveness of the correction assessed immediately. An on-site continuous monitor is useful for demonstrating the effects of technique errors on trace gas levels.

A small hospital might periodically lease an instrument or share one with other hospitals in the area rather than purchase its own.

Equipment for Determining Trace Gas Concentrations

Infrared Analyzers (286, 325)

Each anesthetic gas has a unique set of absorption peaks in the IR spectrum. In an infrared analyzer, a light beam of a certain wavelength is passed through a cell containing the sample to be analyzed. The concentration of the gas can be determined by measuring the amount of light absorbed. These monitors are the most practical for the average hospital because they are reliable, relatively inexpensive, and easy to use. They are very useful for locating leaks, especially those in unusual locations. They give continuous measurements so that exposed personnel and those responsible for air monitoring are given an immediate reading. When operated on battery power, a number of locations can be sampled quickly. A recording attachment may be helpful.

These instruments are most often used for monitoring nitrous oxide concentrations. Unfortunately, carbon dioxide and water vapor in high concentrations will interfere with the analysis. This can be avoided by sampling 6 to 10 inches away from personnel (285). Analyzers capable of measuring halogenated anesthetics are available but have many technical difficulties; alcohols and other substances in the operating room cause interference (325–327).

Dosimeter (286)

Passive dosimeters measure the amount of nitrous oxide that diffuses into a molecular sieve. Analysis (usually by the manufacturer) requires extraction of the nitrous oxide.

Passive dosimeters have many advantages. They can give a time-weighted average concentration for as long as a month. They are convenient to use. They can be made lightweight and compact so that they can be worn for personal sampling.

A variant of the passive dosimeter is the gas cartridge sampler, which is actually a small container that is filled with a sample of operating room air and then sent to the laboratory for analysis.

Active dosimeters depend on energy outside of the absorbing medium to obtain the sample. A pump is used to take in gases that are then stored in a gas-tight bag in an absorbing medium. The samples are aspirated into an analyzer.

Ionizing Leak Detector (171, 328, 329)

The ionizing leak detector (leak meter) consists of three components: an electron capture detector housed within a hand piece and fitted with a probe; a control unit that processes the signal from the detector and displays the output on a meter; and a carrier gas supply. The instrument is compact, relatively inexpensive, portable, and can be operated on batteries.

It is suitable for measuring low concentrations of halogenated agents. However, there may be interference from other halogenated agents in the area, including antibiotic and skin-protection sprays. It is not useful for nitrous oxide detection. It is somewhat unstable in use, requiring frequent zeroing and recalibration (171, 288).

Thermocamera (330–332)

Because nitrous oxide has the ability to absorb IR light, it will absorb the light liberated by a heat screen. An IR camera with a filter allows visualization of dispersed or leaking nitrous oxide. It is sensitive to 100 ppm or more of nitrous oxide. This is not a quantitative meter and is primarily of use when constructing and evaluating scavenging equipment and in producing educational material.

Oxygen Analyzer

An oxygen monitor can be used to check the scavenging system. Using 100% oxygen the sensor is positioned at the interface where overflow would exit into the room. Any increase indicates that anesthetic gas will be released during normal use.

CO₂ Analyzer

The efficacy of scavenging with an open interface can be checked by analyzing the open end of the reservoir for CO_2 (216). If any of the patient's expired gases overflow, CO_2 will be detected.

Sampling Methods

Instantaneous Sampling

Instantaneous (grab, single-shot, periodic, snatch) sampling is performed by drawing a sample of air into a container and subsequently measuring the trace gas concentration. The container must not adsorb or absorb the contaminant or leak. Nylon bags are the preferred storage container when nitrous oxide levels are measured (333).

This method is relatively inexpensive, quick and simple to perform, and does not involve taking bulky equipment into the operating room, but it has some serious disadvantages. A long interval between sampling and reporting makes it difficult to remember the precise circumstances that were in effect when the sample was taken. The effect of corrective measures cannot be immediately assessed. It is of limited value in determining leak sites and assessing correction of leaks. Another serious disadvantage is that each sample represents the level at one location in a relatively small volume and over a very short time period. Failure to sample in the right place at the right time can produce low-exposure level results that are misleading (9). Similarly, a report of a high-exposure level may lead to costly corrective action when, in fact, the measured levels were only momentarily high. One investigation concluded that gradients in operating rooms were sufficiently large to invalidate estimation of personnel exposure from instantaneous samples (334). This disadvantage can be decreased by taking multiple samples, but this increases the expense.

The instantaneous sample is probably best employed for analysis of steady-state contamination, i.e., sampling before starting anesthesia for intermediate pressure leaks or when an equilibrium has been achieved. If good techniques are employed and leakage has been controlled, trace gas levels tend to rise in a fluctuating pattern during the early part of an anesthetic, then roughly equilibrate, reaching a level that represents the net effects of leaks, air conditioning, inflowing gas, scavenging efficiency and personnel movement (334). Under these circumstances an instantaneous sample 30 to 45 minutes after induction is probably a good index of the average trace gas levels (334, 204). If poor techniques are employed and/or no attempt has been made to eliminate leakage, pollution levels will vary markedly and instantaneous samples may be quite misleading. If unacceptably high levels are found, one cannot be sure whether the cause is a leak, poor technique, or a fault in the scavenging system.

When an instantaneous sample is taken, it is important to record the date and time of collection, the work practices (breathing system, fresh gas flow rate, use of mask or tracheal tube, use of ventilator, spontaneous or manually controlled ventilation), the sampling site, and the person administering anesthesia.

Time-Weighted Average Sampling

The toxicity of anesthetics is probably a function of both dose and exposure time. Hence, a method that gives an average exposure level during a period of time (an integrated sample) is of interest. Time-weighted average (TWA) sampling is also called integrated or time-integrated sampling.

TWA samples can be obtained using active dosimetry in which gases are pumped continuously over a period of time into an inert container (327, 335–337) or a tube or other device containing a sorbent (338–343).

Passive dosimetry, which depends on diffusion of gas into a molecular sieve, can be used to obtain time-weighted averages (344, 345). Small, rugged, lightweight dosimeters (diffusive samplers) are available (278, 344, 346). They are unobtrusive, easily attached, and require a minimum of maintenance (157). They must be uncapped at the beginning of each workday and capped at the end of the day (347). They can be used either as personal or area monitors for periods of up to 40 hours (346). They have been found to be quite accurate (344, 346, 348). Separate sampling media have to be used for nitrous oxide and the halogenated agents (2). However, more than one halogenated agent can be measured from one sampler.

Other ways of obtaining a time-weighted average are to average the results of many instantaneous samples, average the concentrations measured at equal time intervals throughout the recorded tracing of a continuous analyzer, and integrate the output of a continuous analyzer (349).

By eliminating errors due to temporal fluctuations, time-weighted average sampling reflects personnel exposure better than instantaneous sampling. It requires only a modest capital investment, and there is a considerable savings of time and labor compared with taking and analyzing multiple instantaneous samples.

There are several disadvantages to this method. One is that it does not help in leak detection or improving work techniques. Delayed results make it difficult to correlate with activities at the time of collection. If concentrations in excess of those recommended are found, one cannot tell whether the problem is technique errors, leaks, or inadequate scavenging.

Continuous Sampling

Continuous (direct-reading, real-time) monitoring is carried out using an infrared analyzer or leak meter. Use of a battery-powered instrument allows easy movement within and between rooms. If a writer is attached and the analyzer is run over a period of time, a time-weighted average sample is obtained (349).

A continuous monitor can be used to detect leaks (by probing about the machine, hoses, wall sockets, etc.) and to determine if a leak has been reduced or eliminated. Furthermore, a continuous analyzer operated while anesthesia is being administered can be used to demonstrate the effects of improper work habits on trace levels and the improvement from modifying those practices.

The convenience and immediate feedback of continuous monitoring are distinct advantages over instantaneous or time-weighted average sampling. When high readings are obtained the causes can usually be determined immediately and corrective measures taken.

One disadvantage of continuous monitors is that the time and expense required to maintain one may make it unsatisfactory for a small facility. In such circumstances, several hospitals might consider sharing an instrument or a manufacturer's service representative might use one during routine quarterly maintenance calls. This method tends to disrupt the operating room routine more than instantaneous or time-weighted average sampling. Finally, rapidly changing concentrations are difficult to interpret in terms of personnel exposure unless integration over time is employed.

End-Tidal Sampling (322, 334, 350–352)

End-tidal samples of gases may be taken from exposed personnel after a period of exposure. With high levels of agents in the atmosphere, some agent may be detectable in the morning from the previous day's exposure (161, 350–354). End-tidal samples are inherently time weighted and show less scatter than time-weighted average samples (355). This method is most suitable for potent halogenated agents. Nitrous oxide is so rapidly absorbed and excreted that its level in end-tidal gas reflects only the most recent exposure of the subject.

The main disadvantage is that collecting end-tidal samples may be disruptive to operating room personnel performing their duties.

Blood or Urine Sampling (158, 322, 350, 351, 354, 356–359)

Samples of venous blood can be drawn from personnel at the end of an exposure period and analyzed. Urinary nitrous oxide has been shown to be a good monitor of the agent in the blood (361, 362). In personnel exposed to high concentrations of potent agents, a detectable amount may be present in the blood or urine in the morning from the previous day's exposure (351, 354).

Agents to be Monitored

Ideally, all gases employed in the conduct of an anesthetic should be measured. Analyzers are available that can scan the infrared spectrum and are programmable to distinguish individual inhalational agents. Likewise, mass spectrometry and gas chromatography can measure all agents. However, it is simpler to monitor a single gas. The NIOSH criteria document (253) does not recommend monitoring of all anesthetic agents but only the one most frequently used.

Nitrous Oxide

Many people believe that nitrous oxide is the most logical agent to monitor because it is administered in higher concentrations than other agents, is easy to measure, and is more likely to be subject to occult leakage than potent agents (285).

Because nitrous oxide and other agents are not separated by buoyancy effects (288, 171), they will be present in a room in the same ratio in which they are introduced. Because of this, many people contend that nitrous oxide can serve as a tracer of other agents administered with it to a degree of accuracy sufficient for routine appraisal of occupational exposure (363). This tracer concept works best under steady-state conditions and low equipment leakage. It does not work well when a vaporizer is being filled or drained, during cardiopulmonary bypass, during induction or recovery from anesthesia, or when there is a nitrous oxide leak or a leak in a vaporizer.

Potent Agents

Monitoring of other agents can be worthwhile (364, 365). Volatile agents can leak independently of nitrous oxide. Analyzers that measure potent agents are more expensive than those that measure only nitrous oxide (286).

Sites to be Monitored

Monitoring should be scheduled so that the work of each anesthesia person and of each operating room is checked while using a mask and a tracheal tube and while using a ventilator. Monitoring should be performed during spontaneous, manually assisted, and manually controlled ventilation. The results of the monitoring should be analyzed and discussed with all parties concerned.

Personal Monitoring

Sampling the zone of exposed personnel is usually considered the preferred method. Anesthesia personnel are considered the most important to monitor, because they usually are exposed to higher concentrations than other operating room personnel (366) and are more likely to remain in the room for the entire duration of anesthesia administration.

Passive dosimeters can be attached to the person's clothing and worn for prolonged periods. Sampling directly in the pathway of the subject's expired air must be avoided if measurement of nitrous oxide by infrared analysis is used.

Area (Room) Sampling

The exhaust grille of the air-conditioning system or the open door will be representative of average personnel exposure if gases are evenly distributed in the room. Fifteen or more air exchanges per hour are sufficient to produce near homogeneity of anesthetic concentrations in all locations except those close to the source of leakage (286, 288, 367). With lower exchange rates, mixing may not be complete and localized areas of high (hot spots) or low (cold spots) concentration may occur. Area sampling may be less disruptive to the operating room routine than personal monitoring.

Postanesthesia Care Units

One study measured concentrations 24 inches over the patient's head (368). A more elaborate method is to take samples 50 cm above the patient's thorax, at the foot end of the bed, and 2 m from the foot end of the bed, all at 180 cm above floor level (369), and multiply these concentrations by how long personnel remained in the different areas. It is suggested that concentrations be measured during the "peak load period" when there are a maximum number of patients exhaling gases.

Frequency of Monitoring

At the initiation of a waste gas control program, frequent monitoring under actual working conditions will be necessary. As experience is gained and equipment is maintained leak tight, the frequency can be decreased. However, whenever concentrations higher than acceptable are found, new equipment is installed, or old equipment is modified, monitoring should be repeated.

The following have been suggested (9):

1. An annual comprehensive survey in which exposure levels are measured, leaks detected and corrected, and time-weighted average exposure levels are calculated or measured.
2. Quarterly follow-up with a less-detailed survey; if there appears to be a problem, a comprehensive survey should be performed to determine causes and assess corrective actions.
3. A repeat comprehensive survey in the event of major changes to the ventilation system, anesthesia equipment, or scavenging systems.

Time-weighted average monitoring of each member of the staff for a short period, such as a week, repeated on a 6-month basis also has been suggested (327).

ROLE OF THE FEDERAL GOVERNMENT (9, 370, 371)

In 1970 the U.S. Congress passed the Occupational Safety and Health Act. It created two separate executive-branch agencies to carry out the provisions of the act: the National Institute for Occupational Safety and Health (NIOSH), an agency with the Centers for Disease Control and Prevention under the Department of Health and Human Services, and the Occupational Safety and Health Administration (OSHA), under the Department of Labor.

OSHA is responsible for enacting job safety and health standards, establishing reporting and recordkeeping procedures, inspecting workplaces, and enforcing the requirements of the act using citations and fines.

NIOSH is responsible for conducting and funding research and education and for preparing criteria documents to be used for the development of standards. Criteria documents prepared by NIOSH are transmitted to the secretary of labor for review by the OSHA staff.

Such a criteria document on trace gases was published and transmitted to OSHA in 1977 (253). The following are important aspects of this document.

1. Although it was maintained that a safe level of exposure to trace anesthetic gases could not be defined, maximum concentrations to which

a worker in the operating room should be exposed were recommended. For halogenated agents used alone this was 2 ppm time-weighted average. For nitrous oxide alone, a time-weighted average exposure limit of 25 ppm was recommended. When halogenated agents are used in combination with nitrous oxide the recommended limits were 25 ppm nitrous oxide and 0.5 ppm of the halogenated agent. For dental facilities a level of 50 ppm nitrous oxide was recommended.

The Ad Hoc Committee of the American Society of Anesthesiologists has suggested that less than 180 ppm nitrous oxide is satisfactory with mask techniques (204). The American Conference on Governmental Industrial Hygienists has suggested limits for some halogenated agents that are higher than those proposed by NIOSH (9).

The United Kingdom Committee for Occupational Safety and Health has established threshold values of 100 ppm for N_2O, 50 ppm for isoflurane and 10 ppm for halothane (5). The Swedish Occupational Health Standards specify that maximum exposure as a time-weighted average over 8 hours must not exceed 100 ppm for nitrous oxide, 5 ppm for halothane, and 10 ppm for enflurane and isoflurane (372). Norway, Denmark, and Italy have set a maximum limit of TWA of 100 ppm for nitrous oxide (373–375), while in the Netherlands it is 25 ppm (374). For halothane the limits are 5 ppm in Germany and 2.5 ppm in the Commonwealth of Independent States (157).

2. Monitoring of exposure levels is recommended in all areas with potential for worker exposure on a quarterly basis and following changes to ventilation systems, anesthetic equipment, or scavenging techniques. Breathing zone or immediate work area samples are most desirable.
3. Results of monitoring and corrective measures are to be maintained and retained for 20 years.
4. Recommendations were made regarding scavenging, ventilation systems, leak testing, and work practices aimed at minimizing employee exposure.
5. Medical surveillance, including comprehensive employee preplacement medical and occupational histories, annual updating of employee

medical histories, and annual physical examinations of employees exposed to waste anesthetic gases is recommended.

6. Employees are to be informed on assignment and at least yearly thereafter of the possible health effects of exposure to trace anesthetics, especially possible effects on reproduction. Appropriate signs and labeling were recommended.

7. Any abnormal outcome of the pregnancies of employees or of their spouses must be documented as part of the employees medical record.

NIOSH participation came to a halt after the transmittal of this document to OSHA. To promulgate this as a standard, OSHA would have to go through an extensive rule-making procedure, including a public comment period. This has not occurred to date.

JOINT COMMISSION ON THE ACCREDITATION OF HEALTHCARE ORGANIZATIONS

The Joint Commission on Accreditation of Healthcare Organizations in 1983 recommended, but did not require, that each anesthesia machine be equipped with a gas-scavenging device. It now recommends, but does not yet require, that monitoring be performed.

MEDICOLEGAL CONSIDERATIONS (376)

Because the NIOSH document does not constitute a promulgated OSHA standard, employers are not obligated to comply with its recommendations. However, the general duty clause of the 1970 act gives OSHA the authority to inspect workplaces to determine whether employers are providing a workplace free from hazards, even in the absence of a relevant standard.

The act gives each employee the right to request an OSHA inspection if the employee believes he or she is in imminent danger from a hazard or OSHA standards are being violated. Several inspections in response to employee complaints were carried out in the 1970s. Fines and citations were issued because employees were exposed to

concentrations of nitrous oxide in excess of the NIOSH recommended levels or because exposure was not reduced to the lowest feasible level (371, 377).

The ASA legal counsel has advised that it is within the right of an employer to refuse to permit an OSHA representative to enter the premises of the hospital or operating room unless that individual has either a search warrant or a court order compelling the inspection. OSHA would need to seek a search warrant from a federal court and show probable cause for making an inspection (377). If faced with a visit from an OSHA representative, obtaining legal counsel is advisable. Failure to demand a search warrant or court order normally would constitute a waiver of any later right to object to the validity of an inspection.

All states have workers' compensation laws so that individuals suffering occupational diseases can collect benefits, irrespective of whether or not the employer's negligence caused the disease. It is possible that a workers' compensation case could arise from an operating room employee suffering from one of the problems described in the first section of this chapter, provided the employee could show that the illness was work connected and that employment in the operating room subjected him or her to special risk in excess of those experienced by the general public.

In most states workers' compensation laws preclude private lawsuits by an employee against his or her employer. However, in addition to making a claim for workers' compensation, an employee can bring a civil suit for damages against a third party (such as an anesthesia provider) whom the employee claims caused injury.

REFERENCES

1. National Institute for Occupational Safety and Health (NIOSH). Alert. Controlling exposure to nitrous oxide during anesthetic administration. DHHS (NIOSH) Publication No. 94–100, April, 1994.

2. Ilsley AH, Plummer JL, Runciman WB, Cousins MJ. Anaesthetic gas analyzers for vaporizer calibration, patient circuit monitoring and determination of environmental waste anaesthetic gas levels. Anaesthesia and Intensive Care 1988;16:35–37.

3. Dang Vu B, Estryn-Behar M, Maillard MF, et al. Theatre staff members and exposure to halogenated agents. Paediatr Anaesth 1992;39:279–284.

4. Wood C, Ewen A, Goresky G. Exposure of operating room personnel to nitrous oxide during paediatric anaesthesia. Can J Anaesth 1992;39:682–686.

5. Hoerauf K, Funk W, Harth M, Hobbhahn J. Occupational exposure to sevoflurane, halothane and nitrous oxide during paediatric anaesthesia. Anaesthesia 1997;52:215–219.

6. Spence AA, Knill-Jones RP. Is there a health hazard in anaesthetic practice? Br J Anaesth 1978;50:713–719.

7. Ferstandig LL. Trace concentrations of anesthetic gases. Acta Anaesthesiol Scand 1982;Suppl75: 38–43.

8. Spence AA. Environmental pollution by inhalation anaesthetics. Br J Anaesth 1987;59:96–103.

9. Anonymous. Personnel exposure to waste anesthetic gases. Health Devices 1983;12:169–177.

10. Mazze RI, Lecky JH. The health of operating room personnel. Anesthesiology 1985;62:226–228.

11. Tannenbaum TN, Goldberg RJ. Exposure to anesthetic gases and reproductive outcome. J Occup Med 1985;27:659–668.

12. Walts LF, Forsythe AB, Moore G. Critique. Occupational disease among operating room personnel. Anesthesiology 1975;42:608–611.

13. Ferstandig LL. Trace concentrations of anesthetic gases. A critical review of their disease potential. Anesth Analg 1978;57:328–345.

14. Ad Hoc Committee on the Effects of Trace Anesthetics on the Health of Operating Room Personnel, American Society of Anesthesiologists. Occupational disease among operating room personnel: a national study. Anesthesiology 1974;41:321–340.

15. Cohen EN, Bellville JW, Brown BW. Anesthesia, pregnancy and miscarriage: a study of operating room nurses and anesthetists. Anesthesiology 1971;35: 343–347.

16. Cohen EN, Brown BW, Wu ML, et al. Occupational disease in dentistry and chronic exposure to trace anesthetic gases. J Am Dent Assoc 1980;10:21–31.

17. Knill–Jones RP, Rodrigues LV, Moir DD, Spence AA. Anaesthetic practice and pregnancy. Lancet 1972;1:1326–1328.

18. Knill–Jones RP, Newman BJ, Spence AA. Anaesthesia practice and pregnancy. Lancet 1975;2:807–809.

19. Mirakhur RK, Badve AV. Pregnancy and anaesthetic practice in India. Anaesthesia 1975;30:18–22.

20. Rosenberg P, Kirves A. Miscarriages among operating theatre staff. Acta Anaesthesiol Scand 1973; Suppl53:37–42.

21. Tomlin PJ. Health problems of anaesthetists and their families in the West Midlands. BMJ 1979;1: 779–784.

22. Guirguis SS, Roy ML, Pelmear PL, Wong L. Health effects associated with exposure to anaesthetic gases in Ontario hospital personnel. Br J Ind Med 1990; 47:490–497.

23. Saurel–Cubizolles MJ, Hays M, Estryn–Behar M. Work in operating rooms and pregnancy outcome among nurses. Int Arch Occup Environ Health 1994; 66:235–241.

24. Klebanoff MA, Shiono PH, Rhoads GG. Spontaneous and induced abortion among resident physicians. JAMA 1991;265:2821–2825.

25. Axelsson G, Rylander R. Exposure to anaesthetic gases and spontaneous abortion: response bias in a postal questionnaire study. Int J Epidemiol 1982;11: 250–256.

26. Ericson A, Kallen B. Survey of infants born in 1973–1975 to Swedish women working in operating rooms during their pregnancies. Anesth Analg 1979; 58:302–305.

27. Ericson HA, Kallen AJB. Hospitalization for miscarriage and delivery outcome among Swedish nurses working in operating rooms 1973–1978. Anesth Analg 1985;64:981–988.

28. Hemminki K, Kyyronen P, Lindbohm M. Spontaneous abortions and malformations in the offspring of nurses exposed to anaesthetic gases, cytostatic drugs, and other potential hazards in hospitals, based on registered information of outcome. J Epidemiol Community Health 1985;39:141–147.

29. Lauwerys R, Siddons M, Misson CB, et al. Anaesthetic health hazards among Belgian nurses and physicians. Int Arch Occup Environ Health 1981;48: 195–203.

30. Pharoah POD, Alberman E, Doyle P. Outcome of pregnancy among women in anaesthetic practice. Lancet 1977;1:34–36.

31. Rosenberg PH, Vanttinen H. Occupational hazards to reproduction and health in anaesthetists and paediatricians. Acta Anaesthesiol Scand 1978;22: 202–207.

32. Buring JE, Hennekens CH, Mayrent SL, et al. Health experiences of operating room personnel. Anesthesiology 1985;62:325–330.

33. Mazze RI. Fertility, reproduction, and postnatal survival in mice chronically exposed to isoflurane. Anesthesiology 1985;63:663–667.

34. Mazze RI, Fujinaga M, Rice SA, et al. Reproductive and teratogenic effects of nitrous oxide, halothane, isoflurane, and enflurane in Sprague–Dawley rats. Anesthesiology 1986; 64:339–344.

35. Wharton RS, Mazze RI, Wilson AI. Reproduction and fetal development in mice chronically exposed to enflurane. Anesthesiology 1981;54:505–510.

36. Strout CD, Nahrwold ML, Taylor MD, et al. Effects

of subanesthetic concentrations of enflurane on rat pregnancy and early development. Environ Health Perspect 1977;21:211–214.

37. Halsey MJ, Green CJ, Monk SJ, et al. Maternal and paternal chronic exposure to enflurane and halothane. fetal and histological changes in the rat. Br J Anaesth 1981;53:203–215.

38. Lansdown ABG, Pope WDB, Halsey MJ, et al. Analysis of fetal development in rats following maternal exposure to subanesthetic concentrations of halothane. Teratology 1976;13:299–303.

39. Pope WDB, Halsey MJ, Phil HD, et al. Fetotoxicity in rats following chronic exposure to halothane, nitrous oxide, or methoxyflurane. Anesthesiology 1978;48:11–16.

40. Vieira E, Cleaton-Jones P, Austin JC, et al. Effects of low concentrations of nitrous oxide on rat fetuses. Anesth Analg 1980;59:175–177.

41. Vieira E, Cleaton-Jones P, Moyes D. Effects of low intermittent concentrations of nitrous oxide on the developing rat fetus. Br J Anaesth 1983;55:67–69.

42. Fujinaga M, Baden JM, Yhap EO, et al. Reproductive and teratogenic effects of nitrous oxide, isoflurane, and their combination in Sprague–Dawley rats. Anesthesiology 1987;67:960–964.

43. Askrog VF, Harvald B. Teratogen effekt of inhalatiosanaestetika. Nord Med 1970;83:498–500.

44. Cohen EN, Brown BW, Bruce DL, et al. A survey of anesthetic health hazards among dentists. J Am Dent Assoc 1975;90:1291–1296.

45. Wyrobek AJ, Brodsky J, Gordon L, et al. Sperm studies in anesthesiologists. Anesthesiology 1981;55:527–532.

46. Baden JM, Land PC, Egbert B, et al. Lack of toxicity of enflurane on male reproductive organs in mice. Anesth Analg 1982;61:19–22.

47. Coate WB, Kapp RW Jr., Lewis TR. Chronic exposure to low concentrations of halothane-nitrous oxide: reproductive and cytogenetic effects in the rat. Anesthesiology 1979;50:310–318.

48. Rowland AS, Baird DD, Weinberg CR, et al. Reduced fertility among women employed as dental assistants exposed to high levels of nitrous oxide. N Engl J Med 1992;327:993–997.

49. Land PC, Owen EL, Linde HW. Morphologic changes in mouse spermatozoa after exposure to inhalational anesthetics during early spermatogenesis. Anesthesiology 1981;54:53–56.

50. Kundomal YR, Baden JM. Inhaled anaesthetics have no effect on fertility in *Drosophila melanogaster*. Br J Anaesth 1985;57:900–903.

51. Wharton RS, Mazze RI, Baden JM, et al. Fertility, reproduction and postnatal survival in mice chronically exposed to halothane. Anesthesiology 1978;48:167–174.

52. Kennedy GL Jr., Smith SH, Keplinger ML, et al. Reproductive and teratologic studies with halothane. Toxicol Appl Pharmacol 1976;35:467–474.

53. Mazze RI, Wilson AI, Rice SA, et al. Reproduction and fetal development in mice chronically exposed to nitrous oxide. Teratology 1982;26:11–16.

54. Kripke BJ, Kelman AD, Shah NK, et al. Testicular reaction to prolonged exposure to nitrous oxide. Anesthesiology 1976;44:104–113.

55. Vieira E, Cleaton–Jones P, Moyes D. Effects of intermittent .5% nitrous oxide/air (v/v) on the fertility of male rats and the post-natal growth of their offspring. Anaesthesia 1983;38:319–323.

56. Corbett TH, Cornell RG, Endres JL, et al. Birth defects among children of nurse-anesthetists. Anesthesiology 1974;41:341–344.

57. Cote CJ. Birth defects among infants of nurse anesthetists. Anesthesiology 1975;42:514–515.

58. Rosenberg PH, Kallio H. Operating-theatre gas pollution and chromosomes. Lancet 1977;2:452–453.

59. Green CJ, Monk SJ, Knight JF, et al. Chronic exposure of rats to enflurane 200 ppm: no evidence of toxicity or teratogenicity. Br J Anaesth 1982;54:1097–1104.

60. Pope WDB, Halsey MJ, Lansdown ABG, et al. Lack of teratogenic dangers with halothane. Acta Anaesthesiol Belg 1975;26 (Suppl):169–173.

61. Wharton RS, Wilson AI, Mazze RI, et al. Fetal morphology in mice exposed to halothane. Anesthesiology 1979;51:532–537.

62. Levin ED, Bowman RE. Behavioral effects of chronic exposure to low concentrations of halothane during development in rats. Anesth Analg 1986;65:653–659.

63. Quimby KL, Katz J, Bowman RE. Behavioral consequences in rats from chronic exposure to 10 ppm halothane during early development. Anesth Analg 1975;54:628–633.

64. Baden JM, Rice SA, Serra M, et al. Thymidine and methionine syntheses in pregnant rats exposed to nitrous oxide. Anesth Analg 1983;62:738–741.

65. Korttila K, Pfaffli P, Linnoila M, et al. Operating room nurses' psychomotor and driving skills after occupational exposure to halothane and nitrous oxide. Acta Anaesthesiol Scand 1978;22:33–39.

66. Gamberale F, Svensson G. The effect of anesthetic gases on the psychomotor and perceptual functions of anesthetic nurses. Work Environ Health 1974;11:108–113.

67. Gambill AF, McCallum RN, Henrichs TF. Psychomotor performance following exposure to trace con-

centrations of inhalation anesthetics. Anesth Analg 1979;58:475–482.

68. Stollery BT, Broadbent DE, Lee WR, et al. Mood and cognitive functions in anaesthetists working in actively scavenged operating theatres. Br J Anaesth 1988;61:446–455.

69. Ayer WA, Russell EA, Ballinger ME, et al. Failure to demonstrate psychomotor effects of nitrous oxide oxygen exposure in dental assistants. Anesth Prog 1978;25:186–187.

70. Bruce DL, Bach MJ. Psychological studies of human performance as affected by traces of enflurane and nitrous oxide. Anesthesiology 1975; 42:194–196.

71. Bruce DL, Bach MJ, Arbit J. Trace anesthetic effects on perceptual cognitive and motor skills. Anesthesiology 1974;40:453–458.

72. Bruce DL, Bach MJ. Effects of trace anaesthetic gases on behavioural performance of volunteers. Br J Anaesth 1976;48:871–875.

73. Smith G, Shirley AW. Failure to demonstrate effect of trace concentrations of nitrous oxide and halothane on psychomotor performance. Br J Anaesth 1977;49:65–70.

74. Cook TL, Smith M, Winter PM, et al. Effect of subanesthetic concentrations of enflurane and halothane on human behavior. Anesth Analg 1978;57:434–440.

75. Cook TL, Smith M, Starkweather JA, et al. Behavioral effects of trace and subanesthetic halothane and nitrous oxide in man. Anesthesiology 1978;49:419–424.

76. Frankhuizen JL, Vlek CAJ, Burm AGL, et al. Failure to replicate negative effects of trace anaesthetics on mental performance. Br J Anaesth 1978;50:229–234.

77. Allison RH, Shirley AW, Smith G. Threshold concentration of nitrous oxide affecting psychomotor performance. Br J Anaesth 1979;51:177–180.

78. Saurel–Cubizolles MJ, Estryn–Behar, Maillard MF, et al. Neuropsychological symptoms and occupational exposure to anaesthetics. Br J Ind Med 1992; 49:276–281.

79. Quimby KL, Aschkenase LJ, Bowman RE, et al. Enduring learning deficits and cerebral synaptic malformation from exposure to 10 ppm of halothane per million. Science 1974;185:625–627.

80. Bruce DL, Eide KA, Smith NJ. A prospective survey of anesthesiologist mortality: 1967–1971. Anesthesiology 1974;41:71–74.

81. Doll R, Peto R. Mortality among doctors in different occupations. BMJ 1977;1:1433–1436.

82. Lew EA. Mortality experience among anesthesiologists: 1954–1976. Anesthesiology 1979; 51:195–199.

83. Linde HW, Mesnick PS, Smith NJ. Causes of death among anesthesiologists: 1930–1946. Anesth Analg 1981;60:1–7.

84. Neil HAW, Fairer JG, Coleman MP, et al. Mortality among male anaesthetists in the United Kingdom, 1957–1983. BMJ 1987;295:360–362.

85. Baden JM, Mazze RI, Wharton RS, et al. Carcinogenicity of halothane in Swiss/ICR mice. Anesthesiology 1979;51:20–26.

86. Eger EI II, White AE, Brown CL, et al. A test of the carcinogenicity of enflurane, isoflurane, halothane, methoxyflurane and nitrous oxide in mice. Anesth Analg 1978;57:678–694.

87. Baden JM, Egbert B, Mazze RI. Carcinogen bioassay of enflurane in mice. Anesthesiology 1982;56:9–13.

88. Corbett TH. Cancer and congenital anomalies associated with anesthetics. Ann N Y Acad Sci 1976;271:58–66.

89. Baden JM, Kundomal YR, Mazze RI, et al. Carcinogen bioassay of isoflurane in mice. Anesthesiology 1988;69:750–753.

90. Baden JM, Kundomal YR, Luttropp ME, et al. Carcinogen bioassay of nitrous oxide in mice. Anesthesiology 1986;64:747–750.

91. Coate WB, Ulland BM, Lewis TR. Chronic exposure to low concentrations of halothane-nitrous oxide. Anesthesiology 1979;50:306–309.

92. Baden JM, Brinkenhoff M, Wharton RS, et al. Mutagenicity of volatile anesthetics: halothane. Anesthesiology 1976;45:311–318.

93. Eger EI. Fetal injury and abortion associated with occupational exposure to inhaled anesthetics. J Am Assoc Nurse Anesth 1991;59:309–312.

94. McCoy EC, Hankel R, Rosenkranz HS, et al. Detection of mutagenic activity in the urine of anesthesiologists: a preliminary report. Environ Health Perspect 1977;21:221–223.

95. Baden JM, Kelley M, Cheung A, et al. Lack of mutagens in urine of operating room personnel. Anesthesiology 1980;53:195–198.

96. Husum B, Wulf HC. Sister chromatid exchanges in lymphocytes in operating room personnel. Acta Anaesthesiol Scand 1980;24:22–24.

97. Husum B, Wulf HC. Niebuhr E. Monitoring of sister chromatid exchanges in lymphocytes of nurse-anesthetists. Anesthesiology 1985;62:475–479.

98. Holmberg K, Lambert B, Lindsten J, et al. DNA and chromosome alterations in lymphocytes of operating room personnel and in patients before and after inhalation anaesthesia. Acta Anaesthesiol Scand 1982;26:531–539.

99. Husum B, Niebuhr E, Wulf HC, et al. Sister chromatic exchanges and structural chromosome aberra-

tions in lymphocytes in operating room personnel. Acta Anaesthesiol Scand 1983;27:262–265.

100. Husum B, Wulf HC, Mathiassen F, et al. Sister chromatid exchanges in lymphocytes of dentists and chairside assistants: no indication of a mutagenic effect of exposure to waste nitrous oxide. Community Dent Oral Epidemiol 1986;14:148–151.

101. Natarajan D, Santhiya ST. Cytogenetic damage in operation theatre personnel. Anaesthesia 1990; 54: 574–577.

102. Sardas S, Cuhruk H, Karakaya AE, et al. Sister-chromatic exchanges in operating room personnel. Mutat Res 1992; 279:117–120.

103. White AE, Takehisa S, Eger EI, et al. Sister chromatid exchanges induced by inhaled anesthetics. Anesthesiology 1979;50:426–430.

104. Waskell L. Lack of mutagenicity of two possible metabolites of halothane. Anesthesiology 1979;50: 9–12.

105. Waskell L. A study of the mutagenicity of anesthetics and their metabolites. Mutat Res 1978; 57:141–153.

106. Sturrock J. Lack of mutagenic effect of halothane or chloroform on cultured cells using the azaguanine test system. Br J Anaesth 1977;49:207–10.

107. Basler A, Rohrborn G. Lack of mutagenic effects of halothane in mammals in vivo. Anesthesiology 1981; 55:143–147.

108. Baden JM, Kundomal YR. Mutagenicity of the combination of a volatile anaesthetic and nitrous oxide. Br J Anaesth 1987;59:772–775.

109. Kramers PGN, Burm AGL. Mutagenicity studies with halothane in *Drosophila melanogaster*. Anesthesiology 1979;50:510–513.

110. Edmunds HN, Baden JM, Simmon VF. Mutagenicity studies with volatile metabolites of halothane. Anesthesiology 1979;51:424–429.

111. Garro AJ, Phillips RA. Mutagenicity of the halogenated olefin, 2-bromo-2-chloro-1,1-difluoroethylene, a presumed metabolite of the inhalation anesthetic halothane. Environ Health Perspect 1977;21: 65–69.

112. Sachdev K, Cohen EN, Simmon VF. Genotoxic and mutagenic assays of halothane metabolites in *Bacillus subtilis* and *Salmonella typhimurium*. Anesthesiology 1980;53:31–39.

113. Sturrock JE. No mutagenic effect of enflurane on cultured cells. Br J Anaesth 1977;49:777–779.

114. Baden JM, Kelley M, Wharton RS, et al. Mutagenicity of halogenated ether anesthetics. Anesthesiology 1977;46:346–350.

115. Baden JM, Kelley M, Mazze RI, et al. Mutagenicity of inhalation anesthetics: trichlorethylene, divinyl ether, nitrous oxide, and cyclopropane. Br J Anaesth 1979; 51:417–421.

116. Knill–Jones RP. Comparative risk of hepatitis in doctors working within hospitals and outside hospitals. Digestion 1974;10:359–360.

117. Nunn JF, Sharer N, Royston D, et al. Serum methionine and hepatic enzyme activity in anaesthetists exposed to nitrous oxide. Br J Anaesth 1982;54: 593–597.

118. Belfrage S, Ahlgren I, Axelson S. Halothane hepatitis in an anaesthetist. Lancet 1966;2:1466–1467.

119. Johnston CI, Mendelsohn F. Halothane hepatitis in a laboratory technician. Aust N Z J Med 1971;2: 171–173.

120. Klatskin G, Kimberg DV. Recurrent hepatitis attributable to halothane sensitization in an anesthetist. N Engl J Med 1969;280:515–522.

121. Lund I, Skulberg A, Helle I. Occupation hazard of halothane. Lancet 1974;2:528.

122. Ghoneim MM, Delle M, Wilson WR, et al. Alteration of warfarin kinetics in man associated with exposure to an operating-room environment. Anesthesiology 1975;43:333–336.

123. Harman AW, Russell WJ, Frewin DB, et al. Altered drug metabolism in anaesthetists exposed to volatile anaesthetic agents. Anaesthesia and Intensive Care 1978;6:210–214.

124. Plummer JL, Hall P de la M, Jenner MA, et al. Effects of chronic inhalation of halothane, enflurane, or isoflurane in rats. Br J Anaesth 1986;58:517–23.

125. Plummer JL, Hall P de la M, Cousins MJ, et al. Hepatic injury in rats due to prolonged sub-anaesthetic halothane exposure. Acta Pharmacol Toxicol 1983; 53:16–22.

126. Clark GC, Kesterson JW, Coombs DW, et al. Comparative effects of repeated and prolonged inhalation exposure of beagle dogs and cynomolgus monkeys to anaesthetic and subanaesthetic concentrations of enflurane and halothane. Acta Anaesthesiol Scand 1979;Suppl71:1–11.

127. Nunn JF. Clinical aspects of the interaction between nitrous oxide and vitamin B_{12}. Br J Anaesth 1987; 59:3–13.

128. DeZotti R, Negro C, Gobbato F. Results of hepatic and hemopoietic controls in hospital personnel exposed to waste anesthetic gases. Int Arch Occup Environ Health 1983;52:33–41.

129. Salo M, Rajamaki A, Nikoskelainen J. Absence of signs of vitamin B_{12}-nitrous oxide interaction in operating theatre personnel. Acta Anaesthesiol Scand 1984;28:106–8.

130. Armstrong P, Rae PWH, Gray WM, et al. Nitrous oxide and formiminoglutamic acid: excretion in surgical patients and anaesthetists. Br J Anaesth 1991; 66:163–9.

131. Sweeney B, Bingham RM, Amos RJ, et al. Toxicity of bone marrow in dentists exposed to nitrous oxide. Br Med J 1985;291:567–569.

132. Baden JM, Egbert B, Rice SA. Enflurane has no effect on haemopoiesis in mice. Br J Anaesth 1980;52: 471–474.

133. Cleaton-Jones P, Austin JC, Banks D, et al. Effect of intermittent exposure to a low concentration of nitrous oxide on haemopoiesis in rats. Br J Anaesth 1977;49:223–226.

134. Layzer RB. Myeloneuropathy after prolonged exposure to nitrous oxide. Lancet 1978;2:1227–1230.

135. Gutmann L, Johnsen D. Nitrous oxide-induced Myeloneuropathy: report of cases. J Am Dent Assoc 1981; 103:239–241.

136. Brodsky JB, Cohen EN, Brown BW, et al. Exposure to nitrous oxide and neurologic disease among dental professionals. Anesth Analg 1981;60:297–301.

137. Dyck P, Grina A, Lambert EH, et al. Nitrous oxide neurotoxicity studies in man and rat. Anesthesiology 1980;53:205–208.

138. Beall GN, Nagel EL, Matsui Y. Immunoglobulins in anesthesiologists. Anesthesiology 1975;42:232.

139. Bruce DL. Immunologically competent anesthesiologists. Anesthesiology 1972;37:76–78.

140. Salo M, Vapaavuori M. Peripheral blood t- and b-lymphocytes in operating theatre personnel. Br J Anaesth 1976;48:877–880.

141. Ziv Y, Shohat B, Baniel J, et al. The immunologic profile of anesthetists. Anesth Analg 1988;67: 849–851.

142. Peric M, Vranes Z, Marusic M. Immunological disturbances in anaesthetic personnel chronically exposed to high occupational concentrations of nitrous oxide and halothane. Anaesthesia 1991;46:531–537.

143. Spence AA, Cohen EN, Brown BW, et al. Occupational hazards for operating room-based physicians. Analysis of data from the United States and the United Kingdom. JAMA 1977;238:955–959.

144. Lattey M. Halothane sensitization. A case report. Can Anaesth Soc J 1970;17:648–649.

145. Plummer JL, Sandkson CH, Ilsley AH, et al. Attitudes of anaesthetists and nurses to anaesthetic pollution. Anaesthesia and Intensive Care 1987; 15: 411–420.

146. Schwettmann RS, Casterline CL. Delayed asthmatic response following occupational exposure to enflurane. Anesthesiology 1976;44:166–169.

147. Pitt EM. Halothane as a possible cause of laryngitis in an anaesthetist. Anaesthesia 1974;29:579–580.

148. Boyd CH. Ophthalmic hypersensitivity to anaesthetic vapours. Anaesthesia 1972;27:456–457.

149. Dadve AV, Mirakhur RK. Ophthalmic hypersensitivity to anaesthetic vapours. Anaesthesia 1973;28: 338–339.

150. Elder BF, Beal H, DeWald W, et al. Exacerbation of subclinical myasthenia by occupational exposure to an anesthetic. Anesth Analg 1971;50:383–387.

151. Bodman R. Skin sensitivity to halothane vapour. Br J Anaesth 1979;51:1092.

152. Soper LE, Vitez TS, Weinberg D. Metabolism of halogenated anesthetic agents as a possible cause of acneiform eruptions. Anesth Analg 1973;52:125–127.

153. McNamee R, Keen RI, Corkill CM. Morbidity and early retirement among anaesthetists and other specialists. Anaesthesia 1987;42:133–140.

154. Arnold WP. Application of OSHA standard to waste anesthetic gases. American Society of Anesthesiologists Newsletter 1992;56(8):23.

155. Lecky JH. Anesthetic pollution in the operating room: a notice to operating room personnel. Anesthesiology 1980;52:157–159.

156. Davenport HT, Halsey MJ, Wardley–Smith B, et al. Occupational exposure to anaesthetics in twenty hospitals. Anaesthesia 1980;35:354–359.

157. Gardner RJ. Inhalation anaesthetics—exposure and control: a statistical comparison of personal exposures in operating theatres with and without anaesthetic gas scavenging. Ann Occup Hyg 1989;33:159–173.

158. Krapez JR, Saloojee Y, Hinds CJ, et al. Blood concentrations of nitrous oxide in theatre personnel. Br J Anaesth 1980;52:1143–1148.

159. Nikki P, Pfaffli K, Ahlman K, et al. Chronic exposure to anaesthetic gases in the operating theatre and recovery room. Ann Clin Res 1972;4:266–272.

160. Yoganathan S, Johnston IG, Parnell CJ, et al. Determination of contamination of a chemical warfare-proof operating theatre with volatile anaesthetic agents and assessment of anaesthetic gas scavenging systems. Br J Anaesth 1991;67:614–617.

161. Whitcher CE, Cohen EN, Trudell JR. Chronic exposure to anesthetic gases in the operating room. Anesthesiology 1971;35:348–353.

162. Oulton JL. Operating-room venting of trace concentrations of inhalation anesthetic agents. Can Med Assoc J 1977;116:1148–1151.

163. McIntyre JWR, Pudham JT, Jhsein HR. An assessment of operating room environment air contamination with nitrous oxide and halothane and some scavenging methods. Can Anaesth Soc J 1978;25: 499–505.

164. Parbrook GD, Still DM, Halliday MM, et al. The reduction of nitrous oxide pollution in relative analgesia. Br Dent J 1981;150:128–130.

165. Henry RJ, Primosch RE. Influence of operatory size and nitrous oxide concentration upon scavenger effectiveness. J Dent Res 1991;70(9):1286–1289.

166. American Society for Testing and Materials. Standard specification for anesthetic equipment—scavenging systems for anesthetic gases (ASTM F1343-91). West Conshohocken, PA: ASTM, 1991.

167. Inhalational anaesthesia systems—Part 3: Anaesthetic gas scavenging systems—transfer and receiving systems (ISO8835). Geneva: International Standards Organization. 1997.

168. Flowerdew RMM. A hazard of scavenger port design. Can Anaesth Soc J 1981;28:481–483.

169. Tavakoli M, Habeeb A. Two hazards of gas scavenging. Anesth Analg 1978;57:286–287.

169a. Gill-Rodriguez JA. A modified MIE Superlite exhaust valve incorporating a positive pressure relief valve. Anaesthesia 1984;39:1237–1239.

170. Albert CA, Kwan A, Kim C, et al. A waste gas scavenging valve for pediatric systems. Anesth Analg 1977;56:291–292.

171. U.S. Department of Health Education and Welfare. Development and evaluation of methods for the elimination of waste anesthetic gases and vapors in hospitals (DHEW [NIOSH] Publication No. 75–137). Washington, DC: US Government Printing Office, 1975.

172. Brinklov MM, Andersen PK. Gas evacuation from paediatric anaesthetic systems. Br J Anaesth 1978;50:305.

173. Cestone KJ, Ryan WP, Loving CD. An anesthetic gas scavenger for the Jackson–Rees system. Anesthesiology 1976;55:881–882.

174. Emralino CQ, Bernhard WN, Yost L. Overflow-gas scavenger for Jackson-Rees anesthesia system. Respir Care 1978;23:178–179.

175. Flowerdew RMM. Coaxial scavenger for paediatric anaesthesia. Can Anaesth Soc J 1979;26:367–369.

176. Houghton A, Taylor PB. Problems with high-flow scavenging system. Anaesthesia 1983;38:292.

177. Keneally JP, Overton JH. A scavenging device for the T-piece. Anaesthesia and Intensive Care 1977;5:267–268.

178. Karski J, Sych M. A simple device designed to protect operating theatres against atmospheric pollution by volatile anaesthetics. Anaesth Res Intensive Ther 1976;4:61–64.

179. Maver E. Extractors for anaesthetic gases. Anaesthesia and Intensive Care 1975;3:348–350.

180. Oh TH, McGill WA, Becker MJ, Epstein BS. Scavenging pediatric circuits through an adult circle system. Anesthesiology 1980;53:S324.

181. Paul DL. An antipollution device for use with the Jackson–Rees modification of the Ayre's T-piece. Anaesthesia 1987;42:439–440.

182. Nott MR. A paediatric scavenging valve. Anaesthesia 1988;43:67–68.

183. Spargo PM, Apadoo A, Wilton HJ. An improved antipollution device for the Jackson–Rees modification of the Ayre's T-piece. Anaesthesia 1987;42:1240–1241.

184. Sik MJ, Lewis RB, Eveleigh DJ. Assessment of a scavenging device for use in paediatric anaesthesia. Br J Anaesth 1990;64:117–123.

185. Whitcher C. Waste anesthetic gas scavenging—indications and technology (ASA Refresher Course No. 126). Park Ridge, IL: ASA, 1974.

186. Whitcher CE. Control of occupational exposure to inhalational anesthetics—current status (ASA Refresher Course No. 205). Park Ridge, IL: ASA, 1977.

187. Weng J, Smith RA, Balsamo JJ, et al. A method of scavenging waste gases from the Jackson–Rees system. Anesth Rev 1980;7:35–38.

188. Chan MSH. A new T-piece scavenging system. Anaesthesia and Intensive Care 1993;21:899.

189. van Hasselt G, Phillips J. T-piece scavenging: simple alternatives. Anaesthesia 1994;49:263–264.

190. Hatch DJ, Miles R, Wagstaff M. An anaesthetic scavenging system for paediatric and adult use. Anaesthesia 1980;35:496–499.

191. Steward DJ. An anti-pollution device for use with the Jackson–Rees modification of the Ayre's T-Piece. Can J Anaesth 1972;19:670–671.

192. Chan MSH, Kong AS. T-piece scavenging—the double-bag system. Anaesthesia 1993;48:647.

193. Kumar CM. Another antipollution device for the Jackson–Rees modification of Ayre's T-piece system. Anaesthesia 1991;46:792–793.

194. Bray RJ. Another antipollution device for the Jackson–Rees modification of Ayre's T-piece. Anaesthesia 1992;47:174.

195. Baraka A, Muallem M. Scavenging by the double T-piece circuit. Anaesthesia 1993;48:1116–1117.

196. Steven IM. A scavenging system for use in paediatric anaesthesia. Anaesthesia and Intensive Care 1990;18:238–240.

197. Bernow J, Bjordal J, Wiklund KE. Pollution of delivery ward air by nitrous oxide. Effects of various modes of room ventilation, excess and close scavenging. Acta Anaesthesiol Scand 1984;28:119–123.

198. Nitka AC, O'Riordan EF, Julien RM. A new technique of scavenging exhaled nitrous oxide. Anesthesiology 1986;65:314–316.

199. Corn SB. Evaluation of the anesthetic scavenging hood. Anesthesiology 1995;83:A393.

200. Weber GM, Unterberger J, Gangoly W. Reduced exposure to halothane and nitrous oxide by operating personnel during induction of anesthesia in children using double mask system. Anesthesiology 1991;75:A927.

201. Jastak JT. Nitrous oxide in dental practice. Int Anesthesiol Clin 1989;27:92–97.

202. Railton R, Fisher J. Low flow active antipollution systems. An evaluation of two systems with automatic ventilators. Anaesthesia 1984;39:904–907.

203. Hoerauf K, Harth M, Wild K, et al. Occupational exposure to desflurane and isoflurane during cardiopulmonary bypass: is the gas outlet of the membrane oxygenator an operating theatre pollution hazard? Br J Anaesth 1997;78:378–380.

204. Ad Hoc Committee on Effects of Trace Anesthetics on Health of Operating Room Personnel, American Society of Anesthesiologists. Waste gases in operating room air: a suggested program to reduce personnel exposure. Park Ridge, IL: ASA, 1981.

205. Lawson D, Jelenich S. Capnographs: a new operating room hazard? Anesth Analg 1985;64:378.

206. Yamashita M, Shirasaki S, Matsuki A. A neglected source of nitrous oxide in operating room air. Anesthesiology 1985;62:206–207.

207. Tessler MJ, Kleiman SJ, Wiesel S. Nitrous oxide levels in the operating room: the effects of scavenging the Ohmeda 5200 capnometer. Can J Anaesth 1991;38: A60.

208. Conley RJ. Scavenging of capnometers. Anesth Analg 1986;65:102–103.

209. Wray RP. A source of nonanesthetic nitrous oxide in operating room air. Anesthesiology 1980; 52:88–89.

210. Anonymous. Update: nitrous oxide exhausted from cryosurgical units. Health Devices 1981;9:180.

211. Abadir AR. A simple gas scavenging hood for anesthesia machines. Journal of Clinical Monitoring 1992;8:168.

212. Sarma VJ, Leman J. Laryngeal mask and anaesthetic waste gas concentrations. Anaesthesia 1990;45: 791–792.

213. Carlsson P, Ljungqvist B, Hallen B. The effect of local scavenging on occupational exposure to nitrous oxide. Acta Anaesthesiol Scand 1983; 27:470–475.

214. Nilsson K, Sonander H, Stenqvist O. Close scavenging of anaesthetic gases during mask anaesthesia. Acta Anaesthesiol Scand 1981;25:421–426.

215. Houldsworth HB, O'Sullivan JO, Smith M. Dynamic behavior of air break receiver units. Br J Anaesth 1983;55:661–670.

216. Paloheimo M, Salanne SO. Open scavenging systems. Acta Anaesthesiol Scand 1979;23:596–602.

217. Moyes DG, Samson HH. Evaluation of a scavenging device for use with automatic ventilators. S Afr Med J 1981;59:178–180.

218. Jorgensen S, Jacobsen F. Uncalibrated anaesthetic scavenging systems with open reservoirs. Anaesthesia 1982;37:833–835.

219. Gray WM. Scavenging equipment. Br J Anaesth 1985;57:685–695.

220. Mostafa SM, Natrajan KM. Hydrodynamic evaluation of a new anaesthetic gas scavenging system. Br J Anaesth 1983;55:681–686.

221. Enderby DH, Booth AM, Churchill–Davidson HC. Removal of anaesthetic waste gases. An inexpensive antipollution system for use with pipeline suction. Anaesthesia 1978;33:820–826.

222. Houldsworth HB, O'Sullivan J, Smith M. An improved air break receiver unit. A design suited to high-vacuum scavenging systems. Br J Anaesth 1983; 55:671–680.

223. Anonymous. Anesthesia scavengers. Health Devices 1983;11:267–286.

224. Eisenkraft JB, Sommer RM. Flapper valve malfunction. Anesth Analg 1988;67:1132.

225. Petty C. Scavenger is often a neglected safety device. Anesthesia Patient Safety Foundation Newsletter 1992;7:28.

226. Cicman J, Himmelwright C, Skibo V, et al. Operating Principles of Narkomed Anesthesia Systems. Telford, PA: North American Drager, 1993.

227. Asbury AJ, Hancox AJ. The evaluation and improvement of an anti-pollution system. Br J Anaesth 1977; 49:439–446.

228. Armstrong RF, Kershaw EJ, Bourne SP, et al. Anaesthetic waste gas scavenging systems. Br Med J 1977; 1:941–943.

229. Bruce DL. A simple way to vent anesthetic gases. Anesth Analg 1973;52:595–598.

230. Bethune DW, Collis JM. Anaesthetic practice. Pollution in operating theatres. Biomed Eng 1974;9: 157–159.

231. Hawkins TJ. Anaesthetic gas scavenging systems. Anaesthesia 1984;39:190.

232. Mehta S, Behr G, Chari J, et al. A passive method of disposal of expired anaesthetic gases. Br J Anaesth 1977;49:589–593.

233. Mehta S. Terminal gas-exhaust valve for a passive disposal system. Anaesthesia 1977;32:51–52.

234. Vickers MD. Pollution of the atmosphere of operating theatres. Important notice. Anaesthesia 1975;30: 697–699.

235. Hagerdal M, Lecky JH. Anesthetic death of an experimental animal related to a scavenging system malfunction. Anesthesiology 1977;47:522–523.

236. Alexander KD, Stewart NF, Oppenheim RC, et al. Adsorption of halothane from a paediatric T-piece circuit by activated charcoal. Anaesthesia and Intensive Care 1977;5:218–222.

237. Enderby DH, Bushman JA, Askill S. Investigations of some aspects of atmospheric pollution by anaesthetic

gases. II: aspects of adsorption and emission of halothane by different charcoals. Br J Anaesth 1977;49: 567–573.

238. Hawkins TJ. Atmospheric pollution in operating theatres. Anaesthesia 1973;28:490–500.

239. Kim BM, Sircar S. Adsorption characteristics of volatile anesthetics on activated carbons and performance of carbon canisters. Anesthesiology 1977;46: 159–165.

240. Murrin KR. Atmospheric pollution with halothane in operating theatres. A clinical study using activated charcoal. Anaesthesia 1975;30:12–17.

241. Maggs FAP, Smith ME. Adsorption of anaesthetic vapours on charcoal beds. Anaesthesia 1976; 31: 30–40.

242. Murrin KR. Adsorption of halothane by activated charcoal. Further studies. Anaesthesia 1974; 29: 458–461.

243. Vaughan RS, Mapleson WW, Mushin WW. Prevention of pollution of operating theatres with halothane vapour by adsorption with activated charcoal. BMJ 1973;1:727–729.

244. Vaughan RS, Willis BA, Mapleson WW, et al. The Cardiff Aldavac anaesthetic-scavenging system. Anaesthesia 1977;32:339–343.

245. Capon JH. A method of regenerating activated charcoal anaesthetic adsorbers by autoclaving. Anaesthesia 1974;29:611–614.

246. Hojkjaer V, Larsen VH, Severinsen I, et al. Removal of halogenated anaesthetics from a closed circle system with a charcoal filter. Acta Anaesthesiol Scand 1989;33:374–378.

247. LeDez KM. Snedden W, Au J. A simple system using activated charcoal to scavenge anesthetic vapours in remote locations. Can J Anaesth 1995;42:A12.

248. Wright BM. Vacuum pipelines for anaesthetic pollution control. Br Med J 1978;1:918.

249. Abramowitz M, McGill WA. Hazard of anesthetic scavenging device. Anesthesiology 1979;51:276.

250. Parbrook GD, Mok IB. An expired gas collection and disposal system. Br J Anaesth 1975;47:1185–1193.

251. Lai KM. A flow-inducer for anaesthetic scavenging systems. Anaesthesia 1977;32:794–797.

252. Standard for Health Care Facilities, Quincy, MA: NFPA 1996.

253. U.S. Department of Health Education and Welfare. Criteria for a recommended standard: occupational exposure to waste anesthetic gases and vapors (DHEW (NIOSH) Publication No. 77–140). Washington, DC: US Government Printing Office, 1977.

254. Ilsley AH, Crea J, Cousins MJ. Assessment of waste anaesthetic gas scavenging systems under simulated conditions of operation. Anaesthesia and Intensive Care 1980;8:52–64.

255. Lecky JH. The mechanical aspects of anesthetic pollution control. Anesth Analg 1977;56:769–774.

256. Anonymous. Waste anesthetic gas, Part II. Technol for Anesth 1995;16(2):1–5.

257. Stone PA, Asbury AJ, Gray WM. Use of scavenging facilities and occupational exposure to waste anaesthetic gases. Br J Anaesth 1988;61:111P.

258. Connell GR, Mangar D. Is your scavenger system functional. Anesth Analg 1992;75:1075.

259. Barnett R, Gallant B, Fossey S, et al. Nitrous oxide environmental pollution. A comparison between face mask, laryngeal mask and endotracheal intubation. Can J Anaesth 1992;39:A151.

260. Lambert–Jensen P, Christensen NE, Brynnum J. Laryngeal mask and anaesthetic waste gas exposure. Anaesthesia 1992;47:697–700.

261. Torda TA, Jones R, Englert J. A study of waste gas scavenging in operating theatres. Anaesthesia and Intensive Care 1978;6:215–221.

262. Hovey TC. A gas scavenger system. J Am Assoc Nurse Anesth 1977;45:170–177.

263. Cramond T, Mead P. Non-rebreathing valve assembly. Anaesthesia and Intensive Care 1986;14: 465–468.

264. Reiz S, Gustavisson A-S, Haggmark S, et al. The double mask—a new local scavenging system for anaesthetic gases and volatile agents. Acta Anaesthesiol Scand 1986;30:260–265.

265. Breum NO, Kann T. Elimination of waste anaesthetic gases from operating theatres. Acta Anaesthesiol Scand 1988;32:388–390.

266. Siker D, Escorcia E, Sprung J, et al. Gas flow management during induction influences postintubation inhalational anesthetic concentration and operating room pollution. Anesthesiology 1995;83:A438.

267. Tharp JA. A simple way to limit anesthetic pollution during anesthetic induction. Anesth Analg 1987;66: 198.

268. Stevens WC, Casson H, Joyce JR. Comparison of methods to decrease operating room pollution with anesthetic gases during endotracheal intubation. Anesthesiology 1993;79:A534.

269. Sexton A. The circuit mount. Anaesthesia and Intensive Care 1995;23:754–755.

270. Goldman DB, Mushlin PS. Leakage of anesthetic agent from an Ohmeda Tech IV vaporizer. Anesth Analg 1991;72:567.

271. Davies JM, Strunin L, Craig DB. Leakage of volatile anaesthetics from agent-specific keyed vapourizer filling devices. Can Anaesth Soc J 1982; 29:473–476.

272. Sorensen BH, Thomsen A. Bronchoscopy and nitrous oxide pollution. Eur J Anaesth 1987;4: 281–285.

273. Carden E, Vest HR. Further advances in anesthetic technics for microlaryngeal surgery. Anesth Analg 1974;53:584–587.

274. Becker MJ, McGill WA, Oh TH, et al. The effect of an airway leak on nitrous oxide contamination of the operating room. Anesthesiology 1981;55:A335.

275. Laucks SO. Scavenging waste gases in pediatric patients. Anesthesiology 1983;59:602.

276. Vickery IM, Burton GW. Throat packs for surgery. An improved design based on anatomical measurements. Anaesthesia 1977;32:565–572.

277. Virtue RW, Escobar A, Modell J. Nitrous oxide levels in operating room air with various gas flows. Can Anaesth Soc J 1979;26:313–318.

278. Kim JS, Aldrete JA, Kullavanijaya T. Measurements of exposure to N_2O by personal dosimeters: comparison using different gas flows. Circular 1987;4:31–33.

279. Imberti R, Preseglio I, Imbriani M, et al A. Low-flow anaesthesia reduces occupational exposure to inhalation anaesthetics. Environmental and biological measurements in operating room personnel. Acta Anaesthesiol Scand 1995;39:586–591.

280. Ewen A, Sheppard SD, Goresky GV, et al. Occupational exposure to nitrous oxide during paediatric anaesthesia: a comparison of two induction techniques. Can J Anaesth 1989;36:S132–S133.

281. Albert SN, Kwan AM, Dadisman JW Jr. Leakage in anesthetic circuits. Anesth Analg 1977;56:878.

282. Berner O. Concentration and elimination of anaesthetic gases in operating theatres. Acta Anaesthesiol Scand 1978;22:46–54.

283. Whitcher CE. Methods of control. In: Cohen EN, ed. Anesthetic exposure in the workplace. Littleton, MA: PSG, 1980:117–148.

284. Stringer BW. Scavenging adaptor misconnection. Anaesthesia and Intensive Care 1982;10:169.

285. Berner O. Anaesthetic apparatus leakages. A possible solution. Acta Anaesthesiol Scand 1973; 17:1–7.

286. Whitcher C, Piziali RL. Monitoring occupational exposure to inhalation anesthetics. Anesth Analg 1977; 56:778–785.

287. Whitcher C. Controlling occupational exposure to nitrous oxide. In: Eger EI, ed. Nitrous oxide/N_2O. New York: Elsevier, 1985:3133–3137.

288. Piziali RL, Whitcher C, Sher R, et al. Distribution of waste anesthetic gases in the operating room air. Anesthesiology 1976;45:487–494.

289. Langley DR, Steward A. The effect of ventilation system design on air contamination with halothane in operating theatres. Br J Anaesth 1974;46:736–741.

290. Male CG. Theatre ventilation. A comparison of design and observed values. Br J Anaesth 1978;50:1257–1263.

291. Russell WJ, Webb RK, van der Walt JH, et al. Problems with ventilation: an analysis of 2000 incident reports. Anaesthesia and Intensive Care 1993;21:617–620.

292. Mann ES, Sprague DH. An easily overlooked malassembly. Anesthesiology 1982;56:413–414.

293. Holly HS, Eisenman TS. Hazards of an anesthetic scavenging device. Anesth Analg 1983;62:458–460.

294. Davies G, Tarnawsky M. Letter to the editor. Can Anaesth Soc J 1976;23:228.

295. Mantia AM. Gas scavenging systems. Anesth Analg 1982;61:162–164.

296. Burns THS. Pollution of operating theatres. Anaesthesia 1979;34:823.

297. Hamilton RC, Byrne J. Another cause of gas-scavenging-line obstruction. Anesthesiology 1979; 51:365–366.

298. Malloy WF, Wightman AE, O'Sullivan D, et al. Bilateral pneumothorax from suction applied to a ventilator exhaust valve. Anesth Analg 1979;58:147–149.

299. Rendell-Baker L. Hazard of blocked scavenge valve. Can Anaesth Soc J 1982;29:182–183.

300. O'Connor DE, Daniels BW, Pfitzner J. Hazards of anaesthetic scavenging: case reports and brief review. Anaesthesia and Intensive Care 1982;10:15–19.

301. Farquhar-Thomson DR, Goddard JM. The hazards of anaesthetic gas scavenging systems. Anaesthesia 1996;51:860–862.

302. Sainsbury DA. Scavenging misconnection. Anaesthesia and Intensive Care 1985;13:215–216.

303. Phillips S. Scavenging hazard. Anaesthesia and Intensive Care 1991;19:615.

304. Nunn G. Hazards of scavenging devices. Anaesthesia 1996;51:404–405.

305. Anonymous. Scavenging gas from membrane oxygenators. Technol for Anesth 1987;8(5):6–7.

306. Anonymous. Use of inadequate (old) anesthesia scavenger interfaces. Technol for Anesth 1994;14(8):1–2.

307. Schreiber P. Anesthesia systems. Telford, PA: North American Drager, 1984.

308. Smith DG. Anaesthetic gas scavenging systems. Anaesthesia 1985;40:90.

309. Gray WM, Hall RC, Carter KB, et al. Medishield AGS system and servo 900 ventilators. Anaesthesia 1984; 39:790–794.

310. Blackstock D, Forbes M. Analysis of an anaesthetic gas scavenging system hazard. Can J Anaesth 1989; 36:204–208.

311. Lanier WL. Intraoperative air entrainment with Ohio Modulus anesthesia machine. Anesthesiology 1986; 64:266–268.

312. Mostafa SM, Sutclffe AJ. Antipollution expiratory

valves. A potential hazard. Anaesthesia 1982; 37: 468–469.

313. Mor ZF, Stein ED, Orkin LR. A possible hazard in the use of a scavenging system. Anesthesiology 1977; 47:302–303.

314. Patel KD, Dalal FY. A potential hazard of the Drager scavenging interface system for wall suction. Anesth Analg 1979;58:327–328.

315. Sivalingam P, Hyde RA, Easy WR. An unpredictable and possibly dangerous hazard of an anaesthetic scavenging system. Anaesthesia 1997; 52:609–610.

316. Seymour A. Possible hazards with an anaesthetic gas scavenging system. Anaesthesia 1982; 37: 1218–1219.

317. Milliken RA. Hazards of scavenging systems. Anesth Analg 1980;59:162.

318. Sharrock NE, Gabel RA. Inadvertent anesthetic overdose obscured by scavenging. Anesthesiology 1978; 49:137–138.

319. Heard SO, Munson ES. Ventilator alarm nonfunction associated with a scavenging system for waste gases. Anesth Analg 1983;62:230–232.

320. Kam PCA, Kam AC, Thompson JF. Noise pollution in the anaesthetic and intensive care environment. Anaesthesia 1994;49:982–986.

321. Halsey MJ. Occupational health and pollution for anaesthetics. A report of a seminar. Anaesthesia 1991; 46:486–488.

322. Hallen B, Ehrner–Samuel H, Thomason M. Measurements of halothane in the atmosphere of an operating theatre and in expired air and blood of the personnel during routine anaesthetic work. Acta Anaesthesiol Scand 1970;14:17–27.

323. Halsey MJ, Chand S, Dluzewski AR, et al. Olefactory thresholds: detection of operating room contamination. Br J Anaesth 1977;49:510–511.

324. Sutton BA, Shephard JN, Hall JA, et al. Exhaust gas monitoring, safety and the integrity of gas supply in cardiopulmonary bypass. J Cardiothorac Vascul Anesth 1994;8:29.

325. Ilsley AH, Crea J, Cousins MJ. Evaluation of infrared analysers used for monitoring waste anaesthetic gas levels in operating theatres. Anaesthesia and Intensive Care 1980;8:436–440.

326. Halliday MM, Carter KB, Davis PD, et al. Survey of operating room pollution with an N.H.S. district. Lancet 1979;1:1230–1232.

327. Campbell D, Davis PD, Halliday MM, et al. Comparison of personal pollution monitoring techniques for use in the operating room. Br J Anaesth 1980;52: 885–892.

328. Holmes CM. Pollution in operating theatres. Part 2. The solution. N Z Med J 1978;87:50–53.

329. Knights KM, Strunin JM, Strunin L. Measurement of low concentrations of halothane in the atmosphere using a portable detector. Lancet 1975;1:727–728.

330. Allander C, Carlsson P, Hallen B, et al. Thermo camera, a macroscopic method for the study of pollution with nitrous oxide in operating theatres. Acta Anaesthesiol Scand 1981;25:21–24.

331. Carlsson P, Ljungqvist B, Allander C, et al. Thermo camera studies of enflurane and halothane vapours. Acta Anaesthesiol Scand 1981;25:315–318.

332. Carlsson P, Hallen B, Hallonsten A, et al. Thermo camera studies of nitrous oxide dispersion in the dental surgery. Scand J Dent Res 1983;91:224–230.

333. Austin JC, Shaw R, Crichton R, et al. Comparison of sampling techniques for studies of nitrous oxide pollution. Br J Anaesth 1978;50:1109–1112.

334. Beynen FM, Knopp TJ, Rehder K. Nitrous oxide exposure in the operating room. Anesth Analg 1978; 57:216–223.

335. Davenport HT, Halsey MJ, Wardley–Smith FB, Wright BM. Measurement and reduction of occupational exposure to inhaled anesthetics. BMJ 1976; 2: 1219–1221.

336. Gray WM, Burnside GW. The evacuated canister method of personal sampling. An assessment of its suitability for routine monitoring of operating theatre pollution. Anaesthesia 1985;40:288–294.

337. Austin JC, Shaw R, Moyes D, et al. A simple air sampling technique for monitoring nitrous oxide pollution. Br J Anaesth 1981;53:997–1003.

338. Burm AG, Spierdijk J. A method for sampling halothane and enflurane present in trace amounts in ambient air. Anesthesiology 1979;50:230–233.

339. Carter KB, Halliday MM. A personal air sampling pump for hospital operating staff. J. Med Eng Technol 1978;2:310–312.

340. Dupressoir CAJ. A practical apparatus for measuring average exposure of operating theatre personnel to halothane. Anaesthesia and Intensive Care 1975;3: 345–347.

341. Choi-Lao AT. Trace anesthetic vapors in hospital operating-room environments. Nurs Res 1981;30: 156–161.

342. Hunter L. An occupational health approach to anaesthetic air pollution. Med J Aust 1976;1:465–468.

343. Halliday MM, Carter KB. A chemical adsorption system for the sampling of gaseous organic pollutants in operating theatre atmospheres. Br J Anaesth 1978; 50:1013–1018.

344. Bishop EC, Hossain MA. Field comparison between two nitrous oxide (N_2O) passive monitors and conventional sampling methods. Am Ind Hyg Assoc J 1984;45:812–816.

345. Cox PC, Brown RH. A personal sampling method for the determination of nitrous oxide exposure. Am Ind Hyg Assoc J 1984;45:345–350.

346. Ward BG. Development and application of a long dynamic range nitrous oxide monitoring system. Am Ind Hyg Assoc J 1985;46:697–703.

347. Aclerman J. Monitoring waste nitrous oxide. AORN J 1985; 41:895–898.

348. Whitcher C. Clinical evaluation of two dosimeters for monitoring occupational exposure to N_2O. Anesthesiology 1984;61:A169.

349. Mcgill WA, Rivera O, Howard R. Time-weighted average for nitrous oxide: an automated method. Anesthesiology 1980;53:424–426.

350. Korttila K, Pfaffli P, Ertama P. Residual nitrous oxide in operating room personnel. Acta Anaesthesiol Scand 1978;22:635–639.

351. Pfaffli P, Nikki P, Ahlman K. Halothane and nitrous oxide in end-tidal air and venous blood of surgical personnel. Ann Clin Res 1972;4:273–277.

352. Corbett TH. Retention of anesthetic agents following occupational exposure. Anesth Analg 1973; 52:614–618.

353. Anonymous. Workshop on anesthetic pollution. Anesthesiol Rev 1977;4:25–34.

354. Nikki P, Pfaffli P, Ahlman K. End-tidal and blood halothane and nitrous oxide in surgical personnel. Lancet 1972;2:490–491.

355. Salamonsen LA, Cole WJ, Salamonsen RF. Simultaneous trace analysis of nitrous oxide and halothane in air. Br J Anaesth 1978;50:221–227.

356. Hillman KM, Saloojee Y, Brett II, et al. Nitrous oxide concentrations in dental surgery. Atmospheric and blood concentrations of personnel. Anaesthesia 1981;36:257–262.

357. Imbriani M, Ghittori S, Pezzagno G, et al. Evaluation of exposure to isoflurane (Forane): Environmental and biological measurements in operating room personnel. J Toxicol Environ Health 1988;25:393–402.

358. Imbriani M, Ghittori S, Pezzagno G, et al. Nitrous oxide (N_2O) in urine as biological index of exposure in operating room personnel. Appl Ind Hyg 1988;3:223–226.

359. Imbriani M, Ghittori S, Zadra P, et al. Biological monitoring of the occupational exposure to halothane (Fluothane) in operating room personnel. Am J Ind Med 1991;20:103–112.

360. Imbriani M, Ghittori S, Pezzagno G, et al. Biological monitoring of occupational exposure to enflurane (Ethrane) in operating room personnel. Arch Environ Hlth 1994;49:135–140.

361. Sonander H, Stenqvist O, Nilsson K. Exposure to trace amounts of nitrous oxide. Br J Anaesth 1983;55:1225–1229.

362. Sonander H, Stenqvist O, Nilsson K. Urinary N_2O as a measure of biologic exposure to nitrous oxide anaesthetic contamination. Ann Occup Hyg 1983;27:73–79.

363. Whitcher C. Correspondence. Anesthesiol Rev 1976; 3:41–42.

364. Milliken RA. A plea for monitoring both halogenated and non-halogenated anesthetic agents in the operating room. Anesthesiol Rev 1976;3:29–31.

365. Ackerman J. Monitoring waste nitrous oxide. One medical center's experience. AORN J 1985;41:895–898.

366. Gray WM. Occupational exposure to nitrous oxide in four hospitals. Anaesthesia 1989;44:511–514.

367. Draft report on anesthetic waste gas: scavenging for Ministry of Health. Ontario, Canada: October 1977.

368. Bruce DL, Linde HW. Halothane content in recovery room air. Anesthesiology 1972;36:517–518.

369. Berner O. Concentration and elimination of anaesthetic gases in recovery rooms. Acta Anaesthesiol Scand 1978;22:55–57.

370. Geraci CL Jr. Operating room pollution: governmental perspectives and guidelines. Anesth Analg 1977; 56:775–777.

371. Mazze RI. Waste anesthetic gases and the regulatory agencies. Anesthesiology 1980;52:248–256.

372. Anonymous: Scavenging systems to comply with "stiff laws" regulating trace gas exposure in OR described. Anesthesiol News, Aug 14, 1984.

373. Lambert–Jensen P, Christensen NE, Brynnum J. Laryngeal mask and anaesthetic waste gas exposure. Anaesthesia 1992;47:697–700.

374. Borm PJ, Kant I, Houben G, et al. Monitoring of nitrous oxide in operating rooms: identification of sources and estimation of occupational exposure. J Occup Med 1990;32:1112–1116.

375. Gardner RJ. Inhalation anaesthetics—exposure and control: a statistical comparison of personal exposures in operating theatres with and without anaesthetic gas scavenging. Ann Occup Hyg 1989;33:159–173.

376. Mondry GA. Medical-legal implications. In: Cohen EN, ed. Anesthetic exposure in the workplace. Littleton, MA: PSG, 1980:163–182.

377. Anonymous. OSHA inspections of hospital operating rooms. American Society of Anesthesiologists Newsletter 1980;44:7.

QUESTIONS

1. Trace gases of which of the following have been shown to have an effect on anesthesia personnel performance in the operating room.
   A. Halothane
   B. Nitrous oxide
   C. Enflurane
   D. Isoflurane
   E. None of these

2. Which of the following anesthetic agents is most likely to be associated with spontaneous abortions in animals?
   A. Halothane
   B. Nitrous oxide
   C. Enflurane
   D. Isoflurane
   E. Sevoflurane

Each question below contains four suggested answers of which one or more is correct. Choose the answer:

A. if 1, 2, and 3 are correct
B. if 1 and 3 are correct
C. if 2 and 4 are correct
D. if 4 is correct
E. if 1, 2, 3 and 4 are correct.

3. The following measures are necessary to eliminate trace gases in the operating room
   1. A scavenging system
   2. Work techniques
   3. Elimination of leaks
   4. The room air conditioning system

4. Gas collecting devices need to be attached to
   1. Anesthesia breathing systems
   2. Pump oxygenators
   3. Anesthesia agent monitors
   4. Ventilators

5. Open interfaces include
   1. A bag with valves for air intake or gas relief
   2. Tube within a tube
   3. A pressure relief valve in the disposal tubing
   4. T-tube

6. Parts of the scavenging system connected by the transfer tubing include
   1. The interface and an adsorption device
   2. The interface and ventilator
   3. The interface and the ventilation system
   4. The interface and the APL valve

7. Passive disposal assemblies include
   1. The room ventilation system
   2. Piped vacuum system
   3. Piping directly to atmosphere
   4. Duct system with a fan

8. Possible problems associated with the use of piped suction systems for gas disposal include
   1. Inadequate number of outlets
   2. Damage to the suction pump
   3. Vacuum system overload
   4. Exposure of personnel in other parts of the facility

9. Gas disposal devices that employ a mechanical system include
   1. Piping to atmosphere
   2. Active duct systems
   3. Adsorption devices
   4. Suction systems

10. Components connected by the gas disposal tubing include
    1. The interface and an adsorption device
    2. The interface and the suction system
    3. The interface and the ventilation system
    4. The interface and the APL valve

11. The following work practices will reduce exposure of operating room personnel to trace anesthetic gases
    1. Use of cuffed tracheal tubes
    2. Use of high fresh gas flows
    3. Disconnecting the nitrous oxide sources when the machine is not in use
    4. Use of insufflation techniques

12. Maximum time-weighted average concentrations to which a worker in the operating room should be exposed

according to the Occupational Safety and Health Administration include
1. 5 ppm for halogenated agents
2. 2 ppm for halogenated agents
3. 180 ppm for nitrous oxide
4. 25 ppm for nitrous oxide

13. Hazards associated with scavenging equipment include
    1. Negative pressure in the breathing system
    2. Misconnections
    3. Barotrauma
    4. Ventilator malfunction

14. Sampling methods for determining trace gas concentrations include:
    1. Single shot
    2. Time-weighted average
    3. End-tidal sampling
    4. Urine sampling

15. Size(s) of the inlet and outlet fittings of the transfer tubing include
    1. 15 mm
    2. 19 mm
    3. 22 mm
    4. 30 mm

16. Ways in which leak sites can be identified include
    1. Application of a 50% soap solution to a component
    2. Testing the capacity of the machine to sustain pressure
    3. Using a nitrous oxide analyzer to check suspected sites
    4. Turning on the nitrous oxide cylinder and watching the pressure drop

17. When the intermediate pressure system is checked for leaks
    1. The pre-use machine checkout will reveal even small leaks
    2. The bag port and the Y piece should be occluded
    3. The vaporizers should be in the OFF position

4. The leak rate should be less than 1 liter per minute

18. Concerning the room air conditioning system for gas disposal
    1. Air exchanges should be 25 to 35 per hour
    2. Recirculating systems are less effective than nonrecirculating systems
    3. The flow should be upward rather than downward
    4. The anesthesia machine should be placed near the exhaust grill

19. Problems which could cause positive pressure in the breathing system include
    1. Occlusion of the gas disposal assembly
    2. Misassembly of the connection to the gas disposal system
    3. Incorrect assembly of the positive pressure relief valve
    4. Application of subambient pressure to the APL valve

20. Concerning monitors which can be used for detection of trace gases
    1. Infrared analyzers are most often used to measure volatile agents
    2. The ionizing leak detector is best suited to measure nitrous oxide
    3. The Thermo camera can provide quantitative measurement of nitrous oxide
    4. An oxygen analyzer can be used to monitor the scavenging system interface

ANSWERS

1.	E	11.	B
2.	B	12.	C
3.	E	13.	E
4.	E	14.	E
5.	C	15.	C
6.	C	16.	A
7.	B	17.	C
8.	E	18.	C
9.	C	19.	E
10.	A	20.	D

Hazards of Anesthesia Machines and Breathing Systems

I. Hypoxia
  A. Hypoxic Inspired Gas Mixture
    1. Incorrect Gas Supplied
      a. Piping System
      b. Cylinders
      c. Cross-Overs in the Anesthesia Machine
    2. Hypoxic Mixture Delivered
      a. Flow Control Malfunction
      b. Incorrect Flowmeter Settings
      c. Incorrect Flowmeter Readings
      d. Inaccurate Flowmeter
    3. Loss of Oxygen to Atmosphere
    4. Air Entrainment
  B. Hypoxia Secondary to Hypoventilation
    1. Causes
      a. Insufficient Gas in the Breathing System
        (1) Low Inflow
          (a) Pipeline Problems
          (b) Cylinder Problems
          (c) Machine Problems
            ((1)) Obstruction
            ((2)) Leaks
            ((3)) Loss of Gas Supply from the Anesthesia Machine
          (d) Problems with the Fresh Gas Supply
        (2) Excessive Outflow
          (a) Breathing System Leaks
          (b) Disconnections
          (c) Negative Pressure Applied to the Breathing System
          (d) Improper Adjustment to the APL Valve

      b. Blockage of Inspiratory Pathway
    2. Detection
    3. Response
      a. Check Ventilator Settings
      b. Check Ventilator Bellows
        (1) Ventilator Bellows Does not Move
        (2) Ventilator Bellows Fills but Fails to Compress Fully
        (3) Ventilator Bellows Fails to Fill
  C. Incorrect Placement of PEEP Valve
II. Hypercapnia
  A. Hypoventilation
  B. Inadvertent Administration of Carbon Dioxide
  C. Rebreathing without Removal of Carbon Dioxide
    1. Absorbent Failure
    2. Bypassed Absorbent
    3. Unidirectional Valve Problems
    4. Problems with Nonrebreathing Valves
    5. Inadequate Fresh Gas Flow to a Mapleson System
    6. Improper Assembly of Bain System
    7. Excessive Dead Space
III. Hyperventilation
IV. Excessive Airway Pressure
  A. Modifying Factors
  B. Causes
    1. High Inflow
    2. Low Outflow
      a. Obstruction in the Expiratory Limb
      b. Obstruction at the Ventilator
      c. Obstruction at the APL Valve

HAPPY IS HE who gains wisdom from another's mishaps.

Although enormous strides have been made in improving the safety of anesthesia apparatus, reports of problems continue to appear. Studies have shown that human error is more frequent than equipment failure (1–7).

This chapter will principally examine hazards of anesthesia machines and breathing systems from the perspective of their effect on the patient. Many examples are given, but this should not be considered a complete listing of all possible dangers. Many hazards involve older apparatus that may have been modified and is no longer sold or serviced by the manufacturer.

HYPOXIA
Hypoxic Inspired Gas Mixture
Incorrect Gas Supplied
Piping System

Crossovers between oxygen and other gases may occur anywhere in a piped system. Most commonly the transposition is in the piping itself (8, 9). During or following construction or repair, a pipeline may be filled with air or nitrogen rather than oxygen (10). Such a line must be purged thoroughly with oxygen before use. An incorrect gas may be installed at the central supply (11–14).

Incorrect outlets may be installed inside the operating room (OR) (15–19). An incorrect connector may be placed on a hose (20–23) or the pipeline inlet of the anesthesia machine (18). Quick-connect fittings may be damaged or poorly designed so that an incorrect connection can be made (24). Connections between piped gases can occur in peripheral equipment and result in the oxygen pipeline being contaminated with another gas if the pressure of that gas is higher than that of oxygen (25–28). An air flowmeter may have an oxygen outlet connector (29, 30).

Gas crossovers are particularly hazardous as the first instinct of the anesthesia provider presented with a hypoxemic patient is to supply 100% oxygen. If a crossover or contamination has occurred, simply opening an oxygen cylinder on the anesthesia machine will not be effective. The oxygen hose must be disconnected from the wall outlet.

Cylinders

It is possible for a cylinder labeled *oxygen* to contain another gas (31, 32). A cylinder may be painted a color other than that normally used. Particular care should be taken with cylinders in other countries, because four different colors (green, white, blue, and black) are used around the world for oxygen (33). In a cylinder containing a mixture of two gases, incomplete mixing may result in a hypoxic mixture being delivered (34, 35). Such a cylinder may require 45 minutes of rotating before mixing is complete.

Despite almost universal use of the Pin Index Safety System, reports of incorrect cylinders being connected to yokes continue to appear (36–41). An incorrect yoke block may be inserted (42, 43). A pin may become unscrewed from the yoke (44).

Crossovers in the Anesthesia Machine

Crossovers between oxygen and other gases can occur inside the anesthesia machine (47, 48).

Hypoxic Mixture Delivered

Flow Control Valve Malfunction

Damage to the oxygen flow control valve can result in low oxygen flow (45–50). Damage to the flow control valve for another gas may result in excessive flow of that gas relative to that of oxygen.

Incorrect Flowmeter Settings

Most anesthesia machines manufactured before 1979 do not have an oxygen–nitrous oxide interlock or proportioning system to prevent the user from dialing a hypoxic fresh gas flow. On these machines a hypoxic mixture can be caused by closing, partly or fully, the flow control valve for oxygen while allowing the nitrous oxide flow to continue (51–54). On machines manufactured after 1979 there may be problems with the minimum oxygen ratio device (55–58), or the machine may have additional gases that are not incorporated into the safety system.

Oxygen flow can be inadvertently lowered (or the flow of another gas increased) if the flow control knob is inadvertently rotated by an item on the surface below (59) or by a hose or wire allowed to drape around it. With some flowmeters, in-and-out movement of the flow control valve can change the flow significantly (60). Someone helping to move the machine could grab a flow control valve knob and change the flow (Fig. 13.1). Various devices have been developed to protect flow control valves (see Figure 4.31).

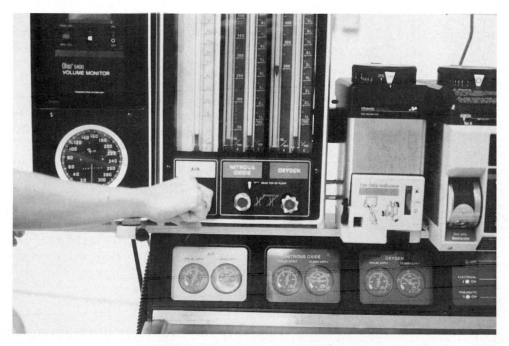

FIGURE 13.1.   A dangerous practice. The flow control knob may look like a good thing to grab to someone moving an anesthesia machine. Flows may be altered in the process.

Incorrect Flowmeter Reading

On some older machines, the flowmeter indicator can disappear from view at the top of the tube when the flow of gas exceeds the maximum scale calibration. Such a flowmeter is very similar in appearance to one with the indicator resting at the bottom. If the flowmeter is for a gas other than oxygen, a hypoxic mixture may result.

If an air flowmeter is present on a machine, dialing air instead of oxygen can result in a hypoxic mixture (61). To prevent this, most modern anesthesia machines do not allow administration of air and nitrous oxide without oxygen flow (see Fig. 4.28).

Inaccurate Flowmeter

Flowmeter inaccuracies are common. Causes include dirt, grease, or oil on the indicator or tube; a stuck or damaged indicator; misalignment of the tube; static electricity; improper calibration; the stop at the top of the tube falling down onto the indicator (Fig.13.2); and transposition of indica-

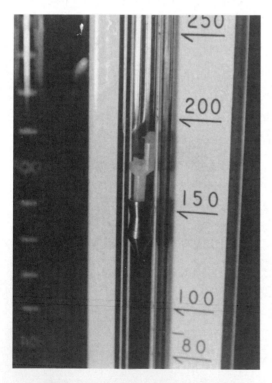

FIGURE 13.2. The stop at the top of the flowmeter tube has broken off and fallen onto the indicator. The flowmeter will read less than the actual flow.

tor, scale, or tube (62–67). This can sometimes be detected by an indicator not rotating or lying at an angle in the tube.

Loss of Oxygen to Atmosphere

If there is a leak at the top of the oxygen flowmeter tube, oxygen will be preferentially lost, even if the oxygen flowmeter is downstream of the other flowmeters (65–77). The position of the indicator may not be affected. Often the defect cannot be seen until the tube is disassembled.

Other leaks in the anesthesia machine can result in hypoxia, the magnitude of which will depend on the size of the leak and its location (74–76, 78–86). It is important to use a yoke plug in any yoke not containing a cylinder so that gas will not leak out if a flow control valve is left open.

Air Entrainment

If the pressure in the breathing system falls below atmospheric levels, air may be drawn into the system through a leak or disconnection and dilute the oxygen concentration. Subatmospheric pressure may be caused by the inspiratory effort of the patient, suction applied to an enteric tube inadvertently placed in the tracheobronchial tree or to the working channel of a fiberscope in the airway, a problem with the scavenging system, a ventilator with a hanging bellows, or a sidestream gas analyzer with a low fresh gas flow (87–91).

In a ventilator powered by air, air may enter the system through a hole in the bellows. Air used to reduce the fogging of a lens on a bronchoscope may dilute the inspired oxygen (92).

If it is suspected that the pipeline oxygen system is delivering less than 100% oxygen, it is important to open an oxygen cylinder *and* to disconnect the oxygen pipeline hose. If the pipeline hose is not disconnected, gas from the piping system will still be delivered. If the cause of a low oxygen concentration is not obvious and the situation is not corrected by disconnecting the oxygen pipeline hose and opening an oxygen cylinder, the patient should ventilated with room air.

Hypoxia Secondary to Hypoventilation

Problems with equipment can result in inadequate or total failure of ventilation.

Causes

Insufficient Gas in the Breathing System
Low inflow.

PIPELINE PROBLEMS. Loss of pipeline oxygen pressure was discussed in Chapter 2, "Medical Gas Piping Systems." Causes include damage during construction, debris left in the line following installation, unannounced system shutdown, regulator malfunction, malfunction of the central supply system, disruption of the line between the central supply and the healthcare facility, failure of a compressor due to an electrical storm, fires, and closure of an isolation valve (22, 93–96). A station outlet may become blocked or not accept quick connector (97, 98).

A hose may develop a leak (99, 100), become blocked (101), or develop a kink that obstructs gas flow (102). The anesthesia machine may roll over a hose, occluding gas flow (103). The check valve in the pipeline inlet at the back of the machine may malfunction, blocking flow (104).

If piped oxygen pressure is lost, an oxygen cylinder should be opened and the pipeline hose disconnected from the wall to prevent flow from the cylinder into the pipeline. To minimize oxygen usage, the ventilator should be turned off, manual or spontaneous ventilation instituted, and the fresh gas flow lowered.

If opening an oxygen cylinder does not repressurize the anesthesia machine, there is a problem in the intermediate pressure system of the machine, unless the cylinder is empty or not connected properly (103). A resuscitation bag should be used to ventilate the patient until another machine can be obtained.

CYLINDER PROBLEMS. A cylinder may be delivered empty or with an inoperable valve or blocked valve outlet (105–107).

Before a cylinder can be used it must be correctly installed on the machine. Frequently, the most inexperienced person in the OR is told, without any instructions, to replace an empty cylinder. He or she may fail to crack the valve; install it without a washer, with a damaged washer, or with two washers; fail to remove the dust protection cap (Fig 13.3); or fail to check to see that the cylinder is full. Another error is screwing the retaining screw of the yoke into the safety-relief de-

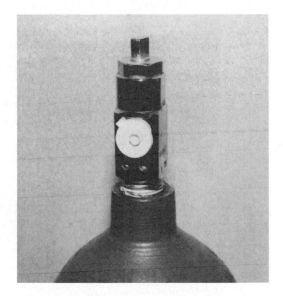

FIGURE 13.3. Failure to remove the dust protection cap from a cylinder before installing it on a machine caused a portion of the cap to be pushed into the cylinder valve port, and this blocked the exit of gas from the cylinder.

vice on the cylinder (108). It is sometimes possible to spot an incorrectly placed cylinder simply by looking at it. An improperly installed cylinder may hang at an angle instead of parallel to the machine (Fig. 13.4).

The fact that a full cylinder is present on an anesthesia machine does not mean that there will be oxygen available when needed. First, there must be a means of opening the cylinder. A good practice is to chain a handle to each machine so that it will always be there when needed.

A cylinder can empty and there may not be another cylinder available to replace it. If there is a single yoke for oxygen, the cylinder should be full before starting a case and there should be a supply of oxygen close at hand (109). The anesthesia provider must be watchful of the cylinder pressure gauge to determine the remaining oxygen in the cylinder.

MACHINE PROBLEMS

OBSTRUCTION. Obstruction to gas flow in the anesthesia machine resulting from problems in the oxygen flush valve, flow control valve, and vaporizer connections have been reported (110–113).

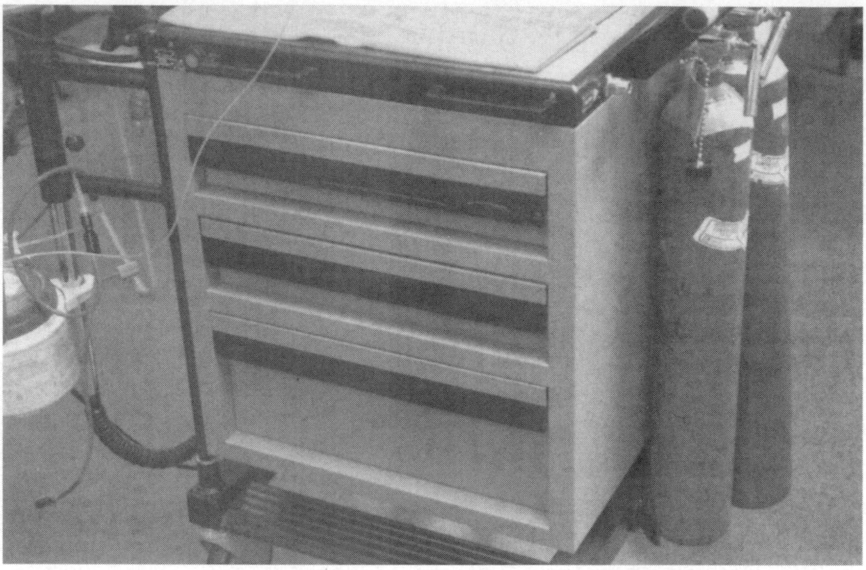

FIGURE 13.4. A sure sign that a cylinder is not correctly fitted in its yoke is that it hangs at an angle to the machine rather than perpendicular to the floor.

Other reported causes include the leaflet from a check valve (114) and a foreign body (115).

LEAKS. If the check valve in the pipeline inlet of the anesthesia machine fails, gas may flow into the room (if the pipeline hose is disconnected) or into the piping system (if the hose is connected) (116, 117). A leaking or broken flowmeter tube or an open flow control valve with an opening to atmosphere upstream of the flowmeter can result in loss of gas (77).

Leaks can occur in the piping of the machine (118, 119) or at a loose or defective vaporizer connection (120–135). Leaks can occur at a loose, defective, or absent vaporizer filler cap or drain screw (136–138) (Fig. 13.5); or in the vaporizer itself (139). Some machines are designed so that when a vaporizer is removed, a manifold cap must be placed where the vaporizer was situated (see Figure 5.44). Failure to do so will result in a major leak. The pressure relief device on the machine may vent fresh gas if resistance downstream causes the pressure to rise (140, 141).

LOSS OF GAS SUPPLY FROM THE ANESTHESIA MACHINE. The main On-Off switch on the machine may be accidentally turned to the Off position (142, 143).

PROBLEMS WITH THE FRESH GAS SUPPLY. The fresh gas supply hose can become detached (88, 107,

144) or occluded (96, 145–151) or can develop a leak (152). A component placed in the fresh gas line can develop a leak or become disconnected. The inner tube of the Bain system, which carries the fresh gas flow, can become obstructed (153–155).

Excessive outflow

BREATHING SYSTEM LEAKS. Most breathing system leaks are too small to be of clinical significance, but some are large enough that the patient cannot be ventilated adequately, especially if low fresh gas flows are used. Leaks also cause pollution of OR air (see Chapter 12, "Controlling Trace Gas Levels").

A common location for leaks in the circle system is the absorber. If the canisters do not fit together properly or the top and bottom do not seal well, a large leak can result (156, 157). Accidental disengagement of a canister can occur (96, 158–160). Humidifiers, breathing tubes, elbow adapters, bags, temperature probe sites, connectors for respiratory gas analyzers or pressure monitors, bag-ventilator selector valves, filters, heat and moisture exchangers (HME), oxygen analyzers, adjustable pressure-limiting (APL) valves, fresh gas tubing and Y pieces have all been reported as sources of leaks (96, 161–190) (Fig.

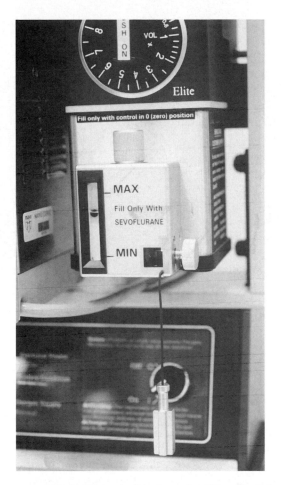

FIGURE **13.5.** When the block on the filling block is not in place, there will be a leak when the vaporizer is turned on.

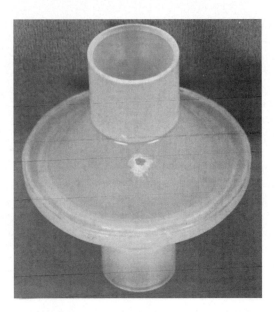

FIGURE **13.6.** Parts of the breathing system may have holes in them when they are received from the manufacturer.

13.6). A reservoir bag mount may break (191, 192). A heated humidifier may burn a hole in a breathing tube (193–196).

The APL valve may fail to close (197–200). Newer bag-ventilator selector valves cause the APL valve to be excluded from the system when switched to the automatic mode (see Chapter 8, "Breathing Systems III: Circle System"). On machines where the APL valve is not excluded, the user may forget to close it when switching to automatic ventilation.

Leaks may occur in a ventilator (201, 202) or its attachment to the breathing system (203–205). Loss of gas will occur if the pilot line becomes disconnected or kinked during expira-

tion, the spill valve ruptures or becomes stuck in the open position, or the exhaust valve malfunctions (206–210). A bag/ventilator switch placed in the ventilator position with no ventilator in place will result in a large leak (211).

A defective nonrebreathing valve or misassembly of a manual resuscitator can result in part or all of the volume leaving the bag escaping to atmosphere (212–214).

Most leaks can be detected by checking before use. During a case, leaks may be indicated by a low expired volume, an increase in end-tidal carbon dioxide, or an increase in inspired nitrogen during spontaneous ventilation. With a standing bellows ventilator, the bellows may not return to its fully expanded position (215) and there may be a change in the sound of the ventilator. A low airway pressure monitor may detect a leak but cannot be relied on.

When a leak is suspected, a systematic search of the anesthesia machine and breathing system should be made, following the route of gas travel. It may be easier to detect a leak if gloves are removed (183).

DISCONNECTIONS (216). A disconnection is an unintended separation of components in a breathing system. Studies show that disconnections are the most common type of preventable anesthetic mishap involving equipment (1, 2, 157, 217). Most breathing system connectors are slip fittings that rely on friction to hold them together. They will come apart if sufficient tension is applied. Drapes may make it difficult to see a disconnection (218).

Disconnections can occur anywhere in the breathing system. The most common site is between the breathing system and tracheal tube connector (1, 219). Other common sites are the common gas outlet, the end of the ventilator hose, and the connection of the tubing to an airway pressure monitor or aspirating respiratory gas monitor. Disconnections are often associated with interference to the breathing system by a third party and with surgery on the head and neck (157).

Disconnections can be made less frequent by making secure connections. Connectors with lugs or other features that make them easy to grip may be easier to tighten. Wrung (push-and-twist) connections are much stronger than those made with a straight push and metal-to-metal or plastic-to-plastic joints are stronger than metal-to-plastic joints (220). Antidisconnect devices for use in breathing systems have been described (216, 221). Locking connectors use a mechanical means to ensure the connectors do not separate under any force found during use. Many believe that they should not be used at the connection between the tracheal tube connector and the breathing system, reasoning that it is safer for such a joint to come apart under tension than for the tracheal tube to be pulled out of the patient (222). Also, it may be necessary to make a disconnection rapidly at this point for suctioning or to relieve a high pressure in the breathing system. Latching connectors are similar to locking connectors but are designed to "break away" at a certain disconnection force (216).

Adhesive tape is sometimes used to prevent disconnections. Unfortunately, this can prevent visual detection of a disconnection, inhibit reconnection, and form an obstruction (216).

NEGATIVE PRESSURE APPLIED TO THE BREATHING SYSTEM. If the negative pressure inlet valve of a closed scavenging interface or the opening to atmosphere of an open interface becomes blocked, or the interface is omitted, a subatmospheric pressure may be transmitted across the APL valve to the breathing system (223–228).

If suction is applied to the working channel of a fiberscope passed into the airway or an enteric tube that has entered the trachea rather than the esophagus, respiratory gases will be removed rapidly from the lung and breathing system (90, 229–231).

IMPROPER ADJUSTMENT OF THE APL VALVE. When manually controlled or assisted ventilation is used, gas is vented from the system during inspiration (unless a closed system technique is used). Part of the gas displaced from the bag goes into the patient and the rest is discharged from the breathing system. The person squeezing the bag may find it difficult to estimate how much gas is entering the patient and how much is escaping to atmosphere. Hypoventilation can occur if too much gas escapes through the valve.

Blockage of the Inspiratory Pathway

Partial or complete blockage between the reservoir bag or ventilator and the patient can result in hypoventilation. Causes include manufacturing defects; water, blood, and/or secretions; and foreign bodies (171, 232–239). Connecting a flow direction–sensitive component such as a positive end–expiratory pressure (PEEP) valve or humidifier in the inspiratory limb of a breathing system in reverse will result in no flow (240). If the bag-ventilator selector valve is left in the wrong position, complete obstruction to gas flow will result.

Breathing tubes can become obstructed from kinking or twisting (241) (Fig. 13.7) as can the neck of the reservoir bag (Fig. 13.8). A heated humidifier may cause the tubing to melt and become obstructed (242) (Fig. 13.9).

With obstruction, the peak pressure recorded on the breathing system manometer may be increased. The travel of the ventilator bellows will be reduced, but not totally eliminated. An airway pressure monitor may or may not alarm, depending on the locations of the occlusion and the airway pressure sensor.

Hypoventilation secondary to ventilator problems is discussed in Chapter 11, "Anesthesia Ventilators." Causes include cycling failure, leaks of driving or breathing system gas, inaccurate settings, and the ventilator being turned off.

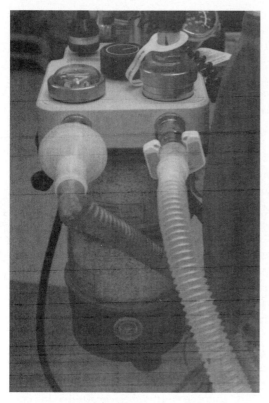

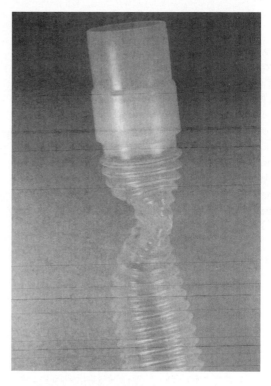

FIGURE 13.9. Contact with a heated humidifier can cause a breathing tube to melt and become obstructed.

FIGURE 13.7. Kinking of a breathing tube.

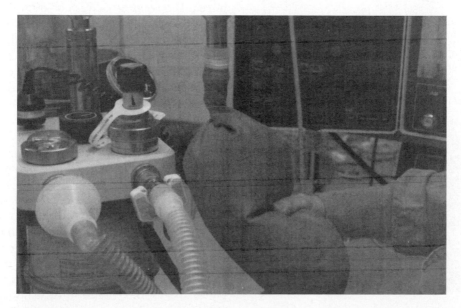

FIGURE 13.8. Twisting has caused this bag to become obstructed. Many bags have a guard in the neck to prevent this.

Detection

Vigilance aids used to detect hypoventilation include airway pressure and carbon dioxide monitors and respirometers. They are discussed in Chapter 18, "Anesthesia Gas Monitoring" and Chapter 19, "Airway Pressure, Volume, and Flow Measurements." An oxygen analyzer may detect some disconnections (157, 243, 244) but should not be relied on because it is effective in only a limited set of circumstances. The low temperature alarm on a heated humidifier may signal loss of gas flow in the breathing system (157). Because any single monitoring modality may fail to detect a problem (245–249), it is advisable to use more than one. Use of multiple monitors enhances vigilance and diagnostic utility (250).

Response (250, 251)

It is assumed that the anesthesia provider has available a resuscitation bag (Fig. 13.10) that can

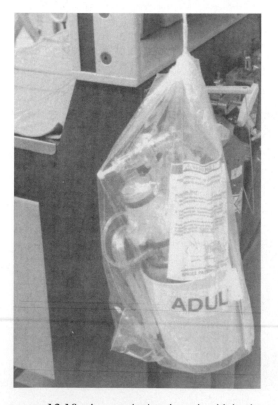

FIGURE 13.10. A resuscitation bag should be kept readily available in each OR for use in emergencies.

be connected by a source of oxygen to ventilate the patient and that this will be used if necessary. If ventilation appears to be inadequate, the following steps should be taken.

Check the Ventilator Settings

A quick glance at the ventilator settings should be made to determine if they are correct.

Check the Ventilator Bellows

Ventilator bellows does not move. Failure of the ventilator to cycle means that the driving gas supply has been shut off or the electrical power has failed or been turned off. If the ventilator cannot be turned on, manual ventilation should be instituted.

Ventilator bellows fills but fails to compress fully. If the bellows fills but fails to compress fully, there is obstruction to ventilation or a leak in the ventilator. The ventilator should be turned off and the bag-ventilator selector valve checked to make certain it is set for automatic ventilation. If it is, the user should immediately disconnect the tracheal tube connector from the breathing system. If this results in an outrush of gas, there is an obstruction in the expiratory pathway.

If disconnection of the tracheal tube does not result in an outrushing of gas, the user should attach a resuscitation bag and ventilate the patient. If the tracheal tube is obstructed, it should be replaced. If there is no outrush of gas with disconnection and the tracheal tube is not blocked, manual ventilation should be attempted. If the reservoir bag fills and the patient can be ventilated, the problem is related to the ventilator. Common causes are a disconnection of the ventilator hose and a leak in the bellows. If there is obstruction to ventilation it is in the inspiratory limb between the reservoir bag and the patient connection.

Ventilator bellows fails to fill. If the bellows does not fill, the flowmeters on the anesthesia machine should be checked. If low flows are being used, they should be increased. Often this will correct the problem. If the flowmeter indicators are at the bottom of their tubes, an oxygen cylinder should be turned on and the oxygen pipeline hose disconnected. If the indicators return to their normal positions, the problem is in the pipeline supply. If they do not return to their normal positions, there is a problem in the machine and a new machine should be obtained.

If the flowmeter indicators are at their normal positions, the operator should perform a rapid visual scan for disconnections in the breathing system, starting with the patient connection and proceeding through the entire system. The cuff on the tracheal tube should be checked. If the problem is not found, a switch should made to manual ventilation. If the reservoir bag fails to fill, the fresh gas supply hose should be checked for a leak, disconnection, or obstruction. Deliberately kinking the fresh gas supply hose should cause the flowmeter indicators to fall. If they do not, there is a leak in the machine. If the reservoir bag fills with use of the oxygen flush but does not stay filled when ventilation of the patient is attempted, there is excessive outflow from the breathing system. A systematic check should be made, starting with the fresh gas supply hose and moving around the entire system, looking for a leak, an open APL valve, disconnection, or source of negative pressure. The tracheal tube should be disconnected from the breathing system and the patient connection port occluded. Applying positive pressure to the reservoir bag may make it possible to audibly locate the source of outflow. Equipment such as a humidifier that can be easily taken out of the system should be removed. This may eliminate the leak.

Incorrect Placement of a PEEP Valve

Low levels of PEEP may be beneficial in improving low arterial oxygen tension levels. If a bidirectional PEEP valve is incorrectly placed against the direction of flow or a unidirectional PEEP valve is placed in the inspiratory limb oriented with the flow, PEEP will not be applied to the patient's airway, although gas flow will not be obstructed.

HYPERCAPNIA
Hypoventilation

Causes of hypoventilation are discussed under Hypoxia.

Inadvertent Administration of Carbon Dioxide (252)

In some countries, it is not uncommon to have a carbon dioxide cylinder and flowmeter on an anesthesia machine. The flowmeter may be accidentally turned on and this may not be noticed, especially when the indicator is at the top of the tube (253). An apparently OFF flowmeter may leak carbon dioxide into the breathing system. (254) In one reported case, a nitrous oxide hose was connected to the carbon dioxide station outlet (255). A cylinder may be mistakenly filled with carbon dioxide (256)

Rebreathing without Removal of Carbon Dioxide
Absorbent Failure

Hypercarbia can occur if channeling allows gases to bypass the absorbent (96, 257). Fluorescent lights in an OR can deactivate the indicator around the outside of the canister so it does not change color when exhausted (258). Cases have been reported in which the absorbent did not contain an indicator (259).

Bypassed Absorbent

Some older absorbers are fitted with a bypass that allows some or all of the gases to bypass the absorbent. Accidental activation of this bypass can lead to inadvertent hypercarbia. The partial bypass on one older absorber is located on the side of the absorber opposite from where the user normally stands (Fig.13.11). It is easy to miss seeing that the valve is in the bypass position unless a special effort is made to check it. The absorber may be defective so that gas flow is not directed through the absorbent (260).

If channels develop in the absorbent, gas may pass through the canister without contacting any active absorbent. This will result in increased carbon dioxide in the inspiratory gas. Hypercarbia due to problems with the absorbent or absorber should be corrected by increasing the fresh gas flow. Other problems, such as an incompetent unidirectional valve will not be corrected by this maneuver (261).

Unidirectional Valve Problems

Correct movement of gases in a circle system depends on proper functioning of the unidirectional valves. If they do not close properly, rebreathing will occur. The disc or seat may become displaced, wet, sticky, or damaged so that the disc will not seat properly (96, 261–271) (Fig. 13.12).

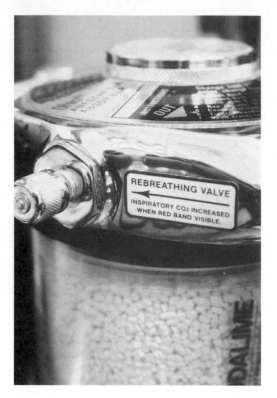

FIGURE 13.11. The partial bypass on this absorber is on the opposite side of the absorber from where anesthesia personnel normally stand and is not easily seen. A special effort should be made to check it.

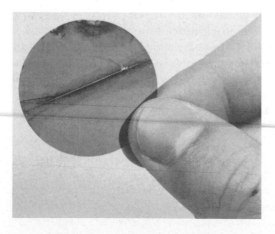

FIGURE 13.12. Damaged unidirectional valve leaflet.

A disc may not be replaced after removal for cleaning or servicing.

Problems with Nonrebreathing Valves

Improper assembly or sticking of nonrebreathing valves can result in partial or total rebreathing. This is discussed more fully in Chapter 9, "Manual Resuscitators."

Inadequate Fresh Gas Flow to a Mapleson System

In systems without carbon dioxide absorption a low fresh gas flow can result in dangerous rebreathing (see Chapter 7, "Breathing Systems II: Mapleson Systems"). Reported causes include the flow being set too low, a leak or obstruction in the machine, common gas outlet, fresh gas supply line or a vaporizer, and an empty cylinder (114, 167, 272–274). In systems in which the fresh gases are delivered to the distal end of the system by an inner tube, rebreathing will occur if the inner tube is avulsed, damaged, kinked, or omitted; has a leak at the machine end; or does not extend to the patient port (Fig. 13.13) (154, 266–274).

Improper Assembly of the Bain System

Cases of incorrect assembly of the Bain system have been reported (275–284). In one case, the fresh gas supply tube was connected to the pressure manometer while the manometer was connected to the inflow orifice. In the other case, the system was assembled without the inner tube. In both cases the entire hose became dead space.

Excessive Dead Space

An increase in dead space will increase rebreathing, especially in small patients (Fig. 13.14). One possible source is the HME. These come in a variety of sizes and if a large one is used on a patient with a small tidal volume, dangerous rebreathing may occur (285). Hypercarbia is best detected using capnometry. Inspired carbon dioxide will be zero if hypoventilation is the sole cause of hypercarbia. Inadvertent administration of carbon dioxide and rebreathing without carbon dioxide removal will result in an inspired concentration greater than zero. See Chapter 18, "Anesthesia

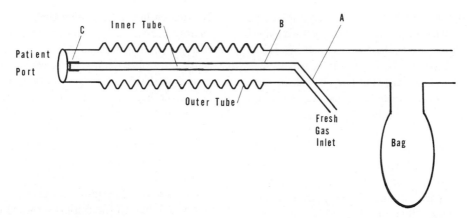

FIGURE 13.13.   Possible problems with the inner tube of the Bain system that can result in hypercarbia. **A,** the fresh gas supply tube can become detached; **B,** the inner tube can become kinked or develop a leak; and **C,** the inner tube may not extend to the patient port.

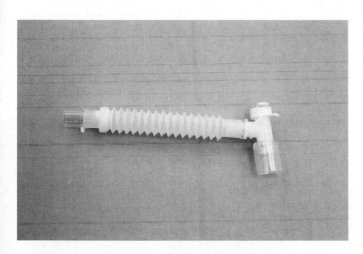

FIGURE 13.14. Increased dead space between the breathing system and the patient can result in serious hypercarbia in pediatric patients and spontaneous breathing adults.

Gas Monitoring," for a full discussion of CO_2 monitoring.

HYPERVENTILATION

A hole or tear in the bellows can cause inadvertent hyperventilation (286–288). This can be detected by an increased oxygen concentration if oxygen is the driving gas (or a decreased concentration if air is used).

EXCESSIVE AIRWAY PRESSURE (289)

In addition to interfering with ventilation, a high pressure can cause barotrauma and adverse effects on the cardiovascular system. Neurological changes and otorrhagia have been reported (290, 291). A hyperinflated lung may interfere with surgery (292).

Modifying Factors

The rate and extent of the pressure rise are important and will be affected by a number of factors, including the reservoir bag, the volume and compliance of the system, the fresh gas flow, and use of a cuffed or uncuffed tracheal tube, mask or laryngeal mask airway (LMA). The most important of these is the bag.

The pressure in the breathing system is normally limited to 50 cm H_2O by the reservoir bag. When an automatic ventilator is in use, the bellows buffers increase in pressure. Exclusion of the bag or bellows from the system removes this buffering capacity so that dangerously high pressures may be reached rapidly if there is coincidental obstruction to the outflow of gases from, or high inflow into, the system. The most common cause of exclusion of the bag is obstruction of the expiratory limb upstream of the bag (see below). The bag may be obstructed by kinking at its neck (293) (see Fig. 13.11). A bag/ventilator switch placed in the ventilator position with no ventilator in place and a blocked ventilator port has been reported (211).

Unfortunately, an anesthesia provider who finds a reservoir bag that is not filled may incorrectly assume that there is a leak in the system and operate the oxygen flush in an attempt to compensate for the leak (289).

Another factor that can affect the rate of pressure rise is an uncuffed tracheal tube or a tracheal tube whose cuff is not inflated to a high pressure. Adjusting cuff pressure to less than 34 cm H_2O will allow it to act as a safety valve for excessive pressure in the airway. Disconnection of components cannot be relied on to provide pressure relief because the pressures required for disconnection are far in excess of those that cause injury (220).

Causes

High Inflow

If the oxygen flush valve sticks in the on position, 35 to 75 l/min will be delivered. On some older anesthesia machines, the oxygen flush valves could be locked in the flush position. Oxygen flush valves on newer machines are designed to close automatically, but can fail (294–296). With some oxygen flush valves, it is possible for personnel accidentally to actuate them with their bodies. Other equipment may cause the flush valve to stick in the on position (297–300).

Activation of the oxygen flush valve during the inspiratory phase of the ventilator cycle will cause a large volume of gas to be added to the inspired tidal volume. This will result in a greatly increased pressure (301, 302).

Low Outflow

Buildup of pressure will occur when there is obstruction to the outflow of gases from the breathing system while inflow continues.

Obstruction in the Expiratory Limb

As noted above, exclusion of the bag from the breathing system results in loss of its buffering capacity. Thus obstruction of the expiratory limb is particularly hazardous if it occurs upstream of the reservoir bag. The expiratory pathway can be obstructed by foreign bodies (including ampoules, coins, plastic wraps, discs, tape, and caps) (303–307), water (308) or equipment defects or misassembly (302, 309–314). A PEEP valve may stick or become obstructed (315–317).

The expiratory breathing tube may be connected by mistake to the outlet of the APL valve (318–322), the ventilator spill valve (323), or the ventilator port of a bag-ventilator selector valve. A unidirectional PEEP valve placed backward in the expiratory limb (324, 325) or attached in reverse to the expiratory port of a manual resuscitation bag (326) will cause complete obstruction to flow.

Obstruction can result from the seals on a disposable absorbent package not being removed, from occlusions in the holes in the top and bottom panels or from compacted absorbent (96, 327–331) (Fig. 13.15).

The expiratory limb of a T-piece system can become obstructed by the user's finger, kinking, external compression, misassembly, or adhesive (332–334). Cases have been reported in which

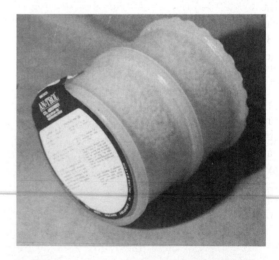

FIGURE 13.15. Prepacked absorbent container. Failure to remove the label from the top and/or bottom will result in obstruction to flow through the absorber.

the leaflet from a unidirectional valve was lost during servicing (335, 336). It was later found obstructing the connection to the bag mount. If a pediatric breathing system with an adapter that has the fresh gas inlet protruding near the end is used with a "low dead space" tracheal tube connector, the fresh gas supply tube may closely approximate or even press against the end of the connector, causing partial or complete obstruction of the exhalation pathway (337–340). The same problem has been reported with a bronchoscope (341).

Obstruction at the Ventilator

If the ventilator spill valve becomes stuck, the pressure in the breathing system will rise (208, 342–345). Blockage of the exit of driving gas from the bellows housing may occur (346).

Obstruction at the APL Valve

Omission, malfunction, or blockage of an APL valve may occur (289, 293, 347). The user may fail to open the valve when switching from controlled to spontaneous ventilation. With some APL valves, subambient pressure from an active scavenging system will cause the valve to close, preventing gas from flowing out of the breathing system (348–351).

Obstruction in the Scavenging System

The scavenging system is essentially an extension of the breathing system. Obstruction between the APL valve in the breathing system or the spill valve in the ventilator and the interface can prevent gas from leaving the breathing system (350, 352–354). The transfer tubing may be connected to an incorrect site (355–357).

Problems with Nonrebreathing Valves in Resuscitators

A sudden high inflow of gas or a quick squeeze or bump on the bag of a resuscitator may generate sufficient pressure to lock the nonrebreathing valve in the inspiratory position (358). Continuing inflow will cause a rise in pressure. Incorrect assembly or malfunction of a nonrebreathing valve may result in obstruction to exhalation (359–362).

Unintentional PEEP

An external PEEP valve may be left in the circuit and not removed or an integral PEEP valve may be left in the On position at the end of a case and not noticed by the next user (363) (Fig. 13.16). With older breathing systems, the airway pressure gauge is located on the absorber side of the unidirectional valves and PEEP cannot be observed on the gauge (325). With these systems, PEEP may be inadvertently set too high (292).

PEEP may be caused by water condensed in the tubing connecting the ventilator to the breathing system (364).

Misconnection of Oxygen Tubing

Misconnection of an oxygen tubing or mask directly to an indwelling tracheal or tracheostomy tube or laryngeal mask without provision for venting has occurred, with disastrous results (365–373) (Fig. 13.17). Another cause is connection to a T-piece with a closed expiratory limb (374).

Detection

When an automatic ventilator is used, it is essential that the chest wall motion, deflections on the breathing system pressure gauge, tidal and minute volumes registered on a respirometer, and breath sounds be carefully monitored. Observation of the airway pressure waveform, if available, can also help to detect some problems. The ventilator may change sound with stacked breaths. A continuing or high airway pressure alarm may alert the operator of the hazard. The capnograph may show an ascending limb with a prolonged rise time and no plateau.

Response

If there is a pressure buildup in the system, a disconnection should be made IMMEDIATELY at the tracheal tube connector. Ventilation can be carried on with a resuscitation bag until the problem is diagnosed and corrected. Time spent looking for the cause of the problem may result in ever increasing pressure.

INHALATION OF A FOREIGN SUBSTANCE

Absorbent Dust

Inhalation of absorbent dust can cause bronchospasm, laryngospasm, cough, decreased compliance, and burns of the patient's face (375, 376). This can be avoided by using a filter on the inspira-

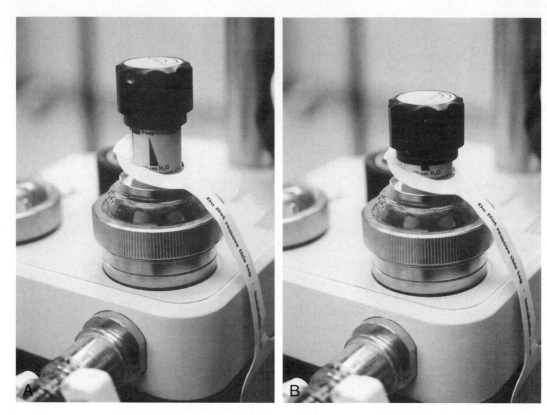

FIGURE 13.16. **A,** positive end–expiratory pressure (PEEP) valve with 0 PEEP. **B,** same valve with PEEP. Note how similar in appearance they are.

tory side of the circle system, placing the reservoir bag on the inspiratory limb, releasing the pressure at the APL valve when checking for leaks (377), tapping each canister to remove dust before it is put into the absorber, and not overfilling canisters (378).

Ethylene Oxide and Glycol (See Chapter 27, "Cleaning and Sterilization")

If equipment sterilized with ethylene oxide is not aerated adequately, residual ethylene oxide can be inhaled. When equipment is cleaned, water may remain. If wet equipment is sterilized with ethylene oxide, ethylene glycol, a toxic substance, will be formed and may subsequently be inhaled.

Contaminants in Medical Gases

Reported contaminants in medical gases include water, oil, hydrocarbons, higher oxides of nitrogen, and metallic fragments (105, 379–391). Bacteria may be found, especially in compressed air (392–395).

Parts of Breathing System Components

Part of a breathing system component may become detached. Reported cases have involved parts of the sampling site for an aspirating respiratory gas monitor (396, 397), an APL valve (398), an oxygen sensor (399), and HMEs (400, 401). Some manufacturers plate the inside surfaces of components with materials that may flake off (402, 403).

Foreign Bodies

A number of foreign bodies have been found in breathing systems (235, 236, 238, 239, 303–306, 404–406). Often these enter during cleaning.

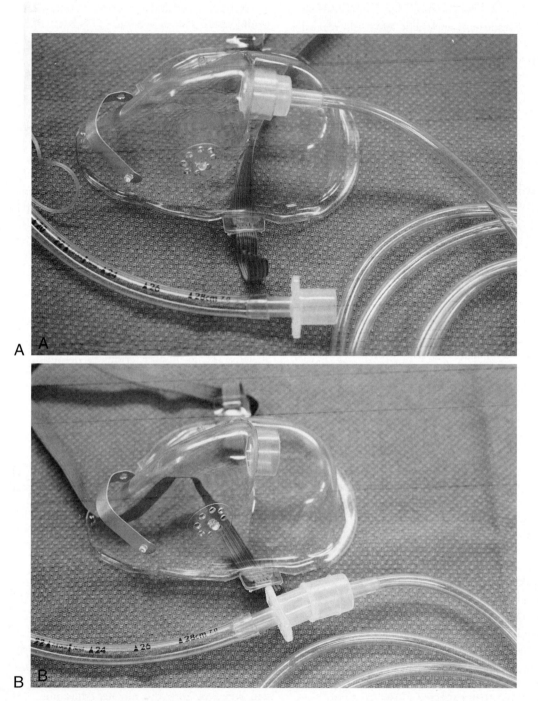

FIGURE 13.17.   **A,** the oxygen tubing is attached to the mask. **B,** the adapter has become detached from the mask and is attached to the tracheal tube connector. There is no way for the gas to escape.

ANESTHETIC AGENT OVERDOSAGE

An overdose of anesthetic agent can result in severe cardiovascular depression. See Chapter 5, "Vaporizers," for a more complete discussion of overdosage caused by vaporizer malfunction.

Tipping of a Vaporizer

If a vaporizer charged with liquid is tipped or agitated, a very high concentration may be delivered when the vaporizer is turned on (407).

Vaporizer or Nitrous Oxide Inadvertently Turned On

Previous use of the machine by a colleague or servicing by a technician can result in the control dial on a vaporizer being left in the on position (408–410). Someone helping to move the machine may grasp a control dial, inadvertently turning it on. Most newer vaporizers have locks to prevent a vaporizer from being turned on inadvertently.

Inadvertent administration of anesthetic agents may occur if gas from the main flowmeters is used to supply supplementary oxygen (411).

Incorrect Agent

If an agent is incorrectly placed in a vaporizer designed for an agent with a lower vapor pressure and/or a higher minimum alveolar concentration (MAC) value, a hazardously high concentration may be delivered (412–414). Examples include placing isoflurane or halothane in a vaporizer designed for enflurane or placing halothane in a vaporizer designed for isoflurane.

Improper Vaporizer Installation

If a vaporizer is located in the fresh gas supply tube, there will be a higher-than-usual flow of gas through the vaporizer after the oxygen flush is activated (415). If such a vaporizer is connected so that the flow is reversed, the concentration of vapor coming from the vaporizer may be considerably higher than expected (416).

Early versions of the Select-A-Tec mounting system had the entry and exit tubings in close proximity (Fig. 13.18A). This made it possible to connect the inlet tubing to the outlet and vice versa. If this occurred, flow through the vaporizer would be reversed and an increased concentration would result. Newer versions (Fig. 13.18B) have the outlet on the opposite end of the mounting device, making it extremely unlikely that this problem could occur.

Overfilled Vaporizer

Most vaporizers are designed so that they cannot be overfilled. Agent-specific filling devices prevent overfilling by connecting the air intake in the bottle to the inside of the vaporizing chamber. However, this safety feature can be overridden by slightly unscrewing the bottle adapter or turning the concentration dial on during filling (417).

When an overdose of anesthetic agent is suspected, the patient should be disconnected from the breathing system and ventilated using a resuscitation bag.

INADEQUATE ANESTHETIC AGENT

Although not delivering enough anesthetic agent is usually not as serious as delivering too much, serious morbidity can result (418).

Decreased Nitrous Oxide Flow

Loss of pipeline nitrous oxide caused by leaks, freezing of regulators, improper maintenance, depletion of a system too small to meet demand, and deliberate tampering have been reported (22, 419–421). Cylinder supplies can also fail. An obstruction or leak in the anesthesia machine may cause the nitrous oxide flow to decrease (422).

Another potential problem is the inadvertent use of air instead of nitrous oxide (423).

Unexpectedly High Oxygen Concentration

If a connection between the nitrous oxide and oxygen sources occurs in either the pipeline system or the anesthesia machine, and the oxygen pressure is higher than that of nitrous oxide, oxygen will flow into the nitrous oxide line (424, 425). An inward leak of oxygen downstream of the vaporizers will dilute volatile agents as well as nitrous oxide (426).

Accidental activation of the oxygen flush may occur (295, 298, 427–430). Repeated use of the

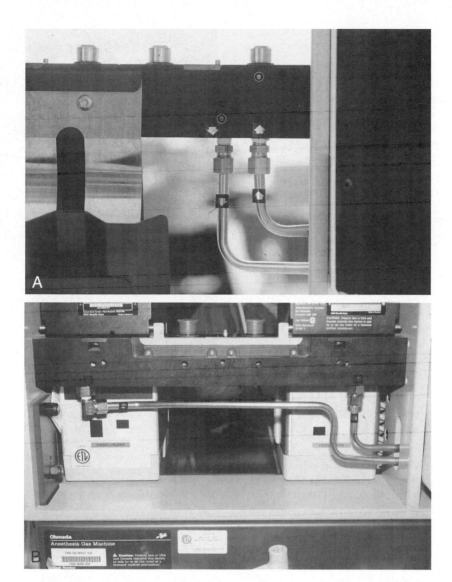

FIGURE 13.18. Select-A-Tec System. **A,** older version with adjacent inlet and outlet tubes. **B,** newer system with tubes separated.

oxygen flush to keep the reservoir bag filled can lead to patient awareness (296, 431, 432).

Leak in Vaporizer

A leak in a vaporizer caused by a loose or absent filler cap or keyed filler block, or a defect in the inflow or outflow connections can cause a low concentration to be delivered. A vaporizer selector or interlock device can malfunction in such a way that no vapor is delivered, although the vaporizer appears to be situated normally (433).

Empty Vaporizer

Another cause of underdosage is a vaporizer that runs empty (418). Cases have been reported in which a fluid level was visible in the sight glass of a vaporizer when the vaporizer was empty (434).

Incorrect Agent in Vaporizer

If a vaporizer designed for use with a highly volatile agent is filled with one of low volatility, the patient will fail to receive the concentration expected (412, 413). Examples include placing isoflurane or enflurane in a vaporizer designed for halothane and placing enflurane in a vaporizer designed for isoflurane.

Incorrect Vaporizer Setting

An incorrect setting of a vaporizer control or flowmeter can be a cause of underdosage. It is important to check settings frequently during a case because they can be altered without the operator's knowledge. It is not uncommon to forget to turn on a vaporizer after filling it during use.

Incorrect Vaporizer Mounting

Malfunction of a vaporizer mounting mechanism can result in a lower-than-expected vapor output (435–437).

Damaged Vaporizer

Damage to a vaporizer may occur if water or other substances are allowed to enter the vaporizing chamber (Fig. 13.19).

Air Entrained into the Breathing System

If a patient is breathing spontaneously, the negative pressure generated during inspiration may cause air entrainment through a leak or disconnection. Negative pressure can also be caused by a ventilator that has a hanging bellows or a negative pressure phase (438) or by an active scavenging system (87).

Dilution by Ventilator Driving Gas

Driving gas (oxygen or air) can enter the breathing system if the bellows is improperly connected or has a hole (286, 288, 439–443).

Air Added from Light Source

A stream of air used to reduce fogging of a lens may cause dilution of the inhaled anesthetic agents (92).

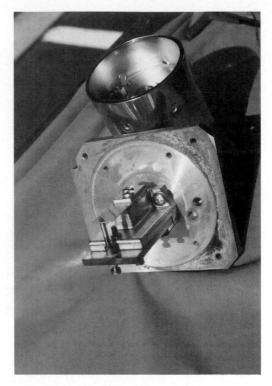

FIGURE 13.19. Foreign substances in the vaporizing chamber have caused corrosion of the internal parts of the vaporizer.

INADVERTENT EXPOSURE TO VOLATILE AGENTS

It is possible that halothane-related hepatitis or malignant hyperthermia may be triggered by small amounts of agent present in a machine and breathing system even if the vaporizers are turned off (433, 444–449).

When a patient with a history of one of these entities must be anesthetized, a machine should be prepared for use by removing all vaporizers (unless the machine isolates the vaporizers from the gas circuit when all vaporizers are in the off position). It has been shown that there is less background contamination if the vaporizers have been removed than if they are just kept in the OFF position (450). Removal also prevents the anesthesia provider from inadvertently turning on a vaporizer. Other necessary actions include changing the absorbent, replacing the fresh gas supply hose, using new disposable tubings and bag, and flushing with a high flow of oxygen for 20 minutes (451–455).

Should an episode of malignant hyperthermia occur during administration of anesthesia and the department has a machine from which vaporizers have been removed and that has been thoroughly flushed of volatile agents, it should be substituted for the machine in use. A fresh breathing system should be used. If the department does not have such a machine, the following measures should be taken to reduce the inhaled concentration of volatile anesthetic (451, 453).

1. Change the breathing system hoses and bag.
2. Change the fresh gas supply hose.
3. Change the absorbent.
4. Use very high flows of oxygen.
5. Insert a charcoal filter on the inspiratory port of the absorber.
6. Avoid using a contaminated ventilator.
7. Remove vaporizers from the machine if they are mounted on a system which allows the anesthesia provider to remove vaporizers.

FIRES AND EXPLOSIONS

Although flammable anesthetics have disappeared from ORs, perioperative fires continue to occur. They can have devastating consequences and typically come as a complete surprise to the staff (456). Many of the fuels present in the OR include plastics that produce dense black smoke when ignited. The smoke may be toxic as well as an impediment to safe evacuation of the patient and staff from the room. Tracheal tube fires during laser procedures are discussed in Chapter 17, "Tracheal Tubes."

Factors

Three ingredients (the fire triangle) must be present for a fire to occur: a gas to support combustion, a source of ignition, and a flammable substance. Head and neck surgery offers a particularly good opportunity for all three to be in close proximity.

Gas to Support Combustion

An oxygen-enriched atmosphere will cause materials that are flammable in air to ignite more easily and burn more vigorously and will lower the ignition threshold for some materials. Because oxygen is heavier than air, it collects in low-lying areas. Some materials such as some drape fabrics, absorb oxygen and retain it for some time. Dilution of oxygen with nitrogen (air) and/or helium will reduce the potential for combustion.

Air will support combustion because it contains oxygen. Nitrous oxide supports combustion and in the process releases the energy of its formation, providing increased heat.

Source of Ignition

A common source of ignition is the electrosurgical unit or a hot-wire cautery tip (457, 458). Other reported sources include defibrillators, laser beams, resectoscopes, OR lights, heat lamps, endoscopic light sources and cables, heated probes, drills and burs, argon beam coagulators, defective electrical equipment, and static electricity (456, 459–465).

A heated wire breathing tubing can ignite the breathing hose if it is used outside its suggested range of flows or minute volumes or the heated breathing circuit and the humidifier are electrically incompatible (196, 466–468). Another source of heat is adiabatic compression of a gas in a regulator. Pieces of Teflon tape, chips from seal materials, hydrocarbon contaminants, and other materials may be ignited (469–471).

A Combustible Substance

A number of articles used in or near the patient can serve as the flammable material. These include (but are not limited to) tracheal and tracheostomy tubes, tape, oxygen cannulae and tubings, breathing tubes and bags, sponges, eye patches, masks, nasogastric tubes, lubricants and ointments, drapes, covers, airways, paper products, blood pressure cuffs, tourniquets, gloves, stethoscope tubing, throat packs, egg crate foam mattresses, gowns, masks, hoods, and cleaning and prepping solutions and sprays (457, 460, 472–500). Disposable drapes may be particularly difficult to extinguish because they are water repellent (486). Once ignited they burn rapidly (493).

Measures to Prevent Fires

1. High-pressure oxygen equipment should not be contaminated with oil, grease, or other

combustible materials. Such equipment should not be cleaned with a flammable agent such as alcohol.

2. A cylinder should always be opened slowly to allow dissipation of heat as the gas is recompressed.

3. Oxygen should be administered only when indicated and in no higher a concentration than is needed (as guided by oxygen saturation monitoring).

4. Use of air for insufflating under drapes should be considered. If oxygen must be used, a barrier should be established between the oxygen-enriched atmosphere and the surgical field, if possible. An attempt should be made to prevent oxygen and oxygen–nitrous oxide mixtures from being vented near a source of ignition. When there must be an oxygen-rich environment near a heat source, using wet, sterile towels, packers, or sponges or nonflammable drapes around the surgical site can prevent ignition of materials near the site (457, 501). A local scavenging system will help to remove the gases from the vicinity of the surgery.

5. Hair near the operative site (e.g., eyebrows, mustaches) should be made nonflammable by coating it thoroughly with a water-soluble lubricating jelly or soaking with saline (464).

6. When diathermy is used in the oral cavity, the oxygen level should be minimized by using a cuffed tracheal tube (483). If an uncuffed tube must be used, a moist pharyngeal pack will reduce the flow of gases into the cavity (502). Gauze or packs to be used in the oral cavity should be moistened with a nonflammable liquid.

7. Water-based prep solutions should be used. If a flammable solution must be used, draping should be delayed to allow the vapor to dissipate (503).

8. Flammable liquids and sprays should be handled in such a way that pooling or saturation of drapes is avoided.

9. All aerosols should be considered flammable and the use of electrosurgery delayed for several minutes following their application.

10. The electrosurgical unit should function properly and have a proper dispersive (ground plate) circuit. This will shorten the required duty cycle and minimize heating of the tip. The electrosurgery unit with the lowest tip temperature that is effective for a given use should be used (504). Use of bipolar rather than unipolar electrodes will reduce the current density in the tissues surrounding the active electrode (502).

11. Nitrogen or air rather than oxygen should be used for powering surgical tools.

12. Metal breathing system components may prevent the spread of a fire (505).

13. Unnecessary foot switches should be removed to prevent accidental device activation (503).

14. Only the breathing tube and heating circuit labeled for use with a specific humidifier should be used. Heated breathing circuits should not be covered with sheets, blankets, towels, clothing or other material. They should not rest on other surfaces such as the patient, OR table, blankets, or medical equipment. Instead a boom arm or tube tree should be used to support them. A heated-wire breathing circuit should not be turned on until flow has been initiated.

15. The best available grade of fire/laser-proof drapes should be used when exposure to ignition is possible.

16. During a tracheostomy, the tracheal tube cuff should be filled with saline (500).

Preparation for Fires (456, 503, 506)

Surgical teams should be trained in and practice drills for keeping minor fires from getting out of control and managing fires that do get out of control. They should know the location and proper use of fire-fighting tools; medical gas valves; heating, ventilation and air-conditioning controls; electrical supply switches; and the fire alarm and communication systems. Fire extinguishers should be located in convenient, easy-to-reach locations that are known by all OR staff, who should be well-trained in how to use them. It has been recommended that a halon fire extinguisher be kept in every OR (507, 501). Keeping fire blankets should be considered.

Action in Case of a Fire (503, 507, 509)

If a fire occurs, infection control takes second place to controlling the fire. The following steps should be taken.

1. Burning material on or in the patient should be removed and extinguished. A small area of burning can be patted out with a gloved hand or nonflammable liquid (e.g., saline from a basin on the scrub table). Larger areas can be smothered with a blanket or wet towel. If the fire is under and in the drape and the drape is water resistant, water and extinguishing materials poured on the drapes will be ineffective (510). The most effective method is to pull the burning materials away from the patient.
2. If electrical equipment is involved, the power supply should be disconnected before using water to fight the fire, or a carbon dioxide or dry chemical extinguisher should be used (511).
3. The flow of oxygen, nitrous oxide, or air to any equipment involved should be turned off if this can be accomplished without injury to personnel. The shutoff valves to the room should be closed. The patient should be ventilated with air and intravenous anesthetics used to maintain anesthesia. Cylinder valves should be closed and all cylinders removed from the area.
4. The patient and staff should be evacuated if the fire and smoke are excessive. However, it may be more hazardous to move the patient than to attempt to extinguish or contain the fire. The attending physician must determine which step would present the lesser hazard.
5. The fire alarm should be sounded.
6. The doors should be closed to contain the smoke and isolate the fire.
7. Whatever steps are necessary to protect or evacuate patients in adjacent areas should be taken.
8. Fire fighters should be directed to the site of the fire. Involved materials and devices should be saved for later investigation.

PHYSICAL DAMAGE

Many anesthesia machines are piled high with monitors and other equipment. It is frequently

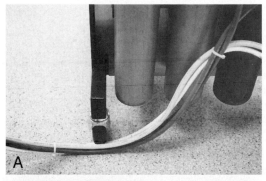

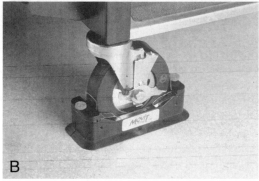

FIGURE 13.20. **A,** If the machine's wheels go over the hoses, the machine will be tipped. **B,** This device allows easier movement of the machine by pushing hoses out of the way. (Courtesy of Movit Inc.)

necessary to alter the position of the machine. Moving this equipment can present a danger to the OR personnel. If a wheel contacts a hose (Fig. 13.20*A*) while the machine is moving it can cause it to tip, spilling equipment onto the floor. Devices to push the hoses away from the wheel are available (Fig. 13.20*B*).

LATEX ALLERGY (512–519)

Latex sensitivity has become a major concern in the medical community as health care workers are confronted with a dramatically increased incidence of reactions not only among patients but also among themselves.

Sources of Latex

Latex is found throughout the industrialized environment. In the OR environment it is found in gloves; tracheal tubes; face masks; mask straps; airways; wrappers on trays; laryngoscope bulb gaskets; skin temperature monitors; bite blocks; teeth protectors; breathing tubes; reservoir bags; ventilator hoses; ventilator bellows; resuscitation bags (black, reusable); blood pressure cuffs, tubings and inflation bulbs; intravenous tubing injection ports; medication vials; syringe plungers; intravenous bag and medical vial needle ports; tape and other adhesives (e.g., Esmarch bandages, Band-Aids); elastic bandages (ace wraps); dressings (e.g., Coban); rubber pads; protective sheets; drains; electrode pads; circulating fluid warming blankets; some cast material; pulmonary artery catheter balloons; epidural adaptors; IV medication pump cassettes; electrocardiogram (ECG) electrodes and pads; finger cots; ostomy bags; intestinal and stomach tubes; rubber bands; chest tube drainage system tubing; condom urinals; urinary and nephrostomy catheters; adhesive drapes; nipples; instrument mats; specimen traps; catheter bag straps; dilating catheters; and the elastic in items ranging from molded surgical masks, head coverings and booties to diapers.

Latex allergens are adsorbed onto the powder inside gloves. When donned or discarded, these powders disperse into the air with the possibility of inhalation, inoculation of the open wound, and contamination of surgical field instruments. Even in OR where laminar air flow devices are used, latex aeroallergens are present in high quantities. They are carried throughout the environment by ventilation air exchange systems as well as by settling on clothing and equipment.

Outside the health care setting, latex is found in toys, condoms, diaphragms, balloons, hot water bottles, erasers, shoe soles, motorcycle handgrips, squash equipment., pacifiers, bottle nipples, household rubber gloves and carpet padding (518).

Individuals at Increased Risk

Anyone with frequent exposure to latex-containing materials is at risk for the development of latex allergy. Children and younger adults are more likely to become latex-sensitive compared to the general population.

The incidence is highest in patients requiring multiple operations along with repetitive urinary catheterizations. This includes patients with neurologically impaired bladders such as those suffering a spinal cord injury, and patients with myelodysplasia, congenital orthopedic defects, and congenital genitourinary tract abnormalities (520). Other groups include patients who undergo repeated esophageal dilations, patients having frequent vaginal exams (particularly those going through an in vitro fertilization program) who are examined with a latex-covered ultrasound probe (521) and patients undergoing barium edema procedures with a latex balloon tip. Other at-risk patients include those who in their daily activities (farming, housework) use latex gloves and individuals with prior reactions to latex-containing devices. Many report swelling or itching of hands or other areas after contact with rubber gloves, condoms, diaphragms, toys or other rubber products. or swelling or itching of the lips or mouth from blowing up balloons or after dental examinations.

The majority of latex-sensitive people has a history of atopy (seasonal allergic asthma, allergic rhinitis, contact dermatitis, hay fever) or multiple positive skin tests in atopy screening. Some have a history of anaphylactic reaction in the past.

Cross reactivity has been demonstrated between latex and foods such as bananas, avocados, peaches, chestnuts, kiwi fruit, passion fruit, nectarines, papaya, celery, peanuts, cherries, strawberries, plums, and tomatoes (512, 515). There may be cross sensitivity between latex and ficus, bluegrass and ragweed (517).

Factory workers with occupational exposure to latex, especially those in the rubber industry or the manufacturing of latex products (gloves, catheters, etc.) are another group at higher risk of latex allergy.

Finally, health care workers must be considered at increased risk. Certain individuals within the medical profession—those who wear latex gloves on a regular basis (surgeons, anesthesia providers, OR nurses, dental personnel, medical laboratory technicians)—are more likely to become latex sensitive than other health care workers. Housekeeping staff who frequently use latex gloves also have a high incidence.

Clinical Picture

Symptoms can appear anywhere from 5 to 290 minutes after secondary exposure has occurred.

The most common sign is diffuse or patchy eczema on any part of the skin in contact with a latex product. This may last 30 minutes to 2 hours after exposure has ceased. The clinical syndrome ranges from contact dermatitis through a spectrum of more severe allergic disturbances to life-threatening anaphylaxis. A number of case reports describe severe intraoperative anaphylaxis associated with contact of surgical gloves with the peritoneum and viscera.

Prevention (515)

If patients requiring surgery have confirmed latex sensitivity or convincing histories of latex reactions, avoidance of latex-containing products is mandatory. Procedures on all patients with spina bifida, regardless of history, should be performed in a latex-free environment.

The Food and Drug Administration (FDA) requires all medical products that contain latex that come directly or indirectly into contact with the body during use to bear labels stating that the product contains latex and to declare that latex may cause allergic reactions in some individuals. The term "hypoallergenic" is no longer used for medical devices. At present there is no test that can adequately determine the level of latex proteins in a product and there is no manufacturing process that can reduce the level below the minimum required to produce a reaction in some people. Therefore the term "hypoallergenic" is meaningless when applied to latex-containing devices.

The latex-sensitive patient should be scheduled as the first case of the day with all latex-containing materials (gloves, blood pressure cuff and tubing, etc.) removed the preceding night to minimize exposure to aerosols. Some health care facilities have established a specific OR where all latex-containing materials are banned. Appropriate personnel (e.g., anesthesia, OR, pharmacy, postanesthesia care unit (PACU) staff) should be notified to ensure that appropriate measures are taken. Latex-sensitive signs, reminding medical personnel of the situation, should be posted on all entrances to that operating room. Traffic in the room should be kept to a minimum.

A cart containing non–latex alternative supplies is a good idea. Guidelines for latex safe technique and a list of latex free equipment should be perma-nently attached to this cart. Latex-sensitive patient packages containing breathing tubes, reservoir bag, filter, mask, and head strap are available.

No latex-containing items (i.e., gowns, hats, boots, compression stockings) should be placed on the patient.

Intravenous tubing with no injection ports should be used or all latex injection ports should be taped to prevent inadvertent puncture. Stopcocks or one-way valves should be used for push and piggyback medications. Intravenous fluid or commercially prepared medication bags should be pierced through the intravenous tubing port, not the latex injection port.

Although reactions to rubber syringe plungers have been reported, no problems have so far been described if the medications are freshly drawn and immediately administered. However, glass syringes offer an attractive alternative. Totally plastic syringes are now availale (515, 522).

Rubber stoppers on vials of drugs should not be pierced. Drugs should be drawn after the rubber stopper has been removed from the opened vial.

Lyophilized drugs should be reconstituted using a syringe, not shaken in a multidose vial and withdrawn using a filter. A high-efficiency filter should be used at the patient port to protect the patient from airborne latex allergens.

It may not be possible to entirely avoid some rubber-containing anesthetic equipment—rubber bellows, diaphragms, valves, tubings. However, when these parts of equipment do not come into contact with the patient and have been previously washed, no complications have resulted (519).

Latex-free equipment including face masks, airways, mask straps, tracheal tubes, bag-valve-mask units, reservoir bags, ECG electrodes and pads, stethoscopes, pulse oximetry sensors, esophageal stethoscopes, nasogastric and suction tubes, tape, and breathing tubes should be used. All gloves should be non-latex. If an epidural catheter adaptor contains latex, it should be replaced using a blunt, latex-free, needle adaptor.

Contact of blood pressure cuffs can be prevented by wrapping the area under the cuff with soft cotton. A nonlatex glove can be used as a tourniquet.

From the surgical point of view, use of nonlatex

gloves, drains, and catheters is mandatory. Special precautions should be undertaken to avoid latex-based equipment such as instrument mats, rubber-shod clamps, vascular tags, bulb syringes, rubber bands, and Band-aids. A non-latex glove can be used as a Penrose drain.

REFERENCES

1. Cooper JB, Newbower RS, Long CD, et al. Preventable anesthesia mishaps: a study of human factors. Anesthesiology 1978;49:399–406.
2. Cooper JB, Newbower RS, Kitz RJ. An analysis of major errors and equipment failures in anesthesia management. Considerations for prevention and detection. Anesthesiology 1984;60:34–42.
3. Craig J, Wilson ME. A survey of anaesthetic misadventures. Anaesthesia 1981;36:933–936.
4. Currie M. A prospective survey of anaesthetic critical events in a teaching hospital. Anaesthesia and Intensive Care 1989;17:403–411.
5. Desmonts JM. Role of equipment failure in the causation of anaesthetic morbidity and mortality: results from the French national survey and comparison with the Boston study. Eur J Anaesth 1987;4:200–203.
6. Kumar V, Barcellos WA, Mehta MP, et al. Analysis of critical incidents in a teaching department for quality assurance. A survey of mishaps during anaesthesia. Anaesthesia 1988;43:879–883.
7. Short TG, O'Regan A, Lew J, et al. Critical incident reporting in an anaesthetic department quality assurance programme. Anaesthesia 1992;47:3–7.
8. Emmanuel ER, Teh JL. Dental anaesthetic emergency caused by medical gas pipeline installation error. Aust Dent J 1983;28:79–81.
9. Sato T. Fatal pipeline accidents spur Japanese standards. Anesthesia Patient Safety Foundation Newsletter 1991;6:14.
10. McAleavy JC. Believe your monitors. Anesthesiology 1993;79:409–410.
11. Smith FP. Multiple deaths from argon contamination of hospital oxygen supply. J Forensic Sci 1987;32:1098–1102.
12. Holland R. Foreign correspondence: "wrong gas" disaster in Hong Kong. Anesthesia Patient Safety Foundation Newsletter 1989;4:26.
13. Anonymous. Puritan–Bennett quick connect valves for medical gases. Canadian medical devices alert warns of possible cracks. Biomedical Safety & Standards 1984;14:52–53.
14. Bernstein D, Rosenberg A. Intraoperative hypoxia from nitrogen tanks with oxygen fittings. Anesth Analg 1997;84:225–227.
15. Anonymous. Old-style Chemetron central gas outlets. Health Devices 1981;10(9):222–223.
16. Anonymous. Crossed connections in medical gas systems. Technology for Anesthesia 1984;5(3):3.
17. Anonymous. Crossed N_2O and O_2 lines blamed for outpatient surgery death. Biomedical Safety and Standards 1992;22:14.
18. Downing JW. Safety of anaesthetic machines. South Afr Med J 1981;30:815.
19. Krenis LJ, Berkowitz DA. Errors in installation of a new gas delivery system found after certification. Anesthesiology 1985;62:677–678.
20. Spurring PW, Shenolikar BK. Hazards in anaesthetic equipment. Br J Anaesth 1978;50:641–645.
21. Robinson JS. A continuing saga of piped medical gas supply. Anaesthesia 1979;34:66–70.
22. Feeley TW, Hedley–Whyte J. Bulk oxygen and nitrous oxide delivery systems: design and dangers. Anesthesiology 1976;44:301–305.
23. Anonymous. The Westminster inquiry. Lancet 1977;2:175–176.
24. Lane GA. Medical gas outlets—a hazard from interchangeable "quick connect" couplers. Anesthesiology 1980;52:86–87.
25. Carley RH, Houghton IT, Park GR. A near disaster from piped gases. Anaesthesia 1984;39:891–893.
26. Karmann U, Roth F. Prevention of accidents associated with air–oxygen mixers. Anaesthesia 1982;37:680–682.
27. Thorp JM, Railton R. Hypoxia due to air in the oxygen pipeline. Anaesthesia 1982;37:683–687.
28. Ziecheck HD. Faulty ventilator check valves cause pipeline gas contamination. Respiratory Care 1981;26:1009–1010.
29. Anonymous. Patient receives air instead of oxygen: Canadian safety alert. Biomedical Safety & Standards 1991;21:97–98.
30. O'Connor CJ, Hobin KF. Bypassing the diameter-indexed safety system. Anesthesiology 1989;71:318–319.
31. Boon PE. C-size cylinders. Anaesthesia and Intensive Care 1990;18:586–587.
32. Jawan B, Lee JH. Cardiac arrest caused by an incorrectly filled oxygen cylinder. A case report. Br J Anaesth 1990;64:749–751.
33. Rendell–Baker L. Problems with anesthetic gas machines and their solutions. In: Rendell–Baker L, ed. Problems with anesthetic and respiratory therapy equipment. Int Anesthesiol Clin 1982;20(3):1–82.
34. Anonymous. Cylinders with unmixed helium/oxygen. Technology for Anesthesia 1990;10(10):4.
35. Orr IA, Hamilton L. Entonox hazard. Anaesthesia 1985;40:496.

36. Sim P. Entonox hazard: a reply. Anaesthesia 1985; 40:496.

37. Anonymous. Misconnection of oxygen regulator to nitrogen cylinder could cause death. Biomedical Safety & Standards 1988;18:90–91.

38. Anonymous. Nonstandard user modification of gas cylinder pin indexing. Technology for Anesthesia 1989;10(2):2.

39. Goebel WM. Failure of nitrous oxide and oxygen pin-indexing. Anesth Prog 1980;27:188–191.

40. Jayasuriya JP. Another example of Murphy's law—mix up of pin index valves. Anaesthesia 1986; 41:1164.

41. Mead P. Hazard with cylinder yoke. Anaesthesia and Intensive Care 1981;9:79–80.

42. MacMillan RR, Marshall MA. Failure of the pin index system on a Cape Waine ventilator. Anaesthesia 1981; 36:334–335.

43. Fuller WR, Kelly R, Russell WJ. Pin-indexing failure. Anaesthesia and Intensive Care 1985;13:440–441.

44. Youatt G, Love J. A funny yoke: tale of an unscrewed pin. Anaesthesia and Intensive Care 1981;9:178.

45. Spurring PW, Shenolikar BK. Hazards in anaesthetic equipment. Br J Anaesth 1978;50:641–645.

46. Bonsu AK, Stead AL. Accidental cross-connection of oxygen and nitrous oxide in an anaesthetic machine. Anaesthesia 1983;38:767–769.

47. Beudoin MG. Oxygen needle valve obstruction. Anaesthesia and Intensive Care 1988;16:130–131.

48. Khalil SN, Neuman J. Failure of an oxygen flow control valve. Anesthesiology 1990;73:355–356.

49. Rung GW, Schneider AJL. Oxygen flowmeter failure on the North American Drager Narkomed 2A anesthesia machine. Anesth Analg 1986;65:211–212.

50. Kalil SN, Neuman J. Failure of an oxygen flow control valve. Anesthesiology 1990;73:355–356.

51. Anonymous. Oxygen deprivation alleged in $2.5 million negligence suit. Biomedical Safety & Standards 1981;11:53.

52. McGarry PMF. Anaesthetic machine standard. Can Anaesth Soc J 1978;25:436.

53. Wyant GM. Some dangers in anaesthesia. Can Anaesth Soc J 1978;25:71–72.

54. Jenkins IR. A "too close to door" knob. Anaesthesia and Intensive Care 1991;19:614.

55. Richards C. Failure of a nitrous oxide-oxygen proportioning device. Anesthesiology 1989;71:997–999.

56. Goodyear CM. Failure of nitrous oxide-oxygen proportioning device. Anesthesiology 1990;72: 397–398.

57. Lohmann G. Fault with an Ohmeda Excel 410 machine. Anaesthesia 1991;46:695.

58. Kidd AG, Hall I. Fault with an Ohmeda Excel 210 anaesthetic machine. Anaesthesia 1994;49:83.

59. Henling CE, Diaz JH. The cluttered anesthesia machine—a cause for hypoxia. Anesthesiology 1983;58: 288–289.

60. Linton RAF, Foster CA, Spencer GT. A potential hazard of oxygen flowmeters. Anaesthesia 1982;37: 606–607.

61. Russell WJ. The danger of air on anaesthetic machines. Anaesthesia and Intensive Care 1988;16:499.

62. Battig CG. Unusual failure of an oxygen flowmeter. Anesthesiology 1972;37:561–562.

63. Chadwick DA. Transposition of rotameter tubes. Anesthesiology 1974;40:102.

64. Hodge EA. Accuracy of anaesthetic gas flowmeters. Br J Anaesth 1979;51:907.

65. Kelley JM, Gabel RA. The improperly calibrated flowmeter—another hazard. Anesthesiology 1970; 33:467–468.

66. Thomas D. Interchangeable rotameter tubes. Anaesthesia and Intensive Care 1983;11:385–386.

67. Szocik JF. Preoperative hypoxemia. Anesth Analg 1993;76:681–682.

68. Hutton P, Boaden RW. Performance of needle valves. Br J Anaesth 1986;58:919–924.

69. Chi OZ. Another example of hypoxic gas mixture delivery. Anesthesiology 1985;62:543–544.

70. Riendl J. Hypoxic gas mixture delivery due to malfunctioning inlet port of a Select-a-Tec vaporizer manifold. Can J Anaesth 1987;34:431.

71. Chung DC, Jing QC, Prins L, et al. Hypoxic gas mixtures delivered by anaesthetic machines equipped with a downstream oxygen flowmeter. Can Anaesth Soc J 1980;27:527–530.

72. Dudley M, Walsh E. Oxygen loss from rotameter. Br J Anaesth 1986;58:1201–1202.

73. Russell WJ. Hypoxia from a selective oxygen leak. Anaesthesia and Intensive Care 1984;12:275–276.

74. McHale S. A critical incident with the Ohmeda Excel 410 machine. Anaesthesia 1991;46:150.

75. Powell J. Leak from an oxygen flow meter. Br J Anaesth 1981;53:671.

76. Wishaw K. Hypoxic gas mixture with Quantiflex monitored dial mixer and induction room safety. Anaesthesia and Intensive Care 1991;19:127.

77. McHale S. A critical incident with the Ohmeda 410 machine. Anaesthesia 1991;46:150.

78. Hanning CD, Kruchek D, Chunara A. Preferential oxygen leak—an unusual case. Anaesthesia 1987;42: 1329–1330.

79. Moore JK, Railton R. Hypoxia caused by a leaking rotameter—the value of an oxygen analyser. Anaesthesia 1984;39:380–381.

80. Julien RM. Potentially fatal machine fault. Anesthesiology 1983;58:584–585.

81. Cole AGH, Thompson JB, Fodor IM, et al. Anaesthetic machine hazard from the selectatec block. Anaesthesia 1983;38:175–177.

82. Lenoir RJ, Easy WR. A hazard associated with removal of carbon dioxide cylinders. Anaesthesia 1988; 43:892–893.

83. McQuillan PJ, Jackson IJB. Potential leaks from anaesthetic machines. Anaesthesia 1987;42: 1308–1312.

84. Williams AR, Hilton PJ. Selective oxygen leak. A potential cause of patient hypoxia. Anaesthesia 1986; 41:1133–1134.

85. Wilson A. Dangerous leak. Anaesthesia and Intensive Care 1990;18:575.

86. Stoneham MD, Ismail F, Sansome AJ. Leakage of fresh gas from vacant CO_2 cylinder yoke. Anaesthesia 1993;48:730–731.

87. Lanier WL. Intraoperative air entrainment with Ohio Modulus anesthesia machine. Anesthesiology 1986; 64:266–268.

88. Ghanooni S, Wilks DH, Finestone SC. A case report of an unusual disconnection. Anesth Analg 1983;62: 696–697.

89. Ditchik J, Herr GP. Can we do without O_2 analyzers? Anesthesiology 1984;61:629–630.

90. Eisenkraft, J B. Complications of anesthesia delivery systems. ASA Annual Refresher Courses, 1996, New Orleans.

91. Walker T. Another problem with a circle system. Anaesthesia 1996;51:89.

92. Mostello LA, Patel RI. Dilution of anesthetic gases by a new light source for bronchoscopy. Anesthesiology 1986;65:445.

93. Russell WG. Oxygen supply at risk. Anaesthesia and Intensive Care 1985;13:216–217.

94. Johnson DL. Central oxygen supply versus mother nature. Respiratory Care 1975;20:1043–1044.

95. Newson AJ, Dyball LA. A visual monitor for piped oxygen supply systems to anaesthetic machines. Anaesthesia and Intensive Care 1978;6:146–148.

96. Webb RK, Russell WJ, Klepper I, et al. Equipment failure: an analysis of 2000 incident reports. Anaesthesia and Intensive Care 1993;21:673–677.

97. Anderson B, Chamley D. Wall outlet oxygen failure. Anaesthesia and Intensive Care 1987;15:468–469.

98. Chung DC, Hunter DJ. The quick-mount pipeline connector. Failure of a "fail-safe" device. Can Anaesth Soc J 1986;33:666–668.

99. Ewart IA. An unusual cause of gas pipeline failure. Anaesthesia 1990;45:498.

100. Lacoumenta S, Hall GM. A burst oxygen pipeline. Anaesthesia 1983;38:596–597.

101. Craig DB, Culligan J. Sudden interruption of gas flow through a Schrader oxygen coupler unit. Can Anaesth Soc J 1980;27:175–177.

102. Muir J, Davidson-Lamb R. Apparatus failure—cause for concern. Br J Anaesth 1980;52:705–706.

103. Anderson WR, Brock–Utne JG. Oxygen pipeline supply failure. A coping strategy. Journal of Clinical Monitoring 1991;7:39–41.

104. Varga DA, Guttery JS, Grundy BL. Intermittent oxygen delivery in an Ohmeda Unitrol anesthesia machine due to a faulty O-ring check valve assembly. Anesth Analg 1987;66:1200–1201.

105. Feeley TW, Bancroft ML, Brooks RA, et al. Potential hazards of compressed gas cylinders: a review. Anesthesiology 1978;48:72–74.

106. Blogg CE, Colvin MP. Apparently empty oxygen cylinders. Br J Anaesth 1977;49:87.

107. Singleton RJ, Lucbrook GL, Webb RK, et al. Physical injuries and environmental safety in anaesthesia: an analysis of 2000 incident reports. Anaesthesia and Intensive Care 1993;21:659–663.

108. Milliken RA. An explosion hazard due to an imperfect design. Arch Surg 1972;105:125–127.

109. McDade W, Ballantyne JC. Potential risk associated with anesthesia machines with single oxygen cylinders. Journal of Clinical Anesthesia 1996;8: 260–261.

110. Fitzpatrick G, Moore KP. Malfunction in a needle valve. Anaesthesia 1988;43:164.

111. McMahon DJ, Holm R, Batra MS. Yet another machine fault. Anesthesiology 1983;58:586–587.

112. Boscoe MJ, Baxter RCH. Failure of anaesthetic gas supply. Anaesthesia 1983;38:997–998.

113. From R, George GP, Tinker JH. Foregger 705 malfunction resulting in loss of gas flow. Anesthesiology 1984;61:321–322.

114. Chang JL, Larson CE, Bedger RC, et al. An unusual malfunction of an anesthetic machine. Anesthesiology 1980;52:446–447.

115. Wan YL, Swan M. Exotic obstruction. Anaesthesia and Intensive Care 1990;18:274.

116. Bamber PA. Possible safety hazard on anaesthetic machines. Anaesthesia 1987;42:782.

117. Heine JF, Adams PM. Another potential failure in an oxygen delivery system. Anesthesiology 1985;63: 335–336.

118. Nuttall GA, Baker RD. Internal common gas line disconnect. Anesthesiology 1993;79:605–607.

119. Kua JSE, Tan I. A rare cause of oxygen failure. Anaesthesia 1994;49:650–651.

120. Capan L, Ramanathan S, Chalon J, et al. A possible hazard with use of the Ohio Ethrane Vaporizer. Anesth Analg 1980;59:65–68.

121. Forrest T, Childs D. An unusual vaporiser leak. Anaesthesia 1982;37:1220–1221.

122. Pyles ST, Kaplan RF, Munson ES. Gas loss from Ohio Modulus vaporizer selector-interlock valve. Anesth Analg 1983;62:1052.

123. Loughnan TE. Gas leak associated with a selectatec. Anaesthesia and Intensive Care 1988;16:501.

124. Van Besouw JP, Thurlow AC. A hazard of free-standing vaporizers. Anaesthesia 1987;42:671.

125. Qadri AM. Unusual detection of an old problem. Anaesthesia 1988;43:611.

126. Berry PD, Ross DG. Missing O-ring causes unrecognized large gas leak. Anaesthesia 1992;47:359.

127. Patterson KW, Kean PK. Hazard with a Boyle Vaporizer. Anaesthesia 1991;46:152–153.

128. Wraight WJ. Another failure of Selectatec block. Anaesthesia 1990;45:795.

129. Hogan TS. Selectatec switch malfunction. Anaesthesia 1985;40:66–69.

130. Jove F, Milliken RA. Loss of anesthetic gases due to defective safety equipment. Anesth Analg 1983;62:369–370.

131. Jablonski J, Reynolds AC. A potential cause (and cure) of a major gas leak. Anesthesiology 1985;62:842–843.

132. Childres WF. Malfunction of Ohio Modulus anesthesia machine. Anesthesiology 1982;56:330.

133. Carter JA, McAtteer P. A serious hazard associated with the Fluotec Mark 4 vaporizer. Anaesthesia 1984;39:1257–1258.

134. Powell JF, Morgan C. Selectatec gas leak. Anaesthesia and Intensive Care 1993;21:891–892.

135. Jablonski J, Reynolds AC. A potential cause (and cure) of a major gas leak. Anesthesiology 1985;62:842.

136. Anonymous. Anesthesia unit vaporizers. Technology for Anesthesia 1987;7:4.

137. Dolan PF. Vaporizer leak. Anesthesiology 1978;49:302.

138. Cooper PD. A hazard with a vaporizer. Anesthesia 1984;39:935.

139. Rosenberg M, Solod E, Bourke DL. Gas leak through a Fluotec Mark III Vaporizer. Anesth Analg 1979;58:239–240.

140. Beavis R. Boyles machine. Anaesthesia and Intensive Care 1983;11:80.

141. Kataria B, Price P, Slack M. Delayed filling of the breathing bag due to a portable vaporizer. Anesth Analg 1987;66:1055.

142. Pomykala Z. Schecter H. Design flow in an anesthesia machine. Anesthesiology 1992;77:399–400.

143. Maurer WG. A disadvantage of similar machine controls. Anesthesiology 1991;75:167–168.

144. Okell RW. Chain of errors. Anaesthesia 1989;44:703–704.

145. Friesen RM. Safety of anaesthetic machines. Can J Anaesth 1989;36:364.

146. Goldman JM, Phelps RW. No flow anesthesia. Anesth Analg 1987;66:1339.

147. Mantia AM. A defective Washington T-piece. An example of inevitable failure and lessons to be learned. Anesthesiology 1983;59:167–168.

148. Milliken RA, Bizzarri DV. An unusual cause of failure of anesthetic gas delivery to a patient circuit. Anesth Analg 1984;63:1047–1048.

149. Anonymous. Anesthesia breathing circuits and fresh gas elbows recalled. Biomedical Safety & Standards 1989;19:19.

150. Bissonnette B, Roy WL: Obstruction of fresh gas flow in an Ayre's T-piece. Can Anaesth Soc J 1986;33:535–536.

151. Silver L, Lopes N, Brock-Utne J. Raising the operating table causing a sudden anesthesia system obstruction. Anesth Analg 1996;82:1107–1108.

152. Miguel R, Vila H. Machine wars. Another cause of pressure loss in the anesthesia machine. Anesthesiology 1992;77:398–399.

153. Goresky GV. Bain circuit delivery tube obstructions. Can J Anaesth 1990;37:385.

154. Inglis MS. Torsion of the inner tube. Br J Anaesth 1980;52:705.

155. Forrest PR. Defective anaesthetic breathing circuit. Can J Anaesth 1987;34:541–542.

156. Kshatri AM, Kingsley CP. Defective carbon dioxide absorber as a cause for a leak in a breathing circuit. Anesthesiology 1996;84:475–476.

157. Russell WJ, Webb RK, van der Walt JH, et al. Problems with ventilation: an analysis of 2000 incident reports. Anaesthesia and Intensive Care 1993;21:617–620.

158. Anonymous. Anesthesia machine owners alerted to potential breathing circuit leak. Biomedical Safety & Standards 1989;19:122.

159. Birch AA, Fisher NA. Leak of soda lime seal after anesthesia machine check. J Clin Anesth 1989;1:474–476.

160. Anderson TY. Failure to ventilate. Anaesthesia and Intensive Care 1993;21:898.

161. Brown MC, Burris WR, Hilley MD. Breathing circuit mishap resulting from Y-piece disintegration. Anesthesiology 1988;69:436–437.

162. Colavita RD, Apfelbaum JL. An unusual source of leak in the anesthesia circuit. Anesthesiology 1985;62:208–209.

163. Cullingford D. Broken yoke. Anaesthesia and Intensive Care 1985;13:442.

164. Cooper MG, Vouden J, Rigg D. Circuit leaks. Anaesthesia and Intensive Care 1987;15:539–540.

165. Ferderbar PJ, Kettler RE, Jablonski J, et al. A cause of breathing system leak during closed circuit anesthesia. Anesthesiology 1986;65:661–663.

166. Kemen M, Desai K, Roizen MF, et al. Over fifty percent of disposable circuits leak. Anesth Analg 1990; 70:S194.

167. Lamarche Y. Anaesthetic breathing circuit leak from cracked oxygen analyzer sensor connector. Can Anaesth Soc J 1985;32:682–683.

168. Mantia AM. Faulty Y-piece. Anesth Analg 1981;60: 121–122.

169. Lee O, Sommer RM. Pressure monitoring hose causes leak in anesthesia breathing circuit. Anesth Analg 1991;73:365.

170. Poulton TJ. Unusual corrugated tubing leak. Anesth Analg 1986;65:1365.

171. Prasad KK, Chen L. Complications related to the use of a heat and moisture exchanger. Anesthesiology 1990;72:958.

172. Patil AR. Melting of anesthesia circuit by humidifier. Anesth Prog 1989;36:63–65.

173. Raja SN, Geller H. Another potential source of a major gas leak. Anesthesiology 1986;64:297–298.

174. Sosis MB, Payne MN. Another cause for a leak in a disposable breathing circuit. Anesthesiology 1989; 71:806.

175. Shampaine EL, Helfaer M. A modest proposal for improved humidifier design. Anesth Analg 1991;72: 130–131.

176. Biro P. Unusual cause for a circle system leak. Anesth Analg 1996;83:196.

177. Denman W, Collier BB. An inappropriate use of tape. Anaesthesia 1990;45:794–795.

178. Edge G, Papee E. An unsuspected source of breathing system failure. Anaesthesia 1994;49:827–828.

179. Feinglass NG, Dorsch JA. Disposable circuit disconnects. Anesthesiology 1993;79:1449–1450.

180. Horton RG. Exhale spill valve failure. Anaesthesia and Intensive Care 1994;22:233–234.

181. Koehli N. Defective feed mount. Anaesthesia 1992; 47:354–355.

182. Lacoux PA, Christie G. Leaking Datex sampling set for the end-tidal CO_2 monitor. Anaesthesia 1992;47: 173.

183. Lam WH, Evans JM. Rubber gloves and anaesthetic gas leak. Anaesthesia 1996;51:1075.

184. Malhotra V, Bradley E. Broken inner sleeve of a Y-connector: course of a circuit leak and a potential foreign body aspiration. Anesth Analg 1993;76: 1169–1170.

185. Needleman S, Kaplan RF. Unusual source of air leak in a pediatric anesthesia breathing circuit. Anesth Analg 1995;81:654.

186. Reinhart DJ, Friz R. Undetected leak in corrugated circuit tubing in compressed configuration. Anesthesiology 1993;78:218.

187. Richardson J, Bickford–Smith PJ. Covert breathing system failure. Anaesthesia 1993;48:541.

188. Wang J-S, Hung W-T, Lin C-Y. Leakage of disposable breathing circuits. J Clin Anesth 1992;4: 111–115.

189. Williams N. A leaky circuit. Anaesthesia 1996;51: 406–407.

190. Yassin K, Gibbons JJ. A hidden leak in the circle system. Anesth Analg 1991;73:236.

191. Stevenson PH, McLeskey CH. Breakage of a reservoir bag mount, an unusual anesthesia machine failure. Anesthesiology 1980;53:270–271.

192. Milliken RA. Bag mount detachment. A function of age? Anesthesiology 1982;56:154.

193. Wood D, Boyd M, Campbell C. Insulation of heated wire circuits. Anesth Analg 1992;74:471.

194. Mizutani AR, Ozaki G, Rusk R. Insulation of heated wire circuits. In response. Anesth Analg 1992;74: 472.

195. Sprague DH, Maccioli GA. Disposable circuit tubing melted by heated humidifier. Anesth Analg 1986;65: 1247.

196. Wood D, Boyd M, Campbell C. Insulation of heated wire circuits. Anesth Analg 1992;74:471.

197. Brown CQ, Canada ED, Graney WF. Failure of Bain circuit breathing system. Anesthesiology 1981;55: 716–717.

198. Breen DP. Failure of a valve in a Bain system. A dangerous design? Anaesthesia 1990;45:417.

199. Miller DC, Collins JW, Wallace L. Failure of the expiratory valve on a Bain System. Anaesthesia 1990;45: 992.

200. Nelson RA, Snowdon SL. Failure of an adjustable pressure limiting valve. Anaesthesia 1989;44: 788–789.

201. Judkins KC, Safe M. Routine servicing of the Cape-Wane Ventilator. Anaesthesia 1983;38:1102.

202. Ripp CH, Chapin JW. A bellow's leak in an Ohio anesthesia ventilator. Anesth Analg 1985;64:942.

203. Hutchinson BR. An unusual leak. Anaesthesia and Intensive Care 1987;15:355.

204. Rolbin S. An unusual cause of ventilator leak. Can Anaesth Soc J 1977;24:522–524.

205. Wolf S, Watson CB, Clark P. An unusual cause of leakage in an anesthesia system. Anesthesiology 1981;55:83–84.

206. Choi JJ, Guida J, Wu W. Hypoventilatory hazard of an anesthetic scavenging device. Anesthesiology 1986;65:126–127.

207. Eisenkraft JB, Sommer RM. Flapper valve malfunction. Anesth Analg 1988;67:1132.

208. Eisenkraft JB. Potential for barotrauma or hypoventilation with the Drager AV-E ventilator. J Clin Anesth 1989;1:452–456.

209. Sommer RM, Bhalla GS, Jackson JM, et al. Hypoventilation caused by ventilator valve rupture. Anesth Analg 1988;67:999–1001.

210. Khalil SN, Gholston TK, Binderman J, et al. Flapper valve malfunction in an Ohio closed scavenging system. Anesth Analg 1987;66:1334–1336.

211. Anonymous. Risk of barotrauma and/or lack of ventilation on ventilatorless anesthesia machines. Technology for Anesthesia 1994;14(9):2–3.

212. Munford BJ, Wishaw KJ. Critical incidents with nonrebreathing valves. Anaesthesia and Intensive Care 1990;18:560–563.

213. Oliver JJ, Pope R. Potential hazard with silicone resuscitators. Anaesthesia 1984;39:933–934.

214. Anonymous. Valve component on resuscitation kits may leak. Biomedical Safety & Standards 1989;19:35–36.

215. Graham DH. Advantages of standing bellows ventilators and low-flow techniques. Anesthesiology 1983;58:486.

216. Adams AP. Breathing system disconnections. Br J Anaesth 1994;73:46–54.

217. Heath ML. Accidents associated with equipment. Anaesthesia 1984;39:57–60.

218. Brahams D. Two locum anaesthetists convicted of manslaughter. Anaesthesia 1990;45:981–982.

219. Neufeld PD, Johnson DL. Results of the Canadian Anaesthetists' Society opinion survey on anaesthetic equipment. Can Anaesth Soc J 1983;30:469–473.

220. Neufeld PD, Johnson DL, deVeth J. Safety of anaesthesia breathing circuit connectors. Can Anaesth Soc J 1983;30:646–652.

221. Blatt D. Breathing circuit disconnects, leaks could be prevented with locking pin. Anesthesia Patient Safety Foundation Newsletter 1995;10:20.

222. Eck J, Jantzen J-PAH. To disconnect is better than to extubate. Anesthesiology 1992;76:483–484.

223. Blackstock D, Forbes M. Analysis of an anaesthetic gas scavenging system hazard. Can J Anaesth 1989;36:204–208.

224. Morr ZF, Stein ED, Orkin LR. A possible hazard in the use of a scavenging system. Anesthesiology 1977;47:302–303.

225. Mostafa SM, Sutcliffe AJ. Antipollution expiratory valves. A potential hazard. Anaesthesia 1982;37:468–469.

226. Seymour A. The need for care in using electric warming blankets. Anaesthesia 1982;37:1218–1219.

227. Patel KD, Dalal FY. A potential hazard of the Drager scavenging interface for wall suction. Anesth Analg 1979;58:327–328.

228. Jones D. An unusual cause of a leak from an anaesthetic machine. Anaesthesia 1995;50:751.

229. Hodgson CA, Mostafa SM. Riddle of the persistent leak. Anaesthesia 1991;46:799.

230. Stirt JA, Lewenstein LN. Circle system failure induced by gastric suction. Anaesthesia and Intensive Care 1981;9:161–162.

231. Lee T, Schrader MW, Wright BD. Pseudo-failure of mechanical ventilator caused by accidental endobronchial nasogastric tube insertion. Respiratory Care 1980;25:851–853.

232. Anonymous. Breathing-circuit connectors blocked by plastic membrane. Biomedical Safety & Standards 1991;21:91.

233. Anonymous. Valves, positive end expiratory pressure. Technology for Anesthesia 1991;11(12):11.

234. Anonymous. Videotape explains OR fires. Technology for Anesthesia 1992;13:7.

235. Gallacher BP, Kelly M, Mora RR. Failure to ventilate due to glass ampule fragment occlusion of the breathing circuit. Anesthesiology 1997;87:180.

236. Krensavage TJ, Richards E. Sudden development of anesthesia circuit obstruction by an end-tidal CO_2 cap in the gas sampling elbow. Anesth Analg 1995;81:204–213.

237. Marshall FPF. Kinked inner tube of coaxial breathing system. Br J Anaesth 1993;71:171.

238. Platt ND. Unusual cause of obstructed airway. Anaesthesia 1993;48:540–541.

239. Wilkes PRH. Bain circuit occluded by foreign body. Can J Anaesth 1994;41:137–139.

240. Cameron AE, Power I, Tierney B. Portex swivel connector hazard. Anaesthesia 1984;39:496.

241. Crowhurst P. Mishaps with the Mera-F circuit. Anaesthesia and Intensive Care 1987;15:121–122.

242. Shroff PK, Skerman JH. Humidifier malfunction—a cause of anesthesia circuit occlusion. Anesth Analg 1988;67:710–711.

243. McGarrigle R, White S. Oxygen analyzers can detect disconnections. Anesth Analg 1984;63:464–465.

244. Meyer RM. A case for monitoring oxygen in the expiratory limb of the circle. Anesthesiology 1984;61:374.

245. Spurring PW, Small LFG. Breathing system disconnections and misconnections. Anaesthesia 1983;38:683–688.

246. Heath ML. Accidents associated with equipment. Anaesthesia 1984;39:57–60.

247. Levins RA, Francis RI, Burnley SR. Failure to detect disconnection by capnography. Anaesthesia 1989;44:79.

248. Morrison AB. Failure to detect anesthetic circuit disconnections. Canadian "medical devices alert" issued

by HPB. Biomedical Safety and Standards 1981;11: 28.

249. Slee TA, Pavlin EG. Failure of low pressure alarm associated with the use of a humidifier. Anesthesiology 1988;69:791–793.

250. Raphael DT. An algorithmic response for the breathing system low-pressure alarm conditions. Progress in Anesthesiology 1997;11:219–244.

251. Raphael DT, Weller RS, Doran DJ. A response algorithm for the low-pressure alarm condition. Anesth Analg 1988;67:876–883.

252. Barry JES, Adams A. Inadvertent administration of carbon dioxide. Surv Anesth 1991;35:368–374.

253. Dinnick DP. Accidental severe hypercapnia during anaesthesia. Br J Anaesth 1968;40:36–45.

254. Todd DB. Dangers of CO_2 cylinders on anaesthetic machines. Anaesthesia 1995;50:911–912.

255. Klein SL, Lilburn JK. An unusual case of hypercarbia during general anaesthesia. Anesthesiology 1980;53: 248–250.

256. Holland R. Foreign correspondence. Another "wrong gas" incident in Hong Kong. Anesthesia Patient Safety Foundation Newsletter 1991;6:9.

257. Whitten MP, Wise CC. Design faults in commonly used carbon dioxide absorbers. Br J Anaesth 1972; 44:535–537.

258. Andrews JJ, Johnston RV, Bee DE, et al. Photodeactivation of ethyl violet. A potential hazard of sodasorb. Anesthesiology 1990;72:59–64.

259. Detmer MD, Chandra P, Cohen PJ. Occurrence of hypercarbia due to an unusual failure of anesthetic equipment. Anesthesiology 1980;52:278–279.

260. Loughman E. Defective soda lime canisters. Anaesthesia and Intensive Care 1990;18:275.

261. Aung SM, Ramez–Salem M, Podraza AG, et al. An unusual cause of carbon dioxide rebreathing in a circle absorber system. Anesth Analg 1994;78: 1027–1028.

262. Parry TM, Jewkes DA, Smith M. A sticking flutter valve. Anaesthesia 1991;46:229.

263. Nunn BJ, Rosewarne FA. Expiratory valve failure. Anaesthesia and Intensive Care 1990;18:273–274.

264. Anonymous. Anesthesia gas absorber check valves may "stick open." Biomedical Safety & Standards 1990;20:156.

265. Fogdall RP. Exacerbation of iatrogenic hypercarbia by PEEP. Anesthesiology 1979;51:173–175.

266. Pyles ST, Berman LS, Modell JH. Expiratory valve dysfunction in a semiclosed circle anesthesia circuit—verification by analysis of carbon dioxide waveform. Anesth Analg 1984;63:536–537.

267. Kim JM, Kovac AL, Mathewson HS. Incompetency of unidirectional dome valves. A multi-hospital study. Anesth Analg 1985;64:237.

268. Rosewarne F, Wells D. Three cases of valve incompetence in a circle system. Anaesthesia and Intensive Care 1988;16:376–377.

269. Whalley DG. Malfunctioning unidirectional valves of Ohmeda series 5 and 5A carbon dioxide absorbers. Can J Anaesth 1988;35:668–669.

270. Dzwonczyk D, Dahl MR, Steinhauser R. A defective unidirectional dome valve was not discovered during normal testing. J Clin Eng 1991;16:485–4890.

271. Hornbein TF, Glauber DT. Inadvertent inspiration of carbon dioxide. Anesthesiology 1984;61:114.

272. Berner MS. Profound hypercapnia due to disconnection within an anaesthetic machine. Can J Anaesth 1987;34:622–626.

273. Dunn AJ. Empty tanks and Bain circuits. Can Anaesth Soc J 1978;25:337.

274. Skilton R, Kumar R. A new source of gas leak from an Ohmeda Excel 410 machine. Anaesthesia 1995; 50:266–267.

275. Breen M. Letter to the editor. Can Anaesth Soc J 1975;22:247.

276. Hannallah R, Rosales JK. A hazard connected with re-use of the Bain's circuit: a case report. Can Anaesth Soc J 1974;21:511–513.

277. Naqvi NH. Torsion of inner tube. Br J Anaesth 1981; 53:193.

278. Peterson WC. Bain circuit. Can Anaesth Soc J 1978; 25:532.

279. Mansell WH. Spontaneous breathing with the Bain circuit at low flow rates: a case report. Can Anaesth Soc J 1976;23:432–434.

280. Fukunaga AF. Torsion and disconnection of inner tube of coaxial breathing circuit. Br J Anaesth 1981; 53:1106–1107.

281. Roberts PJ. Unattached inner coaxial tube. Anaesthesia 1987;42:1128.

282. Read PJH, Lukey R. Potential hazard of the Kendall "Bain" circuit. Anaesthesia and Intensive Care 1989; 17:510.

283. Wildsmith JAW, Grubb DJ. Defective and misused co-axial circuits. Anaesthesia 1977;32:293.

284. Paterson JG, Vanhooydonk V. A hazard associated with improper connection of the Bain breathing circuit. Can Anaesth Soc J 1975;22:373–377.

285. Raju R. Humidifier-induced hypercarbia. Anaesthesia 1987;42:672–673.

286. Rigg D, Joseph M. Split ventilator bellows. Anaesthesia and Intensive Care 1985;13:213.

287. Podraza A, Salem MR, Harris TL, et al. Effects of bellows leaks on anesthesia ventilator function. Anesth Analg 1991;72:S215.

288. Waterman PM, Pautler S, Smith RB. Accidental ventilator-induced hyperventilation. Anesthesiology 1978;48:141.

289. Newton NI, Adams AQ. Excessive airway pressure during anesthesia. Anaesthesia 1978;33:689–699.

290. Dogu TS, Davis HS. Hazards of inadvertently opposed valves. Anesthesiology 1970;33:122–123.

291. Weaver LK, Fairfax WR, Greenway L. Bilateral otorrhagia associated with continuous positive airway pressure. Chest 1988;93:878–879.

292. Mayle LL, Reed SJ, Wyche MQ. Excessive airway pressures occurring concurrently with use of the Fraser Harlake PEEP valve. Anesthesiol Rev 1990; 17:41–44.

293. Thompson PW. Prevention of the hazard of excessive airway pressure. Anaesthesia 1979;34:593.

294. Bailey PL. Failed release of an activated oxygen flush valve. Anesthesiology 1983;59:480.

295. Puttick N. Hazard from the oxygen flush control. Anaesthesia 1986;41:222–224.

296. McCrirrick A, Warwick JP, Thomas TA. Capnography and awareness. Anaesthesia 1992;47:1102–1103.

297. Anderson EC, Rendell-Baker L. Exposed O_2 flush hazard. Anesthesiology 1982;56:328.

298. Cooper CMS. Capnography. Anaesthesia 1987;42:1238–1239.

299. Hanafiah Z, Sellers WFS. Nudging the emergency oxygen. Anaesthesia 1991;46:331.

300. Morris S, Barclay K. Oxygen flush buttons: more critical incidents. Anaesthesia 1993;48:1115–1116.

301. Andrews JJ. Understanding anesthesia ventilators (ASA Refresher Course #242). Park Ridge, IL: ASA, 1990.

302. Anonymous. Barotrauma from anesthesia ventilators. Technology for Anesthesia 1988;9(5):1–2.

303. Alston RP. Expiratory obstruction in a circle system. Anaesthesia 1987;42:1120.

304. Bishay EG, Echiverri E, Abu–Zaineh M, et al. An unusual cause for airway obstruction in a young healthy adult. Anesthesiology 1984;60:610–611.

305. Hindman BJ, Sperring SJ. Partial expiratory limb obstruction by a foreign body abutting upon an Ohio 5400 volume monitor sensor. Anesthesiology 1986; 65:349–350.

306. Jack TM. An unusual cause of complete expiratory obstruction. Anaesthesia 1987;42:564.

307. Davies JR. Misuse of adhesive tape. Anaesthesia 1988;43:841.

308. Hilgenberg JC, Burke BC. Positive end-expiratory pressure produced by water in the condensation chamber. Anesth Analg 1985;64:541–543.

309. Anonymous. Dryden anesthesia breathing circuits. Technology for Anesthesia 1988;8(9):4–5.

310. Register SD. Detection of defective equipment by proper preanesthetic checks. Anesthesiology 1985; 62:546–547.

311. Smith CE, Otworth JR, Kaluszyk P. Bilateral tension pneumothorax due to a defective anesthesia breathing circuit filter. J Clin Anesth 1991;3:229–234.

312. Anonymous. Anesthesia death related to "wet" oxygen filters. Biomedical Safety & Standards 1993;23: 11–12.

313. Barton RM. Detection of expiratory antibacterial filter occlusion. Anesth Analg 1993;77:197.

314. McEwan AI, Dowell L, Karis JH. Bilateral tension pneumothorax caused by a blocked bacterial filter in an anesthesia breathing circuit. Anesth Analg 1993; 76:440–442.

315. Anagnostou JM, Hults SL, Moorthy SS. PEEP valve barotrauma [Letter]. Anesth Analg 1990;70:674–675.

316. Anonymous. Valves, positive end expiratory pressure. Technology for Anesthesia 1991;11(12):11.

317. Rek RM, Dimas S, Reynolds J, Shapiro BA. Technical aspects of positive end-expiratory pressure (PEEP). Part II. PEEP with positive-pressure ventilation. Respiratory Care 1982;27:1490–1504.

318. Flowerdew RMM. A hazard of scavenger port design. Can Anaesth Soc J 1981;28:481–483.

319. Holley HS, Eisenman TS. Hazards of an anesthetic scavenging device. Anesth Analg 1983;62:458–460.

320. Mann ES, Sprague DH. An easily overlooked malassembly. Anesthesiology 1982;56:413–414.

321. Stevens IM. Hazardous misconnection. Anaesthesia and Intensive Care 1988;16:374–375.

322. Tavakoli M, Habeeb A. Two hazards of gas scavenging. Anesth Analg 1978;57:286–287.

323. Edwards ND. Another misconnection. Anaesthesia 1988;43:1066.

324. Anonymous. PEEP valves in anesthesia circuits. Health Devices 1983;13:24–25.

325. Cooper JB. Unidirectional PEEP valves can cause safety hazards. Anesthesia Patient Safety Foundation Newsletter 1990;5:28–29.

326. Arellano R, Ross D, Lee K. Inappropriate attachment of PEEP valve causing total obstruction of ventilation bag. Anesth Analg 1987;66:1050–1051.

327. Feingold A. Carbon dioxide absorber packaging hazard. Anesthesiology 1976;45:260.

328. Anonymous. Sodasorb prepack CO_2 absorption cartridges. Health Devices 1988;17:35–36.

329. Anonymous. Sodasorb prepack safety advisory. Lexington, MA: WR Grace and Co., March 6, 1992.

330. Norman PH, Daley MD, Walker JR, et al. Obstruction due to retained carbon dioxide absorber canister wrapping. Anesth Analg 1996;83:425–426.

331. Ransom ES, Norfleet EA. Obstruction due to retained carbon dioxide absorber canister wrapping. Anesth Analg 1997;84:703.

332. Anonymous. Dupaco bag tail scavenging valves. Technology for Anesthesia 1983;4(6):1–2.

333. Prince GD. Nichols BJ. Kinked breathing systems—again. Anaesthesia 1989;44:792.

334. Munro HM. An accident with the Lack system. Anaesthesia 1990;45:601–602.

335. Anonymous. CO_2 absorber subject of class I recall; firm disputes FDA designation for anesthesia device component. Biomedical Safety & Standards 1983;13: 98–99.

336. Dean HN, Parsons DE, Raphaely RC. Case report. Bilateral tension pneumothorax from mechanical failure of anesthesia machine due to misplaced expiratory valve. Anesth Analg 1971;50:195–198.

337. Goldsmith M. FDA issues pediatric respiratory device alert. JAMA 1983;250:2264.

338. Anonymous. Incompatability of Nellcor ADAP-PS gas sampling Tee and Dryden CPRAM breathing circuit. Technology for Anesthesia 1989;10(5):6–8.

339. Branson R, Lam AM. Increased resistance to breathing: a potentially lethal hazard across a coaxial circuit-connector coupling. Can J Anaesth 1987;34: S90–S91.

340. Villforth JC. FDA safety alert. Breathing system connectors. Rockville, MD: U.S. Food and Drug Administration, September 2, 1983.

341. Sloan IA, Ironside NK. Internal mis-mating of breathing system components. Can Anaesth Soc J 1984;31:576–578.

343. Anonymous. Pre-use testing prevents "helpful" reconnection of anesthesia components. Technology for Anesthesia 1987;8(1):1–2.

344. Henzig D. Insidious PEEP from a defective ventilator gas evacuation outlet valve. Anesthesiology 1982;57: 251–252.

345. Chaney MA. Delivery of excessive airway pressure to a patient by the anesthesia machine. Anesth Analg 1993;76:1166–7.

346. Roth S, Tweedie E, Sommer RM. Excessive airway pressure due to a malfunctioning anesthesia ventilator. Anesthesiology 1986;65:532–534.

347. Burgess RW. Blockage of spill valve. Anaesthesia and Intensive Care 1986;14:327–328.

348. Sharrock ME, Leith DE. Potential pulmonary barotrauma when venting anesthetic gases to suction. Anesthesiology 1977;46:152–154.

349. Rendell–Baker L. Hazard of blocked scavenging valve. Can Anaesth Soc J 1982;29:182–183.

350. O'Conner DE, Daniels BW, Pfitzner J. Hazards of anaesthetic scavenging: case reports and brief review. Anaesthesia and Intensive Care 1982;10:15–19.

351. Malloy WF, Wrightman AE, O'Sullivan D, et al. Bilateral pneumothorax from suction applied to a ventilator exhaust valve. Anesth Analg 1979;58:147–149.

352. Davies G, Tarnawsky M. Letters to the Editor. Can Anaesth Soc J 1976;23:228.

353. Hamilton RC, Byrne J. Another cause of gas scavenging-line obstruction. Anesthesiology 1979;51: 365–366.

354. Hagerdal M, Lecky JH. Anesthetic death of an experimental animal related to a scavenging system malfunction. Anesthesiology 1977;47:522–523.

355. Hayes C. An interesting misconnection. Anaesthesia 1991;46:508–509.

356. Sainsbury DA. Scavenging misconnection. Anaesthesia and Intensive Care 1985;13:215–216.

357. Phillips S. Scavenging hazard. Anaesthesia and Intensive Care 1991;19:615.

358. Anonymous. Improperly cleaned resuscitator valves may stick and block airway. Biomedical Safety & Standards 1991;21:105–107.

359. Dolan PF, Shapiro S, Steinbach RB. Valve misassembly—manually operated resuscitation bag. Anesth Analg 1981;60:66–67.

360. Klick JM, Bushnell LS, Bancroft ML. Barotrauma, a potential hazard of manual resuscitators. Anesthesiology 1978;49:363–365.

361. Jumper A, Desai S, Liu P, et al. Pulmonary barotrauma resulting from a faulty Hope II resuscitation bag. Anesthesiology 1983;58:572–574.

362. Pauca AL, Jenkins TE. Airway obstruction by breakdown of a nonrebreathing valve. How foolproof is foolproof? Anesth Analg 1981;60:529–531.

363. Markovitz BP, Silverberg M, Godinez RI. Unusual cause of an absent capnogram. Anesthesiology 1989; 71:992–993.

364. Highley DA. Condensation. Anaesthesia 1994;49: 1101.

365. Katz L, Crosby JW. Accidental misconnections to endotracheal and tracheostomy tubes. Can Med Assoc J 1986;135:1149–1151.

366. Wasserberger J, Ordog GJ, Turner AF, et al. Iatrogenic pulmonary overpressure accident. Ann Emerg Med 1986;15:947–951.

367. Onsiong MK. Potential hazard of Hudson facemask. Anaesthesia 1988;43:907.

368. Newton NI. Supplementary oxygen—potential for disaster. Anaesthesia 1991;46:905–906.

369. Davies JR. A false compatibility. Anaesthesia 1991; 46:991.

370. Davies JR. A false compatibility. Anaesthesia 1992; 47:991.

371. Dubinsky IL. Near death caused by accidental misconnection to an endotracheal tube. Can Med Assoc J 1987;137:1105–1106.

372. Wasserberger J, Ordog GJ. Why endotracheal and oxygen tubing might be misconnected. Can Med Assoc J 1988;139:372.

373. Grime PD, Malins TJ. Hazard warning. A case of post-operative pulmonary barotrauma. Br J Oral Maxillofac Surg 1991;29:183–184.

374. Giesecke AH, Skrivanek GD. Respiratory obstruction in the recovery room. Anesth Analg 1992;75:639.

375. Davis R. Soda lime dust. Anaesthesia and Intensive Care 1979;7:390.

376. Lauria JI. Soda-lime dust contamination of breathing circuits. Anesthesiology 1975;42:628–629.

377. Ribak B. Reducing the soda lime hazard. Anesthesiology 1975;43:277.

378. Goodie D, Stewart I. Ulco carbon dioxide absorber. Anaesthesia and Intensive Care 1991;19:609–610.

379. Tingay MG, Ilsley AH, Willis RJ, et al. Gas identity hazards and major contamination of medical gas system of a new hospital. Anaesthesia and Intensive Care 1978;6:202–209.

380. Dinnick OP. Medical gases—pipeline problems. Eng Med 1979;8:243–247.

381. Anonymous. Oxygen cylinders recalled because of oil contamination. Biomedical Safety & Standards 1991; 21:20.

382. Russell WJ. Industrial gas hazard. Anaesthesia and Intensive Care 1985;13:106.

383. Eichorn JH, Bancroft ML, Laasberg LH, et al. Contamination of medical gas and water pipelines in a new hospital building. Anesthesiology 1977;46: 286–289.

384. Gilmour IJ, McComb C, Palahniuk RJ. Contamination of a hospital oxygen supply. Anesth Analg 1990; 71:302–304.

385. Coveler LA, Lester RC. Contaminated oxygen cylinder. Anesth Analg 1989;69:674–676.

386. Clutton–Brock J. Two cases of poisoning by contamination of nitrous oxide with higher oxides of nitrogen during anaesthesia. Br J Anaesth 1967;39: 388–392.

387. Moss E, Nagle T. Medical air systems are complex, usually poorly understood. Anesthesia Patient Safety Foundation Newsletter 1996;11:18–21.

388. Gilmour IJ, McComb C, Palahniuk RJ. Contamination of a hospital oxygen supply. Anesth Analg 1990; 71:302–304.

389. Anonymous. Oxygen system contamination probed in patient deaths. Biomedical Safety & Standards 1996;26:57–58.

390. Moss E. Hospital deaths reportedly due to contaminated O_2. American Society of Anesthesiologists Newsletter 1996;11:13–18.

391. Moss E. Dangers seen possible from contaminated medical gases. Anesthesia Patient Safety Foundation Newsletter 1993;8:6–7.

392. Bjerring P, Oberg B. Bacterial contamination of compressed air for medical use. Anaesthesia 1986;41: 148–150.

393. Bjerring P, Oberg B. Possible role of vacuum systems and compressed air generators in cross-infection in the ICU. Br J Anaesth 1987;59:648–650.

394. Oberg B, Bjerring P. Comparison of microbiological contents of compressed air in two Danish hospitals. Effect of oil and water reduction in air-generating units. Acta Anaesth Scand 1986;30:305–308.

395. Warren RE, Newsom SWB, Matthews JA, et al. Medical grade compressed air. Lancet 1986;1:1438.

396. Anonymous. Device safety alert. Anesthesia gas elbow component may separate. Biomedical Safety & Standards 1989;19:90.

397. Paulus DA. Drilling remnants in elbow adapters. Anesth Analg 1986;65:824.

398. Oh T. Bagging a foreign body. Anaesthesia and Intensive Care 1978;6:89–91.

399. Ross A. Oxygen analyser hazard. Anaesthesia and Intensive Care 1986;14:466–467.

400. Taylor BL, Rainbow C, Ford D. Debris in a breathing system. Anaesthesia 1989;44:702.

401. James PD, Gothard JWW. Possible hazard from the inserts of condenser humidifiers. Anaesthesia 1984; 39:70.

402. Gold MI. Defect in a T-fitting connection. Anesthesiology 1980;52:184.

403. Wald A, Mercurio A. Blistering of epoxy material of Narco Airshields ventilator Anesthesiology 1983;58: 390.

404. Williams EL, Reede L. One cap too many. Anesth Analg 1987;66:1340–1341.

405. Nimmagadda UR, Salem MR, Klowden AJ, et al. An unusual foreign body in the left main bronchus after open heart surgery. Anesth Analg 1989;68:803–805.

406. Siler JN, Neumann G. Latex glove hazard. Anesthesia Patient Safety Foundation Newsletter 1992;7:11.

407. Scott DM. Performance of BOC Ohmeda Tec 3 and Tec 4 vaporizers following tipping. Anaesthesia and Intensive Care 1991;19:441-3.

408. Riley RH, Hammond KA, Currie MS. "Hazards" of oxygen therapy during spinal anaesthesia. Anaesthesia 1991;46:421.

409. Williams L, Barton C, McVey JR, et al. A visual warning device for improved safety. Anesth Analg 1986; 65:1364.

410. Currie M, Mackay P, Morgan C, et al. The "wrong drug" problem in anaesthesia: an analysis of 2000 incident reports. Anaesthesia and Intensive Care 1993;21:596–601.

411. Woehlick HJ. Hazards of supplying supplemental oxygen through main gas flowmeters. Anesthesiology 1993;78:401–402.

412. Bruce DL, Linde HW. Vaporization of mixed anesthetic liquids. Anesthesiology 1984;60:342–346.

413. Chilcoat RT. Hazards of mis-filled vaporizers. Summary tables. Anesthesiology 1985;63:726–727.

414. Martin S. Hazards of agent-specific vaporizers. A case report of successful resuscitation after massive isoflurane overdose. Anesthesiology 1985;62:830–831.

415. Kelly DA. Free-standing vaporizers. Anaesthesia 1985;40:661–663.

416. Railton R, Inglis MD. High halothane concentrations from reversed flow in a vaporizer. Anaesthesia 1986;41:672–673.

418. Lewyn MJ. Patient wins damages for injury secondary to "light" anesthesia. Anesth Malprac Protector 1991;3:109–113.

419. Francis RN. Failure of nitrous oxide supply to theatre pipeline system. Anaesthesia 1990;45:880–882.

420. Yogananthan S. Failure of nitrous oxide supply. Anaesthesia 1990;45:897.

421. Paul DL. Pipeline failure. Anaesthesia 1989;44:523.

422. Comber REH. Penlon rotameter block failure. Anaesthesia and Intensive Care 1990;18:141–142.

423. James RH. Rotameter sequence—a variant of "read the label." Anaesthesia 1996;51:87–88.

424. Craig DB, Longmuir J. An unusual failure of an oxygen fail-safe device. Can Anaesth Soc J 1971;18:576–577.

425. Puri GD, George MA, Singh H, et al. Awareness under anaesthesia due to a defective gas-loaded regulator. Anaesthesia 1987;42:539–540.

426. Anonymous. Internal leakage from anesthesia unit flush valves. Health Devices 1981;10:172.

427. Brahams D. Anaesthesia and the law. Awareness and pain during anaesthesia. Anaesthesia 1989;44:352.

428. Judkins KC. BOC Boyle M anaesthetic machine—a modification. Anaesthesia 1983;38:387–388.

429. Paymaster NJ. Inadvertent administration of 100% oxygen during anaesthesia. Br J Anaesth 1978;50:1268.

430. Dodd KW. Inadvertent administration of 100% oxygen during anaesthesia. Br J Anaesth 1979;51:573.

431. Longmuir J, Craig DB. Misadventure with a Boyle's gas machine. Can Anaesth Soc J 1976;23:671–673.

432. Peters KR, Wingard DW. Anesthesia machine leakage due to misaligned vaporizers. Anesth Rev 1987;14:36–39.

433. Duncan JAT. Select-a-tec switch malfunction. Anaesthesia 1985;40:911–924.

434. Barcroft JP. Is there liquid in the vaporizer? Anaesthesia 1989;44:939.

435. Cudmore J, Keogh J. Another Selectatec switch malfunction. Anaesthesia 1990;45:754–756.

436. Lamberty JM, Lerman J. Intraoperative failure of a fluotec Mark II vapourizer. Can Anaesth Soc J 1984;31:687–689.

437. Maltby JR. Intraoperative failure of a Fluotec Mark II vapourizer. Can Anaesth Soc J 1985;32:200.

438. Bookallil MJ. Entrainment of air during mechanical ventilation. Br J Anaesth 1967;39:184.

439. Baraka A, Muallem M. Awareness during anaesthesia due to a ventilator malfunction. Anaesthesia 1979;34:678–679.

440. Longmuir J, Craig DB. Inadvertent increase in inspired oxygen concentration due to defect in ventilator bellows. Can Anaesth Soc J 1976;23:327–329.

441. Love JB. Misassembly of a Campbell ventilator causing leakage of the driving gas to a patient. Anaesthesia and Intensive Care 1980;8:376–377.

442. Hillyer KW, Johnston RR. Unsuspected dilution of anesthetic gases detected by an oxygen analyzer. Anesth Analg 1978;57:491–492.

443. Marsland AR, Solomos J. Ventilator malfunction detected by O_2 analyser. Anaesthesia and Intensive Care 1981;9:395.

444. Varma RR, Whitesell RC, Iskandarani MM. Halothane hepatitis without halothane. Role of inapparent circuit contamination and its prevention. Hepatology 1985;5:1159–1162.

445. Ellis FR, Clarks IMC, Modgill EM, et al. New causes of malignant hyperpyrexia. Br Med J 1975;1:575.

446. Bridges RT. Vaporizers—serviced and checked? Anaesthesia 1991;46:695–697.

447. Cook TL, Eger EI, Behl RS. Is your vaporizer off? Anesth Analg 1977;56:793–800.

448. Robinson JS, Thompson JM, Barratt RS. Inadvertent contamination of anaesthetic circuits with halothane. Br J Anaesth 1977;49:745–753.

449. Ritchie PA, Cheshire MA, Pearce NH. Decontamination of halothane from anaesthetic machines achieved by continuous flushing with oxygen. Br J Anaesth 1988;60:859–863.

450. Ritchie PA, Cheshire MA, Pearce NH. Decontamination of halothane from anaesthetic machines achieved by continuous flushing with oxygen. Br J Anaesth 1988;60:859–863.

451. Beebe JJ, Sessler KI. Preparation of anesthesia machines for patients susceptible to malignant hyperthermia. Anesthesiology 1988;69:395–400.

452. McGraw TT, Keon TP. Malignant hyperthermia and the clean machine. Can J Anaesth 1989;36:530–532.

453. Cooper JB, Philip JH. More on anesthesia machines and malignant hyperpyrexia. Anesthesiology 1989;70:561–562.

454. Samulksa HM, Ramaiah S, Noble WH. Unintended

exposure to halothane in surgical patients. halothane washout studies. Can Anaesth Soc J 1972;19:35–41.

455. Gilly H, Weindlmayr–Goettel M, Koberl H, et al. Anaesthetic uptake and washout characteristics of patient circuit tubing with special regard to current decontamination techniques. Acta Anaesthesiol Scand 1992;36:621–627.

456. ECRI. Understanding the fire hazard. Technology for Anesthesia 1992;12(9):1–6.

457. Axelrod EH, Kusnetz AB, Rosenberg MK. OR fires initiated by hot wire cautery. Anesthesiology 1993; 79:1123–1126.

458. Mandych A, Mickelson S, Amis R. OR fire. Arch Otolaryngol Head Neck Surg 1990;116:1452.

459. Anderson EF. A potential ignition source in the operating room. Anesth Analg 1976;55:217–218.

460. Rita L, Seleny F. Endotracheal tube ignition during laryngeal surgery with resectoscope. Anesthesiology 1982;56:60–61.

461. Anonymous. Hazard: unshielded radiant heat sources. Technology for Anesthesia 1984;5(1,2): 1–2.

462. Anonymous. Laser starts fire in OR. Technology for Anesthesia 1988;8:3–4.

463. Willis MJ, Thomas E. The cold light source that was hot. Gastrointest Endosc 1984;30:117–118.

464. Epstein RH, Brummett RR Jr., Lask GP. Incendiary potential of the flash-lamp pumped 585-nm tunable dye laser. Anesth Analg 1990;71:171–175.

465. Wegrzynowicz ES, Jensen NF, Pearson KS, et al. Airway fire during jet ventilation for laser excision of vocal cord papillomata. Anesthesiology 1992;76: 468–469.

466. Burlington DB. FDA safety alert. Hazards of heated-wire breathing circuits. Rockville, MD: Food and Drug Administration, July 14, 1993.

467. Anonymous. Incompatibility of disposable heated-wire breathing circuits and heated-wire humidifiers. Technology for Anesthesia 1993;14, 2:4–5.

468. Anonymous. Anesthesia breathing circuits may overheat and melt tubing. Biomedical Safety & Standards 1994;24:85.

469. Anonymous. Oxygen regulator fire caused by use of two yoke washers. Technology for Anesthesia 1990; 11(5):1–2.

470. Garfield JM, Allen GW, Silverstein P, et al. Flash fire in a reducing valve. Anesthesiology 1971;34: 578–579.

471. Newton BE, Langford RK, Meyer GR. Promoted ignition of oxygen regulators In: Stoltzful JM, Benz FJ, Stradling JS, eds. Flammability and sensitivity of

materials in oxygen-enriched atmospheres. Vol. 4. Philadelphia: ASTM, 1989;241–266.

472. Perel A, Mahler Y, Davidson JT. Combustion of a nasal catheter carrying oxygen. Anesthesiology 1976; 45:666–667.

473. Anonymous. Infant dies after OR flash fire. Biomedical Safety & Standards 1988;18:154.

474. Anonymous. Use of acetone and "eggcrate" mattress cited in OR fire. Indiana hospitals advised to review internal policies. Biomedical Safety & Standards 1989;19:26.

475. Ashcraft KE, Golladay ES, Guinee WS. A surgical field flash fire during the separation of dicephalus dipus conjoined twins. Anesthesiology 1981;55: 457–458.

476. Anonymous. Fires during surgery of the head and neck area. Health Devices Alerts 1980;4:3–4.

477. Bowdle TA, Glenn M, Colston H, et al. Fire following use of electrocautery during emergency percutaneous transtracheal ventilation. Anesthesiology 1987;66:697–698.

478. Collee GG. A fire in the mouth. Anaesthesia 1984; 39:936.

479. Datta TD. Flash fire hazard with eye ointment. Anesth Analg 1984;63:700–701.

480. Gupte SR. Gauze fire in the oral cavity: a case report. Anesth Analg 1972;51:645–646.

481. Gibbs JM. Combustible plastic drape. Anaesthesia and Intensive Care 1983;11:176.

482. Simpson JI, Wolf GL. Endotracheal tube fire ignited by pharyngeal electrocautery. Anesthesiology 1986; 65:76–77.

483. Wong A, Macdonald M, Walker P, et al. Diathermy-induced airway fire during tonsillectomy. Anesthesiology 1992;77:A1060.

484. Anonymous. Laser-ignited latex glove causes airway fire. Biomedical Safety & Standards 1992;22:51.

485. Magruder GB, Gruber D. Fire prevention during surgery. Arch Ophthalmol 1970;84:237.

486. Milliken RA, Bizzarri DV. Flammable surgical drapes—a patient and personnel hazard. Anesth Analg 1985;64:54–67.

487. Milliken RA, Bizzarri DV. Combustible plastic drape. Anaesthesia and Intensive Care 1984;12:275.

488. Marsh B, Riley RH. Double-lumen tube fire during tracheostomy. Anesthesiology 1992;76:480–481.

489. Le Clair J, Gartner S, Halma G. Endotracheal tube cuff ignited by electrocautery during tracheostomy. J Am Assoc Nurse Anesth 1990;58:259–261.

490. Plumlee JE. Operating-room flash fire from use of cautery after aerosol spray: a case report. Anesth Analg 1973;52:202–203.

491. Schettler WH. Correspondence. Anesth Analg 1974; 53:288–289.

492. Simpson JI, Wolf GL. Flammability of esophageal stethoscopes, nasogastric tubes, feeding tubes, and nasopharyngeal airways in oxygen-and nitrous oxide-enriched atmospheres. Anesth Analg 1988;67: 1093–1095.

493. Ott AE. Disposable surgical drapes—a potential fire hazard. Obstet Gynecol 1983;61:667–668.

494. Bennett JA, Agree M. Fire in the chest. Anesth Analg 1994;78:406.

495. Bortolussi ME, Hunter JG. Fire hazard of the ophthalmic cautery. Plast Reconstr Surg 1989;83:753.

496. Curtin JW. The disposable cautery: a fire hazard. Plast Reconstr Surg 1989;84:853.

497. Ally A, McIlwain M, Duncavage JA. Electrosurgery-induced endotracheal tube ignition during tracheotomy. Ann Otol Rhinol Laryngol 1991;100:31–33.

498. Marsh B, Riley RH. Double-lumen tube fire during tracheostomy. Anesthesiology 1992;76:480–481.

499. Wood DK. Thermocautery causes a gauze pad fire. JAMA 1993;270:2299–2300.

500. Wilson PTJ, Igbaseimokumo U, Martin J. Ignition of the tracheal tube during tracheostomy. Anaesthesia 1994;49:734–735.

501. Lake CH. From the literature. ECRI review explains, warns of OR fires. Anesthesia Patient Safety Foundation Newsletter 1991;6:46.

502. Sommer RM. Preventing endotracheal tube fire during pharyngeal surgery. Anesthesiology 1987;66: 439.

503. Anonymous. Preventing, preparing for, and managing surgical fires. Health Devices 1992;21,1:24–31.

504. Chestler RJ, Lemke BN. Intraoperative flash fires associated with disposable cautery. Ophthalmic Plast Recon Surg 1989;5:194–195.

505. Sosis M, Braverman B, Ivankovich AD. Metal anesthesia circuit components stop laser fires. Anesthesiology 1991;75:A396.

506. Moxon MA, Reading ME, Ward MB. Fire in the operating theatre. Evacuation pre-planning may save lives. Anaesthesia 1986;41:543–546.

507. McCranie J. Fire safety in the OR. Today's O.R. Nurse 1994;1:33–37.

508. Reference deleted.

509. National Fire Protection Association. Health care facilities. Suggested procedures in the event of a fire or explosion, anesthetizing locations (NFPA 99.1990). Quincey, MA: NFPA, 1990:182–184.

510. Bruner JMR. Fire in the OR. American Society of Anesthesiologists Newsletter 1990;54:22–25.

511. The Compressed Gas Association. Handbook of compressed gases. 3rd ed. New York: Van Nostrand Reinhold, 1990.

512. Hamid RKA. Latex allergy. Diagnosis, management and safe equipment. 1995 ASA Refresher Courses, Atlanta.

513. Anonymous. Latex sensitivity among health care workers. Technology for Anesthesia 1994;14(10): 1–7.

514. Randel GI. Latex allergy: who is next? American Society of Anesthesiologists Newsletter 1997;61,5: 14–17.

515. Mostello LA. The clinical significance and management of latex allergy. 1996 ASA Annual Refresher Courses, New Orleans.

516. Konrad C, Fieber T, Gerber H, et al. The prevalence of latex sensitivity among anesthesiology staff. Anesth Analg 1997;84:629–633.

517. Kam PCA, Lee MSM, Thompson JF. Latex allergy: an emerging clinical and occupational health problem. Anaesthesia 1997;52:570–575.

518. Bernstein M. An overview of latex allergy and its implications for emergency nurses. J Emerg Nurs 1996; 22:29–36.

519. Holzman RS. Latex allergy: an emerging OR problem. Anesth Analg 1993;76:635–641.

520. Porri F, Pradal M, Lemiere C, et al. Association between latex sensitization and repeated latex exposure in children. Anesthesiology 1997;86:599–602.

521. Ballantyne JC, Brown E. Latex anaphylaxis: another case, another cause. Anesth Analg 1995;81: 1303–1304.

522. Kubasiewicz MK. Latex allergy and nonlatex syringes. Anesth Analg 1996;83:1352.

QUESTIONS

Each question below contains four suggested answers of which one or more is correct.
Choose the answer:
A if 1, 2, and 3 are correct
B if 1 and 3 are correct
C if 2 and 4 are correct
D if 4 is correct
E if 1, 2, 3 and 4 are correct.

1. Hypercarbia due to an incompetent unidirectional valve can be distinguished from that due to exhausted absorbent by
   1. The shape of the CO_2 waveform
   2. An increase in inspired carbon dioxide
   3. Absence of heat in the absorber
   4. Increasing the fresh gas flow

2. Causes of air entrainment include:
   1. Suction applied to a N-G tube curled in the esophagus
   2. Malfunction of the interface of the scavenging system
   3. Use of a mainstream gas analyzer
   4. A leak in the ventilator bellows

3. What course of action should be taken if a gas crossover in the pipeline system is suspected?
   1. Use the oxygen flush on the machine to purge the crossed gas
   2. Disconnect the pipeline and open an oxygen cylinder
   3. Turn up the flowmeter for the crossed gas and turn off the oxygen flowmeter
   4. Use a resuscitation bag to ventilate with room air

4. Worldwide, an oxygen cylinder should be painted
   1. Black
   2. White
   3. Blue
   4. Green

5. Which safety mechanism(s) are used to prevent hypoxic mixtures being delivered when flowmeters are incorrectly set
   1. Oxygen failure safety valve
   2. Oxygen analyzer
   3. Oxygen pressure failure alarm

4. Proportioning system

6. What is the result of a leak in the air flowmeter if air is in the middle flowmeter position if nitrous oxide and oxygen are in use?
   1. The oxygen concentration will be higher than would be expected
   2. Air would be entrained into the fresh gas flow
   3. The nitrous oxide concentration would be less than expected
   4. No effect on oxygen since the air flowmeter is not in use

7. Which measures should be taken in the event of the loss of the oxygen pipeline supply?
   1. Use low fresh gas flows
   2. Turn the ventilator off
   3. Disconnect the machine from the central supply
   4. Open an oxygen cylinder

8. A leak in the breathing system must be suspected if
   1. The end-tidal carbon dioxide begins to increase
   2. The inspired nitrogen increases during spontaneous ventilation
   3. A standing ventilator bellows fails to return to the top of its housing
   4. The FiO_2 begins to decrease during controlled ventilation

9. Which situations would result a negative pressure in the breathing system
   1. A nasogastric tube placed in the trachea
   2. Suction applied to a working channel of a fiberscope
   3. Malfunction of valves in a closed scavenging interface
   4. Loss of oxygen pressure to the machine

10. An obstruction in the breathing system may cause
   1. An increase in the peak breathing system pressure
   2. Activation of the high pressure alarm
   3. Hypoventilation

4. Decreased movement of the ventilator bellows

11. Which monitors are reliable detectors of hypoventilation?
    1. Carbon dioxide
    2. Airway pressure
    3. Respirometer
    4. Oxygen analyzer

12. What problems should be suspected if there is carbon dioxide in the inspiratory gas?
    1. Absorber in the bypass position
    2. Inadequate fresh gas flow to a circle breathing system
    3. Incompetent unidirectional valves
    4. Excess carbon dioxide production

13. Situations that could result in excessive airway pressure include
    1. Malfunction of the APL valve
    2. Using the oxygen flush during inspiration with a mechanical ventilator
    3. Obstruction in the scavenging sytem
    4. A PEEP valve placed in the expiratory limb

14. Anesthetic agent overdosage may be caused by
    1. Isofluane in an halothane vaporizer
    2. Reversed flow through a vaporizer
    3. Enflurane in an isoflurane vaporizer
    4. Overfilled vaporizer

15. Which situations could result in a lower than expected anesthetic level
    1. Enflurane in a isoflurane vaporizer
    2. Leak in a ventilator bellows
    3. Vaporizer leak
    4. Air from a light source

16. Which gases will support combustion?
    1. Oxygen
    2. Nitrous Oxide
    3. Air

4. Nitrogen

17. Which patients are at increased risk for latex allergic reactions?
    1. Those with congenital orthopedic defects
    2. Those with congenital urologic deformities
    3. Those who undergo repeated esophageal dilations
    4. Patients in an in vitro fertilization program

18. Which symptoms should suggest possible latex allergy?
    1. Seasonal allergic asthma
    2. Swelling of the mouth when blowing up rubber balloons
    3. Sensitivity to kiwi fruit
    4. Past history of an anaphylactic reaction

19. What precautions can be taken if a patient is suspected to be latex sensitive?
    1. Using nonlatex-containing devices when possible
    2. Wrapping the arm before applying a blood pressure cuff
    3. Using glass syringes
    4. Using hypoallergenic medical devices

ANSWERS

1. D	11. A
2. C	12. B
3. C	13. A
4. E	14. C
5. C	15. E
6. B	16. A
7. E	17. E
8. A	18. E
9. A	19. A
10. E	

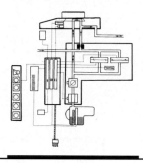

AIRWAY EQUIPMENT

Face Masks and Airways

FACE MASKS

The face mask (face piece) allows administration of gases from the breathing system without introducing any apparatus into the patient.

General Description

A face mask may be constructed of clear plastic, an elastomeric material, or a combination of these.

Body

The body constitutes the main part of the mask. A transparent body allows observation of the patient for vomitus, secretions, blood, lip color, and condensation of exhaled moisture and may be better accepted by a conscious patient (1).

A malleable body may allow a better fit to the face and reduced dead space.

Seal

The seal (rim, flap) is the part of the mask that comes in contact with the face. Two general types are used. One is a pad (cushion) that is often inflatable or filled with a material that will conform to the face when pressure is applied. It may be high-

volume, low pressure or high-volume, low pressure. The second type is a flange that is a noninflatable flexible extension of the body.

Connector

The connector (orifice, collar) is at the opposite side from the seal. It consists of a thickened fitting with a 22 mm internal diameter. A ring with hooks (Fig. 14.1) may be placed around the connector to allow a mask strap to be attached.

Specific Masks

Masks come in a variety of sizes and shapes (Figure 14.1). An assortment should be kept readily available, because none will fit every face well.

Anatomical Mask

The anatomical mask (Fig. 14.2) has a slightly malleable rubber body, a sharp notch for the nose

FIGURE 14.1. Clear, disposable masks. (**A** courtesy of SIMS Inc. **B** courtesy of Rusch Inc.)

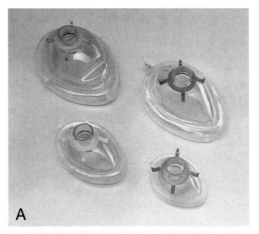

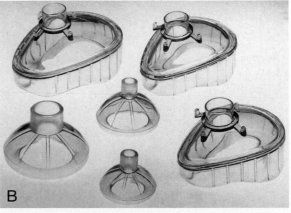

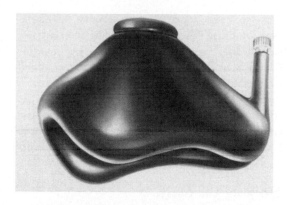

FIGURE 14.2. Anatomical mask (also known as Connell Mask or Form-It). (Courtesy of Ohio Medical Products, a division of Airco, Inc.)

and a curved chin section. The low-volume high-pressure cushion may be factory sealed or have a nipple for inflation with additional air.

Rendell-Baker-Soucek Mask

The Rendell-Baker-Soucek (RBS) mask (Fig. 14.3A.), which is designed for the pediatric patient, has a triangular body. It has a low dead space (2, 3). Some of these masks are scented and may have a pacifier (Fig. 14.3B). This mask has been used to administer positive pressure ventilation to patients with tracheostomies (4, 5).

Patil–Syracuse Endoscopic Mask (6, 7)

The Patil (intubating) mask (Fig. 14.4) allows oral or nasal fiberoptic intubation through a port/diaphragm in body of the mask. This pro-

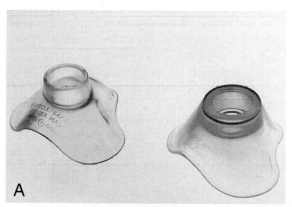

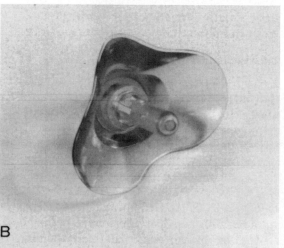

FIGURE 14.3. Rendell–Baker-Soucek masks. **A,** Clear plastic version. **B,** With pacifier. (**A** is courtesy of Rusch Inc. **B** is courtesy of Ohio Medical Products, a division of Airco, Inc.)

vides a seal, allowing positive pressure ventilation with a fiberscope in place. A cap for covering the port is attached to the mask. Use of the mask requires two operators: one to perform the intubation and one to maintain the airway, mask fit, and ventilation (8).

Scented Masks

Since face masks are often used for inhalational induction of anesthesia or for preoxygenation prior to induction, efforts have been made to

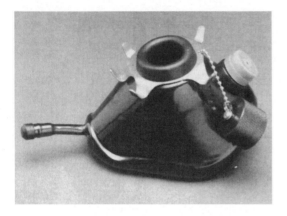

FIGURE 14.4. Patil–Syracuse endoscopic mask. (Courtesy of Mercury Medical.)

make this experience more acceptable to the patient by using scents to camouflage the odors of inhalational agents. The scent may be incorporated into the mask by the manufacturer or added by the anesthesia provider (9–12) (Fig. 14.5). Some masks are color coded according to the scent. In a study of adult patients, most found a scented mask more acceptable than an unscented one (13). The ethyl alcohol in some fruit flavors may affect the accuracy of some gas monitors (14).

Holding the Mask

The face mask should form a tight seal on the patient's face while fitting comfortably in the user's hand. A poor fit requires the anesthesia provider to maintain steady pressure. This may lead to cramped hands and tired muscles and limits the ability to perform other tasks. Failure to obtain a tight fit with spontaneous respiration will result in air dilution (15). This can be compensated for to some extent by increasing the fresh gas flow, but this is wasteful and contaminates the room with anesthetic gases. In addition, the reservoir bag no longer serves as a means of monitoring ventilation. With assisted or controlled ventilation adequate gas exchange may be impossible with a poor mask fit.

There are several methods of holding a mask

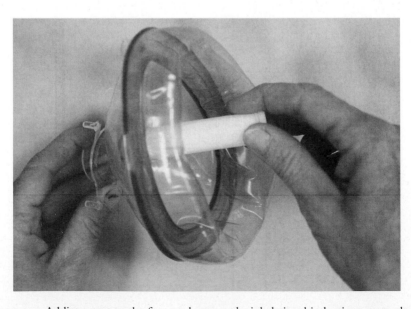

FIGURE 14.5. Adding scent to the face mask may make inhalational inductions more pleasant.

to maintain an open airway and a tight seal. A commonly used method is shown in Figure 14.6. The thumb and index finger of the left hand are on the body of the mask on opposite sides of the connector. These push downward to hold the mask to the face and prevent leaks. Additional downward pressure can be exerted by the anesthesiologist's chin on the mask elbow. The remaining three fingers are placed on the mandible or the inferior part of the mask. It is important that there

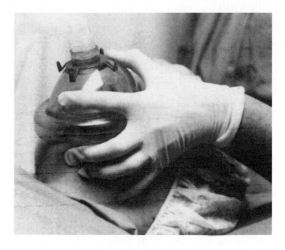

FIGURE 14.6. Holding the mask with one hand.

be no pressure applied to soft tissues of the patient's face or neck, as this may decrease patency of the airway. Care should be taken that there is no pressure on the eyes. If airway patency is not a problem, the fingers can be extended to the right side of the mask, so that the proximal interphalangeal joints of the fingers and the distal interphalangeal joint of the thumb are at the midline of the mask, allowing the pads of the fingers to put pressure on the right side of the mask (16).

A second method can be used to open any but the most difficult airway and obtain a tight fit (Fig. 14.7). It requires two hands so a second person is necessary if assisted or controlled respiration is used. The thumbs are placed on either side of the body of the mask. The index fingers are placed under the angles of the jaw. The mandible is lifted and the head extended. If a leak is present, downward pressure on the mask can be increased by the anesthesia provider's chin on the mask elbow (see Fig. 14.7B).

Another method is to have one individual stand at the head of the patient and perform a jaw thrust at the angle of the left mandible while the right hand compresses the reservoir bag (17). The second person stands at the patient's shoulder, facing the first individual. This person's right hand covers the left hand of the first person and the left

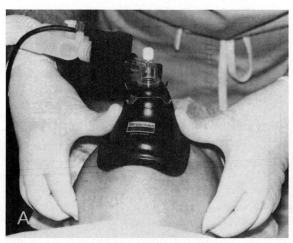

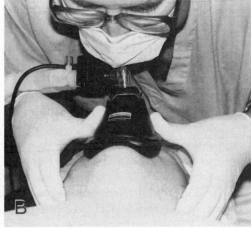

FIGURE 14.7. **A,** Holding the mask with two hands. Also shown is the Esmarch–Heiberg maneuver, which involves dorsiflexion at the atlantooccipital joint and protrusion of the mandible anteriorly by exerting a for-

ward thrust on the rami. **B,** The anesthesiologist's chin on the mask elbow helps create a better seal between the mask and the patient's face.

hand achieves right-sided jaw thrust and mask seal.

Another technique has been described using a triangular-shaped mask in edentulous patients (18). The patient's mouth is opened and the inferior margin of the mask is placed between the gingiva of the maxilla and mandible, then the mouth is closed. Mandibular protrusion occurs as the superior angle of the mask is rotated posteriorly to form a seal between the mask and the maxillary and nasal surfaces of the face.

Correct use of a face mask starts with selection of the appropriate size and shape. This may require some trial and error. The smallest mask that will do the job is the most desirable because it will cause the least increase in dead space, will usually be easiest to hold, and will be less likely to result in pressure on the eyes.

A variety of facial characteristics (fat, emaciated, and edentulous faces and those with prominent nares, burns, flat noses, receding jaws, beards, drainage tubes in the nose) will be encountered in clinical practice. The edentulous patient presents the most common problem. There is loss of bone of the alveolar ridge, causing a loss of distance between the points where the mask rests on the mandible and the nose. Furthermore, the buccinator muscle loses its tone in these patients. The cheeks sag, creating gaps between them and the mask. Alveolar process resorption results in a shrinking of the corners of the mouth. Means to improve mask fit include inserting an oral airway, leaving the patient's dentures in place, packing the cheeks with gauze sponges, and inserting the inferior margin of the mask between the gingiva of the maxilla and mandible (18). Other techniques include hooking the mask beneath the mandible rather than in front of the chin and gathering the cheek in the left hand and sliding the mask to the right side of the face.

Patients with facial deformities are particularly challenging. Application of the mask rotated 180° has been used for children with certain facial deformities (19) and patients with acromegaly (20). Various methods have been described for patients with beards (21–23).

If the mask is too small with an oral airway in place, the oral airway should be removed and a nasal airway used. If a mask is too long, the face can be elongated by inserting an oral airway.

Dead Space

The face mask and its adaptor normally constitute the major part of the mechanical dead space. Although the entire volume of the face mask must be considered as potential dead space, channeling of gas currents may reduce the actual dead space (24). Dead space may be decreased by increasing the pressure on the mask, changing the volume of the cushion, using a smaller mask, extending the separation of the inspiratory and expiratory channels close to or into the mask, and blowing a jet of fresh gas into the mask.

Mask Straps

A mask strap (mask holder, inhaler retainer, head strap, head harness, mask harness, mask retainer, headband, head-restraining strap) helps to hold the mask firmly on the face. Its use may decrease leaks. A typical mask strap consists of thin strips arranged in a circle with four or six projections (Fig. 14.8). The head rests in the circle and the straps attach around the mask connector.

The precise application of the straps (crossed versus uncrossed) is a matter of individual preference and may be the best result of a trial-and-error process (16).

The straps at the jaw may tend to pull the jaw posteriorly. Crossing the two lower straps under the chin may result in a better fit and counteract the pull of the upper straps so that there is less tendency for the mask to creep up above the bridge of the nose (25). Another method is to insert a tongue depressor transversely under the straps below the jaw (26).

Care must be taken that the straps are no tighter than necessary to achieve a seal to avoid pressure damage from the mask or the straps. They should be released periodically and the mask moved slightly. Gauze sponges placed between the straps and the skin will help to protect from excessive pressure. Another danger of mask straps is that should vomiting or regurgitation occur, it takes longer to remove the mask.

Particular care needs to be paid to maintaining the airway when using a mask strap as obstruction

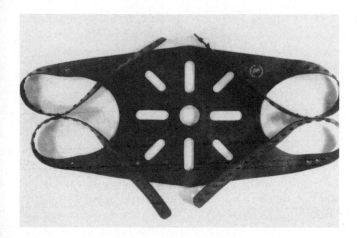

FIGURE 14.8. Mask strap.

is more likely to go unrecognized than when the mask is being held by hand.

Advantages and Disadvantages

Advantages

Use of a face mask is associated with a lower incidence of sore throat and requires less anesthetic depth than use of an LMA or tracheal tube. Also muscle relaxants do not need to be used. For short cases, the face mask may be the most cost-efficient choice of airway management (27).

Disadvantages

With a face mask the anesthesia provider's hands are tied up and higher fresh gas flows are often needed. Remote airway access (magnetic resonance imaging and computerized tomography scans) is difficult to perform. Compared to patients managed with an LMA, patients managed with a face mask have more episodes of oxygen desaturation, require more intraoperative airway manipulations and present more difficulties in maintaining an airway (28, 29).

Complications

Skin Problems

Dermatitis may occur if the patient is allergic to the material from which the mask is made (30). The pattern of the dermatitis follows the area of contact between the mask and skin. Chemical or gas sterilization can leave a residue that can cause a reaction (31, 32). Necrosis of the skin has been

reported following prolonged mask application in the presence of hypotension (33).

Nerve Injury

Pressure from a mask or mask strap may result in pressure injury to underlying nerves. Forward displacement of the jaw may cause nerve injury from stretching. Fortunately, the sensory and motor dysfunctions reported have been transient (34–39). If excessive pressure on the face or extreme forward displacement of the jaw must be exerted, tracheal intubation or use of a laryngeal mask should be considered. The mask should be removed from the face periodically and readjusted to make certain that continuous pressure is not applied to one area.

Aspiration of Gastric Contents

A mask does not protect the tracheobronchial tree from aspiration of gastric contents. Ventilation with a mask may cause air to enter the stomach, increasing the risk of regurgitation.

Foreign Body Aspiration

Certain masks designed to facilitate fiberoptic intubation have a thin diaphragm through which the tracheal tube is inserted. It is possible for this diaphragm to rupture during insertion of the tube and a piece to be pushed into the patient's tracheobronchial tree. (40–44)

Eye Injury

Chemicals that enter the mask cushion during cleaning and disinfection can come into contact with the eye when the mask is applied to the face (45–48). Pressure on the medial angles of the eyes and supraorbital margins may result in edema of the eyelids, chemosis of the conjunctiva, pressure on the supraorbital or supratrochlear nerve, corneal injury, and temporary blindness due to occlusion of the central retinal artery (49). A corneal abrasion may be caused by a face mask inadvertently placed on an open eye (50). A check should always be made that the eyes are fully closed.

Manufacturing Defects

A mask on which a plastic membrane occluded the connector has been reported (51). Another mask had a metal wire sticking out of it (52).

Movement of the Cervical Spine

Mask ventilation moves the cervical spine more than any commonly used method of tracheal intubation (53).

Latex Allergy

If rubber is a component of a face mask, a serious reaction can occur in the patient with latex allergy (54, 55). This is discussed more fully in Chapter 13, "Hazards of Anesthesia Machines and Breathing Systems." Because of the seriousness of this problem, it is recommended that non-latex masks be used whenever possible.

Lack of Correlation between Arterial and End-Tidal CO$_2$

Estimation of arterial carbon dioxide partial pressure by monitoring end-tidal carbon dioxide tension is somewhat unreliable with a face mask, particularly with small tidal volumes (56, 57).

Environmental Pollution

Studies show that use of a face mask is associated with greater operating room pollution with anesthetic gases and vapors than use of a tracheal tube or laryngeal mask (58, 59). Pollution can be reduced by use of a close active scavenging device (60, 61).

User Fatigue

Holding a mask securely onto the face and at the same time maintaining the correct position of the jaw can be difficult and may result in operator

fatigue. Failure to maintain the correct jaw position may result in loss of airway patency or gastric distention.

AIRWAYS
Purpose (62, 63)

A fundamental responsibility of the anesthesia provider is to maintain a patent airway. Failure to do so can result in brain damage or death.

Figure 14.9A shows the normal unobstructed airway in a supine patient. The air passage has a rigid posterior wall, supported by the cervical vertebrae, and a collapsible anterior wall, consisting of the tongue and epiglottis. Figure 14.9B shows the most common cause of airway obstruction.

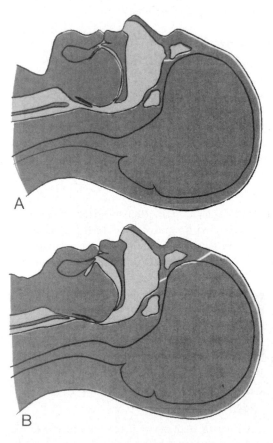

FIGURE 14.9. **A,** The normal airway. The tongue and other soft tissues are forward, allowing an unobstructed air passage. **B,** the obstructed airway. The tongue and epiglottis fall back to the posterior pharyngeal wall, occluding the airway. (Courtesy of V. Robideaux, MD.)

The muscles of the floor of the mouth and pharynx supporting the tongue relax, and the tongue and epiglottis fall back into the posterior pharynx, occluding the airway. The purpose of an airway is to lift the tongue and epiglottis away from the posterior pharyngeal wall and prevent them from obstructing the space above the larynx. Use of maneuvers such as dorsiflexion at the atlanto-occipital joint and protrusion of the mandible anteriorly may still be necessary to ensure a patent airway (63).

Unlike other maneuvers to maintain a patent airway, including chin lift, jaw thrust, and tracheal intubation, insertion of an airway does not cause movement of the cervical spine (64).

Types

Oropharyngeal Airways

Figure 14.10 shows an oropharyngeal (oral) airway in place. The bite portion is between the teeth and lips and the flange is outside the lips. The pharyngeal end rests between the posterior wall of the oropharynx and the base of the tongue and, by pressure along the base of the tongue, pulls the epiglottis forward.

In addition to helping maintain an open airway, an oropharyngeal airway may be used to prevent a patient from biting and occluding an oral tracheal tube, protect the tongue from biting, fa-

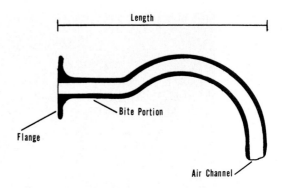

FIGURE 14.11. Oropharyngeal airway. All oral airways have a flange to prevent overinsertion, a straight bite block portion and a curved section.

cilitate oropharyngeal suctioning, obtain a better mask fit, and provide a pathway for insertion of tubular devices into the esophagus or pharynx. Its use has not been associated with an increased incidence of sore throat or other related symptoms (65, 66) or bacteremia (67).

Description

An oropharyngeal airway (Fig. 14.11) may be made of elastomeric material or plastic. It has a flange at the buccal end to prevent it from moving back into the mouth. The flange may also serve as a means to fix the airway in place. The bite portion is straight and fits between the teeth or gums. It must be firm enough that the patient cannot close the lumen by biting. The curved portion extends backward to correspond to the shape of the tongue and palate.

The American standard (68) specifies that the size of oral airways be designated by a number that is the length in centimeters (Figure 14.11).

Specific Airways

Guedel airway. The Guedel airway (Fig. 14.12) has a large flange, a reinforced bite portion, and a tubular channel. A modification of this airway to aid flexible fiberoptic intubation in children has been described (69).

Berman airway (70). The Berman airway (Figs. 14.10 and 14.11) has a center support and open sides. The center support may have openings. There is a flange at the buccal end.

Patil–Syracuse oral airway. The Patil–Syracuse oral (Patil endoscopic) airway was designed to aid fiberoptic intubation (7). It has lateral suction

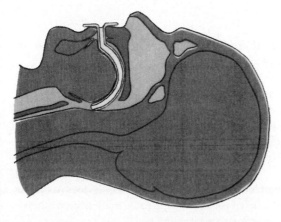

FIGURE 14.10. Oropharyngeal airway in place. The airway follows the curvature of the tongue, pulling it and the epiglottis away from the posterior pharyngeal wall and providing a channel for air passage. (Courtesy of V. Robideaux, MD.)

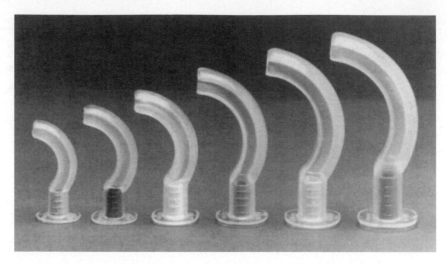

FIGURE 14.12. Guedel airways. The bite portions are color coded to provide easy identification of size. (Courtesy of Mercury Medical.)

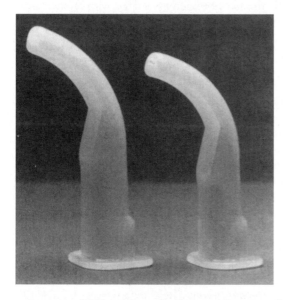

FIGURE 14.13. Williams airway intubators. (Courtesy of Mercury Medical.)

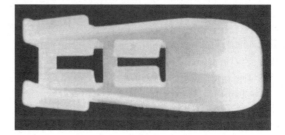

FIGURE 14.14. Ovassapian fiberoptic intubating airway. (Courtesy of A. Ovassapian, MD.)

channels and a central groove on the lingual surface to allow passage of a fiberscope. A slit in the distal end allows the fiberscope to be manipulated in the anteroposterior direction but limits lateral movement.

Williams airway intubator (71, 72). The Williams airway intubator was designed for blind orotra-

cheal intubations (73). It can also be used in fiberoptic intubations or as an oral airway.

The airway, shown in Figure 14.13, is plastic and available in two sizes, #9 and #10, which will admit up to an 8.0 or 8.5 mm tracheal tube, respectively. The tracheal tube connector should be removed during intubation, because it will not pass through the airway.

The proximal half is cylindrical, while the distal half is open on its lingual surface. It does not allow the tip of the fiberscope to be maneuvered anteroposteriorly or laterally.

Ovassapian fiberoptic intubating airway (74). The Ovassapian intubating airway (Fig. 14.14) was designed for use during fiberoptic intubation. It has a flat lingual surface which gradually widens

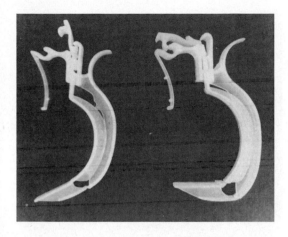

FIGURE 14.15. Tongue-retracting airways. The airway on the right is in the retracted position.

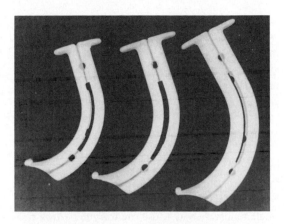

FIGURE 14.16. Berman intubation pharyngeal airways.

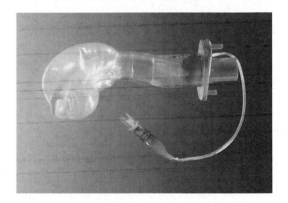

FIGURE 14.17. Cuffed oropharyngeal airway (COPA). (Courtesy of Mallinckrodt Medical, Inc.)

at the distal end. At the buccal end are two vertical side walls. Between the side walls are a pair of guide walls that curve toward each other. The guide walls are flexible and permit removal of the airway from around the tracheal tube. The proximal half is tubular so it can function as a bite block. The distal half is open posteriorly to provide an open space in which the fiberscope can be maneuvered. It will accommodate a tracheal tube up to 9.0 mm internal diameter.

Tongue retracting airway. The tongue retracting airway is shown in Figure 14.15. It has a latching mechanism that allow the pharyngeal tip to be manipulated so that it moves the tongue anteriorly.

Berman intubating/pharyngeal airway. The Berman intubating/pharyngeal airway (Berman II) (Fig. 14.16) is tubular along its entire length. It is open on one side so that it can be split and removed from around a tracheal tube. It can be used the same way as an oral airway or as an aid to fiberoptic or blind orotracheal intubation (75).

Cuffed oropharyngeal airway (COPA). The COPA (Fig. 14.17) is a Guedel airway with an inflatable cuff designed to seal the oropharynx. It has an integral bite block and a 15-mm connector for attachment to the breathing circuit. It is intended for maintaining the airway during short procedures in patients at low risk for aspiration. When the cuff is inflated, it displaces the base of the tongue, forming a low pressure seal with the

pharynx and elevates the epiglottis from the posterior pharyngeal wall to provide an open airway. It is available in several sizes.

It is inserted in a similar manner to an oropharyngeal airway. The cuff is inflated with 25 to 40 cc of air. Some patients may required additional support (head lift, chin lift, jaw thrust, CPAP) to maintain an open airway (76). The airway should not be removed until swallowing and cough reflexes are restored. The cuff should not be deflated prematurely since secretions above the cuff could cause airway obstruction.

Contraindications to use include the need for inspiratory pressures higher than 20 cm H_2O, high risk of aspiration, when it is anticipated that the patient will undergo extreme flexion of the head or position changes (e.g, to a lateral or prone position) during use, and procedures that will involve the use of a laser or electrosurgical device in the immediate area of the device. It should not be used in patients with grossly abnormal airways. It does not protect the airway from aspiration.

Insertion

Pharyngeal and laryngeal reflexes should be depressed before placement of an oral airway to avoid coughing or laryngospasm.

Selection of the correct size is important. Too small an airway may cause the tongue to kink and force part of it against the roof of the mouth, causing obstruction. Too large an airway may cause obstruction by displacing the epiglottis posteriorly and may traumatize the larynx. The correct size can be estimated by holding the airway next to the patient's mouth. The tip should rest cephalad to the angle of the mandible. The best criterion for proper size and position of the airway is unobstructed gas exchange. If the airway repeatedly comes out of the mouth, it should be removed and reinserted or a different size tried.

Wetting or lubricating the airway may facilitate insertion. The jaw is opened with the left hand. The teeth or gums are separated by pressing the thumb against the lower teeth or gum and the index or third finger against the upper teeth or gum.

One method of insertion is shown in Figure 14.18. The airway is inserted with its concave side facing the upper lip. When the junction of the bite portion and the curved section is near the incisors, the airway is rotated 180° and slipped behind the tongue into the final position.

An alternate method of insertion is shown in Figure 14.19. A tongue blade may be used to push forward and depress the tongue. The airway is inserted with the concave side toward the tongue. As it is advanced, it is rotated to slide around behind the tongue.

Use with Fiberoptic Endoscopes

An adhesive transparent dressing can be used over an airway designed to aid in fiberoptic intubation to provide a tight seal and allow for positive pressure ventilation (77).

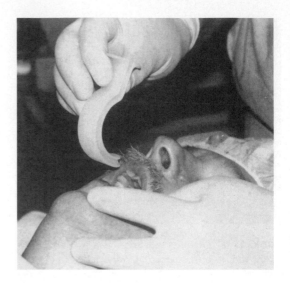

FIGURE 14.18. Insertion of oral airway. The airway is inserted 180° from the final resting position.

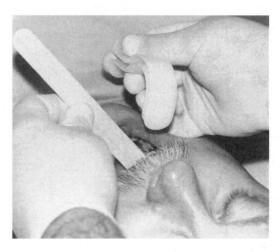

FIGURE 14.19. Alternative method of inserting an oral airway. A tongue blade is used to displace the tongue forward.

Bite Block

A bite block (gag, mouth prop) is placed between the teeth or gums to prevent them from occluding a tracheal tube or damaging a fiberscope and to keep the mouth open for suctioning. It also is used during electroconvulsive therapy and in unconscious individuals to protect the

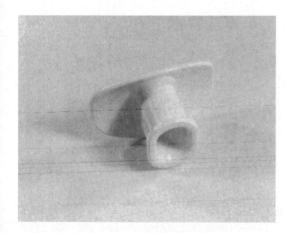

FIGURE 14.20. Bite block. This is placed between the teeth or gums (preferably in the molar area) to prevent occlusion of a tracheal tube or damage to a fiberoptic endoscope or to keep the mouth open for suctioning.

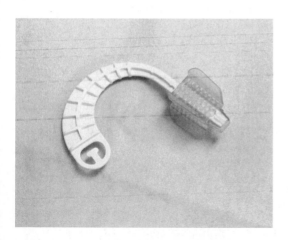

FIGURE 14.21. This bite block is designed to be placed between the molar teeth with the flat portion extending toward the side of the face. The flat portion is used to grip for insertion and removal.

tongue and lips. Because a bite block does not extend into the pharynx, it is usually less irritating than an oral airway. A bite block may be placed between the molar teeth.

A variety of bite blocks has been developed (Figs. 14.20–14.22). Some have a channel for gas passage. Many have an attached string that can be pinned to the patient's gown or taped to the skin

so that it can be easily retrieved. The curved portion of an oral airway can be removed or shortened, leaving the remaining portion as a bite block. (78, 79). A barrel of a plastic syringe fitted around the tracheal tube may be used (80). A gauze sponge roll may serve as a bite block. A bite block may be part of a device used to secure a tracheal tube.

Nasopharyngeal Airways

A nasopharyngeal airway (nasal airway, nasal trumpet) is shown in position in Figure 14.23.

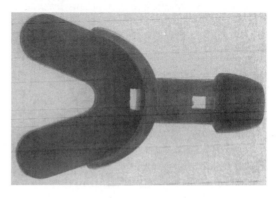

FIGURE 14.22. Oberto mouth prop, which is used for protecting the teeth during electroconvulsive therapy. (Courtesy of Rusch Inc.)

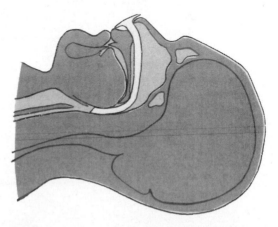

FIGURE 14.23. The nasopharyngeal airway in place. The airway passes through the nose and extends to just above the epiglottis. (Courtesy of V. Robideaux, MD.)

The pharyngeal end should be below the base of the tongue but above the epiglottis (81).

A nasal airway is better tolerated in the patient with intact airway reflexes than an oral airway. It is preferable if the patient's teeth are loose or in poor condition, or there is trauma or pathology of the oral cavity and can be used when the mouth cannot be opened.

Contraindications to the use of a nasopharyngeal airway include hemorrhagic disorders; anticoagulants or a coagulopathy; a basilar skull fracture; pathology, sepsis, or deformity of the nose or nasopharynx; or a history of nosebleeds requiring medical treatment.

There is no evidence that nasal airways cause significant bacteremia. (67, 82).

Nasopharyngeal airways have been used during and after pharyngeal surgery (83, 84), in infants with Pierre Robin syndrome (85), to apply continuous positive airway pressure (86), to facilitate suctioning (87), as a guide for a fiberscope (87), to treat singultus (hiccups), as a guide for a nasogastric tube (88, 89), to dilate the nasal passages in preparation for nasotracheal intubation (88) and as a means to maintain the airway and administer anesthesia during dental surgery (90).

General Description

A nasopharyngeal airway resembles a shortened tracheal tube with a flange or movable disk at the outside end to prevent it from passing into the naris. Some come with a safety pin to be inserted into the flange (91). On some models the flange is movable. The American standard (68) requires that the size of a nasopharyngeal airway be designated by a number expressing the inside diameter in millimeters.

Specific Airways

A variety of nasopharyngeal airways is available. Some are shown in Figure 14.24.

Linder nasopharyngeal airway (92, 93). The Linder nasopharyngeal airway (Fig. 14.25) is plastic with a large flange. The distal end is even cut rather than beveled. The airway is supplied with an introducer, which has a balloon on its tip. The balloon can be inflated and deflated by attaching a syringe to the one-way valve at the other end of the introducer.

Before insertion, the introducer is inserted into the airway until the tip of the balloon is just past the end. Air is injected through the one-way valve until the tip of the balloon is inflated to approximately the outside diameter of the tube. The com-

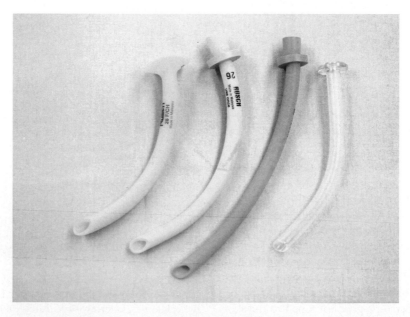

FIGURE 14.24. Nasopharyngeal airways. The one on the right does not contain latex.

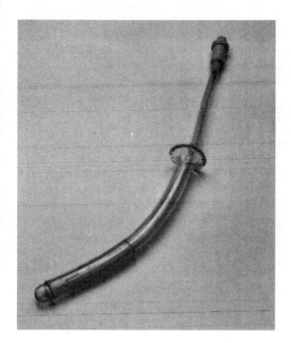

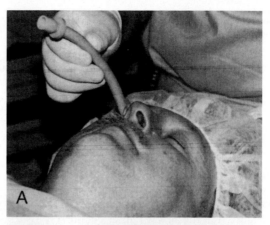

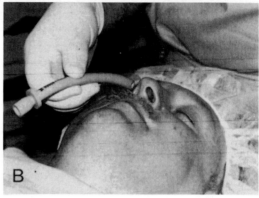

FIGURE 14.25. Linder nasopharyngeal airway. (Courtesy of Polamedco, Inc.)

plete assembly is lubricated, then inserted through the nostril. After it is in place, the balloon is deflated and the introducer removed.

Cuffed nasopharyngeal airway (94–97). The cuffed nasopharyngeal (pharyngeal) airway is similar to a shortened cuffed tracheal tube. It is inserted through the nose into the pharynx, the cuff inflated, then pulled back until resistance is felt.

Insertion

Although the correct length of a nasal airway for a patient has been stated to correlate with simple external measurements of the face and neck, studies indicate a correlation only with the patient's height (81). For children, diameters are the same as for tracheal tubes. For adult males, the diameter should be 7.0–7.5 mm and for female 6.5–7 mm (98).

Before insertion, the nasal airway should be lubricated thoroughly along its entire length. Each side of the nose should be inspected for size, patency, and the presence of polyps. Vasoconstrictors may be applied before insertion to reduce trauma.

The nasopharyngeal airway should be inserted

FIGURE 14.26. Insertion of a nasal airway. **A,** Correct method: the airway is inserted perpendicularly, in line with the nasal passage. **B,** Incorrect method: the airway is being pushed away from the air passage and into the turbinates.

as shown in Figure 14.26A. The airway is held in the hand on the same side as it is to be inserted with the bevel against the septum and gently advanced posteriorly while rotating back and forth gently. If resistance is encountered during insertion, the other nostril or a smaller size should be used. Figure 14.26B shows an incorrect method for inserting the airway. The airway is being pushed toward the roof of the nose.

The airway may be adjusted to fit the pharynx by sliding it in or out. If the tube is inserted too deeply, laryngeal reflexes may be stimulated; if too short, airway obstruction will not be relieved.

Binasal Airway (99–103)

The binasal airway (Fig. 14.27) consists of two nasal airways joined together by a connection that

FIGURE 14.27. The binasal airway. (Courtesy of Rusch, Inc.)

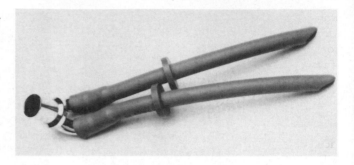

has an adaptor for attachment to the breathing system. After the airway is inserted, the soft tissues often seal the hypopharynx, permitting assisted or controlled respiration. Excess gas will overflow through the mouth. These devices have been used to maintain ventilation during oral fiberoptic endoscopy (7) and to administer continuous positive pressure (86).

Complications

Airway Obstruction (63)

Misplacement of nasopharyngeal and oropharyngeal airways is common (63, 81). The tip of an airway can press the epiglottis against the posterior pharyngeal wall and cover the laryngeal aperture (104). If an oropharyngeal airway is incorrectly inserted or is too small it may push the tongue into the posterior pharynx, obstructing the airway (63). With a nasopharyngeal airway, movement of the neck in rotation or anteroposteriorly may result in obstruction of the lumen (105). Use of a fenestrated airway may overcome this problem.

A foreign body can enter an airway and cause complete or partial obstruction (106, 107). The lumen of a nasopharyngeal airway may be compressed in the nose (81).

A nasopharyngeal airway can perforate the retropharyngeal space. The space can then expand and cause airway obstruction (108).

Damage to the Tongue

Massive tongue edema, either unilateral or bilateral, can occur following surgery, especially in the sitting position, and can result in airway obstruction (109, 110). Pressure from an oral airway may be a contributing factor. To prevent this complication, the oral airway should not be left in

place for an extended period or should be withdrawn until its tip functions as a bite block between the teeth. Excessive flexion of the head and neck should be avoided, and the head and neck checked frequently during long cases for edema or ecchymoses.

Care should be taken that the tongue is not caught between the teeth and the airway.

Trauma

Injuries to the nose and posterior pharynx are potential complications of nasal airways. Epistaxis is usually self-limiting but can present a serious problem in patients with bleeding disorders or who are receiving anticoagulants. Pharyngeal perforation and retropharyngeal abscess formation can occur (108). The lip or tongue may be caught between the teeth and an oral airway and traumatized by biting. This may go unrecognized if a mask is in place.

Central Nervous System Trauma

Use of a nasal airway in a patient with a basilar skull fracture can result in its entering the anterior cranial fossa (111).

Uvular Edema

Uvular edema apparently caused by entrapment of the uvula between the hard palate and an oropharyngeal airway has been reported (112).

Dental Damage (113, 114)

Teeth can be damaged or avulsed if the patient bites down hard on an oral airway (115, 116). Oral airways should be avoided if there is evidence of periodontal disease, teeth weakened by caries or restorations, crowns, fixed partial dentures, pronounced proclination (the front teeth having a forward inclination and overlapping the lower front teeth) or isolated teeth. In these cases, use of a nasopharyngeal airway and/or a bite block between the back teeth may be preferable.

Laryngospasm and Coughing

Insertion of an airway before establishment of adequate depth of anesthesia may cause coughing or laryngospasm, especially if it contacts the epiglottis or vocal cords.

Ulceration and Necrosis

Ulceration of the nose or tongue can occur if an airway remains in place for a long period of time (117).

Retention, Aspiration or Swallowing of the Airway

Part or all of an airway may become displaced into the pharynx, tracheobronchial tree, or esophagus (118–125). This may be difficult to detect. It is important to inspect all items of equipment after they have been used in the upper airway to ensure that no part is missing.

Devices Caught in Airway

When an esophageal stethoscope was removed from a patient with an oral airway in place, the cuff became detached (126). It was postulated that it got caught in the side grooves of the airway.

A case has been reported in which a fiberscope inadvertently traversed a fenestrated oral airway, making passage of a tracheal tube impossible (127).

Equipment Failure

An oral airway may fracture at the connection between the bite portion and the curved section (128).

Cardiovascular Response

Studies have shown a significant increase in heart rate and blood pressure following insertion of an oral airway (129).

Latex Allergy

If an airway has rubber in it, a severe reaction may occur if the patient has an allergy to latex (54). See Chapter 13, "Hazards of Anesthesia Machines and Breathing Systems" for more details on this problem.

Gastric Distention

A nasopharyngeal airway that is too long may enter the esophagus with the associated problem of gastric distention (81).

REFERENCES

1. Carson KD, Moriarty DC. Teaching airway management skills—use of a clear PVC face mask. Anaesthesia 1995;50:571.
2. Rendell–Baker L, Soucek DH. New paediatric face masks and anaesthetic equipment. Br Med J 1962;1:1690.
3. Palme C, Nystrom B, Tunell R. An evaluation of the efficiency of face masks in the resuscitation of newborn infants. Lancet 1985;1:207–210.
4. Aghdami A, Ellis R, Rah KH. A pediatric face mask can be a useful aid in lung ventilation on postlaryngectomy patients. Anesthesiology 1985;63:335.
5. Northwood D, Wade MJ. Novel use of the Rendell–Baker Soucek mask. Anaesthesia 1991;46:319.
6. Mallios C. A modification of the Laerdal anesthesia mask for nasotracheal intubation with the fiberoptic laryngoscope. Anaesthesia 1980;35:599–600.
7. Patil V, Stehling LC. Zauder HL, et al. Mechanical aids for fiberoptic endoscopy. Anesthesiology 1982;57:69–70.
8. Rogers SN, Benumof JL. New and easy techniques for fiberoptic endoscopy-aided tracheal intubation. Anesthesiology 1983;59:569–572.
9. Hinkle AJ. Scented masks in pediatric anesthesia. Anesthesiology 66:104–5, 1987.
10. Mather C. "Smelly agents." Anaesthesia 1993;48:540.
11. Mayhew JF. "Smelly agents." Anaesthesia 1993;49:1021.
12. Yamashita M, Motokawa K. "Fruit-flavored" mask induction for children. Anesthesiology 1986;64:837.
13. Carson K. Patients prefer scented face masks. Can J Anaesth 1995;42:482–483.
14. Yashita M, Tsuneto S. "Normac" falsely recognizes "fruit extract" as an anesthetic agent. Anesthesiology 1987;66:97.
15. McGowan P, Skinner A. Preoxygenation—the importance of a good face mask seal. Br J Anaesth 1995;75:777–778.
16. McGee JP, Vender JS. Nonintubation management of the airway. In Clinical procedures in anesthesia and intensive care. JL Benumof ed., Philadelphia, PA: JB Lippincott Co, 1992:89–114.

17. Benumof JL. Definition and incidence of the difficult airway. In Airway management. principles and practice, JL Benumof, ed. St. Louis, MO: Mosby, 1996: 121–125.

18. Lanier WL. Improving anesthesia mask fit in edentulous patients. Anesth Analg 1987;66:1053.

19. Diaz JH. A new transparent disposable plastic face mask for children and adults. Anesthesiology 1993; 78:1195–1196.

20. Edmondson WC, Rushton A. The upside down facemask again. Anaesthesia 1992;47:361.

21. Lawes EG, Murrell D. An airtight seal for the bearded face. Anaesthesia 1985;40:1142.

22. Mortimer AJ. An airtight seal between facemask and beard. Anaesthesia 1986;41:670–671.

23. Seavell CR, Priestley GS, Solving a hairy problem. Anaesthesia 1995;50:271.

24. Clarke AD. Potential deadspace in an anaesthetic mask and connectors. Br J Anaesth 1958;30: 176–181.

25. Chander S. A new head strap. Anesth Analg 1980; 59:457–458.

26. Jeal DE. Head strap modification. Anesth Analg 1980;59:809–8010.

27. Macario A, Chang PC, Stempel DB, et al. A cost analysis of the laryngeal mask airway for elective surgery in adult outpatients. Anesthesiology 1995;83: 250–257.

28. Johnston DF, Wrigley SR, Robb PJ, et al. The laryngeal mask airway in paediatric anaesthesia. Anaesthesia 1990;45:924–927.

29. Smith I, White PF. Use of the laryngeal mask airway as an alternative to a face mask during outpatient arthroscopy. Anesthesiology 1992;77:850–855.

30. Begenau VG. Allergic dermatitis due to rubber: report of case. Anesthesiology 1951;12:771–772.

31. Anonymous. Physician and the law. Anesth Analg 1970;49:889.

32. Potgieter SV, Mostert JW. A hazard associated with the use of a face mask: case report. S A Med J 1959; 33:989–990.

33. Smurthwaite GJ, Ford P. Skin necrosis following continuous positive pressure with a face mask. Anaesthesia 1993;48:147–148.

34. Azar I, Lear E. Lower lip numbness following anesthesia. Anesthesiology 1986;65:450–451.

35. Ananthanarayan C, Rolbin SH, Hew E. Facial nerve paralysis following mask anaesthesia. Can J Anaesth 1988;35:102–103.

36. Glauber DT. Facial paralysis after general anesthesia. Anesthesiology 1986;65:516–517.

37. Barron DW. Supra-orbital neurapraxia. Anaesthesia 1955;10:374.

38. Keats AS. Post-anaesthetic cephalagia. Anaesthesia 1956;11:341–343.

39. James FM. Hypesthesia of the tongue. Anesthesiology 1975;42:359–360.

40. Zornow MH, Mitchell MM. Foreign body aspiration during fiberoptic assisted intubation. Anesthesiology 1986;64:303.

41. Davis K. Alterations to the Patil–Syracuse mask for fiberoptic intubation. Anesth Analg 1992;74: 472–473.

42. Waring PH, Vinik HR. A potential complication of the Patil–Syracuse endoscopy mask. Anesth Analg 1991;73:668–669.

43. Williams L, Teague PD, Nagia AH. Foreign body from a Patil–Syracuse mask. Anesth Analg 1991;73: 359–360.

44. Thomas JC. An alternative diaphragm for Patil–Syracuse masks. Anesth Analg 1992;74:473.

45. Anonymous. Allegedly defective anesthetic mask blamed in eye injury suit. Biomedical Safety & Standards 1985;15:109.

46. Durkan W, Fleming N. Potential eye damage from reusable masks. Anesthesiology 1987;67:444.

47. Murray WJ. A case of eye injury from a reusable anesthetic mask. Anesthesiology 1988;68:302.

48. Murray WJ, Ruddy MP. Toxic eye injury during induction of anesthesia. South Med J 1985;78: 1012–1013.

49. Munn KA, Williams RT, Shafto CM. Transient unilateral blindness following general anaesthesia: Case report. Can J Anaesth 1978;25:433–435.

50. Snow JC, Kripke BJ, Norton ML, et al. Corneal injuries during general anesthesia. Anesth Analg 1975; 54:465–467.

51. Cook WP, Gravenstein JS. Breathing circuit occlusion due to a defective paediatric face mask. Can J Anaesth 1988;35:205–206.

52. Gordon HL, Tweedie IE. Facemask hazard. Anaesthesia 1989;44:84.

53. Hauswald M, Sklar DR, Tandberg D, et al. Cervical spine movement during airway management. Cinefluoroscopic appraisal in human cadavers. Am J Emerg Med 1991;9:535–538.

54. Parisian S. Latex allergies causing more anesthesia problems. Anesthesia Patient Safety Foundation Newsletter 1992;7:1.

55. McKinstry LJ, Fenton WJ, Barrett P. Anaesthesia and the patient with latex allergy. Can J Anaesth 1992; 39:587–589.

56. Ivens D, Berborgh C, Phan Thi H, et al. The quality of breathing and capnography during laryngeal mask and facemask ventilation. Anaesthesia 1995;50: 858–862.

57. Ivens D, Verborgh C, Phan Thi H, et al. The quality of breathing and capnography during laryngeal mask and facemask ventilation. Anaesthesia 1995;50: 858–862.

58. Barnett R, Gallant B, Fossey S, et al. Nitrous oxide environmental pollution. A comparison between face mask, laryngeal mask and endotracheal intubation. Can J Anaesth 1992;39:A151.

59. Sarma VJ, Leman J. Laryngeal mask and anaesthetic waste gas concentrations. Anaesthesia 1990;45: 791–792.

60. Carlsson P, Ljungqvist B, Hallen B. The effect of local scavenging on occupational exposure to nitrous oxide. Acta Anaesth Scand 1983;27:470–475.

61. Sik MJ, Lewis RB, Eveleigh DJ. Assessment of a scavenging device for use in paediatric anaesthesia. Br J Anaesth 1990;64:117–123.

62. Boidin MP. Airway patency in the unconscious patient. Br J Anaesth 1985;57:306–310.

63. Marsh AM, Nunn JF, Taylor SJ, et al. Airway obstruction associated with the use of the Guedel airway. Br J Anaesth 1991;67:517–523.

64. Aprahamian C, Thompson B, Finger WA, et al. Experimental cervical spine injury model. Evaluation of airway management and splinting techniques. Ann Emerg Med 1984;13:584–587.

65. Browne B, Adams CN. Postoperative sore throat related to the use of a Guedel airway. Anaesthesia 1988; 43:590–591.

66. Monroe MC, Gravenstein N, Saga–Rumley S. Postoperative sore throat. Effect of oropharyngeal airway in orotracheally intubated patients. Anesth Analg 1990;70:512–516.

67. Ali MT, Tremewen DR, Hay AJ, et al. The occurrence of bacteremia associated with the use of oral and nasopharyngeal airways. Anaesthesia 1992;47: 153–155.

68. American Society for Testing and Materials. Standard specification for anesthetic equipment—oropharyngeal and nasopharyngeal airways (F 1573–95). West Conshohocken PA: ASTM, 1995.

69. Wilton NCT. Aids for fiberoptically guided intubation in children. Anesthesiology 1991;75:549–550.

70. Berman RA, Lilienfeld SM. To the editor. Anesthesiology 1950;11:136–137.

71. Palazzo MGA, Soltice NJ. A new aid to fiberoptic bronchoscopy. Anaesthesia and Intensive Care 1983; 11:388–389.

72. Williams RT. Comments from an experienced user of the airway intubator. Anesthesiology 1984;61: 108–109.

73. Williams RT, Harrison RE. Prone tracheal intubation simplified using an airway intubator. Can Anaesth Soc J 1981;28:288–289.

74. Ovassapian A, Dykes HM. The role of fiber-optic endoscopy in airway management. Semin Anesth 1987; 6:93–104.

75. Berman RA. A method for blind oral intubation of the trachea or esophagus. Anesth Analg 1977;56: 866–867.

76. Berry A, Brimacombe J. An evaluation of the cuffed oropharyngeal airway (COPA). Anaesthesia and Intensive Care 1997;25:173.

77. McAlpine G, Williams RT. Fiberoptic assisted tracheal intubation under general anesthesia with IPPV. Anesthesiology 1987;66:853.

78. Chaffe A, Street MN. A modified airway. Anaesthesia 1988;43:611.

79. Schwartz AJ, Dougal RM, Lee KW. Modification of oral airway as a bite block. Anesth Analg 1980;59: 225.

80. Samra SK. Endotracheal tube in place passing through bite block. Anesth Analg 1981;60:66.

81. Stoneham MD. The nasopharyngeal airway. Assessment of position by fiberoptic laryngoscopy. Anaesthesia 1993;48:575–580.

82. Rooney R, Crummy EJ, McShane AJ. Bacteraemia following nasopharyngeal airway insertion. Anaesthesia 1992;47:1099.

83. Stallings JO, Lines J. Use of nasopharyngeal tubes as aids to lateral port construction and maintenance of the airway in pharyngeal flap surgery. Plast Reconstr Surg 1976;58:379–380.

84. Donnelly J, Thirlwell J. Nasopharyngeal airway in infants after palatal surgery. Br J Anaesth 1992;67:227.

85. Heaf DP, Helms PJ, Dinwiddie R, et al. Nasopharyngeal airways in Pierre Robin syndrome. J Pediatr 1982;100:698–703.

86. Young ML, Hanson C. An alternative to tracheostomy following transsphenoidal hypophysectomy in a patient with acromegaly and sleep apnea. Anesth Analg 1993;76: 446–449.

87. Wanner A, Zighelboim A, Sackner MA. Nasopharyngeal airway: a facilitated access to the trachea. For nasotracheal suction, bedside bronchofiberscopy, and selective bronchography. Ann Intern Med 1971;75: 593–595.

88. Lewis JD. Facilitation of nasogastric and nasotracheal intubation with a nasopharyngeal airway. Am J Emerg Med 1986;4:426.

89. Shetty S, Henthorn RW, Ganta R. A method to reduce nasopharyngeal trauma from nasogastric tube placement. Anesth Analg 1994;78:410–411.

90. Bagshaw ONT, Southee R, Ruiz K. A comparison of the nasal mask and the nasopharyngeal airway in paediatric chair dental anaesthesia. Anaesthesia 1997; 52:786–796.

91. Mobbs AP. Retained nasopharyngeal airway. A reply. Anaesthesia 1989;44:447.

92. Gallagher WJ, Pearce AC, Power SJ. Assessment of a new nasopharyngeal airway. Br J Anaesth 1988;60: 112–115.

93. Long TMW. Atraumatic nasopharyngeal intubation for upper airway obstruction. Anaesthesia 1988;43: 510–511.

94. Boheimer NO, Feldman SA, Soni N. A self-retaining nasopharyngeal airway. Anaesthesia 1990;45:72–73.

95. Feldman SA, Fauvel NJ, OOI R. The cuffed pharyngeal airway. European J Anaesth 1991;8:291–295.

96. Ralston S, Wright E, Charters P. Cuffed nasopharyngeal tube and upper airway obstruction. Br J Anaesth 1993;71:759P.

97. Ralston SJ, Charters P. Cuffed nasopharyngeal tube as "dedicated airway" in difficult intubation. Anaesthesia 1994;49:133–136.

98. Patrick MR. Airway manipulations. In Hazards and complications of anaesthesia. Taylor TH, Major E, eds., Edinburgh: Churchill Livingstone, 469–502.

99. Elam JO, Titel JH, Feingold A, et al. Simplified airway management during anesthesia or resuscitation: a binasal pharyngeal system. Anesth Analg 1969;48: 307–316.

100. Feingold A, Runyan NJ. Experience with the latex binasal pharyngeal airway. Anesth Analg 1973;52: 263–266.

101. Komesaroff D. An unusual indication for the double nasopharyngeal airway: a case report. Anesth Analg 1971;50:240–243.

102. Weisman H, Weis TW, Elam JO, et al. Use of double nasopharyngeal airways in anesthesia. Anesth Analg 1969;48:356–361.

103. Weisman H, Bauer RO, Huddy RA, et al. An improvised binasopharyngeal airway system for anesthesia. Anesth Analg 1972;51:11–13.

104. Brown TCK. The airway in mucopolysaccharidoses. Anaesthesia and Intensive Care 1984;12:178.

105. Inkster S. The fenestrated nasopharyngeal airway. Anaesthesia 1995;50:567.

106. McNicol LR. Unusual cause of obstructed airway in a child. Anaesthesia 1986;41:668–669.

107. Walker MB. An unusual destination for oral premedication. Anaesthesia 1994;49:839.

108. Baumann RC, MacGregor DA. Dissection of the posterior pharynx resulting in acute airway obstruction. Anesthesiology 1995;82:1516–1518.

109. Drummond JC. Anesthesia for posterior fossa procedures. ASA Annual Refresher Courses, 1994.

110. Haynes GR, Gramling–Babb P, Baker JD III. Fatal outcome of postoperative macroglossia as a complication of a craniotomy. Am J Anesth 1995;22:41–44.

111. Muzzi DA, Losasso TJ, Cucchiara RF. Complication from a nasopharyngeal airway in a patient with a basilar skull fracture. Anesthesiology 1991;74:366–368.

112. Shulman MS. Uvular edema without endotracheal intubation. Anesthesiology 1981;55:82–83.

113. Clokie C, Metcalf I, Holland A. Dental trauma in anaesthesia. Can J Anaesth 1989;36:675–680.

114. Burton JF, Baker AB. Dental damage during anaesthesia and surgery. Anaesthesia and Intensive Care 1987;15:262–268.

115. Pollard BJ, O'Leary J. Guedel airway and tooth damage. Anaesthesia and Intensive Care 1981;9:395.

116. Solazzi RW, Ward RJ. The spectrum of medical liability cases. Int Anesthesiol Clin 1984;22:43–59.

117. Moore MW, Rauscher LA. A complication of oropharyngeal airway placement. Anesthesiology 1977;47: 526.

118. Anonymous. Nasopharyngeal airway. Biomedical Safety & Standards 1984;14:111–112.

119. Daly SM, Weinberg B, Murphy RJC, et al. Unrecognized aspiration of an oropharyngeal airway. Pediatr Radiol 1983;13:227–228.

120. Howat DDC. Disposable nasopharyngeal airways—a potential hazard. Anaesthesia 1982;37:101.

121. Hayes JD, Lockrem JD. Aspiration of a nasal airway: a case report and principles of management. Anesthesiology 1985;62:534–535.

122. Ho G, Weinger MB. Unusual complication of nasotracheal suctioning. Anesthesiology 1993;79:630.

123. Milam MG, Miller KS. Aspiration of an artificial nasopharyngeal airway. Chest 1988;93:223–224.

124. Zaltzman J, Ferman A. An acute life-threatening complication caused by a Guedel airway. Crit Care Med 1987;15:1074.

125. Smith BL. Retained nasopharyngeal airway. Anaesthesia 1989;44:447.

126. Gandhi S, Dhamee MS. Detachment of an esophageal stethoscope cuff-possible role of an oral airway. Anesthesiology 1983;58:202.

127. Topf AI, Complication associated with the use of an oral airway. Anesthesiology 1996;84:485.

128. Lloyd–Williams R. Fractured airways. Anaesthesia and Intensive Care 1985;13:335–336.

129. Hickey S, Cameron AE, Asbury AJ. Cardiovascular response to insertion of Brain's laryngeal mask. Anaesthesia 1990;45:629–633.

QUESTIONS

Each question below contains four suggested answers of which one or more is correct. Choose the answer:

A. if 1, 2, and 3 are correct
B. if 1 and 3 are correct
C. if 2 and 4 are correct
D. if 4 is correct
E. if 1, 2, 3 and 4 are correct

1. Complications associated with use of a face mask include:
   1. Movement of the cervical spine
   2. Facial nerve injury
   3. Chemical irritation of the eyes
   4. Sinusitis

2. Which maneuvers can be used to secure a patent airway?
   1. Jaw thrust
   2. Posterior protrusion of the mandible
   3. Chin lift
   4. Posterior flexion of the atlanto-occipital joint

3. Airways developed to aid in fiberoptic intubation include
   1. Patil–Saracuse
   2. Williams
   3. Ovassapian
   4. Tongue retracting airway

4. Contraindications to the use of nasal airways include
   1. Hemorrhagic disorders
   2. Sepsis
   3. Basilar skull fracture
   4. Seizure disorders

5. Which external measurements correlate with the proper length of a nasal airway?
   1. Tip of nose to 2 cm above the thyroid cartilage
   2. The distance from the tip of the thumb to the tip of the index finger measured to the hand and back
   3. Tip of the earlobe to cricoid cartilage
   4. The patient's height

6. Complications associated with the use of oral airways include
   1. Swelling of the tongue
   2. Edema of the uvula
   3. Ulceration of the tongue
   4. Swallowing of the airway

ANSWERS

1. A	**4.** A
2. B	**5.** D
3. A	**6.** E

Laryngeal Mask Airways

C. Leakage
D. Learning Curve
E. Need to Educate Postanesthesia Care Unit Nurses
F. Loss of Airway Management Skills
G. Loss of Tactile Monitoring
H. Less Reliable Airway

The laryngeal mask airway (LMA, laryngeal mask, LM, Brain Mask Airway, BMA, Brain laryngeal mask, BLM, BLA) is designed to secure the airway by establishing an end-to-end circumferential seal around the laryngeal inlet with an inflatable cuff (Fig. 15.1) (1). It is a useful advance in airway management, filling a niche between the face mask and tracheal tube in terms of both anatomical position and degree of invasiveness.

DESCRIPTION
Standard Laryngeal Mask Airway

The LMA consists of a curved tube (shaft) connected to an elliptical spoon-shaped mask (cup) at a 30° angle (Fig. 15.2). There are two flexible vertical bars at the entry of the tube into the mask to prevent obstruction of the tube by the epiglottis. The mask is surrounded by an inflatable cuff. An inflation tube and self-sealing pilot balloon are attached to the proximal wider end of the mask. A black line running longitudinally along the pos-

terior aspect of the tube helps to orient it after placement. At the machine end of the tube is a standard 15-mm connector. The LMA is made from medical-grade silicone to withstand repeated steam autoclaving and contains no latex.

The laryngeal mask is available in seven sizes, as shown in Table 15.1. Disposable LMAs are available for sizes 3–5. More than one size should always be available because the correct size cannot always be predicted correctly. When there is doubt, a larger rather than a smaller size should be chosen for the first attempt (2, 3).

TABLE 15.1. **Available Laryngeal Mask Airways**

Size	mm	cm	Patient Size
1	5.25/8.2	8	Neonates/Infants up to 5 kg
1.5	6.1/9.6	10	Infants between 5–10 kg
2	7.0/11.0	11.0	Infants/children between 10–20 kg
2.5	8.4/13.0	12.5	Children between 20–30 kg
3	10/15	16	Children and small adults over 30 kg
4	10/15	16	Normal adults*
5	11.5/16.5	18	Large adults*

* A very approximate guide is to use a size 4 for patients weighing 50–79 kg and a size 5 for individuals over 70 kg.

FIGURE **15.1.** The laryngeal mask in place. The tip of the mask rests against the upper esophageal sphincter while the sides face the pyriform fossae.

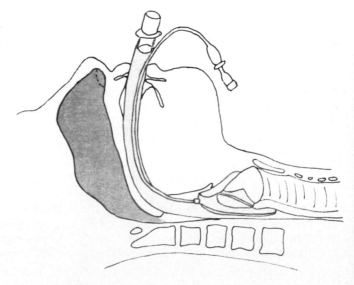

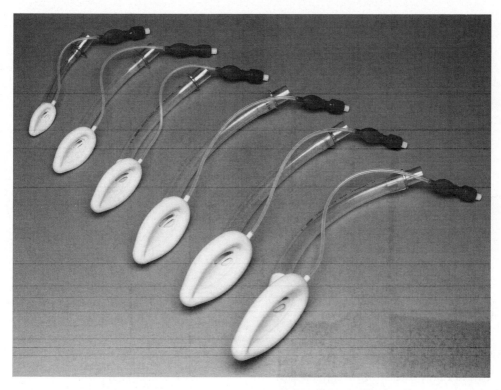

FIGURE 15.2. Laryngeal mask airways. Note the bars at the junction of the tube and the mask. (Courtesy of Gensia Pharmaceuticals Inc.)

Flexible Laryngeal Mask Airway

The flexible (wire-reinforced, reinforced) laryngeal mask (FLMA) (Fig. 15.3) differs from the standard version in that it has a flexible, wire-reinforced tube. It is available in sizes 2, 2½, 3, 4, and 5. The size of the cuff is the same as with standard LMAs. In each size the tube is longer and has a smaller diameter than the standard LMA.

The flexible tube can be bent to any angle. This allows it to be positioned away from the surgical field without occluding the lumen or losing the seal against the larynx. (4, 5) It is less likely to be displaced during rotation of the head or repositioning of the tube than the standard LMA.

The wire reinforcement makes the tube more resistant to kinking and compression than the standard LMA but does not prevent obstruction from biting. While it is more resistant to obstruction during oropharyngeal instrumentation, compression of the tube between the lower teeth

and the blade of a Boyle Davis gag has been reported (6–9).

The small diameter of the tube limits the size of bronchoscope or tracheal tube that can be passed through it and causes increased resistance to flow, making it unsuitable for prolonged spontaneous ventilation. It is also unsuitable for magnetic resonance imaging (MRI) scanning (10).

Short Tube Laryngeal Mask

The short tube (ST) laryngeal mask has a tube that is 2 cm shorter than a standard LMA (4). Only size #3 is available.

Other

A single-use (disposable) standard LMA is available in sizes 3, 4, and 5.

An intubating LMA with a shorter, wider bore tube and a metal handle (Fig. 15.4) is available in sizes 3, 4, and 5. It will permit intubation with a tracheal tube up to 8.0 mm.

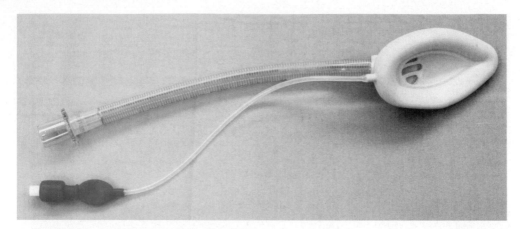

FIGURE **15.3.** Flexible laryngeal mask airway. The wire-reinforced tube is longer and has a smaller diameter than the standard laryngeal mask airway (LMA).

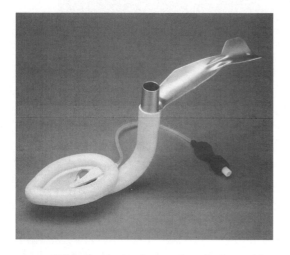

FIGURE **15.4.** Intubating laryngeal mask airway. Note that the tube is shorter and wider and has a metal handle. (Courtesy of LMA North America.)

USE

An LMA of the chosen size plus one size smaller and larger should always be immediately available. The syringe used to inflate the LMA should contain only air. Use of a syringe that contains organic substances such as propofol may result in damage to the LMA (11).

Inspection Before Use

Before it is used, the LMA should be inspected carefully. The first step is to examine the tube. It should be transparent so that particles or fluids within it can be seen. The interior should be free from obstruction or foreign particles. The exterior should be examined to ensure that it is free from cracks, abrasions, or foreign material. The tube should be flexed 180°. Kinking should not occur. The tube should not be bent beyond 180° since this could cause permanent damage. The flexible mask should be examined to make sure that the reinforcing wire is wholly contained within the wall of the tube.

The next test is to examine the mask aperture. The bars should be probed gently to make certain they are not damaged and the space between is free from particulate matter.

The next step is to check the function of the valve. Air is withdrawn from the cuff so that the walls are flattened against each other. Excessive force should be avoided. The syringe is removed from the inflation valve and the cuff observed to ensure that it remains deflated. If it reinflates, there is a faulty valve or leaking cuff and the LMA should not be used. Replacement valves are available from the manufacturer.

The next step is to inflate the cuff with the maximum amount of air the cuff should contain. These volumes are given in Table 15.2.

After the cuff is filled, it should hold pressure for at least 2 minutes. If not, the LMA should not be used.

The integrity of the cuff should be verified by

inflating it temporarily with a volume of air 50% greater than the recommended maximum volume. These volumes are given in Table 15.3. Any herniation, thinning of the wall, or asymmetry is an indication to discard the LMA. There are also maximum diameter values for the cuff. These are listed in Table 15.3. The LMA should not be used if any of the measurements exceeds its maximum permitted value.

The next step is to check the pilot balloon diameter. With the cuff 50% overinflated, the balloon should be elliptical, not spherical. The transverse diameter should not exceed 14.5 mm at its widest point. Excessive width of the pilot balloon indicates weakness and imminent rupture.

The last step is to check the 15-mm connector. It should fit tightly and not pull out easily.

Preparation of Mask

The cuff should be fully deflated with a dry syringe to form a flat oval disc by pressing the

hollow side down firmly against a clean, hard, flat surface with a finger pressing the tip flat (Fig. 15.5) (12, 13). This is done so that during insertion the tip forms a smooth, thin, relatively stiff wedge capable of passing behind the epiglottis even when it is lying against the posterior pharyngeal wall. The deflated cuff should be wrinkle free to facilitate its passage and avoid bruising tissues. If the edges are irregular, there is more likelihood

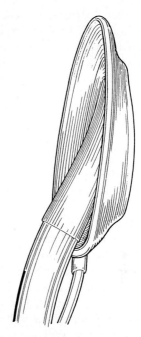

FIGURE 15.5. The laryngeal mask ready for insertion. The cuff should be deflated tightly with the rim facing away from the mask aperture. There should be no folds near the tip. (Courtesy of Gensia Pharmaceuticals Inc.)

TABLE 15.2. Recommended Cuff Inflation Volumes

Mask Size	Inflation Volume
1	Up to 4
1.5	Up to 7
2	Up to 10
2.5	Up to 14
3	Up to 20
4	Up to 30
5	Up to 40

* Recommended cuff inflation volumes. These are the maximum amounts that should be injected into the cuff. In practice it is rarely necessary to inflate with the full amount and a "just seal" volume should be sought.

TABLE 15.3. Maximum Cuff Dimensions

Mask Size	Air Volume (ml)	Maximum Bulge of Cuff Tip (mm)	Maximum Bulge of Wide End of Cuff (mm)	Maximum Transverse Diameter of Cuff (mm)
1	6	7.8	8.6	26.3
1.5	10	9.5	10.2	32.6
2	15	11.5	13.0	39.0
2.5	21	13.0	14.5	45.0
3	30	14.8	16.6	51.2
4	45	17.0	19.0	58.5
5	60	21.1	22.4	68.3

that the mask will curl and not seal properly. Special deflation tools are available from the manufacturer and this use may result in a better shape for insertion (14).

Lubrication should be applied to the posterior surface of the cuff just before insertion, taking care to avoid getting lubricant on the anterior surface. The manufacturer recommends water-soluble jelly and does not recommend analgesic-containing gels or sprays (15, 16). Studies show that lubrication with lidocaine gel or spray will result in a lower incidence of retching and coughing on emergence (17, 18). However, another study showed increased intra- and postoperative problems (19). Lubricants or sprays containing silicone may cause the mask to soften and swell (3, 15).

Insertion

Insertion of the LMA requires that airway reflexes be obtunded by general or topical anesthesia or muscle relaxants. Muscle relaxants are usually not necessary. Intact airway reflexes may cause gagging, laryngospasm, recurrent swallowing, or vomiting. If general anesthesia is used, insertion requires a depth similar to that necessary for insertion of an oropharyngeal airway but not as deep as is needed for tracheal intubation (20). Absence of a motor response to a jaw thrust is a reliable method for assessing the adequacy of anesthesia for LMA insertion (21). Application of topical spray to the posterior pharyngeal wall will result in fewer attempts for successful insertion and less coughing and gagging (22, 23).

Standard Technique (13)

The standard insertion technique involves using a midline or slightly diagonal approach with the cuff fully deflated. The head should be extended and the neck flexed (sniffing position) (12). This position is best maintained during insertion by having the non-intubating hand stabilize the occiput (Fig. 15.6). The LMA can be inserted without placing the head in this position (24). The neutral position may cause a small decrease in successful placement compared to the standard sniffing position (25, 26).

The mouth may be allowed to fall open or may be held open by an assistant during insertion of the mask into the mouth.

The tube portion is grasped as if it were a pen, with the index finger pressing on the point where the tube joins the mask (Fig. 15.6). With the aperture facing anteriorly (and the black line facing the patient's upper lip), the tip of the cuff is placed against the inner surface of the upper incisors or gums. At this point the tube should be parallel to the floor rather than vertical (12). The jaw should be released during further insertion.

The mask is pressed back against the hard palate to keep it flattened as it is advanced into the oral cavity, using the index finger to push upward against the palate. This means that the direction of applied pressure is different from the direction in which the mask moves (27). If resistance is felt, the tip may have folded over on itself or impacted on an irregularity or the posterior pharynx. In this case a diagonal shift in direction is often helpful, or a gloved finger may be inserted behind the mask to lift it over the obstruction (15). If at any time during insertion the mask fails to stay flattened out or it starts to fold back, it should be withdrawn and reinserted.

A change of direction can be sensed as the mask tip encounters the posterior pharyngeal wall and follows it downward. By withdrawing the other fingers as the index finger is advanced and slight pronation of the forearm it is often possible to insert the mask fully into position with a single movement (Fig. 15.7). If not, hand position is changed for the next movement. The tube is grasped with the other hand, straightened slightly, and then pressed down with a single, quick but gentle movement until a definite resistance is felt (Fig. 15.8). This may coincide with anterior displacement of the larynx (28).

Application of cricoid pressure, especially two handed, may reduce the rate of successful placement (25, 29–36). If the first attempt at insertion is unsuccessful, cricoid pressure should be transiently released as the mask is moving downward during a second attempt (37).

When initial insertion is unsuccessful a number of maneuvers may be helpful, including inserting the LMA from the side of the mouth; pulling the tongue forward; a jaw thrust; repositioning the head; insertion with the lumen facing backwards then rotating it 180° as it enters the pharynx (see below); applying continuous positive airway pres-

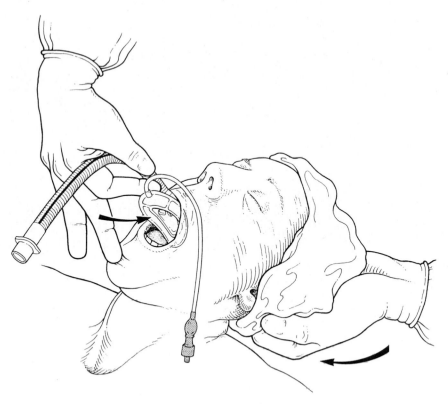

FIGURE **15.6.**   Initial insertion of the laryngeal mask. Under direct vision, the mask tip is pressed upward against the hard palate. The middle finger may be used to push the lower jaw downward. The mask is pressed upward as it is advanced into the pharynx to ensure that the tip remains flattened and avoids the tongue. The jaw should not be held open once the mask is inside the mouth. The non-intubating hand can be used to stabilized the occiput. (Courtesy of Gensia Pharmaceuticals Inc.)

sure; slight lateral rotation of the mask; partial inflation of the cuff; insertion of a finger behind the mask to act as a guide; use of a laryngoscope, oral airway, stylet or bougie; and pressing the tip anteriorly toward the bowl as the cuff is deflated (15, 38–56). In a patient with a restricted mouth opening, an alternative method is to pass the LMA behind the molar teeth and then maneuver the tubular part forward to lie centrally (57).

The mask is now in place, resting on the floor of the hypopharynx. The pliable cuff allows it to conform to the contours of this area. The sides face the pyriform fossae and the upper border of the cuff is behind the base of the tongue (Figs. 15.1 and 15.9). The tip of the epiglottis may rest either within the bowl of the mask or under the proximal cuff at an angle determined by the extent to which passage of the mask has deflected it

downwards (13, 32, 46, 52, 58–62). In some cases, the upper part of the esophagus lies within the rim of the mask. Studies have shown that satisfactory function may be achieved even when positioning is not ideal (46, 52, 62–67).

The longitudinal black line on the shaft should lie in the midline facing the upper lip. Any deviation may indicate misplacement of the cuff.

The cuff should then be inflated over 3 to 5 seconds without holding the tube unless the position is obviously unstable (e.g., in edentulous patients with slack tissues). The recommended maximum cuff inflation volumes are given in Table 15.2. If a smaller volume will provide a seal, the lesser amount should be used (68–70). Insertion of greater-than-recommended volumes into the cuff will not improve the seal against the larynx, because it reduces the cuff's ability to conform to

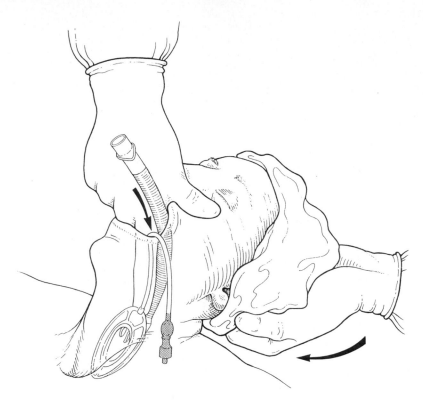

FIGURE 15.7. By withdrawing the other fingers and with a slight pronation of the forearm, it is usually possible to push the mask fully into position in one fluid movement. Note that the neck is kept flexed and the head extended. (Courtesy of Gensia Pharmaceuticals Inc.)

the shape of the laryngeal inlet. Inflation of the cuff usually causes slight upward movement of the entire LMA and a slight bulging at the front of the neck is commonly seen. If the laryngeal mask is too large or too much air is injected into the cuff, the mask may come out of the hypopharynx.

After the cuff is inflated, the tube should be connected to the breathing system and either spontaneous or gentle positive pressure ventilation initiated. Indications of correct positioning include normal breath sounds; normal chest movement; an expired CO_2 waveform; normal excursions of the reservoir bag; and absence of stridor, intercostal recession, use of accessory muscles of respiration, tracheal tug, or out-of-phase respiratory movements of the chest, abdomen, or reservoir bag. A fiberscope can be inserted through the tube to confirm the position and rule out airway obstruction. The position can also be confirmed by X-ray or MRI. An esophageal detector device can be used (71–73), although its utility has been questioned (74) and it may give inaccurate results in pediatric patients (75).

If the airway is obstructed, it may be the result of incorrect positioning of the mask, down folding of the epiglottis, or closure of the glottic sphincter. In most cases the obstruction can be eliminated by removing and reinserting the mask. Another method is to lift the anterior neck structures using a gloved hand inserted into the mouth, deflating the cuff and rotating the mask 360° around its tube axis (76). Another method is to digitally pull the epiglottis straight (77). Manipulation of the jaw or repositioning of the head usually does not help to relieve airway obstruction.

A leak can be detected by listening through a stethoscope over the trachea (78). The LMA may leak slightly for the first three or four breaths before settling into position (15, 79–81). It may be possible to improve the seal by adding more air

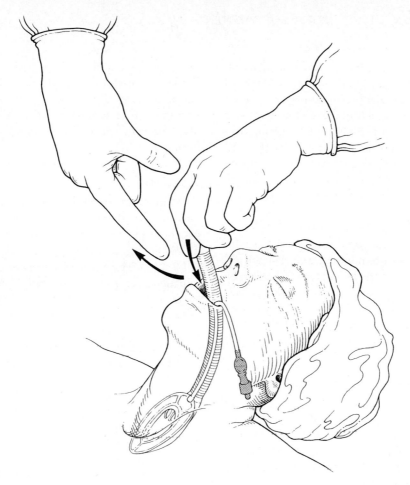

FIGURE 15.8. The laryngeal mask is grasped with the other hand and the index finger withdrawn. The hand holding the tube presses gently downward untilresistance is encountered. (Courtesy of Gensia Pharmaceuticals Inc.)

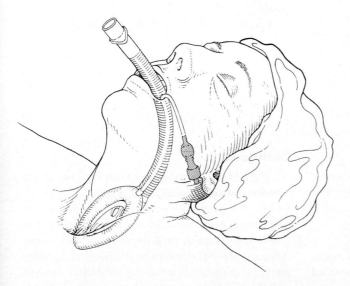

FIGURE 15.9. The laryngeal mask in place. (Courtesy of Gensia Pharmaceuticals Inc.)

to the cuff (if the maximum recommended volume has not been injected), or flexing the head 10 to 20° (82). Higher pressures may be achieved by pressing on either side of the midline just above the thyroid cartilage (83–86) or by applying continuous forward pressure on the LMA (87). If, despite these efforts, adequate ventilation without a leak cannot be achieved, the device should be withdrawn and reinserted or a larger LMA used.

180 Degree Technique (42, 50, 60, 88)

Another technique is to insert the LMA with the laryngeal aperture pointing cephalad and rotate it 180° as it enters the pharynx. Insertion by this method is nearly as satisfactory as the standard insertion and may be especially useful in pediatric patients but when in place, 23.3% of the LMAs placed using this technique had some residual rotation (63).

Partial Inflation

Another technique is to partially inflate the cuff before insertion. This has been found to increase the success rate in some studies (18, 51, 89–91) and may result in less sore throat (92). However, the incidence of down folding and trapping of the epiglottis is increased (63).

Technique with Wire-Reinforced LMA

The wire-reinforced LMA is more difficult to insert than the standard device. The manufacturer recommends that it be held between the thumb and index finger at the junction of the tube and cuff and positioned by inserting the index finger to its fullest extent into the oral cavity until resistance is encountered. It may be easier to insert using the thumb, index, and middle fingers at the junction of the tube and bowl, then using the index and middle finger to advance it into the hypopharynx (93). Use of a stylet or other device inserted into the tube to stiffen it has been recommended (12, 94–100). A modified Magill's forceps or other device may be helpful (101, 102).

Awake Placement

The laryngeal mask can be inserted in an awake patient following topical anesthesia of the upper airway (103–112). This may be useful when management of the airway is expected to be difficult or the patient is at increased risk for aspiration of gastric contents. It may be helpful to partially inflate the cuff to simulate a bolus of food (113). Mask insertion should be coordinated with swallowing.

Fixation

A bite block or roll of gauze should be inserted into the mouth beside the tube to prevent the patient from biting the tube and to improve stability (12). Various other devices have been used (114–117). The best device will vary from patient to patient, according to the state of dentition, the surgical procedure, and the fixation technique (13). An oropharyngeal airway is not satisfactory because both it and the LMA are designed to be placed in the midline and the tip might compromise the LMA cuff or cause compression of the tube.

The tube should be secured with tape, taking care that the tube does not become twisted. This can be accomplished by affixing the tape first to the maxilla, winding it over the cephalad side of the tube and down around the caudal side to fix the tube and bite block firmly to each other, and then affixing it to the opposite maxilla. Further security can be provided by separate taping from zygoma to zygoma under the mandible (118) or around the neck (119, 120). A tracheal tube holder may be used (121).

Bending of the tube against its natural curvature may cause dislodgment or kinking unless a wire-reinforced LMA is used. The LMA should be fixed to the breathing system below the chin. Traction from the breathing system should be avoided and several methods to achieve this have been suggested (119, 122).

Maintenance

The LMA can be used with standard breathing systems, including low flow or closed systems (123). During maintenance, patency of the airway and correct orientation of the mask should be verified at regular intervals. A depth of anesthesia adequate to prevent reaction to the surgical stimulus must be maintained until the surgery is finished (124). If laryngospasm, wheezing, swallowing, coughing, straining, or breath holding occurs, anesthesia should be deepened or muscle relaxants administered. An aerosol can be administered using an LMA (125).

Patients can be positioned prone or on the side with the LMA in place (84, 126), but this should be attempted only after considerable experience with the device because changing position can result in loss of seal. The LMA should not be rotated, but the tube can be slid from one side of the mouth to the other without disturbing the position of the cuff against the larynx (15).

The LMA can be used with controlled (including mechanical) or spontaneous ventilation. It has been used for pressure support ventilation (127).

If controlled ventilation is used, the peak inspiratory pressure should be monitored. It should below 25 cm H_2O. Higher pressures may result in leakage of gas around the mask, gastric distention, operating room pollution, and oxygen leakage during laser surgery (80, 128–133). Changes in the ventilatory pattern to increase frequency and reduce tidal volume and use of muscle relaxants may result in a lower peak pressure. A sudden increase in leakage often signals the need for more muscle relaxation, although other causes such as displacement of the LMA and airway obstruction also need to be considered.

The patient's upper abdomen should be periodically observed for signs of distention. If high pressures are required, consideration should be given to exchanging the LMA for a tracheal tube (134).

During maintenance, intracuff pressure will vary. Nitrous oxide and carbon dioxide can diffuse into the cuff so that intracuff pressure and volume increase (135–139). The increase is self limiting over a 1- to 2-hour period (129, 140), but may cause airway obstruction (139). Use of nitrous oxide for cuff inflation produces unpredictable results (141, 142).

Cuff pressure can be checked by feeling the tension in the pilot balloon or by monitoring with a pressure transducer (13). A spherical pilot balloon is an indication that there is too much gas in the cuff (15). The manufacturer and others recommend monitoring the intracuff pressure and reducing excessive pressure by deflating the cuff. However, this could lead to a flood of secretions

under the mask. There is no agreement on what pressure should be maintained. Suggestions include 60 cm H_2O (70), less than 30 torr (142a), less than 22 torr (143–145), and just seal (146). A pressure of less than 10 cm H_2O may not prevent contamination of the larynx with oropharyngeal secretions (147).

Emergence

It is important that the bite block or roll of gauze be left in place until the LMA is removed to maintain patency of the LMA and prevent damage to it. The LMA is tolerated well even at light levels of anesthesia and can be left in place during emergence. Keeping the LMA in place during transfer to the postanesthesia care unit (PACU) will maintain a patent airway, while leaving the anesthesia provider's hands free for other tasks. During recovery, supplementary oxygen can be delivered with the LMA in place using a T-piece or other device (148–152). Respiration may be assisted manually by intermittently occluding the T-piece (13).

Some recommend that the LMA be left in position until full recovery of airway reflexes has occurred and the patient can phonate or open his mouth on command (12, 13, 15, 153). This will ensure maintenance of a secure airway until the laryngeal reflexes have returned. The onset of swallowing is a useful predictor that such a level of wakefulness is imminent. The patient should be left undisturbed until the reflexes are restored, except to administer oxygen and perform monitoring. The patient should not be turned onto his or her side, unless there is an important indication (such as regurgitation or vomiting), because this may cause premature rejection of the LMA. It is not necessary to remove secretions from the upper pharynx because they will not enter the larynx provided the cuff is not deflated or the LMA removed before the patient is able to swallow effectively. If the patient is swallowing prior to removal, secretions that have accumulated above the mask can be withdrawn with the LMA or swallowed. Suctioning through the LMA should not be performed unless there is evidence of gastric contents in the tube.

Patients will often remove the LMA themselves (153). A restless, struggling patient is not an indication for removal. Coughing should not necessarily be an indication for removal.

Some have recommended that the LMA be removed while the patient is under deep anesthesia (154–156). This should not be done in a patient known to be difficult to intubate. In children, some studies show fewer respiratory complications with removal at deep levels of anesthesia. (157–159) while others show no difference (160). The LMA should not be removed during light levels of general anesthesia. If swallowing and cough reflexes are not present, secretions in the upper pharynx may flood into the larynx, provoking laryngeal spasm, coughing or gagging.

Tracheal Intubation

The LMA can facilitate tracheal intubation by serving as a conduit through which a tracheal tube, stylet, or fiberscope is passed. It serves to position the device centrally over the laryngeal aperture. The 30° angle between the tube and cuff was chosen because it was found to be optimal for intubation through the LMA (160).

Passage of a tracheal tube or fiberscope may be aided by removal of the bars at the junction of the tube and mask (161, 162).

Oxygen and other gases may be administered by positive pressure ventilation or during spontaneous ventilation and the adequacy of respiration may be monitored by capnography during intubation.

It is important to understand the relative dimensions of the tracheal tube and LMA so the proper size tube and fiberscope can be selected. These are given in Table 15.4.

Use of the laryngeal mask to facilitate tracheal intubation presents several problems. With a standard tracheal tube the cuff may lie between the vocal cords when the tracheal tube is fully inserted through the LMA. This is made worse by neck extension. Deeper placement can be achieved by using an extra-long tracheal tube (163–171), shortening the LMA tube (172, 173), removing the connector from the LMA, deflating the LMA cuff (174, 175), or using a split LMA (161, 176). The ST-LMA, which has a tube 2 cm shorter than a conventional LMA may be useful.

It may be helpful to pass the tracheal tube through the same size LMA outside the patient

TABLE 15.4. Maximum Sized–Tracheal Tubes and Fiberscopes That Can Fit in an LMA

Mask Size	Largest Tracheal Tube that Fits into LMA (i.d. in mm)	Largest Fiberscope that Fits into Tracheal Tube (OD in mm)*
1	3.5	2.7
1.5	4.0	3.0
2	4.5	3.5
2.5	5.0	4.0
3	6.0 cuffed	5.0
4	6.0 cuffed	5.0
5	7.0 cuffed	7.3

* One study indicates that larger fiberscopes can be accomodated (187).

and note or mark the position on the shaft of the LMA when the tracheal tube tip passes through the LMA aperture.

Head position is important in successful intubation. The classic sniffing position should be tried first. If this is not successful, varying degrees of neck flexion and extension may be helpful (177).

Cricoid pressure may make passage of a tracheal tube more difficult (32, 34, 36), so if intubation is initially unsuccessful and intubation is deemed vital, a second attempt should be made with transient release of cricoid pressure.

It is difficult to perform tracheal intubation through the LMA when the epiglottis is present in the passage. This may be less likely when a jaw thrust or head extension is used.

Another problem that may occur is inadvertent extubation when the LMA is removed. Many users prefer to leave both devices in place (178, 179). If this is done, the protruding end of the tracheal tube should be stabilized (180). Another solution is to use another same size or slightly smaller tracheal tube to hold the tracheal tube steady as the LMA is withdrawn over it (181–185). An LMA may be modified by splitting the tube and cuff so that it can be easily removed over the tracheal tube (186).

If the LMA must be removed after intubation, a fiberscope, jet stylet, or tube exchanger may be passed through the tracheal tube to facilitate reintubation should extubation accidentally occur during removal of the LMA.

Blind

Blind intubation through the LMA has been performed in both adults and children. The success rate may be as high as 96%, depending on technique, time available, experience, the number of attempts made, and the equipment chosen (36, 168, 177, 188). The brand of tracheal tube used may play a role in the success of blind tracheal intubation through the LMA (177). The success rate in patients with limited neck motion is lower than those with normal anatomy.

Because down folding of the epiglottis can impair blind intubation, it has been recommended that intubation through the LMA always be preceded by fiberoptic assessment of epiglottis position (189).

The LMA is inserted in the standard way and the cuff inflated. The tracheal tube should be well lubricated and rotated 15 to 90° counterclockwise as it is advanced down the LMA tube to prevent the bevel from catching on the bars at the junction of the tube and mask (190, 191). Once through the bars, the tracheal tube is rotated anteriorly, and the neck is extended to enable the tip to pass anterior to the arytenoids. The tracheal tube is then advanced until resistance is felt. The head is then flexed, permitting further passage of the tube into the trachea. A variety of head maneuvers may be attempted if this routine fails. Auscultation of the end of the tube may be useful during spontaneous breathing.

Alternatively, the LMA may be loaded with a lubricated tracheal tube with the tip oriented at the level of the bars so that when pushed down, it will pass smoothly through the middle aperture (6). The tracheal tube cuff is inflated and the tracheal tube marked where it emerges from the LMA connector and 3 cm above. The LMA is inserted in the usual manner and the cuff inflated. The tracheal tube cuff is then deflated and the tracheal tube pushed down while simultaneously extending the head, until resistance is felt. If resistance is felt before the 3 cm mark is reached, epiglottic impaction is likely. The tracheal tube should be withdrawn to the first mark, the LMA tube pressed downward, and the intubation attempt repeated. If resistance is felt at or beyond the 3 cm mark, impaction of the tube tip against

the anterior laryngeal or tracheal wall is likely. Downward pressure should be released, and the neck flexed, then the tracheal tube pushed down again.

After insertion, the tracheal tube cuff should be inflated and the tube connected to the breathing system and a CO_2 monitor used to confirm intratracheal placement. If the trachea is not entered initially, it is likely that the LMA is not well situated over the laryngeal aperture or the aperture is blocked by the epiglottis. Adjustments in the patient's position should be made. If the tube still does not enter the trachea, it should be withdrawn until the bevel is just behind the aperture bars. The LMA cuff should be deflated, and the LMA pushed a little farther into the hypopharynx. This maneuver may cause elevation of the down folded epiglottis. The tracheal tube is then pushed through the bars.

The LMA can be used to guide a bougie or exchange catheter blindly into the trachea (39, 109, 192–197). Success rates using an exchange catheter with a straight distal tip are lower than with an angulated bougie or blind insertion of a tracheal tube (192). Passage of the bougie may be easier if its angulated end is made to point anteriorly until it passes through the grill of the mask, then rotated 180° (198).

Disadvantages of the blind technique are that it may be time consuming, may result in trauma, and there is a risk of esophageal intubation (6, 199).

Fiberscope Guided

The laryngeal mask has proved equal or superior to other devices designed to aid with intubation using a fiberscope (200, 201). This method of intubation has been used in infants as small as 3.6 kg (202).

Direct-vision–guided techniques have a higher success rate than blind and are associated with less risk of trauma or esophageal intubation. Less neck movement may be required. The fiberscope has been used to aid intubation via the LMA when blind passage of a tracheal tube or bougie has failed (203, 204) and in patients in whom neck movement needs to be avoided (105).

The LMA may be modified to aid in fiberoptic intubation by splitting the tube along its entire length, shortening its length or removing the bars at the opening to the mask (161, 172, 176, 186, 205).

The LMA is inserted in the usual manner. Use of a tracheal tube connector with a rubber seal allows leisurely inspection of the tracheobronchial tree while keeping the patient asleep. The fiberscope, with a well-lubricated tracheal tube and a fully deflated cuff threaded over its shaft, is advanced through the vocal cords and into the trachea, and the tracheal tube passed over the scope into the trachea. The tube should be rotated as it is advanced.

Fiberscope size is important, especially in small patients. The maximum diameters of scopes for various size tracheal tubes are given in Table 15.4. Smaller tracheal tubes are easier to place correctly than larger ones (206). After placement, the tracheal tube may be replaced by a larger one using a tube exchanger.

A fiberscope may be used to insert a bougie or other guide into the trachea through an LMA (173, 197, 207–212). After the guide is placed, the LMA is removed and a tracheal tube advanced over the guide. This technique allows placement of a larger tracheal tube and avoids the problem of accidental extubation when the LMA is removed.

Retrograde

The LMA can be used to facilitate tracheal intubation using a retrograde wire technique (213). The guidewire is inserted through the cricothyroid membrane and passed cephalad. A guide catheter is then threaded antegrade over the wire. The LMA is then removed and a tracheal tube passed over the catheter.

Awake

The LMA can be used to aid tracheal intubation in awake patients after the larynx has received adequate topical anesthesia. This technique may be used in patients in whom awake intubation is indicated, such as those with mediastinal masses, those known to be difficult to intubate and those at high risk for aspiration of gastric contents (104).

Nasotracheal Intubation

The LMA has been used to facilitate nasotracheal intubation (214). The LMA was inserted

and a catheter placed in the trachea. Another catheter was inserted into the nose and brought out through the mouth. The LMA was removed with the catheters in place. Both catheters were sutured together and traction applied to the nasal catheter so that the curve in the mouth was removed. The tracheal tube was then inserted over the catheters into the larynx.

Another method is to cut a window in the posterior aspect of the tube near the mask and remove the aperture bars (215). A fiberscope mounted with a tracheal tube is inserted via the nose through the window in the LMA and into the trachea.

Finally one may insert the LMA, then partially withdraw the cuff into the oropharynx where it can supply fresh gas to the spontaneously breathing patient (216). Nasotracheal intubation is then accomplished using a fiberscope.

Insertion of a Nasogastric Tube

A nasogastric tube is best placed before LMA insertion. However, it is possible to pass one during anesthesia by slightly deflating the cuff and using a forceps to push the tube down behind the mask.

CARE OF THE LARYNGEAL MASK

As soon as possible after use, the LMA should be gently cleaned with soap and warm water. Prior immersion in an 8.4% solution of bicarbonate will help dissolve secretions (12). A pipe-cleaner type brush should be inserted through the distal aperture to clean out the shaft. The inflation valve should not be exposed to any cleaning solution (15). The LMA should be dried, then placed in a pouch and stored with other LMAs to avoid damage by contact with sharp instruments (16).

The LMA can be autoclaved at temperatures up to 138°C (274°F) (12, 15, 16). Higher temperature can cause the tube to become brittle and fragmentation may occur. As much air as possible should be removed from the cuff shortly before autoclaving (217, 218). Residual air will expand in the heat and may damage the cuff, valve or pilot balloon (218–220).

Liquid chemical agents or ethylene oxide should not be used to clean or sterilize the LMA as they are adsorbed onto the silicone, and can cause pharyngitis and laryngitis as well as shorten the life of the LMA (12, 15, 221).

PHYSICAL CONSIDERATIONS
Cuff Pressure

The pressure on the mucosa beneath the fully inflated cuff may be greater than capillary pressure (129, 137, 138), raising concerns about ischemic damage to the mucosa or reflex relaxation of the lower esophageal sphincter (222). A relationship between cuff pressure and pharyngeal morbidity has not yet been established. There is evidence that the pharynx may adapt to the LMA cuff (137, 142).

Dead Space

The dead space associated with the LMA is less than with a face mask but greater than with a tracheal tube in place.

Resistance to Flow and Work of Breathing

Resistance to breathing is an important consideration with the LMA because it is frequently used with spontaneous respiration. While the LMA itself offers less resistance than a corresponding tracheal tube, total respiratory resistance and work of breathing are similar since the larynx is not bypassed (108, 223–226). The work of breathing through the LMA is similar to that with a face mask unless there is difficulty maintaining a patent airway with the face mask. The reinforced LMA imposes significantly greater resistance than the standard LMA (4, 187).

USEFUL SITUATIONS

The LMA has been used for a wide variety of procedures, but it is probably best suited to short cases, making it especially useful for outpatient surgery. It has proved useful in patients who need multiple anesthetics over a short period of time. The maximum duration for which the LMA can be safely used is not yet known. It has been used for surgical procedures lasting up to 8 hours (227, 228). It has been used in the ICU to provide respiratory support for 10–24 hrs with no apparent problems (229).

Indications for use include routine, elective cases where tracheal intubation is not required or

is required only because the surgery interferes with maintenance of the airway with a face mask.

Use of a Face Mask Difficult

In patients in whom maintenance of a clear airway might be difficult, such as edentulous patients or those with facial injuries, facial contours not suited to a face mask, or beards, it may be easier to maintain a satisfactory airway with the LMA. Studies comparing the use of the LMA with a face mask show fewer episodes of desaturation and less difficulty in maintaining an airway with the LMA (230–232).

Patients with facial burns often require multiple anesthetics. Use of a face mask in these patients is difficult and often painful. Also excessive handling of the facial burns can cause infection and delay healing. The LMA may prove useful in these patients (233). However, it is not appropriate to use the LMA to secure the airway in a patient with upper airway burns.

Other patients in whom a laryngeal mask is useful are those in whom it is difficult to obtain a good seal with the face mask, those undergoing laser treatment of the face, and patients in whom airway obstruction occurs when a face mask is used (110, 234–236).

Difficult Airway

The LMA may be useful in patients with airway distortion secondary to tumor (237), fracture of the larynx (238), congenital problems (39, 110, 162, 239–245), facial injuries (246), hematoma, abscess (247), laryngeal polyposis (248, 249), tonsillar hypertrophy (250), upper airway obstruction due to residual neuromuscular blockade (251), limited mouth opening (57, 195, 252, 253), poor mobility of the neck or presence of a cervical collar (24, 194, 252, 254–257), and instability of the cervical spine (24, 26, 105, 258–260).

Failed Intubation

In cases of inability to intubate or ventilate the patient, the LMA may be useful and even lifesaving by using it either as the primary means of maintaining an airway or to facilitate passage of a tracheal tube (175, 211, 243, 246, 249, 252, 261–278). For this reason it is recommended that an LMA be immediately available whenever a "cannot intubate/cannot ventilate" scenario is possible. The American Society of Anesthesiologists' Task Force on Management of the Difficult Airway has incorporated the LMA into the difficult airway algorithm (168).

Securing the airway with an LMA will allow ventilation while definitive management such as intubation through the LMA is planned or the patient is allowed to awaken. The LMA should be considered prior to using transtracheal ventilation or establishing a surgical airway.

Studies differ on whether the ease of insertion and adequate function of the LMA are independent of Mallampatti and Cormack and Lehane scoring (188, 279–281). Although fiberoptic laryngoscopy is usually considered to be the technique of choice in cases of anticipated difficult intubation, the LMA may be the only practical option in some cases. In these circumstances the patient should not be paralyzed and it is preferable to place the LMA while the patient is awake (282).

Ophthalmic Surgery

The LMA has been used for ophthalmological procedures. Studies have shown that intraocular pressure is lower during induction and emergence when an LMA is used compared to a tracheal tube (283–288), although one study found intraocular pressure was the same with both techniques (289). The ability of patients to tolerate the LMA at lighter levels of anesthesia should reduce the likelihood of coughing intraoperatively. Intraocular pressure remains lower during recovery from anesthesia with an LMA (286, 290)

Reservations have been expressed about use of the LMA in ocular surgery (291, 292). Use of a reinforced LMA is advisable. Dislodgment during intraocular surgery has been reported (293, 294) and must be prevented by careful fixation and maintenance of an adequate depth of anesthesia and muscle relaxation (295). It is essential to prevent coughing, especially when the eye is open.

Tracheal and Pulmonary Pathology

The LMA is a suitable device for patients with respiratory disease who do not require high airway pressures. Asthmatics and other patients with re-

active airways disease are at increased risk of bronchospasm during manipulations of the airway. Because the LMA is less invasive than a tracheal tube, the risk of bronchospasm should be lower. However, the LMA is unsuitable for the patient with acute asthma requiring high airway pressures.

The LMA may offer benefits in infants with bronchopulmonary dysplasia (296–298) and patients with chronic obstructive pulmonary disease (299).

The laryngeal mask has been used to diagnose laryngomalacia and tracheobronchomalacia in children (236, 300). However, its use in patients with collapsible airways has been questioned (301).

In the patient with tracheal stenosis, minimal interference with airflow and avoidance of further damage to the trachea are essential. Placement of a tracheal tube through the stenotic area may be technically difficult, will reduce the diameter of the trachea, and may cause trauma. Such a patient may be successfully managed using the laryngeal mask (85, 302, 303). Since the diameter of the tube of the laryngeal mask is larger than the tracheal tube and the trachea is not intubated, the increase in airway resistance with the LMA is small. Stent placement for a tracheal stenosis using the LMA has been described (304, 305). Controlled ventilation may be used if the stenosis is not so pronounced that high pressures are needed to inflate the lungs (301). Spontaneous ventilation has also been used. Failure of the LMA in patients with tracheal stenosis where tracheal intubation had failed has been reported (306).

Compression of the trachea by a mediastinal mass can cause problems similar to tracheal stenosis. Both mediastinoscopy and thoracotomy have been performed in this situation with the LMA and spontaneous ventilation (307, 308). However, use of the LMA in patients with mediastinal masses has been questioned since it cannot prevent airway collapse and the use of high inflation pressures with it is not recommended (301).

The LMA has been used for standard (242, 265, 269, 309) and percutaneous dilational tracheostomy (310, 311). Use of the LMA eliminates the need to share the trachea with the surgeon. It also allows visualization of the trachea with a fiberscope during the procedure.

The LMA has been used as a blocker to prevent loss of gas from the trachea during a tracheoplasty (312) and for laser treatment and resection of a tracheal tumor (313).

Thyroid Surgery

The LMA has been used for surgery on the thyroid. The cuff displaces the gland anteriorly, facilitating surgical access (15). Because damage to the recurrent laryngeal nerve is a complication of thyroid surgery, it may be desirable to stimulate that nerve during surgery and observe the motion of the vocal cords by inserting a fiberscope through the LMA (12, 314–322).

Possible problems with this technique include displacement of the mask and laryngospasm (316, 323). Topical application of lidocaine has been recommended to prevent laryngospasm (324). Tracheal deviation and narrowing should be considered relative contraindications to use of the LMA in thyroid surgery (316).

Other Head and Neck Surgery

The LMA has been used for a variety of ear-nose-throat (ENT) procedures, including laryngoscopy and microsurgical procedures on the larynx (300, 325, 326), nasal and pharyngoplastic surgery (327–329), myringotomies (230, 232), adenoidectomy and tonsillectomy (7, 8, 232, 330–332) and dental procedures (330, 333–337). It has been used as the primary airway and to facilitate intubation in patients with Pierre–Robin (110, 162, 239, 241, 242, 244, 245) and Treacher Collins syndromes (243).

It may be preferable to use the reinforced LMA in some of these situations (330, 332). Because it has a narrower tube and can be moved easily within the mouth, it provides better surgical access than the standard LMA. Kinking of the LMA tube, which can be a problem during intraoral procedures, especially when a mouth gag is used, occurs less often when a reinforced LMA is used.

The LMA cuff acts as a throat pack, preventing aspiration of blood, teeth, and secretions (6, 8, 332, 338). If the cuff is dislodged, however, aspiration is possible. Further protection may be obtained by inserting an oropharyngeal pack or positioning a suction catheter in the groove between the mask and the tube of the LMA (339). A pack may help to secure the LMA internally (340).

How well the LMA protects the trachea from matter from above is controversial. Although one study showed that dye instilled into the pharynx outside the LMA cannot be detected inside the LMA mask (341), another found staining inside the mask in 10% of patients (342). In another study, blood was not detected on the tracheal side of the LMA following nasal polypectomy or antral washout (327). The LMA appears to offer better protection than an uncuffed tracheal tube (332) but offers no protection from reflux of gastric contents, including blood and irrigation fluid swallowed during surgery.

The LMA offers many advantages for this type of surgery. The head can be turned to either side without loss of airway, although extreme flexion may cause obstruction (15). In a comparative study between the nasal mask and the LMA, there was less hypoxia and a better seal with the LMA (333). The frequency of postoperative stridor, laryngospasm, and oxygen desaturation is reduced by use of the LMA for tonsillectomy in children (8).

Pathology in the mouth or pharynx is a relative contraindication to use of the LMA. Placement is sometimes difficult in patients with large tonsils (49, 343). Caution must be taken when moving the tube not to displace the LMA or allow it to rotate. Compression of the LMA tube between the teeth and mouth gag may occur (7, 8). The LMA may get caught in the groove of the tongue blade, which can lead to premature removal at the end of the procedure (232). This can be avoided by coating the groove with a lubricant jelly.

Pediatric Patients

The LMA can be used in children, including small infants. It may be particularly helpful with children in whom unusual anatomy makes tracheal intubation difficult.

Because the epiglottis in children is relatively large and floppy, the likelihood of its being within the mask is greater (46, 49, 52, 344). This may make blind intubation or intubation over a bougie or guide wire passed blindly through the LMA difficult (88).

Studies show fewer hypoxic episodes and improved surgical conditions in children ventilated with the LMA compared to a face mask (230). In children with bronchopulmonary dysplasia, the LMA can maintain a satisfactory airway with fewer adverse respiratory effects than a tracheal tube (298). However, some studies found a tendency for the LMA position to deteriorate after initial satisfactory placement in infants (60, 66).

The LMA has been used for neonatal resuscitation in infants as small as 1.2 kg and neonates with abnormal airways (87, 242, 345–348) Disadvantages include inability to remove meconium and the inability to administer high pressures (349). This may make it unsuitable for resuscitation of premature newborns or ones who require high airway pressures.

The LMA has been used for children having anesthesia for radiotherapy who require multiple anesthetics over a short period of time (350–352).

Tracheal Suctioning

The laryngeal mask can be used to aid tracheal suctioning without resorting to intubation or tracheostomy (353).

Professional Singers

The laryngeal mask may be especially useful for professional singers and speakers in whom laryngeal complications of intubation would be most serious (354, 355). The LMA causes less change in vocal function than tracheal intubation (356).

Remote Anesthesia Provider

Situations in which the anesthesia provider must be away from the patient, including diagnostic imaging and radiotherapy procedures, can often be managed using a laryngeal mask (10, 98, 126, 350, 352, 357, 358). If these require that the patient be placed in an awkward position, the reinforced LMA may be useful.

MRI poses some special problems. Because some of the inflation valves contain metallic material, it may be necessary to remove the valve and knot the pilot tube (359). Special LMAs with valves that do not contain ferrous material are available (12). If the reinforced LMA is used, the metal coil produces a large black hole in the image in the area surrounding the airway as well as a

deterioration of the image further out (10). The LMA may not be suitable if magnetic resonance spectroscopy is performed because the resonance of some silicone-containing materials compromises interpretation of the scans (360). The flexible LMA will cause distortion of the image in the area surrounding the airway.

Supplementation of Regional Block

In cases where the surgery outlasts a regional block or only a partial block is present, supplementation with light general anesthesia may be desirable. In addition, many patients cannot tolerate prolonged surgery under regional anesthesia. The LMA has been used for these cases (228, 361, 362). It allows a lighter level of anesthesia than would be required with a tracheal tube.

Resuscitation

Resuscitation requires rapid attainment of a clear airway and administration of oxygen. Tracheal intubation is the technique of choice, but it requires skill and even then can be very difficult or impossible. Successful use of the LMA during cardiac arrest has been reported (363–365). The presence of an LMA does not hinder identification of the carotid pulse (366).

Non-anesthesia personnel can learn the insertion technique easily. Better ventilation can be achieved than with a face mask (367, 368). Satisfactory chest expansion has been shown to be present in 86% of patients in whom the LMA was placed by non-anesthesia personnel (369).

One problem with using the LMA for resuscitation is that often the patient has a full stomach and the LMA cannot offer full protection from aspiration. The LMA must not be considered a substitute for a tracheal tube if someone present has the ability to place a tracheal tube.

Out-of-Hospital Use

The LMA has been used in out-of-hospital situations, including emergency care and transportation. It has been used during helicopter transfer of patients (370, 371). The laryngeal mask has proved useful in patients with cervical spine injury and those trapped in positions which do not lend themselves to tracheal intubation (372).

Paramedics and respiratory therapists acquire

skill more rapidly and have a higher rate of successful placement with the LMA than a tracheal tube (373–375).

Obstetrics

Because the risk of aspiration of gastric contents is high in the obstetrical patient, its routine use is not recommended (376). However, if intubation cannot be performed and an adequate airway cannot be achieved with a face mask, the LMA may be lifesaving (266, 270, 276, 377–381). For this reason, and because the incidence of failed intubation in the obstetric population is higher than in the general population, it is recommended that the laryngeal mask be kept in the obstetric operating room. However, it may not always be effective (382).

In the obstetric patient who can be ventilated using a face mask while cricoid pressure is continuously applied, placement of the LMA may have little benefit and might induce vomiting and aspiration. Cricoid pressure might have to be momentarily released to allow successful insertion of the LMA.

The laryngeal mask has been inserted using topical anesthesia and used to facilitate tracheal intubation in a parturient (383).

Laser Surgery

The LMA has been used for laser surgery to the face (384, 385), the pharynx (386), and the carina (303). During facial surgery, use of the LMA markedly decreases the leakage of gases compared with that of a face mask. However, when positive pressure ventilation is employed, leakage around the cuff may occur.

Studies show that the LMA is more resistant to perforation by lasers than PVC tracheal tubes (387). However, because fires have such serious consequences, it has been recommended that when a laser is used, the shaft of the LMA tube be wrapped in a laser-resistant material, the cuff be protected with gauze, and a saline solution used to fill it (386, 388, 389). It may be prudent not to use a gauze bite-block when a laser is used (385).

Fiberoptic Laryngoscopy and Bronchoscopy

The LMA has been used to aid diagnostic and therapeutic fiberoptic airway endoscopy in adults and children by directing the fiberscope to the glottis (58, 303, 315, 321, 390–399). Bronchial lavage has been performed using a fiberscope via a laryngeal mask (400). Use of a connector incorporating a rubber seal will permit passage of the fiberscope without loss of seal so ventilation can be maintained and monitored. The LMA offers less resistance than a tracheal tube. Also, it allows the laryngeal opening and vocal cord function to be assessed. The reinforced laryngeal mask airway is not suitable for fiberoptic examinations because of the narrowness of the tube and because the internal wire may be damaged (187).

Laparoscopy

Use of the LMA for laparoscopic procedures is controversial. Studies suggest that the LMA is safe for gynecologic laparoscopy (277, 401–403). However, there have been reports of aspiration in patients undergoing laparoscopy and upper abdominal surgery with the LMA (404).

Neurosurgery

It has been used for patients undergoing ventriculoperitoneal shunts (405) and intracranial surgery (406, 407).

Extubation

It may be desirable to extubate certain patients who are still deeply anesthetized (408–411) These include patients with reactive airways disease, patients who have undergone intracranial surgery and patients with coronary artery disease. The LMA can be substituted for the tracheal tube while the patient is still in a deep plane of anesthesia or before antagonism of neuromuscular blockade (412).

Ventilatory Support without Tracheal Intubation

The LMA can be used for short-term airway maintenance (251, 413) or application of continuous positive airway pressure (414, 415).

Access to the Upper Gastrointestinal Tract

The LMA can be used to direct a gastroscope or nasogastric tube into the esophagus (416, 417).

COMPLICATIONS

The incidence of complications is related to the experience and expertise of the clinician (418). Problems are more likely to occur during induction or emergence from anesthesia (418).

Aspiration of Gastric Contents

The LMA does not form an airtight seal around the larynx and cannot be relied on to protect the tracheobronchial tree from the contents of the gastrointestinal tract as reliably as a cuffed tracheal tube (404, 419–426). Studies suggest an incidence of aspiration of 1 in 5000 uses (427). Although in some cases the distal part of the cuff will provide some protection by obstructing the upper esophagus, in others the esophagus communicates directly with the airway (32). A reduction in lower esophageal sphincter tone may occur when a laryngeal mask is used (428, 429). However, the upper esophageal sphincter remains competent and can prevent regurgitation in the absence of neuromuscular block (430). Postoperative laryngeal competence is not impaired by the LMA (431).

Many reported cases of aspiration with the LMA are associated with use in inappropriate patients. However, aspiration in fasted patients with no predisposing factors during elective procedures has been reported. There appears to be no increased risk of aspiration with controlled versus spontaneous ventilation or in the pediatric population (13).

Regurgitation usually provides little warning, with the first indication often the appearance of gastric secretions in the tube. Fortunately most of the reported cases have had favorable outcomes because the regurgitated material was not aspirated or the aspiration was relatively mild.

Failed intubation and the full stomach pose a difficult problem. In the event of a failed intubation in a patient for whom there is a significant risk of aspiration and in whom ventilation can be maintained with a face mask while cricoid pressure is applied, it may be safer to continue with the face mask and cricoid pressure rather than try to insert the LMA (29, 432). If maintenance of a clear airway is impossible, LMA insertion is an alternative to cricothyroid puncture. Use of cricoid pressure may make positioning of the LMA more difficult and may decrease the success of ventilation (25, 29, 30, 32–36, 433). It may be necessary to momentarily relax cricoid pressure during LMA insertion. The LMA does not decrease the effectiveness of cricoid pressure (434, 435) so it should be reapplied and maintained after LMA insertion unless it interferes with ventilation.

If gastric contents are seen in the laryngeal mask the patient should be placed in the 30° head-down position, the LMA left in situ, anesthesia deepened and the breathing system disconnected temporarily to allow drainage. The lateral position has no apparent advantage since regurgitated fluid is prevented from escaping via the pharynx. 100% oxygen should be supplied. Forceful ventilation attempts should be avoided and small tidal volumes delivered. Suctioning should be performed via the LMA, preferably using a fiberscope. The LMA should be replaced with a tracheal tube if aspiration has occurred.

Techniques to minimize the incidence of aspiration include limiting elective use of the LMA to fasting patients who are not at increased risk for gastroesophageal reflux. Gastric distention, which has been implicated as a factor in aspiration, can occur with intermittent positive pressure ventilation (128, 133, 418). This can be minimized by using the correct size mask, avoiding under- or overinflation of the cuff, careful positioning and fixation, maintenance of an adequate depth of anesthesia and relaxation throughout surgery, and low inflation pressures. Use of low tidal volumes and low inspiratory flow rates will help keep peak airway pressure low. The mean pressure at which gastric insufflation occurs is 28 cm H_2O with a range of 19 to 41 cm H_2O using size 4 and 5 LMAs (13). Epigastric auscultation should be performed to ensure that gastric insufflation is not occurring. A nasogastric tube may be used but may not always be helpful (297, 436).

During spontaneous respiration, it is important to maintain an adequate level of anesthesia as gastric distention due to recurrent swallowing can occur when anesthesia is too light (437).

Foreign Body Aspiration

A foreign body may become entrapped in the LMA tube (438, 439). Such an object may be subsequently aspirated or cause airway obstruction.

Airway Obstruction

Causes of complete or partial airway obstruction while using a laryngeal mask include malpositioning, back folding of the distal cuff, rotation of the LMA, back folding of the epiglottis, forward displacement of the postcricoid area, infolding of the aryepiglottic folds, obstruction of the laryngeal opening by the distal cuff, kinking of the tube (98, 440–443), increased cuff volume, lubricant applied to the mask aperture, a faulty LMA (444, 445), the presence of a foreign body, and laryngospasm (60, 62, 337, 446, 447). While the head can be turned to either side without loss of the airway, extreme flexion may cause obstruction (15). Maneuvers that may help to relieve obstruction include minor adjustments of the jaw or the LMA, protrusion of the mandible, head extension, repositioning of the LMA, repacking, and unkinking of the LMA tube (60).

The reported incidence of laryngospasm is 1 to 3% and may occur anytime during the perioperative period (60, 323, 448–452). Stridor has been reported as long as 2 days following uneventful use of an LMA (453, 454). Laryngospasm is usually the result of inadequate anesthetic depth. It may also be caused by lubricant on the anterior surface of the mask. It can be treated by increasing the depth of anesthesia, muscle relaxants, or continuous pressure.

Overdistension of the cuff can cause obstruction (455, 456) so it is important not to exceed the recommended volumes. Cases of obstruction during use where slight deflation of the cuff relieved the obstruction have been reported (135, 139). It is thought that nitrous oxide diffused into the cuff and increased its volume so that it encroached on the laryngeal inlet.

Biting on the tube can cause obstruction. This can be avoided by using a bite block or gauze roll and leaving it in place until the LMA is removed. Mouth gags used for surgery may cause obstruction of the tube portion (7, 457).

Airway obstruction may be caused by rotation of the LMA so that the inflated rim occludes the larynx (81, 458, 459). Rotation can be detected by checking for the black line, which should face the upper lip.

Application of cricoid pressure may cause airway obstruction with the laryngeal mask in place (433), as may downward pressure on the mandible by the surgeon (460).

If airway obstruction develops, rapid use of fiberoptic endoscopy may help differentiate the various causes and guide appropriate management (447, 461, 462).

Injury to the Airway

The oral and pharyngeal mucosa may be injured during insertion of the LMA. Injuries of the epiglottis, posterior pharyngeal wall, uvula, soft palate, and tonsils have been reported (54, 449, 463–468). A hematoma above the vocal cords has been reported in a patient with a bleeding diathesis (469).

Cyanosis of the tongue has been reported (470). Replacement of the LMA with a smaller size corrected the problem.

Dislodgment

Accidental dislodgment can occur (293, 418, 460). A correctly placed LMA may be forced upwards out of the hypopharynx if cricopharyngeal muscle tone is permitted to increase or the cuff becomes overinflated. If the LMA has come out only a short distance, it can often be pushed back into place (15). Persistent difficulty in keeping the inflated LMA in position may be solved by using a different size, reducing the cuff volume, elevating the mandible, or using a different head position.

Damage to the LMA

The LMA may break apart (471–476). This is usually the result of using it beyond its useful life span. The tube can be transected by the teeth (477). Disconnection of the tube and mask portions of the LMA can occur (472). The cuff or pilot tube may be torn on a tooth or damaged by a surgeon (11, 478–483). If the LMA does break in situ, it should be remembered that often the patient can still be ventilated by the application of a face mask (13).

Laryngopharyngeal Complaints

The incidence of sore throat following use of the LMA has been reported to be between 0% and 28% (28, 78, 84, 231, 289, 403, 449, 450, 484–490). Use of an insertion aid and cuff deflation may lower the incidence (488, 491). The incidence increases with the duration of LMA use (492). Studies differ on the effect of intracuff pressure on the incidence of sore throat (490, 493, 494).

Dysphagia is seen more frequently with use of the LMA than a tracheal tube (490).

Mild dysphonia is common following use of the LMA, but less common than with a tracheal tube (490). Severe dysphonia due to recurrent nerve palsy or arytenoid dislocation associated with use of the LMA has been reported (495, 496).

Failure of Cuff to Inflate or Deflate

In one reported case the pilot tube became stuck between the patient's teeth so that the cuff could not be inflated (497). In another case the pilot tube became looped around the mask aperture bars (498).

Nerve Injury

Palsies of the hypoglossal (499, 500), recurrent laryngeal (70, 495, 501–504) and lingual (505, 506) nerves have been reported after use of an LMA.

Bronchospasm

Bronchospasm associated with the use of the laryngeal mask has been reported (448, 507). A bronchodilator aerosol can be administered through the LMA (125).

Pulmonary Edema

Pulmonary edema has been reported following insertion of a laryngeal mask (508). In these cases, insertion was difficult and associated with obstruction before proper placement was achieved.

Other

Transient swelling of the parotid glands (509) and tongue (510) has been reported following use of an LMA.

Presence of an LMA may displace mobile landmarks used to cannulate the internal jugular vein (511).

ADVANTAGES
Ease of Insertion

An outstanding feature of the LMA is that it provides a rapid clear airway rapidly in the vast majority of patients and is both faster and easier to insert than a tracheal tube. The insertion technique is simple and even those with little or no experience in its use are usually successful at inserting it correctly. The training for proper insertion is neither long nor elaborate. People who are not skilled at intubation have a high success rate with the laryngeal mask (375, 512, 513).

Reported first-time insertion rates in adults vary from 76 to 96% in adults (28, 78, 128, 159, 374, 375, 449, 450, 484, 514–516). Slightly lower rates may occur with pediatric patients (46, 49, 61, 66, 159, 230, 350, 448, 451, 517–519). Studies show an unobstructed airway can be achieved in more than 90% of cases (49, 52, 60, 159, 230, 231, 350, 449, 450, 484, 515, 518–521). With experience the success rate increases and may exceed 99% (188, 277, 418).

The LMA can be inserted from the side or in front of the patient or with the patient in the lateral or prone positions (522–524). This makes it useful for maintaining the airway after accidental extubation when the patient is in an unconventional position (525).

It has been used in out-of-hospital care when access to the patient was so limited that it was impossible to insert a tracheal tube (372). A cervical collar or manual in-line stabilization do not appear to interfere with successful placement (24, 26).

Smooth Awakening

The LMA allows a smoother awakening than a tracheal tube with fewer episodes of desaturation, interrupted spontaneous breathing, coughing, laryngospasm and hypertension (8, 49, 286, 526). Emergence and recovery times are shorter (231, 527). Patients who have had an LMA require less analgesia during recovery (486).

Low Operating Room Pollution

There is less operating room pollution with the LMA than with a face mask (80, 130, 450, 528–531). However, when positive pressure ventilation is employed, N_2O levels increase and may reach as high as 280 ppm (532). Use of a close (local) scavenging device will lower the levels of trace anesthetic gases to those associated with tracheal intubation.

Avoiding the Complications of Intubation

While blood pressure and heart rate increase after placement of the laryngeal mask, these increases are similar to those found during insertion of an oral airway and less marked and of shorter duration than those associated with tracheal intubation (285, 286, 289, 486, 533–538). There is minimal increase in intraocular pressure following insertion.

Less anesthesia is needed to tolerate a laryngeal mask than a tracheal tube (20, 539, 540). Neither laryngoscopy nor the use of a neuromuscular blocking agent is required, thus preventing associated problems such as muscle pains and trauma to the lips, gums, and teeth.

Since it is not introduced into the trachea, the diameter of the latter is not compromised. This allows ventilation with low pressures when using intermittent positive-pressure ventilation. Laryngeal edema and trauma and postoperative laryngeal incompetence should not occur.

The incidence of sore throat following its use is lower than that following tracheal tube insertion. The incidence of bacteremia is low (541, 542).

The time needed for insertion is usually less than that for tracheal intubation (373–375). Inadvertent bronchial or esophageal intubation cannot occur.

In patients with tracheal stents, use of an LMA avoids disturbing the stent (543, 544).

Because it minimizes stimulation of the airways, especially below the glottis, it is less likely to precipitate bronchospasm. The incidence of coughing, straining and breath holding during emergence is reduced (285, 289).

Ease of Use

Because there is no need to support the jaw or hold a face mask, the user's hands are free for other tasks. Airway deterioration due to user fatigue is eliminated. Intraoperative airway manipulations, difficulty in maintaining a patent airway, and hypoxemia are less common with the LMA than a face mask (230, 231, 332, 545).

Avoiding the Complications Associated with Face Masks

The LMA avoids many of the complications associated with use of a face mask, including leakage of gas, dermatitis, and injury to the eyes, teeth, and nerves of the face (384, 546). It is not necessary to use a mask strap.

Protection from Barotrauma

Barotrauma is a potential problem with tracheal tubes because of the tight seal inside the trachea. This is less likely with the laryngeal mask because of the tendency to leak at high pressures (547).

Cost Effectiveness

While the initial price of an LMA is high compared to a disposable face mask or tracheal tube, if it is reused enough times, it may be a cost-effective choice (532, 548, 549). Many authors report its use when recycled 200–250 times (219, 550). Its lifespan is prolonged by careful use, strict adherence to cleaning and sterilization procedures, and avoiding forceful removal through partially clenched teeth (13). There are savings from reduced use of muscle relaxants, volatile anesthetics, narcotics, airways, suction tubing and suckers; potentially increased patient turnover; reduced postoperative morbidity; and reduced postoperative analgesic requirements. It can be used with low fresh gas flows (123).

Accidental disposal of LMAs can be costly. This can be minimized with in-service education of the staff. Some form of accountability may be desirable.

DISADVANTAGES
Certain Unsuitable Situations

The LMA should not be used in situations associated with an increased risk of aspiration (full stomach, previous gastric surgery, gastroesophageal reflux, obesity, diabetic gastroparesis, dementia, trauma, opiate medications, increased intestinal pressure) unless other techniques for securing the airway have failed.

Many authors believe this device should not be used for a cholecystectomy because the high intra-abdominal pressures may increase the risk of regurgitation of gastric contents and reduce compliance of the lungs.

The patient with glottic or subglottic airway obstruction, such as tracheomalacia or external compression of the trachea, should not be managed with a laryngeal mask because it cannot prevent collapse of the trachea (301, 551).

Supraglottic pathology such as a cyst, abscess, hematoma, or tissue disruption can make proper positioning difficult or impossible (552), although the LMA has proved useful in upper airway obstruction caused by supraglottic edema or a thyroglossal tumor (249, 269). It may be more appropriate to use alternative insertion techniques, depending on the nature of the pathology (13).

The LMA should not be used in obstetrical patients except when intubation and manual ventilation with a face mask are not possible.

In certain patients the LMA may be difficult or impossible to insert. These include those with an angle between the oral and pharyngeal axes of less than 90° at the back of the tongue, limited mouth opening, palatal defects, oropharyngeal masses, hard palate crib for thumb sucking, or sharp edges in the mouth (13, 553).

The LMA is not suitable for patients who require high inflation pressures i.e., those with low compliance or high resistance. This includes patients with obesity, bronchospasm, thoracic trauma, and pulmonary edema or fibrosis. While it has been used during thoracotomy, reinflation of the collapsed portion of the lung may not be possible (515). There is disagreement about the safety of the laryngeal mask for procedures such as laparoscopic surgery, where intra-abdominal pressure is high. Successful use of the LMA in this situation has been reported (277, 402, 403).

Presence of a bleeding disorder is considered a relative contraindication to use of an LMA (469, 554).

Some feel that the LMA is relatively contraindicated in situations where there is restricted access to the airway (12, 555, 556), especially if there is

no guarantee that it can be replaced if it becomes dislodged or should intubation become necessary during the operation. It would be prudent to use spontaneous ventilation and the reinforced LMA in this situation. The LMA has been used in the lateral and prone positions.

Requirement for Paralysis or Obtundation of Airway Reflexes

The LMA cannot be inserted unless the jaw and pharynx are fully relaxed. Coughing, gagging, vomiting, biting, laryngospasm, and bronchospasm can occur in inadequately anesthetized patients. These may be more of a problem in patients with chronic respiratory diseases and heavy smokers (299). Performance of a superior laryngeal nerve block may help to prevent these problems (557).

Leakage

Leakage usually occurs when the peak airway pressure exceeds 20 cm H_2O and increases with peak airway pressure (130). This usually does not prevent effective ventilation but does cause pollution of the operating room air with anesthetic agents

Learning Curve

Although LMA placement is easier to learn than tracheal intubation, skill and confidence in its use require instruction and practice. Studies have shown that the learning curve is relatively short and that a high degree of success can be achieved (418). There is also evidence of a long-term learning curve (188).

Need to Educate Postanesthesia Care Unit Nurses

Personnel caring for the patient in the PACU must be trained to care for a patient with the laryngeal mask in place and when to remove it (153, 558).

Loss of Airway Management Skills

The ability to maintain an adequate airway using a face mask is one of the fundamental skills of anesthetic practice. Increasing dependency on the LMA may result in a lack of experience and skill in using a face mask for prolonged periods or with a difficult airway.

Loss of Tactile Monitoring

While the laryngeal mask frees the anesthesia provider's hands, it distances him or her from the patient and may cause delay in diagnosing a decrement in airway quality.

Less Reliable Airway

The LMA does not secure a clear airway as effectively as a tracheal tube and airway obstruction at the glottic and subglottic levels cannot be prevented. The LMA can be more easily displaced than a tracheal tube and requires correct orientation to function properly. Surgeons must be made aware that movements of the head, neck, or drapes, insertion of a pack, etc., that would be acceptable with a tracheal tube in place may cause displacement of an LMA.

REFERENCES

1. Brain AIJ. The laryngeal mask—a new concept in airway management. Br J Anaesth 1983;55:801–804.
2. Brimacombe JR, Berry AM, Campbell RC, et al. In response. Anesth Analg 1996;83:664.
3. Woods K. Beware of mismatch of cuff/tube on laryngeal mask airway. Anesth Analg 1994;79:604.
4. Al-Hasani A. Resistance to constant air flow imposed by the standard laryngeal mask, the reinforced laryngeal mask airway and RAE tubes. Br J Anaesth 1993;71:594–596.
5. Brimacombe J, Berry A, Verghese C. The laryngeal mask airway: its uses in anesthesiology. Anesthesiology 1994;80:706–707.
6. Brimacombe JR, Berry AM, Brain AIJ. The laryngeal mask airway. Anesth Clin North Am 1995;13:411–437.
7. Heath ML. The reinforced laryngeal mask airway for adenotonsillectomy. Br J Anaesth 1994;72:728–729.
8. Webster AC, Morley–Forster PK, Ganapathy S, et al. Anaesthesia for adenotonsillectomy: a comparison between tracheal intubation and the armored laryngeal mask airway. Can J Anaesth 1993;40:1171–1177.
9. Williams PJ, Bailey PM. The reinforced laryngeal mask airway for adenotonsillectomy. A reply. Br J Anaesth 1994;72:729.
10. Stevens JE, Burden G. Reinforced laryngeal mask air-way and magnetic resonance imaging. Anaesthesia 1994;49:79–80.
11. Wat LI, Brimacombe JR. Laryngeal mask airway longevity and pilot-balloon failure. J Clin Anesth 1997;9:432.
12. Asai T, Morris S. The laryngeal mask airway: its features, effects and role. Can J Anaesth 1994;41:930–960.
13. Brimacombe JR, Brain AIJ. The laryngeal mask airway. A review and practical guide. London: WB Saunders Company, 1997.
14. Brimacombe J, Brain AIJ, Branagan H, et al. Optimal shape of the laryngeal mask cuff: the influence of three deflation techniques. Anaesthesia 1996;51:673–676.
15. Brain AIJ, Denman WT, Goudsouzian NG. Laryngeal Mask Airway Instruction Manual, 1995.
16. Brimacombe JR. The laryngeal mask airway in the USA. Anesthesiology News 1996;22:38, 41–43.
17. Chan ST, Tham CS. The effects of 2% lignocaine gel on incidence of retching with the use of the laryngeal mask airway. Anaesthesia 1995;50:257–258.
18. O'Neill B, Templeton JJ, Caramico L, et al. The laryngeal mask airway in pediatric patients: factors affecting ease of use during insertion and emergence. Anesth Analg 1994;78:659–662.
19. Keller C, Sparr HJ, Brimacombe JR. Laryngeal mask lubrication. A comparative study of saline versus 2% lignocaine gel with cuff pressure control. Anaesthesia 1997;52:592–597.
20. Taguchi M, Watanabe S, Asakura N, et al. End-tidal sevoflurane concentrations for laryngeal mask airway insertion and for tracheal intubation in children. Anesthesiology 1994;81:628–631.
21. Drage MP, Nunez J, Vaughan RS, et al. Jaw thrusting as a clinical test to assess the adequate depth of anaesthesia for insertion of the laryngeal mask. Anaesthesia 1996;51:1167–1170.
22. Cook TM, Seavell CR, Cox CM. Lignocaine to aid the insertion of the laryngeal mask airway with thiopentone. A comparison between topical and intravenous administration. Anaesthesia 1996;51:787–790.
23. Glaisyer HR, Parry M, Bailey PM. Topical lignocaine for laryngeal mask airway insertion. Anaesthesia 1996;51:1187.
24. Pennant JH, Pace NA, Gajraj NM. Role of the laryngeal mask airway in the immobile cervical spine. J Clin Anesth 1993;5:226–230.
25. Asai T, Barclay K, Power I, et al. Cricoid pressure impedes placement of the laryngeal mask airway. Br J Anaesth 1995;74:521–525.
26. Brimacombe J, Berry A. Laryngeal mask airway insertion. A comparison of the standard versus neutral position in normal patients with a view to its use in

cervical spine instability. Anaesthesia 1993;48:670–671.

27. Brain AIJ. Modification of laryngeal mask insertion technique in children. Anesth Analg 1995;81:212.

28. Reddy SVG, Win N. Brain laryngeal mask—study in 50 spontaneously breathing patients. Singapore Med J 1990;31:338–340.

29. Ansermino JM, Blogg CE. Cricoid pressure may prevent insertion of the laryngeal mask airway. Br J Anaesth 1992;69:465–467.

30. Asai T, Barclay K, Power I, et al. Cricoid pressure impedes placement of the laryngeal mask airway and subsequent tracheal intubation through the mask. Br J Anaesth 1994;72:47–51.

31. Aoyama K, Takenaka I, Sata T, et al. Cricoid pressure impedes positioning and ventilation through the laryngeal mask airway. Can J Anaesth 1996;43:1035–1040.

32. Brimacombe J. Cricoid pressure and the laryngeal mask airway. Anaesthesia 1991;46:986–987.

33. Brimacombe J, Berry A, White A. Single- compared with double-handed cricoid pressure for insertion of an LMA [Letter]. Br J Anaesth 1994;72:732–734.

34. Brimacombe J, White A, Berry A. Effect of cricoid pressure on ease of insertion of the laryngeal mask airway. Br J Anaesth 1993;71:800–802.

35. Brimacombe JR, Berry AM. Cricoid pressure. Can J Anaesth 1997;44:414–425.

36. Heath ML, Allagain J. Intubation through the laryngeal mask. A technique for unexpected difficult intubation. Anaesthesia 1991;46:545–548.

37. Brimacombe J, Berry A, White A. An algorithm for use of the laryngeal mask airway during failed intubation in the patient with a full stomach. Anesth Analg 1993;77:398–399.

38. Aoyama K, Takenaka I, Sata T, et al. The triple airway manoeuvre for insertion of the laryngeal mask airway in paralyzed patients. Can J Anaesth 1995;42:1010–1016.

39. Chadd GD, Crane DL, Phillips RM, et al. Extubation and reintubation guided by the laryngeal mask airway in a child with the Pierre–Robin syndrome. Anesthesiology 1992;76:640–641.

40. Fukatome T. Correct positioning of the epiglottis for application of the Brain laryngeal mask airway. Anaesthesia 1995;50:818–819.

41. Leader GL. Facilitation of the insertion of the laryngeal mask. Anaesthesia 1991;46:987.

42. Chow BFM, Lewis M, Jones SEF. Laryngeal mask airway in children: insertion technique. Anaesthesia 1991;46:590–591.

43. Cass L. Inserting the laryngeal mask. Anaesthesia and Intensive Care 1991;19:615.

44. Dingley J, Asai T. Insertion methods of the laryngeal mask airway. A survey of current practice in Wales. Anaesthesia 1996;51:596–599.

45. Elwood T, Cox RG. Laryngeal mask insertion in pediatric patients is facilitated with a laryngoscope. Anesth Analg 1995;80:S114.

46. Goudsouzian NG, Denman W, Cleveland R, et al. Radiologic localization of the laryngeal mask airway in children. Anesthesiology 1992;77:1085–1089.

47. Garcia–Pedrajas F, Monedero P, Carrascosa F. Modification of Brain's technique for insertion of laryngeal mask airway. Anesth Analg 1994;79:1024–1025.

48. Jenkins J. The laryngoscope and the laryngeal mask airway. Anaesthesia 1993;48:735.

49. Mason DG, Bingham RM. The laryngeal mask airway in children. Anaesthesia 1990;45:760–763.

50. McNicol LR. Insertion of the laryngeal mask airway in children. Anaesthesia 1991;46:330.

51. Newman PTF. Insertion of a partially inflated laryngeal mask airway. Anaesthesia 1991;46:235.

52. Rowbottom SJ, Simpson DL, Grubb D. The laryngeal mask airway in children. A fibreoptic assessment of positioning. Anaesthesia 1991;46:489–491.

53. Sing G. The laryngeal mask airway and the Guedel airway. Anaesthesia 1994;49:171.

54. van Heerden PV, Kirrage D. Large tonsils and the laryngeal mask airway. Anaesthesia 1989;44:703.

55. Maroof M, Khan RM. LMA and the stylet: a source of new strength for the old mask. Anesth Analg 1993;76:1162.

56. Cino PJ, Webster AC. Laryngeal mask insertion—a useful tip. Anaesthesia 1993;48:1012.

57. Maltby JR, Loken RG, Beriault MT, et al. Laryngeal mask airway with mouth opening less than 20 mm. Can J Anaesth 1995;42:1140–1142.

58. DuPlessis MC, Barr AM, Verghese C, et al. Fibreoptic bronchoscopy under general anaesthesia using the laryngeal mask airway. Eur J Anaesth 1993;10:363–365.

59. Grebenik CR, Ferguson C. In reply. Anesthesiology 1990;73:1054.

60. Mizushima A, Wardall GJ, Simpson DL. The laryngeal mask airway in infants. Anaesthesia 1992;47:849–851.

61. McLeod DH, Narang VPS. Functional and anatomical assessment of the laryngeal mask airway in infants and children. Anaesthesia and Intensive Care 1992;20:109.

62. Nandi PR, Nunn JF, Charlesworth CH, et al. Radiological study of the laryngeal mask. Eur J Anaesth 1991;4(suppl):33–39.

63. Brimacombe J, Berry A. Insertion of the laryngeal mask airway—a prospective study of four techniques. Anaesthesia and Intensive Care 1993;21:89–92.

64. Ball AJ. Laryngeal mask misplacement—a nonproblem. Anesth Analg 1995;81:204.

65. Molloy AR. Unexpected position of the laryngeal mask airway. Anaesthesia 1991;46:592.

66. Mizushima A, Wardall GJ, Simpson DL. The laryngeal mask airway in infants. Anaesthesia 1992;47:849–851.

67. Gurpinar A, Yavascaoglu B, Korfall G, et al. Fibreoptic assessment of positioning of the laryngeal mask airway in children. Br J Anaesth 1996;76:96.

68. Asai T, Morris S. Inflation of the cuff of the laryngeal mask. Anaesthesia 1994;49:1098–1099.

69. Brain AIJ. Course of the hypoglossal nerve in relation to the position of the laryngeal mask airway. Anaesthesia 1995;50:82–83.

70. Brain AIJ. Pressure in laryngeal mask airway cuffs. Anaesthesia 1996;51:603.

71. Ainsworth QP, Calder I. The esophageal detector device and the laryngeal mask. Anaesthesia 1990;45:794.

72. Reference deleted.

73. Wafai Y, Salem MR, Tertaglione A, et al. Facilitation of positioning of the laryngeal mask airway by the self-inflating bulb. Anesthesiology 1994;81:A628.

74. Asai T. The oesophageal detector device is not useful for the laryngeal mask. Anaesthesia 1995;50:175.

75. Burnett YL, Brennan MP, Salem MR. Comparison of end-tidal CO_2, fiberoptic scope, self-inflating bulb, and chest wall movement for correct laryngeal mask placement in pediatric patients. Anesthesiology 1994;81:A1388.

76. Adejumo SWA, Davies MW. The laryngeal mask airway—another trick. Anaesthesia 1996;51:604.

77. Charters P. Digital exploration and the laryngeal mask. Anaesthesia 1996;51:990.

78. Miranda AF, Reddy VG. Controlled ventilation with Brain laryngeal mask. Med J Malaysia 1990;45:65–69.

79. Alexander CA, Leach AB, Thompson AR, et al. Use your Brain. Anaesthesia 1988;43:893–894.

80. Lambert–Jensen P, Christensen NE, Brynnum J. Laryngeal mask and anaesthetic waste gas exposure. Anaesthesia 1992;47:697–700.

81. Maltby JR. The laryngeal mask airway. Anesth Rev 1991;18:55–57.

82. Isserles SA, Rozenberg B. LMA—reduction of gas leak. Can J Anaesth 1995;42:449.

83. Brain AIJ. Three cases of difficult intubation overcome by the laryngeal mask airway. Anaesthesia 1985;40:353–355.

84. Brain AL, McGhee TD, McAteer EJ, et al. The laryngeal mask airway. Development and preliminary trials of a new type of airway. Anaesthesia 1985;40:356–361.

85. Asai T, Fujise K, Uchida M. Use of the laryngeal mask in a child with tracheal stenosis. Anesthesiology 1991;75:903–904.

86. Brimacombe J, Berry A. Leak reduction with the laryngeal mask airway—the application of external neck pressure. Can J Anaesth 1996;43:537.

87. Paterson SJ, Byrne PJ, Molesky MG, et al. Neonatal resuscitation using the laryngeal mask airway. Anesthesiology 1994;80:1248–1253.

88. Haynes SR, Morton NS. The laryngeal mask airway: a review of its use in paediatric anaesthesia. Paediatr Anaesth 1993;3:65–73.

89. Matta BF, Marsh DS, Nevin M. Laryngeal mask airway: a more successful method of insertion. J Clin Anesth 1995;7:132–135.

90. Navaratnam S, Taylor S. The laryngeal mask—another insertion technique. Anaesthesia and Intensive Care 1993;21:250.

91. Southern DA, Lake APJ, Wadon AJ. The laryngeal mask—a modification in its use and design. Anaesthesia 1992;47:530.

92. Wakeling HG, Butler PJ, Baxter PJC. The laryngeal mask airway: a comparison between two insertion techniques. Anesth Analg 1997;84:S278.

93. Brimacombe J, Berry A. The flexible, reinforced tube LMA—initial experience. Anaesthesia and Intensive Care 1993;21:379.

94. Asai T, Stacey M, Barclay K. Stylet for reinforced laryngeal mask airway. Anaesthesia 1993;48:636–637.

95. Brimacombe J, Berry A. Stylet for reinforced laryngeal mask [Reply]. Anaesthesia 1993;48:637.

96. Bapat PP. The Bosworth introducer and the flexible reinforced laryngeal mask airway. Anaesthesia 1997;52:713–714.

97. Harris S, Perks D. Introducer for the reinforced laryngeal mask airway. Anaesthesia 1997;52:607–608.

98. Moylan SL, Luce MA. The reinforced laryngeal mask airway in paediatric radiotherapy. Br J Anaesth 1993;71:172.

99. Philpott B, Renwick. An introducer for the flexible laryngeal mask airway. Anaesthesia 1993;48:174.

100. Palmer JHM. Introducing the re-inforced laryngeal mask airway. Anaesthesia 1994;49:1098.

101. Bosworth A, Jago RH. The Bosworth introducer for use with the flexible reinforced laryngeal mask airway. Anaesthesia 1997;52:281–282.

102. Welsh BE. Use of a modified Magill's forceps to place a flexible laryngeal mask. Anaesthesia 1995;50:1002–1003.

103. Asai T. Use of the laryngeal mask for tracheal intubation in patients at increased risk of aspiration of gastric contents. Anesthesiology 1992;77:1029–1030.

104. Reference deleted.

105. Asai T. Fiberoptic tracheal intubation through the laryngeal mask in an awake patient with cervical spine injury. Anesth Analg 1993;77:404.

106. Brain AIJ. The development of the laryngeal mask—a brief history of the invention, early clinical studies and experimental work from which the laryngeal mask evolved. Eur J Anaesth 1991;4(Suppl):5–17.

107. Brimacombe J. The laryngeal mask airway: use in the management of stridor. Anaesthesia and Intensive Care 1992;20:117–118.

108. Ferguson C, Herdman M, Evans K, et al. Flow resistance of the laryngeal mask in awake subjects. Br J Anaesth 1991;66:440P.

109. McCrirrick A, Pracilio JA. Awake intubation: a new technique. Anaesthesia 1991;46:661–663.

110. Markakis DA, Sayson SC, Schreiner MS. Insertion of the laryngeal mask airway in awake infants with the Robin sequence. Anesth Analg 1992;75:822–824.

111. Sellers WFS, Edwards RJ. Awake intubation with Brain laryngeal airway. Anaesthesia and Intensive Care 1991;19:473.

112. Williams PJ, Bailey PM. Management of failed oral fibreoptic intubation with laryngeal mask airway insertion under topical anaesthesia. Can J Anaesth 1993;40:287.

113. Brimacombe JR, Berry A. Active swallowing to aid LMA insertion in awake patients. Anesth Analg 1994; 78:1029.

114. Brimacombe J, Berry A. Translucent vinyl tubing—an alternative bite guard for the LMA. Anaesthesia and Intensive Care 1993;21:893.

115. Marks LF. Protection of the laryngeal mask airway. Anaesthesia 1990;45:259.

116. Maltby JR, Loken RG, Low JS. Bite guard for laryngeal mask airway. Anaesthesia 1993;48:273.

117. Townsend M, Frew RM, Hoyle JR. Bite block for the laryngeal mask airway. Anaesthesia 1995;50:918.

118. Bremner WGM. Fixing the laryngeal mask airway during eye surgery. Anaesthesia 1993;48:542.

119. Conacher ID. A method of fixing of laryngeal mask airways. Anaesthesia 1993;48:638.

120. Nott MR. A tie for the laryngeal mask airway. Anaesthesia 1993;48:1013.

121. Worsley MH, Howie CCM. Fixation of the laryngeal mask airway. Anaesthesia 1990;45:1001.

122. Bignell S, Brimacombe J. LMA stability and fixation. Anaesthesia and Intensive Care 1994;22:746.

123. Mollhoff T, Burgard G, Prien T. Low-flow and minimal-flow anesthesia and the laryngeal mask airway. Anesthesiology 1995;83:A499.

124. Brimacombe JR, Berry A. Monitoring anesthetic depth during laryngeal mask anesthesia. J Clin Anesth 1994;6:525–526.

125. Spain BT, Riley RH, Salbutamol via the LMA for relief of bronchospasm. Anaesthesia 1992;47:1107.

126. Ngan Kee WD. The laryngeal mask airway and intraocular surgery. Anaesthesia 1992;47:446–447.

127. Capdevila X, Biboulet P, Vallce M, et al. Pressure support ventilation with a laryngeal mask airway during general anesthesia. Anesthesiology 1995;83: A1226.

128. Devitt JH, Wenstone R, Noel AG, et al. The laryngeal mask airway and positive-pressure ventilation. Anesthesiology 1994;80:550–555.

129. Epstein RH, Ferouz F, Jenkins MA. Airway sealing pressures of the laryngeal mask airway in pediatric patients. J Clin Anesth 1996;8:93–98.

130. Fullekrug B, Pothmann W, Werner C, et al. The laryngeal mask airway: anesthetic gas leakage and fiberoptic control of positioning. J Clin Anesth 1993; 5:357–363.

131. Gursoy F, Algren JT, Skjonsby BS. Positive pressure ventilation with the laryngeal mask airway in children. Anesth Analg 1996;82:33–38.

132. Weiler N, Latorre F, Eberle B, et al. Respiratory mechanics, gastric insufflation pressure, and air leakage of the laryngeal mask airway. Anesth Analg 1997;84: 1025–1028.

133. Wittmann PH, Wittmann FW. Laryngeal mask and gastric dilatation. Anaesthesia 1991;46:1083.

134. Brimacombe J, Berry A. The laryngeal mask airway in elective difficult intubation. J Clin Anesth 1994; 6:450–451.

135. Collier C. A hazard with the laryngeal mask airway. Anaesthesia and Intensive Care 1991;19:301.

136. Lumb AB, Wrigley MW. The effect of nitrous oxide on laryngeal mask cuff pressure. Anaesthesia 1992; 47:320–323.

137. Marjot R. Pressure exerted by the laryngeal mask airway cuff upon the pharyngeal mucosa. Br J Anaesth 1993;70:25–29.

138. O'Kelly SW, Heath KJ, Lawes EG. A study of laryngeal mask inflation. Pressures exerted on the pharynx. Anaesthesia 1993;48:1075–1078.

139. Wright ES, Filshie J, Dark CH. Laryngeal mask cuff pressure and nitrous oxide. Anaesthesia 1992;47: 713–714.

140. Brimacombe J, Berry A. Laryngeal mask airway cuff pressure and position during anaesthesia lasting one to two hrs. Can J Anaesth 1994;41:589–593.

141. Brimacombe J, Berry A. Laryngeal mask airway cuff pressure and position: the effect of adding nitrous oxide to the cuff. Anesthesiology 1994;80:957–958.

142. Gursoy F, Algren JT, Skjonsby BS. The effect of nitrous oxide (N_2O) on laryngeal mask airway (LMA) volume and pressure in children. Anesthesiology 1994;81:A1320.

142a. Marjot R. Laryngeal mask cuff pressures. Anaesthesia 1994;49:447.

143. Fawcett WJ, Daya H, Weir N. Recurrent laryngeal nerve palsy and the laryngeal mask airway. Anaesthesia 1996;51:708.

144. Morris GN, Marjot R. Laryngeal mask airway performance: effect of cuff deflation during anaesthesia. Br J Anaesth 1996;76:456–458.

145. Marjot RM, Morris G. Optimal intracuff pressures with the laryngeal mask. Br J Anaesth 1996;77:296.

146. Brimacombe J, Berry A. Laryngeal mask cuff pressure [Reply]. Anaesthesia 1994;49:447–448.

147. Brimacombe J, Berry A, Brain AIJ. Optimal intracuff pressures with the laryngeal mask. Br J Anaesth 1996; 77:295–296.

148. Broadway PJ, Royle P. Supplementary oxygen and the laryngeal mask airway. Anaesthesia 1990;45: 792–793.

149. Dashfield AK, Langton JA, Johnston CG, et al. Two oxygen delivery devices compared in a modified laryngeal mask airway. Can J Anaesth 1997;44: 572–573.

150. Goodwin APL. Postoperative oxygen via the laryngeal mask airway. Anaesthesia 1991;46:700.

151. Kennedy R, Meyer M, Joyce C. Supplemental oxygen using a laryngeal mask airway. Anaesthesia and Intensive Care 1992;20:118.

152. Lewis RP, Porter M. Supplementary oxygen and the laryngeal mask airway. Anaesthesia 1991;46:70.

153. Brimacombe J. The laryngeal mask airway: tool for airway management. J Post Anesth Nurs 1993;8: 88–95.

154. Erskine RJ, Rabey PG. The laryngeal mask airway in recovery. Anaesthesia 1992;47:354.

155. Edwards ND. Lignocaine gel and the laryngeal mask airway. Anaesthesia 1995;50:746–747.

156. Gataure PS, Latto IP, Rust S. Complications associated with removal of the laryngeal mask airway: a comparison of removal in deeply anesthetized versus awake patients. Can J Anaesth 1995;42:1113–1116.

157. Kitching AJ, Walpole AR, Blogg CE. Removal of the laryngeal mask airway in children: anaesthetized compared with awake. Br J Anaesth 1996;76:874–876.

158. Laffon M, Plaud B, Dubousset A-M, et al. Removal of laryngeal mask airway; airway complications in children, anesthetized versus awake. Paediatr Anaesth 1994;4:35–37.

159. McGinn G, Haynes SR, Morton NS. An evaluation of the laryngeal mask airway during routine paediatric anaesthesia. Paediatr Anaesth 1993;3:23–28.

160. Splinter WM, Reid CW. Removal of the laryngeal mask airway in children: deep anesthesia versus awake. J Clin Anesth 1997;9:4–7.

161. Brimacombe J, Johns K. Modified intravent LMA. Anaesthesia and Intensive Care 1991;19:607.

162. Hansen TG, Joensen H, Henneberg SW, et al. Laryngeal mask airway guided tracheal intubation in a neonate with the Pierre–Robin syndrome. Acta Anaesthesiol Scand 1995;39:129–131.

163. Asai T. Tracheal intubation through the laryngeal mask airway. Anesthesiology 1996;85:439.

164. Alfery DD. The laryngeal mask airway and the ASA difficult airway algorithm [Letter]. Anesthesiology 1996;85:685.

165. Choi JE, Leal YR, Johnson MD. Fiberoptic intubation through the laryngeal mask airway. J Clin Anesth 1996;8:687–688.

166. Silk JM, Hill HM, Calder I. The distance between the grille of the laryngeal mask airway and the vocal cords. Anaesthesia 1994;49:170.

167. Ullman DA. Laryngeal mask airway and the ASA difficult airway algorithm: III. Anesthesiology 1996;85: 686.

168. Benumof JL. Laryngeal mask airway and the ASA difficult airway algorithm. Anesthesiology 1996;84: 686–699.

169. Pennant JH, Joshi GP. Intubation through the laryngeal mask airway. Anesthesiology 1995;83:891–892.

170. Preis CA, Preis IS. Oversize endotracheal tubes and intubation via laryngeal mask airway. Anesthesiology 1997;87:187.

171. Yamashita M. Longer tube length eases endotracheal intubation via the laryngeal mask airway in infants and children. J Clin Anesth 1997;9:432–433.

172. Goldie AS, Hudson I. Fibreoptic tracheal intubation through a modified laryngeal mask. Paediatr Anaesth 1992;2:343–344.

173. Haxby EJ, Liban JB. Fibreoptic intubation via laryngeal mask in an infant with Goldenhar syndrome. Anaesthesia and Intensive Care 1995;23:753.

174. Asai T, Latto IP, Vaughan RS. The distance between the grille of the laryngeal mask airway and the vocal cords. Is conventional intubation through the laryngeal mask safe? Anaesthesia 1993;48:667–669.

175. Biro P, Kaplan V, Bloch KE. Anesthetic management of a patient with obstructive sleep apnea syndrome and difficult airway access. J Clin Anesth 1995;7: 417–421.

176. Darling JR, Keohane M, Murray JM. A split laryngeal mask as an aid to training in fibreoptic tracheal intubation. Anaesthesia 1993;48:1079–1082.

177. Lim SL, Tay DHB, Thomas E. A comparison of three types of tracheal tube for use in laryngeal mask assisted blind orotracheal intubation. Anaesthesia 1994;49:255–257.

178. Ball DR. Tolerance of the laryngeal mask airway. Anesth Analg 1997;84:469.

179. Kessell G, Gray C. Tolerance of the laryngeal mask airway. Anesth Analg 1997;84:469–470.

180. Roth DM, Benumof JL. Intubation through a laryngeal mask airway with a nasal RAE tube: stabilization of the proximal end of the tube. Anesthesiology 1996;85:1220.

181. Breen PH. Simple technique to remove laryngeal mask airway "guide" after endotracheal intubation. Anesth Analg 1996;82:1302.

182. Chadd GD, Walford AJ, Crane DL. The 3.5/4.5 modification for fiberscope-guided tracheal intubation using the laryngeal mask airway. Anesth Analg 1992;75:307–308.

183. Reynolds PI, O'Kelly SW. Fiberoptic intubation and the laryngeal mask airway. Anesthesiology 1993;79:1144.

184. Theroux MC, Kettrick RG, Khine HH. Laryngeal mask airway and fiberoptic endoscopy in an infant with Schwartz–Jampel syndrome. Anesthesiology 1995;82:605.

185. Zagnoev M, McCloskey J, Martin T. Fiberoptic intubation via the laryngeal mask airway. Anesth Analg 1994;78:813–814.

186. Maroof M, Siddique MS, Khan RM. Modified laryngeal mask as an aid to fiberoptic endotracheal intubation. Acta Anaesthesiol Scand 1993;37:124.

187. Brimacombe J, Dunbar–Reid K. The effect of introducing fibreoptic bronchoscopes on gas flow in laryngeal masks and tracheal tubes. Anaesthesia 1996;51:923–928.

188. Brimacombe J. Analysis of 1500 laryngeal mask uses by one anaesthetist in adults undergoing routine anaesthesia. Anaesthesia 1996;51:76–80.

189. Dubreuil M, Ecoffey C. Laryngeal mask guided tracheal intubation in paediatric anaesthesia. Paediatr Anaesth 1992;2:344.

190. Brain AIJ. Further developments of the laryngeal mask. Anaesthesia 1989;44:530.

191. Heath ML. Endotracheal intubation through the laryngeal mask—helpful when laryngoscopy is difficult or dangerous. Eur J Anaesth 1991;4(Suppl):41–45.

192. Brimacombe J, Berry A. Placement of a Cook airway exchange catheter via the laryngeal mask airway. Anaesthesia 1993;48:351–352.

193. Carey MF, Smith J, Cooney CM. Laryngeal mask to aid tracheal intubation. Anaesthesia 1991;46:1083.

194. Silk JM, Hill HM, Calder I. Difficult intubation and the laryngeal mask. Eur J Anaesth 1991;4(Suppl):47–51.

195. Chadd GD, Ackers JWL, Bailey PM. Difficult intubation aided by the laryngeal mask airway. Anaesthesia 1989;44:1015.

196. Higgins D, Astley BA, Berg S. Guided intubation via the laryngeal mask. Anaesthesia 1992;47:816.

197. Hornbein TF, Turnquist K, Freund P. Another way through a laryngeal mask airway. Anesthesiology 1995;83:880.

198. Allison A, McCrory J. Tracheal placement of a gum elastic bougie using the laryngeal mask airway. Anaesthesia 1990;45:419–420.

199. Asai T, Vaughan RS. Misuse of the laryngeal mask airway. Anaesthesia 1994;49:467–469.

200. Crichlow A, Locken R, Todesco J. The laryngeal mask airway and fibreoptic laryngoscopy. Can J Anaesth 1992;39:742–744.

201. Hapberg C, Abramson D, Chelly J. A comparison of fiber optic orotracheal intubation using two different intubating conduits. Anesthesiology 1995;83:A1220.

202. Johnson CM, Sims C. Awake fibreoptic intubation via laryngeal mask in an infant with Goldenhar's syndrome. Anaesthesia and Intensive Care 1994;22:194–197.

203. Smith JE, Sherwood NA. Combined use of a laryngeal mask airway and fibreoptic laryngoscope in difficult intubation. Anaesthesia and Intensive Care 1991;19:471–472.

204. Denman WT, Gouldsouzian NG. Position of the laryngeal mask airway. Anesthesiology 1992;77:401–402.

205. Brimacombe J. The split laryngeal mask airway. Anaesthesia 1993;48:639.

206. Koga K, Asai T, Vaughan RS. Effect of the size of a tracheal tube and the efficacy of the use of the laryngeal mask for fibrescope-aided tracheal intubation. Anaesthesia 1997;52:131–135.

207. Atherton DPL, O'Sullivan E, Lowe D, et al. A ventilation-exchange bougie for fibreoptic intubations with the laryngeal mask airway. Anaesthesia 1996;51:1123–1126.

208. Hasham F, Kumar CM, Lawler PGP. The use of the laryngeal mask airway to assist fibreoptic orotracheal intubation. Anaesthesia 1991;46:891.

209. Hasan MA, Black AE. A new technique for fibreoptic tracheal intubation in children. Anaesthesia 1994;49:1031–1033.

210. Heard CMB, Caldicott LD, Fletcher JE, et al. Fiberoptic-guided endotracheal intubation via the laryngeal mask airway in pediatric patients: a report of a series of cases. Anesth Analg 1996;82:1287–1289.

211. Kadota Y, Oda T, Yoshimura N. Application of a laryngeal mask to a fiberoptic bronchoscope-aided tracheal intubation. J Clin Anesth 1992;4:503–504.

212. Logan S, Charters P. Laryngeal mask and fibreoptic tracheal intubation. Anaesthesia 1994;49:543–544.

213. Harvey SC, Fishman RL, Edwards SM. Retrograde intubation through a laryngeal mask airway. Anesthesiology 1996;85:1503–1504.

214. Thomson KD. A blind nasal intubation using a laryngeal mask airway. Anaesthesia 1993;48:785–787.

215. Marjot R, Cook TM, Baylis R. Teaching fibreoptic nasotracheal intubation via the laryngeal mask airway. Anaesthesia 1996;51:511–512.

216. Alexander R, Moore C. The laryngeal mask airway and training in nasotracheal intubation. Anaesthesia 1995;50:350–351.

217. Brain AIJ. Autoclaving laryngeal masks. Anesth Analg 1994;79:199.

218. Brimacombe J. Spontaneous reinflation characteristics of the laryngeal mask airway. Can J Anaesth 1993; 40:873.

219. Biro P. Damage to laryngeal masks during sterilization. Anesth Analg 1993;77:1079.

220. Brimacombe J. Laryngeal mask residual volume and damage during sterilization. Anesth Analg 1994;79: 391.

221. Shannon PE, Steel D. Potential hazard from incorrect cleaning of laryngeal mask airway. Anaesthesia 1996; 51:603–604.

222. Thomson SJ, Healy M, Littlejohn IH. Nitrous oxide and laryngeal mask cuff pressure. Anaesthesia 1992; 47:815.

223. Bhatt SB, Kendall AP, Lin ES, et al. Resistance and additional inspiratory work imposed by the laryngeal mask airway. Anaesthesia 1992;47:343–347.

224. Berry AM, Verghese C. Changes in pulmonary mechanics during IPPV with the laryngeal mask airway compared to the endotracheal tube. Anesth Analg 1994;78:S38.

225. Boisson–Bertrand D, Hannhart B, Rousselot JM, et al. Comparative effects of laryngeal mask and tracheal tube on total respiratory resistance in anaesthetised patients. Anaesthesia 1994;49:846–849.

226. Joshi GP, Morrison SG, Miciotto CJ, et al. Evaluation of work of breathing during anesthesia: use of laryngeal mask airway versus tracheal tube. Anesthesiology 1994;81:A1449.

227. Brimacombe J, Archdeacon J. The LMA for unplanned prolonged procedures. Can J Anaesth 1995; 42:1176.

228. Brimacombe J. Shorney N. The laryngeal mask airway and prolonged balanced regional anaesthesia. Can J Anaesth 1993;40:360–364.

229. Arosio EM, Conci F. Use of the laryngeal mask airway for respiratory distress in the intensive care unit. Anaesthesia 1995;50:635–636.

230. Johnston DF, Wrigley SR, Robb PJ, et al. The laryngeal mask airway in paediatric anaesthesia. Anaesthesia 1990;45:924–927.

231. Smith I, White PF. Use of the laryngeal mask airway as an alternative to a face mask during outpatient arthroscopy. Anesthesiology 1992;77:850–855.

232. Ruby RRF, Webster AC, Morley–Forster PK, et al. Laryngeal mask airway in paediatric otolaryngologic surgery. J Otolaryngol 1995;24:288–291.

233. Russell R, Judkins KC. The laryngeal mask airway and facial burns. Anaesthesia 1990;45:894.

234. Garbin GS, Bogetz MS, Grekin RC, Frieden IJ. The laryngeal mask as an airway during laser treatment of post wine stains. Anesthesiology 1991;75:A953.

235. Michel MZ, Stubbing JF. Laryngeal mask airway and laryngeal spasm. Anaesthesia 1991;46:71.

236. Smith TGC, Whittet H, Heyworth T. Laryngomalacia—a specific indication for the laryngeal mask. Anaesthesia 1992;47:910.

237. Sarma VJ. The use of a laryngeal mask airway in spontaneously breathing patients. Acta Anaesthesiol Scand 1990;34:669–672.

238. O'Kelly SW, Reynolds PI, Collito M. The use of fiberoptic endoscopy and laryngeal mask airway in securing the traumatized airway in the pediatric patient. Am J Anesthesiol 1995;22:152–153.

239. Beveridge ME. Laryngeal mask anaesthesia for repair of cleft palate. Anaesthesia 1989;44:656–657.

240. Bailey C, Chung R. Use of the laryngeal mask airway in a patient with Edward's syndrome. Anaesthesia 1992;47:713.

241. Baraka A. Laryngeal mask airway for resuscitation of a newborn with Pierre–Robin syndrome. Anesthesiology 1995;83:645–646.

242. Denny NM, Desilva KD, Webber PA. Laryngeal mask airway for emergency tracheostomy in a neonate. Anaesthesia 1990;45:895.

243. Ebata T, Nishiki S, Masuda A, et al. Anaesthesia for Treacher Collins syndrome using a laryngeal mask airway. Can J Anaesth 1991;38:1043–1045.

244. Mecklem D, Brimacombe JR, Yarker J. Glossopexy in Pierre–Robin sequences using the laryngeal mask airway. J Clin Anesth 1995;7:267–269.

245. Wheatley RS, Stainthorp SF. Intubation of a one-day-old baby with Pierre–Robin syndrome via a laryngeal mask. Anaesthesia 1994;49:733.

246. Allen JG, Flower EA. The Brain laryngeal mask. An alternative to difficult intubation. Br Dent J 1990; 168:202–204.

247. Brimacombe J, Berry A, Van Duren P. Use of a size 2 LMA to relieve life-threatening hypoxia in an adult with quinsy. Anaesthesia and Intensive Care 1993; 21:475–476.

248. Pennant JH, Gajraj NM, Yamanouchi KJ. The laryngeal mask airway and laryngeal polyposis. Anesth Analg 1994;78:1206–1207.

249. King CJ, Davey AJ, Chandradeva K. Emergency use of the laryngeal mask airway in severe upper airway obstruction caused by supraglottic oedema. Br J Anaesth 1995;75:785–786.

250. Biro P, Shahinian H. Management of difficult intubation caused by lingual tonsillar hyperplasia. Anesth Analg 1994;79:389.

251. Kumar CM. Laryngeal mask airway for inadequate reversal. Anaesthesia 1990;45:792.

252. Cork R, Monk JE. Management of a suspected and unsuspected difficult laryngoscopy with the laryngeal mask airway. J Clin Anesth 1992;4:230–234.

253. Thompson KD, Ordman AJ, Parkhouse N, et al. Use of the Brain laryngeal mask airway in anticipation of difficult tracheal intubation. Br J Plast Surg 1989;42:478–480.

254. Aziz ES, Thompson AR, Baer S. Difficult laryngeal mask insertion in a patient with Forestier's disease. Anaesthesia 1995;50:370.

255. Dimitriou VM, Voyagis GS, Malefaki A. Use of the LMA for management of difficult airway due to extensive facial and neck contracture. Anesthesiology 1997;86:1011–1012.

256. Defalque RJ, Hyder ML. Laryngeal mask airway in severe cervical ankylosis. Can J Anaesth 1997;44:305–307.

257. Smith BL. Brain airway in anaesthesia for patients with juvenile chronic arthritis [Letter]. Anaesthesia 1988;43:421.

258. Kiyama S. Intubation via a laryngeal mask airway and cervical spine surgery. Anaesthesia 1995;50:83.

259. Logan A. Use of the laryngeal mask in a patient with an unstable fracture of the cervical spine. Anaesthesia 1991;46:987.

260. Pennant JH, Gajraj NM, Pace NA. Laryngeal mask airway in cervical spine injuries. Anesth Analg 1992;75:1074.

261. Aye T, Milne B. Use of the laryngeal mask prior to definitive intubation in a difficult airway: a case report. J Emerg Med 1995;5:711–714.

262. Baraka A. Laryngeal mask airway in the cannot-intubate, cannot-ventilate situation. Anesthesiology 1993;79:1151–1152.

263. Brimacombe J, Berry A. The laryngeal mask airway for obstetric anaesthesia and neonatal resuscitation. Int J Obstet Anesth 1994;3:211–218.

264. Calder I, Ordman AJ, Jacklowski A, et al. The Brain laryngeal mask airway. An alternative to emergency tracheal intubation. Anaesthesia 1990;45:137–139.

265. Lee JJ, Yau K, Barcroft J. LMA and respiratory arrest after anterior cervical fusion. Can J Anaesth 1993;40:395–396.

266. Chadwick IS, Vohra A. Anaesthesia for emergency caesarean section using the Brain laryngeal airway. Anaesthesia 1989;44:261–262.

267. Castresana MR, Cancel AR, Stefansson S, et al. Use of the laryngeal mask airway during thoracotomy in a paediatric patient with Cri-du-Chat syndrome. Anesth Analg 1994;78:817.

268. De Mello WF, Kocan JM. The laryngeal mask in failed intubation. Anaesthesia 1990;45:689–690.

269. Dalrymple G, Lloyd E. Laryngeal mask: a more secure airway than intubation. Anaesthesia 1992;47:712–713.

270. McClune S, Regan M, Moore J. Laryngeal mask airway for caesarean section. Anesthesia 1990;45:227–228.

271. McNamara JT, Fisher WJ. The laryngeal mask airway and the multiple injured patient. Anaesthesia 1996;51:97–98.

272. Nath G, Major V. The laryngeal mask in the management of a paediatric difficult airway. Anaesthesia and Intensive Care 1992;20:518–520.

273. Owen G, Browning S, Davies CA, et al. The laryngeal mask. Br Med J 1993;306:580.

274. Priscu V, Priscu L, Soroker D. Laryngeal mask for failed intubation in emergency Caesarean section. Can J Anaesth 1992;39:893.

275. Ravalia A, Goddard JM. The laryngeal mask and difficult tracheal intubation. Anaesthesia 1990;45:168.

276. Storey J. The laryngeal mask for failed intubation at caesarean section. Anaesthesia and Intensive Care 1992;20:118–119.

277. Verghese C, Brimacombe JR. Survey of laryngeal mask airway usage in 11,910 patients: safety and efficacy for conventional and nonconventional usage. Anesth Analg 1996;82:129–133.

278. White A, Sinclair M, Pillai R. Laryngeal mask airway for coronary artery bypass grafting. Anaesthesia 1991;46:1083.

279. Asai T. The view of the glottis at laryngoscopy after unexpectedly difficult placement of the laryngeal mask. Anaesthesia 1996;51:1063–1065.

280. Brimacombe J, Berry A. Mallampati classification and laryngeal mask airway insertion. Anaesthesia 1993;48:347.

281. McCrory CR, Moriarty DC. Laryngeal mask airway positioning is related to Mallampati grading in adults. Anesth Analg 1995;81:1001–1004.

282. Asai T, Morris S. Elective use of the laryngeal mask in patients with difficult airways. Can Anaesth Soc J 1993;40:1221–1222.

283. Barclay K, Wall T, Asai T. Intra-ocular pressure changes in patients with glaucoma. Comparison between the laryngeal mask airway and tracheal tube. Anaesthesia 1994;49:159–162.

284. Demiralp S, Ates Y, Yorukoglu D, et al. Laryngeal mask airway does not increase intraocular pressure regardless of the induction method. Br J Anaesth 1996;76:96.

285. Holden R, Morsman CDG, Butler J, et al. Intra-ocular pressure changes using the laryngeal mask airway and tracheal tube. Anaesthesia 1991;46:922–924.

286. Lamb K, James MFM, Janicki PK. The laryngeal mask airway for intraocular surgery: effects on intraocular pressure and stress responses. Br J Anaesth 1992;69:143–147.

287. Watcha MF, White PF, Tychsen L, et al. Comparative effects of laryngeal mask airway and endotracheal tube insertion on intraocular pressure in children. Anesth Analg 1992;75:355–360.

288. Whitford AM, Hone SW, O'Hare B, et al. Intra-ocular pressure changes following laryngeal mask airway insertion: a comparative study. Anaesthesia 1997;52:794–796.

289. Akhtar TM, McMurray P, Kerr WJ, et al. A comparison of laryngeal mask airway with tracheal tube for intra-ocular ophthalmic surgery. Anaesthesia 1992;47:668–671.

290. Myint Y, Singh AK, Peacock JE, et al. Changes in intra-ocular pressure during general anaesthesia. A comparison of spontaneous breathing through a laryngeal mask with positive pressure ventilation through a tracheal tube. Anaesthesia 1995;50:126–129.

291. McCartney CA, Wilkinson DJ. The laryngeal mask airway and intra-ocular surgery. Anaesthesia 1992;47:445.

292. Rabey PG, Murphy PJ. The laryngeal mask airway and intra-ocular surgery. Reply. Anaesthesia 1992;47:445–446.

293. Haden RM, Pinnock CA, Campbell RL. The laryngeal mask for intraocular surgery. Br J Anaesth 1993;71:772–775.

294. Ripart J, Cohendy R, Eledjam J-J. The laryngeal mask and intraocular surgery. Br J Anaesth 1993;70:704.

295. Holden R, Morsman D, Butler J, et al. The laryngeal mask airway and intra-ocular surgery. Anaesthesia 1992;47:446.

296. Webster AC, Reid WD, Siebert LF, et al. Laryngeal mask airway for anaesthesia for cryopexy in low birth weight infants. Can J Anaesth 1995;42:361–362.

297. Lonnqvist PA. Successful use of laryngeal mask airway in low-weight ex-premature infants with bronchopulmonary dysplasia undergoing cryotherapy for retinopathy of the premature. Anesthesiology 1995;83:422–424.

298. Ferrari LR, Goudsouzian NG. The use of the laryngeal mask airway in children with bronchopulmonary dysplasia. Anesth Analg 1995;81:310–313.

299. Gunawardene RD. Laryngeal mask and patients with chronic respiratory disease. Anaesthesia 1989;44:531.

300. Lawson R, Lloyd–Thomas AR. Three diagnostic conundrums solved using the laryngeal mask airway. Anaesthesia 1993;48:790–791.

301. Asai T, Morris S. The laryngeal mask and patients with 'collapsible' airways. Anaesthesia 1994;49:169–170.

302. Asai T, Fujise K, Uchida M. Laryngeal mask and tracheal stenosis. Anaesthesia 1993;48:81.

303. Slinger P, Robinson R, Shennib H, et al. Case Conference. Alternative technique for laser resection of a carinal obstruction. J Cardiothorac Vasc Anesth 1992;6:749–755.

304. Catala JC, Pedrajas FG, Carrera J, et al. Placement of an endotracheal device via the laryngeal mask airway in a patient with tracheal stenosis. Anesthesiology 1996;84:239–240.

305. Van De Putte P, Martens P. Anaesthetic management for placement of a stent for high tracheal stenosis. Anaesthesia and Intensive Care 1994;22:619–621.

306. Kokkinis K, Papageorgiou E. Failure of the laryngeal mask airway (LMA) to ventilate patients with severe tracheal stenosis. Resuscitation 1995;30:21–22.

307. Hattamer SJ, Dodds TM. Use of the laryngeal mask airway to manage a patient with anterior mediastinal mass. Anesth Analg 1995;80:SCA139.

308. West KJ, Ahmed MI. The laryngeal, mask airway in mediastinoscopy. Anaesthesia 1993;48:826–827.

309. Thomson KD. Laryngeal mask airway for elective tracheostomy. Anaesthesia 1992;47:76.

310. Dexter TJ. The laryngeal mask airway: a method to improve visualization of the trachea and larynx during fibreoptic assisted percutaneous tracheostomy. Anaesthesia and Intensive Care 1994;22:35–39.

311. Brimacombe J, Clarke G, Simons S. The laryngeal mask airway and endoscopic guided percutaneous tracheostomy. Anaesthesia 1994:49:358–359.

312. Eckhardt WF III, Forman S, Denman W, et al. Another use for the laryngeal mask airway: as a blocker during tracheoplasty. Anesth Analg 1995;80:622–624.

313. Divatia JV, Sareen R, Upadhye SM, et al. Anaesthetic management of tracheal surgery using the laryngeal mask airway. Anaesthesia and Intensive Care 1994;22:69–73.

314. Akhtar TM. Laryngeal mask airways and visualization of vocal cords during thyroid surgery. Can J Anaesth 1991;38:140.

315. Dich–Nielsen JO, Nagel P. Flexible fibreoptic bronchoscopy via the laryngeal mask. Acta Anaesthesiol Scand 1993;37:17–19.

316. Greatorex RA, Denny NM. Application of the laryngeal mask airway to thyroid surgery and the preservation of the recurrent laryngeal nerve. Ann Roy Coll Surg Eng 1991;73:352–354.

317. Hobbiger HE, Allen JG, Greatorex RG, et al. The laryngeal mask airway for thyroid and parathyroid surgery. Anaesthesia 1996;51:972–974.

318. Maroof M, Siddique M, Khan RM. Post-thyroidectomy vocal cord examination by fibrescopy aided by the laryngeal mask airway. Anaesthesia 1992;47:445.

319. Maroof M, Khan RM, Cooper T, et al. Post thyroidectomy vocal cord examination using LMA aided fiberscopy. Anesthesiology 1993;79:A1083.

320. Stott S, Riley R. Visualising the airway after thyroidectomy. Anaesthesia and Intensive Care 1994;22:121.

321. Tanigawa K, Inoue Y, Iwata S. Protection of recurrent laryngeal nerve during neck surgery: a new combination of neutracer, laryngeal mask airway, and fibreoptic bronchoscope. Anesthesiology 1991;74:966–967.

322. Goldik Z, Lazarovici H, Baron E, et al. Continuous fibreoptic video laryngoscopy through the laryngeal mask during thyroidectomy. Br J Anaesth 1995;74:13.

323. Charters P, Cave–Bigley D, Roysam CS. Should a laryngeal mask be routinely used in patients undergoing thyroid surgery. Anesthesiology 1991;75:918–919.

324. Tanigawa K, Inoue Y, Iwata S. In reply. Anesthesiology 1991;75:918–919.

325. Briggs RJS, Bailey P, Howard DJ. The laryngeal mask: A new type of airway in anesthesia for direct laryngoscopy. Otol Head Neck Surg 1992;107:603–605.

326. Brimacombe J, Sher M, Laing D, et al. The laryngeal mask airway: a new technique for fiberoptic guided vocal cord biopsy. J Clin Anesth 1996;8:273–275.

327. Daum REO, O'Reilly BJ. The laryngeal mask airway in ENT surgery. J Laryngol Otol 1992;106:28–30.

328. Sher M, Brimacombe J, Laing D. Anaesthesia for laser pharyngoplasty—a comparison for laser pharyngoplasty—a comparison of the tracheal tube with the reinforce laryngeal mask airway. Anaesthesia and Intensive Care 1995;23:149–153.

329. Williams PJ, Thompsett C, Bailey PM. Comparison of the reinforced laryngeal mask airway and tracheal intubation for nasal surgery. Anaesthesia 1995;50:987–989.

330. Alexander CA. A modified Intravent laryngeal mask for ENT and dental anaesthesia. Anaesthesia 1990;45:892–893.

331. Fiani N, Scandella C, Giolitto N, et al. Comparison of reinforced laryngeal mask vs endotracheal tube in tonsillectomy. Anesthesiology 1994;81:A491.

332. Williams PJ, Bailey PM. Comparison of the reinforced laryngeal mask airway and tracheal intubation for adenotonsillectomy. Br J Anaesth 1993;70:30–33.

333. Bailie R, Barnett MB, Fraser JF. The Brain laryngeal mask. A comparative study with the nasal mask in paediatric dental outpatient anaesthesia. Anaesthesia 1991;46:358–360.

334. Brimacombe J, Berry A. The laryngeal mask airway for dental surgery—a review. Aust Dent J 1995;40:10–14.

335. Kendall N. The Brain laryngeal mask. An alternative to difficult intubation. Br Dent J 1990;168:278.

336. Noble H, Wooller DJ. Laryngeal masks and chair dental anaesthesia. Anaesthesia 1991;46:591.

337. Young TM. The laryngeal mask in dental anaesthesia. Eur J Anaesth (Suppl) 1991;4:53–59.

338. Williams PJ, Bailey PM. Laryngeal mask airway: defining the limits. Can J Anaesth 1993;40:901.

339. Ravalia A, Steele A. Reinforced laryngeal mask airway and nasal surgery. Anaesthesia 1996;51:286.

340. Christie IW. A means of stabilizing laryngeal mask airways during dental procedures. Anaesthesia 1996;51:604.

341. John RE, Hill S, Hughes TJ. Airway protection by the laryngeal mask. A barrier to dye placed in the pharynx. Anaesthesia 1991;46:366–367.

342. Samarkandi AH, Ali MS, Elgammal M, et al. Airway protection by the laryngeal mask airway in children. MEJ Anesth 1995;13:107–113.

343. Van Heerden PV, Kirrage D. Large tonsils and the laryngeal mask airway. Anaesthesia 1989;44:703.

344. Denman W, Goudsouzian NG, Cleveland R, et al. The position of the laryngeal mask airway by magnetic resonance imaging. Anesthesiology 1991;75:A1045.

345. Brimacombe J. Use of the laryngeal mask airway in very small neonates. Anesthesiology 1994;81:1302.

346. Brimacombe J, Gandini D. Paediatric airway management. Br J Hosp Med 1995;53:175.

347. Brimacombe J, Gandini D. Resuscitation of neonates with laryngeal mask airway—a caution. Pediatrics 1995;95:453–454.

348. Paterson SJ, Byrne PJ. Time required to insert laryngeal mask airway in neonates requiring resuscitation. Anesthesiology 1995;82:318.

349. Brimacombe J, Berry A. The laryngeal mask airway—a consideration for the neonatal resuscitation programme guidelines? Can J Anaesth 1995;42:88–89.

350. Grebenik CR, Ferguson C, White A. The laryngeal mask airway in pediatric radiotherapy. Anesthesiology 1990;72:474–477.

351. Taylor DH, Child CSB. The laryngeal mask for radiotherapy in children. Anaesthesia 1990;45:690.

352. Waite K, Filshie J. The use of a laryngeal mask airway for CT radiotherapy planning and daily radiotherapy. Anaesthesia 1990;45:894.

353. Lim W. Yet another use for the laryngeal mask. Anaesthesia 1992;47:175–176.

354. Harris TM, Johnston DF, Collins SRC, et al. A new general anaesthetic technique for use in singers. The Brain laryngeal mask airway versus endotracheal intubation. J Voice 1990;4:81–85.

355. Sofair E, The professional singer with a difficult airway. Anesthesiology News 1993;20:4–10.

356. Lee SK, Hong KH, Choe H, et al. Comparison of the effects of the laryngeal mask airway and endotracheal intubation on vocal function. Br J Anaesth 1993;71:648–650.

357. Rafferty C, Burke AM, Cossar DF, et al. Laryngeal mask and magnetic resonance imaging. Anaesthesia 1990;45:590–591.

358. Taylor DH, Child CSB. The laryngeal mask for radiotherapy in children. Anaesthesia 1990;45:690.

359. Langton JA, Wilson I, Fell D. Use of the laryngeal mask airway during magnetic resonance imaging. Anaesthesia 1992;47:532–533.

360. Fairfield JE. Laryngeal mask and magnetic resonance—a caution. Anaesthesia 1990;45:995.

361. Lauretti GR, Mattos AL, Garcia LV, et al. Comparison of anesthetic spent between laryngeal mask airway and endotracheal tube in paediatric anesthesia under caudal blockade. Paper presented at the American Society of Regional Anesthesia meeting, 1994.

362. Murdoch L, Rubin A. Use of the Brain laryngeal mask in balanced regional anaesthesia. Anaesthesia 1989;44:616.

363. Leach A, Alexander CA, Stone B. The laryngeal mask in cardiopulmonary resuscitation in a district general hospital: a preliminary communication. Resuscitation 1993;65:245–248.

364. Kokkinis K. The use of the laryngeal mask airway in CPR. Resuscitation 1993;27:9–12.

365. Samarkandi AH, Seraj MA, El Dawlatly A, et al. The role of laryngeal mask airway in cardiopulmonary resuscitation. Resuscitation 1994;28:103–106.

366. Mather C, O'Kelly S. The palpation of pulses. Anaesthesia 1996;51:189–191.

367. Alexander R, Hodgson P, Lomax D, et al. A comparison of the laryngeal mask airway and Guedel airway, bag and facemask for manual ventilation following formal training. Anaesthesia 1993;48:231–234.

368. Martin PD, Cyna AM, Hunter WAH, et al. Training nursing staff in airway management for resuscitation. A clinical comparison of the facemask and laryngeal mask. Anaesthesia 1993;48:33–37.

369. Study group. The use of the laryngeal mask airway by nurses during cardiopulmonary resuscitation. Anaesthesia 1994;49:3–7.

370. Brimacombe JR, De Maio B. Emergency use of the laryngeal mask airway during helicopter transfer of a neonate. J Clin Anesth 1995;7:689–690.

371. Brimacombe JR, Gandini D. The laryngeal mask airway for helicopter transportation of neonates. Med J Aust 1995;162:56.

372. Greene MK, Rosen R, Hinchley G. The laryngeal mask airway. Two cases of prehospital trauma care. Anaesthesia 1992;47:688–689.

373. Reinhart DJ, Simmons G. Comparison of placement of the laryngeal mask airway with endotracheal tube by paramedics and respiratory therapists. Ann Emerg Med 1994;24:260–263.

374. Davies PRF, Tighe SQM, Greenslade GL, Evans GH. Laryngeal mask airway and tracheal tube insertion by unskilled personnel. Lancet 1990;336:977–979.

375. Pennant JH, Walker MB. Comparison of the endotracheal tube and laryngeal mask in airway management by paramedical personnel. Anesth Analg 1992;74:531–534.

376. Freeman R, Baxendale B. Laryngeal mask airway for caesarean section. Anaesthesia 1990;45:1094.

377. Davies JM, Weeks S, Crone LA. Failed intubation at caesarean section. Anaesthesia and Intensive Care 1991;19:303.

378. Gataure PS, Hughes JA. The laryngeal mask airway in obstetrical anaesthesia. Can J Anaesth 1995;42:130–133.

379. Hasham FM, Andrews PJD, Juneja MM, et al. The laryngeal mask airway facilitates intubation at cesarean section. A case report of difficult intubation. Int J Obstet Anesth 1993;2:181–182.

380. Hawthorne L, Wilson R, Lyons G, et al. Failed intubation revisited: 17-year experience in a teaching maternity unit. Br J Anaesth 1996;76:680–684.

381. McFarlane C. Failed intubation in an obese obstetric patient and the laryngeal mask. Int J Obstet Anesth 1993;2:183–185.

382. Christian AS. Failed obstetric intubation. Anaesthesia 1990;45:995.

383. Godley M, Reddy ARR. Use of LMA for awake intubation for Caesarean section. Can J Anaesth 1996;43:299–302.

384. Epstein RH, Halmi BH. Oxygen leakage around the laryngeal mask airway during laser treatment of port-wine stains in children. Anesth Analg 1994;78:486–489.

385. McCulloch T, Jones M, O'Neill A. Safety of the laryngeal mask for laser treatment of port-wine stains. Anaesthesia and Intensive Care 1997;25:189–190.

386. Brimacombe J, Sher M, Berry A. The reinforced la-

ryngeal mask airway for laser pharyngoplasty. Anaesthesia 1993;48:1105.

387. Brimacombe J. The incendiary characteristics of the laryngeal and reinforced laryngeal mask airway to CO_2 laser strike—a comparison with two polyvinyl chloride tracheal tubes. Anaesthesia and Intensive Care 1994;22:694–697.

388. Pennant JH, Gajraj NM. Lasers and the laryngeal mask airway. Anaesthesia 1994;49:448–449.

389. Pandit JJ, Chambers P, O'Malley S. KTP laser-resistant properties of the reinforced laryngeal mask airway. Br J Anaesth 1997;78:594–600.

390. Brimacombe J, Newell S, Swainston T, et al. A potential new technique for awake diagnostic bronchoscopy—use of the laryngeal mask airway. Med J Aust 1992;156:876–877.

391. Brimacombe J. Laryngoscopy through the LMA—a useful skill to acquire. Anaesthesia and Intensive Care 1992;20:535.

392. Brimacombe J, Tucker P, Simons S. The laryngeal mask airway for awake diagnostic bronchoscopy—a study of 200 consecutive patients. Eur J Anaesth 1995;12:357–361.

393. Llagunes J, Rodriguez–Hesles C, Catala JC, et al. Therapeutic fibreoptic bronchoscopy in critically ill patients via laryngeal mask. Anaesthesia and Intensive Care 1996;24:396–397.

394. McNamee CJ, Meyns B, Pagliero KM. Flexible bronchoscopy via the laryngeal mask: a new technique. Thorax 1991;46:141–142.

395. Tuck M, Phillips R, Corbett J. LMA for fibreoptic bronchoscopy. Anaesthesia and Intensive Care 1991; 19:472–473.

396. Moloney GM, Oabaru N. Intraoperative bronchoscopy during thoracotomy through an LMA in an infant. Anaesthesia and Intensive Care 1997;25: 310–311.

397. Brimacombe JR. LMA in awake fibreoptic bronchoscopy. Anaesthesia and Intensive Care 1991;19:472.

398. Rowbottom SJ, Morton CPJ. Diagnostic fibreoptic bronchoscopy using the laryngeal mask. Anaesthesia 1991;46:161.

399. Tuck M, Phillips R, Corbett J. LMA for fiberoptic bronchoscopy. Anaesthesia and Intensive Care 1991; 19:472–473.

400. Yahagi N, Kumon K, Tanigami H. Bronchial lavage with a fibreoptic bronchoscope via a laryngeal mask airway in an infant. Anaesthesia 1994;49:450.

401. Bapat PP, Verghese C. Laryngeal mask airway and the incidence of regurgitation during gynecological laparoscopies. Anesth Analg 1997;85:139–143.

402. Goodwin APL, Rowe WL, Ogg TW. Day case laparoscopy. A comparison of two anaesthetic techniques using the laryngeal mask during spontaneous breathing. Anaesthesia 1992;47:892–895.

403. Swann DG, Spens H, Edwards SA, Chestnut RJ. Anaesthesia for gynaecological laparoscopy—a comparison between the laryngeal mask airway and tracheal intubation. Anaesthesia 1993;48:431–434.

404. Griffin RM, Hatcher IS. Aspiration pneumonia and the laryngeal mask airway. Anaesthesia 1990;45: 1039–1040.

405. Agarwal A, Shobhana N. LMA in neurosurgery. Can J Anaesth 1995;42:750.

406. Agarwal A, Rajan S. The LMA in intracranial aneurysm surgery. Can J Anaesth 1995;42:1176–1177.

407. Hagberg C, Berry J, Haque S. The laryngeal mask airway for awake craniotomy in pediatric patients. Anesthesiology 1995;83:A184.

408. Nair I, Bailey PM. Use of the laryngeal mask for airway maintenance following tracheal extubation. Anaesthesia 1995;50:174–175.

409. Groudine SB, Sandison MR. Pressure support ventilation with the laryngeal mask airway: a method to manage severe reactive airway disease postoperatively. Can J Anaesth 1995;42:341–343.

410. Silva LCE, Brimacombe JR. Tracheal tube/laryngeal mask exchange for emergence. Anesthesiology 1996; 85:218.

411. Taylor JC, Bell GT. An asthmatic weaned from a ventilator using a laryngeal mask. Anaesthesia 1995;50: 454–455.

412. George SL, Blogg CE. Role of the LMA in tracheal extubation? Br J Anaesth 1994;72:610.

413. Glaisyer HR, Parry M, Lee J, et al. The laryngeal mask airway as an adjunct to extubation on the intensive care unit. Anaesthesia 1996;51:1187–1188.

414. Groudine SB, Lumb PD. Noninvasive ventilatory support with the laryngeal mask airway. A preliminary report. Am J Anesth 1996;23:124–128.

415. Glaisyer HR, Parry M, Bailey PM. The LMA for the application of postoperative CPAP. Can J Anaesth 1997;44:784–785.

416. Brimacombe J. Laryngeal mask airway for access to the upper gastrointestinal tract. Anesthesiology 1996;84:1009–1010.

417. Gajraj NM. Use of the laryngeal mask airway during oesophago-gastro-duodenoscopy. Anaesthesia 1996; 51:991.

418. Lopez–Gil M, Brimacombe J, Cebrian J, et al. Laryngeal mask airway in pediatric practice. A prospective study of skill acquisition by anesthesia residents. Anesthesiology 1996;84:807–811.

419. Alexander R, Arrowsmith JE, Frossard RJ. The laryngeal mask airway: safe in the X-ray department? Anaesthesia 1993;48:734.

420. Akhtar TM, Street MK. Risk of aspiration with the laryngeal mask. Br J Anaesth 1994;72:447–450.

421. Brain AIJ. The laryngeal mask and the oesophagus. Anaesthesia 1991;46:701–702.

422. Nanji GM, Malt JR. Vomiting and aspiration pneumonitis with the laryngeal mask airway. Can J Anaesth 1992;39:69–70.

423. Cyna AM, MacLeod DM. The laryngeal mask: cautionary tales. A reply. Anaesthesia 1990;45:167.

424. Koehli N. Aspiration and the laryngeal mask airway. Anaesthesia 1991;46:419.

425. Maroof M, Khan RM, Siddique MS. Intraoperative aspiration pneumonitis and the laryngeal mask airway. Anesth Analg 1993;77:409–410.

426. Koehli N. Aspiration and the laryngeal mask airway. Anaesthesia 1991;46:419.

427. Brimacombe JR, Berry A. The incidence of aspiration associated with the laryngeal mask airway: a meta-analysis of published literature. J Clin Anesth 1995; 7:297–305.

428. Barker P, Langton JA, Murphy PJ, et al. Regulation of gastric contents during general anaesthesia using the laryngeal mask airway. Br J Anaesth 1992;69: 314–315.

429. Rabey PG, Murphy PJ, Langton JA, et al. Effect of the laryngeal mask airway on the lower oesophageal sphincter pressure in patients during general anaesthesia. Br J Anaesth 1992;69:346–348.

430. Vanner RG. Regurgitation and the laryngeal mask airway. Br J Anaesth 1993;70:380–381.

431. Stanley GD, Bastianpillai BA, Mulcahy K, et al. Postoperative laryngeal competence. The laryngeal mask airway and tracheal tube compared. Anaesthesia 1995;50:985–986.

432. Ansermino JM, Blogg CE, Carrie LES. Failed tracheal intubation at Caesarean section and the laryngeal mask. Br J Anaesth 1992;68:118.

433. Brimacombe J, Berry A. Mechanical airway obstruction after cricoid pressure with the laryngeal mask airway. Anesth Analg 1994;78:604–605.

434. Asai T, Barclay K, McBeth C, et al. Cricoid pressure applied after placement of the laryngeal mask prevents gastric insufflation but inhibits ventilation. Br J Anaesth 1996;76:772–776.

435. Strang TI. Does the laryngeal mask airway compromise cricoid pressure? Anaesthesia 1992;47: 829–831.

436. Graziotti PJ. Intermittent positive pressure ventilation through a laryngeal mask airway. Is a nasogastric tube useful? Anaesthesia 1992;47:1088–1090.

437. Brimacombe JR. Laryngeal mask anaesthesia and recurrent swallowing. Anaesthesia and Intensive Care 1991;19:275–276.

438. Conacher ID. Foreign body in a laryngeal mask airway. Anaesthesia 1991;46:164.

439. Riley RH, Browning FS. Another foreign body in a laryngeal mask airway. Anaesthesia 1996;51: 286–287.

440. Dempsey GA, Barrett PJ. Hazard with the reinforced laryngeal mask airway. Anaesthesia 1995;50: 660–661.

441. Goldberg PL, Evans PF, Filshie J. Kinking of the laryngeal mask airway in two children. Anaesthesia 1990;45:487–488.

442. Herrick MJ, Kennedy DJ. Airway obstruction and the laryngeal mask airway in paediatric radiotherapy. Anaesthesia 1992;47:910.

443. Wilson IG, Eastley R. A modification of the laryngeal mask airway. Anesthesiology 1991;74:1157.

444. Handsworth JL. Faulty laryngeal mask. Anaesthesia and Intensive Care 1996;24:728–729.

445. Schwab C, Prevedoros H. LMA obstruction. Anaesthesia and Intensive Care 1997;25:89.

446. Brimacombe JR. The laryngeal mask airway. A review for the nurse anesthetist. J Am Assoc Nurse Anesth 1992;60:490–499.

447. Dubreuil M, Janvier G, Dugrais G, et al. Uncommon laryngeal mask obstruction. Can J Anaesth 1992;39: 517–518.

448. Dubruil M, Laffon M, Plaud B, et al. Complications and fiberoptic assessment of size 1 laryngeal mask airway. Anesth Analg 1993;76:527–529.

449. McCrirrick A, Ramage DTO, Pracilio JA, et al. Experience with the laryngeal mask airway in two hundred patients. Anaesthesia and Intensive Care 1991;19: 256–260.

450. Sarma VJ. The use of a laryngeal mask airway in spontaneously breathing patients. Acta Anaesthesiol Scand 1990;34:669–672.

451. Fawcett WJ, Ravilia A, Radford P. The laryngeal mask airway in children. Can J Anaesth 1991;38:685–686.

452. Wilkinson PA. The laryngeal mask: cautionary tales. Anaesthesia 1990;45:167.

453. Thomas DG, Moloney JT. Stridor after removal of laryngeal mask. Anaesthesia and Intensive Care 1991; 19:300–301.

454. Nair I, Thompsett C. Laryngeal mask airway and late postoperative stridor. Anaesthesia 1994;49: 449–450.

455. Boge E, Brandis K. Testing the laryngeal mask. Anaesthesia and Intensive Care 1995;23:751–752.

456. Welsh BE. Will we ever learn? Anaesthesia 1990;45: 892.

457. Williams PJ, Bailey PM. The reinforced laryngeal mask airway for adenotonsillectomy. Br J Anaesth 1994;72:729.

458. O'Connor B. Rotation of the laryngeal mask airway. Anaesthesia 1994;49:169.

459. Ravalia D, Kumar N. Rotation of reinforced laryngeal mask airway. Anaesthesia 1994;49:541–542.

460. Quinn AC, McAteer EM, Moss E, et al. The reinforced laryngeal mask airway for dento-alveolar surgery. Br J Anaesth 1996;77:185–188.

461. Brimacombe J, Berry A. Laryngeal mask airway and pulmonary edema: III. Anesthesiology 1993;79:185.

462. Payne J. The use of the fiberoptic laryngoscope to confirm the position of the laryngeal mask. Anaesthesia 1989;44:865.

463. Miller AC, Bickler P. The laryngeal mask airway. Anaesthesia 1991;46:659–660.

464. McKinney B, Grigg R. Epiglottitis after anaesthesia with a laryngeal mask. Anaesthesia and Intensive Care 1995;23:618–619.

465. Marjot R. Trauma to the posterior pharyngeal wall caused by a laryngeal mask airway. Anaesthesia 1991;46:589–590.

466. Connolly AAP. Laryngeal mask airway in ENT surgery. J Laryngol Otol 1992;106:479.

467. Lee JJ. Laryngeal mask and trauma to uvula. Anaesthesia 1989;44:1014.

468. Van Dongen VCP, Langemeijer JJM. Anaesthesia 1994;49:1097–1098.

469. Thompsett C, Cundy JM. Use of the laryngeal mask airway in the presence of a bleeding diathesis. Anaesthesia 1992;47:530–531.

470. Wynn JM, Jones KL. Tongue cyanosis after laryngeal mask airway insertion. Anesthesiology 1994;80:1403.

471. Crawford M, Davidson G. A problem with a laryngeal mask airway. Anaesthesia 1992;47:76.

472. Khoo ST. The laryngeal mask airway—an unusual complication. Anaesthesia and Intensive Care 1993;21:249–250.

473. Squires SJ. Fragmented laryngeal mask airway. Anaesthesia 1992;47:274.

474. Vickers R, Springer A, Hindmarsh J. Problem with the laryngeal mask airway. Anaesthesia 1992;47:639.

475. Woodforth IJ. The safe life of reusable airway devices. Anaesthesia and Intensive Care 1994;22:318–319.

476. Zavattaro M. LMA failure. Anaesthesia and Intensive Care 1996;24:119.

477. Kramer–Kilper OT. Removal of laryngeal mask airway during light anaesthesia. Anaesthesia 1992;47:816.

478. Pennant JH, Gajraj NM, Griffith K. Puncture of the laryngeal mask airway cuff. Anaesthesia 1994;49:448.

479. Hardingham M, Hills MM. The laryngeal mask. Br Med J 1993;306:508–509.

480. Kalapac S. Donald A, Brimacombe J. Laryngeal mask biopsy! Anaesthesia and Intensive Care 1996;24:283.

481. McLure HA. Dental damage to the laryngeal mask. Anaesthesia 1996;51:1078–1079.

482. Neunam PTF. Dental damage to the laryngeal mask. Anaesthesia 1997;52:283.

483. Short JA, Melillo EP. Damage to a laryngeal mask during tonsillectomy. Anaesthesia 1997;52:507.

484. Brodrick PM, Webster NR, Nunn JF. The laryngeal mask airway. Anaesthesia 1989;44:238–241.

485. Alexander CA, Leach AB. Incidence of sore throats with the laryngeal mask. Anaesthesia 1989;44:791.

486. Cork RC, Depa RM, Standen JR. Prospective comparison for use of the laryngeal mask and endotracheal tube for ambulatory surgery. Anesth Analg 1994;79:719–727.

487. Denny NM, Gadelrab R. Complications following general anaesthesia for cataract surgery: a comparison of the laryngeal mask airway with tracheal intubation. J Roy Soc Med 1993;86:521–522.

488. Dingley J, Whitehead MJ, Wareham K. A comparative study of the incidence of sore throat with the laryngeal mask airway. Anaesthesia 1994;49:251–254.

489. Splinter WM, Smallman B, Rhine EJ, et al. Postoperative sore throat in children and the laryngeal mask airway. Can J Anaesth 1994;41:1081–1083.

490. Rieger A, Brunne N, Hass I, et al. Laryngo-pharyngeal complaints following laryngeal mask airway and endotracheal intubation. J Clin Anesth 1997;9:42–47.

491. Lacroix O, Billard V, Bourgain JL, et al. Prevention of postoperative sore throat during use of the laryngeal mask airway. Br J Anaesth 1996;76:16.

492. Foley EP, O'Neill BL, Chang AS. The effect of duration of LMA exposure on the incidence of postoperative pharyngeal complaints. Anesth Analg 1995;80:S130.

493. Burgard G, Moellhoff TM, Prien T. The effect of laryngeal mask cuff pressure on postoperative sore throat incidence. J Clin Anesth 1996;8:198–201.

494. Rieger A, Brunne B, Striebel HW. Intracuff pressures do not predict laryngopharyngeal discomfort after use of the laryngeal mask airway. Anesthesiology 1997;87:63–67.

495. Cros AM, Pitti R, Conil C, et al. Severe dysphonia after use of a laryngeal mask airway. Anesthesiology 1997;86:498–500.

496. Rosenberg MK, Rontal E, Rontal M, et al. Arytenoid cartilage dislocation caused by a laryngeal mask airway treated with chemical splinting. Anesth Analg 1996;83:1335–1336.

497. George A. 'Failed' cuff inflation of a laryngeal mask. Anaesthesia 1994;49:80.

498. Richards JT. Pilot tube of the laryngeal mask airway. Anaesthesia 1994;49:450.

499. King C, Street MK. Twelfth cranial nerve paralysis following use of a laryngeal mask airway. Anaesthesia 1994;49:786–787.

500. Nagai K, Sakuramoto C, Goto F. Unilateral hypoglossal nerve paralysis following the use of the laryngeal mask airway. Anaesthesia 1994;49:603–604.

501. Inomata S, Nishikawa T, Suga A, et al. Transient bilateral vocal cord paralysis after insertion of a laryngeal mask airway. Anesthesiology 1995;82:787–788.

502. Lloyd Jones FRE, Hegab A. Recurrent laryngeal nerve palsy after laryngeal mask airway insertion. Anaesthesia 1996;51:171–172.

503. Morikawa M. Vocal cord paralysis after use of the LM. J Clin Anesth 1992;12:1194.

504. Daya H, Fawcett W, Weir N. Vocal fold palsy after use of the laryngeal mask airway. J Laryngol Otol 1996;110:383–384.

505. Ahmad NS, Yentis SM. Laryngeal mask airway and lingual nerve injury. Anaesthesia 1996;51:707–708.

506. Laxton CH, Kipling R. Lingual nerve paralysis following the use of the laryngeal mask airway. Anaesthesia 1996;51:869–870.

507. Cook T. Bronchospasm and the laryngeal mask airway. Anaesthesia 1994;49:82.

508. Ezri T, Priscu V, Szmuk P, et al. Laryngeal mask and pulmonary edema [Letter]. Anesthesiology 1993;78: 219.

509. Harada M. Transient swelling of the parotid glands following laryngeal mask airway. Can J Anaesth 1992; 39:745–746.

510. Maltby JR, Elwood T, Price B. Acute transient unilateral macroglossia following use of a LMA. Can J Anaesth 1996;43:94–95.

511. Nandwani N, Fairfield MC, Krarup K, et al. The effect of laryngeal mask airway insertion on the position of the internal jugular vein. Anaesthesia 1997;52: 77–83.

512. De Mello WF, Ward P. The use of the laryngeal mask airway in primary anaesthesia. Anaesthesia 1990;45: 793–794.

513. Stone BJ, Leach AC, Alexander CA, et al. The use of the laryngeal mask airway by nurses during cardiopulmonary resuscitation. Anaesthesia 1994;49:3–7.

514. Bailey AR, Hett DA. The laryngeal mask airway in resuscitation. Resuscitation 1994;28:107–110.

515. Maltby JR, Loken RG, Watson NC. The laryngeal mask airway. Clinical appraisal in 250 patients. Can J Anaesth 1990;37:509–513.

516. Tolley PM, Watts ADJ, Hickman JA. Comparison of the use of the laryngeal mask and face mask by inexperienced personnel. Br J Anaesth 1992;69: 320–321.

517. Lopez–Gill M, Brimacombe J. Safety and efficacy of the laryngeal mask airway. A prospective survey of 1400 children. Anaesthesia 1996;51:969–972.

518. Efrat R, Kadari A, Katz S. The laryngeal mask airway in pediatric anesthesia: experience with 120 patients undergoing elective groin surgery. J Pediatr Surg 1994;29:206–208.

519. Ravalia A, Fawcett W, Radford P. The Brain laryngeal mask airway in paediatric anaesthesia. Anesth Analg 1991;72:S220.

520. Haynes SR, Allsop JR, Gillies GWA. Arterial oxygen saturation during induction of anaesthesia and laryngeal mask insertion. Prospective evaluation of four techniques. Br J Anaesth 1992;68:519–522.

521. Verghese C, Smith TGC, Young E. Prospective survey of the use of the laryngeal mask airway in 2359 patients. Anaesthesia 1993;48:58–60.

522. McCaughey W, Bhanumurthy S. Laryngeal mask placement in the prone position. Anaesthesia 1993; 48:1104–1105.

523. Milligan KA. Laryngeal mask in the prone position. Anaesthesia 1994;49:449.

524. Riley RH, Swan HD. Value of the laryngeal mask airway during thoracotomy. Anesthesiology 1992; 77:1051.

525. Goldik Z, Mecz Y, Bornstein J, et al. LMA insertion after accidental extubation. Can J Anaesth 1995;42: 1065.

526. Joshi GP, Morrison SG, Gairaj NM, et al. Hemodynamic changes during emergence from anesthesia: use of the laryngeal mask airway versus endotracheal tube. Anesth Analg 1994;78:S185.

527. Joshi GP, Taylor-Kennedy L, Hyun J, et al. Effects of airway device on recovery following outpatient surgery: use of an LMA versus tracheal tube. Anesthesiology 1996;85:A47.

528. Cameron AE, Sievert J, Asbury AJ, et al. Gas leakage and the laryngeal mask airway. A comparison with the tracheal tube and facemask during spontaneous ventilation using a circle breathing system. Anaesthesia 1996;51:1117–1119.

529. Hoerauf KH, Koller C, Jakob W, et al. Isoflurane waste gas exposure during general anaesthesia: the laryngeal mask compared with tracheal intubation. Br J Anaesth 1996;77:189–193.

530. Sarma VJ, Leman J. Laryngeal mask and anaesthetic waste gas concentrations. Anaesthesia 1990;45: 791–792.

531. Barnett R, Gallant B, Fossey S, et al. Nitrous oxide environmental pollution. A comparison between face mask, laryngeal mask, and tracheal intubation. Can J Anaesth 1992;39:A151.

532. Pennant JH, White PF. The laryngeal mask airway—its uses in anesthesiology. Anesthesiology 1993;79:144–163.

533. Dyer RA, Llewellyn RL, James MFM. Total intravenous anaesthesia with propofol and the laryngeal mask for orthopaedic surgery. Br J Anaesth 1995;74: 123–128.

534. Wood MLB, Forrest ETS. The haemodynamic response to the insertion of the laryngeal mask airway: a comparison with laryngoscopy and tracheal intubation. Acta Anaesthesiol Scand 1994;38:510–513.

535. Fujii Y, Tanaka Y, Toyooka H. Circulatory responses to laryngeal mask airway insertion or tracheal intubation in normotensive and hypertensive patients. Can J Anaesth 1995;42:32–36.

536. Wilson IG, Fell D, Robinson SL, et al. Cardiovascular responses to insertion of the laryngeal mask. Anaesthesia 1992;47:300–302.

537. Braude N, Clements EAF, Hodges UM, et al. The pressor response and laryngeal mask insertion. Anaesthesia 1989;44:551–554.

538. Hickey S, Cameron AE, Asbury AJ. Cardiovascular response to insertion of Brain's laryngeal mask. Anaesthesia 1990;45:629–633.

539. Wilkins CJ, Cramp PGW, Staples J, et al. Comparison of the anesthetic requirement for tolerance of laryngeal mask airway and endotracheal tube. Anesth Analg 1992;75:794–797.

540. Inagaki Y, Joshi GP, Wat L, et al. Comparison of airway devices for ambulatory anesthesia: LMA versus tracheal tube. Anesth Analg 1997;84:S7.

541. Stone JM, Karallliedde LD, Carter ML, et al. Bacteremia and insertion of laryngeal mask airways. Anaesthesia 1992;47:77.

542. Brimacombe J, Shorney N, Swainston R, et al. The incidence of bacteraemia following laryngeal mask insertion. Anaesthesia and Intensive Care 1992;20: 484–486.

543. Hester ZR, Jones DE, Johnson JG, et al. Anesthesia in a patient with a tracheal stent and for placement of tracheobronchial stents. Am J Anesth 1996;23: 297–300.

544. Lau S, Pinosky ML, Cooke JE, et al. The laryngeal mask airway in a patient with an endotracheal stent. Am J Anesth 1995;22:318–320.

545. Watcha MF, Garner FT, White PF, et al. Laryngeal mask airway versus face mask and Guedel airway during pediatric myringotomy. Arch Otol Head Neck Surg 1994;120:877–880.

546. Alexander R. The laryngeal mask airway and ocular injury. Can J Anaesth 1993;40:901–902.

547. Brimacombe J, Berry A. Barotrauma and the laryngeal mask airway. Anaesthesia 1994;49:1009.

548. Macario A, Chang PC, Stempel DB, et al. A cost analysis of the laryngeal mask airway for elective surgery in adult outpatients. Anesthesiology 1995;83: 250–257.

549. Joshi GP, Smith I, Watcha MF, et al. A model for studying the cost-effectiveness of airway devices: laryngeal mask airway vs tracheal tube. Anesth Analg 1995;80:S219.

550. Leach AB, Alexander CA. The laryngeal mask—an overview. Eur J Anaesth 1991;4:19–31.

551. Maltby JR. The laryngeal mask airway in anaesthesia. Can J Anaesth 1994;41:888–893.

552. Evans A. Difficulty in inserting a laryngeal mask airway. Anaesthesia 1995;50:468–469.

553. Ishimura H, Minami K, Sata T, et al. Impossible insertion of the laryngeal mask airway and oropharyngeal axes. Anesthesiology 1995;83:867–869.

554. Brimacombe J. Laryngeal mask and bleeding diathesis. Anaesthesia 1992;47:1004–1005.

555. Elias M. Laryngeal mask airway and radiotherapy in the prone position. Anaesthesia 1992;47:1005.

556. Lim W, Cone AM. Laryngeal mask and the prone position. Anaesthesia 1994;49:542.

557. Dasey N, Mansour N. Coughing and laryngospasm with the laryngeal mask. Anaesthesia 1989;44:865.

558. Brimacombe J, Berry A, Fletcher D. To the editor. J Post Anesth Nurs 1993;8:236–237.

QUESTIONS

Each question below contains four suggested answers of which one or more is correct. Choose the answer:

A if 1, 2, and 3 are correct
B if 1 and 3 are correct
C if 2 and 4 are correct
D if 4 is correct
E if 1, 2, 3 and 4 are correct.

1. Uses for the flexible LMA include
   1. Intubation through the LMA
   2. MRI scanning
   3. Situations where low resistance to flow is needed
   4. Surgical procedures around the head and neck

2. Checking the LMA before use should include the following:
   1. The inflated cuff should hold pressure for at least 2 minutes
   2. Air should be forcibly withdrawn to reveal leaks in the cuff
   3. The bars should be probed to be certain they are intact
   4. The tube should be flexed more than 180°

3. To prepare the LMA for use
   1. Both sides of the cuff should be lubricated
   2. The cuff should be wrinkle free
   3. Lubricants that contain silicone are recommended
   4. The cuff should form a stiff wedge

4. Maneuvers helpful if there is difficulty inserting the LMA include
   1. Inserting the LMA backwards
   2. Positive pressure ventilation
   3. Insertion from the side of the mouth
   4. Two-handed cricoid pressure

5. When cleaning and sterilizing the LMA
   1. It should first be washed with soap and water
   2. It can be sterilized using the steam autoclave
   3. Ethylene oxide should not be used
   4. The LMA can be soaked in liquid chemical agents for up to 30 minutes

6. Which statements are correct?
   1. Dead space is greater with the LMA than the face mask
   2. The pharynx adapts to the shape of the LMA cuff
   3. The reinforced LMA offers less resistance to breathing than the standard version
   4. The work of breathing with the LMA is similar to that associated with a tracheal tube

7. Clinical situations considered to be indications for use of the laryngeal mask include
   1. Failed intubation
   2. Facial burns
   3. Professional singer
   4. Limited mouth opening

8. When an LMA is to be used for ophthalmologic surgery,
   1. Intraocular pressure is lower during induction and emergence than with a tracheal tube
   2. The LMA is more likely to be dislodged during surgery than a tracheal tube
   3. There is less likelihood of coughing during the surgical procedure
   4. The standard LMA should be used

9. Pulmonary and tracheal problems for which the LMA may be useful include
   1. Chronic obstructive pulmonary disease
   2. Mediastinal mass with tracheal compression
   3. Tracheal stenosis
   4. Acute asthmatic attack

10. Procedures to be performed if gastric contents appear in the LMA include
    1. 30° head down position
    2. Removal of the LMA for suctioning
    3. Insertion of a tracheal tube if aspiration has occurred
    4. Placement of the patient in the lateral position

11. What measures should be taken to minimize the incidence of aspiration?
    1. The LMA cuff should be overinflated by 10 cc
    2. Low tidal volumes should be used
    3. Inflation pressure should be kept to less than 41 cm H_2O
    4. A level of anesthesia adequate to prevent swallowing should be maintained

12. Causes of airway obstruction associated with the LMA include

    1. Back folding of the distal cuff
    2. Laryngospasm
    3. Obstruction of the laryngeal opening by the distal cuff
    4. Overdistension of the cuff

ANSWERS

1.	D	7.	E
2.	B	8.	A
3.	C	9.	B
4.	A	10.	B
5.	A	11.	C
6.	C	12.	E

Laryngoscopes

LARYNGOSCOPES ARE USED to view the larynx and adjacent structures, most commonly for the purpose of inserting a tube into the tracheobronchial tree. They range from simple rigid blades to complex fiberoptic apparatus. The wide range of devices available attests to the many and diverse difficulties encountered in placing tubes correctly.

THE RIGID LARYNGOSCOPE

Most laryngoscopes in use today consist of a handle plus detachable blade. The light source is energized when the blade and handle are locked in the working position.

Description

Standards for the connection between the handle and the blade for blades that have a lamp include ASTM F965 and ISO 7376-1 (1, 2). ASTM F1195 and ISO 7376-3 cover fittings for laryngoscopes that are fiberoptic illuminated (3, 4). They provide methods of identifying compatible blades and handles by a circumferential band of color between the hook-on fitting and the midpoint of the handle. The dimensions of the fittings for each color system are specified in the standards.

Handle

The handle provides the power source for the light. Most often this is disposable batteries. Handles with rechargeable batteries are available. Fiberoptic-illuminated laryngoscopes may use a remote light source (5). Most handles are designed to accept either fiberoptic-illuminated or lamp-in-bulb blades, but some can engage either.

A hook-on (hinged folding) connection between the handle and blade is most commonly used. The handle is fitted with a hinge pin that fits a slot on the base of the blade. This allows quick and easy attachment and detachment.

Handles designed to accept blades that have a light bulb have a metallic contact, which completes an electrical circuit when the handle and blade are in the working position. Handles containing batteries and using fiberoptic illumination contain a halogen lamp bulb. When the handle and blade are locked in the working position, an activator switch is depressed. This provides a connection between the bulb and the batteries. A halogen lamp bulb has a useful life three times that of light bulbs used in other laryngoscopes. Studies have shown that the illumination is better with lamp-in-blade than fiberoptic systems (6–9). Use of mains power may improve the brightness (7, 5).

Handles are available in several sizes (Fig. 16.1). Short handles may be advantageous for patients in whom the chest and/or breasts contact the handle during use, when cricoid pressure is being applied or when the patient is in a body cast (10). Other techniques for handling this situation include inserting the blade laterally into the

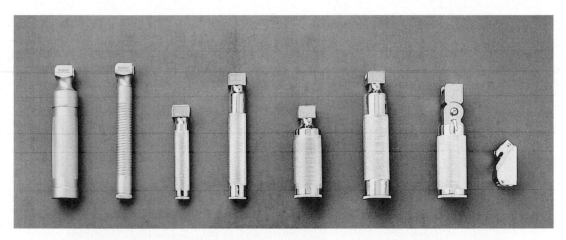

FIGURE 16.1.   Laryngoscope handles. The Patil–Syracuse handle is the second from the right. The Howland lock, shown on the far right, fits between the handle and the blade by means of hook-on connections on both parts. It changes the angle between the handle and the blade. (Courtesy of Rusch Inc.)

mouth, advancing it halfway into the mouth and rotating it back to the normal position (11, 12), and inserting a detached blade into the mouth and then attaching the handle (13, 14).

Although most blades form a right angle with the handle when ready for use, the angle may also be acute or obtuse. An adapter may be fitted between the handle and the blade to allow the angle to be altered (15–17) (Fig. 16.1). The Patil–Syracuse handle (Fig. 16.2) can be positioned and locked in four different positions (18).

Blade

The blade is the rigid component that is inserted into the mouth. When a blade is available in more than one size, the blades are numbered, with the number increasing with size. Disposable blades are available (Fig. 16.3).

The blade is composed of several parts, including the base, heel, tongue, flange, web, tip, and light source (Fig. 16.4).

The base is the part that attaches to the handle. It has a slot for engaging the hinge pin of the handle. The proximal end of the base is called the heel.

The tongue (spatula) is the main shaft. It serves to compress and manipulate the soft tissues (especially the tongue) and lower jaw. The long axis of the tongue may be straight or curved in part or

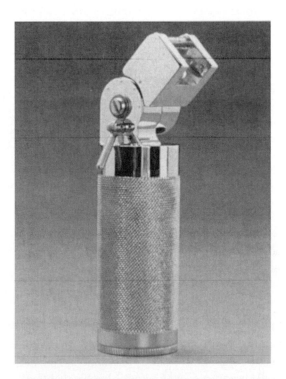

FIGURE 16.2.   Patil-Syracuse handle. With this handle, the blade can be adjusted and locked in four different positions (180°, 135°, 90°, or 45°). Courtesy of Mercury Medical.

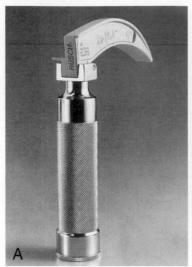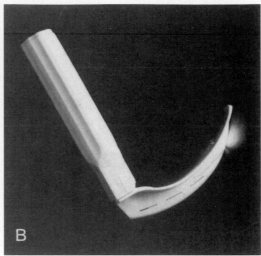

FIGURE 16.3. **A,** Disposable blade attached to reusable handle. **B,** Disposable handle and blade. (Courtesy of Rusch Inc. and Vital Signs.)

all of its length. Blades are commonly referred to as curved or straight, depending on the predominant shape of the tongue.

The flange projects off the side of the tongue and is connected to it by the web. It serves to guide instrumentation and deflect tissues out of the line of vision. The flange determines the cross-sectional shape of the blade. The vertical height of the cross-sectional shape of a blade is sometimes referred to as the "step" (19).

The tip (beak) contacts either the epiglottis or the vallecula and directly or indirectly elevates the epiglottis. It is usually blunt and thickened to decrease trauma.

The blade may have a lamp (bulb) (Fig. 16.5) or a fiberoptic bundle that transmits light from a source in the handle (Fig. 16.6). The lamp screws into a socket that has a metallic contact. On most blades the socket is located near the tip. On some blades it is in the base. When the blade is snapped into place, electrical contact with the batteries in the handle is made. The socket is subject to soiling by fluids that can affect the electrical contacts, causing the light to fail. A fiberoptic-illuminated blade has an encased fiberoptic bundle that transmits light from a source in the handle or base of the blade. Because there is no bulb or electrical contact in the blade, cleaning and sterilization are easier and the laryngoscope is more reliable. Even if the light is left on for an extended period of time, the blade stays cool. The ASTM (3) standard requires fiberoptic-illuminated blades to have a color coded mark on the heel.

In most cases, use of a laryngoscope presents little or no difficulty to the experienced operator, and skill is of more importance than the type of blade employed. There are, however, situations in which a certain blade is particularly advantageous (20). This has led to the development of a number of blades. The blades discussed here are commercially available in the United States. A number of other blades has been described in the literature.

Macintosh Blade (21, 22)

The Macintosh blade (Fig. 16.4) is one of the most popular. The tongue has a smooth, gentle curve that extends to the tip. There is a flange at the left to push the tongue out of the way. In cross-section, the tongue, web, and flange form a reverse Z. Numerous modifications have been suggested (23–30).

The number 4 blade may be more useful than the number 3 in normal and large adults because the tallest portion of the blade will often lie outside the mouth during intubation (31).

CURVED
(MACINTOSH)

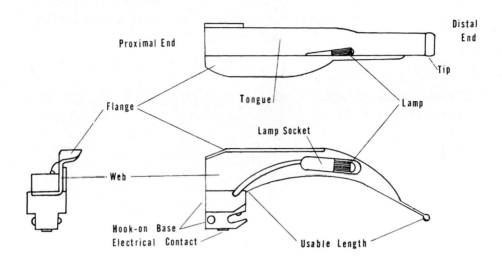

STRAIGHT
(MILLER)

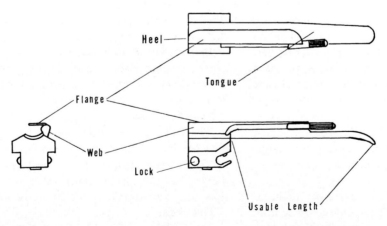

FIGURE 16.4. The parts of the Macintosh (**top**) and the Miller (**bottom**) blades are illustrated. The tip is the distal end of the blade intended for insertion into the patient. The proximal end is the part closest to the handle. Redrawn from a drawing in Committee, American National Standards Institute. Draft standard, laryngoscopes for tracheal intubation (Z-79). Philadelphia: ASTM.

FIGURE **16.5.** Left-handed Macintosh blade. (Courtesy of Penlon Ltd.)

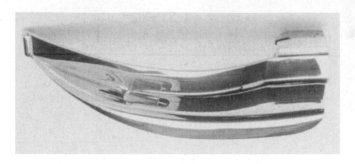

FIGURE **16.6.** English Macintosh blade. (Courtesy of Welch Allyn, Inc.)

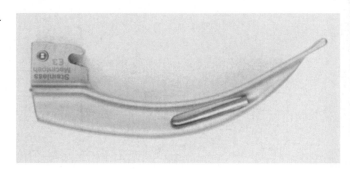

Left-Handed Macintosh Blade (32)

The left-handed Macintosh blade (Fig. 16.5) has the flange on the opposite side from the usual Macintosh blade. This blade may be useful for abnormalities of the right side of the face or oropharynx, left-handed persons, intubating in the right lateral position, and positioning a tracheal tube directly on the left side of the mouth (33, 34).

English Macintosh

The English Macintosh (Fig. 16.6) is similar to the conventional Macintosh except the flange is curved and lower at the handle end.

Polio Blade

The polio blade (Fig. 16.7) is also a modification of the Macintosh. The blade is offset from the handle at an obtuse angle to allow intubation of patients in iron lung respirators or body jackets, and intubating patients after the anesthesia screen is in place. It is also useful for obese patients and those with breast hypertrophy, kyphosis with severe barrel chest deformity, short neck, or restricted neck mobility (35, 36). Disadvantages of this blade are that little force can be applied and control is minimal (13).

Improved Vision Macintosh Blade (37)

The improved vision (I.V.) Macintosh blade (Fig. 16.8) is similar to the standard version except that the midportion of the tongue is concave.

Oxiport Macintosh (Mac/Port)

The oxiport Macintosh blade (Fig. 16.9) is a conventional Macintosh blade with a tube to deliver oxygen.

Tull Macintosh

The Tull (suction) blade (Fig. 16.10) is a modified Macintosh that has a suction port near the tip. The suction channel extends next to the handle and has a finger-controlled valve so that suction can be controlled by the laryngoscopist.

Fink Blade

The Fink blade (Fig. 16.11) is another modification of the Macintosh. The tongue is wider and has a sharper curve at the distal end. The height of the flange is reduced, especially at the proximal end. The light bulb is placed farther forward than on the Macintosh.

Bizzarri–Giuffrida Blade (38)

The Bizzarri–Giuffrida blade (flangeless Macintosh) (Fig. 16.12) is a modified Macintosh.

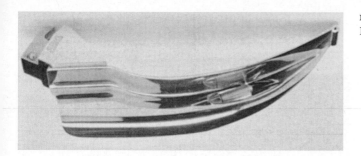

FIGURE 16.7. The polio blade. (Courtesy of Penlon Ltd.)

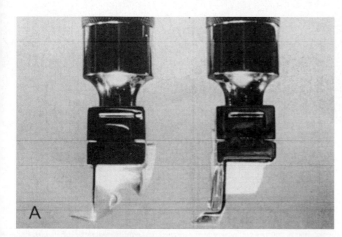

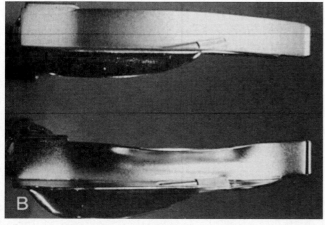

FIGURE 16.8. A, The improved vision (I.V.) Macintosh blade (**left**) and the conventional Macintosh blade (right). Note the improved vision when the blade is viewed from the proximal end. B, Conventional Macintosh blade (**top**) and the I.V. Macintosh blade (**bottom**). On the I.V. Macintosh, the midportion of the spatula is concave. (Courtesy of Gabor B. Racz, M.D.)

FIGURE 16.9. The oxiport Macintosh blade. (Courtesy of Mercury Medical.)

FIGURE **16.10.** Tull (suction) Macintosh and Miller blades. The finger-controlled valve allows suction to be regulated by the laryngoscopist. (Courtesy of Mercury Medical.)

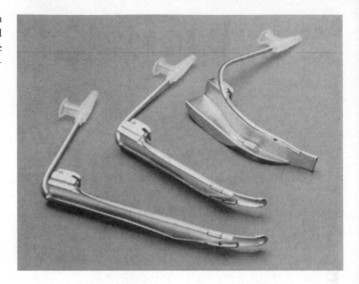

FIGURE **16.11.** The Fink blade. Note that the tongue is more curved at the tip and the flange is reduced at the proximal end compared with the Macintosh blade. The light bulb is placed nearer the distal end. (Courtesy of Puritan–Bennett Corp.)

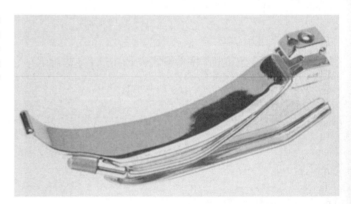

FIGURE **16.12.** The Bizzarri–Giuffrida blade. (Courtesy of Puritan-–Bennett Corp.)

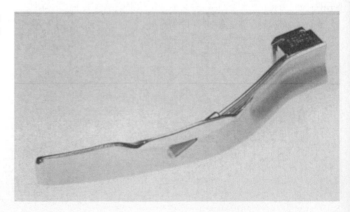

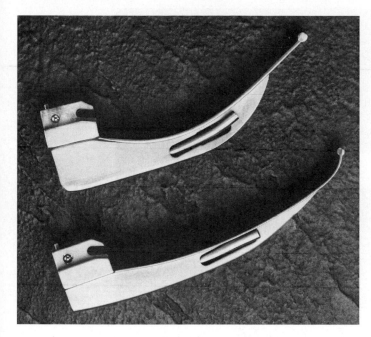

FIGURE **16.13.** Upsher low profile (ULP) blade. At top is a standard Macintosh blade. The bottom is a ULP blade.

The flange is removed, except for a small part that encases the light bulb. This was done to attempt to limit damage to the upper teeth. The blade is particularly designed for patients with a limited mouth opening, prominent incisors, receding mandible, short thick neck, or anterior larynx.

ULP

The ULP (Upsher low profile) (Fig. 16.13) is a modified Macintosh blade with a low flange and a fairly straight proximal section that leads to a tip with a significant curve. This configuration is designed for insertion into a small mouth.

Upsher ULX Macintosh blade

The ULX blade (Fig. 16.14) has a little more curve than the standard Macintosh blade.

Miller Blade (39)

The Miller (Figs. 16.4 and 16.15) is one of the most popular blades. The tongue is straight with a slight upward curve near the tip. In cross-section the flange, web, and tongue form a C with the top fattened. Some versions of the blade have the lamp socket on the tongue, whereas other versions have it on the web. The lamp may be on either the right or left side of the blade. Several modifications have been described in the literature (39–41).

In comparing force and torque exerted during intubation using the Macintosh and Miller blades, it was found that force was lower and head extension was less with the Miller (42).

Oxiport Miller Blade (43–46)

The oxiport Miller (Miller/port, oxyscope) blade (Fig. 16.16) has a built-in tube that allows delivery of oxygen or other gases during intubation. It may also be used for suction. Insufflation of oxygen during intubation using this blade has been found to lessen oxygen desaturation in spontaneously breathing anesthetized patients (47, 48).

Tull Miller Blade

The Tull (suction) Miller blade is a standard Miller blade with a suction tube whose port ends near the tip of the blade (see Fig. 16.10). Near the handle is a finger-controlled port that allows control of suction.

Mathews Blade

The Mathews blade (Fig. 16.17) is straight with a wide and flattened petalloid configuration tip. It is designed for difficult nasotracheal intubations.

Wisconsin Blade

Unlike the Miller blade, the Wisconsin blade's tongue has no curve (Fig. 16.18). The flange is curved to form two-thirds of a circle in cross-

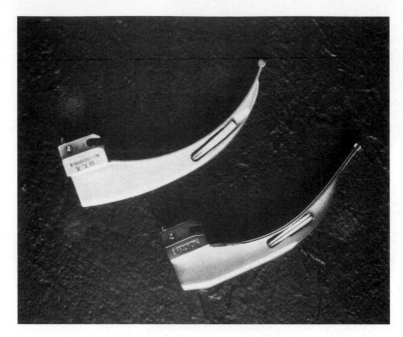

FIGURE 16.14. ULX blade. The ULX is at the top. A standard Macintosh blade is at the bottom. (Courtesy of Mercury Medical.)

FIGURE 16.15. The Miller blade. (Courtesy of Penlon Ltd.)

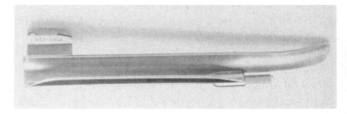

section. The depth of the flange is small at the proximal end and wider in the distal portion.

Wis–Foregger Blade (49)

The Wis–Foregger (Fig. 16.19) is a modification of the Wisconsin blade with a straight tongue and a flange that expands slightly toward the distal end. The distal portion of the blade is wider and formed slightly to the right.

Wis–Hipple Blade

The Wis–Hipple (Fig. 16.20) is also a modified Wisconsin blade. The tongue is straight, and the flange is large and circular. Compared with the Wisconsin blade, the flange is straighter and runs parallel to the tongue and the tip is wider. It is designed primarily for use in infants.

Schapira Blade (50)

The Schapira blade (Fig. 16.21) is a straight blade with a tip that curves upward. The vertical component is minimal. The blade is designed to facilitate intubation by cradling the tongue and pushing it to the left side of the mouth.

Alberts Blade

The Alberts blade (Fig. 16.22) combines characteristics of the Miller and Wis–Hipple blades with a cutaway flange to increase visibility. There is a recess to facilitate insertion of a tracheal tube.

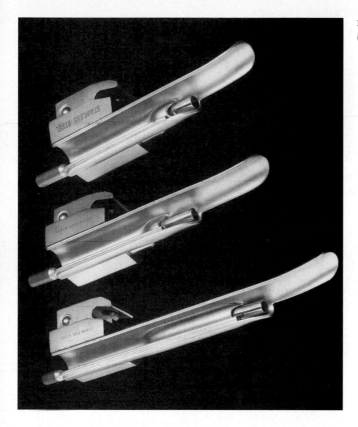

FIGURE **16.16.** Oxiport Miller blades. (Courtesy of Rusch Inc.)

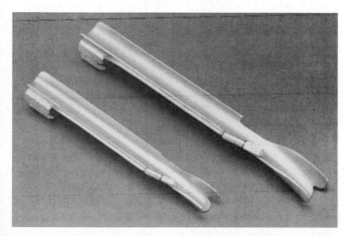

FIGURE **16.17.** The Mathews blade. (Courtesy of Mercury Medical.)

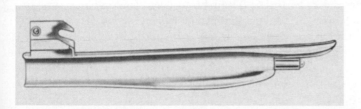

FIGURE **16.18.** The Wisconsin blade. (Courtesy of Ohio Medical Products, a division of Airco, Inc.)

FIGURE **16.19.** The Wis–Foregger blade. (Courtesy of Puritan–Bennett Corp.)

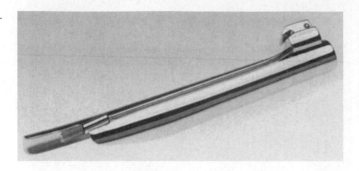

FIGURE **16.20.** The Wis–Hipple blade. (Courtesy of Puritan–Bennett Corp.)

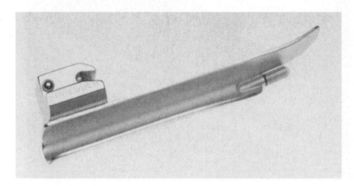

FIGURE **16.21.** The Schapira blade. (Courtesy of Puritan–Bennett Corp.)

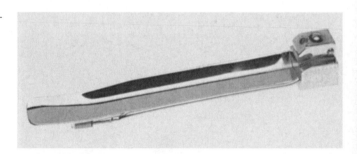

The blade forms a 67° angle with the handle. It is used for pediatric patients.

Michaels Blade

The Michaels blade (Fig. 16.22) differs from the Alberts blade only in that it forms a 93° angle with the handle.

Soper Blade (51)

The Soper blade (Fig. 16.23) combines the Z shape on the flange of the Macintosh blade with a straight blade. It has a slot built into the tip, which is intended to prevent the epiglottis from slipping off the blade.

Heine Blade

The Heine (Propper) blade (Fig. 16.24) is straight with a slight upward curve at the tip. The flat flange is curved away from the blade. It is useful for children with large tongues.

Snow Blade (52)

The Snow blade (Fig. 16.25) is a hybrid blade consisting of a Miller tongue and a Wis–Foregger flange. It is curved 1 inch from the tip.

Flagg Blade (53)

The Flagg blade (Fig. 16.26) has a straight tongue. The flange has a C shape that gradually decreases in size as it approaches the distal end.

Guedel Blade

The Guedel blade (Fig. 16.27) is a straight blade on which the tongue is set at a 72° angle to the handle. The flange has the shape of a U on its side. The light is close to the tip, which has an uptilt of 10°.

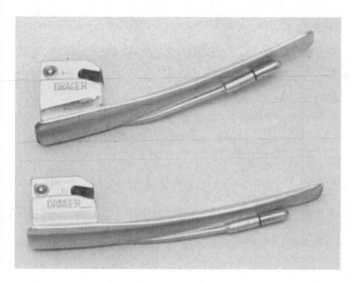

FIGURE 16.22. The Alberts (**top**) and Michaels (**bottom**) blades. The Alberts blade offers a sharp 67° angle, whereas the Michaels blade has a slight 93° angle. (Courtesy of North American Drager.)

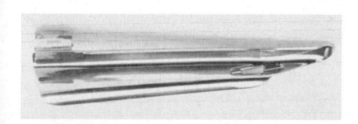

FIGURE 16.23. The Soper blade. (Courtesy of Penlon Ltd.)

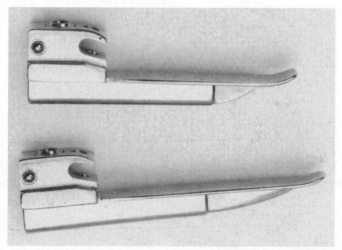

FIGURE 16.24. Heine blades. (Courtesy of Propper Manufacturing Co., Inc.)

FIGURE **16.25.** The Snow blade. (Courtesy of Air Products and Chemicals, Inc.)

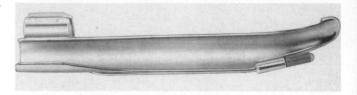

FIGURE **16.26.** The Flagg blade. (Courtesy of Ohio Medical Products, a division of Airco, Inc.)

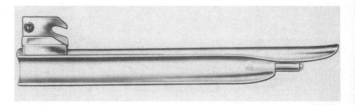

FIGURE **16.27.** The Guedel blade. (Courtesy of Penlon Ltd.)

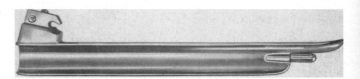

FIGURE **16.28.** The Bennett blade. (Courtesy of Puritan–Bennett Corp.)

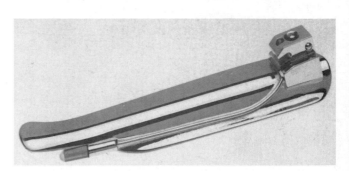

FIGURE **16.29.** The Eversole blade. (Courtesy of Puritan–Bennett Corp.)

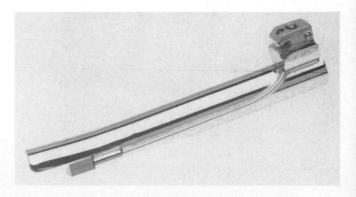

Bennett Blade

The Bennett blade (Fig. 16.28) is a modification of the Guedel blade. It also forms an acute angle with the handle. The upper part of the flange has been omitted.

Eversole Blade

The Eversole blade (Fig. 16.29) has a straight tongue. The flange forms a *C* with the tongue and web near the proximal end. Midway to the tip the upper flange tapers.

Seward Blade (54)

The Seward blade (Fig. 16.30) has a straight tongue with a curve near the tip. It has a small reverse *Z*-shaped flange. The blade is useful for nasotracheal intubation because its shape allows a Magill forceps to be introduced with minimal loss of view (55). It is intended for use in children less than 5 years old.

Phillips Blade (56)

The Phillips blade (Fig. 16.31) is straight with a low flange and a curved tip similar to a Miller blade. The light bulb is on the left side of the blade.

Racz–Allen Blade (57)

The Racz–Allen blade is straight with a curved tip. The proximal portion of the blade flexes to relieve pressure on the teeth. The vertical portion is hinged and held in position by a spring. The spring allows lateral deflection of the vertical por-tion without occluding the view. Exposure is improved by tilting the handle of the laryngoscope to the left. The hinged portion is concave along its length. The tongue surface is rough and unpolished to reduce slippage.

Robertshaw Blade (58)

The Robertshaw blade (Fig. 16.32) has a straight tongue with a gentle curve near the tip. It is designed to lift the epiglottis indirectly. The flange is extended to the left. The blade was designed for infants and children. It has been found to be useful for nasotracheal intubation because it allows a Magill forceps to be introduced with minimal loss of view (55).

Oxford Infant Blade (59)

The Oxford infant blade (Fig. 16.33) has a straight tongue that curves up slightly at the tip. It has a *U* shape at the proximal end with the bottom limb of the *U* decreasing toward the tip so that the distal part is open. It tapers from a maximum width at the proximal end to the tip. Although intended primarily for newborns, it can be used for children up to the age of 4.

Bainton Blade (60)

The Bainton blade (Fig. 16.34) has a straight tongue. The distal 7-cm section is tubular so that it is protected from obstruction by edematous tissue, blood, secretions, intraoral masses, and scar tissue and has an intraluminal light source. The

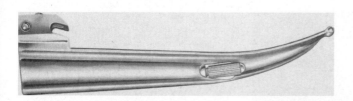

FIGURE 16.30. The Seward blade. (Courtesy of Penlon Ltd.)

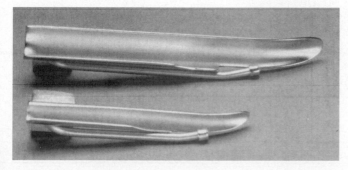

FIGURE 16.31. Phillips blades. (Courtesy of Mercury Medical.)

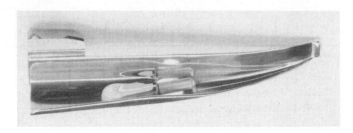

FIGURE **16.32.** The Robertshaw blade. (Courtesy of Penlon Ltd.)

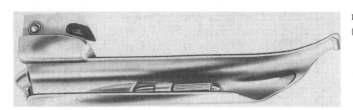

FIGURE **16.33.** The Oxford infant blade. (Courtesy of Penlon Ltd.)

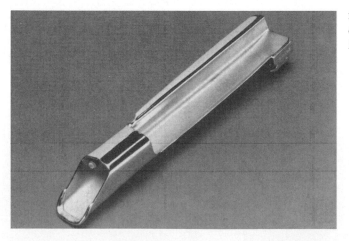

FIGURE **16.34.** The Bainton blade. Note the distal tubular section. (Courtesy of Mercury Medical.)

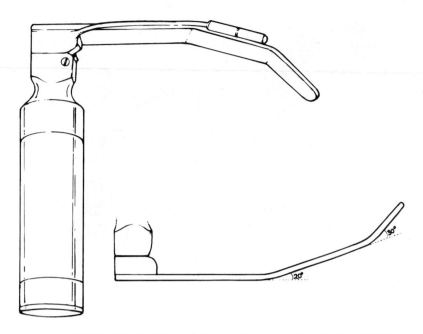

FIGURE 16.35. The double-angle blade. (Courtesy of Jay J. Choi, M.D.)

tip is beveled at a 60° angle to create an oval opening at the distal end of the tube. A tracheal tube of 8 mm or less can be inserted through the tubular lumen without significantly obstructing vision.

The Bainton blade is designed for patients with right-sided or circumferential pharyngeal lesions. The tubular portion can displace tissues circumferentially and thus overcome this problem.

A modified two-piece tubular pharyngolaryngoscope is also available. The two parts of the blade are held together by a screw during intubation. A tracheal tube is placed intraluminally into the glottis, then the two pieces are dismantled for removal from around the tube.

Double-Angle Blade (61, 62)

The spatula of the double-angle (Choi) blade (Fig. 16.35) has two incremental angulations, 20° and 30°, to improve lifting of the epiglottis and reduce the need to tilt the blade posteriorly. The spatula and tip form a wide, flat surface. The bulb is located on the left edge of the blade between the two curvatures. The flange has been eliminated. The blade may be especially useful for the patient with an anterior larynx. Because there is no flange, there is more room to pass the tracheal tube than with a straight blade.

Blechman Blade

The Blechman blade (Fig. 16.36) is a modification of the Macintosh-style blade, with the tip angled sharply to elevate the epiglottis. The flange has been removed near the handle end of the blade.

Belscope Blade (63, 64)

The Belscope blade (Fig. 16.37) is bent forward 45° near its midpoint. It also has an offset handle. The tip is beaded on the underside. The blade is designed to be used like a straight blade, with the tip lifting the epiglottis. It is available in several lengths.

When a satisfactory view of the larynx cannot be obtained, a prism of transparent acrylic can be attached to the blade just proximal to the angle (Fig. 16.35*B*). Condensation of moisture on the prism can be prevented by applying an antifog preparation to the leading and trailing surfaces of the prism and/or warming the prism before use. Another measure to prevent fogging is to direct a continuous flow of oxygen over the prism through a suction catheter taped to the blade (65). Because the image of the larynx is rotated, the user's head must be moved higher and further forward than when the prism is omitted.

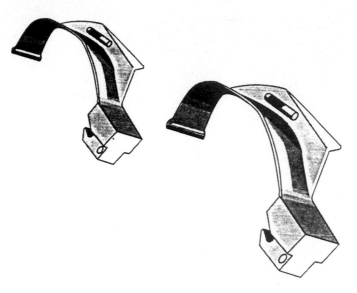

FIGURE **16.36.** Blechman blade. (Courtesy of Mercury Medical.)

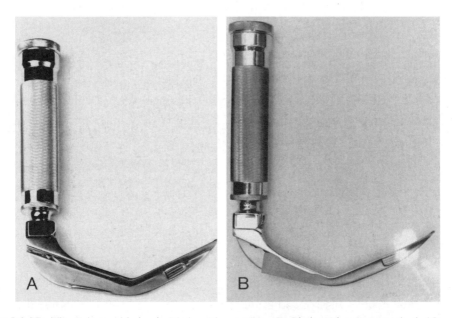

FIGURE **16.37.** The Belscope blade. **A,** Blade without prism. **B,** Blade with prism attached. (Courtesy of Dr. Paul Bellhouse.)

The Belscope provides a greater distance between the posterior end of the blade and the upper teeth, making it less likely to contribute to dental damage than other blades (66).

Several studies have shown an improved view of the larynx could be obtained with this blade compared to other blades (66–69).

This blade feels different from other blades so practice is necessary to acquire proficiency (62, 70). Intubation may take longer and be less successful when the prism is used (71).

Cranwall Blade

The Cranwall blade (Fig. 16.38) has a curved tip like a Miller blade. There is a reduced flange

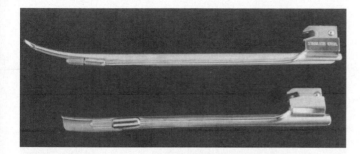

FIGURE **16.38.** Cranwall (**top**) and White-head (**bottom**) blades. (Courtesy of Bay Medical, Inc.)

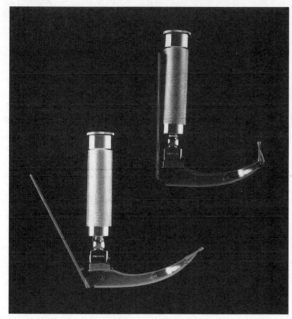

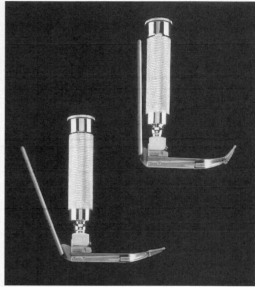

FIGURE **16.39.** CLM (Corazzelli, London, McCoy) blades. **Left,** Curved. **Right,** Straight. (Courtesy of Mercury Medical.)

to decrease the potential for damage to the upper teeth.

Whitehead Blade

The Whitehead blade (Fig. 16.38) is a modification of the Wis–Foregger blade. The flange is reduced in height and open proximally and distally.

CLM Blade (72, 73)

On the CLM (Corazzelli, London, McCoy) (McCoy, Articulating, Levering, ALB) laryngoscope blade (Fig. 16.39) the distal end is hinged so that the tip is movable. A lever is attached to the proximal end of the blade. When the lever is pushed toward the handle, the tip of the blade is flexed. A pediatric version using a Seward-type blade and adult versions using Miller and Macin-tosh blades are available. The tip is less rounded than on the usual Macintosh blade (74). It can also be used as an ordinary blade.

This laryngoscope has been reported to be helpful when a difficult intubation is encountered (74–80). It has been recommended where minimal neck movement is desirable (81–83). It may result in less pressure on the teeth during intubation (84). However, in patients in whom the view is satisfactory with the Macintosh blade, use of the McCoy may make the view worse (74).

Studies have shown that use of the McCoy blade results in significantly less force being applied and a reduction in the stress response compared to the Macintosh blade (85–87).

FIGURE **16.40.** The Huffman prism. (Courtesy of Penlon Ltd.)

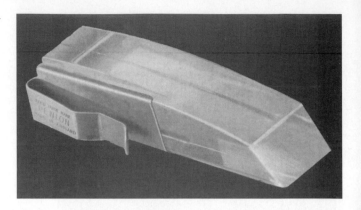

Huffman Prism and Prism Laryngoscope Blade (88–90)

The Huffman prism and prism laryngoscope blade are designed to provide an indirect view of the larynx in patients in whom direct exposure is difficult. The prism is a block of Plexiglas shaped to fit on the proximal end of a No. 3 Macintosh blade (Fig. 16.40). It is fastened onto the blade with a steel clip. The ends are polished to produce optically flat surfaces. A refraction of 30° in the line of sight is provided, thereby bringing into view structures within a few millimeters of the tip of the blade. The image is right side up. It is necessary to warm the prism before use to prevent condensation.

The prism laryngoscope blade has the prism built into the blade. An additional 20° refraction from right to left is added, because the prism is to the left of the midline. The prism laryngoscope blade allows either conventional direct exposure of the larynx or indirect viewing through the prism.

Techniques of Use

The optimal position for laryngoscopy in most patients is flexion of the lower cervical spine and extension of the head at the atlantooccipital level, the so-called sniffing position. The lower portion of the cervical spine can be maintained in a position of flexion by use of a small pillow under the head. Extension of the atlantooccipital joint is achieved by pressure on the top of the head and/or upward traction on the upper teeth or gums by the laryngoscopist's hand (91). In children, it

may be unnecessary to flex the lower cervical vertebrae, and in neonates it may be necessary to elevate the shoulders.

The laryngoscope handle is held in the left hand. Moistening or lubricating the blade will facilitate insertion if the mouth is dry. In some situations the chest will impinge on the handle, making insertion of the blade difficult. In these cases, a short handle may be used, the blade may be inserted sideways (11, 12), or the blade may be inserted and then attached to the handle (13, 14).

The fingers of the right hand are used to open the mouth and spread the lips. In patients with dentition, the optimum opening of the mouth is often achieved with a thumb-over-index-finger approach, with the index finger on the maxillary dentition as far to the right as possible and the thumb placed on the lower teeth (92).

The blade is inserted at the right side of the mouth. This reduces the likelihood that the incisor teeth will be damaged and helps push the tongue to the left. The blade is advanced on the side of the tongue toward the right tonsillar fossa, so that the tongue lies on the left side of the blade. The right hand keeps the lips from getting caught between the teeth or gums and the blade. If the tongue is slippery, placement of tape on the lingual surface of the blade may be helpful (93). When the right tonsillar fossa is visualized, the tip of the blade is moved toward the midline. The blade is then advanced behind the base of the tongue, elevating it, until the epiglottis comes into view.

There are two methods for elevating the epiglottis, depending on whether a straight or curved blade is being used.

Straight Blade

The straight blade is shown in position for intubation in Figure 16.41*A*. The tip is alternately advanced and the handle rotated backward until the epiglottis is exposed. The blade is then made to scoop under the epiglottis and lift it anteriorly. The vocal cords should be identified. Displacement of the larynx by external backward upward and rightward pressure (BURP) on the thyroid cartilage may improve visualization of the glottis (94–98).

If the blade is advanced too far, it will result in elevation of the larynx as a whole rather than exposure of the vocal cords. Occasionally, the blade will expose the esophagus. It should then be withdrawn slowly. If it is withdrawn too far,

the tip of the epiglottis will be released and flip over the glottis.

The straight blade can also be inserted into the vallecula (the angle made by the epiglottis with the base of the tongue) and used in the same manner as a curved blade.

Another technique using a straight blade has been reported to be successful after failure with a Macintosh blade (99). A Miller blade is passed from the right corner of the mouth into the groove between the tongue and the tonsil using leftward and anterior pressure to displace the tongue to the left of the laryngoscope and to maintain the tongue in this position. The blade is advanced, the epiglottis identified and the tip of the blade is passed posterior to the epiglottis. Next, the blade is lifted anteriorly, elevating the epiglottis directly so that the glottis is exposed. The blade is then moved toward the midline push-

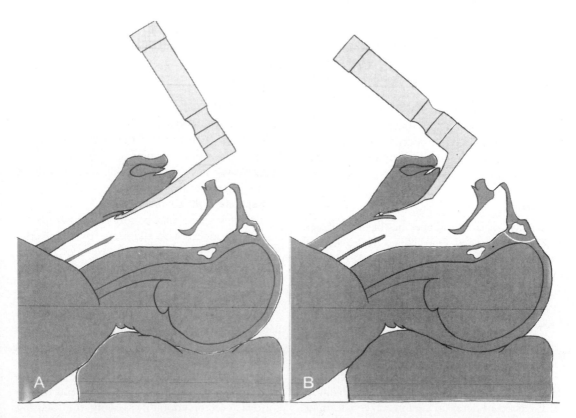

FIGURE 16.41.   A, Intubation with a straight laryngoscope blade. The tip of the blade picks up the epiglottis. **B,** Intubation with the curved laryngoscope blade. The epiglottis is below the tip of the blade. A small pillow under the head allows better visualization on the larynx. (Courtesy of Vance Robideaux, MD)

ing the tongue to the left. An assistant may be needed to retract the corner of the mouth so that the tracheal tube can be manipulated into place (99).

Curved Blade

Figure 16.41*B* shows the curved blade in position. After the epiglottis is seen, the blade is advanced until the tip fits into the vallecula. Traction is then applied along the handle, at right angles to the blade to move the base of the tongue and the epiglottis forward. The glottis should come into view. It is important that the handle not be pulled backward. This will cause the tip to push the larynx upward and out of sight and could cause damage to the teeth or gums. Displacement of the larynx by external BURP on the thyroid cartilage may improve visualization of the glottis (94–98).

A curved blade can be used as a straight blade, lifting the epiglottis directly, if it is long enough (100).

Use of laryngoscopes during magnetic resonance imaging (MRI) creates special problems (101). Plastic laryngoscopes are available, but the batteries in the handle still cause a pull from the magnetic field. Laryngoscopes have been modified to operate from a DC source connected to the MRI machine (102). A special cable with nonmagnetic connectors is used to connect the laryngoscope to the power source.

Cleaning

Cleaning of laryngoscopes has been a subject of debate for several years. Since blades are inserted into the mouth and often stimulate bleeding, there is potential for cross-infection among patients. The handle, while not in direct contact with the patient, may also be contaminated with blood or secretions.

Reprocessing

Recommended cleaning procedures including washing the blade and liquid chemical sterilization are discussed in detail in Chapter 27, "Cleaning and Sterilization." Some blades can be steam autoclaved.

Disposable Equipment

Disposable laryngoscope blades and handles are available (Fig. 16.3). When the entire blade and handle are disposable the battery and/or light source are usually reusable. Disposable laryngoscope covers are available (Fig. 16.42).

Disposable Sheaths

Disposable sheaths that cover the blade or the entire blade and handle are available.

FLEXIBLE FIBEROPTIC ENDOSCOPE (103)

Uses of flexible fiberoptic endoscopy include placement of and evaluation of the positions of tracheal, double-lumen, tracheostomy, and nasogastric tubes, larangeal mask airways (LMAs), and bronchial blockers; repositioning, changing or checking the patency of tubes; evaluation of the airway, and locating and removing secretions (103–111).

Description (103, 112, 113)

The fiberscope is composed of several parts, including the light source, handle, and flexible insertion portion (Fig. 16.43).

Light Source

Handle with Batteries

A handle with batteries that uses a low-power halogen light bulb is compact, convenient, and inexpensive. However, the illumination will be weaker than that from a separate source.

Separate Light Source

The light source may be contained in a separate box and connected to the scope by a universal (light transmission) cord. This produces a bright light without much heat.

Handle

The handle, or body, is the part held in the hand during use. It houses the batteries, if they are used as the power source, or there may be an adapter to a high-intensity remote light source. Other parts of the handle include the eyepiece, focusing ring, working channel port, and the tip control lever or knob. By turning the focusing (adjusting) ring, the image just in front of the tip of the scope can be brought into focus. Often a

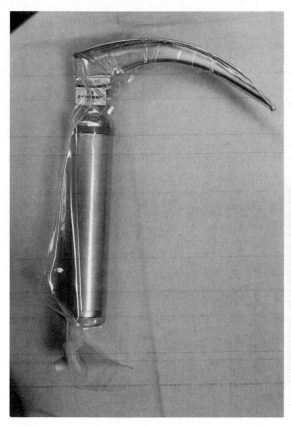

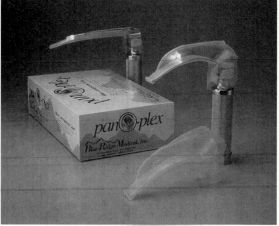

FIGURE **16.42.** Disposable laryngoscope covers. **Left,** the cover ensheathes both the blade and the handle. **Right,** only the blade is covered. (Courtesy of Blue Ridge Products.)

camera adapter or teaching attachment can be fitted to the eyepiece.

The tip (bending, angulation) control lever or knob may be on the side of the body, or a thumb-controlled lever system on the back section of the handle. By turning this, the tip of the insertion cord can be flexed or extended in one plane. A full range of motion can be achieved by rotating the entire instrument. Many fiberscopes have a tip-locking lever to lock the bending tip at a desired position.

The connection of the handle to the insertion portion is usually tapered to hold a tracheal tube.

Insertion Cord

The insertion cord (shaft, tube) is the long portion of the fiberscope that is inserted into the patient and over which tracheal tubes are passed. It contains one image-transmitting bundle, one or two light-conducting bundles, two angulation wires, and may contain a working channel. These are surrounded by a protective wire mesh and vinyl covering. This portion is fully submersible, which facilitates cleaning. Circular white markings indicate depth of insertion.

The outside diameter of the insertion cord determines the size of the smallest tracheal tube that can be used. The inside diameter of the tracheal tube should be at least 1 mm larger than the diameter of the insertion cord (103). If the tube is passed through the nose, a difference of 2 mm is appropriate (114). Fiberscopes as thin as 1.8 mm OD are available. These allow intubation with a tracheal tube as small as 3.0 mm ID (115, 116).

The length of the insertion cord varies. For tracheal intubation in adults, a 50-cm insertion cord

FIGURE **16.43.** Flexible fiberoptic laryngo-scope. Light is supplied from a separate source. The lever on the handle controls deflection of the tip in two directions. Two ports attach to the working channel. One is for insufflation or injection and one for suctioning. (Courtesy of Olympus Corp.)

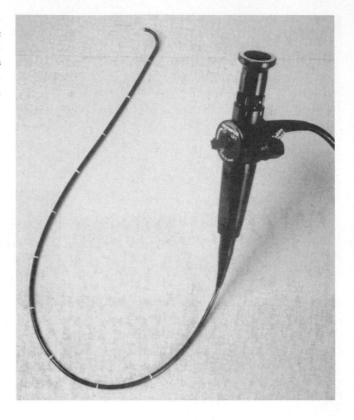

is usually sufficient. To allow placement of double-lumen bronchial tubes and nasotracheal intubation, 55 to 60 cm are needed.

Image-Conducting Bundle

The image-conducting (optic fiber, image transmission, image guide) bundle transmits the image from the distal lens to the eyepiece. These fibers are arranged so that the relationship of one fiber to the other is the same at each end of the bundle. Such a bundle is called *coherent* and allows transmission of a clear image. A lens at the distal end allows the image transmitted by the fibers to be focused. Except at the ends where the fibers are fused for strength, the bundle is flexible. However, the fibers are delicate and breakage may occur. When broken, a fiber will no longer pass its image and the viewer will see a black dot in that fiber's location.

Light-Conducting Fiber Bundle

The light-conducting fiber (light guide, light transmission) bundle can transmit light from a powerful source without producing dangerous heating. Unlike the image-conducting bundle, the fibers are not arranged in a precise manner. This is known as an *incoherent* bundle.

Working Channel

Although the working (suction, injection) channel is optional, most scopes have one extending the length of the scope. This can be used for suctioning, injection of saline or medications, insufflation of gases, and passage of other instruments (such as forceps, brushes or guidewires) (117).

Tip Flexion Cables

Two tip flexion cables (angulation wires, control wires, tip-bending control wires) connecting the tip to the bending knob on the handle are placed along the sides of the insertion cord.

Endoscopic Accessories

Accessory devices to protect the fiberscope from the teeth, keep it in the midline and carry it forward to the vicinity of the larynx are often used. These are discussed in Chapter 14, "Face Masks and Airways." A nipple from a baby bottle may be used in an awake infant (118). Intubation using an LMA is discussed in Chapter 15, "The Laryngeal Mask Airway."

Techniques of Use (103, 110, 113, 119, 120)

A full discussion of fiberoptic techniques is beyond the scope of this book. Only the basics will be mentioned.

It can be inserted either nasally or orally, in awake or anesthetized patients who are either breathing spontaneously or being ventilated. Although fiberoptic intubation can be done in unconscious individuals, most authors recommend that where possible it be performed in the awake patient using sedation and topical anesthesia. Loss of consciousness is associated with a loss of tone in the submandibular muscles that directly support the tongue and indirectly support the epiglottis. Various methods of ventilation can be employed during use of a fiberscope (103, 121–134). Complications of insufflating oxygen through the working channel include gastric distention and rupture (135) and subcutaneous emphysema (136).

Practice is needed to learn to manipulate the tip control while advancing the scope. Nevertheless, facility with this instrument can be achieved without an inordinate expenditure of time or effort. As experience is gained, the average time required for intubation will decrease. Rather than making first attempts with a difficult intubation, facility should be developed first with an intubation mannequin or animal model then with awake, spontaneously breathing patients in whom no difficulty with intubation is anticipated.

Because this instrument is expensive and delicate, great care must be taken not to damage it. A minor blow can break glass fibers. Care must be taken to avoid forceful bending of the cord, especially the distal end. A blow to the distal end may crack the objective lens. The insertion portion must not be withdrawn or advanced with the distal tip angulated.

Before use, the light and suction sources should be tested. The tip should be treated with anti-fogging solution or placed in warm water (not saline) for several minutes before use. Alter-

natively, the tip of the scope can be briefly held against the buccal mucosa to warm the lens. The light source should be connected and tested. The focusing ring should be adjusted by viewing small print at a distance of 2 to 3 cm. The outside of the flexible portion should be coated with a lubricating gel, but the lubricant should not contact the lens.

Generally the proximal control section of the scope is held in one hand with the index finger on the suction port and the thumb on the lever that regulates angulation of the distal tip. The other hand holds the shaft of the scope distally and guides its advance. Because the cables are not strong enough to lift, part, or dislodge tissues, it is important to have an air space at the end of the tip. In the anesthetized patient, visualization is often difficult or impossible unless some means to expand the pharynx is used. This may be accomplished by having a second person pull the tongue anteriorly or elevate the jaw. Occasionally, it may be necessary to lift the larynx by grasping it externally. Alternately, a modified surgical tongue retractor or a rigid laryngoscope can be used to push the tongue forward (137, 138). The awake patient can be asked to stick out his or her tongue, which is then held gently between gauze by an assistant.

Disorientation in the airway is best resolved by withdrawing the tip a bit and examining the area with gentle up and down tip deflection, by rotating the scope, or by alternately advancing the tip and withdrawing it slightly. If the view is consistently foggy or hazy, irrigation with saline and suction will usually resolve this problem. Adherent secretions may require withdrawal of the entire instrument and mechanical cleaning of the tip with a moist gauze. Insufflation of oxygen serves the dual purpose of maintaining the distal lens clear from secretions and increasing the oxygen concentration at the end of the fiberscope.

Occasionally a tracheal tube will fail to pass over the fiberscope into the trachea. Flexible spiral-wound tubes may more easily follow the curves of the fiberscope as it passes through the glottis and trachea (139–142). If an obstruction is encountered, the tracheal tube should be rotated counterclockwise 90°, then again advanced (143–145). If the tube does not advance smoothly, the tongue and epiglottis should be elevated by pushing or pulling the mandible forward, pulling the tongue forward, or using a tongue retractor or rigid laryngoscope (146). Application of external pressure to the larynx also may assist tube advancement (147).

Attempting to pass a relatively large tracheal tube over a small scope may result in a lower rate of successful intubation and a longer duration of intubation (148, 149). One solution is to interpose a smaller tracheal tube between the fiberscope and the larger tracheal tube (149, 150).

If the tip of the fiberscope protrudes through the Murphy eye of the tracheal tube, it may not be possible to slip the tube off the endoscope or to withdraw the fiberscope from the tracheal tube (151–153). The fiberscope and tracheal tube should be withdrawn together as a unit. To avoid this problem, the tracheal tube should be threaded onto the fiberscope before endoscopy or the fiberscope should be advanced through the tube under direct vision, identifying both the side and distal openings and taking care to pass the fiberscope through the distal one. The tip of the endoscope should be in the neutral position as the tracheal tube is advanced and the fiberscope is withdrawn.

A variety of techniques is available, the choice often being a matter of personal preference. The first is to thread a tracheal or double-lumen tube with the lumen lubricated over the cord until it abuts the handle, advance the flexible portion until the tip enters the trachea, then thread the tube over the flexible portion.

With the second technique, the tracheal tube is first advanced into the pharynx so that it acts as a guide to bring the tip of the scope close to the entrance of the larynx. The fiberscope is passed through the tube and into the trachea, then the tube is threaded over the flexible portion.

A third technique is to use the fiberscope to place a guide wire or stylet into the trachea under direct vision (154–158). The fiberscope is withdrawn and a tracheal tube passed over the guide wire into the trachea.

Another approach is to position the fiberscope near the laryngeal entrance, then separately advance the tracheal tube until it can be visualized through the fiberscope. The tube is then advanced under direct fiberoptic vision. This is useful for patients who require a tube too small to fit on a fiberscope (159, 160). A variant of this technique is to pass a guide into the larynx under direct vision from the fiberoptic scope (161). The tracheal tube is then passed over the guide into the trachea.

The fiberoptic endoscope can be used in a manner similar to a lighted intubation stylet (162, 163).

A technique for pediatric patients involves threading a tracheal tube of a size larger than can be accommodated by the trachea over the fiberscope until it impacts in the larynx (164). The fiberscope is then removed and a tube changer slipped through the tube and into the trachea. The tracheal tube is then removed and a smaller tracheal tube threaded over the tube changer into the trachea.

Oral Intubation (165)

Oral intubation is considered more difficult than intubation by the nasal route. The optic tip enters the larynx at an acute angle to the glottis whereas via the nasal route it is at an oblique angle (166).

Optimal positioning for fiberoptic laryngoscopy by the oral route includes extension of the cervical spine rather than flexion as recommended for direct laryngoscopy (167, 168). Intubation may be easier if used with an accessory that will protect the instrument from the patient's teeth, guide it into the midline, and keep the tongue from falling backward. These are discussed in Chapter 14, "Face Masks and Airways." In some cases it is helpful to have an assistant gently retract the tongue. A rigid laryngoscope may be used to direct the fiberscope near the glottis (169).

The fiberscope is placed in the midline and advanced under direct vision, curving downward at the posterior pharyngeal wall, seeking the epiglottis. It is important that the laryngoscope be kept in the midline as it is advanced. When the epiglottis has been located, the fiberscope tip is rotated downward so that it passes beneath the epiglottis and is then turned upward until the vocal cords are seen. The tip is then passed between the cords and advanced several centimeters into the trachea. For bronchial intubation, the tip is advanced to view the carina, then into the desired mainstem bronchus.

With the tip of the fiberscope in place, the lubricated tracheal tube is advanced over the scope which functions as a stylet. The bevel of the tube should be oriented in an anteroposterior direction parallel to the vocal cords and advanced through the glottis during a deep inspiration. The fiberscope should be used to verify that the tip of the tube is correctly positioned, then withdrawn, leaving the tube in place.

The fiberscope can be used to convert a nasal intubation to an oral intubation. It is used to follow the tube to the larynx. At this point, the scope is manipulated anteriorly between the tracheal tube and the aryepiglottic fold towards the anterior commissure. After it is passed into the trachea, the nasal tube is withdrawn and the oral tube inserted over the scope (170).

Nasal Intubation (165, 171)

Fiberoptic nasotracheal intubation is usually easier than orotracheal intubation because midline positioning is easier to maintain, the patient cannot bite the scope, and the anatomy of the nasopharynx naturally directs the tube into the trachea.

Several techniques have been used (172). (1) A nasopharyngeal airway is inserted, then replaced with the nasotracheal tube introduced until its enters the nasopharynx. (2) A nasopharyngeal airway is inserted, then removed and a fiberscope loaded with a tracheal tube introduced. (3) The fiberscope with a tube loaded can be introduced through a slit nasal airway which is removed before passage of the tracheal tube (173). (4) The airway may be accessed through an anesthetic mask designed to accommodate the fiberscope.

It is important to use the most patent nares. The tube may be compressed in the nose so that it will not accommodate the laryngoscope, even when the tube lumen would otherwise be adequate (174).

Difficulty in advancing the tube over the fiberscope is usually the result of the tip hanging up on the epiglottis (144) or an arytenoid (174, 175). The tube should be withdrawn, rotated 90 to 180°, then advanced. If it still does not advance smoothly, the epiglottis should be moved anteriorly by elevating the mandible or external pressure applied on the larynx.

Retrograde-Assisted Fiberoptic Intubation

A fiberoptic scope can be used to assist retrograde intubation (176, 177). A wire is inserted into the trachea and advanced until it exits the nostril or mouth. At this point, the wire is inserted into the working channel of a flexible fiberscope. The fiberscope with a tracheal tube threaded over it is then advanced past the vocal cords and the wire is withdrawn. The scope is then advanced further and the tube advanced over the fiberscope.

Tracheal Tube Exchange (107)

To exchange a tracheal tube, the new tube is threaded over the fiberscope. In one technique, the insertion portion of the fiberscope is advanced into the tube to be replaced (178). As the old tube is pulled out, it is cut and removed from around the fiberscope. The new tube is then advanced into place over the fiberscope. In an alternative technique, the malfunctioning tube is visualized in the pharynx using the fiberscope and followed down to the level of the vocal cords (107, 179). It may be advisable to insert a jet stylet catheter through the old tracheal tube before removing it to allow for ventilation or reintubation over it if the new tracheal tube cannot be passed into the trachea (178). The cuff on the malfunctioning tube is then deflated and the fiberscope advanced through the space around the tube past the cords. The old tube is gently removed and the new one advanced over the fiberscope into position.

As an Adjunct to Extubation

The fiberscope has been used to evaluate a difficult extubation (180). Another use is in extubating patients who would be difficult to reintubate (181). The fiberscope is inserted through the tube and the tube withdrawn from the larynx. The working channel is used to insufflate oxygen. If the patient is unable to maintain a patent airway, the tube can be reinserted over the fiberscope.

Advantages

The fiberscope can be used to intubate patients who are difficult or impossible to intubate with a rigid laryngoscope (104, 115, 154, 158, 182–192). Its use has been recommended in patients with unstable cervical spines and those at high risk of dental damage. It can be used in cases where the patient cannot be placed in the supine position (193).

Disadvantages

Compared with a rigid laryngoscope, the flexible fiberoptic endoscope (fiberscope) is more expensive, fragile, and difficult to use and clean. Fiberoptic techniques require more time than conventional intubation. It requires considerable experience and maintenance of skills.

A major impediment to its successful use is the presence of significant amounts of blood and/or secretions (62).

If oxygen is insufflated through the working channel and the tip of the scope is in the esophagus, gastric distention and rupture may occur (135).

Cleaning (103)

Cleaning procedures will vary with the particular scope being used. It is important to read the instruction manual carefully because improper care can cause extensive and expensive damage to the scope. Most scopes are sterilized with chemical sterilants. Cleaning methods are discussed in more detail in Chapter 27, "Cleaning and Sterilization."

LIGHTED INTUBATION STYLET

The lighted intubation stylet (lightwand, flexible; lighted stylet; Trach light; illuminating or lighted intubating stylet) uses transillumination of the neck to guide the placement of a tracheal tube. The larynx is not visualized.

Description (194)

Several lightwands are available commercially (Figs. 16.44 and 16.45). Each has a handle containing the power control circuitry and batteries and a malleable wand section with a light at the end. The wand section may be disposable and detachable from the handle. On later models the shaft and bulb are encased in a plastic covering to prevent detachment of the bulb (195). Some have a fiberoptic lighting system. Some have a retractable but malleable inner stylet. Some have a means to secure the tube to the lightwand. One has a tip which can be manipulated during insertion into the trachea. Pediatric lightwands that can accommodate tubes as small as 3.5 mm are available (196).

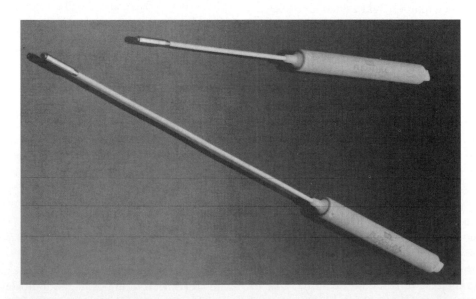

FIGURE 16.44. Lighted intubation stylets. There is a light bulb at the tip of the malleable stylet. (Courtesy of Concept Inc.)

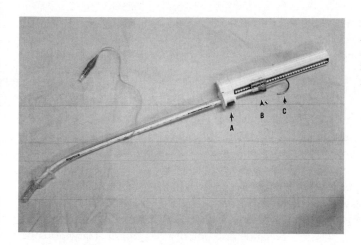

FIGURE **16.45.** Lighted intubation stylet. **A,** Locking device for the tracheal tube connector. **B,** Control for moving the lightwand inside the tracheal tube. **C,** Control for the retractable stylet.

A catheter may be threaded under the casing and used to administer topical anesthesia (197).

Techniques of Use (194, 198–206)

Intubation with a lighted stylet can be performed under general anesthesia or in an awake patient following topical anesthesia of the airway. A lubricated lightwand (with a lubricated stylet) is passed through a transparent tracheal tube so that the light is just short of the end of the tube. The tube should be firmly attached. The tube-stylet is bent to the desired shape, usually 90° (207). For oral intubation a hockey stick bend is placed in the distal portion beginning just proximal to the proximal end of the tube cuff (62, 194, 204). Care should be taken not to bend the stylet at the point at which the bulb meets the shaft (203). It may be useful to measure the mandibular-hyoid distance by placing the index, middle, and ring fingers if necessary between the submental area of the mandible and the hyoid bone (208). The index finger is then placed at the junction of the light bulb and stylet, and the bend is made at the finger corresponding to the previous measurement.

The operator may stand at the head or to the side of the patient's head. It is useful to lower the bed as far as practical. The head should be in a neutral or extended position (194). In obese patients or patients with an extremely short neck, placing a pillow under the shoulders and neck may be useful. The mouth is opened and the tongue and, if possible, the mandible pulled forward. A

bite block may be inserted to prevent the patient from biting the tube-stylet. A Williams airway intubator (see Chapter 14, "Face Masks and Airways") may be used to keep the device in the midline (209). The room lights should be dimmed or the anterior neck shaded in obese patients or those with thick necks. The jaw is grasped and lifted upward using the thumb and index finger of the intubator's non-dominant hand.

The lightwand is illuminated and the tube-lightwand inserted in the midline of the oral cavity. It is then advanced into the hypopharynx using a gentle rocking motion. As the tube-stylet is advanced, its position can be discerned by observing the transillumination of the soft tissues of the neck. The intensity of the illumination may be increased by applying cricoid pressure. If resistance is felt, the lightwand-tube should be rocked backward and the tip redirected toward the thyroid prominence using the glow of the light as a guide.

A well-defined bright glow in the midline slightly below the thyroid prominence can be seen when the lightwand-tube enters the glottic opening. The stylet, if present, should be pulled back several centimeters and the tube-lightwand advanced so that the glow rests at the level of the sternal notch (210). Following release of the locking device, the lightwand is withdrawn from the tracheal tube.

A very diffuse or absent light means the esophagus has been entered (63, 195). This can be corrected by lifting the stylet to bring the tip more anterior (208). With placement in the pyriform fossa, a glow will be seen to the side of the midline. Bright transillumination high in the neck near the hyoid occurs if the stylet is in the vallecula. It may be necessary to flex the neck or to use a jaw lift to allow the tube to enter the trachea.

A digital technique can also be used. Gloved fingers are inserted into the mouth and the tongue and jaw pulled forward (203). The tube and stylet are slid along the tongue and guided into the trachea. The patient with a clenched jaw can be intubated by retracting the cheek and inserting the lightwand from the right side through a gap behind the latter-most teeth (211).

Nasal intubation can be performed using a lighted stylet (194, 212, 213). The trocar should be removed so that the lightwand is more flexible (194) and the styletted tube should be shaped as an open letter C (207). The lightwand-tube is inserted through the nostril and advanced gently. If resistance is felt, the device should be withdrawn slightly and the tip redirected toward the thyroid prominence. A faint glow above the thyroid prominence indicates that the tip of the device is in the vallecula. A jaw lift helps to elevate the epiglottis and enhances passage of the device under it. Alternatively, the patient's neck can be flexed while advancing the device. This technique has been found to be more successful than blind nasotracheal intubation (214).

This technique has been used successfully in pediatric patients (196, 215). A shoulder roll and slight head extension should be used to project the thyroid cartilage anteriorly. An anterior jaw lift will elevate the relatively long epiglottis.

The lighted stylet can be used to intubate through a laryngeal mask (216). The lighted stylet has been recommended as an adjunct to direct laryngoscopy with a conventional laryngoscope (217). The lighted stylet is placed in the tracheal tube. This results in increased airway illumination.

The lighted stylet can be used to determine the location of the distal end of the tracheal tube (195, 218). The distance to the end of the tube is determined then the lighted stylet is placed in the tube to the correct depth. If the light is seen at 1 to 2 cm below the sternal notch the tube is correctly placed.

Advantages (194, 219)

Intubation using a lightwand is a simple and easy-to-learn technique. It is associated with a low incidence of mucosal injury, sore throat, and dental trauma compared to laryngoscopy (219). Other advantages include rapidity of intubation and ability to intubate without movement of the head or neck.

The technique is easily learned, can be performed with cricoid pressure, is effective when blood and/or secretions are present, and can be used in uncooperative patients (220). It may be especially useful when anatomical abnormalities preclude insertion of a conventional laryngoscope or extension of the head and in patients with extensive dental work or poor teeth (206, 221–223). It has been used successfully with rapid sequence induction and in patients who are difficult to intubate with conventional direct laryngoscopy (196, 203, 204, 206, 222–227). Use of the lighted intubation stylet has been found to be superior to blind techniques for both oral and nasal intubations (201, 214).

It is possible to use the device from the front or side of the patient so the technique can be used in cramped quarters such as hallways and helicopters (194, 203). It will rapidly and reliably distinguish intratracheal from inadvertent esophageal placement (95). It can be used in pediatric patients (222, 226, 228, 229). The equipment is simple, inexpensive, reusable, reliable, compact, lightweight, easily cleaned, portable, and reasonably durable.

No significant problems with this method have been noted when it was compared with the conventional laryngoscopic methods, although more attempts before successful intubation may be required (200, 206, 208, 230, 231). The lightwand may be less stimulating to the patient than the conventional laryngoscope (232, 233). There may be less trauma and sore throat (212, 219).

Disadvantages

Anything that interferes with transmission of the light from the neck (anterior neck scarring, flexion contractions, a beard, excessive adipose tissue, midline neck tumors or swellings, covering of the bulb with blood and/or secretions) will decrease the effectiveness of the technique (62, 63, 204).

It should not be used in patients with known abnormalities of the upper airway such as tumors, polyps, infection, upper airway trauma, or a foreign body. Since this is a blind technique, unsuspected pathology or a foreign body may not be detected. Older lightwands require low ambient light for use.

Experience and practice in routine cases are needed for successful use in the occasional difficult case.

Hazards

Detachment of the bulb or lens has been reported (200, 207, 209, 234, 235). Fracture of the device near the handle has been reported (236). Inadequate lubrication was blamed. There is the potential for trauma in the upper airway associated with its use. Two cases of arytenoid dislocation have been reported (237, 238). It is not uncom-

mon to cause some bleeding in the larynx with this technique. If this technique fails, the presence of blood in the larynx makes fiberoptic techniques more difficult.

THE BULLARD LARYNGOSCOPE (239)

Description

The Bullard laryngoscope (Fig. 16.46) has a rigid anatomically-shaped blade. Fiberoptic bundles for illumination and operator viewing are housed in a sheath on the posterior aspect of the blade. A viewing arm with eyepiece extends at a 45° angle from the handle. A snap-on diopter for users with uncorrected vision is available. Later versions have an eyepiece that can be focused.

Three sizes are available: pediatric, pediatric long, and adult (Fig. 16.46). The pediatric version is used for babies. The pediatric long version is used for patients up to 8 to 10 years of age. The adult version is intended for adults and children

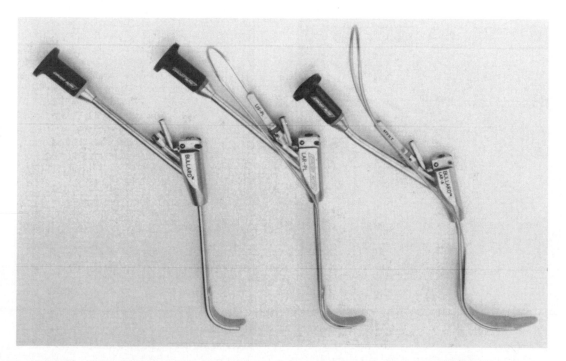

FIGURE 16.46. Bullard laryngoscopes. **Left,** Pediatric version without stylet. **Middle,** Pediatric long version with introducing stylet in place. **Right,** Adult version with introducing stylet in place. The handle contains batteries that power a halogen light bulb. Note that the curve of the adult blade differs from the other two. (Courtesy of Circon Acmi, a division of Circon Corp.)

over 8 to 10 years. The blade on the adult version has a deeper curve than on the pediatric versions. A plastic tip extender is available to lengthen the tip of the adult blade. This is useful for intubating male patients but is usually not necessary for females. The handle may contain batteries and a halogen bulb and/or have an adaptor for a flexible cable that is connected to a high intensity light source (halogen or xenon). Light from the source is transmitted to the distal blade via the fiberoptic bundle.

A working (suction/insufflation) channel extends from the body of the scope to the point where the light bundles end at the tip. The end nearest the handle has two openings. One has a Luer lock connector for attachment of a medication syringe. It can be used for suction, insufflation of oxygen, or administration of local anesthetics or saline during laryngoscopy. The other port has the attachment for the introducing stylet. Two stylets are available.

Introducing (Intubating) Stylet

This stylet (Fig. 16.47) is thin with a curve to the left at approximately 20° near the tip to bring the end of the stylet into the field of vision and facilitate passage of the tracheal tube into the laryngeal inlet. It attaches near the base of the viewing arm with a spring-loaded, locking mechanism. Studies have shown that use of this stylet results in fewer attempts at intubation and faster intubations than other methods (62, 240, 241).

Multifunctional Stylet

The multifunctional stylet (Figs 16.48, 16.49, and 16.50) consists of a long hollow tube which is curved at the tip to direct the tube into the field of vision. It may attach to the viewing arm using a screw clamp. Its hollow core can serve as a guide by threading a flexible fiberscope, a tracheal tube exchanger, or a small catheter through it. It is somewhat less maneuverable than the introducing stylet.

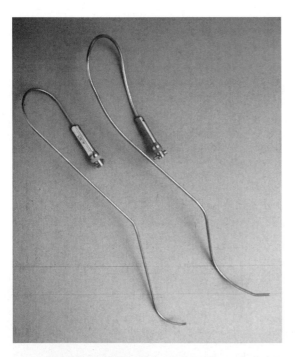

FIGURE 16.47. Introducing stylets for Bullard laryngoscope. The adult version is on the left and the pediatric version on the right. (Courtesy of Circon Acmi, a division of Circon Corp.)

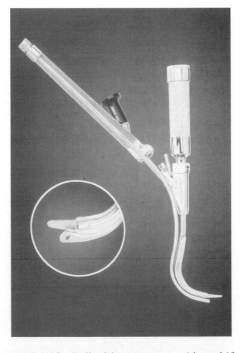

FIGURE 16.48. Bullard laryngoscope with multifunctional stylet. The insert shows the tip with stylet and tracheal tube in place. (Courtesy of Circon Acmi, a division of Circon Corp.)

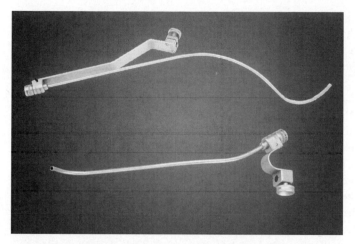

FIGURE 16.49. Multifunctional stylets with screw clamps. Adult version on top. The pediatric version on the bottom. Note the end of the lumen through which a catheter can be inserted. (Courtesy of Circon Acmi, a division of Circon Corp.)

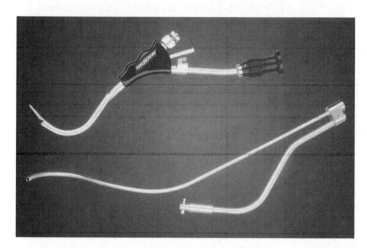

FIGURE 16.50. Newer version (Elite) of Bullard laryngoscope. The handle has been reshaped. There is a built-in focus adjustment in the eyepiece. On the viewing arm adjacent to the handle is a spring-loaded mechanism to hold the multifunctional stylet, which is shown below. This Bullard laryngoscope is fully immersible. (Courtesy of Circon Acmi, a division of Circon Corp.)

Techniques of Use (239–242)

Bullard laryngoscopy can be performed in the awake patient with topical anesthesia or in an anesthetized patient either paralyzed or breathing spontaneously (243, 244). If the topical anesthesia is not satisfactory, local anesthesia can be sprayed through the working channel. Before use, the image bundle window at the distal end of the sheath should be wiped clean.

Jet ventilation can be administered using the working channel (245–248). For patients who are breathing spontaneously, connecting oxygen to the working channel can provide extra oxygenation (241, 249). It will also will help to blow secretions away from the vision bundles and prevent fogging (249). Suction can also be applied to the channel.

Intubation can be accomplished with a styletted tracheal tube, a tracheal tube with a directional tip or one of the Bullard stylets. A reinforced (anode) tracheal tube may be used (250). If the pediatric introducing stylet or the multifunctional stylet is used, the tracheal tube connector must be removed before it is back loaded over the stylet.

Before the tracheal tube is placed on the stylet, a small amount of lubricant should be applied to the stylet and the tube. The adult tracheal tube is threaded over the lubricated stylet so that the tip of the stylet protrudes through the Murphy eye.

The pediatric and multipurpose stylets should be positioned near the tip of the tracheal tube but not protruding through the end.

The stylet-tracheal tube combination is fastened to the laryngoscope. This brings the vertical part of the stylet behind and to the right side of the laryngoscope in the groove formed by the blade anteriorly and by the lens housing in the middle. When properly loaded, the tip of the introducing stylet should be visible at the four o'clock position through the eyepiece or video camera. The tip of the multipurpose stylet may not be visible.

The user is positioned at patient's head, and the scope held in the left hand with the handle horizontal. The patient's head is kept in the neutral position.

Oral Intubation

Either by manually opening the mouth or with the aid of a tongue blade, the blade is inserted midline in the oral cavity, with the handle horizontal. The handle sometimes impinges upon the chest during insertion, especially in obese patients (251). In these cases it must be removed prior to insertion and reconnected after the laryngoscope is positioned in the pharynx.

As the blade is advanced, the handle is rotated to the vertical position so that the blade slides over the tongue. Once the blade has been rotated around the tongue, upward movement along the axis of the handle is exerted to visualize the larynx. It is best not to look through the eyepiece until the laryngoscope is in place. If properly placed, either the epiglottis or the glottis should come into view through the eyepiece. Occasionally it may be necessary to slightly displace the blade posteriorly and then lift vertically to optimize visualization. The blade can be used to directly or indirectly lift the epiglottis.

In some cases the tip of the tracheal tube will impact on the right arytenoid (252). If this occurs, the scope and stylet should be repositioned to the left. If this does not work, another maneuver is to rotate the tube 180° on the stylet, positioning the end of the bevel near the blade and having the tip of the stylet protrude through the central opening of the tracheal tube (252). If the tube passes through the vocal cords but cannot be ad-

vanced past the level of the cricoid cartilage, the laryngoscope should be angled slightly forward.

Introducing Stylet

Once the larynx is visualized, the stylet tip is manipulated until it points between the cords. Under visualization, the tube is advanced off the stylet until the cuff passes beyond the vocal cords. The laryngoscope and stylet are then removed. If the tube does not enter the larynx, the tube and stylet must be withdrawn and the tube again placed over the stylet before another attempt at intubation is made.

Multipurpose Stylet

Once the larynx is visualized, the tube should be advanced until it is visible. If possible, the tube should be advanced between the vocal cords. If this is not possible a catheter can sometimes be threaded through the stylet into the larynx. The tracheal tube is then advanced over the catheter. The tracheal tube is then threaded over the catheter into the larynx.

The Bullard laryngoscope can also be used for oral intubation without a stylet by passing a catheter through the channel where the introducing stylet would attach (253, 254).

Nasotracheal Intubation

For nasotracheal intubation, no stylet is used. A directional tip tracheal tube may be especially useful in this situation (255–257). The larynx is visualized using the Bullard laryngoscope; the patient's head position and the thyroid cartilage are manipulated to allow the tube to be advanced between the vocal cords (258).

Another method of nasal intubation was used in an infant with Treacher-Collins syndrome (259). The patient was first intubated orally. A small tube changing catheter was placed through the nose and under direct vision manipulated alongside the orotracheal tube. The oral tube was removed and a nasal tube passed over the catheter into the larynx.

Advantages

This laryngoscope is useful in patients who are difficult to intubate, including those in whom head and neck movement is limited or undesirable, those with limited mouth opening, facial fractures and the morbidly obese (241, 250,

260–264). Its use results in less cervical spine movement than conventional laryngoscopy (264, 265). Compared with flexible fiberoptic intubation the Bullard laryngoscope provides quicker intubation in patients with cervical spine disease (244, 266, 267).

Other advantages include rapidity of intubation, low risk of failed intubation or trauma to the lips and teeth, and less discomfort in the awake patient than direct laryngoscopy (246).

The laryngoscope is rugged and less likely to be damaged than flexible fiberoptic scopes.

Its use causes less cardiovascular instability than the Macintosh blade with conventional intubation techniques (268).

Disadvantages

Disadvantages include that practice is needed to achieve proficiency. The equipment is expensive. Cleaning is somewhat complicated. Use of tracheal tubes larger than 7.5 mm may cause the introducing stylet to be displaced posteriorly, so that less of it can be seen (269).

Certain tracheal tubes (e.g., the metallic laser tube) will not fit over the stylet. In these cases another tube can be inserted using the Bullard and a tube exchanger used to insert the desired tube.

WUSCOPE (270, 271)
Description

The WuScope (Fig. 16.51) combines a rigid, tubular, anatomically-shaped blade and a separate flexible fiberscope. The blade gives the fiberscope its maneuverability.

Flexible Fiberscope Portion

The fiberscope has light- and image-transmitting fiberoptic bundles and tip deflection control. The same fiberscope is compatible with the large adult and adult blades and the handle with or without the extender. A light transmission cable can be attached to a fiberoptic light source.

Blade Portion

The blade portion has three detachable stainless steel parts: handle, main blade and bivalve ele-

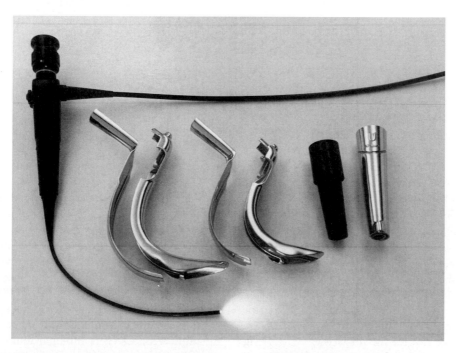

FIGURE 16.51. WuScope. Shown from left to right are the fiberscope, the large-adult bi-valve element, the large-adult main blade, the adult bi-valve element, the adult main-blade, the extender and the handle. (Courtesy of ACHI Corporation.)

FIGURE **16.52.** Three channels of the Wu Blade for the suction catheter and tracheal tube, fiberscope and oxygen.

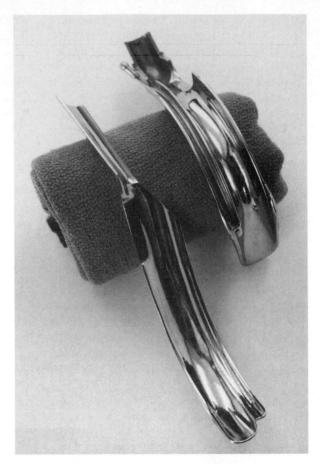

ment. The bivalve element can be attached or released from the handle and the distal main blade by separate interlocking mechanisms.

The handle is a cone-shaped tube that receives the fiberscope at the top and connects to the main blade at the base. The handle-to-blade angle is 110°. An extender that adjusts the length of the fiberscope insertion portion for the adult blade so that one fiberscope will be compatible with various sized blades is available.

The main blade and bivalve element are anatomically shaped. Each has corresponding grooves that form a larger passageway for a suction catheter and the tracheal tube and a smaller one for the fiberscope (Fig. 16.52). An oxygen channel is alongside the slot for the fiberscope.

Different sizes of the main blade and bivalve element are designed to be interchangeable with the handle. The adult blade for use in a small or medium adult can accommodate a tracheal tube up to 8.5 mm while the large-adult blade can contain a 9.0 mm tube.

Techniques for Use

The WuScope can be used to facilitate intubation in the awake or anesthetized patient. The patient's head should be in the neutral position.

The components are assembled (Figs. 16.53 and 16.54). If the adult blade is used, the extender should be attached to the handle. The tracheal tube should be lubricated and inserted until the Murphy eye is just beyond the distal edge of the bi-valve element. The suction catheter should also be lubricated. Oxygen tubing should be connected to the oxygen channel. Anti-fogging solution should be applied to the fiberscope lens.

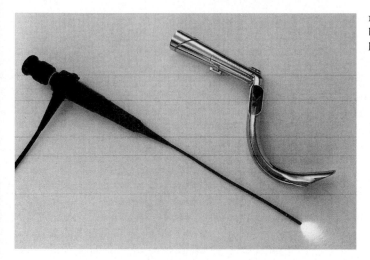

FIGURE 16.53. WuScope partially assembled, showing fiberscope and assembled handle, blade, and bivalve element.

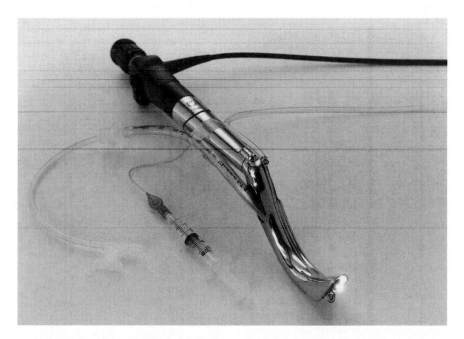

FIGURE 16.54. Fully assembled WuScope with a tracheal tube in the tracheal tube passage, a suction catheter in the tracheal tube lumen, and oxygen tubing connected to the oxygen port.

Orotracheal Intubation

Holding the metal portion of the handle, the scope is inserted into the patient's mouth in the midline much like an oropharyngeal airway. The handle is gradually rotated towards the operator as the distal main blade glides over the tongue.

The operator looks through the eyepiece and identifies the uvula, posterior pharyngeal wall, and epiglottis as the scope is advanced towards the larynx. If the epiglottis blocks the view, the device may be withdrawn slightly and re-advanced to lift up the epiglottis. The suction catheter in the tracheal tube passageway can be used to remove excessive blood or secretions.

When the larynx comes into view the suction catheter is advanced from the tracheal tube lumen into the glottis. Then, with the catheter acting as a guide the position of the distal main blade is adjusted, if necessary, to align the tracheal tube with the glottic opening. Once the tube is properly positioned, it is advanced over the suction catheter into the trachea. The bi-valve element is removed first. Then the handle, main blade and fiberscope are removed as one unit, leaving the tracheal tube in place.

Nasotracheal Intubation

For nasotracheal intubation, the bi-valve element is not attached to the scope. After a tracheal tube is passed into the oropharynx through the nostril, the scope is positioned inside the mouth in a similar manner to oral intubation. The concave undersurface of the distal main blade is directed to straddle the tracheal tube and guide it towards the larynx. The tracheal tube is advanced into the trachea and the device removed from the mouth.

Advantages

This device has been used successfully in difficult-to-intubate patients (270, 271). Its tubular structure protects the fiberoptic lens from blood, secretions, or redundant soft tissue. This may make it especially useful in the patient with airway obstruction due to hematoma or edema.

The head can be maintained in the neutral position. The handle-to-blade angle facilitates entry in obese patients and those with barrel chests, short necks, or large breasts. There is no need for head extension or tongue lifting. Minimal jaw opening is necessary.

No forceps or stylet is needed so the risk of airway injury is low. Suctioning and administration of oxygen can be performed simultaneously.

It is compatible with regular tracheal tubes, the Univent tube, and double-lumen tubes.

Disadvantages

This device may not be useful in a patient with a severely limited mouth opening.

The flexible fiberscope portion can be damaged during cleaning or storage. Time and experience are necessary to achieve proficiency in its use.

UPSHERSCOPE (272)
Description

The UpsherScope (Fig. 16.55) consists of a C-shaped metal blade shaped to approximate the curve of the oropharynx. The open part of the C to the right is the delivery slot, which ends about one inch from the end of the blade. The distal part of the blade has a slight curve. To the left are two tubes which carry fiberoptic bundles. Both bundles end at the point where the semicircular channel ends. Proximally, the viewing bundle terminates in an eyepiece with a focusing ring while the light bundle makes contact with the fiberoptic light source at the handle.

The blade may be attached to a regular Upsher handle or a special fiberoptic handle that contains the batteries and light or has an adapter which connects to an independent light source.

Techniques for Use

Prior to intubation, the viewing fiberoptic bundle should be treated with an anti-fogging solution. Use of an antisialagogue will minimize secretions. The tracheal tube is lubricated and placed in the delivery slot with the tip not quite protruding from the distal end of the channel. The blade is clipped to the handle and the viewing lens focused.

The scope is passed into the mouth much like an oral airway, aiming to pick up the epiglottis by a scooping motion. Head and neck flexion will increase the probability of success. Under vision, the tip of the scope is positioned in front of the larynx. The tube is then advanced in the channel and observed to pass between the vocal cords. The scope is then removed from the tube and withdrawn from the mouth.

If the tube impacts the right arytenoid, this can often be corrected by rotating the tracheal tube 180° in the channel, further flexion of the head on the neck, modification of the vector of lift, rotation of the tip of the scope to the left or right, or passage of a guide with subsequent passage of the tracheal tube over it (272).

In practice, the blade sometimes rolls off the

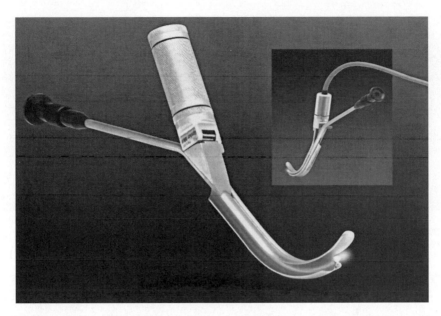

FIGURE 16.55. UpsherScope. The larger photograph shows the delivery slot for the tracheal tube. The blade is attached to a conventional Upsher handle. The inset show the opposite site of the blade with the eyepiece. A fiberoptic cable from the light source is attached to the handle. (Courtesy of Mercury Medical.)

tongue to the side. When this occurs, a paramedian approach should be attempted.

Advantages

This device is useful to intubate patients with difficult airways within a reasonable time (272). It can be used with all sizes of adult tracheal tubes.

Disadvantages

The UpsherScope demonstrated no advantages over conventional laryngoscopy in routine intubation (273). The time needed to perform intubation and the number of attempts were significantly longer and higher with the UpsherScope. The UpsherScope is not suitable for nasotracheal intubation.

FLEXGUIDE (INTUBATING FIBERSCOPE)

The Flexguide (intubating fiberscope) (Fig. 16.56) is a combination flexible stylet and fiberscope. The stylet can be manipulated 120° upwards and downwards. The light bundle can connect to most common light sources.

TOOTH PROTECTORS

Tooth protectors (mouth guards, mouth protectors, dentguards) are placed over the upper teeth to protect them from damage by the laryngoscope blade. They also prevent the blade from getting caught in a gap between teeth. Use of a protector does not guarantee avoidance of dental trauma (274). Although it will prevent direct trauma to the surface of the teeth, it cannot prevent transmission of pressure to the roots.

Tooth protectors are available in different designs (Fig. 16.57). and are fashioned from a variety of materials (275–277). A tooth protection device may be attached to the laryngoscope blade (278–281).

These devices may make it harder to visualize the larynx and may inhibit insertion of the tracheal tube because of lack of space (274). They slightly increase the time of intubation (282). Cutting off part of the right side of the protector or using a transparent protector may decrease these problems (274, 283). It may be necessary to remove the protector before intubation can be accomplished.

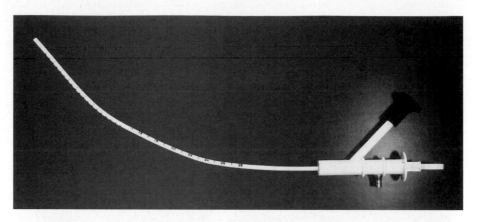

FIGURE 16.56. Intubating fiberscope. (Courtesy of Scientific Sales International, Inc.)

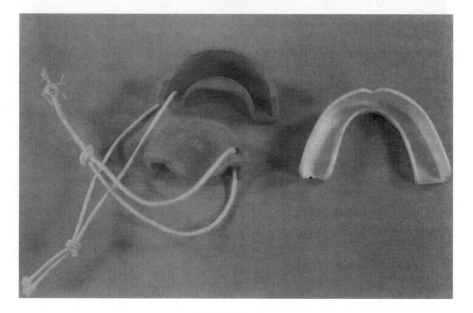

FIGURE 16.57. Tooth protectors.

COMPLICATIONS OF LARYNGOSCOPY
Dental Injury (284)

Damage to teeth, gums, or dental prostheses constitutes the most frequent anesthesia-related claim (285). In addition to cosmetic disfigurement and discomfort there may be pulmonary complications if the dislodged tooth or fragment is aspirated. Profuse bleeding may result (286).

A tooth or prosthetic device may be chipped, broken, loosened, or avulsed. The teeth most

likely to be damaged are those that have been restored or weakened by periodontal disease (287). The upper incisors are most frequently involved (288). This usually is caused by using the teeth as a fulcrum point for the laryngoscope while elevating the epiglottis.

The condition of each patient's teeth should be carefully assessed preoperatively to identify possible problems. Inquiry should be made concerning vulnerable dental repair work or loose or carious teeth. Anatomical conditions of the mouth and pharynx that can cause difficulty in exposing the larynx should be noted. The patient should be advised beforehand if there is likely to be a problem. A suture may be placed around a loose tooth to prevent it from entering the airway should it become dislodged.

In patients 4 to 11 years old, the deciduous teeth may be easily dislodged. If such teeth are loose, removal before or during anesthesia may be indicated.

When there are gaps between the upper front teeth, a portion of a tracheal tube or other device may be used to bridge the gap (289, 290) or a tooth protector may be used. Keeping partial upper dentures in place may prevent the laryngoscope from slipping into gaps between teeth.

If a tooth, fragment, or dental appliance is dislodged, prevention of foreign body aspiration should be of major concern. An immediate search should be conducted, starting with an examination of the oral cavity and the area surrounding the patient's head. X-rays of the chest and neck must be taken if the fragment is not found (291).

Different types of tooth damage may occur (292). These require different treatments. A qualified dentist or oral surgeon should be consulted. If a tooth is avulsed, immediate replacement in its original position and stabilization will increase the chances of successful replantation (293).

Tooth protectors may prevent dental damage. Placing adhesive tape on the flange of the blade has also been reported to be effective (294).

Damage to Soft Tissues and Nerves

Reported injuries to the upper airway include abrasion, hematoma, and laceration of the lips, tongue, palate, pharynx, hypopharynx, larynx, and esophagus (203, 295–301). One common occurrence is rolling of the lower lip between the teeth and the laryngoscope blade as the blade is inserted. As the blade is inserted, the right hand should retract the lower lip. The lingual nerve may be injured (302–305). Massive tongue swelling following laryngoscopy has been reported (306, 307).

Patients with temporomandibular joint derangement sometimes report that the problem began following general anesthesia (307).

Injury to Cervical Spinal Cord

Aggressive positioning of the head for intubation, especially extension of the head or neck, has the potential to cause damage in the patient with an unstable cervical spinal such as those with congenital weaknesses, malformations, fractures, or dislocations of cervical vertebrae; or other conditions such as osteoporosis, connective tissue disease, or tumor (265, 308–314).

There are no data to suggest that any mode of airway intervention is superior to another in decreasing secondary injury or improving outcome (316, 317). There is evidence that in-line immobilization reduces spinal movement and the likelihood of secondary injury (261, 265, 316–322).

Suggested methods for reducing cervical spine movement include use of the Bullard laryngoscope, the CLM blade, and the lightwand.

Circulatory Changes

Laryngoscopy may result in significant hemodynamic changes, although these changes are less than those associated with tracheal intubation (268, 323–326). These changes may be less with use of the CLM blade, lighted stylet, or flexible fiberscope.

Swallowing or Aspiration of a Foreign Body

Cases have been reported in which the bulb from a laryngoscope was aspirated during intubation (200, 203, 209, 234, 235, 327, 328). A portion of the diaphragm of a Patil–Syracuse mask may enter the airway (329–331).

It is important to make every effort to find these foreign bodies. If they cannot be found in the oral cavity or around the patient's head, X-rays of the chest and neck should be taken.

Shock and/or Burn

If a laryngoscope light, which is left on, contacts the patient's skin, a burn may result (332). Malpositioning of a blade on the handle can produce a short circuit, which leads to rapid heating of the handle (333). The tip of a fiberscope connected to a powerful light source may be hot enough to produce a burn (334, 335).

Laryngoscope Malfunction

The most common malfunction of the laryngoscope is failure of the light to illuminate. This may be the result of a defective power source, lamp, or socket, or poor contact between the blade and handle. Fiberoptic laryngoscopes are more reliable, because the useful light of a halogen lamp is longer than an ordinary light bulb and the lamp is usually in the handle rather than the blade.

Breakage of the various parts of the blade and handle have been reported (336–344).

A preuse check will detect most malfunctions. An extra handle and blade should always be immediately available. Neglecting to observe these precautions could spell disaster, especially when a rapid sequence induction is being performed.

REFERENCES

1. American Society for Testing and Materials. Standard specification for rigid laryngoscopes for tracheal intubation. Hook-on fittings for laryngoscope handles and blades with lamps (F965-85 reapproved 1993). West Conshohocken, PA: ASTM, 1993.
2. International Standards Organization. Laryngoscopic fittings.—Part 1: Conventional hook-on type handle—blade fittings (ISO 7376-1:1994). Geneva Switzerland: ISO, 1994.
3. American Society for Testing and Materials. Standard specification for rigid laryngoscopes for tracheal intubation. Hook-on fittings for fiber illuminated blades and handles (F1195-88 reapproved 1993). West Conshohocken, PA: ASTM, 1993.
4. International Standards Organization. Laryngoscopic fittings—Part 3: Fibre-illuminated re-usable rigid laryngoscopes (ISO 7376-3:1996). ISO: Geneva, 1996.
5. Greenblatt GM. Fiberoptic illuminating laryngoscope with remote light source—further development. Anesth Analg 1981;60:841–842.
6. Bjoraker DG, Gibby GL. Comparison of lamp-in-blade and fiberoptic laryngoscope illumination. Anesthesiology 1992;77:A518.
7. Skilton RWH, Parry D, Arthurs GJ, et al. A study of the brightness of laryngoscope light. Anaesthesia 1996;51:667–672.
8. Fletcher J. Laryngoscope light intensity. Can J Anaesth 1995;42:259–260.
9. Tousignant G, Tessler MJ. Light intensity and area of illumination provided by various laryngoscope blades. Can J Anaesth 1994;41:865–869.
10. Datta S, Briwa J. Modified laryngoscope for endotracheal intubation of obese patients. Anesth Analg 1981;60:120–121.
11. King H, Wang L, Khan AK. A modification of laryngoscopy technique. Anesthesiology 1986;65:566.
12. Thomas DV. Difficult tracheal intubation in obstetrics. Anaesthesia 1985;40:307.
13. Bourke DL, Lawrence J. Another way to insert a Macintosh blade. Anesthesiology 1983;59:80.
14. Gandhi SK, Burgos L. A technique of laryngoscopy for difficult intubation. Anesthesiology 1986;64: 528–529.
15. Dhara SS, Cheong TW. An adjustable multiple angle laryngoscope adaptor. Anaesthesia and Intensive Care 1991;19:243–245.
16. Jellicoe JA, Harris NR. A modification of a standard laryngoscope for difficult tracheal intubation in obstetric cases. Anaesthesia 1984;39:800–802.
17. Yentis SM. A laryngoscope adaptor for difficult intubation. Anaesthesia 1987;42:764–766.
18. Patil VU, Stehling LC, Zauder HL. An adjustable laryngoscope handle for difficult intubations. Anesthesiology 1984;60:609.
19. Cooper SD. The evolution of upper-airway retraction: new and old laryngoscopy blades in airway management. In: Benumof JL, ed. Airway management: principles and practice. St. Louis: Mosby, 1996; 374–411.
20. McIntyre JWR. Laryngoscope design and the difficult adult tracheal intubation. Can J Anaesth 1989;36: 94–98.
21. Macintosh RR. A new laryngoscope. Lancet 1943;1: 205.
22. Jephcott A. The Macintosh laryngoscope. A historical note on its clinical and commercial development. Anaesthesia 1984;39:474–479.
23. Campbell NN, Millar R. Modification of laryngoscope for nasogastric intubation. Anaesthesia 1985; 40:703–704.
24. Callander CC, Thomas J. Modification of Macintosh laryngoscope for difficult intubation. Anaesthesia 1987;42:671–672.
25. Gabrielczyk MR. A new integrated suction laryngoscope. Anaesthesia 1986;41:970–971.
26. Ibler M. Modification of Macintosh laryngoscope blade. Anesthesiology 1983;58:200.
27. Kessel J. A laryngoscope for obstetrical use. An obstetrical laryngoscope. Anaesthesia and Intensive Care 1977;5:265–266.
28. Mazumder JK. Laryngoscope blade with suction unit. Can Anaesth Soc J 1979;26:513–514.
29. McWhinnie F. Modification of laryngoscope for nasogastric intubation. Anaesthesia 1986;41:218–219.

30. Buck MJL, Snijders CJ, van der Vegt MH, et al. Reshaping the Macintosh blade using biomechanical modelling. A prospective comparative study in patients. Anaesthesia 1997;52:662–667.

31. Relle A. Laryngoscope design. Can J Anaesth 1994; 41:162–163.

32. Pope ES. Left handed laryngoscope. Anaesthesia 1960;15:326–328.

33. McComish PB. Left sided laryngoscopes. Anaesthesia 1965;20:372.

34. Lagade MRG, Poppers PJ. Use of the left-entry laryngoscope blade in patients with right-sided oro-facial lesions. Anesthesiology 1983;58:300.

35. Lagade MRG, Poppers PJ. Revival of the polio laryngoscope blade. Anesthesiology 1982;57:545.

36. Weeks DB. A new use of an old blade. Anesthesiology 1974;40:200–201.

37. Racz GB. Improved vision modification of the Macintosh laryngoscope. Anaesthesia 1984;39: 1249–1250.

38. Bizzarri DV, Giuffrida JG. Improved laryngoscope blade designed for ease of manipulation and reduction of trauma. Anesth Analg 1958;37:231–232.

39. Miller RA. A new laryngoscope. Anesthesiology 1941;2:317–320.

40. Jones RDM. Lamp placement and the Miller I laryngoscope blade. Anesthesiology 1985;62:207.

41. Rokowski WJ, Gurmarnik S. Laryngoscope blades modified for neonates and infants. Anesth Analg 1983;62:241–242.

42. Hastings RH, Hon ED, Nghiem C, et al. Force and torque vary between laryngoscopists and laryngoscope blades. Anesth Analg 1996;82:462–468.

43. Cork RC, Woods W, Vaughn RW, et al. Oxygen supplementation during endotracheal intubation of infants. Anesthesiology 1979;51:186.

44. Diaz JH. Further modifications of the Miller blade for difficult pediatric laryngoscopy. Anesthesiology 1984;60:612–613.

45. Wung J, Stark RI, Indyk L, et al. Oxygen supplement during endotracheal intubation of the infant. Pediatrics 1977;59:1046–1048.

46. Hencz P. Modified laryngoscope for endotracheal intubation of neonates. Anesthesiology 1980;55:84.

47. Ledbetter JL, Rasch DK, Pollard TG, et al. Reducing the risks of laryngoscopy in anaesthetised infants. Anaesthesia 1988;43:151–153.

48. Todres ID, Crone RK. Experience with a modified laryngoscope in sick infants. Crit Care Med 1981;9: 544–545.

49. Portzer M, Wasmuth CE. Endotracheal anesthesia using a modified Wis–Foregger laryngoscope blade. Cleve Clin Q 1959;26:140–143.

50. Schapira M. A modified straight laryngoscope blade designed to facilitate endotracheal intubation. Anesth Analg 1973;52:553–554.

51. Soper RL. A new laryngoscope for anaesthetists. Br Med J 1947;1:265.

52. Snow JC. Modification of laryngoscope blade. Anesthesiology 1962;23:394.

53. Flagg P. Exposure and illumination of the pharynx and larynx by the general practitioner. A new laryngoscope designed to simplify the technique. Arch Laryngol 1928;8:716–717.

54. Seward EH. Laryngoscope for resuscitation of the newborn. Lancet 1957;2:1041.

55. Hatch DJ. Paediatric anaesthetic equipment. Br J Anaesth 1985;57:672–674.

56. Phillips OC, Duerksen RL. Endotracheal intubation. A new blade for direct laryngoscopy. Anesth Analg 1973;52:691–698.

57. Racz GB, Allen FB. A new pressure-sensitive laryngoscope. Anesthesiology 1985;62:356–358.

58. Robertshaw FL. A new laryngoscope for infants and children. Lancet 1962;2:1034.

59. Bryce–Smith R. A laryngoscope blade for infants. Br Med J 1952;1:217.

60. Bainton CR. A new laryngoscope blade to overcome pharyngeal obstruction. Anesthesiology 1987;67: 767–770.

61. Choi JJ. A new double-angle blade for direct laryngoscopy. Anesthesiology 1990;72:576.

62. Benumof JL. Management of the difficult adult airway. Anesthesiology 1991;75:1087–1110.

63. Mayall RM. The Belscope for management of the difficult airway. Anesthesiology 1992;76:1059–1060.

64. Bellhouse CP. An angulated laryngoscope for routine and difficult tracheal intubation. Anesthesiology 1988;69:126–129.

65. Bucx MJL, Droogers W, Mallios C. A method to prevent clouding of the Belscope prism. Anaesthesia and Intensive Care 1994;22:320.

66. Watanabe S, Akihiko S, Asakura N, et al. Determination of the distance between the laryngoscope blade and the upper incisors during direct laryngoscopy: comparisons of a curved, an angulated straight, and two straight blades. Anesth Analg 1994;79:638–641.

67. Sultana A, Simmons M, Gatt S. The "Belscope"— A new angulated laryngoscope: randomized, prospective, controlled comparison with the Macintosh laryngoscope. Anaesthesia and Intensive Care 1994; 22:98.

68. Taguchi N, Watanabe S, Kumagai M, et al. Radiographic documentation of increased visibility of the larynx with a Belscope laryngoscope blade. Anesthesiology 1994;81:773–775.

69. Mayall RM. The Belscope for management of the difficult airway. Anesthesiology 1992;76:1059–1060.

70. Hodges UM, O'Flaherty D, Adams AP. Tracheal intubation in a mannikin: comparison of the Belscope with the Macintosh laryngoscope. Br J Anaesth 1993;71:905–907.

71. Gajraj NM, Chason DP, Shearer VE. Cervical spine movement during orotracheal intubation: comparison of the Belscope and Macintosh blades. Anaesthesia 1994;49:772–774.

72. London RA. The articulating laryngoscope blade. Am J Anesth 1995;22:300–32.

73. McCoy EP, Mirakhur RK. The levering laryngoscope. Anaesthesia 1993;48:516–519.

74. Cook TM, Tuckeyy JP. A comparison between the Macintosh and the McCoy laryngoscope blades. Anaesthesia 1996;51:977–980.

75. Chadwick IS, McCluskey A. Another trachea intubated with the McCoy laryngoscope. Anaesthesia 1995;50:571.

76. Ward M. The McCoy levering laryngoscope blade. Anaesthesia 1994;49:357–358.

77. Farling PA. The McCoy levering laryngoscope blade. Anaesthesia 1994;49:358.

78. Johnston HML, Rao U. The McCoy levering laryngoscope blade. Anaesthesia 1994;49:358.

79. Tuckey JP, Cook TM, Render CA. An evaluation of the levering laryngoscope. Anaesthesia 1996;51:71–73.

80. Morley H. The McCoy laryngoscope and difficult intubation. Anaesthesia and Intensive Care 1996;24:620–621.

81. Gabbott DA. Laryngoscopy using the McCoy laryngoscope after application of a cervical collar. Anaesthesia 1996;51:812–814.

82. Laurent SC, de Melo AE, Alexander–Williams JM. The use of the McCoy laryngoscope in patients with simulated cervical spine injuries. Anaesthesia 1996;51:74–75.

83. Uchida T, Hikawa Y, Saito Y, et al. The McCoy levering laryngoscope in patients with limited neck extension. Can J Anaesth 1997;44:674–676.

84. Haridas RP. The McCoy levering laryngoscope blade. Anaesthesia 1996;51:91.

85. Castano J, Castillo J, Escolano F, et al. Cardiovascular response to laryngoscopy: a comparison between the McCoy and Macintosh blade. Br J Anaesth 1996;76:17–18.

86. McCoy EP, Mirakhur RK, Rafferty C, et al. A comparison of the forces exerted during laryngoscopy. The Macintosh versus the McCoy blade. Anaesthesia 1996;51:912–915.

87. McCoy EP, Mirakhur RK, McCloskey BV. A comparison of the stress response to laryngoscopy. The Macintosh versus the McCoy blade. Anaesthesia 1995;50:943–946.

88. Huffman J. The application of prisms to curved laryngoscopes: a preliminary study. J Am Assoc Nurse Anesth 1968;35:138–139.

89. Huffman J, Elam JO. Prisms and fiber optics for laryngoscopy. Anesth Analg 1971;50:64–67.

90. Huffman J. The development of optical prism instruments to view and study the human larynx. J Am Assoc Nurse Anesth 1970;38:197–202.

91. Murrin KR. Intubation procedure and causes of difficult intubation. In: Latto IP, Rosen M, eds. Difficulties in tracheal intubation. London: Bailliere Tindall, 1985:75–89.

92. Brown A, Norton ML. Instrumentation and equipment for management of the difficult airway. In: Norton ML, Brown ACD, eds. Atlas of the difficult airway. A source book. St. Louis: Mosby Year Book, 1991:24–32.

93. Moynihan P. Modification of pediatric laryngoscope. Anesthesiology 1982;56:330.

94. Knill RL. Difficult laryngoscopy made easy with a "BURP." Can J Anaesth 1993;40:279–282.

95. Relle A. Difficult laryngoscopy—"BURP." Can J Anaesth 1993;40:798–799.

96. LaLande P, Knill RL. "BURP" is more effective than backward pressure on the thyroid cartilage in managing difficult laryngoscopy. Can J Anaesth 1994;41:A65.

97. Takahata O, Kubota M, Mamiya K, et al. The efficiency of the "BURP" maneuver during a difficult laryngoscopy. Anesth Analg 1997;84:419–421.

98. Benumof JL, Cooper SD. Quantitative improvement in laryngoscopic view by optimal external laryngeal manipulation. J Clin Anesth 1996;8:136–140.

99. Henderson JJ. The use of paraglossa straight blade laryngoscopy in difficult tracheal intubation. Anaesthesia 1997;52:552–560.

100. Eldor J, Gozal Y. The length of the blade is more important than its design in difficult tracheal intubation. Can J Anaesth 1990;37:268.

101. Patteson SK, Chesney JT. Anesthetic management for magnetic resonance imaging: problems and solutions. Anesth Analg 1992;74:121–128.

102. Karlik SJ, Heatherley T, Pavan F, et al. Patient anesthesia and monitoring at a 1,5-T MRI installation. Magn Reson Med 1988;7:210–221.

103. Ovassapian A. Fiberoptic endoscopy and the difficult airway. Philadelphia: Lippincott–Raven, 1996.

104. Divatia JV, Upadhye SM, Sareen R. Fiberoptic intubation in cicatricial membranes of the pharynx. Anaesthesia 1992;47:486–489.

105. Ovassapian A, Schrader C. Fiber-optic-aided bronchial intubation. Semin Anesth 1987;6:133–142.

106. Slinger PD. Fiberoptic bronchoscopic positioning of double-lumen tubes. J Cardiothorac Anesth 1989;3:486–496.

107. Rosenbaum SH, Rosenbaum LM, Cole RP, et al. Use of the flexible fiberoptic bronchoscope to change endotracheal tubes in critically ill patients. Anesthesiology 1981;54:169–170.

108. Watson CB. Use of fiberoptic bronchoscope to change endotracheal tube endorsed. Anesthesiology 1981;55:476–477.

109. Ovassapian A, Dykes HM. The role of fiber-optic endoscopy in airway management. Semin Anesth 1987;6:93–104.

110. Marks JD, Bainton CD. Practical aspects of fiberoptic laryngobronchoscopy. Int Anesth Clin 1994;32:31–46.

111. McNamara J, Chisholm DG. Use of a fibreoptic intubating laryngoscope to replace a misplaced tracheostomy tube. Anaesthesia 1996;51:894.

112. Dierdorf SF. Types and physics of fiberscopes. In: Roberts JT, ed. Fiberoptics in anesthesia [Special issue]. Anesth Clin North Am 1991;9:19–42.

113. Roberts JT. Preparing to use the flexible fiber-optic laryngoscope. J Clin Anesth 1991;3:64–75.

114. Wang JF, Reves JG, Corssen G. Use of the fiberoptic laryngoscope for difficult tracheal intubation. Ala J Med Sci 1976;13:247–251.

115. Kleeman P, Jantzen JAH, Bonfils P. The ultra-thin bronchoscope in management of the difficult paediatric airway. Can J Anaesth 1987;34:606–608.

116. Laravuso RB, Perloff WH. Difficult pediatric intubation. Anesthesiology 1986;64:668–669.

117. Cherian MN, Mathews MP. Use of an infant feeding tube in fibreoptic intubation. Anaesthesia and Intensive Care 1995;23:524–525.

118. Goskowicz R, Colt HG, Voulelis LD. Fiberoptic tracheal intubation using a nipple guide. Anesthesiology 1996;85:1210–1211.

119. Morris IR. Fibreoptic intubation. Can J Anaesth 1994;41:996–1008.

120. Randell T, Hakala P. Fibreoptic intubation and bronchofiberscopy in anaesthesia and intensive care. Acta Anaesthesiol Scand 1995;39:3–16.

121. Patil VU, Stehling NC, Zauder HL. Fiberoptic endoscopy in anesthesia. Chicago: Year Book Medical Publishers, 1983.

122. Cooper DW, Long GT. Difficult fiberoptic intubation in an intellectually handicapped patient. Anaesthesia and Intensive Care 1992;20:227–229.

123. Baraka A. Transtracheal jet ventilation during fiberoptic intubation under general anesthesia. Anesth Analg 1986;65:1091–1092.

124. Lu GP, Frost EAM, Goldiner PL. Another approach to the problem airway. Anesthesiology 1986;65:101–102.

125. Patil V, Stehling LC, Zauder HL, et al. Mechanical aids for fiberoptic endoscopy. Anesthesiology 1982;57:69–70.

126. Rogers SN, Benumof JL. New and easy techniques for fiberoptic endoscopy-aided tracheal intubation. Anesthesiology 1983;59:569–572.

127. Wangler MA, Weaver JM. A method to facilitate fiberoptic laryngoscopy. Anesthesiology 1984;61:111.

128. Maroof M, Khan RM, Bonsu A, et al. A new solution to fibreoptic intubation in the presence of blood and secretions. Can J Anaesth 1995;42:177–178.

129. Nagaro T, Hamami G, Takasaki Y, et al. Ventilation via a mouth mask facilitates fibreoptic nasal tracheal intubation in anesthetized patients. Anesthesiology 1993;78:603–604.

130. Imai M, Kommotsu O. A new adapter for fiberoptic endotracheal intubation for anesthetized patients. Anesthesiology 1989;70:374–375.

131. McAlpine G, Williams RT. Fiberoptic assisted tracheal intubation under general anesthesia with IPPV. Anesthesiology 1987;66:853.

132. Soroker D, Ezri T, Szmuk P. Fiberoptic bronchoscopy in a patient requiring continuous positive airway pressure. Anesthesiology 1995;82:797–798.

133. Chen L, Sher SA, Aukburg SJ. Continuous ventilation during transnasal fiberoptic bronchoscope-aided tracheal intubation. Anesth Analg 1996;82:674.

134. Sivarajan M, Stoler E, Kil HK, et al. Jet ventilation using fiberoptic bronchoscopes. Anesth Analg 1995;80:384–387.

135. Hershey MD, Hannenberg AA. Gastric distention and rupture from oxygen insufflation during fiberoptic intubation. Anesthesiology 1996;85:1479–1480.

136. Richardson MG, Dooley JW. Acute facial, cervical, and thoracic subcutaneous emphysema: a complication of fiberoptic laryngoscopy. Anesth Analg 1996;82:878–880.

137. Childress WF. New method for fiberoptic endotracheal intubation of anesthetized patients. Anesthesiology 1981;55:595–596.

138. Johnson C, Hunter J, Ho E, et al. Fiberoptic intubation facilitated by a rigid laryngoscope. Anesth Analg 1991;72:714.

139. Calder I. When the endotracheal tube will not pass over the flexible fiberoptic bronchoscope. Anesthesiology 1992;77:398.

140. Brull SJ, Wiklund R, Ferris C, et al. Facilitation of fiberoptic orotracheal intubation with a flexible tracheal tube. Anesth Analg 1994;78:746–748.

141. Erb T, Frei FJ. The 'railroaded' tube—always successful? Anaesthesia 1995;50:659–660.

142. Tan I. Easier fibreoptic intubation. Anaesthesia 1994; 49:830–831.

143. Schwartz D, Johnson C, Roberts J. A maneuver to facilitate flexible fiberoptic intubation. Anesthesiology 1989;71:470–471.

144. Katsnelson T, Frost EAM, Farcon E, et al. When the endotracheal tube will not pass over the flexible fiberoptic bronchoscope. Anesthesiology 1992;76: 151–152.

145. Thorin D, Rosselet P, Ravussin P, et al. Impact of the endotracheal tube on glottic and supraglottic structures during orotracheal fiberoptic intubation. Br J Anaesth 1995;74:13.

146. Couture P, Perreault C, Girard D. Fiberoptic bronchoscopic intubation after induction of general anaesthesia: another approach. Can J Anaesth 1992;39:99.

147. Bond A. Assisting fiberoptic intubation. Anaesthesia and Intensive Care 1992;20:247–248.

148. Hakala P, Randell T. Comparison between two fiberscopes with different diameter insertion cords for fibreoptic intubation. Anaesthesia 1995;50:735–737.

149. Marsh NJ. Easier fiberoptic intubations. Anesthesiology 1992;76:860–861.

150. Rosenblatt WH. Overcoming obstruction during bronchoscope-guided intubation of the trachea with the double setup endotracheal tube. Anesth Analg 1996;83:175–177.

151. Ovassapian A. Failure to withdraw flexible fiberoptic laryngoscope after nasotracheal intubation. Anesthesiology 1985;63:124–125.

152. MacGillivray RG, Odell JA. Eye to eye with Murphy's Law. Anaesthesia 1986;41:334.

153. Nichols KP, Zornow MH. A potential complication of fiberoptic intubation. Anesthesiology 1989;70: 562–563.

154. Howardy–Hansen P, Berthelsen P. Fiberoptic bronchoscopic nasotracheal intubation of a neonate with Pierre-Robin syndrome. Anaesthesia 1988;43: 121–122.

155. Scheller JG, Schulman SR. Fiberoptic bronchoscopic guidance for intubating a neonate with Pierre-Robin syndrome. J Clin Anesth 1991;3:45–47.

156. Gerrish SP, Weston GA. The use of a biopsy brush wire as a bronchoscope guide. Anaesthesia 1986;41: 444.

157. Suriani RJ, Kayne RD. Fiberoptic bronchoscopic guidance for intubating a child with Pierre-Robin Syndrome. J Clin Anesth 1992;4:258.

158. Telford RJ, Searle JF, Boaden RW, et al. Use of a guide wire and a ureteral dilator as an aid to awake fibreoptic intubation. Anaesthesia 1994;49: 691–693.

159. Skinner AC. Glottic illumination by fibrescope. Anaesthesia 1983;38:1100–1101.

160. Alfery DD, Ward CF, Harwood IR, et al. Airway management for a neonate with congenital fusion of the jaws. Anesthesiology 1979;51:340–342.

161. Gouverneur J-M, Veyckemans F, Licker M. Using an ureteral catheter as a guide in difficult neonatal fiberoptic intubation. Anesthesiology 1987;66: 436–437.

162. Foster CA. An aid to blind nasal intubation in children. Anaesthesia 1977;32:1038.

163. Stone DJ. Another use for the fiberoptic bronchoscope. Anesthesiology 1987;67:608.

164. Berthelsen P, Prytz S, Jacobsen E. Two-stage fiberoptic nasotracheal intubation in infants: a new approach to difficult pediatric intubation. Anesthesiology 1985;63:457–458.

165. Dellinger RP. Fiberoptic bronchoscopy in adult airway management. Crit Care Med 1990;18:882–887.

166. Sia RL, Edens ET. How to avoid problems when using the fibre-optic bronchoscope for difficult intubations. Anaesthesia 1981;36:74–75.

167. Shorten GD, Ali HH, Roberts JT. Assessment of patient position for fiberoptic intubation using video laryngoscopy. Anesth Analg 1991;72:S253.

168. Roberts JT, Ali HH, Shorten GD, et al. Why cervical flexion facilitates laryngoscopy with a Macintosh laryngoscope, but hinders it with a flexible fiberscope. Anesthesiology 1990;73:A1012.

169. Ross DG. Fiberoptic intubation and double-lumen tubes. Anaesthesia 1990;45:895.

170. Smith JE. Intraoperative nasotracheal to orotracheal tube change in a patient with Klippel-Feil syndrome. Anaesthesia and Intensive Care 1996;24:120.

171. Delaney KA, Hessler R. Emergency flexible fiberoptic nasotracheal intubation: A report of 60 cases. Ann Emerg Med 1988;17:919–926.

172. Boysen PG. Fiberoptic instrumentation for airway management. ASA Refresher Courses 1993; Washington DC.

173. Patil VU. Oral and nasal fiberoptic intubation with a single lumen tube in fiberoptics in anesthesia. In: Roberts JT, ed. Fiberoptics in anesthesia [Special issue]. Anesth Clin North Am 1991;9:83–96.

174. Nakayama M, Kataoka N, Usui Y, et al. Techniques of nasotracheal intubation with the fiberoptic bronchoscope. J Emerg Med 1992;10:729–734

175. Hughes S, Smith JE. Nasotracheal tube placement over the fibreoptic laryngoscope. Anaesthesia 1996; 51:1026–128.

176. Audenaert SM, Montgomery CL, Stone B, et al. Retrograde-assisted fiberoptic tracheal intubation in children with difficult airways. Anesth Analg 1991;73: 660–664.

177. Bissinger U, Guggenberger H, Lenz G. Retrograde-

guided fiberoptic intubation in patients with laryngeal carcinoma. Anesth Analg 1995;81:408–410.

178. Benumof JL. Additional safety measures when changing endotracheal tubes. Anesthesiology 1991;75:921–922.

179. Halebian P, Shires T. A method of replacement of the endotracheal tube with continuous control of the airway. Surg Gynecol Obstet 1985;161:285–286.

180. Nakagawa H, Komatsu R, Hayashi K, et al. Fiberoptic evaluation of the difficult extubation. Anesthesiology 1995;82:785–786.

181. Wheeler S, Gaughan S, Benumof JL. Use of the fiberoptic bronchoscope as a jet stylet. Anesthesiology Rev 1993;20:16–17.

182. Daum REO, Jones DJ. Fiberoptic intubation in Klippel-Feil syndrome. Anaesthesia 1988;43:18–21.

183. Hemmer D, Lee T, Wright BD. Intubation of a child with a cervical spine injury with the aid of a fiberoptic bronchoscope. Anaesthesia and Intensive Care 1982;10:163–165.

184. Keenan MA, Stiles CM, Kaufman RL. Acquired laryngeal deviation associated with cervical spine disease in erosive polyarticular arthritis. Use of fiberoptic bronchoscope in rheumatoid disease. Anesthesiology 1983;58:441–448.

185. Ovassapian A, Land P, Schaffer MF, et al. Anesthetic management for surgical corrections of severe flexion deformity of the cervical spine. Anesthesiology 1983;58:370–372.

186. Ovassapian A, Doka JC, Romsa DE. Acromegaly: use of fiberoptic laryngoscopy to avoid tracheostomy. Anesthesiology 1981;54:429–430.

187. Rashid J, Warltier B. Awake fiberoptic intubation for a rare cause of upper airway obstruction: an infected laryngocele. Anaesthesia 1989;44:834–836.

188. Stella JP, Kageler WV, Epker BN. Fiberoptic endotracheal intubation in oral and maxillofacial surgery. J Oral Maxillofac Surg 1986;44:923–925.

190. Finer NN, Muzyka D. Flexible endoscopic intubation of the neonate. Pediatr Pulmonol 1992;12:48–51.

191. Ranasinghe DN, Calder I. Large cervical osteophyte—another use of difficult flexible fibreoptic intubation. Anaesthesia 1994;49:512–514.

192. Wilder RT, Belani KG. Fiberoptic intubation complicated by pulmonary edema in a 12-year-old child with Hurler syndrome. Anesthesiology 1990;72:205–27.

193. Neal MR, Groves J, Gell IR. Awake fibreoptic intubation in the semi-prone position following facial trauma. Anaesthesia 1996;51:1053–1054.

194. Hung OR, Stewart RD. Lightwand intubation. I—A new lightwand device. Can J Anaesth 1995;42:820–825.

195. Stewart RD, LaRosee A, Stoy WA, et al. Use of a

lighted stylet to confirm correct endotracheal tube placement. Chest 1987;92:900–93.

196. Schreiner MS. Difficult airway and intubation. STA Interface 1994;5,4:19.

197. Higgins MS, Wherry TJ. Topical anesthesia of the airway using the lighted stylet. Anesthesiology 1993;79:1148.

198. Ainsworth QP, Howells TH. Transilluminated tracheal intubation. Br J Anaesth 1989;62:494–497.

199. Ducrow M. Throwing light on blind intubation. Anaesthesia 1978;33:827–829.

200. Ellis DG, Jakymec A, Kaplan RM, et al. Guided orotracheal intubation in the operating room using a lighted stylet. A comparison with direct laryngoscopic technique. Anesthesiology 1986;64:823–826.

201. Fox DJ, Castro T, Rastrelli AJ. Comparison of intubation techniques in the awake patient. The Flexilum surgical light (lightwand) versus blind nasal approach. Anesthesiology 1987;66:69–71.

202. Mehta S. Transtracheal illumination for optimal tracheal tube placement. A clinical study. Anaesthesia 1989;44:970–972.

203. Vollmer TP, Stewart RD, Paris PM, et al. Use of a lighted stylet for guided orotracheal intubation in the pre-hospital setting. Ann Emerg Med 1985;14:324–328.

204. Weis FR, Hatton MN. Intubation by use of the lightwand: experience in 253 patients. J Oral Maxillofac Surg 1989;47:577–580.

205. Hung OR, Murphy M. Lightwands, lighted-stylets and blind techniques of intubation. Anesth Clin North Am 1995;13:477–489.

206. Hung OR, Pytka S, Morris I, et al. Lightwand intubation. II.—Clinical trial of a new lightwand for tracheal intubation in patients with difficult airways. Can J Anaesth 1995;42:826–830.

207. Boerner TF. Innovations in lighted stylet intubation. Anesthesiology News, March 1996;22:32–34.

208. Ellis DG, Stewart RD, Kaplan RM, et al. Success rates of blind orotracheal intubation using a transillumination technique with a lighted stylet. Ann Emerg Med 1986;15:138–142.

209. Williams RT, Stewart RD. Transillumination of the trachea with a lighted stylet. Anesth Analg 1986;65:542–543.

210. Stewart RD, LaRosee A, Kaplan RM, et al. Correct positioning of an endotracheal tube using a flexible lighted stylet. Crit Care Med 1990;18:97–99.

211. Hartman RA, Castro T, Matson M, –. Rapid orotracheal intubation in the clenched-jaw patient. A modification of the lightwand technique. J Clin Anesth 1992;4:245–246.

212. Hung OR, Lung KE, Multari J. Clinical trial of a

new lightwand device for nasotracheal intubation in surgical patients. Can J Anaesth 1993;40:A57.

213. Verdile VP, Heller MB, Paris PM, et al. Nasotracheal intubation in traumatic craniofacial dislocation. use of the lighted stylet. Am J Emerg Med 1988;6:39–41.

214. Verdile VP, Chiang J-L, Bedger R, et al. Nasotracheal intubation using a flexible lighted stylet. Ann Emerg Med 1990;19:506–510.

215. Fisher QA, Tunkel DE. Endoscopic analysis of factors in successful pediatric lightwand intubation. Anesthesiology 1995;83:A498.

216. Asai T, Latto IP. Use of the lighted stylet for tracheal intubation via the laryngeal mask airway. Br J Anaesth 1995;75:503–504.

217. Crosby ET. Lighting the way in emergency airway care. Can J Anaesth 1994;41:78.

218. Devine W, Lang D, Wafai Y, et al. Use of the lighted flexguide for optimal tracheal tube placement in critically ill patients. Anesthesiology 1995;83:A267.

219. Hung OR, Pytka S, Morris I, et al. Clinical trial of a new lightwand device (Trachlight) to intubate the trachea. Anesthesiology 1995;83:509–514.

220. Weis FR. Light-wand intubation for cervical spine injuries. Anesth Analg 1992;74:622.

221. Graham DH, Doll WA, Robinson AD, et al. Intubation with lighted stylet. Can J Anaesth 1991;38:261–262.

222. Rayburn RL. Lightwand intubation. Anaesthesia 1979;34:677–678.

223. Graham DH, Doll WA, Robinson AD, et al. Intubation with lighted stylet. Can J Anaesth 1991;38:261–262.

224. Culling RD, Mongan P, Castro T. Lightwand guided rapid sequence orotracheal intubation. Anesthesiology 1989;71:A994.

225. Robelen GT, Shulman MS. Use of the lighted stylet for difficult intubation in adult patients. Anesthesiology 1989;71:A438.

229. Holzman RS, Nargozian CD, Florence B. Lightwand intubation in children with abnormal upper airways. Anesthesiology 1988;69:784–787.

226. Fox DJ, Matson MD. Management of the difficult pediatric airway in an austere environment using the lightwand. J Clin Anesth 1990;2:123–125.

227. Iseki K, Watanabe K, Iwama H. Use of the Trachlight (for intubation in the Pierre-Robin syndrome. Anaesthesia 1997;52:801.

228. Reference deleted.

230. Knight RG, Castro T, Rastrelli AJ, et al. Arterial blood pressure and heart rate response to lighted stylet or direct laryngoscopy for endotracheal intubation. Anesthesiology 1988;69:269–272.

231. Kashin BA, Wynands JE. A comparison of haemody-namic changes during lighted stylet or directed laryngoscopy for endotracheal intubation. Can J Anaesth 1989;36:S72–S73.

232. Hung OR, Pytka S, Murphy ME, et al. A comparison of haemodynamic changes in patients undergoing laryngoscopic or lightwand orotracheal intubation. Can J Anaesth 1993;40:A71.

233. Hung OR, Pytka S, Murphy MF, et al. Comparative hemodynamic changes following laryngoscopic or lightwand intubation. Anesthesiology 1993;79:A497.

234. Stone DJ, Stirt JA, Kaplan MJ, et al. A complication of lightwand-guided nasotracheal intubation. Anesthesiology 1984;61:780–781.

235. Dowson S, Greenwald KM. A potential complication of lightwand-guided intubation. Anesth Analg 1992;74:169.

236. Cohn AI, Joshi S. Lighted stylet intubation: greasing your way to success Anesth Analg 1994;78:1205–1206.

237. Debo RF, Colonna D, Dewerd G, et al. Cricoarytenoid subluxation: complication of blind intubation with a lighted stylet. Ear Nose Throat J 1989;68:517–520.

238. Szigeti CL, Baeuerle JJ, Mongan PD. Arytenoid dislocation with lighted stylet intubation: Case report and retrospective review. Anesth Analg 1994;78:185–196.

239. Bjoraker DG. The Bullard intubation laryngoscopes. Anesthesiol Rev 1990;17:64–70.

240. Gaughan SD, Benumof JL, Ozaki GT. Evaluation of the Bullard laryngoscope with the new intubating stylet. Anesthesiology 1992;77:A512.

241. Cooper SD, Benumof JL, Ozaki GT. Evaluation of the Bullard laryngoscope using the new intubating stylet: comparison with conventional laryngoscope. Anesth Analg 1994;79:965–970.

242. Borland LM, Casselbrant M. The Bullard laryngoscope. A new indirect oral laryngoscope (pediatric version). Anesth Analg 1990;70:105–108.

243. Nakatsuka M. Combined use of high frequency jet ventilation with Bullard intubating laryngoscope for difficult airway and intubation. Anesthesiology 1993;79:A1085.

244. Cohn AI, King WH. Awake intubation of the adult trachea using the Bullard laryngoscope. Can J Anaesth 1995;42:246–248.

245. Cohn AI, Zornow MH. Awake endotracheal intubation in patients with cervical spine disease: a comparison of the Bullard laryngoscope and the fiberoptic bronchoscope. Anesth Analg 1995;81:1283–1286.

246. D'Alessio JG. The Bullard laryngoscope as jet ventilator. Anesth Analg 1995;81:435.

247. Mendel P, Bristow A. Anaesthesia for procedures on the larynx and pharynx. The use of the Bullard laryngoscope in conjunction with high-frequency jet ventilation. Anaesthesia 1993;48:253–255.

248. Weeks DB, Bland KB, Koufman JA. Jet venturi ventilation via the Bullard laryngoscope. Anesthesiology 1993;79:866–867.

249. Crosby ET. Techniques using the Bullard laryngoscope. Anesth Analg 1995;81:1314.

250. Adamo AK, Katsnelson T, Rodriquez ED, et al. Intraoperative airway management with pan-facial fractures. Alternative approaches. J Cranio-Maxillofacial Trauma 1996;2:30–35.

251. Neubarth J. New power source for Bullard laryngoscope. Anesth Analg 1994;79:1021.

252. Katsnelson T, Farcon E, Schwalbe SS, et al. The Bullard laryngoscope and the right arytenoid. Can J Anaesth 1994;41:552–553.

253. Baraka A, Muallem M, Sibai AN. Facilitation of difficult tracheal intubation by the fiberoptic Bullard laryngoscope. Middle East J Anesthesiol 1991;11:73–77.

254. Patil VU, Lopez CJ, Romano DJ. Use of an 8-F catheter to assist with Bullard laryngoscopy in intubating the trachea. Anesthesiology 1996;85:440–441.

255. Shigematsu T, Miyazawa N, Yorozu T. Nasotracheal intubation using Bullard laryngoscope. Can J Anaesth 1991;38:798.

256. Katsnelson T, Straker T, Farcon E, et al. The Bullard laryngoscope and a "Directional Tip" RAE tube. J Clin Anesth 1996;8:80–81.

257. Shigematsu T, Miyazawa N, Kobayashi M, et al. Nasal intubation with Bullard laryngoscope. A useful approach for difficult airways. Anesth Analg 1994;79:132–135.

258. Shigematsu T, Miyazawa N, Yorozu T. Nasotracheal intubation using Bullard laryngoscope. Can J Anaesth 1991;38:798.

259. Brown RE, Vollers JM, Rader GR, et al. Nasotracheal intubation in a child with Treacher Collins syndrome using the Bullard intubating laryngoscope. J Clin Anesth 1993;5:492–493.

260. Baraka A, Muallem M, Sibai AN, et al. Bullard laryngoscopy for tracheal intubation of patients with cervical spine pathology. Can J Anaesth 1992;39:513–514.

261. Grande CM, Barton CR, Stene JK. Appropriate technique for airway management of emergency patients with suspected spinal cord injury. Anesth Analg 1988;67:714–715.

262. Cohn AI. Bullard laryngoscopes, apples and oranges, and coin tosses. Anesth Analg 1995;81:425.

263. Ghouri AF, Bernstein CA. Use of the Bullard laryngoscope in patients with maxillofacial injuries. Anesthesiology 1996;84:490.

264. Cohn AI, Hart RT, McGraw SR, et al. The Bullard laryngoscope for emergency airway management in a morbidly obese parturient. Anesth Analg 1995;81:872–873.

265. Hastings RH, Marks JD. Airway management for trauma patients with potential cervical spine injuries. Anesth Analg 1991;73:471–482.

266. Hastings RH, Vigil AC, Hanna R, et al. Cervical spine movement during laryngoscopy with the Bullard, Macintosh, and Miller laryngoscopes. Anesthesiology 1995;82:859–869.

267. Cohn AI, Hokanson JA, Zornow MH. Awake fiberoptic endotracheal intubation with cervical spine disease: a comparison of techniques. Anesthesiology 1996;83:A497.

268. Katsnelson T, Farcon E, Darvishzadeh S, et al. Cardiovascular effects of Bullard laryngoscopy. Anesthesiology 1994;81:A495.

269. Katsnelson T, Farcon E, Cosio M, et al. The Bullard laryngoscope and size of the endotracheal tube. Anesthesiology 1994;81:261–262.

270. Wu T-L, Chou H-C. A new laryngoscope. The combination intubating device. Anesthesiology 1994;81:1085–1087.

271. Wu T-L, Chou H-C. Use of the WuScope in the trauma patient. Anesthesiology News, October 1995;21:40–42.

272. Pearce AC, Shaw S, Macklin S. Evaluation of the Usherscope. A new rigid fibrescope. Anaesthesia 1996;51:561–564.

273. Fridrich F, Kraft P, Krenn CG, et al. Randomized, controlled trial on fibreoptic orotracheal intubation using the UpsherScope. Br J Anaesth 1997;78:11.

274. Aromaa U, Pesonen P, Linko K, et al. Difficulties with tooth protectors in endotracheal intubation. Acta Anaesthesiol Scand 1988;32:304–307.

275. Davis FO, DeFreece AB, Shroff PF. Custom-made plastic guards for tooth protection during endoscopy and orotracheal intubation. Anesth Analg 1971;50:203–26.

276. Evers W, Racz GB, Glazer J, et al. Orahesive as a protection for the teeth during general anaesthesia and endoscopy. Can Anaesth Soc J 1967;14:123–128.

277. Rosenberg M, Bolgla J. Protection of teeth and gums during endotracheal intubation. Anesth Analg 1968;47:34–36.

278. Haddy S. Protecting teeth during endotracheal intubation. Anesthesiology 1989;71:810–811.

279. Hohmann JE. Practice gems. Welcome Trends Anesthesiol 1992;10:10.

280. Lisman SR, Shepherd NJ, Rosenberg M. A modified laryngoscope blade for dental protection. Anesthesiology 1981;55:190.

281. Nique TA, Bennett CR, Altop H. Laryngoscope modification to avoid trauma due to laryngoscopy. Anesth Prog 1982;29:47–49.

282. Brosnan CM, Fadford P. Does the routine use of toothguard cause intubation to be more difficult. A randomised controlled trial. Br J Anaesth 1997;78:10–11.

283. Beneby G. The use of a transparent mouthguard at induction. Anaesthesia 1989;44:705.

284. Herlich A, Garber JG, Orkin FK. Dental and salivary gland complications. In: Gravenstein N, Kirby RR, eds. Complications in anesthesiology. Philadelphia: Lippincott–Raven, 1996;163–173.

285. Rosenberg M. Anesthesia-induced dental injury. Int Anesthesiol Clin 1989;27:120–125.

286. Lopes J, Ortega RA. Difficult ventilation caused by profuse hemorrhage after dislodging a tooth. Anesth Analg 1993;76:1373–1374.

287. Burton JF, Baker AB. Dental damage during anaesthesia and surgery. Anaesthesia and Intensive Care 1987;15:262–268.

288. Lockhart PB, Feldbau EV, Gabel RA, et al. Dental complications during and after tracheal intubation. J Am Dent Assoc 1986;112:480–483.

289. Fry ENS. A lead tooth-bridge. Br J Anaesth 1974;46:543.

290. Sniper W. Filling a gap. Br J Anaesth 1984;56:313–314.

291. Siek GW, Bjorkman LL. Missed pharyngeal foreign body. JAMA 1978;239:722.

292. Clokie C, Metcalf I, Holland A. Dental trauma in anaesthesia. Can J Anaesth 1989;36:675–680.

293. Kainuma M, Yamada M, Miyake T. Early application of the cross-suture splint to teeth avulsed at tracheal intubation. Anesthesiology 1996;84:1516.

294. Ghabash MB, Matta MS, Mehanna CB. Prevention of dental trauma during endotracheal intubation. Anesth Analg 1997;84:230–231.

295. Hawkins DB, Seltzer DC, Barnett TE, et al. Endotracheal tube perforation of the hypopharynx. West J Med 1974;120:282–286.

296. Hirsch IA, Reagan JO, Sullivan N. Complications of direct laryngoscopy. Anesthesiol Rev 1990;17:34–40.

297. Hawkins DB, House JW. Postoperative pneumothorax secondary to hypopharyngeal perforation during anesthetic intubation. Ann Otol 1974;93:556–557.

298. McGoldrick KE, Donlon JV. Sublingual hematoma following difficult laryngoscopy. Anesth Analg 1979;58:343–344.

299. Roberts J. Fundamentals of tracheal intubation. New York: Grune & Stratton, 1983.

300. Stauffer JL, Petty TL. Accidental intubation of the pyriform sinus. A complication of "roadside" resuscitation. JAMA 1977;237:2324–2325.

301. Wolf AP, Kuhn FA, Ogura JH. Pharyngeal-esophageal perforations associated with rapid oral endotracheal intubation. Ann Otol 1972;81:258–261.

302. Teichner RL. Lingual nerve injury: a complication of orotracheal intubation. Br J Anaesth 1971;43:413–414.

303. Jones BC. Lingual nerve injury: a complication of intubation. Br J Anaesth 1971;43:730.

304. Loughman E. Lingual nerve injury following tracheal intubation. Anaesthesia and Intensive Care 1983;11:171.

305. Silva DA, Colingo KA, Miller R. Lingual nerve injury following laryngoscopy. Anesthesiology 1992;76:650–651.

306. Grigsby EJ, Lennon RL, Didier EP, et al. Massive tongue swelling after uncomplicated general anaesthesia. Can J Anaesth 1990;37:825–826.

307. Upton LG. Oral and maxillofacial surgical considerations in the difficult airway. In: Norton, ML, Brown ACD, eds. Atlas of the difficult airway. A source book. St. Louis: Mosby Year Book, 1991;129–144.

308. Blanc VF, Tremblay NAG. The complications of tracheal intubation. A new classification with a review of the literature. Anesth Analg 1974;53:202–213.

309. Aprahamian C, Thompson B, Finger WA, et al. Experimental cervical spine injury model. Evaluation of airway management and splinting techniques. Ann Emerg Med 1984;13:584–587.

310. Doolan LA, O'Brian JF. Safe intubation in cervical spine injury. Anaesthesia and Intensive Care 1985;13:319–324.

311. Stout DM, Bishop MJ. Perioperative laryngeal and tracheal complications of intubation. Probl Anesth 1988;2:225–234.

312. Fitzgerald RD, Krafft P, Skrbensky G, et al. Excursions of the cervical spine during tracheal intubation: blind oral intubation compared with direct laryngoscopy. Anaesthesia 1994;49:111–115.

313. Hastings RH, Kelley SD. Neurologic deterioration associated with airway management in a cervical spine-injured patient. Anesthesiology 1993;78:580–583.

314. Swain PD, Todd MM, Traynelis VC, et al. Cervical spine motion with direct laryngoscopy and orotracheal intubation. Anesthesiology 1996;85:26–36.

315. Suderman VS, Crosby ET, Lui A. Elective oral tracheal intubation in cervical spine-injured adults. Can J Anaesth 1991;38:785–789.

316. Majernick TG, Bieniek R, Houston JB, et al. Cervical spine movement during orotracheal intubation. Ann Emerg Med 1986;15:417–420.

317. Hastings RH, Marks JD. Airway management for trauma patients with potential cervical spine injuries. Anesth Analg 1991;73:471–482.

318. Bivins HG, Ford S, Bezmalinovic Z, et al. The effect of axial traction during orotracheal intubation of the trauma victim with an unstable cervical spine. Ann Emerg Med 1988;17:25–29.

319. Criswell JC, Parr MJA. Emergency airway management in patients with cervical spine injuries. Anaesthesia 1994;49:900–903.

320. Hastings RH, Wood PR. Head extension and laryngeal view during laryngoscopy with cervical spine stabilization maneuvers. Anesthesiology 1994;80:825–8231.

321. Heath KJ. The effect on laryngoscopy of different cervical spine immobilization techniques. Anaesthesia 1994;49:843–845.

322. Scott RC, Field JM. Orotracheal intubation and cervical spine injury. Anaesthesia 1995;50:567.

323. Schrader S, Ovassapian A, Dykes MH, et al. Cardiovascular changes during awake rigid and fiberoptic laryngoscopy. Anesthesiology 1987;67:A28.

324. Norris TJ, Baysinger CL. Heart rate and blood pressure response to laryngoscopy. The influence of laryngoscopic technique. Anesthesiology 1985;63:560.

325. Cozanitis DA, Nuuttila K, Merrett JD, et al. Influence of laryngoscope design on heart rate and rhythm changes during intubation. Can Anaesth Soc J 1984;31:155–159.

326. Bucx MJL, Van Geel RTM, Scheck PAE, et al. Cardiovascular effects of forces applied during laryngoscopy. The importance of tracheal intubation. Anaesthesia 1992;47:1029–133.

327. Johnson JD, Love JD. Lights out! A preventable complication of endotracheal intubation. Chest 1985;87:701–702.

328. Perel A, Katz E, Davidson JT. Fiberbronchoscopic retrieval of an aspirated laryngoscope bulb. Intensive Care Med 1981;7:143–144.

329. William L, Teague PO, Nagia AH. Foreign body from a Patil-Syracuse mask. Anesth Analg 1991;73:359–360.

330. Waring PH, Vinik HR. A potential complication of the Patil-Syracuse endoscopy mask. Anesth Analg 1991;73:668–669.

331. Zornow MH, Mitchell MM. Foreign body aspiration during fiberoptic—assisted intubation. Anesthesiology 1986;64:303.

332. Toung TJK, Donham RT, Shipley R. Thermal burn caused by a laryngoscope. Anesthesiology 1981;55:184–185.

333. Siegel LC, Garman JK. Too hot to handle. A laryngoscope malfunction. Anesthesiology 1990;72:1088–1089.

334. Willis MJ, Thomas E. The cold light-source that was hot. Gastrointest Endosc 1984;30:117–118.

335. Can der Walt JH, Gassmanis K. Skin burns from a cold light source. Anaesthesia and Intensive Care 1990;18:113–115.

336. Daley H, Amoroso P. Dangerous repairs. Anaesthesia 1991;46:997.

337. Desmeules H, Tremblay P. Laryngoscope blade breakage during intubation. Can J Anaesth 1988;35:202–203.

338. Smith MB, Camp P. Broken laryngoscope. Anaesthesia 1989;44:179.

339. Rocco M, Chatwani A, Shupak R. Laryngoscope handle malfunction. Anesthesiology 1986;65:107.

340. Vernon JM. A broken laryngoscope. Anaesthesia 1990;45:697.

341. Anonymous. Disposable laryngoscope blades may break during use. Biomedical Safety & Standards 1994;24:101–102.

342. Gibson S, Kelly K. Paediatric laryngoscope blade failure. Anaesthesia and Intensive Care 1996;24:724–725.

343. Hodges UM. Damage to a laryngoscope. Anaesthesia 1988;43:711.

344. Krishna M. A potential complication associated with laryngoscope. Anesth Analg 1997;84:938–939.

QUESTIONS

1. The best position for intubating an adult patient using a rigid laryngoscope is with
   1. The shoulders elevated
   2. Flexion of the lower cervical spine and extension of the head
   3. Flat on the bed
   4. Pressure exerted on the top of the head

2. Techniques for inserting a tracheal tube with a flexible fiberoptic laryngoscope include:
   1. Visualizing the larynx with the fiberoptic scope, placing the scope into the larynx, and sliding the tracheal tube over the scope
   2. Placing a bougie in the trachea under direct vision using the fiberoptic scope and then inserting the tube over the bougie
   3. Placing the tracheal tube into the pharynx as a guide for placement of the fiberoptic scope and then advancing the scope and then the tube into the larynx
   4. Placing the trachea tube into the larynx with a blind technique and checking its position with the fiberscope

3. If the tracheal tube cannot be advanced into the trachea, the following maneuvers may be helpful
   1. Withdrawing the tube and turning it 180°
   2. Applying external pressure on the larynx
   3. Elevation of the mandible
   4. Placing the head in the chin up position

4. Reported complications associated with laryngoscopy include
   1. Tooth damage
   2. Protrusion of the fiberoptic scope through the Murphy eye
   3. Damage to the cervical spinal cord
   4. Damage to the recurrent laryngeal nerve

5. The best illumination with rigid laryngoscope blades is provided
   1. Using mains electrical power
   2. Using fiberoptics to transmit the light from the handle
   3. With the bulb near the tip of the blade
   4. Using a halogen bulb

6. Which maneuvers are useful for nasal intubation with a fiberoptic scope?
   1. Using a nasopharyngeal airway to dilate the nose
   2. Introducing the tube through a specially designed mask
   3. Using a slit nasopharyngeal airway to introduce the tube
   4. Introducing the fiberscope orally and using it to guide the tube from the nose

7. If a tracheal tube hangs up when introduced over a fiberscope, what techniques may be used to correct the problem?
   1. Applying pressure to the larynx
   2. Rotating the tube 90 to 180°
   3. Elevating the mandible
   4. Use of a flexible, wire-reinforced tracheal tube

ANSWERS

1. C		**5.** B	
2. A		**6.** E	
3. A		**7.** E	
4. A			

CHAPTER
17

Tracheal Tubes

2. Low-Pressure, High-Volume Cuff
3. Sponge Cuff
G. Securing the Tube
H. Changing the Tube
    I. Removing the Tube

IV. Perioperative Complications
A. Trauma
B. Failure to Achieve a Satisfactory Seal
C. Intubation of the Esophagus
    1. Direct Visualization
    2. Feel of the Reservoir Bag
    3. Chest Wall Motion
    4. Auscultation
    5. Sounds of Air around the Tube
    6. Epigastric Distention
    7. Moisture Condensation in the Tracheal Tube
    8. Gastric Contents in Tracheal Tube
    9. Oxygenation
    10. Chest X-Ray
    11. Palpation of Suprasternal Notch
    12. Measuring Amount of Cuff Inflation Needed to Cause a Seal
    13. Use of a Fiberscope
    14. Tactile Confirmation
    15. Esophageal Detector Device
    16. Sonic Detection
    17. Ultrasound
    18. Intentional Bronchial Intubation
    19. Passing Introducer through the Tracheal Tube
    20. Tracheal Intubation during Intubation
    21. Roll Test
    22. Pressure- and Flow-Volume Loops
    23. Tracheal Illumination
    24. Exhaled Carbon Dioxide
D. Swallowed Tracheal Tube
E. Inadvertent Bronchial Intubation
    1. Auscultation for Bilateral Breath Sounds
    2. Visualization of Symmetrical Chest Expansion
    3. Chest X-Ray
    4. Tube Position at the Lips/Nostril
        a. Adult Patients
        b. Pediatric Patients
            (1) Oral Intubation
            (2) Nasotracheal Intubation
    5. Placement of the Cuff Just Below the Vocal Cords
    6. Guide Marks on the Tracheal Tube
    7. Breath Sounds
    8. Fiberscope through the Tube

9. Palpation of Anterior Neck
10. Fluid in Cuff
11. Magnetically Detectable Metallic Element
12. Monitoring Expired Carbon Dioxide
13. Lighted Intubation Stylet
14. Illumination by a Fiberoptic Strand
15. Pressure- and Flow-Volume Loops
16. Transcutaneous Oxygen Monitor or Pulse Oximetry
F. Foreign Body Aspiration
G. Leak while the Tube Is in Place
H. Airway Perforation
I. Murphy Eye Complications
J. Laser-Induced Tracheal Tube Fire
    1. Physics of Lasers
        a. Laser Medium
        b. The Optical Cavity
        c. Pumping Source
        d. Light Guide
    2. Types
        a. Carbon Dioxide Laser
        b. Nd-YAG Laser
        c. KTP Laser
        d. Argon Laser
    3. Fires
    4. Minimizing Risk
        a. Low Inspired Oxygen Concentration
        b. Laser Protocol
        c. Filling Cuff with Saline
        d. Protective Wrappings
        e. Use of Special Tubes
        f. Use of Positive End-Expiratory Pressure
        g. Other
    5. Action in Case of Fire
K. Cautery-induced Tracheal Tube Fire
L. Tracheal Tube Obstruction
    1. Causes
        a. Biting
        b. Kinking
        c. Material in the Lumen of the Tube
        d. Spiral Embedded Tubes
        e. Bevel Abutting against the Tracheal Wall
        f. Obstruction by the Cuff
        g. External Compression
        h. Defective Connector
    2. Prevention
    3. Diagnosis and Treatment
M. Aspiration of Gastric Contents
    1. Use of Low-Pressure Cuffs

THE TRACHEAL TUBE (endotracheal tube, intra-tracheal tube, and catheter) is inserted into the trachea and is used to conduct gases and vapors to and from the lungs.

GENERAL PRINCIPLES
Resistance and Work of Breathing

A tracheal tube places a mechanical burden on the spontaneously breathing patient (1–5). It adds more resistance and is a more important factor in determining the work of breathing than the breathing system (6–8).

Several factors help to determine the resistance to gas flow imposed by a tracheal tube.

Internal Diameter

The single most important factor is the internal diameter (ID) of the tube and its connector. A tube with a thick wall will offer more resistance than a thin-walled tube with the same outer diameter. The wall thickness:tube diameter ratio is greater in small tubes, leading to a relatively higher increase in airway resistance after intubation in children (9). Resistance will be increased if a suction catheter, fiberscope, or other device is passed through the tube or secretions line in the inner wall, because this decreases the size of the lumen (10, 11). Double-lumen bronchial tubes offer high resistance because of the small diameters of their lumens.

Length

Decreasing tube length lowers its resistance, but the decrease is much less than could be accomplished by increasing the ID (5, 12–14). Disposable tubes are usually supplied longer than needed and may be cut to a more suitable length to reduce resistance.

Configuration

Abrupt changes in direction and diameter increase resistance (13, 15, 16). A preformed tube offers more resistance than a tube with gentler curves (9). Kinking increases resistance.

Curved connectors offer more resistance than straight ones (17). A gently curved connector offers less resistance than a right-angled one. The resistance of swivel connectors is similar to that of curved connectors (18).

Gas Density

Decreasing the density of the gas flowing through the tube (e.g., by including helium in the inspired gases) will reduce resistance (5, 12).

Dead Space

The tracheal tube and connector constitute mechanical dead space, which was discussed in Chapter 6, "Breathing Systems I: General Considerations." Because the volume of a tracheal tube and its connector is usually less than that of the natural passages, dead space is normally reduced by intubation. In pediatric patients, however, long tubes and connectors may increase the dead space. Special low-volume pediatric connectors are available.

TRACHEAL TUBES

Materials of Construction (19–21)

The material from which a tracheal tube is manufactured should have the following characteristics:

1. Low cost
2. Lack of tissue toxicity
3. Transparency
4. Ease of sterilization and durability with repeated sterilizations (unless disposable)
5. Nonflammability
6. A smooth, nonwettable surface inside and outside to prevent secretion buildup, allow easy passage of a suction catheter or bronchoscope, and prevent trauma
7. Sufficient body to maintain its shape during insertion and prevent occlusion by torsion, kinking, or compression by the cuff or external pressure
8. Sufficient strength to allow thin wall construction
9. Thermoplasticity to conform to the patient's anatomy when in place
10. Nonreactivity with lubricants and anesthetic agents

To date, no substance with all of the above traits has been found. This section will describe some of the substances that have been used for tubes and some of the problems encountered.

For many years, tracheal tubes were made from rubber. These tubes can be cleaned, sterilized, and reused multiple times. However, they are not transparent, harden and become sticky with age, have poor resistance to kinking, become clogged by inspissated secretions more easily than plastic tubes, and do not soften appreciably at body temperature. Latex allergy is another possible problem (22).

At present, polyvinyl chloride (PVC) is the substance most widely used in disposable tracheal tubes. It is relatively inexpensive and compatible with tissues. Tubes made from PVC have less tendency to kink than rubber tubes. They are stiff enough for intubation at room temperature but soften at body temperature, so that they tend to conform to the anatomy of the patient's upper airway, reducing pressure at points of contact. A polyvinyl chloride tube may be refrigerated to

make it more firm for intubation or warmed prior to use to facilitate placement over a fiberscope (23). They have a smooth surface that facilitates passage of a suction catheter or bronchoscope. Their transparency permits observation of the tidal movement of respiratory moisture as well as objects or materials in the lumen.

Silicone is used in the manufacture of some tracheal tubes. Although more expensive than PVC, many products made from it can be sterilized and reused.

Some materials used in the manufacture of tracheal tubes in the past have shown evidence of tissue toxicity. To meet the American Society for Testing and Materials (ASTM) standard (21), materials must pass a United States Pharmacopeia (USP) implantation test in which the material to be tested is implanted in the paravertebral muscle of a rabbit. Tissue reaction is then compared with a control. Other test methods, including cell cultures, may be used, provided they yield equivalent results. The marking *F-29* or *I.T.* on a tube is evidence that the tube material has been tested and no evidence of toxicity found.

Tube Design (19)

An ASTM standard (21) contains requirements and recommendations for tracheal tubes, including the material from which the tube is constructed, the inside diameter, length, inflation system, cuff, radius of curvature, markings, Murphy eye, packaging, and labeling. A separate standard (24) covers the testing of the shafts of tracheal tubes for laser resistance.

A typical tracheal tube is shown in Figure 17.1. The ASTM standard specifies a radius of curvature of 140 ± 20 mm. The internal and external walls should be circular. A tube whose lumen is oval or elliptic in shape is more prone to kinking than one that is round.

The machine (proximal) end receives the connector and projects from the patient. It should be possible (and is often necessary when received from the manufacturer) to shorten this end. The patient (tracheal or distal) end is inserted into the trachea. It usually has a slanted portion called the bevel. The angle of the bevel is the acute angle between the bevel and the longitudinal axis of the tracheal tube (Fig. 17.1). The tracheal tube standard specifies a bevel angle of $38 \pm 10°$ (21). The

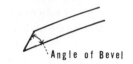

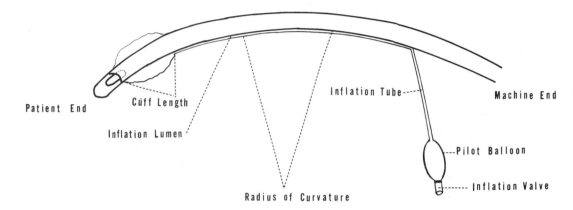

FIGURE 17.1. Cuffed Murphy tracheal tube.

opening of the bevel faces left when viewing the tube from its concave aspect. This is because most often the tube is introduced from the right. Having the bevel facing left facilitates visualization of the larynx as the tube is being inserted.

Figure 17.1 shows a hole through the tube wall on the side opposite to the bevel. This is known as a Murphy eye, and a tube with this feature is called a Murphy or Murphy-type tube (25). The purpose of the eye is to provide an alternate pathway for gas flow if the bevel is occluded (26). Some authors think that having the eye is a disadvantage, because secretions may accumulate there (27). Forceps, tube changers, and fiberscopes have been inadvertently advanced through a Murphy eye (28–31). Some tubes have a second eye on the bevel side. This may provide a measure of safety should the tube accidentally advance into the right mainstem bronchus. Tracheal tubes lacking the Murphy eye are known as Magill or Magill-type tubes (Fig. 17.1). Lack of a Murphy eye allows the cuff to be placed closer to the tip. This may decrease the chances of inadvertent bronchial intubation and may reduce injury to the trachea (32).

The ASTM standard (21) requires that a radiopaque marker be placed at the patient end or along the entire length of the tube to aid in determination of tube position after intubation. A barium sulfate stripe significantly lowers the temperature at which ignition of the tube occurs and thus increases the risk of fire (33).

Special Tubes
Cole Tube (34)

The Cole tube is shown in Figure 17.2. The patient end is smaller in diameter than the rest of the tube. Cole tubes are sized according to the ID of the tracheal portion.

The shoulder, the portion at which the transition from the oral portion to the laryngotracheal portion occurs, provides some protection against inadvertent bronchial intubation. The tube should not, however, be inserted so far that the widened portion contacts the larynx, because this could result in damage to the larynx (35).

Some studies have found that the resistance offered by the Cole tube is less than that of comparable tubes of constant lumen (17, 36). Others have found that resistance is higher with Cole tubes (16). The wide bore section increases dead space slightly, but this is believed to be insignificant (36).

A disadvantage of this tube is that it cannot be

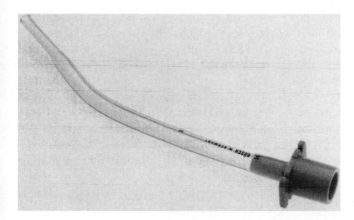

FIGURE **17.2.** Cole tracheal tube. These tubes are sized according to the intratracheal portion. Note that the tube's size is designated by the French scale. (Courtesy of Rusch, Inc.)

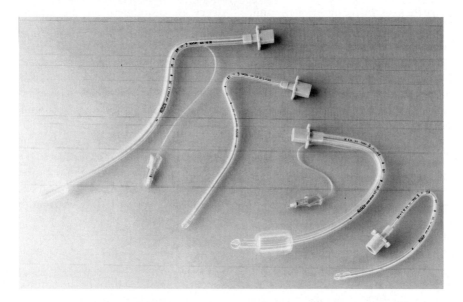

FIGURE **17.3.** Preformed tubes. At left are two nasal tubes, one cuffed and one uncuffed; at right two oral tubes. (Courtesy of Rusch Inc.)

used nasally because the larger segment will not pass through an infant's nares. It has been recommended that this tube be used for resuscitation, but not for long-term intubation (37).

Preformed Tubes (38, 39)

Some tracheal tubes are preformed to facilitate surgery about the head and neck. One of these is the RAE (Ring-Adair-Elwin) tube. (Fig. 17.3). There is a preformed bend in the tube that may be temporarily straightened.

Nasal and oral versions are available in various sizes and cuffed and uncuffed versions. As the di-

ameter increases, the length and distance from the distal tip to the curve also increase. Frequently there is a mark at the bend. In the majority of cases when this mark is at the teeth or naris, the tube will be satisfactorily positioned in the trachea, if the proper size tube for the patient was selected. This is only a guide and should not be used as the sole criterion for judging correct positioning of the tube.

The nasal preformed tube has a curve opposite to the curvature of the oral tube, so that when in place, the outer portion of the tube is directed over the patient's forehead. This helps to reduce pressure on the nares. This tube may be useful for oral intubation of patients who are to be in the prone position (40) or undergoing otolaryngologic procedures (41).

The oral preformed tubes are shorter than nasal ones. The external portion is bent at an acute angle so that when in place, it rests on the patient's chin.

These tubes are easy to secure and their use may reduce the risk of unintended extubation (9). The curve allows the breathing system connection to be placed away from the surgical field during operations around the head without use of special connectors and helps to protect against kinks. The long length may make them useful for insertion through an laryngeal mask airway (LMA) (42, 43).

Disadvantages of preformed tubes include difficulty in passing a suction catheter down them. In critical situations, suctioning can be accomplished by cutting the tube at the preformed curvature and reinserting the connector into the cut end (41). They offer more resistance than comparably sized conventional tubes (9, 44). Since they are designed to fit the average patient, a tube may be either too long or too short for a given patient (45–47). When selecting tube size, reference to height and weight may be more useful than age in years, and the user should always be alert to the possibility of bronchial intubation or accidental extubation (48).

Spiral Embedded Tubes

The spiral embedded (flexo metallic, armored, reinforced, anode, metal spiral, and woven) tube has a metal or nylon spiral-wound reinforcing wire covered internally and externally by rubber, PVC, or silicone (Fig. 17.4). The spiral may not extend into the distal and proximal ends. The connector is frequently bonded to the tube.

Spiral embedded tubes are especially useful in situations where bending or compression of the tube is likely to occur, as in head and neck surgery. Another use is surgery on the trachea. A sterile spiral embedded tube can be placed in the trachea by the surgeon.

The primary advantage of these tubes is resistance to kinking and compression (49). The portion of the tube outside the patient can be angled away from the surgical field without kinking (50).

This may make them useful in patients with tracheostomies (51). In one study, use of a spiral embedded silicone tube resulted in less pressure on the larynx than any other type of tube tested (52). A spiral embedded tube has been found to pass more easily over a fiberscope than a tube with a preformed curve (53, 54).

There are a number of problems with these tubes. A forceps and/or a stylet will often be needed for intubation. The tube may rotate on the stylet during insertion. Insertion through the nose is difficult and sometimes impossible. Because of the spiral, these tubes cannot be shortened. The elastic recoil force may increase the tendency to dislodge from the secured position; suturing to the patient is often performed for this reason.

There are numerous reports of respiratory obstruction with spiral embedded tubes (55–69). Most have been with tubes that have been resterilized. For this reason, it is recommended that these tubes not be reused.

If ventilation beyond the operating room setting is anticipated, a spiral embedded tube should be exchanged for a conventional tube (70, 71).

Cases have been reported in which patients bit the tube, causing it to be permanently deformed and resulting in obstruction (72–76). Some spiral embedded tubes have an external covering over the bite portion (Fig. 17.4, bottom picture). Cuff deflation occurs relatively frequently (68). Another problem is failure of the cuff to deflate as a result of debris in the pilot tubing or double layering of the cuff (68).

RAE-Flex Tube

This tube (Fig. 17.5) has a conventional patient segment and a spiral-reinforced proximal segment.

Carden Bronchoscopy Tube

The Carden bronchoscopy tube (Fig. 17.6) is designed for fiberoptic bronchoscopy. The machine end is wider than the patient end. The larger diameter of the machine end decreases the increase in resistance caused by passage of the bronchoscope. The tube is made of silastic and can be sterilized and reused. It is sized by the ID at the patient end.

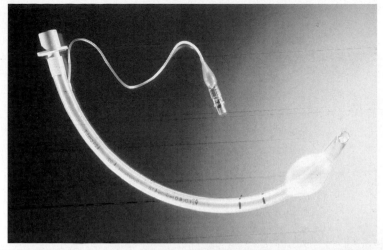

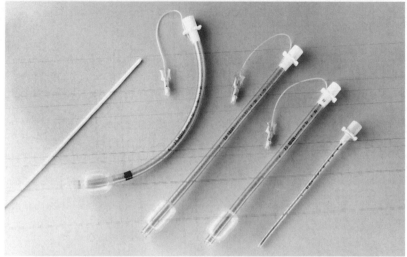

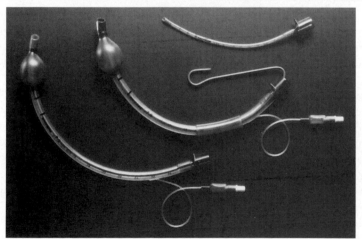

FIGURE 17.4. Spiral embedded tracheal tubes. **Top,** Note the reference marks near the patient end of the tubes to aid in positioning with respect to the vocal cords. (Courtesy of Mallinckrodt Medical Inc.) **Middle,** Note that the tube on the left has a single reference mark. (Courtesy of Rusch Inc.) **Bottom,** The middle tube has a reinforcing covering over the bite area. Note again the referencing marks. (Courtesy of Kendall Healthcare Products Co.)

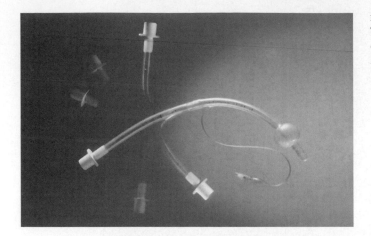

FIGURE **17.5.** RAE-Flex Tracheal Tube. The proximal portion of the tube is spiral embedded. (Courtesy of Mallinckrodt Medical Inc.)

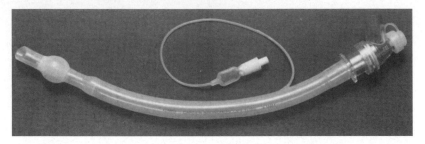

FIGURE **17.6.**   Carden bronchoscopy tube. The larger diameter of the part of tube that lies outside the larynx and trachea reduces resistance to gas flow. (Courtesy of Xomed-Trease.)

Carden Laryngoscopy Tube (77, 78)

The Carden laryngoscopy tube (Fig. 17.7) is used for microlaryngeal surgery. It is less than 7 cm long. It is made from silicone and has a low-pressure cuff and a jet tube built into the side. It can be sterilized for reuse.

This tube is difficult to insert. Various methods have been described (77–82). After insertion, the cuff is inflated to hold it in position. Intermittently jetting gases into the tube causes intermittent inflation of the patient's lungs. Because the jet is mounted in the tube, there is little or no Venturi effect (78). The patient can passively exhale through the tube and the cords during the non-inflation phases. To remove the tube, the cuff is first deflated, and then the jet is activated. This causes the tube to be blown from the trachea (83).

Use of this tube with a jetting device usually results in a good operating field for the surgeon. The gas passing out through the cords during both inflation and exhalation tends to blow blood and debris out of the operating field and away from the lungs. Work below the level of the cords can be performed by placing the tube below the lesion in the trachea (78).

Problems include accidental dislodgement, cephalad movement, and difficulty with removal (84). Respiratory obstruction can occur before the surgeon places the scope and maintains a clear airway or if the cords are allowed to close (82, 85). Obstruction will prevent gas from exiting the lung and can result in high pressures in the lower airway.

Gastric bleeding has been reported after a Carden tube was inadvertently placed in the esophagus and jet ventilation initiated (86, 87).

Hunsaker Mon-Jet Ventilation Tube

This tube (Fig. 17.8) is laser-resistant and designed for subglottic jet ventilation. It is compati-

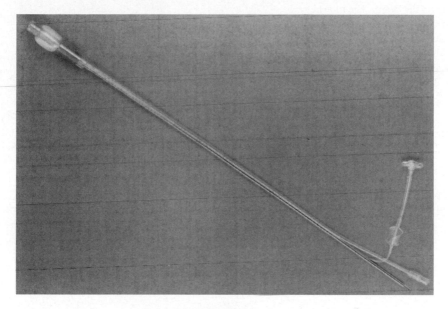

FIGURE 17.7. Carden laryngoscopy tube.

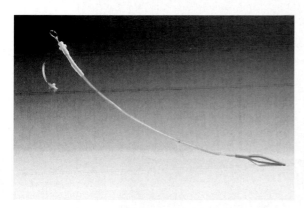

FIGURE 17.8. Hunsaker Mon-Jet Ventilation Tube.

ble with carbon dioxide (CO_2), neodymium-yttrium aluminum-garnet (Nd-YAG), argon and Holmium lasers. The outer diameter is 3 mm and it has an integral lumen for monitoring airway pressure and respiratory gases. The patient end has a balloon designed to center the tube.

Injectoflex

The injectoflex (Fig. 17.9, middle) is used for laryngeal microsurgery. It is a silicone tube with an embedded wire spiral and a short cuff. The cuff inflation and jet (insufflation) lumens are joined

in a sheath with a malleable introducer. The introducer remains in place during the procedure.

Laryngectomy Tube (88)

Laryngectomy tubes with a J configuration (Fig 17.9, left) are designed for insertion into a tracheotomy. This allows the part of the tube external to the patient to be directed away from the surgical field. The tip may be short and/or without a bevel to avoid inadvertent advancement into a bronchus.

The curve may need to be straightened to facilitate insertion. The tube can be secured by suturing or taping it to the chest wall (88).

A case of obstruction of this tube has been reported (89). The soft cuff and short distance between the cuff and distal tip of the tube may cause the bevel to abut against the wall of the trachea.

Microlaryngeal Tracheal Surgery Tube (90)

The microlaryngeal tracheal surgery (laryngeal tracheal surgery [LTS] or microlaryngeal tracheal [MLT]) tracheal tube (Fig. 17.10) is available with an ID of 4, 5, or 6 mm. The cuff diameter is that of a standard 8-mm ID tube. One version has a yellow cuff.

FIGURE 17.9. Left, laryngectomy tube. **Middle,** Injectoflex tube, which is used for procedures on the larynx. The tube has an embedded metal spiral. The insufflation lumen and cuff inflation tube are combined in one sheath with the malleable introducer. **Right,** spiral embedded tube. (Courtesy of Rusch Inc.)

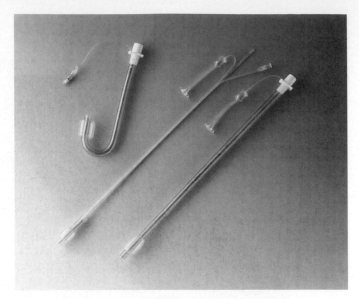

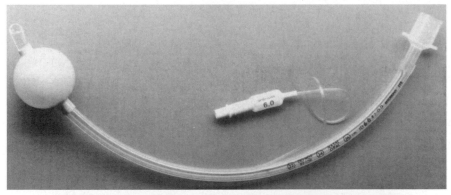

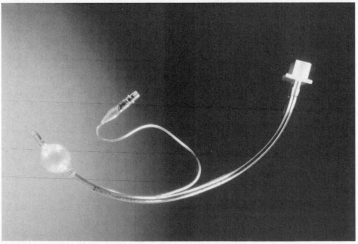

FIGURE 17.10. Tubes for microlaryngeal tracheal surgery. **Top,** The cuff on this tube is colored yellow for greater visibility. (Courtesy of Sheridan Catheter Corp.) **Bottom,** similar tube with an uncolored cuff. (Courtesy of Mallinckrodt Medical, Inc.)

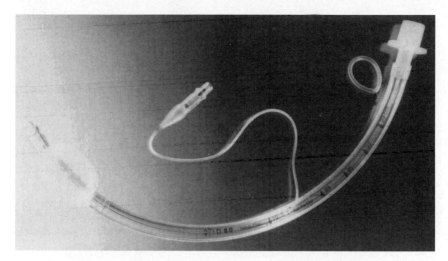

FIGURE 17.11.   Endotrol tracheal tube. The ring is attached to the tip by a cable-like mechanism that allows the tip to be maneuvered. (Courtesy of Mallinckrodt Anesthesiology Division, Mallinckrodt Medical, Inc.)

This tube is designed for microlaryngeal or tracheal surgery or for patients whose airway has been narrowed to such an extent that a normal-size tracheal tube cannot be inserted. The small diameter provides better visibility and access to the surgical field. Problems with a tube having such a small bore include the dangers of incomplete exhalation and occlusion. These tubes are not safe for use with lasers.

Endotrol Tracheal Tube

The Endotrol tracheal tube (Fig. 17.11) provides a means to control the direction of the tip using a ring loop. Pulling on the ring decreases the radius of distal end of the tube via a cable mechanism so that the tip moves anteriorly. This may make the tube useful during certain difficult intubations (91). This tube may be useful in blind intubations (92–94).

In one reported case, obstruction to gas flow was noted after the tube had been inserted nasally (95). The pull ring was exerting tension on the pull wire, causing the tip of the tube to abut against the tracheal wall. Cutting the pull ring alleviated the tension and the obstruction.

Tubes with Extra Lumen(s)

Tubes with one or more separate lumens terminating near the tip are available (Fig. 17.12). They are useful for respiratory gas sampling, suctioning, airway pressure monitoring, injection of fluids and drugs, and jet ventilation.

A number of problems is associated with these tubes (96). The sampling tube must be securely stabilized to minimize tension on the tube and avoid kinking or accidental extubation. The port of the extra lumen can become obstructed by secretions, blood, etc.

Laser-Shield II Tracheal Tube

The Laser-Shield II (Fig. 17.13) is made from silicone with an inner aluminum wrap and a Teflon outer wrap. It is designed for use with CO_2 and KTP (potassium-titanyl-phosphate) lasers. There is 1 cm of unprotected silicone tubing above the cuff. The part of the tube distal to the cuff also is unprotected. The cuff contains methylene blue crystals. Cottonoids for wrapping around the cuff are supplied with each tube. These must be moistened and kept moist during the entire procedure.

Studies have shown that the wrapped portion of the shaft is not penetrated by a CO_2 or Nd-YAG laser, but the overlying Teflon may be vaporized (97, 98). Exposure of the unprotected parts of the tube proximal and distal to the cuff can result in rapid combustion. Blood on the outside of the tube does not affect the protection from combustion with the CO_2 laser (99).

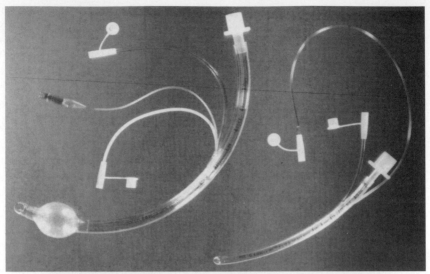

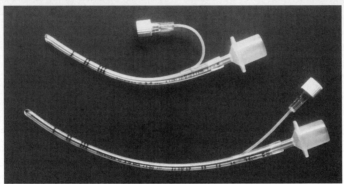

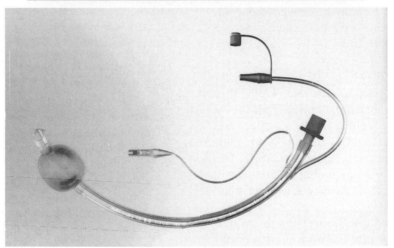

FIGURE 17.12. Tubes with additional lumen(s). These tubes have a main lumen for ventilation of the patient and one or more additional lumens for monitoring, irrigation, pressure monitoring, suctioning, and/or ventilation. **Top,** These tubes have two additional lumens. The clear lumen is used for jet ventilation and administration of oxygen during suctioning and bron- choscopy. The opaque lumen can be used for irrigation and sampling of gases from the trachea. (Courtesy of Mallinckrodt Anesthesiology Division, Mallinckrodt Medical, Inc. **Middle,** Pediatric tubes with monitoring lumens. (Courtesy of Kendall Healthcare Products Co.) **Bottom,** Tube with lumen designed for subglottic suc- tioning. (Courtesy of Mallinckrodt Medical, Inc.)

Laser-Flex Tracheal Tube (100)

The Laser-Flex tube (Fig. 17.14) is a flexible stainless-steel tube with a smooth surface and a matte finish to reflect a de-focused laser beam. It is designed for use with CO_2 and KTP lasers. The wall of the tube is thicker than that of most other tubes (101). The adult version has two PVC cuffs and a PVC tip with a Murphy eye. The two cuffs are inflated using separate inflation tubes, which run along the inside of the tube. The distal cuff can be used if the proximal one is damaged by the laser. Small uncuffed tubes are available.

The cuffs should be filled with saline. The distal cuff should be filled first until sealing occurs, then the proximal cuff filled with saline colored with methylene blue (102).

Studies show that the shaft holds up well when exposed to a CO_2 or KTP laser but not the Nd-YAG laser (101, 103–106). Blood on the outside of the tube renders it less resistant to combustion with the CO_2 laser (99). The cuff and distal tip are vulnerable to all lasers. In a study of damage from reflected CO_2 laser beams from laser-resistant and foil-wrapped tubes, it was found that the danger was least with this tube (107).

Reported problems with the Laser-Flex tube include stiffness and roughness (106). It cannot be trimmed but can be bent and will hold its shape. The double cuff adds to the time of intubation and extubation. The large external diameter can be a problem in small patients (101). In one reported case, great difficulty was experienced in removing the cuffed tube because of a subglottic mass (108). The small ID may significantly restrict the flow of ventilatory gases (109).

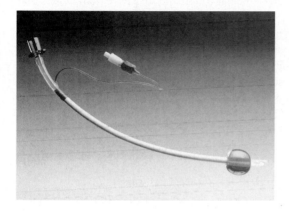

FIGURE 17.13. Laser-shield II tracheal tube. (Courtesy of Xomed-Trease.)

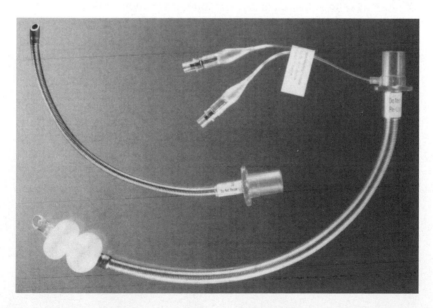

FIGURE 17.14. Laser-flex tracheal tubes. The adult tube has two cuffs. The distal cuff can be used if the proximal one is damaged. (Courtesy of Mallinckrodt Medical, Inc.)

Sheridan Laser Trach Tube

The Sheridan laser tube (Fig. 17.15) is a red rubber tube wrapped with copper foil tape. This is over wrapped with water-absorbent fabric which should be saturated with water prior to use. There is a copper band at the cuff-tube junction. Three radiopaque pledgets designed to be placed above the cuff are provided with each tube. It is designed for use with a CO_2 or KTP laser. It has been shown to perform well with the CO_2 but not the Nd-YAG laser (110). A disadvantage is that it has a thick wall (111).

Norton Tube (100, 112)

The Norton tube is a reusable, flexible, spiral-wound metal tube with a stainless-steel connector

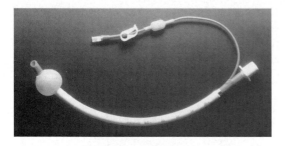

FIGURE 17.15. Sheridan laser trach tube. The outer fabric should be saturated before use. (Courtesy of Kendall Healthcare Products Co.)

and thick walls designed for laser surgery. The exterior of the tube has a matte finish to decrease reflection of the laser beam. It has no cuff. A separate cuff may be placed over the distal tip or packing can be used to achieve a seal. Studies show this tube is acceptable for use with KTP, Nd-YAG, and CO_2 lasers (106).

There are a number of problems with this tube. Its flexible coils are not airtight and angulation can result in a large leak (113). The tube's exterior is somewhat rough and may have sharp edges that could cause tissue damage (114). The large external diameter and stiffness may make surgical exposure and positioning of an operating laryngoscope difficult (115). The tube tends to twist on the stylet during intubation (106). It requires special ventilating techniques when used without a cuff. If it is used with a separate cuff, the cuff and its inflating tube can be ignited and may or may not remain attached to the tube.

Bivona Fome-Cuf Laser Tube

The Bivona Fome-Cuf laser tube has an aluminum and silicone spiral with a silicone covering (Fig. 17.16). It is marketed for use with the CO_2 laser. It has a self-inflating cuff that consists of a polyurethane foam sponge with a silicone envelope. The cuff must be deflated before intubation or extubation (116). The cuff should be filled with

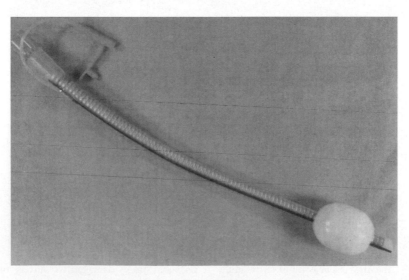

FIGURE 17.16. Bivona Fom-Cuf laser tube.

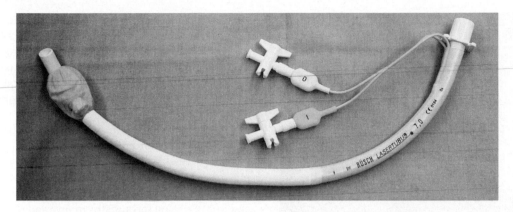

FIGURE **17.17.** Lasertubus. The inflation tubes have stopcocks.

saline during use. The cuff retains its shape and maintains a seal when it is punctured (106). The inflation tube runs along the exterior of the tube and is colored black so that it can be positioned away from areas where the laser will be used (100).

A fire can result when a CO_2 laser operating at high power is applied to this tube (104). Damage also occurs when it is exposed to a Nd-YAG or KTP laser (103, 106, 117). When burned, the silicone covering forms an ash that sloughs off and is left in the trachea, but most of the tube stays intact (106).

A high incidence of sore throats has been noted with this tube (118). If the inflation tube is severed or the cuff punctured, the cuff cannot be deflated.

Lasertubus

This tube (Fig. 17.17) is white rubber with a cuff-within-a-cuff. If the outer cuff is perforated by the laser beam, the trachea will still be sealed by the inner cuff. The pilot balloons are marked *i* (inner) and *o* (outer) to identify which cuff they are connected to. The manufacturer recommends that the inner cuff be filled with air and the outer cuff with water or saline. The tube shaft has a Merocel sponge covering approximately 17 cm in length proximal to the cuff. It is recommended that this be moistened before use with saline. This tube is recommended for use with argon, Nd-YAG, and CO_2 lasers.

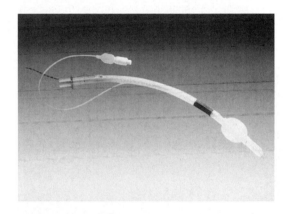

FIGURE **17.18.** Electromyogram (EMG) reinforced tube. Note the surface electrodes and electrode leads. (Courtesy of Xomed Surgical Products, Inc.)

EMG Reinforced Tracheal Tube

This tube (Fig. 17.18) is designed to monitor vocal cord and recurrent laryngeal nerve electromyogram (EMG) activity during surgery. It has a cuff, two channels of surface electrodes, and a pair of recording electrode leads that are connected to a monitor.

ILM ETT and ET Stabilizer

The ILM ETT (intubating laryngeal mask endotracheal tube) and ET (endotracheal) tube (Fig. 17.19) is designed to be inserted through the intubating laryngeal mask (see Chapter 15, "The Laryngeal Mask Airway"). The patient end

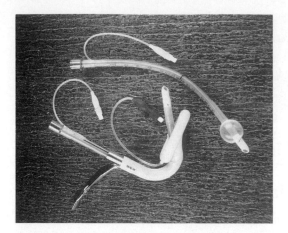

FIGURE **17.19.** ILM-ETT. The black circle near the middle of the tube will be at the end of the connector when the tip of the tube is at the entrance to the bowl of the mask. (Courtesy of LMA North America.)

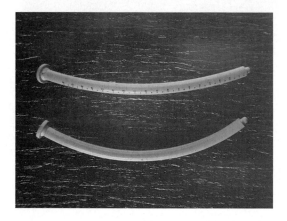

FIGURE **17.20.** Endotracheal (ET) Stabilizer. (Courtesy of LMA North America.)

has a blunt tip with a short bevel and a Murphy eye. Figure 17.20 shows the tube stabilizer. It is used to stabilize and extend the tube while the LMA is being removed.

Combitube (119)

The Combitube (Fig. 17.21) has two separate lumens. This allows ventilation with either esophageal or tracheal placement. Two black rings aid proper placement with respect to depth of insertion and should be situated at approximately the teeth or gums. One lumen is longer proximally and has an occluded distal tip. The other lumen

has a patent tip. It is possible to ventilate the trachea (with tracheal placement) or suction gastric contents (with esophageal placement) through this lumen. The proximal pharyngeal cuff is inflated with 100 ml of air. The distal cuff requires only 10 to 15 ml. There are eight ventilating eyes (holes) between the cuffs.

Blind insertion usually results in a high probability (94% to 98%) of esophageal placement (Fig. 17.22). In this case, the anesthesia breathing system is connected to the longer lumen. Air is prevented from entering the stomach by the distal cuff and from escaping through the mouth and nose by the pharyngeal cuff, so it goes into the trachea. Should the tube enter the trachea, the breathing system is attached to the shorter lumen, and the device used the same as a standard tracheal tube.

There needs to be a means to determine if the distal lumen is in the esophagus or the trachea. The esophageal detector device and the colorimetric carbon dioxide detector have been recommended (120–123).

When the Combitube was compared to a tracheal tube, effectiveness of ventilation appeared to be comparable and intubation time shorter (124–128). It has been recommended for airway management in the difficult-to-intubate patient and emergency situations where personnel trained in tracheal intubation are not available (126, 129, 130). It has been successfully used by non-anesthesia personnel (128, 131). It is included in the Guidelines for Advanced Cardiac Life Support of the American Heart Association and Practice Guidelines for Management of the Difficult Airway of the American Society of Anesthesiologists (132, 133). It has been used in the esophagus for up to 8 hours (134). There is a report of successful use of this tube in a patient who had a wooden splinter through the mouth partially blocking the pharynx (135). It has been used in cases of cervical hematomas causing upper airway obstruction (133), in a patient with excessive pharyngeal bleeding after thrombolytic therapy (136), and in patients in whom tracheal intubation failed (120, 132). It has also been used for ventilation during tracheotomy (137).

Cases have been reported where the patient was unable to be ventilated with the Combitube in spite of placement as described in the directions for use (138). The tube was found to be too deep so that the upper cuff obstructed the tracheal

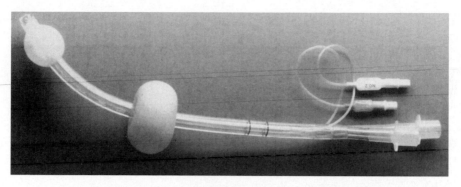

FIGURE 17.21. Combitube. Note the ventilating eyes between the two cuffs. (Courtesy of Sheridan Catheter Corp.)

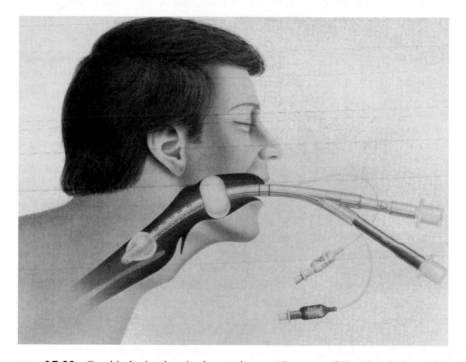

FIGURE 17.22. Combitube in place in the esophagus. (Courtesy of Sheridan Catheter Corp.)

lumen. Pulling the tube backward 3 cm remedied the problem.

Advantages include easy and blind insertion. The insertion technique does not require moving the head and neck. By pressing against the hard palate, the pharyngeal cuff may anchor the device in place, making it difficult to dislodge (139). In maxillofacial trauma the device may help in the tamponade of bleeding from intraoral lacerations

(139). A disadvantage is that in the esophageal position, suctioning of tracheal secretions is impossible.

Tube Size

Different methods have been used for sizing tracheal tubes. Current standards designate tracheal tube size by the ID in millimeters (21). The French scale size (3 times the external diameter

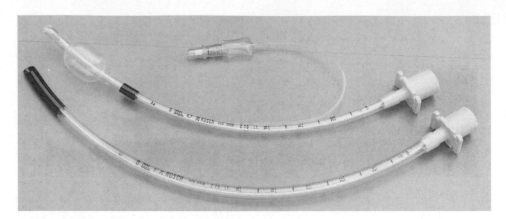

FIGURE **17.23.** Typical tracheal tube markings. The dark marking at the patient end of the bottom tube and the mark above the cuff on the top tube are to aid in proper placement with respect to the vocal cords. The internal and external diameters as well as the size in French scale are shown. (For example, on the top tube, the internal diameter is 5, the external diameter is 6.7, and the French scale size is 20.) Z-79 and IT both indicate that the tube material has passed the tissue toxicity test. Length from the patient tip is marked in centimeters.

in millimeters) may still be listed in catalogs and on packages and is used on some tubes (Fig. 17.23). Because of variations in wall thickness, tubes having the same ID may have different external diameters (140, 141).

The ASTM standard (21) requires tube size to be marked between the cuff and the take-off point of the inflation tube for cuffed tubes (see Fig. 17.4). For uncuffed tubes, the size marking should be toward the patient end (see Fig. 17.3). Some manufacturers also put the tube size on the pilot balloon so the size can be determined when the tube is in the patient. The standard also specifies that tubes size 6.0 and smaller show the external diameter in millimeters (see Figs. 17.3 and 17.8). Many manufacturers also mark this on larger tubes (see Fig. 17.3).

Tube Length

The ASTM standard (21) specifies minimum tube length, which increases as ID increases. Most manufacturers supply tubes longer than the minimum required by the standard.

Tube Markings

Typical tracheal tube markings, shown in Figure 17.23, are situated on the beveled side of the tube above the cuff and read from the patient to the machine end. The following are required by the ASTM (21) standard:

1. The words *oral* or *nasal* or *oral/nasal*
2. Tube size in ID (ID) in millimeters
3. The outside diameter (OD) for size six and smaller
4. The name or trademark of the manufacturer or supplier
5. The notation *F-29* or *Z-79* or *IT,* which indicates that the tube has passed the tissue toxicity test
6. Length (depth) markings in centimeters measured from the patient end
7. A cautionary note such as "Do not reuse" or "Single use only," if the tube is disposable
8. A radiopaque marker at the patient end or along the full length

Other markings not in conflict with the above may be applied.

Many tubes have lines or rings to help position the tube with respect to the vocal cords (Fig. 17.17; see also Fig. 17.4). The distal portions of some pediatric tubes are colored to aid in positioning.

Cuff Systems

A cuff system consists of the cuff itself plus an inflation system, which typically includes an inflation lumen in the wall of the tube, an external inflation tube, a pilot balloon, and an inflation valve (see Fig. 17.1). The purpose of the cuff system is to provide a seal between the tube and tracheal wall to prevent passage of pharyngeal contents into the trachea and ensure that no gas leaks past the cuff during positive pressure ventilation. The cuff also serves to center the tube in the trachea so that its tip is less likely to traumatize the mucosa.

Cuff

The cuff is an inflatable sleeve near the patient end of the tube. The cuff material should be strong and tear resistant but thin, soft, and pliable. Cuffs are usually made of the same material as the tracheal tube. Cuff materials are subject to the same tissue-testing requirements as the tube itself.

The ASTM standard (21) specifies the maximum distance from the tip of the tube to the machine end of the cuff. This varies with tube size. If this distance is too long, the tip could rest on the carina while the cuff impinged on the vocal cords. The standard also requires that the bonded edge of the cuff not encroach on the Murphy eye, if present; that the cuff not herniate over the tube tip under normal conditions of use; and that the cuff inflate symmetrically.

Cuff Pressures

Intracuff pressure and pressure on the tracheal wall. A high cuff pressure prevents aspiration, ventilatory leaks, and eccentric positioning of the tube in the trachea but can cause damage to the trachea. A low cuff pressure minimizes tracheal damage and can act to relieve excessive airway pressure but may result in aspiration, leaks, and eccentric positioning of the tube.

It is desirable that the cuff seal the airway without exerting so much pressure on the trachea that its circulation is compromised or the trachea is dilated. Most authors recommend that the pressure on the lateral tracheal wall measured at end expiration be between 25 and 30 cm H_2O (142–146). If the pressure exceeds 25 cm H_2O, aspiration should not occur, provided the density of the material above the cuff is not greater than

that of water (142, 147). Studies show impaired tracheal blood flow at 30 cm H_2O (144). It may be necessary to use higher pressures when inflating to "just seal" under conditions requiring high ventilatory pressures (148).

Intracuff pressure and use of nitrous oxide. Studies show that the resting intracuff pressure and volume of a cuff inflated with air rise when nitrous oxide is administered (118, 149–158). The increase varies directly with the partial pressure of the nitrous oxide and time, and inversely with cuff thickness. Several methods have been suggested to modify or avoid this increase (159).

1. Filling the cuff with the gas mixture to be used for anesthesia (153, 154, 157, 159–162). This is awkward to perform. A cuff that is at the correct volume will lose volume and may allow a leak when nitrous oxide administration is discontinued or during extracorporeal circulation (163–165).
2. Filling the cuff with saline (166, 167).
3. Monitoring cuff pressure and inflating or deflating the cuff as needed (149, 157, 164).
4. Use of special devices. These are discussed below.

Increases in cuff pressure may also result from pressure from nearby surgical procedures (168) and diffusion of oxygen into the cuff (169).

Low-Volume, High-Pressure Cuff

The low-volume, high-pressure (small resting diameter, low residual volume, low-volume, small, standard, conventional, low-compliance, high-pressure) cuff has a small diameter at rest and a low residual volume (the amount of air that can be withdrawn from the cuff after it has been allowed to assume its normal shape with the inflation tube exposed to atmospheric pressure) (170). It requires a high intracuff pressure to achieve a seal with the trachea. It has a small area of contact with the trachea and distends and deforms the trachea to a circular shape (Fig. 17.24).

Most of the pressure inside this type of cuff is used to overcome cuff wall compliance so that the pressure exerted laterally on the tracheal wall will be less than the intracuff pressure. The intracuff pressure does not change when the tracheal wall

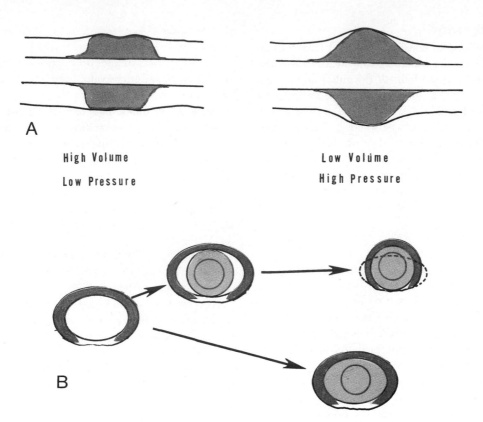

FIGURE 17.24. Relation of different types of cuffs to the trachea. **A,** side view. *Left,* The high-volume, low-pressure cuff has a large area of contact with the trachea. The cuff adapts itself to the irregular tracheal wall. *Right,* The low-volume, high-pressure cuff has a small area of contact with the trachea. It distends the trachea and distorts it to a circular shape. **B,** cross-sectional view. At the *left* is the normal trachea. At the *top,* the low-volume, high-pressure cuff distorts the trachea and makes the tracheal contour the same as the shape of the cuff. At the *bottom,* the soft high-volume, low-pressure cuff conforms to the normal tracheal lumen.

is contacted and does not bear a consistent relationship to tracheal wall pressure.

The pressure on the tracheal wall exerted by such a cuff is difficult to ascertain but will be well above mucosal perfusion pressure (142, 171, 172). Intracuff pressure and the lateral pressure on the tracheal wall increase sharply as increments of air are added to the cuff (173). Use of the largest tracheal tube possible has been advocated, so the cuff will be minimally inflated when a seal is created (173).

These cuffs offer some advantages over low-pressure cuffs. Because they can usually be reused, they are less expensive. They offer better protection against aspiration and better visibility during intubation. Several investigators have reported a lower incidence of sore throat with their use than with high-volume, low-pressure cuffs (118, 174–176). Their use has been recommended in adolescent patients to reduce trauma (177).

The most serious risk associated with high-pressure cuffs is ischemic damage to the trachea following prolonged use. Whether they should be used for short periods of general anesthesia is more controversial. If a tube with a high-pressure cuff is used intraoperatively and the tube must be left in place following surgery or the surgery is expected to last more than a few hours, it should be replaced with a tube with a low-pressure cuff.

High-Volume, Low-Pressure Cuff

A high-volume, low-pressure (large resting diameter; large residual volume; large; high-volume; high-compliance, low-pressure; floppy; low-pressure) cuff has a large resting volume and diameter and a thin compliant wall that allows a seal with the trachea to be achieved without stretching its wall. This type of cuff is floppy and easily deformed. As it is inflated, it first touches the trachea at its narrowest point at that level. As cuff inflation continues, the area of contact becomes larger and the cuff adapts itself to the tracheal surface (173) (see Fig. 17.24). If cuff inflation is continued, the areas in contact will be subject to increasing pressure, and the trachea will be distorted to a circular shape, similar to a high-pressure cuff (178).

Different shapes have been used for the low-pressure cuff (179, 180). A cuff with a short tracheal contact area may have fewer folds and wrinkles when inflated and may be associated with a lower incidence of postoperative sore throat (181). When high airway pressures must be used, a short cuff requires higher intracuff pressures than a cuff with a larger volume, which provides a greater reservoir of gas within the cuff, allowing additional gas to be "milked" into the proximal end of the cuff without increasing the resting cuff pressure (179).

A significant advantage of these cuffs is that provided the cuff wall is not stretched, the intracuff pressure closely approximates that on the wall of the trachea (182–184). Thus it is possible to measure and regulate the pressure exerted on the tracheal mucosa. Cuff pressure can be used to estimate tracheal pressure (185).

The intracuff pressure varies during the ventilatory cycle (178, 179). During spontaneous breathing, airway (and cuff) pressure will be negative during inspiration and positive during exhalation (178). However, if the cuff is located above the thoracic inlet, the intracuff pressure may rise during inspiration (15). With controlled ventilation, when airway pressure exceeds intracuff pressure, positive pressure will be applied to the lower face of the cuff. If the cuff wall is pliable, it will be unable to resist this pressure and will be deformed into a cone shape as the distal portion is compressed and the proximal portion is distended (179). The air in the cuff will be compressed until intracuff pressure equals airway pressure. During exhalation, the intracuff pressure will decrease until its resting pressure is reached. By increasing

its intracuff pressure, the cuff automatically compensates for the increase in airway pressure (self-sealing action). A leak will develop if the diameter of the expanded trachea becomes greater than the diameter of the proximal end of the cuff. At that point, more gas must be added to the cuff to abolish the leak. Unfortunately, this additional cuff inflation will elevate the baseline cuff pressure.

It is desirable that cuff circumference at residual volume be at least equal to the circumference of the trachea (159, 183, 186). If the cuff is smaller, it must be stretched beyond its residual volume to create a seal. At this point, it will act like a high-pressure cuff (179). On the other hand, if the residual diameter of the cuff is much greater than the diameter of the trachea, cuff infolding may occur, with the possibility of aspiration along the folds.

The main advantage of high-volume, low-pressure cuffs is that the risk of significant cuff-induced complications following prolonged intubation is reduced with their use (180, 187, 188). However, tracheal injury can occur even when these cuffs are used properly (189, 190). During hypotension, the mucosal contact pressure that will produce ischemia is reduced (191). A tendency toward tracheal dilatation has been reported (192).

Tubes with these cuffs may be more difficult to insert, as the cuff may obscure the view of the tube tip and larynx so that trauma to the airway may be more common (193, 194). The cuff is more friable and thus more likely to be torn during intubation, especially if forceps are used (195).

The incidence of sore throat is greater than with high-pressure cuffs, unless the cuff is specially designed so that the tracheal contact area is small (118, 174–176, 181). Severe postextubation stridor has been reported with their use (194).

Aspiration can occur past low-pressure cuffs with folds or wrinkles (142, 145, 196–200). This will be increased with spontaneous respiration. Continuous positive airway pressure (CPAP) and positive end–expiratory pressure (PEEP) are protective (200).

It is relatively easy to pass devices such as esophageal stethoscopes, temperature probes, and enteric tubes around low-pressure cuffs (201–208).

There may be a greater likelihood of dislodgement (including extubation) with these cuffs, es-

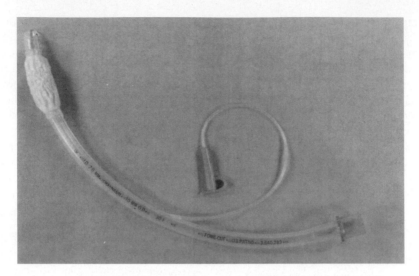

FIGURE 17.25. Tube with deflated foam cuff.

pecially with oral intubation and positive pressure ventilation (65).

One of the biggest problems with use of low pressure cuffs stems from a lack of understanding by the user. There is widespread belief that simply using this type of cuff will prevent high pressures from being exerted on the wall of the trachea. Any cuff, even a so-called low-pressure cuff, can be overfilled or the volume and pressure can increase during use, resulting in high intracuff and tracheal wall pressures (144, 209). The volume of gas necessary to raise the cuff pressure from the point of seal to an unsafe pressure is only 2 to 3 ml (180).

Foam Cuff (151, 210)

The foam (sponge, Fome, Kamen-Wilkinson) cuff has a large diameter, residual volume, and surface area (Fig. 17.25). It is filled with polyurethane foam covered with a sheath. Applying suction to the inflation tube causes the foam to contract. When the negative pressure is released, the cuff expands.

The tube is supplied with a T piece to fit between the connector and the breathing system (Fig. 17.26). When the inflation tube is connected to this T piece, the pressure inside the cuff will follow proximal airway pressure during the ventilatory cycle (151, 210).

Before extubation, the cuff should be collapsed by aspirating then clamping the inflation tube.

Several investigators have found no harmful effects from the gentle removal of the tube without removal of air from the cuff. This permits removal of secretions that have accumulated above the cuff (211). However, damage to the vocal cords is possible.

When in place in the trachea, the degree of expansion of the foam determines the pressure exerted laterally on the tracheal wall (192). The more the foam is expanded, the lower the pressure (210). Thus the pressure on the tracheal wall depends on the relationship between cuff diameter at residual volume and the diameter of the trachea. If too large a cuff is used, the cuff:tracheal wall pressure ratio will be high. If too small a cuff is used, there is risk of aspiration and leaks during positive pressure ventilation.

Diffusion of anesthetic agents into the cuff can occur but will not cause an increase in pressure (149, 151). Cuff pressure is not affected by temperature (212). Use of this cuff obviates the need for measurement of cuff pressure or use of a pressure-regulating device.

It can provide a seal at a low tracheal wall pressure, provided the relationship between the cuff and tracheal diameters is optimal (116, 210, 213). A reduced incidence of tracheal dilatation has been reported with its use (192).

One study found a high incidence of sore

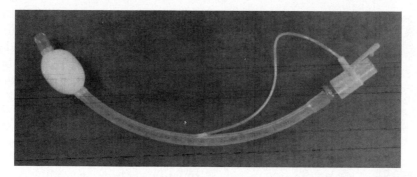

FIGURE 17.26. Tube with inflated foam cuff and a T piece.

throat associated with its use (118), while another found a low incidence compared to air-filled cuffs (212). In two reported cases, the inflation tube was accidentally pulled out at the point of insertion on the tube, making cuff deflation impossible (214, 215).

Inflation System (Fig. 17.1)
Inflation Lumen

The inflation lumen, which connects the inflation tube to the cuff, is located within the wall of the tracheal tube. The ASTM standard (21) requires that it not encroach on the lumen of the tube and recommends that it not bulge outward.

External Inflation Tube

The external inflation tube (cuff tube, pilot tube or line, pilot balloon line, inflating tube, tail) is external to the tube. The ASTM standard (21) requires that its external diameter not exceed 2.5 mm and recommends that it be attached to the tube at a small angle. The standard also specifies the distance from the tube tip to where the tube is attached and requires that the tube extend at least 3 cm beyond the machine end of the tube before a pilot balloon or inflation valve is incorporated.

The inflation tube can become obstructed by kinking or by crushing from a clamp. On spiral embedded tubes, the inflating tube may connect to the inflation lumen above the first spiral ring. If the connector is inserted into the tube far enough to contact the first spiral, it may cause the inflation tube to be blocked (216, 217). This can be remedied by cutting a small V in the connector and inserting the connector so that the inflation

tube passes through the V. Most spiral embedded tubes now have the inflation tube outside the spirals to prevent this problem.

Pilot Balloon

The pilot balloon (bulb, external reservoir, external balloon) may be located near the midpoint of the inflating tube or adjacent to the inflation valve. Its function is to give an indication of inflation or deflation of the cuff.

Inflation Valve

The ASTM standard (21) requires that the external inflation tube either be fitted with an inflation valve with an inlet that will mate with a male luer syringe tip or have a female end capable of accepting a standard luer tip syringe.

The inflation valve is designed so that when the tip of the syringe is inserted into it, a plunger is displaced from its seat and gas can be injected into the cuff. Upon removal of the syringe, the valve seals so that gas cannot escape from the cuff unless something (syringe tip or tip of a pen) is inserted into the valve.

Some tubes may lack an inflation valve. Cuff inflation is maintained by application of a clamp to the external inflation tube or by placing a plug in its free end.

Devices to Measure Cuff Pressure

Several methods have been used to monitor intracuff pressures continuously or intermittently (143, 218–220). Devices for this purpose are available commercially (Fig. 17.27). If the pressure is measured intermittently, the cuff and manometer should be inflated simultaneously (221).

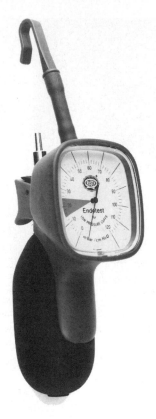

FIGURE 17.27. Device to measure intracuff pressure. (Courtesy of Rusch.)

Devices to Limit Cuff Pressure

Devices that will bleed the cuff when the intracuff pressure rises above a set value have been developed.

Lanz Pressure-Regulating Valve (222–224)

The Lanz pressure-regulating valve (McGinnis balloon system) consists of a very compliant latex pilot balloon inside a transparent plastic sheath with an automatic pressure-regulating valve between the balloon and the cuff (Fig. 17.28). The pilot balloon has three functions: (*a*) an indication of cuff inflation, (*b*) an external reservoir for the cuff, and (*c*) a pressure-limiting device. It is designed to maintain an intracuff pressure of 20 to 25 torr at end expiration while preventing overinflation of the cuff.

The pressure-regulating valve permits rapid gas flow from the balloon to the cuff but only slow flow from the cuff to the balloon. This prevents gas from being squeezed back into the balloon when the airway pressure rises rapidly, so there is no leakage of gas around the cuff during positive pressure ventilation. It also prevents increases in cuff volume and pressure caused by diffusion of nitrous oxide and other gases into the cuff.

As air is injected, the cuff and balloon are inflated in parallel. When the balloon has a stretched appearance, a pressure of approximately 26 to 33 cm H_2O will be present in the cuff. As injection continues, the pilot balloon fills preferentially. The intraballoon pressure remains constant and will not increase until it strikes the confining sheath. Should the trachea expand, air will slowly flow from the balloon into the cuff. The pressure-regulating valve protects against rapid loss of cuff volume into the balloon during inspiration.

This valve has been found by several investigators to be effective in keeping lateral tracheal wall pressure low and preventing increases in pressure due to nitrous oxide (149, 180, 222, 225–227). One study found that to go from the point of tracheal occlusion to an unsafe cuff pressure required 45 ml of air (180). Use of it eliminates the need to measure cuff pressure.

In patients requiring high airway pressures, this system may fail to form a seal with the trachea (143). The cuff may leak, particularly after prolonged use (228). If the balloon is compressed or overinflated, the intracuff pressure will rise (229).

Other (143)

Other mechanisms of automatic cuff pressure control have included a modified epidural syringe (230, 231), pneumatic devices (143, 232), a water column (233, 234), an automatic tourniquet system (235), and electropneumatic devices (219, 236–238). Several of these devices are available commercially, but variability may limit their usefulness (239).

Tracheal Tube Connectors

The tracheal tube connector (union) serves to attach the tube to the breathing system. It may be made of plastic or metal. The dimensions of the connector are set by an ASTM standard (240).

The end that fits into the tube is called the patient (distal) end, and the size of the connector is designated by the ID of this end in millimeters.

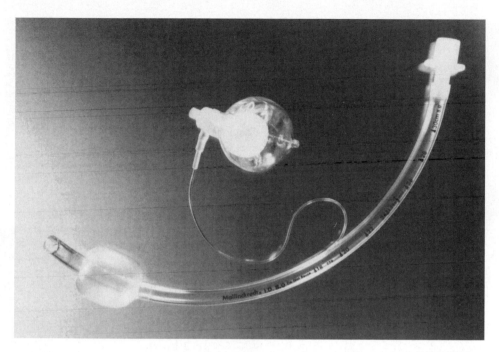

FIGURE 17.28. Lanz pressure-regulating valve. The pilot balloon is confined inside a transparent plastic sheath. There is a pressure-regulating valve between the pilot balloon and the cuff. Air should be injected into the cuff until the pilot balloon is stretched, but it should be smaller than the confining sheath.

The end that connects to the breathing system is the machine (proximal) end and has a 15-mm male fitting.

The connector may have protrusions, lugs, or other features to which elastic bands or other devices may be attached to prevent accidental disconnection from the breathing system, but there is controversy as to their desirability. Some connectors have a port for respiratory gas sampling.

Special connectors with low dead space are available for pediatric use. A hazard is associated with some of these (241, 242). When used in association with a breathing system adapter that has a fresh gas inlet tube that protrudes into the lumen of the adapter, the inlet tube may press against the end of the connector. This can cause partial or complete obstruction of the exhalation pathway.

The connector should be the same size as the tube with which it is intended to mate. This will result in minimal reduction of the lumen and make separation unlikely.

The most commonly used connectors are the straight and 90° curved (right angle). Acute angle connectors with less than a 90° curve (Fig. 17.29)

and flexible connectors (243) are available. A curved or flexible connector may facilitate positioning of the breathing system away from the surgical field. Curved and flexible connectors have two disadvantages: (*a*) they increase resistance (17, 244, 245) and (*b*) they must be removed from the tube when it is desired to insert a stylet or suction catheter.

Many disposable tracheal tubes come with the connector only partly inserted. Before use, it should be fully inserted. Removing it from the tube and wiping the distal end with alcohol will facilitate insertion and cause bonding with the tube. Removal of a connector from the tracheal tube may be facilitated by use of a towel clip (246).

Occasionally, when the connector is firmly seated, the pilot tube may be occluded, making inflation or deflation of the cuff impossible (247).

Laser-Resistant Wraps for Tracheal Tubes
Products

The shafts of tracheal tubes have been wrapped with various materials, including aluminum foil

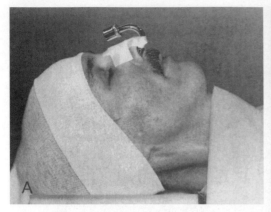
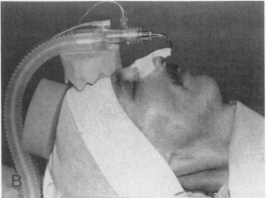
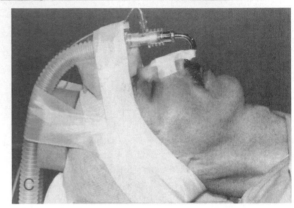

FIGURE **17.29.** Method of securing a nasotracheal tube. **A,** a skull cap is placed around the head. An acute-angle connector is used and taped so that it does not exert pressure on the nasal ala. **B,** foam padding is used to keep the breathing system from exerting pull on the tracheal tube. **C,** tape is added to keep the breathing system firmly in place.

and tape, copper tape, and moist cotton to protect them from laser beams (98, 104, 106, 248–253). Copper foil has been found to protect tubes from CO_2, Nd-YAG, and KTP lasers (103, 104, 106, 248, 254–256). Certain aluminum tapes have been shown to provide adequate protection from the CO_2 laser (98, 103, 104, 254, 255). Although some studies have shown it offers protection against the Nd-YAG laser (98, 106, 248), one study found it did not protect PVC tubes from this laser (106). Blood on the outside of aluminum- or copper-wrapped tubes can compromise protection from combustion (99).

The possibility of changes in the composition of any tape requires that every batch be evaluated for its incendiary characteristics. Every foil- or tape-wrapped tube should be tested with the laser before use (257, 258).

The only product approved by the Food and Drug Administration (FDA) for this purpose is a two-layered sheet of synthetic surgical sponge and adhesive-backed corrugated silver foil (Merocel Laser Guard), which is available in several sizes. It can be applied more quickly to the tracheal tube than foil tapes (249). Before intubation, the tube with wrap is saturated with water or saline. When wet, the sponge and reflective foil act as a heat sink and disperse argon, CO_2, Nd-YAG, and KTP laser beams (106, 259, 260). There is less likelihood of a reflected laser beam causing damage with this product than with foil-wrapped tubes (107). Blood on the coating does not reduce its protective effect (99).

Wrapping Procedure (106, 249, 258)

Some investigators believe that only red rubber tubes should be used for wrapping (106). A burned silicone tube loses its structural integrity, and combustion of a PVC tube will produce toxic gases.

The tube should be cleaned to remove any residue that would prevent the wrap from adhering to it, then thoroughly dried before wrapping.

Painting the tube with tincture of benzoin may strengthen the adhesion of some tapes. The tape should not be wider than ¼ inch (0.6 cm) (106). It should be wrapped in an overlapping spiral starting from just above the cuff and proceeding toward the machine end. The inflation tube should be placed against the tube and wrapped together with it. The cuff should not be wrapped. With an uncuffed tube, the wrapping should extend far enough toward the tip that it will be at least 1 cm below the vocal cords (252, 261). The spiral should overlap by one-third to one-half of the tape width. This allows the tube to be flexed without exposing the underlying tube or breaking or kinking the tape. Applying tension on the tape as it is wrapped around the tube will help it conform to the tube and eliminate kinks, bumps, and wrinkles. The tube should be allowed to retain its manufactured shape.

An alcohol wipe of the wrapped tube will provide disinfection without damaging the tube or tape. Foil-wrapped tubes can be gas sterilized before use without affecting their combustibility (249, 255).

The tube should be inspected for gaps or holes in the wrap before use. Tubes that are not fully protected or that have bumps or wrinkles should not be used.

The cuff remains vulnerable to penetration, and ignition of the tube distal to the cuff may occur (106, 261, 262). Wet cottonoids should be used to protect the cuff, which should be filled with saline (262, 263).

Disadvantages

Wrapping reduces tube flexibility, can predispose to kinking, and may create a rough surface (106, 251, 264). The outer diameter of the tube is increased. Reflection of the laser beam from metallic tape could cause damage to non-targeted tissues (107). The wrapping material may come off and obstruct the airway (265). Errors in wrapping or sharp bends could expose the tube to the laser beam (106). A slight separation or tear in the tape will make the tube vulnerable to ignition. The interior of a tube can be ignited by flaming pieces of tissue in close proximity to or inhaled into the tip of the tube (266, 267).

Wrappings with cotton or sponge material must be kept moist and may ignite if allowed to dry out. An irrigation system has been described (268).

A medicolegal problem is possible if tapes not approved for medical use are used (106). In addition, most manufacturers of standard tracheal tubes state that their tube should not be used with a laser.

It has been recommended that tapes on tracheal tubes be used only as a last resort when other methods of providing laser resistance (laser-resistant tracheal tubes, Merocel wrap, or techniques not using a tracheal tube) are unavailable or cannot be used, such as laser surgery on small patients (106).

USE OF THE TRACHEAL TUBE
Choosing the Tube
Cuffed Versus Uncuffed

In the past, uncuffed tracheal tubes were routinely used in young children. However, studies indicate that use of cuffed tubes is not associated with increased problems (269–272). Advantages of cuffed tubes include improved end-tidal gas monitoring, less risk of aspiration, ability to use high inflation pressures, ability to use lower fresh gas flows, less operating room pollution, and avoidance of repeated laryngoscopy (271, 272). Drawbacks include the need to use a slightly smaller tube, which makes suctioning more difficult and increases resistance, and the risk of overinflation of the cuff, which will result in excessive pressure against the tracheal mucosa.

Size

Smaller-diameter tubes are easier to insert and require less reshaping force to adapt to the patient's airway (273), but they are associated with higher resistance, difficulty in providing adequate tracheobronchial toilet, and increased risk of occlusion and kinking. Passage of a fiberscope may not be possible if the tube is too small (see Chapter 16, "Laryngoscopes").

Larger tubes are associated with less risk of occlusion and lower resistance but may predispose to laryngotracheal injury.

Because no system of choosing the correct size tube is foolproof, the user should always have readily available tubes one size larger and one size smaller than the one chosen. If a difficult intubation is anticipated, a small tube should be used. It has been recommended that a smaller tube be used for children with a history of croup or asthma presenting for routine surgery and for patients with upper airway obstruction caused by laryngotracheobronchitis or epiglottis (274–276).

Cuffed Tubes

With cuffed tubes, the cuff circumference should equal that of the tracheal lumen (186). If the cuff is too small for the trachea, a higher cuff pressure will be needed to achieve a seal, converting the low-pressure cuff into a high-pressure one. If the cuff is too large in relation to the tracheal lumen, it will have folds when it is inflated to occlusion. Aspiration may occur along those folds (277).

One study found that the ideal tube in the average adult would be a 7.5-mm ID tube for women and a 8.5-mm ID tube for men (278). However, there is great variation in sizes and shapes of tracheas in adults (277, 279–281). The transverse dimensions increase with age, but in general, the correlation between age, race, height, weight, body surface area, and tracheal shape or size is poor (277, 279). There is some variation in the cuff circumference of tubes with identical IDs.

Uncuffed Tubes

With uncuffed tubes, a seal is achieved by selection of the size of tube that fits the cricoid ring. There is considerable variation in subglottic size in children and in the external diameters of pediatric tracheal tubes (282).

For prolonged intubation in children, many feel there should be a small leak of gas between the tube and the trachea heard using a stethoscope with the head in the neutral position at a peak pressure of greater than 20 cm H_2O (283–286). The reproducibility of the leak pressure will depend on the degree of neuromuscular blockade and the observer (284, 286).

The following have been used as general guidelines for selection of a tube size in children.

1. One to 6 months—3.0 to 4.0 mm ID
   Six months to 1 year—3.5 to 4.5 mm ID
   Older than 1 year—ID in mm = (16 + age in years) ÷ 4 (273, 287)
2. Premature—gestational age in weeks ÷ 10 + 0.5 = ID in mm (288)
   Younger than 6.5 years—3.5 + age in years ÷ 3 = ID in mm
   Older than 6.5 years—4.5 + age in years ÷ 4 = ID in mm (289)
3. Infants below 1 kg—2.5 mm
   Infants between 1 and 2 kg—3.0 mm
   Infants between 2 and 3 kg—3.5 mm
   Infants over 3 kg—4.0 mm (290)
4. (age + 16)/4 or (age + 18)/4 (291)
5. Choosing a tube whose external diameter is the same width as the distal phalanx of the little or index finger (292, 293). Studies indicate this may be less accurate than other methods (294–296).
6. Use of a measure based on body length (291, 297).

Checking the Tube

Before insertion, the tube should be examined for defects such as splitting, holes, and missing sections (298–300). The cuff, if present, should be inflated and the syringe removed to check for leakage of the inflation valve. If the syringe is left in the valve, the valve housing may crack and leak (301). The cuff should be inspected to make certain it inflates evenly and does not cause the tube lumen to be reduced. It should be left inflated for at least 1 minute to check for a slow leak.

If the tube has a sponge cuff, all the air should be removed by aspiration. The inflation tube should then be closed or clamped off. The cuff should remain collapsed. If it fills, there is a leak, and the tube should be discarded.

The tube should be checked for obstructions. With transparent tubes, simple observation will suffice. With other tubes, the user should look into both ends and/or insert a stylet.

Preparing the Tube

After the sterile wrapper is opened, the tube should be handled only at the connector end. The connector should be inserted as far as possible. Removing it from the tube and wiping the outside with alcohol will make insertion into the tube easier and cause bonding with the tube.

Lubricants have been used on tracheal tubes for many years, although their value has been questioned. Use of a lubricant jelly on a low-pressure, high-volume cuff may decrease aspiration by filling in the folds (198, 200). Only a sterile water-soluble lubricant should be used (302). For oral intubation, only the distal end of the tube should be lubricated. If nasal intubation is planned, lubricant should be placed along the entire length of the tube.

Inserting the Tube

Techniques

Oral Intubation

Oral intubation is generally preferred for general anesthesia and in emergencies because it can be performed more quickly than nasal intubation. It allows passage of a wider and shorter tube with a larger radius of curvature than nasal intubation. This facilitates flexible bronchoscopy and suctioning and lowers resistance to airflow.

Studies comparing orotracheal and nasotracheal intubation in patients requiring ventilatory assistance have found little difference, except that the ease of initial intubation was greater with orotracheal intubation (303, 304). There is less movement of the tube within the trachea with changes in head position with oral intubation (305).

Disadvantages include the possibility of dental and oropharyngeal complications. Oral intubation is usually not well-tolerated by the conscious patient. The patient with an oral tube has difficulty swallowing.

Insertion of the tube is usually easy once the vocal cords are exposed. The tube should be introduced into the right corner of the mouth and directed toward the glottis with the bevel parallel to the vocal cords. If there is movement of the cords, the tube should be inserted during maximum abduction.

A bite block, rolled gauze, or oral airway may be placed between the teeth to prevent the patient from biting down and occluding the lumen.

Nasal Intubation

The nasal route is used for surgical procedures involving the oral cavity, oropharynx, and face, where an oral tube would hinder the surgeon's access to the operative field. Other indications may include an awake or combative patient and patients with neck injuries, mechanical obstruc-

tions to orotracheal intubation, fractured mandibles, and limitations of movement at the temporomandibular joints.

Intubation by the nasal route has many advantages. Fixation of the tube is easier and there may be less risk of inadvertent extubation (65, 306), although a study of long-term intubation found no significant differences between patients who received oral intubation and those with nasal intubation (307). During long-term intubation, oral feedings and oral hygiene are possible. Use of the nasal route eliminates the possibility of tube occlusion by biting.

Disadvantages include the possibility of cosmetic nasal deformities and meteorism with long-term intubation. Smaller tubes must be used, resulting in increased resistance and difficulty in suctioning or using a fiberscope. Intubation takes longer. Nasal bleeding may occur. Nasal intubation has been shown to result in a high incidence of bacteremia (308–311). A high incidence of sinusitis and otitis during and following nasotracheal intubation has been reported (306, 312–326)

Contraindications to nasotracheal intubation include coagulopathy and any mechanical impediment of the nasotracheal route, including polyps, abscesses, and foreign bodies (327). Fracture of the base of the skull is usually considered a contraindication to nasotracheal intubation, although one study concluded that complications of basilar skull fracture are not increased by attempts at nasotracheal intubation (328). Pneumocephalus has been reported after nasal intubation in a patient who had a transnasal repair of the cribriform plate (329).

Before insertion of a nasotracheal tube, there should be local application of a vasoconstrictor. The patency of each nasal cavity should be assessed by having the patient inhale through each nostril separately. Often a tube one size smaller than would be considered optimal for oral intubation is selected to minimize epistaxis. It should be thoroughly lubricated along its entire length with a water-soluble lubricant (302). The tube can be softened by warming it (330).

The patient's head should be put in the usual position for laryngoscopy (see Chapter 16, "Laryngoscopes"). The tube should be inserted into the more patent nostril. Inserting progressively larger lubricated nasal airways will test the patency of the nostril and dilate it (331, 332).

When the tube is inserted, its bevel should face laterally, so as to direct its leading edge away from the turbinates (330, 333). The tube should be directed gently posteriorly until it contacts the posterior pharyngeal wall. Here the natural curve of the tube and the anterior body of the cervical spine will usually direct it anteriorly.

Resistance to passage of the tube may be met at various points along its course. Only gentle pressure should be used. If excessive resistance is encountered, the other nostril or a smaller tube should be tried. Sometimes the tube will impact against the posterior pharyngeal wall and resist attempts to advance it farther. The tube should be pulled back a short distance, and the patient's head extended to facilitate passage beyond this point. It may be useful to withdraw the tube and place a stylet in it, with an acute bend in the distal 1.5 cm of the tube. The tube is inserted until it passes the posterior nasopharynx, then the stylet is withdrawn. Another technique is to pass a small suction catheter through the tube and into the oropharynx (264, 334). The tube can usually be threaded over the catheter, or the tip of the catheter can be picked up and brought out of the mouth. A forward pull on the catheter will usually bring the tip of the tracheal tube forward.

Direct laryngoscopy. After the tube is in the pharynx, the larynx is exposed using a laryngoscope. The tube tip can usually be directed laterally by twisting. The position of the larynx relative to the tube tip may be altered by flexing or extending the neck and/or external pressure on the larynx. If these manipulations do not line up the tube and laryngeal opening, forceps can be used to grasp the tip and direct it through the vocal cords. The cuff should not be grasped as it may be damaged by the forceps.

If the tip passes through the vocal cords but then encounters resistance, it is likely that the curve of the tube is directing the tip into the anterior wall of the larynx. Withdrawing the tube slightly and flexing the neck will usually allow advancement. Other techniques include rotating the tube 180° before pushing it forward, passing a suction catheter through the tube into the larynx

as a guide (335), and inserting a stylet with a bend near the tip (336, 337).

Flexible fiberoptic laryngoscopy. Flexible fiberoptic laryngoscopy is preferred if a conventional rigid laryngoscope cannot be used. Blind nasal intubation may stir up bleeding and ruin the chance to view the larynx through the fiberscope. The technique is described in Chapter 16, "Laryngoscopes."

Blind (338). The blind technique may be useful when direct laryngoscopy or use of a fiberscope would be difficult but it may be associated with more trauma than other techniques.

Blind intubation may be performed under general or local anesthesia. The classical technique of blind nasal intubation requires a spontaneously breathing patient and uses breath sounds as a guide to placement. The patient is placed in the classical intubation position with the neck flexed and the head extended. After the tube is inserted through the nostril, it is advanced blindly. If the patient is breathing spontaneously, breath sounds can be heard as the tip approaches the larynx. When the sounds are at maximal intensity, the tube is gently but swiftly advanced during inspiration. If the sounds suddenly cease but the patient continues to breathe, the tube has passed into a location other than the trachea. Flexion or extension of the head or manipulation of the larynx by external pressure may line up the tube and larynx. The tube tip may be rotated by twisting the tube at the connector end (339). Insertion of a preformed stylet with an anterior curve may help to advance the tip through the vocal cords (336). Inflation of the cuff may help to elevate the tip from the posterior pharyngeal wall and center it (340, 341). The cuff is deflated before the tube is advanced into the trachea (342).

Exhaled CO_2 can aid in performing a blind nasal intubation (342–344). A capnometer or chemical CO_2 detector is attached to the tube as it is being inserted in a spontaneously breathing patient. As the tube approaches the larynx, the end-tidal CO_2 increases, and as it moves away, it decreases. As the tube is advanced and the tip passes between the cords, a normal capnogram is observed.

The Endotrol tube may be useful in blind nasal intubations (92–94).

If the patient is not breathing, certain landmarks on the front of the neck (hyoid bone, notch of the thyroid cartilage, and the cricoid cartilage) can be observed (345). As the tube moves anteriorly, the landmarks are moved by the tip of the tube. The object is to move the tip to the midline at the thyroid angle, where it should enter the larynx. If the tip is above the thyroid cartilage, flexion of the head will move the tip more caudad. If the tip is below the thyroid cartilage, extension of the neck will move it cephalad. If the tip is observed resting laterally, the tube should be withdrawn and twisted to direct it toward the midline. If the tube tip passes the laryngeal inlet but impinges on the anterior trachea, increasing cervical flexion or rotating the tube through 180° may allow it to pass into the trachea.

Retrograde Intubation

When the above techniques do not work, a retrograde intubation technique may be used (346). This may be useful in cases of suspected cervical spine injury or when intubation by other means is unsuccessful. The procedure begins with puncture of the cricothyroid membrane and insertion of a wire or an epidural catheter in a cephalad direction. It is retrieved through the oropharynx then used to guide a tracheal tube into the airway.

Depth of Insertion

The tube should be inserted until the cuff is 2.25 to 2.5 cm below the vocal cords (347). Some manufacturers place a single mark above the proximal end of the cuff and recommend that the tube be advanced until this mark lies at the vocal cords. If no cuff is present, the tube tip should be inserted not more than 1 cm past the cords in children under 6 months, not more than 2 cm past the cords for patients up to 1 year, and not more than 3 to 4 cm past the cords in larger patients. In children, it is possible to pass a tube through the cords but have its passage blocked just below this level. The tube should not be forced, but a smaller tube used instead.

In average-size adult patients, securing the tube at the anterior incisors at 23 cm in males and 21 cm in females will usually avoid bronchial intubation (348, 349). For nasal intubations, 3 cm should be added to these lengths for positioning at the nares. However, caution should be exercised in use of routine depth of insertion since cuffs vary in length (350).

Formulas based on the subject's height may be used (351) or the correct length can be estimated by aligning the proximal end of the cuff externally at the level of the cricoid cartilage and angling the tube anteriorly toward the level of the upper incisors or gums (352).

In children, the optimal depth to which the tracheal tube should be inserted nasally can be estimated by the following formula:

$$L = (3 \times S) + 2$$

where S is the ID of the tube in millimeters and L, the length in centimeters (353).

Checking the Position

After the tube has been inserted, its position should be checked: first to be sure that it is in the tracheobronchial tree and second, that it is neither too deep nor too shallow. Methods to detect intubation of a bronchus or the esophagus are discussed in "Perioperative Complications." After confirmation of correct placement, the portion external to the patient may be shortened to prevent kinking (354).

Inflating the Cuff

Low-Volume, High-Pressure Cuff

A high-pressure cuff should be inflated with the minimal amount of gas that will cause it to seal against the trachea at peak inspiratory pressure. Listening with the unaided ear will often miss small leaks. These can be detected by palpation or auscultation of the suprasternal pretracheal area (355, 356). Inflation until the pilot balloon is tense and/or inflating beyond seal will result in unnecessarily high cuff volume and pressure on the tracheal wall.

Low-Pressure, High-Volume Cuff

With a low-pressure, high-volume cuff, measurement of cuff pressure is necessary to prevent overinflation or under inflation. If a low-pressure cuff is adjusted to the point of just abolishing audible leakage at peak inspiratory pressure, the resulting intracuff pressure may not be high enough to prevent aspiration (357).

The cuff should be inflated to a pressure of 25 to 30 cm H_2O (142, 143). The pressure should be measured and adjusted approximately 10 minutes after the tube has been inserted (358). This delay is necessary to allow for softening of the cuff material at body temperature and for the patient to become settled, because the volume necessary for occlusion will vary with muscle tone. Not measuring the pressure will usually result in a pressure well above those recommended (359).

After cuff pressure has been adjusted, a check should be made to make sure there is no leak at peak airway pressure. If there is a leak and peak airway pressure does not exceed intracuff pressure, the cuff is probably too small for the trachea and a tube with a larger cuff should be used (209).

Cuff pressure should be measured and readjusted frequently. Changes in muscle tone in the trachea and diffusion of gases across the cuff may result in large changes in cuff pressure.

When a tracheal tube with a Lanz pressure-regulating valve is used, the cuff should be inflated until a seal is achieved during peak inspiration. The pilot balloon should be distended but smaller than the confining sheath.

Sponge Cuff

After intubation, the inflation tube should be opened to atmosphere and the cuff allowed to fill with air. The amount of air in the cuff should be ascertained by withdrawal with a syringe. The ability to remove 2 to 3 ml from the smallest cuff or 5 to 6 ml or more from the largest cuff usually signifies that the cuff:tracheal wall pressure ratio will allow adequate mucosal perfusion. If little or no air can be aspirated, the cuff may be too large.

If a leak is present after the cuff has been allowed to expand, wrinkles in the cuff may be present and may be straightened out by injecting 2 or 3 ml of air into the cuff then allowing it to deflate. If the leak persists, consideration should be given to using a larger tube.

Securing the Tube

A securely positioned tracheal tube is essential for safe anesthesia, particularly in pediatric patients in whom the distance from the mid-trachea to the cords or carina is short. If the tube is not well-fixed, there is danger of either unplanned ex-tubation or deeper advancement of the tube. The fixation technique must be appropriate for the nature of the surgery and accessibility of the tube.

Adhesive tape is most commonly used to maintain the tube in the desired position. The part of the tube to which the tape is to be applied should be thoroughly dried. All tapes do not adhere to all tracheal tubes equally well (360, 361), so it is advisable to test available tapes to determine which works best for the chosen tube. Cohesion may be improved by wrapping the tube with a transparent adhesive dressing (360, 362, 363). Use of an adhesive such as tincture of benzoin on the tube and skin may make the tape stick better. Tape should not be placed across the connector in order not to obscure a disconnection or hinder rapid reconnection (364).

The tube may be secured by having the tape completely encircle the head (365, 366). Fixation to both the lower and upper jaws using separate tapes and wrapping twice around the tube and reinforcing these with strips applied longitudinally across the borders of the mouth opening may result in good fixation (361). Splitting the tape longitudinally may increase the likelihood of dislodgement (361).

Use of adhesive tape has the following disadvantages:

1. Some patients have skin conditions that are aggravated by contact with adhesives. Others may have allergic responses.
2. It may interfere with surgery of the head and neck.
3. Many patients have beards or mustaches, making it difficult to attach the tape. In patients with sufficiently long mustache hair, this can be taped around the tracheal tube (367).
4. Oral secretions, sweat, oil, blood, or prep solutions may render the tape ineffective.

For these reasons other materials such as umbilical tape or surgical suture may be used to anchor the tube (368–372). The suture may be passed either around a ring of adhesive tape on the tube or through the wall of the tube and may be anchored by passing it through the gum or around a tooth or by taping it to the skin. Placing a safety pin through the wall of the tube may be helpful.

Because the hair is an insecure medium for fixing a tube, a close-fitting skull cap, elastic net, or a towel taped around the head may be used to provide a firm structure to which to attach tape or ties (Fig. 17.29) (373, 374).

Other methods used to secure the tube include circumpalatal fixation (375), use of liquid silicone foam to form a cast around the tube (376), and use of an umbilical cord clamp to snap around the tube (377). Special devices for securing tracheal tubes without use of adhesives or ties are available commercially and a number have been described in the literature (378–380). A tube holder may be combined with a bite block and/or nasogastric tube holder. The tube may be sutured to the tongue or teeth (380).

With nasal intubation, padding around the tube may help to prevent pressure necrosis (377). Fixation in the direction of the mouth rather than cephalad may decrease the risk of damage to the nasal alae with prolonged intubation (382).

It is important to make sure there is no pull on the tube. Use of a lightweight extension between the tracheal tube connector and the breathing system and/or a tube support may be helpful. Figure 17.29 shows a method of securing the breathing system so that it does not exert pull on a tube inserted nasally.

Changing the Tube (383–386)

There are three general techniques available for changing a tracheal tube: use of a fiberscope, direct laryngoscopy, and use of a tube changer (discussed later in this chapter). Exchange of a tracheal tube using a fiberscope is discussed in Chapter 16, "Laryngoscopes."

Direct laryngoscopy can be used for changing an orotracheal or nasotracheal tube or substituting one for the other. A laryngoscope blade is placed into the mouth and positioned in the hypopharynx. The existing tube is visualized entering the glottis. The replacement tracheal tube is positioned near the glottis, the existing tube pulled out, and the replacement tube inserted. Passage of a jet-stylet tube exchanger through the existing tube and leaving it in place will allow jet ventilation until the new tube enters the trachea (385).

When changing a tracheal tube using a tube exchanger, the lubricated exchanger is inserted into the tube and advanced until it has passed the end of the tube. Most tracheal tube changers have depth marks printed on their sides to aid in precise placement. While the tube changer is held firmly in place, the existing tube is withdrawn. Care must be taken not to alter the position of the changer. The new tracheal tube is then threaded over the tube changer and advanced until it is at the proper depth. Twisting the tube may aid its advancement. The tube changer is then withdrawn. Use of a jet-stylet tube changer allows administration of oxygen, suctioning, and ventilation while the changer is in place (384).

Removing the Tube (387)

The oral airway or bite block should be left in place until after extubation to avoid biting on the tube (388).

Before extubation, the mouth and pharynx should be suctioned and the tape or other fixation device removed. Withdrawing the tube until resistance is met before deflating the cuff may push material that has accumulated above the cuff into the pharynx where it can be removed by suctioning. The patient should be given a large sustained inflation or the adjustable-pressure limiting (APL) valve closed and airway pressure allowed to rise to 5 to 10 cm H_2O. While the lung is near total capacity, the cuff should be deflated using a syringe and the tube removed during inspiration (389, 390). This will blow secretions collected above the cuff into the mouth and pharynx. If a syringe cannot be located, the tip of a pen can be inserted into the valve assembly to deflate the cuff (391). The practice of pulling the pilot balloon and inflation valve from the inflation tube to deflate the cuff should be discouraged as this can cause the inflation tube to seal (392–394).

If the tube cannot be removed easily, the inflating tube should be checked for obstruction, especially at the point where tape was used to hold the tube in place. If the surgery has involved the mouth or thorax, a suture may be around or through the tube or cuff. If the tube is forcibly removed in these circumstances, disastrous consequences may result.

Extubation of a patient who may be difficult to reintubate is best carried out over a jet stylet (395). After the tracheal tube is withdrawn, the catheter may be used as a means of ventilation and/or a guide for reintubation and allow additional time to assess the need for reintubation. After the tracheal tube has been passed over the jet stylet, the jet stylet may be maintained in place while intratracheal placement of the tracheal tube is confirmed by passing the tube exchanger through the self-sealing diaphragm of a fiberoptic elbow adapter. Positive pressure ventilation and carbon dioxide sampling can be performed around the tube exchanger.

If the tracheal tube is to stay in place and nitrous oxide has been in use, the cuff should be evacuated and filled with air to avoid a leak in the postoperative period (165).

PERIOPERATIVE COMPLICATIONS

Trauma

Intubation is often associated with trauma to the structures of the upper and lower airways. One study found that 86% of patients had occult or visible blood after extubation (396). Obviously gloves should be worn whenever the airway is manipulated.

Trauma is often associated with use of excessive force or repeated attempts at intubation. It varies with the skill of the operator, the difficulty of the intubation, and the amount of muscle relaxation. Damage may be increased if a stylet protrudes beyond the end of the tube or through the Murphy eye. Mucosa can be torn when a metal or foil-wrapped tube is used (114, 264). A defective tube may have a barb (336). Plastic tubes become stiffer when cold and this may increase the likelihood of trauma on insertion.

Trauma to the lips, tongue, teeth, nose, pharynx, larynx, trachea, or bronchus may occur. Injuries ranging from simple abrasion to severe laceration and perforation have been reported. The temporomandibular joint can be dislocated (397).

Cases of tracheal, bronchial, esophageal, pharyngeal, nasal fossa, hypopharyngeal, pyriform sinus, and laryngeal perforation have been reported, sometimes with fatal consequences (398–435).

Reported injuries to the larynx include hematomas, contusions, lacerations, puncture wounds, cord avulsions, and fractures (436–439). Arytenoid cartilage dislocation may occur (440–449).

With nasotracheal intubation, abrasion or laceration of the nasal mucosa is common (398, 450, 451). The nasal septum may be dislocated or perforated. Fragments of adenoid tissue, nasal polyps, or tubinates may be dislodged (452–459). Retropharyngeal passage of a tube has been reported (460, 461).

Trauma may also occur during extubation (462).

The best way to avoid trauma is never use more than gentle pressure and avoid patient movement. Stylets should be flexible and never extend beyond the tip of the tube. Use of vasoconstrictors on the nasal mucosa before intubation, warming the tube, and sequential dilatation (inserting progressively larger, lubricated nasal airways) will reduce the trauma associated with nasal intubation (330–332, 463). Tubes used for nasal intubation should be smaller than considered optimal for oral intubation and should be well-lubricated along their entire length. Another possible way to reduce trauma during nasotracheal intubation is to pass a lubricated stylet after spraying the nostrils (464). After visualizing the tip of the stylet in the pharynx, the tracheal tube is threaded over it into the pharynx. The stylet is then withdrawn.

Failure to Achieve a Satisfactory Seal

A leaking cuff or tube may make maintenance of adequate ventilation difficult, fail to protect against aspiration, and make surgery involving the oral cavity difficult.

If the cuff protrudes above the cords, there may be a leak despite a large amount of air being injected into the cuff. Further inflation may seal the leak, but it will gradually return.

During insertion, the cuff, inflation tube, or the tube itself may be torn by a tooth or turbinate, the laryngoscope blade, forceps, or the sharp edge of a stylet or other device (465, 466). High-volume cuffs are more likely to be torn than low-volume ones. A kink in the inflation tube (467, 468) or a problem with the syringe used to inflate the cuff (469, 470) may make it impossible to inflate the cuff. A defect in the tube or eccentric cuff inflation can cause a leak (299, 471). If the compliance of the pilot balloon is greater than that of the cuff, the cuff may empty into it (472). Leaving the inflating syringe attached to the valve assembly may cause a crack in the valve housing, causing a leak (301). Inserting a small tube into a patient with large or highly compliant airways may result in a leak. The connector may be the source of a leak (473, 474).

When a leak is present, laryngoscopy should be performed to determine if the cuff is above the cords. If so, the cuff should be deflated, the tube advanced, and the cuff reinflated. If this fails to solve the problem, the tube should be replaced. If intubation was difficult, consideration should be given to using a tube exchanger or fiberscope for replacing the tube.

Intubation of the Esophagus (475–477)

Esophageal intubation can occur even with an experienced anesthesia provider (473, 478–484). Recognition that this has occurred and prompt correction are necessary to prevent dire consequences.

In most patients, distinguishing esophageal intubation is not difficult. But in some, the signs so closely resemble tracheal placement that they can deceive even a careful, experienced individual. In many of the reported incidents involving esophageal intubation, one or more of the following tests were performed and were misleading.

Direct Visualization

Direct visualization of the tube passing between the vocal cords is one of the most reliable methods. Unfortunately, the glottis often cannot be seen well. Posterior displacement of the tracheal tube with the laryngoscope blade still in the mouth may bring the larynx into view (485, 486). Even after visualization of the tube between the cords, the tube may slip out while the laryngoscope is being withdrawn during removal of the stylet or fixation of the tube.

Feel of the Reservoir Bag

Normal reservoir bag compliance and refilling with manual ventilation are another method. Decreased compliance and expiratory time may be seen with esophageal intubation (487). Unfortunately, this test is unreliable (475, 483, 488–492).

It may be more reliable if performed with no fresh gas flow (493, 494).

A related test is movement of the reservoir bag in time with the patient's spontaneous respiratory efforts. However, tidal volumes have been noted with the tube in the esophagus (483, 488, 489, 491, 495, 496).

Chest Wall Motion

Some users rely on visual and/or manual evidence of chest wall movement during ventilation. Unfortunately, movement of the chest wall simulating ventilation of the lungs can occur with the tube in the esophagus, especially in patients whose respiration is primarily abdominal (475, 488–491, 497–501). Chest wall movement may be difficult to assess in the obese patient or the patient with large breasts. Low lung or chest wall compliance may result in little chest movement, even when the tube is in the trachea (483). Listening through the open end of the tracheal tube while the sternum is abruptly depressed can be misleading (483, 491).

Auscultation

Auscultation should be performed in the midaxillary areas bilaterally, not just the anterior chest. The quality of the sounds is important. A gurgling sound (death rattle) suggests esophageal placement. This test is not reliable, as there are reported cases where normal breath sounds were thought to be heard with esophageal intubation (473, 475, 483, 488, 491, 497, 500–502). With a large intrathoracic hiatal hernia, a gastric pull up, or intrathoracic esophagogastrostomy, sounds that mimic normal breath sounds may be heard (489).

Auscultation of the upper abdomen as well as the lungs has been found to be more reliable than auscultation of the lungs alone (497). Yet such sounds may be confused with breath sounds often heard in the epigastric area in thin individuals and pediatric patients (473, 483, 496).

Sounds of Air around the Tube

With the cuff deflated, the high-pitched sound of air escaping around a tube in the trachea compared with the more guttural sound of leakage around a tube in the esophagus has been used as a distinguishing feature (483). However, if the cuff is near the cricoid cartilage, the distinction in sound may not be present (491).

Epigastric Distention

Some users observe the epigastrium for gastric distention. Unfortunately, the abdomen does not always distend with intermittent gastric inflation and gastric distention can result from mask ventilation before intubation is attempted (475, 490, 491, 499). The presence of a hiatal hernia or intrathoracic gastrointestinal contents may result in the absence of abdominal distention with esophageal intubation (489). A previously placed nasogastric tube may cause decompression of the stomach, and reflux of gases into the esophagus may make gastric filling difficult to distinguish from normal abdominal movements during ventilation.

Moisture Condensation in the Tracheal Tube

Condensation of moisture in a transparent tracheal tube is not reliable since moisture can appear with esophageal intubation (475, 483, 497, 503, 504). But if no water condensation is seen, the tube is almost always in the esophagus.

Gastric Contents in Tracheal Tube

Gastric contents in the tube lumen may indicate misplacement. However, gastric fluid may not appear with esophageal placement and/or may be difficult to distinguish from secretions in the trachea (475, 483).

Oxygenation

Good patient color or satisfactory pulse oximeter readings have been advocated as a means to confirm tracheal placement. However, color changes may be delayed a number of minutes with esophageal intubation if preoxygenation has been performed, and, at that time, a number of other causes for the hypoxemia must be ruled out (475, 483, 505). However, if oxygen saturation improves after intubation, it is likely that the tube is in the tracheobronchial tree (505). The patient can be ventilated using a mask placed over the open tube and mouth. Cyanosis relieved by this maneuver is evidence of tube misplacement (488).

Chest X-Ray

Chest radiography is time consuming and expensive and may not be definitive in determining if the tube is in the esophagus (475, 483, 507–509).

Palpation of Suprasternal Notch

When the cuff is inflated and deflated or the pilot balloon is intermittently squeezed or the tube moved in and out, this should be felt when the neck is palpated suprasternally (510). This test is not always reliable (483, 495, 503, 511, 512).

Measuring Amount of Cuff Inflation Needed to Cause a Seal

Another method is to note the amount of air required to cause the cuff to seal in the trachea. An excessive amount may indicate esophageal placement. However, placement of the cuff at or just above the vocal cords, a tear in the cuff, or failure of the cuff to expand uniformly can also result in the need for high volumes with the tube in the trachea.

Use of a Fiberscope

The tracheal rings can be visualized using a fiberscope. A special adapter with a port will allow ventilation while the examination is carried out. This is a reliable method but requires special instruments, skill, and time and cannot be used with small tubes.

Tactile Confirmation

This test involves placing one hand inside the patient's mouth and the other hand on the neck and confirming that the tube lies immediately anterior to the interarytenoid groove. This test is not totally reliable (513, 514)

Esophageal Detector Device

The esophageal detector device consists of an aspirating component (a syringe or large self-inflating compressible bulb) attached to the tracheal tube using an adapter (515–518). The plunger is withdrawn or the compressed bulb released. If the tube is in the trachea and an airtight seal has been achieved, gas will be aspirated from the patient's lungs without resistance. However, if the tube is in the esophagus, apposition of the walls of the esophagus around the tube will occur. This will occlude the lumen and cause a negative pressure or resistance. As a confirmatory test, the device can be used to inject a bolus of air into the tube while listening over the epigastrium. This will also detect a blocked tracheal tube (516).

This test has a high degree of accuracy even with inexperienced users (516, 519–530). It can be used to detect the position of the Combitube (531). The presence of a nasogastric tube, deflation of the tracheal tube cuff, or prior insufflation of the stomach does not limit its efficacy (429, 532–534). Its accuracy is not affected by lack of pulmonary perfusion. It is faster than most other methods.

There are situations where this device may not confirm placement in the trachea (516, 521, 535). The bulb will not re-expand rapidly in patients with decreased expiratory reserve volume, such as the morbidly obese or pregnant patient and patients with bronchospastic disease, mainstem intubation, tracheomalacia, pulmonary secretions, and upper or lower airway obstructions (527, 536–541). The incidence of false negatives is reduced if the bulb is compressed after connection to the tracheal tube (542). Another source of a false negative is the bevel lying against the tracheal wall (543). This device is unreliable in patients under 1 year of age (544).

Sonic Detection

The Sonomatic Confirmation of Tracheal Intubation (SCOTI) (545) utilizes a sonic technique for detection of tracheal intubation. It is a portable, battery-operated device that depends upon recognition of a resonating frequency that varies according to whether the tracheal tube is in an open (trachea) or closed (esophagus) structure. A liquid crystal display shows a numeric value related to the resonating frequency produced. In addition, there is an audible signal of varying tone and a light-emitting diode that illuminates as red, yellow, or green.

This device must be configured for the individual tracheal tube before each use. One study found that configuration was only successful with certain lengths of conventional tubes and certain sizes of specialized tubes (546). In another study, the device incorrectly identified 1 of 50 tracheal intubations and was unable to identify the position of another (547). It did detect all the esophageal intubations.

Ultrasound

Ultrasound can confirm the placement of a tracheal tube with a foam or fluid-filled cuff (548).

Intentional Bronchial Intubation (549, 550)

With intentional bronchial intubation, the tube is advanced into a mainstem bronchus. The chest is then auscultated during positive pressure ventilation. If breath sounds can be heard on only one side, bronchial intubation has been achieved. With esophageal intubation, the breath sounds are either equal bilaterally or equally diminished or absent on both sides of the chest. This test is not foolproof (549).

Passing Introducer through the Tracheal Tube

A nasogastric tube, introducer, or other device can be passed down the tracheal tube (483, 551). If the tube is in the trachea, it will abut against the carina at 28 to 32 cm in adults. If the tube is in the esophagus, no such resistance will be encountered. Other criteria indicating placement in the trachea include the ability to maintain air entrainment through the open end of the tracheal tube while suction is applied to the tube, the ease of withdrawal of the tube with suction, and the absence of bile or gastric contents in the aspirate (551).

Tracheal Palpation during Intubation

During intubation with gentle palpation in the sternal notch or application of cricoid pressure, a washboard-like sensation can often be appreciated as the tube passes over the tracheal rings (552, 553). This test is not reliable (512).

Roll Test

The "roll test" involves gentle backwards pressure on the cricoid cartilage using two or three fingers and simultaneous side-to-side displacement of the cartilage in an attempt to detect a tracheal tube. If the tracheal tube is in the esophagus, the cricoid cartilage can be rolled over its rounded surface underneath. This test is not reliable (512).

Pressure- and Flow-Volume Loops

Pressure- and flow-volume loops are discussed in Chapter 19, "Airway Pressure, Volume, and Flow Measurements." If the tracheal tube is in the esophagus, the loops will not have their characteristic shapes. The loop will probably be open.

Tracheal Illumination

A light wand (see Chapter 16, "Laryngoscopes") can be passed through the tube and the intensity of transtracheal illumination used to differentiate tracheal from esophageal intubation (554). Obesity and swelling of the neck make this technique difficult.

Exhaled Carbon Dioxide

Analyzing exhaled gases for the presence of carbon dioxide (see Chapter 18, "Anesthesia Gas Monitoring") allows reliable and rapid detection of esophageal intubation (475, 483, 490, 555, 556). Tube placement can be checked on the first few breaths.

There are some special circumstances in which CO_2 may be detected if the tube is in the esophagus (557). Exhaled gases may be forced into the stomach during mask ventilation before intubation. CO_2 can be in the stomach as a byproduct of antacids that have reacted with gastric acid or from ingestion of carbonated beverages. In these cases, the end-tidal CO_2 will be low, the capnograms abnormal in configuration and irregular, and CO_2 levels will rapidly diminish with repeated ventilation. These limitations of CO_2 analysis can be offset by measurement of the volume and temperature of expired gases (558).

CO_2 may not appear despite correct placement with severe bronchospasm or if there is no pulmonary blood flow (492, 552).

It is possible to have CO_2 in the exhaled gases and the tube not be in the trachea. Two cases have been reported where the tube was curled in the pharynx with the Murphy eye at the entrance to the trachea (559, 560).

All of the above methods have both advantages and disadvantages. A high index of suspicion

should be maintained, and more than one of the above methods should always be used.

Swallowed Tracheal Tube

There are a number of case reports of a tracheal tube being lost in the esophagus (561–574). The majority occurred during newborn resuscitation. The tubes were removed and no permanent sequelae occurred.

This complication can be prevented by using a connector that fits firmly into the tube. Bonding between the connector and the tube will be increased if the connector is wiped with alcohol before insertion into the tube. The tube should be long enough that it protrudes from the mouth when correctly placed and firmly secured.

If this complication occurs, removal of the tube need not be immediate. Resuscitation should continue and the patient's condition stabilized.

Inadvertent Bronchial Intubation (47, 575)

In a large study, bronchial intubation was the most common problem involving the tracheal tube (473). In a large study, bronchial intubation accounted for 3.7% of critical incidents (47). A large number of these cases were associated with head or neck surgery, repositioning of the patient and use of pre-formed tubes.

Bronchial placement can lead to atelectasis of the non-ventilated lung and decreased oxygenation. The lung that is ventilated may become hyperinflated, leading to barotrauma and hypotension. A tube inserted into the right main bronchus may occlude the bronchus to the right upper lobe (576). If the tip impinges on the carina, persistent coughing and bucking may occur.

Inadvertent bronchial intubation has been found to occur more frequently during emergency intubations (577, 578) and in pediatric (579, 580) and female (581) patients. A short trachea is associated with a number of pediatric syndromes (582). One study showed that RAE tubes were too long in 32% of children and bronchial intubation occurred in 20% (45).

Usually the tube will enter the right mainstem bronchus. The main reason for this is that the bevel is on the left side of the tube. The tip thus contacts the right side of the carina and is guided into the right mainstem bronchus (583). Non-beveled tubes also tend to enter the right bronchus (584).

Intubation of a bronchus can occur after correct initial placement. If not firmly anchored, the tube may descend into a bronchus as a result of the weight of the attachments, suctioning, movement of the patient's head and/or neck, or general repositioning of the patient. The tube will move caudad with neck flexion, opening of the mouth, and going from an erect to a recumbent position (585–595). Oral tracheal tubes move more with extension than do nasotracheal tubes (596). During laparoscopy, the distance from the cords to the carina is decreased (597–601).

After intubation, an effort should be made to detect bronchial intubation. This should be repeated at intervals, whenever changes in the patient's position are made, and whenever there is any indication of hypoxia. If a patient fails to settle down and continues to cough, it should be suspected that the tube may be irritating the carina.

Several methods have been used to detect bronchial intubation.

Auscultation for Bilateral Breath Sounds

The commonly used method of auscultating the lower and upper peripheral lung fields bilaterally may be misleading as breath sounds can be transmitted to the opposite side of the chest in the presence of bronchial intubation, unless the tube is wedged firmly in a main bronchus (602–603).

Visualization of Symmetrical Chest Expansion

Visualization of symmetrical chest expansion is easily performed but is not reliable.

Chest X-Ray

Chest x-rays are reliable but time consuming and expensive. The tracheal tube standard (21) requires a radiopaque marker at the patient end or along the full length of the tube. Most believe that the tip of the tube should be in the middle third of the trachea with the head in a neutral position (midway between full extension and full flexion) (586, 590, 604). The tip should lie over the second to fourth thoracic vertebrae (492, 586, 605, 606).

In the neonate, infant, and young child, the tip should be 2 cm above the carina with the neck in the neutral position (580, 607). In children approaching 5 to 6 years of age, this distance should be increased to 3.0 cm (607). In adults, the ideal distance is 3, 5, or 7 cm with the neck flexed, neutral, or extended, respectively (581, 586, 605, 608)

Tube Position at the Lips/Nostril

Adult Patients

It is recommended that oral tubes be positioned 21 cm at the teeth (or upper anterior gums in edentulous patients) in normal-size women and 23 cm in normal-size men and that for nasal intubation 3 cm be added to these lengths for positioning at the nostril (348, 552). Studies show this is a better method of preventing bronchial intubation than auscultation of the chest. However, it may result in malpositioning in some patients (581, 609). Another study found that the average distance from the tip of the tracheal tube to the teeth with the tube correctly positioned was 20.2 cm in women and 21.9 cm in men (610).

For patients whose body lengths lie outside the normal range, the tube can be placed alongside the patient's face and neck with the tip at the suprasternal notch. The tube is aligned to conform externally to the position of a nasal or oral tracheal tube. The place on the tube at which the tube intersects with the teeth or gums (oral intubation) or the nares (nasal intubation) is noted, and the tube secured in that position after intubation.

One study determined that the maximum safe tube length at the naris was best determined by measuring the distance between the upper border of the cricoid cartilage and the tip of the xiphoid process (611).

Pediatric Patients

The margin of safety in children is less than in adults. A number of formulas and tables based on body size and gestation age has been developed, including the following:

Oral Intubation

1. Length in centimeters = age/2 + 12 cm (577, 612).

2. Length in centimeters = weight in kilograms/
   5 +12 cm (612).
3. Length in centimeters = height in centime-
   ters/10 + 5 cm (613).
4. Rule of 7-8-9: infants weighing 1 kg are intubated to a depth of 7 cm at the lips; 2-kg infants, to a depth of 8 cm; and 3-kg infants, to
   a length of 9 cm (614).

Equations based on the crown-rump and crown-heel length have been developed (593).

Nasotracheal Intubation

1. $L = (S \times 3) + 2$, where L is the length in
   centimeters and S is the ID of the tube in millimeters (353).
2. Multiplying crown-heel length by 0.21 (615).
3. For total tube length, $0.16 \times$ height in centimeters + 4.5 cm, then leave 2 cm of tube
   outside the nostril of an infant and 3 cm outside for an older child (616).

While use of special formulas will decrease the incidence of this complication, they are based on averages and should not be considered totally reliable (602). Furthermore, tube length markings are not always accurate (617).

Placement of the Cuff Just below the Vocal Cords

Placement of the cuff only a few centimeters past the vocal cords should avoid bronchial intubation in adults.

Guide Marks on the Tracheal Tube

Many tubes have lines or rings to help position the tube with respect to the vocal cords (see Figs. 17.23, 17. 12, and 17.4), and the distal portion of some pediatric tubes is colored (347, 618, 619). Current guide marks vary in their position relative to the cuff and tip of the tube (594). It has been suggested that 3.0 and 3.5 mm tubes be placed with the 3 cm mark at the cords, 4.0, and 4.5 tubes set with the 4 cm mark at the cords, and 5.0 and 5.5 tubes set with the 5 cm mark at the cords (606).

Breath Sounds

The tube can be advanced until unilateral breath sounds and chest movement are observed.

Then the tube is slowly withdrawn, noting the tube length at nares or gum at which symmetrical breath sounds and chest movement return. The tube is then withdrawn an additional 2 cm and secured (607, 620). The head should be in the operative position during these maneuvers.

Fiberscope through the Tube

Passing a fiberscope through the tube is equal in accuracy and faster than a chest x-ray for determining tube position in both adults and pediatric patients (621–623) and more accurate than auscultation (624). The ready availability of fiberscopes in most operating room suites makes this a practical method of checking tube position (625)

Palpation of Anterior Neck

Another method is inflation and deflation of the cuff while palpating the anterior neck (610, 626–628). Alternatively, pressure can be applied to the neck while feeling the pilot balloon for transmitted pulsations with the other hand (479, 629). The lower border of the cuff should be felt just above the suprasternal notch. This method may not be useful in obese patients or with high-volume, low-pressure cuffs (630, 631). Some patients in whom the cuff can be felt by ballottement in the suprasternal notch have bronchial intubation (577).

With uncuffed tubes, the tip of the tube can be palpated during insertion and advancement stopped when the tip has just passed the suprasternal notch (579).

Fluid in Cuff

Injection of fluid into the cuff, followed by gentle compression of the pilot balloon while auscultating over the suprasternal notch is another method (632). The gurgling sound produced is not heard if the tip is in a mainstem bronchus or near the carina.

Magnetically Detectable Metallic Element

A portable locator can be used to detect a metallic element placed near the tip of the tube (633, 634). This method reduces the rate of malpositioning of tubes, but does not eliminate it (633). A thin foil band wrapped around a tracheal tube and detectable by a electronic sensor has also been used to position the tube tip in the mid trachea (631).

Monitoring Expired Carbon Dioxide

Monitoring expired CO_2 may lead to the discovery of bronchial intubation (635–638), but is not a reliable means to detect this problem (47). Either an increase or decrease in end-tidal CO_2 may be seen.

Lighted Intubation Stylet

Inserting a lighted intubation stylet so that the light is at the tip of the tube and positioning the tube so that the maximum transilluminated glow is at the sternal notch can consistently place the tip at a satisfactory level (639).

Illumination by a Fiberoptic Strand

Tracheal tubes in which the tip is illuminated by a fiberoptic strand incorporated into the tube wall and terminating just proximal to the cuff, or near the tip on uncuffed tubes have been used (640, 641). When a light source is connected, a bright transillumination appears distal to the cricoid cartilage.

Pressure and Flow-Volume Loops

Peak inspiratory pressure will usually increase with bronchial intubation. Pressure-volume and flow-volume loops (see Chapter 19, "Airway Pressure, Volume, and Flow Measurements") can detect a bronchial intubation. The pressure-volume loop will show low compliance. If the tube is withdrawn, there will be a marked improvement in compliance if the tube was in a bronchus.

Transcutaneous Oxygen Monitor or Pulse Oximetry

Falls in SpO_2 and transcutaneous oxygen are often seen with bronchial intubation (47, 642). However, desaturation will not necessarily occur even with massive atelectasis (552, 643). If there is arterial desaturation at any stage in an anesthetic, bronchial intubation should be considered (473, 644).

When a tracheal tube is believed to be in a bronchus, the cuff should be deflated, and the tube gently withdrawn, the cuff reinflated, and the position rechecked. If reintubation would be difficult because of the patient's position or because the initial intubation was difficult, consideration should be given to advancing a fiberscope or ventilation catheter into the tube before withdrawing it. If extubation should occur, the tracheal tube can be quickly reinserted. The lungs should then be gently hyperinflated to expand the atelectatic segments. For long-standing atelectasis, bronchoscopy may be required to remove mucous plugs.

Foreign Body Aspiration

During intubation, a variety of materials can be aspirated into the trachea and can cause blockage or check valve obstruction to part of the lungs.

A tracheal tube may dislodge fragments of tissue from the oral cavity, pharynx, or larynx. A tube inserted nasally may dislodge adenoid or nasal tissue during its passage (645). Obstruction of a bronchus by a blood clot following a traumatic intubation has been reported (646).

It is possible for a tracheal tube to become separated from its connector and lost in the trachea or pharynx (647–649). A tube may have the punched-out area forming the Murphy eye still in situ (650–652), and this may be aspirated. A portion or all of a cuff may be left in the airway (653).

Other foreign bodies found in tracheal tubes include cottonoids or pieces of aluminum used to protect the cuff or shaft from a laser beam, the distal portion of a tracheal tube (654, 655), parts of connectors, a cap liner from a tube of anesthetic ointment, parts of sprays and laryngoscopes, teeth, and dentures (253, 265, 654–660).

Careful inspection of equipment before use will help avoid introduction of foreign bodies. The connector should fit firmly in the tracheal tube and the tape or securing device should be attached to the tube, not the connector. When a cuff leaks, it should be carefully examined for missing portions after removal from the patient.

Foreign body aspiration should be suspected whenever obstructive signs or symptoms appear, and an immediate search should be made of the patient's air passages. This should include bronchoscopy if examination above the level of the larynx proves fruitless.

Leak while the Tube Is in Place (661)

The cuff can rupture or become separated from the tube while in place (662–664). Application of lubricant or local anesthetic spray has been associated with cuff leaks (665–667). Puncture of a cuff may occur during intravenous cannulation of the internal jugular or subclavian veins (668, 669) or other nearby procedures (384, 653, 670–682). A laser beam can perforate the cuff and cause a leak (253). An unsatisfactory seal due to chewing gum attached to the cuff has been reported (683).

The inflation system may have a defect (684–691). A common site is at the junction of the pilot tube and main body of the tube. If a device to monitor cuff pressure is left attached to the inflation valve, the valve housing may crack (301).

The connector may leak or separate from the tube (473, 692–694). If there is a covering over this site, the disconnection may not be noticed (695).

The patient may chew a hole in or completely sever a tube (72, 696–698). A tie used to secure the tube may cause damage to the tube (699).

In many cases with leaks the tube shows no evidence of mechanical fault (661). Other causes of leaks include tube malposition (especially the cuff at or above the level of the cords) and eccentric cuff inflation.

When a leak occurs, laryngoscopy should be performed to check the position of the cuff. If it is not completely below the vocal cords, the cuff should be deflated, the tube advanced, then the cuff reinflated. If the problem is in the inflation system, it may be possible to repair the damage or the leak can be bypassed using a three-way stopcock or a needle inserted into the line below the defect (700–704).

If the tube is cut, it may be possible to pass a small uncuffed tube past the cut (680). The small tube can then be used to ventilate the patient until the tube can be changed. In some cases, it may be possible to approximate the ends of the tube and seal the leak (676).

If the cuff is leaking, several alternatives are available:

1. Do nothing (if the leak is small and the patient not in great danger of aspiration). It may be necessary to increase the fresh gas flow to compensate for the leak.
2. Fill the cuff with a mixture of lidocaine jelly and saline (705).
3. Attach a mechanism for maintaining a continuous infusion of gas into the inflation tube. Methods described include an intravenous tubing connected to an air-filled plastic container to which constant external pressure is applied (677), a flowmeter (706, 707), and a system for maintenance of intraocular pressure (708).
4. Reintubation. If this is elected, consideration should be given to use of a tube exchanger or fiberscope.
5. Place a mask over the patient's face and the tube and ventilate.
6. Remove the tube and ventilate with a mask.
7. Use pharyngeal packing to control the leak.
8. Establish an acceptable airway in another fashion (tracheostomy or cricothyroid membrane puncture).

When a tube with a leaking cuff is removed, the damaged cuff should be carefully examined for missing portions.

Airway Perforation

Tracheal or bronchial perforation is a rare but serious complication of intubation (418, 709–715). It is usually associated with preexisting pathology of the airway, use of a stiff tracheal tube, hyperextension of the neck, violent movements of the head and neck, traction on the trachea, or overinflation of the cuff (439). In one case, the trachea was ruptured because the cuff was connected to a jet ventilation device (716). If airway rupture is suspected, it is essential to establish a diagnosis by bronchoscopy.

Murphy Eye Complications

Anything passed down the tracheal tube such as a suction catheter, tube exchanger, or fiberscope can pass through a Murphy eye and become caught (Fig. 17.30). It may be impossible to remove the device without also removing the tracheal tube (717).

Laser-Induced Tracheal Tube Fire

A fire is one of the most serious hazards of laser surgery. All of the three necessary components are present: a combustible substance (tracheal tube), an ignition source (laser), and gas to support combustion (oxygen).

Physics of Lasers (718, 719)

A laser is a source of light that results from the stimulation of atoms, ions, or molecules (the laser medium) by electrical, optical, or thermal energy. The stimulated laser medium gives off energy in the form of light, which is then amplified and emitted as the laser beam. This light has three important characteristics that account for specific interaction between it and tissues: coherence (all waves are in phase in both time and space); collimation (all waves are traveling in parallel directions); and monochromaticity (all waves are of the same wavelength).

A laser system (Fig. 17.31) has four compo-

nents: a laser medium, an optical cavity, a light guide, and a pumping source.

Laser medium. The name of the laser refers to the type of material used as the laser medium. The laser medium, which may be a solid, liquid, or gas, determines the wavelength of the emitted radiation.

The optical cavity. The optical (resonator) cavity provides the environment in which the laser medium is confined. Energy released from the medium travels in all directions. Mirrors are used to reflect and increase the energy of the stimulated emission. One of the mirrors is not 100% reflective and allows the beam to escape.

Pumping source. The pumping source supplies energy to the laser medium. Solid lasers are usually pumped by high-energy photons from a xenon flash lamp. Lasers that use a gaseous medium are pumped by electric discharge through the gas.

Light guide. A light guide directs the laser beam to the surgical site. It may be a hollow tube with mirrors aligned to reflect the beam from its source through the focusing lens. This method is used for wavelengths in the long infrared range such as the CO_2 laser. A flexible fiberoptic guide is used for visible and near-infrared wavelengths.

For surgical procedures that do not require a "no touch" technique, there are special heat-resistant contact probes with a sapphire scalpel. It

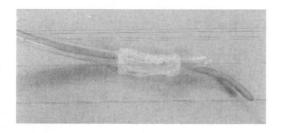

FIGURE 17.30. The tube changer has become caught in the Murphy eye.

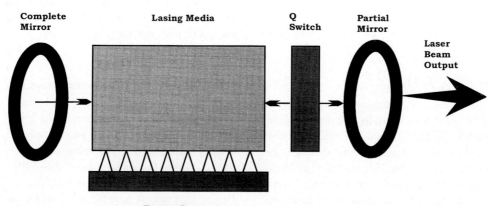

FIGURE 17.31. Laser system. The central component is the laser media which may be a solid, liquid, or gas. The energy pump provides the means to excite the lasing atoms into producing laser light. The mirrors boost lasing efficiency. The mirror on the right is not 100% reflective, allowing the beam to eventually escape.

has a coaxial cooling system which works from compressed gas or a liquid jet.

Types (249, 718, 720)

Carbon Dioxide Laser

The CO_2 laser has been widely used for surgery in the upper airway. The CO_2 laser beam is invisible so it must be used with a helium-neon aiming beam as a marker.

Nd-YAG Laser

In the Nd-YAG laser the medium is a solid rod of material. Its short wavelength allows the beam to be transmitted by fiberoptic fibers. Because it is taken up by pigment, colored markings on tracheal tubes are more likely to be damaged than clear portions (102, 721). Blood or mucus on or in the tracheal tube makes the tube less resistant to the laser beam (721). Fires from a Nd-YAG laser passed through a channel of a flexible bronchoscope have been reported (722–724).

KTP Laser

The KTP laser can be transmitted by fiberoptic bundles. It is often used with a Nd-YAG laser. It passes through clear substances but is absorbed by hemoglobin. Pigments react instantly with the KTP laser.

Argon Laser

The argon laser medium is a gas. This laser has been used during neurosurgery, retinal and otolaryngological surgery, and treatment of cutaneous lesions. It can be transmitted by fiberoptic bundles. Prolonged exposure of PVC or red rubber tubes to the argon laser causes minimal damage (725).

Fires (719, 111)

The cuff, tube, or cottonoids are usually the combustible substance. Initially, the surface of the tube burns. If the burn extends through the tube, the oxygen-enriched gases flowing through the tube may produce a blowtorch-like flame and heat and the products of combustion will be blown into the lungs. If the cuff bursts, oxygen and anesthetic gases will flood the operative site.

The flammability of tubes differs. Polyvinyl chloride tubes do not reflect laser light, nor do they retain and transfer heat. They have a higher index of flammability and so requires a higher concentration of oxygen to sustain a flame than other tubes. Despite the advantages of PVC tubes, they can ignite if excess laser exposure and/or power density occurs, and once ignited, can sustain a torch-like flame.

Red rubber tubes sustain combustion more readily than PVC tubes in room air. Red rubber is thus susceptible to extra luminal fires, but because it is more resistance to the CO_2 laser than PVC, intraluminal fires are less likely to occur. A problem with red rubber tubes is their opacity. Should an intraluminal fire develop, it may go undetected for a longer period of time than with a PVC tube. An advantage to red rubber tubes is that, if ignited, they are less likely than PVC to soften, deform, or fragment.

Silicone, much like red rubber, can ignite in room air. If ignited, it rapidly becomes a brittle ash that crumbles easily.

The cuff is the most vulnerable part of the tracheal tube. It cannot be wrapped, and laser-resistant tubes do not have laser-resistant cuffs.

The tube may be exposed to either the direct or reflected laser beam. Flaming tissue in close proximity to the tube may ignite it (267). The interior surface of a tube can be ignited by burning pieces of tissue inhaled into the tube.

In addition to the tracheal tube, tape that is used to secure the tube can ignite. The more oxygen-enriched the atmosphere is, the more likely this is to occur. Not all tapes combust at the same rate with the CO_2 laser. Ointments and gels do not ignite with the CO_2 laser (726).

Minimizing Risk

Low Inspired Oxygen Concentrations (727)

Nitrogen, air, or helium should be used to reduce the oxygen concentration to the lowest level that will provide acceptable patient oxygenation. Nitrous oxide supports combustion and should not be used as the diluent gas (728–730). While helium may delay ignition better than nitrogen, the fire that occurs may be more severe with helium (731, 732). Using helium does decrease the resistance of the gases passing through the tracheal tube. This is important since smaller tubes are frequently used for laser surgery (733, 734).

Although using low inspired oxygen concentrations will make ignition less likely to occur, it will not totally prevent it. If there is a significant leak, the anesthesia provider may fill the reservoir bag by pushing the oxygen flush (727). This will result in an elevated oxygen concentration. If there is a leak, a more appropriate response would be to increase the fresh gas flow while maintaining the same inspired oxygen concentration or to replace the tracheal tube.

Laser Protocol (719, 727, 735–737)

A laser protocol should be developed and followed in the area where the laser will be used. Lasers should always be kept in the standby mode except when ready to use, so that inadvertent activation does not occur.

Power density (irradiance) is the rate at which laser energy is delivered per unit of irradiated surface in watts per square centimeter (24, 111). The least power density that will do the job should be used.

Filling the Cuff with Saline

If a laser beam penetrates an air-filled cuff, gas can leak into the operative field and, if the oxygen concentration is high, the risk of fire is increased.

Fluid in a cuff acts as a heat sink and makes the cuff less easy to perforate (738, 739). If the cuff is perforated, a jet of fluid may extinguish the fire (740). Addition of methylene blue or other biocompatible and highly visible dye to the saline will help the surgeon to recognize a perforated cuff.

Filling the tracheal tube cuff with a 2% lidocaine jelly-plus-saline mixture not only prevents the cuff from being ignited with the CO_2 laser but has also been found to plug small holes in the cuff which may have resulted from a laser hit (741).

Care must be taken to remove all air from the cuff, because any remaining air will settle in the most superior part of the cuff, which is the part most likely to be hit by the laser beam (102). As a further precaution, cottonoids or pledgets, which must be kept wet, should be placed on the cuff (742). It is important that they be kept moist. Insults from the laser beam may dry them, so that they lose their protective properties. Further hits can cause the cottonoids and/or the cuff to ignite (262). The cottonoids must be carefully retrieved after surgery.

Protective Wrappings

The tube can be covered with a protective wrapping. These were discussed earlier in this chapter.

Use of Special Tubes

Special ready-to-use laser-resistant tubes were discussed earlier in this chapter. Tubes sold for laser use should indicate the type of laser for which they are suited as well as the conditions (power, power density, spot size, and/or oxygen concentration) under which the tube is safe to use. Strict adherence to manufacturer's warnings and directions is highly advisable. A disadvantage is that these tubes are 10 to 30 times more expensive than PVC and red rubber tubes (111).

Use of Positive End-Expiratory Pressure

PEEP can reduce the risk of fire in PVC tubes with the CO_2 laser (743).

Other

The tube should be loosely fixed to the patient so that it can be removed rapidly if necessary (722, 735). The patient should not be excessively draped. Nonflammable drapes and operating room attire should be used. A container of water should be available to douse any flames.

Action in Case of Fire (106, 249, 744)

The entire operating room team should be vigilant whenever the laser is used in or near the airway and well-rehearsed in a protocol to follow in case of a fire.

If a fire occurs, the breathing system should be disconnected from the tracheal tube to stop gas flow. The tube and protective devices should be removed immediately. With plastic tubes, deflation of the saline-filled cuff by aspiration may be faster than cutting the pilot tube (745). With red rubber tubes, unclamping the pilot tube is fastest. The fire should be extinguished with saline or by smothering it with a wet towel. Alcohol or other flammable fluids should not be used.

The airway should be reestablished and the patient ventilated with air until it is certain that nothing remains burning, then 100% oxygen should be used. A search for fragments that remain in the trachea and assessment of damage to the larynx and tracheobronchial tree should be made.

Cautery-Induced Tracheal Tube Fire

Electrocautery is often used in the mouth in proximity to the tracheal tube. If this touches the tracheal tube, a fire can occur (746).

Tracheal Tube Obstruction (473)

One reason for insertion of a tracheal tube is to provide a patent airway. Unfortunately, the tube itself may become the cause of obstruction. In infants and children, serious tracheal tube obstruction occurs in 4% to 5% of intubations (747).

The obstruction can be partial or complete. It is possible to have a ball valve obstruction so that inspiration is unimpeded, but resistance to expiration is increased (58, 748–775).

An obstruction may present as a decrease in compliance, high inspiratory pressures with controlled ventilation, or wheezing resembling bronchospasm (752). Paradoxical movements may be seen in spontaneously breathing patients (439). If the patient inhales against an obstruction, a high negative intrathoracic pressure may be generated. This can result in pulmonary edema (753–755). A problem that permits inhalation but prevents exhalation may present as circulatory collapse or barotrauma (589, 756).

Causes

Biting

Unless protection in the form of an airway or bite block is provided, the patient may bite the tube (69, 72–74, 76, 757, 758). Many of the reported cases involve spiral embedded tubes that were permanently deformed after the bite was released (759–765). An oral airway may not prevent obstruction (762). Care should be taken to prevent the tube from slipping between the molar teeth where occlusion may occur in spite of an airway or bite block. A hemostat applied at 90° to the occlusion may relieve the obstruction (765).

Kinking

Kinking is a relatively common cause of tracheal tube obstruction. Spiral embedded tubes have been used to overcome this problem, but kinking can still occur at the patient end if the connector is not inserted inside the spirals (56).

Kinking may occur where the connector joins the tube due to the weight of bulky connections (766, 767).

Kinking sometimes occurs when the position of the patient's head is changed, especially when the neck is flexed (768–771). It also can occur when a tube is moved from one side of the mouth to other without ensuring that the entire tube has been moved (407).

Tracheal tubes may become entrapped in other equipment in the mouth. Obstruction from a Boyle-Davis mouth gag has been reported (772, 773).

Tubes vary in their resistance to kinking. Smaller tubes kink more readily than larger ones. This can be remedied by placing a larger tube over the small one (774, 775). If a larger tube kinks, a smaller tube may be passed through it (770). A structural fault in the tube such as at the point where the inflating tube enters the wall of the tube (776) or in the intracuff area (777) can predispose to kinking.

When tubes are wrapped for laser surgery, they may become occluded as a result of compression by the foil as the tube accommodates to the curvature of the posterior pharynx (252).

When inserting a tracheal tube through a tracheostomy stoma, the tube may bend back on itself (778)

Material in the Lumen of the Tube

A tracheal tube may be obstructed by dried secretions, blood, pus, debris, tumor, or other tissue (456, 473, 675, 751, 779–791).

Foreign bodies reported in occluded tracheal tubes have included foam rubber from a mask (792), an inflation valve (793), a cleaning brush (794), an adapter from an intravenous set (795), an intravenous needle (796), a stop from a stylet (797), a cork (798), a glass ampule (799), pieces of plastic (750, 800–802), part of a nasogastric tube (802), an oral medication tablet (803), a smaller tracheal tube (804), part of a paper towel (805), part of a sampling tube (473), and dead organisms (806, 807). A manufacturing defect can cause obstruction (808).

The patency of the tubes and connectors should be checked prior to use. Solutions or lubricants that can form film barriers including cellulose products such as lidocaine jelly should be prevented from entering the lumen (809). If it is necessary to reconnect the tracheal tube and connector, these products should not be used.

Spiral Embedded Tubes

In some spiral embedded tubes, the part of the tube distal to the cuff has no spirals. This part may be soft and easily occluded.

Overuse and repeated sterilization of reusable spiral-embedded tubes can predispose to problems. Insertion of a connector can cause the inside of the tube to pucker up and occlude the lumen (810). The inner wall may become detached (59, 811).

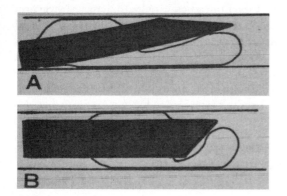

FIGURE 17.32. Two causes of tracheal tube obstruction. **A,** the bevel is pushed against the wall of the trachea by an eccentrically inflated cuff. **B,** the cuff has ballooned over the end of the tube.

During manufacture, air bubbles may form between the layers. If these tubes are gas-sterilized or steam autoclaved with vacuum, blebs may form (66). During anesthesia, nitrous oxide may diffuse into the blebs and cause swelling or gas from the cuff to enter the space between layers. Herniation into the tube lumen will cause obstruction (62, 64, 811–814).

Bevel Abutting against the Tracheal Wall

The bevel may impinge against the wall of the trachea (Figs. 17.32 and 17.33) (56, 129, 473, 748, 785, 815–817). In many of these cases, the cuff inflated eccentrically (see Fig. 17.28). If the tube has a Murphy eye, ventilation may continue (785).

An unusual cause of obstruction involving the Endotrol tube was reported (95). When it was inserted nasally, the loop on the pull cord abutted against the nares, causing the tip of the tube to bend and obstruct against the tracheal wall. The problem was solved by cutting the pull cord.

In infants, when the tube orifice faces in one direction and the infant's head is turned to the other, the orifice may abut against the tracheal wall (818). This occurs more readily with higher tube positions and/or neck flexion. Displacement of the trachea by the aortic arch may cause the bevel to lie against the tracheal wall (819–821).

With Forestier's disease there is hyperostosis of the anterior vertebral body in the cervical and lumbar areas. The osteophytes can cause deviation

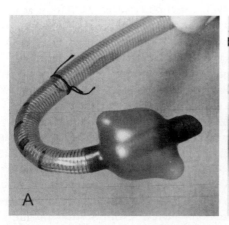
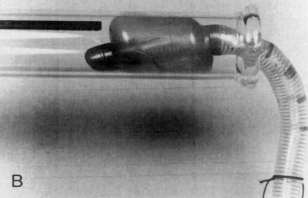

FIGURE 17.33. Tracheal tube obstruction secondary to eccentric cuff inflation. **A,** the cuff as removed from the patient. **B,** when placed in a glass tube, the inflated cuff pushes the bevel toward the wall of the tube.

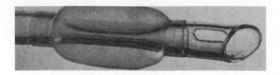

FIGURE 17.34. Reduction of tube lumen by cuff. Inflation of the cuff caused narrowing of the tube lumen.

of the trachea on extension of the neck, directing the bevel against the tracheal wall (822).

Obstruction by the Cuff

It is possible for an inflated cuff to balloon over the tip of the tube (61, 473, 823–825) (see Fig. 17.27). Inflation of the cuff may cause compression of the tube lumen (Fig. 17.34) (69, 826–836). Obstruction from these causes may not occur for some time after initial cuff inflation.

Cases have been reported in which a feeding tube was connected to the cuff inflation system (823, 837, 838). This can cause the cuff to overdistend and obstruct the tube.

External Compression

A case has been reported in which a tube was forced through an obstruction in the nose by a turbinate. This caused lateral compression of the tube (839). Another case of compression occurred when a suction catheter became knotted around a tracheal tube (840). A nearby surgical retractor can cause obstruction (841).

External tracheal tube compression has been reported in a patient with Ludwig's angina (49). In the anatomical abnormality known as "saber-sheath" trachea, the trachea is densely calcified and "C" shaped. In a reported case in which the trachea was intubated with a double-lumen tube, the "C" portion of the trachea obstructed the tracheal lumen (842). Additional air in the tracheal tube cuff might have alleviated the problem (843).

Defective Connector

If the connector is defective or damaged on insertion, it can partially or completely obstruct the lumen (844–850). A connector partially obstructed by plastic film has been reported (851).

Prevention

Prevention of tracheal tube obstruction starts with the choice of tube. Transparent tubes facilitate identification of material or objects blocking the lumen. Use of a fenestrated (Murphy) tube may avoid some cases of obstruction. A spiral embedded tube may be advisable if an operation involves turning the head or other maneuvers that may cause kinking. Spiral embedded tubes should not be reused.

The tracheal tube should be examined carefully before use and the patency of the lumen verified. Foreign bodies and other problems inside the lumen can be detected by inserting a stylet. The cuff should be examined to make certain it is securely attached and inflates symmetrically. The lumen should not be reduced nor should the cuff balloon over the end of the tube when it is inflated. It may be necessary to rotate and examine the tube from several angles to detect obstruction (827). After insertion, the cuff should be inflated as described earlier in this chapter. Cuff pressure should be readjusted frequently, especially if nitrous oxide is used. When an X-ray is taken, the position of the orifice and the configuration of the cuff should be examined.

Biting of the tube may be prevented by using an oral airway or a bite block, maintaining an adequate level of anesthesia, and securing the tracheal tube at the center of the mouth.

Various methods have been described to avoid kinking of the tube due to traction on it (755, 767, 852–854).

Once inserted, the tube should not be withdrawn while the cuff is inflated, as this may cause the cuff to balloon over the end of the tube.

When secretions are heard, they should be removed with a suction catheter. Humidifying the inspired gases will prevent drying of secretions. This is especially important with long intubations and small tubes. Secretions that cannot be removed in this way may be removed using an embolectomy or Foley catheter (855–857).

Diagnosis and Treatment (785)

Early diagnosis is important. Often obstruction occurs slowly as with gradual kinking of the tube. Pressure-volume loops (Chapter 19, "Airway Pressure, Volume, and Flow Measurements") will be altered with obstruction. Peak inspiratory pressure commonly increases with obstruction.

If there is time, the tube should be checked for kinking, either by feeling with a gloved finger or by direct vision using a laryngoscope. Passing a fiberscope down the tube may facilitate diagnosis.

Passage of a suction catheter or stylet down the tube may be helpful. Digital pressure on the site of a kink may relieve the obstruction (856). Alteration of the patient's head position may help. If these simple maneuvers are unsuccessful, the cuff should be deflated and/or the tube rotated.

If the above steps cannot be performed quickly and the patient's condition is deteriorating, the tube should be removed.

Aspiration of Gastric Contents

Although it is generally assumed that a tracheal tube will protect the lungs from the entry of foreign material, aspiration is a common occurrence in patients with artificial airways (858–859A). The incidence is increased by the following.

Use of Low-Pressure Cuffs (198, 199, 859)

The baseline intracuff pressure is significantly lower in high-volume, low-pressure cuffs than low-volume, high-pressure cuffs. Many low-pressure cuffs wrinkle despite proper inflation and fluid can pass along the folds. Infolding can be decreased by increasing the pressure in the cuff, using a thin-walled cuff, and using a tube whose cuff diameter at residual volume approximates the internal diameter of the trachea (142, 145, 186, 198). Lubricant jelly applied to the cuff may fill in the folds (198).

Spontaneous Ventilation (145, 197, 860)

With thin-walled cuffs, a negative airway pressure will be transmitted to the cuff during inspiration. In addition, the trachea tends to dilate during spontaneous inspiration.

Accumulation of Fluid above the Cuff

Frequent suctioning to maintain a clear oropharynx will decrease the pressure exerted by fluid above the cuff. It has been suggested that the cuff be placed just below the vocal cords to reduce the volume of fluid that cannot be removed by suctioning. If the cuff is just below the cords, however, movement of the head may cause the tube to move upward, causing the cuff to exert pressure

on the cords and increasing the risk of inadvertent extubation. Furthermore, a cuff placed just below the cords may compress nerve endings against the thyroid cartilage, resulting in vocal cord paralysis.

Head-Up Position

If the pharynx is filled with fluid when the patient is in a head-up position, the hydrostatic pressure exerted on the cuff will be higher than if the patient is supine.

Use of Uncuffed Tubes (861)

The incidence of aspiration may be as high as 80% in patients with uncuffed tubes (862). PEEP may lower the incidence but cannot totally prevent aspiration (860, 862).

Aspiration can occur upon extubation. Fluid can accumulate above the cuff. Pharyngeal suction may not remove all this fluid and it can find its way into the lungs when the cuff is deflated before extubation. Recommendations to avoid this include withdrawing the inflated cuff until it impinges on the lower surface of the vocal cords, placing the patient in a head down and lateral position before cuff deflation, and deflating the cuff during the application of positive airway pressure to blow material collected above the cuff into the pharynx where it can be removed by suctioning (387).

Aspiration can occur after extubation. Laryngeal function is disturbed for at least 4 hours after tracheal extubation, whether or not residual anesthetic effects are present (863).

Misplacement of Other Equipment into the Trachea

A tracheal tube keeps the glottis open, making it easier to pass other equipment into the tracheobronchial tree (201–203, 205–207, 675, 864). Misplaced items have included nasogastric tubes, esophageal stethoscopes, ECG leads, and temperature probes. If the tube is open there will be loss of gas (865). If suction is attached to the tube, the loss will be magnified.

A case has been reported in which a nasogastric tube previously in the stomach was found in the lung after a tracheal tube was changed (866). It was surmised that the nasogastric tube was pulled out of the stomach during the tube change and entered the trachea beside the tracheal tube.

CT and MRI Scan Artifacts

Artifacts may be seen on a CT scan when radiopaque markers are present on tracheal tubes. Tubes without these markers are available and should be used for this application (867, 868).

The metallic spring in the inflation device of a plastic tube can cause an artifact on an MRI scan (869–871). Repositioning it away from the patient will usually solve the problem.

Wire-reinforced tracheal tubes will cause image distortion when used in an MRI. Nylon reinforced tubes are recommended for this application (872).

Accidental Extubation

Accidental dislocation of a tracheal tube from the trachea is at best a nuisance and at worst a life-threatening emergency. It occurs more commonly in smaller patients (873).

Extension or lateral rotation of the neck can cause cephalad movement of the tube (586, 587, 591, 602, 874). This movement is increased with nasal intubation (305). Certain positions can create a pull on the tube.

Another cause is positioning the cuff between or just below the cords. Distention of the cuff as a result of overinflation or diffusion of nitrous oxide may cause it to herniate upward. This may result in failure to achieve a seal. A likely response is to inject more air into the cuff. If the cuff is at or just above the vocal cords, this may cause the tube to move farther out of the trachea.

Use of antidisconnect devices may increase the danger of inadvertent extubation. It may be preferable for the connection between the tube and the breathing system to give way under strain than to permit the tube to be pulled out.

During insertion, a nasogastric tube may form a knot around the tracheal tube, and the tracheal tube may be removed with it (875, 876). If a mouth gag that has a groove for a tube is used, the tube can become wedged into this groove and it may not be possible to remove the gag without removing the tracheal tube (831).

To prevent dislodgement, the tube should be positioned with the tip in the middle third of the trachea with the neck in a neutral position. It has been suggested that manufacturers place a mark 2 to 4 cm above the proximal end of the cuff for positioning at the vocal cords to ensure placement in the middle third of the trachea (347). Careful observation should be made for leakage, which may indicate that the cuff is located at the level of the vocal cords. A cuff that requires frequent inflation should suggest that it may be situated between instead of below the level of the cords.

Once properly positioned, the tube should be well secured. Fixation to the lower lip may be safer than fixation to the upper lip (874). Pull on the tube should be avoided. Use of an RAE tube may decrease the incidence of accidental extubation (9). Care should be taken to avoid accidental extubation when the patient is repositioned.

Bacteremia

A high incidence of sinusitis and otitis during and following nasotracheal intubation has been reported (306, 308–312, 326, 877, 878). For this reason a head injury is considered a relative contraindication to nasotracheal intubation. Oral intubation is associated with a lower incidence (879). With long-term intubation, the rates of nosocomial sinusitis and pneumonia do not differ significantly between oral and nasal intubation (880).

Difficulty in Extubation

Difficulty in removing a tracheal tube at the end of a procedure is a rare but potentially dangerous problem. The most common cause is failure to deflate the cuff. This is most often due to obstruction of the inflation tube. If the obstruction is distal to the pilot balloon, the balloon will offer no clue that the cuff has not deflated (881). Heat from a laser or a drill may melt the inflating tube, causing it to occlude (528, 882, 883). Biting by the patient may cause the inflating tube to be occluded (214). Some users pull the pilot balloon and inflation valve from the inflation tube to deflate the cuff. This can cause the inflation tube to seal (392–394). The connector may occlude the inflation tube if it fits below the point where the tube leaves the wall of the tracheal tube (216, 247, 884). The pilot tube may be kinked by a retaining bandage (462, 885, 886). Cases of difficult extubation in which the inflating tube became entangled with a nasogastric tube or turbinate have been reported (887, 888).

A fold or flange in the cuff may impede extubation (889–895). With a sponge cuff, deflation will be difficult if the inflation tube is cut or detached (214, 215). A case has been reported in which the cuff of a tracheal tube became transfixed by a tracheostomy tube (671).

Another cause of difficult extubation is surgical transfixation of the tube to adjacent tissues (896–900). In this case, forcibly removing the tube could lead to fatal consequences. If this is the cause of the difficult extubation, the tube will not move up and down easily in the trachea.

Often the cause of a difficult extubation can be detected by using a flexible fiberoptic scope (900).

In cases in which it is impossible to deflate the cuff, a V-shaped cut can be made in the inflation tube to relieve the pressure in the cuff (394). It may be possible to insert a syringe and needle into the stump of the pilot tube and deflate the cuff. If the cuff still remains inflated, the tube should be pulled until the cuff is close to the surface of the vocal cords. A needle can then be inserted through the cricothyroid membrane, puncturing the cuff (901). Alternately, the tube can be withdrawn so that the cuff is seen below the cords and punctured with a sharp object (902). Removal may be aided by relaxing the vocal cords and/or tube rotation (462, 489, 903). Reinsertion, rotation, and traction of the tube or manipulation of the larynx may cause the cuff to smooth out. Skin hooks or forceps may be necessary to free the tube.

Postoperative Sore Throat

Sore throat is common after intubation. The reported incidence varies from 6% to 90% (176, 181, 398, 904–909). It has also been reported in 10 to 22% of unintubated patients (175, 176, 181, 907). Use of a nasogastric tube may also cause a sore throat (910).

Sore throat is more common in females when blood is found in the airway after operations involving the head and neck and when the patient is in the prone position (174, 175, 681, 909, 911, 912). Use of larger tubes is associated with a higher incidence (913–915). Some studies have shown a higher incidence with "difficult" intubation, but other studies have shown no correlation.

Straining on the tube may increase the number of complaints (916). Duration of intubation and age have been found to have little effect (174, 175, 181, 915). Limiting intracuff pressure will decrease the incidence (911, 917).

Studies looking at the effect of topical lidocaine, steroids, and lubricants on the cuff on sore throat offer conflicting evidence (174, 176, 181, 906, 907, 918–923). One study determined that sore throat was less likely if the tube were coated with EMLA cream (a eutectic of 2.5% lidocaine and 2.5% prilocaine) than if lidocaine were used, but there was no difference between the EMLA-treated patients and those who had an untreated tube (924). Most studies show that an increase in cuff-to-trachea contact area increases the incidence of sore throat (118, 178, 181, 502, 915, 920, 925), although one study showed conflicting results (926). The incidence is high with the sponge cuff (118). If the cuff is inflated with a lidocaine solution, the lidocaine will diffuse through the cuff and decrease the incidence and severity of sore throat (927).

Hoarseness after Intubation

The incidence of hoarseness following intubation for surgical procedures has been reported as being between 4 and 67% (914, 918, 921, 928–930). Its incidence may be decreased by using tubes with low-pressure cuffs, smaller tubes, and lubrication with lidocaine jelly (914, 918, 931) and increased with difficult intubation and duration of intubation. Hoarseness that is persistent or that develops later in the postoperative period should be investigated.

Nerve Injuries

Trigeminal, lingual, buccal, and hypoglossal nerve palsies have been reported following short-term intubation (932–935).

Upper Airway Edema

Edema may occur anywhere along the path of the tube, including the tongue, lingual follicles, uvula, epiglottis, aryepiglottic folds, ventricular folds, vocal cords, and the retroarytenoid and subglottic spaces (194, 407, 462, 936–943). The floor of the mouth can swell secondary to purulent sialadenitis from a submandibular duct obstructed by a tracheal tube (944).

Laryngeal edema is also called postintubation croup, uvular edema postintubation inflammation, acute edematous stenosis, stridor, or subglottic edema. The edema encroaches on the airway lumen, increasing airway resistance, especially in the young child, in whom a mild degree of edema may produce a significant reduction in the internal cross-sectional area. Because the cricoid cartilage completely surrounds the subglottic region, no external expansion of the swollen tissues may occur so edema here not infrequently necessitates emergency reintubation or tracheostomy.

Laryngeal edema has a peak incidence between 1 and 4 years of age (945). It is most commonly seen after surgery involving the head and neck and surgery performed with the patient positioned other than supinely. It is more common in adult women than adult men (946). It may manifest itself any time during the first 48 hours after extubation. Usually, the first signs are evident 1 to 2 hours postoperatively. In its mildest form, there is hoarseness or croupy cough. In more severe cases, respiratory obstruction will occur. Decompensation can be rapid.

Inflammation (including preexisting inflammation of the larynx, bacterial contamination, and chemical irritation), mechanical trauma (from inadequate anesthesia or muscle relaxation, roughness, use of too large a tube or motion secondary to movement of the head or neck, bucking, and swallowing), and allergic reactions to the tube itself or materials used in lubrication or sterilization have been postulated as mechanisms.

Prevention begins with avoiding irritant stimuli, particularly an oversized tracheal tube. If there is an upper respiratory infection, use of a face mask or laryngeal mask should be strongly considered. A leak around the tube may help to minimize croup (947). Tubes, sprays, and lubricants used on the tubes should be sterile. Intubation should be atraumatic and adequate anesthetic depth and/ or good muscle relaxation should be maintained to prevent movement of the tube. Movements of the head should be kept to a minimum.

Vocal Cord Dysfunction

Vocal cord paralysis and paresis have been reported after tracheal intubation in spite of the intubation being atraumatic and the site of the surgery remote from the head and neck (438, 657, 948–959). Vocal cord paralysis can be unilateral or bilateral. Most cases resolve spontaneously, usually within days or weeks but it may be long term (959, 960).

Vocal cord dysfunction is more likely to occur in women (961). It has been reported with both high- and low-pressure cuffs. It may originate from pressure exerted by the inflated cuff on branches of the recurrent laryngeal nerve (948, 950, 962, 963). The most susceptible area of the nerve is 6 to 10 mm below the vocal cords (347, 949). Positioning the tube just below the cords may increase the incidence of this problem. High cuff pressure may contribute to the damage.

Ulcerations

Ulcerations (erosions) of the larynx and trachea are common, even when a tube has been in place for only a short time. The incidence and severity increase with the duration of intubation (964).

Ulcers are most commonly found on the posterior parts of the larynx and the anterior and lateral aspects of the trachea at the sites of the cuff and the tube tip (572, 965–967). They vary from superficial lesions involving only the mucosa to deep ones in which the underlying cartilage is exposed. The end result will depend on the location and severity as well as other factors, such as infection, that affect the healing process. If the ulcer is superficial, regeneration to normal epithelium occurs relatively quickly (968). When the damage is deeper, the regeneration follows the same pattern as for the superficial damage but is more protracted. If the ulcer is very deep, scar tissue may form.

Cases of uvular necrosis have been reported (969–971).

Granuloma of Vocal Cord

The incidence of granuloma of the vocal cords (postintubation, contact ulcer, intubation or postanesthesia granuloma) varies from 1 in 800 to 1 in 20,000 intubations. Most cases are in adults, and they are more common in women. The highest incidence is associated with head and neck surgery.

Symptoms include persistent hoarseness, intermittent loss of voice, pain or discomfort in the throat, a feeling of fullness or tension in the throat, chronic cough, hemoptysis, and pain extending to the ear. Some cases are symptomless. Occasionally, respiratory obstruction is seen. Symptoms may start after intubation or may not develop for as long as several months.

A number of prophylactic measures have been suggested, including use of a proper sized tube and gentle intubation as well as avoiding friction between the tube and larynx by a proper depth of anesthesia or use of muscle relaxants. A short period of vocal rest following intubation has been recommended (972).

Persistent hoarseness after intubation warrants laryngeal examination to exclude the presence of a lesion. If the examination reveals ulceration over the vocal processes, the development of a granuloma may be prevented by strict voice rest to allow healing to take place.

Laryngotracheal Membrane

Formation of a laryngotracheal membrane (subglottic membrane, membranous or pseudomembranous laryngotracheitis, or pseudomembrane) is an uncommon but serious and sometimes fatal complication. A portion of the membrane may become detached, leading to sudden respiratory obstruction (973–975). Most cases follow an intubation lasting a few hours. In some cases, the intubation was traumatic, but in others, no problems were encountered. Clinically, the picture is one of respiratory obstruction, resembling laryngeal edema with cough, hoarseness, stridor, dyspnea, and suprasternal retractions. The symptoms typically occur 24 to 72 hours after extubation (973–975).

If this is not immediately and appropriately treated, it may lead to sudden death. Diagnosis is made by laryngoscopy, followed by bronchoscopy. Unless visualization of the larynx is performed, the condition may be erroneously diagnosed as edema, and an unnecessary tracheostomy performed.

Treatment is removal by suction. Removal may not be easy because areas of epithelium still attached to the underlying tissue may be present. If the entire membrane is not removed, it may recur in 24 hours (973).

Glottic and Subglottic Granulation Tissue

Ulcers in the subglottic region may give rise to granulation tissue (15, 194, 976–980). Their principal importance is that they may cause respiratory obstruction. The onset of symptoms may be immediately after extubation or may be delayed for up to several weeks.

Diagnosis is made by laryngoscopy and/or bronchoscopy. Steroids should be administered. Usually, the granulation tissue will regress and may disappear, but occasionally removal is required. Recurrence is quite common.

Nasal Damage

Ulcerations or necrosis of the nasal alae and/or the skin on the bridge of the nose are occasional sequelae of nasotracheal intubation (981, 982). This can be prevented by securing the tube so that there is no undue pressure on the nostril (see Fig. 17.29).

Tracheal Stenosis

While tracheal stenosis is usually thought to be a complication of prolonged tracheal intubation, it may be associated with an intubation as short as 18 hours (983).

Latex Allergy

While most tracheal tubes are made from PVC, some laser tubes are made from latex-containing rubber. A careful history should be taken and proper precautions undertaken if these tubes are used. Latex allergy is discussed in Chapter 13, "Hazards of Anesthesia Machines and Breathing Systems."

DOUBLE-LUMEN TUBES
Indications (921)
Thoracic Procedures

Deflating the lung provides better operating conditions and reduces trauma during thoracic procedures (984–986). The ability to alternate easily and quickly between lung collapse and inflation can help the surgeon visualize lung morphology and facilitates identification of lobar or intersegmental planes. Thoracoscopic procedures require deflation of the lung (987, 988).

Control of Contamination

Use of a DLT can prevent infected material from one lung from contaminating the other lung.

Control of Hemorrhage (774, 780, 990, 991)

When hemorrhage occurs in one lung, a DLT allows ventilation of the unaffected lung to be maintained.

Bronchopleural or Bronchopleuralcutaneous Fistula or Air Cyst (989, 992–996)

A bronchopleural fistula may have such a low resistance to gas flow that most of the tidal volume will flow through it and it will be impossible to ventilate the other lung adequately. A unilateral air cyst or bulla may have a valvular opening and can become overinflated when controlled ventilation is initiated. A DLT allows isolation of the lung or section of lung with the fistula or cyst from the ventilatory volume (997).

Tracheobronchial Tree Disruption

Positive pressure ventilation of a lung with a tracheobronchial tree disruption can result in dissection of gas into the pulmonary interstitial spaces or mediastinum. Use of a DLT allows isolation of the section with the disruption.

Other Indications

Independent (differential) lung ventilation may be useful in the treatment of unilateral pulmonary pathology (998–1002). Unilateral bronchopulmonary lavage and selective pulmonary toilet can be performed using a DLT.

Contraindications

Relative contraindications to the use of DLTs include patients who have a lesion (airway narrowing or endoluminal tumor) somewhere along the pathway of the DLT, small patients in whom a DLT would be too large, patients who will not tolerate being taken off mechanical ventilation even for a short period of time, and those with life-threatening conditions in whom there is insufficient time to insert a DLT. In patients with cystic

fibrosis, it may be difficult to clear the thick secretions from a double lumen tube (1003).

Anatomical Considerations

The right mainstem bronchus is shorter, straighter, and has a larger diameter than the left. It takes off from the trachea at an angle of 25° in adults. The left mainstem bronchus diverges from the median plane at a 45° angle. These angles are slightly larger in children (1004).

These anatomic considerations mean that it is easier to intubate the right mainstem bronchus than the left. However, it is difficult to place a tube in the right mainstem bronchus without obstructing the right upper lobe orifice.

Design
Connector (1001, 1005–1007)

The connector must allow attachment of the two lumens to the breathing system as well as one-lung ventilation, differential ventilation of each lung, application of PEEP to only one lung, differential PEEP to both lungs, and one-lung fiberoptic bronchoscopy. Typical connectors are shown in Figures 17.35, 17.41, 17.47 and 17.48.

Tube

The DLT is essentially two tubes bonded together. Each is designated either right- or left-sided, depending on which mainstem bronchus the bronchial segment is designed to fit. The tracheal lumen is designed to terminate above the carina and the bronchial segment to extend into the appropriate mainstem bronchus. The distal portion of the bronchial segment is angled to fit into a mainstem bronchus.

There may be a carinal hook to aid in proper placement and minimize tube movement after placement. Potential problems with carinal hooks include increased difficulty during intubation, trauma to the airway, malposition of the tube because of the hook, and interference with bronchial closure during pneumonectomy. The hook can break off and become lost in the bronchial tree.

Most manufacturers place radiopaque markers at the bottom of the tracheal cuff or at the end of the tracheal lumen. Other marks may be placed above and below the bronchial cuff. PVC double-lumen tubes are supplied in sterile packages, which include a stylet, connectors, suction catheters, and often a means to supply continuous positive airway pressure.

Cuffs

The tracheal cuff is located just above the tracheal orifice and the bronchial cuff just above the termination of the bronchial segment. Some right-sided DLTs have two bronchial cuffs. The bronchial cuff is shorter than the tracheal cuff. The bronchial cuff for the right-sided tubes varies in shape, depending on the manufacturer. On some tubes, the cuff has a slot to allow ventilation of the right upper lobe. The resting volume and compliance of bronchial cuffs vary (1008, 1009). Most manufacturers color the bronchial cuff blue. Each cuff has its own inflation system marked so that it is easy to determine which cuff is being inflated. If the bronchial cuff is blue, there will usually be blue markings on the pilot balloon and/or the inflation device or they may be colored blue.

Margin of Safety in Positioning Double-Lumen Tubes (1010, 1011)

The length of the tracheobronchial tree between the most distal and proximal acceptable positions for a DLT is called the margin of safety (1010, 1011). It is the length that the tube may be moved without obstructing a conducting airway.

The margin of safety will depend on the length of the lumen into which the cuff is placed and the width of the cuff. If the cuff is narrow or the mainstem bronchus long, the margin of safety will be greater. This does not apply to slotted cuffs where the margin of safety is related to the length of the slot. The margin of safety will be smaller in females, because the mainstem bronchus is shorter.

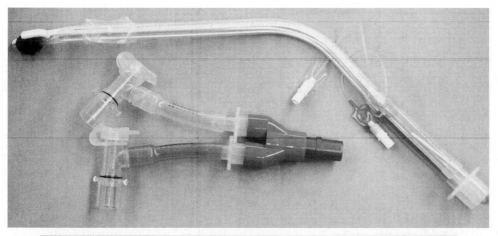

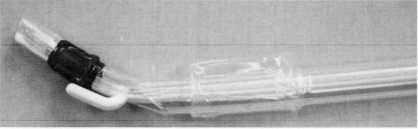

FIGURE 17.35. Carlens double-lumen tube. Top, the connector has ports for fiberscope insertion or suctioning and areas where a clamp can be applied to occlude gas flow. Bottom, note the carinal hook and the blue bronchial cuff.

Left-Sided Tubes

The outermost acceptable position is when the bronchial cuff is just below the carina. If the tube were pulled farther out, the bronchial cuff could obstruct the trachea and/or contralateral (right) mainstem bronchus. The most acceptable distal position is when the tip of the bronchial segment is at the proximal edge of the upper lobe bronchial orifice. Further insertion will result in obstruction

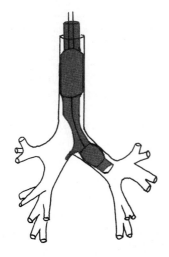

FIGURE 17.36. Carlens tube in place.

of the left upper lobe bronchus. The margin of safety is the difference between these outermost and innermost acceptable positions.

Right-Sided Tubes

The margin of safety is defined somewhat differently for right-sided tubes. A right-sided DLT is acceptably positioned if the right upper lobe ventilation slot is aligned with the right upper lobe orifice. Thus the margin of safety is the length of the ventilation slot minus the diameter of the right upper lobe orifice. The margin of safety is considerably smaller in right-sided tubes than left-sided ones.

Specific Tubes

Because of the anatomical differences between the right and left mainstem bronchi, right- and left-sided tubes differ, notably in the degree of angulation of the bronchial segment and the design of the bronchial cuff. In addition, available tubes have different features and the margin of safety varies with each tube.

Carlens Double-Lumen Tube (1012, 1013)

The Carlens DLT (Figs. 17.35 and 17.36) is intended for insertion into the left main bronchus.

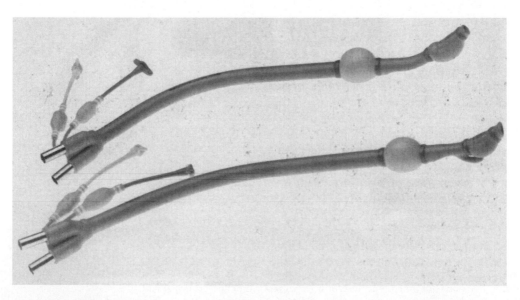

FIGURE 17.37. Red rubber double-lumen tubes. Top, Robertshaw right double-lumen tube (DLT). *Bottom,* White DLT. (Courtesy of Rusch, Inc.)

It has a carinal hook. The margin of safety with a Carlens tube varies from 18 to 23 mm in women and from 22 to 27 mm in men. It is available in both red rubber and polyvinyl chloride.

White Double-Lumen Tube (1014, 1015)

The White DLT (Fig. 17.37) is designed to fit the right mainstem bronchus. It has a carinal hook. The cuff for the right mainstem bronchus is circumferentially superior to the opening to the upper lobe bronchus and continues distally be-

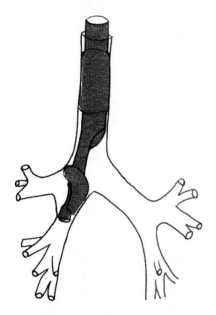

FIGURE 17.38. Polyvinyl chloride Robertshaw right double-lumen tube (DLT). The angle of the bronchial portion is 20°.

hind the opening. It is available in both red rubber and polyvinyl chloride.

Robertshaw Right Double-Lumen Tube

On the Robertshaw right DLT, the angle of the bronchial portion is 20°. It is available in both red rubber and polyvinyl chloride. The bronchial cuff has a slotted opening in its lateral aspect in the red rubber version (Fig 17.37). In the polyvinyl version the bronchial cuff is proximal to the slot on the lateral surface and extends tangentially toward the medial surface (1, 1016) (Figs. 17.38 and 17.39). The margin of safety in positioning a right-sided Robertshaw tube has been reported to be as large as 11 mm (1017) or as little as 1 to 4 mm (1011).

Robertshaw Left Double-Lumen Tube (984, 1018–1020)

The Robertshaw left DLT (Figs. 17.40 and 17.41) differs from the Carlens tube in that the lumens are larger (while the outside diameter is the same) and D shaped, there is no carinal hook, and it has a more molded curvature to prevent kinking. The angle of the bronchial portion is 40°. Studies have found that the margin of safety varies from 12 to 23 mm in females and from 16 to 27 mm in males (1021, 1022). It is available in both red rubber and polyvinyl chloride.

Broncho-Cath Right-Sided Tube

The Broncho-Cath right-sided tube differs from other right-sided DLTs in the design of the bronchial cuff, which has roughly the shape of an S, or slanted doughnut, with the edge of the cuff

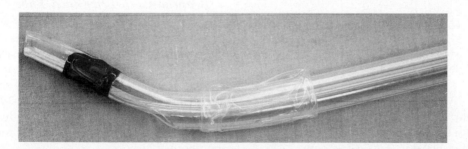

FIGURE 17.39. Polyvinyl chloride Robertshaw right double-lumen tube (DLT).

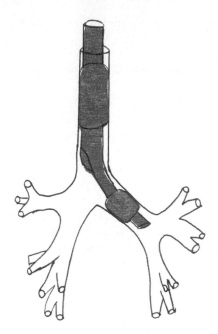

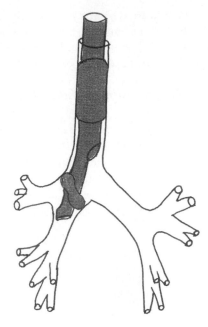

FIGURE **17.40.** Robertshaw left double-lumen tube (DLT). The angle of the bronchial portion is 40°.

FIGURE **17.42.** Broncho-Cath right double-lumen tube (DLT). The bronchial cuff has the shape of an *S* or a slanted doughnut, with the edge of the cuff nearest the right upper lobe bronchus closer to the trachea than the part of the cuff touching the medial bronchial wall. A slot in the tube beyond the cuff corresponds to the opening of the right upper lobe bronchus. Newer versions have no bevel on the bronchial segment.

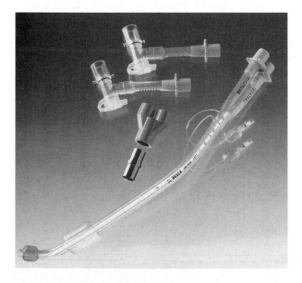

FIGURE **17.41.** Robertshaw left double-lumen tube (DLT). (Courtesy of Rusch Inc.)

to the opening of the upper lobe bronchus (1010). The end of the bronchial segment on newer tubes has no bevel (1023).

The shape of the right bronchial cuff allows the ventilation slot to ride off the right upper lobe orifice, increasing the margin of safety. However, one study found that when this tube was inserted blindly, right upper lobe obstruction occurred in 89% of cases (1016).

Broncho-Cath Left-Sided Tube (984)

The Broncho-Cath left-sided DLT is similar to the right-sided model (Fig. 17.44). It is available with a carinal hook (1024). The bronchial portion of the tube is at an angle of approximately 35°. The margin of safety for placement of this tube has been reported to be approximately 20 mm in men and 15 mm in women in one study (1011) and 21 to 25 in females and 25 to 29 in males in another (1017).

A study comparing this tube with red rubber

nearest the right upper lobe bronchus closer to the trachea than the part of the cuff touching the medial bronchial wall (Figs. 17.42 and 17.43). A slot in the tube just beyond the cuff corresponds

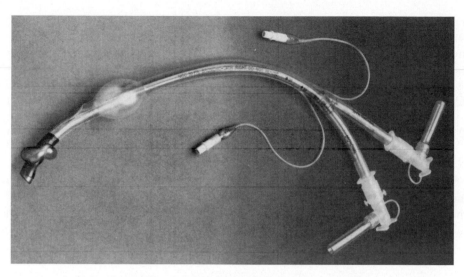

FIGURE 17.43. Broncho-Cath right double-lumen tube (DLT). Newer versions have no bevel at the end of the bronchial segment. (Courtesy of Mallinckrodt Medical, Inc.)

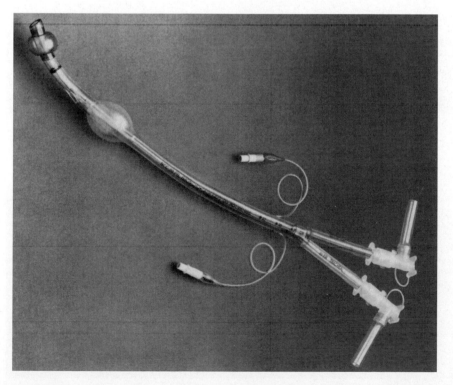

FIGURE 17.44. Broncho-Cath left double-lumen tube (DLT). (Courtesy of Mallinckrodt Medical, Inc.)

Carlens and Robertshaw tubes found that there were fewer difficulties with insertion and fewer complications with the Broncho-Cath tube (984).

There are reports of problems with this tube. There are several reported incidents in which the tip of the bronchial portion abutted the bronchial wall, causing difficulty with ventilation (1025–1027).

Sher-I-Bronch Right-Sided Double-Lumen Tube

The Sher-I-Bronch right-sided DLT has two cuffs on the bronchial segment, proximal and distal to the upper lobe ventilation slot, which is 13 to 14 mm long (Figs. 17.45 and 17.46). In one study comparing the various tubes, the Sher-I-Bronch was found to provide satisfactory ventilation in the greatest number of cases (1028). Another study found that poor lung isolation was more common when this tube was used (1029). A case has been reported in which the tip of this tube became entrapped in the right upper lobe bronchus (1030).

Sher-I-Bronch Left-Sided Double-Lumen Tube

On the Sher-I-Bronch left-sided DLT (Fig. 17.A), the bronchial segment diverges from the

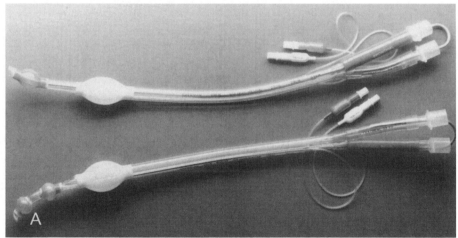

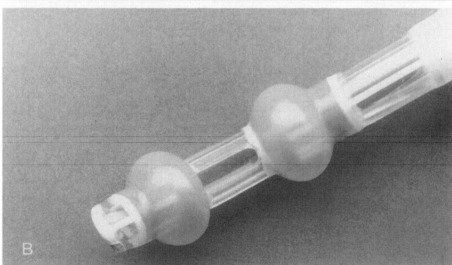

FIGURE **17.45.**   Sher-I-Bronch double-lumen tubes. **A,** *Top,* left-sided tube. *Bottom,* right-sided tube. **B,** close-up of right bronchial segment, showing opening to the right upper lobe. (Courtesy of Sheridan, Inc.)

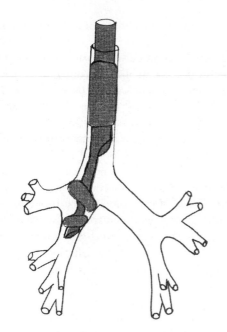

FIGURE 17.46. Sher-I-Bronch right double-lumen tube (DLT). Note the two cuffs proximal and distal to the opening to the right upper lobe.

main tube at an angle of 34°. The average margin of safety is reported to be 14 mm in females and 19 mm in males (1011). One study found that the bronchial cuff on this tube required significantly higher pressures to achieve one-lung isolation than cuffs on other DLTs (1031).

Techniques (1032)

Choice of Tube

Right Versus Left

When surgery is performed on the right lung, a left-sided DLT should be used. Because the margin of safety in positioning a right-sided DLT is so small, use of a right-sided DLT for left lung surgery introduces the risk of either blockade of the right upper lobe or the left lung (1032). For this reason, many people prefer to use a left-sided DLT for left lung surgery (1, 1011, 1017, 1033). During left pneumonectomy, immediately before the left mainstem bronchus is clamped, the DLT can be pulled from the bronchus under the surgeon's guidance and can continue to be used for ventilating the remaining right lung. A disadvantage of this technique is the potential risk of decannulation during surgical manipulations. Be-

cause of this, some anesthesia providers routinely use right-sided DLTs for left thoracotomies (1034).

Many clinicians believe that right-sided DLTs should be used because intubation of the nonoperative bronchus ensures surgical access to the entire left bronchial tree and eliminates the need for intraoperative tube manipulations.

A right-sided DLT must be used for left lung surgery when the following conditions exist: there is rupture of the left mainstem bronchus; a lesion in the left mainstem bronchus or the carina; stenosis or compression of the left mainstem bronchus; or distortion of the left mainstem bronchus by a left lower or upper lobe tumor, causing the left mainstem bronchus to take off from the trachea at a sharp angle (1035).

A left DLT may not provide optimum conditions for ventilation of the residual left lung after previous left upper lobectomy (1036).

Size

A large DLT will result in less resistance to flow, facilitate suctioning, and passage of a fiberscope, and reduce the risk of advancing the DLT too deeply (1037). Less air will be needed in the cuffs, reducing the chance of damage to the airway. If too small a tube is used, the large bronchial cuff seal may force the entire DLT cephalad, making it more difficult to achieve a satisfactory bronchial seal. However, inability to introduce a larger tube through the larynx or past the carina or intrinsic or extrinsic obstruction of the mainstem bronchus to be intubated may necessitate use of a smaller tube.

The correct size may be predicted by measuring the width of the patient's trachea or bronchus from a recent chest x-ray or CT scan (1038, 1039).

Another method is to place the tube on the patient so that the upper edge of the bronchial cuff is 1 cm below the sternal angle and the inserted length of the tube is measured by the distance to the anterior teeth or gums (1040). The correct size tube is one that just passes across the lobe of the ear before bifurcating.

Procedures before Insertion

The tracheal and bronchial cuffs should be inflated and checked for leaks and symmetrical inflation, making certain that each inflation tube is associated with the proper cuff. The tube and stylet should be lubricated, and the stylet placed in the bronchial lumen, making certain it does not extend beyond the tip. The connector should be assembled so that it can be quickly fitted to the tube and the breathing system after intubation.

Insertion

Intubation can be performed under direct vision with a rigid laryngoscope. The tube should be inserted with the bronchial segment concave anteriorly. This places the tube at a 90° angle from where it will eventually rest. After the bronchial cuff has passed the cords, the tube is turned 90° so that the bronchial portion points toward the appropriate bronchus. If the tube is to be placed in the left mainstem bronchus, the head and neck should be rotated to the right before rotating and advancing the tube (1041, 1042). Leaving the stylet in place for the entire intubation procedure rather than removing it once the bronchial cuff has passed the vocal cords will result in a more rapid, accurate placement of the DLT without increasing the incidence of tracheobronchial mucosa injury (1043). Partial inflation of the bronchial cuff may prevent insertion too far (1040, 1044).

A tube with a carinal hook is inserted with the bronchial segment pointing anteriorly until the bronchial cuff passes the cords. The tube is then rotated 180° so that the hook is anterior. After the hook has passed the vocal cords, the tube is rotated 90° so that the bronchial segment is directed toward the appropriate bronchus (1045). The tube is advanced until the hook is engaged by the carina. The hook can be tied closely to the tube with a slip knot to facilitate passage through the larynx, then untied (1046).

The tube is advanced until moderate resistance is encountered. One study found that the average depth of insertion for both male and female patients 170 cm tall was 29 cm and for each 10 cm increase or decrease in height, average placement depth was increased or decreased 1 cm (1047).

A DLT can also be placed by inserting a fiberscope into the bronchial lumen and directing it into the appropriate bronchus under direct vision (1048–1051). This avoids traumatizing the bronchus or inserting the tube too deeply and ensures

that the correct bronchus is intubated on the first attempt.

Another technique is to place a bougie into the correct mainstem bronchus under direct vision using a rigid bronchoscope (1033). The DLT is then inserted over the bougie. A DLT can be placed using a lighted stylet (1052).

Another technique is to advance the tube with the bronchial cuff fully inflated until an increase in resistance to advancement is felt, only one side of the chest moves, and compliance is reduced (1040, 1053). Once the correct bronchus has been identified, the bronchial cuff is deflated completely to allow insertion into the bronchus to a distance of the width of the cuff plus a further 1 cm for a left tube and a further 5 to 10 mm for right-sided tubes.

A double-lumen tube can be inserted into a patient with a tracheostomy (1054–1057). The tracheal cuff may be at the tracheal stoma or lie partly outside the trachea.

Cuff Inflation

Once the tube tip is thought to be in a mainstem bronchus, both cuffs should be inflated. The tracheal cuff should be inflated in a manner similar to that on a tracheal tube.

It is more difficult to inflate the bronchial cuff correctly. An overinflated bronchial cuff may herniate into the trachea, cause the carina to be pushed toward the opposite side, or result in narrowing of the bronchial segment lumen. Studies suggest that when an appropriate-sized tube is used, satisfactory lung collapse can be produced with little or no air in the bronchial cuff (1058). Rarely is more than 3 ml required.

One technique is first to inflate the tracheal cuff. The tracheal lumen is then opened to atmosphere and air injected into the bronchial cuff until there is cessation of leak during positive pressure ventilation. This method may result in excessive pressure in the bronchial cuff (1058, 1059).

A useful technique when the bronchial lumen is in the lung being operated on is to pass a suction catheter through the bronchial lumen when the lung is deflated and leave it until ready for reinflation (1034). This may prevent the bronchial lumen from becoming obstructed by blood or mucus. The catheter must be removed before application of bronchial staples.

Confirmation of Position

It is important to check position after insertion and immediately before initiation of one-lung ventilation since these tubes move during patient positioning, on opening the chest, or during surgical maneuvers (1059–1065).

Auscultatory Techniques (1066)

Left-sided tubes. With the tracheal cuff inflated and the tracheal lumen connected to the breathing system, both lungs should be auscultated in the axillary regions and upper lung fields to detect differences. The bronchial cuff should be inflated and both lumens connected to the breathing system. Auscultation should then be repeated.

Next, the attachment between the breathing system and the tracheal lumen should be occluded with a clamp and the lumen opened to air. Breath sounds should be heard only over the left lung. If breath sounds are heard bilaterally, the tube is too high in the trachea. Both cuffs should be deflated and the tube advanced. If breath sounds are heard only over the right lung, the bronchial lumen is on the right side. If this is the case, both cuffs should deflated, the tube withdrawn until its distal end is above the carina, rotated, then reinserted. The steps outlined above should be repeated.

The attachment to the bronchial lumen is then clamped, the lumen opened to air, and the patient is ventilated through the tracheal lumen. If the tube is in good position, breath sounds should be heard only over the right lung. If there is marked resistance to ventilation, the tube is either too far into the left bronchus or not deep enough. The position can be determined by deflating the bronchial cuff while continuing to ventilate through the tracheal lumen with the bronchial lumen clamped. If the tip is too deep in the left bronchus, breath sounds will be heard only on the left side. If the tube is not deep enough in the bronchus, breath sounds will be present bilaterally. Depending on where breath sounds are heard, the tracheal cuff also should be deflated and the tube pulled back or advanced. Both cuffs should be reinflated and the auscultatory sequence repeated.

One of the lumens should be opened to air

then the connector to that side clamped. Breath sounds should be present on the side that is intended to be ventilated. This should be repeated for the opposite side. If after clamping the left bronchial lumen there is marked resistance to air flow, the tube is either too far into the left lumen or not deep enough (1067). To determine which, the bronchial lumen should be clamped and ventilation through the tracheal lumen continued. If the tube is too deep in the bronchus, breath sounds will be heard only on the left side. If the tube is not deep enough, breath sounds will be heard bilaterally (1067).

Right-sided tubes. Auscultation of a right-sided DLT is similar to that of a left-sided tube. It is especially important to confirm ventilation of the right upper lobe.

Unfortunately, auscultation detects DLT malposition only part of the time because breath sounds can be transmitted from one region of the lung to adjacent areas. Studies have found that over 50% of all left DLTs and over 80% of right DLTs positioned satisfactory by auscultation were found to be inappropriately placed on subsequent fiberoptic surveillance (1061, 1068). However, one study found that this method of placement was not associated with an increased incidence of complications during one-lung ventilation (1029). Another problem with auscultation is that once the patient is prepped and draped, the chest is no longer available for auscultation.

Fiberoptic Techniques (1069)

Fiberoptic bronchoscopy is the most accurate method for determining DLT position (985, 1070, 1071). Many experts feel that the position of a double-lumen tube should be routinely determined in this way. Whenever there is any doubt, this method should be used to check the position (1072). A further advantage is that it can be used to remove blood or secretions (1068).

Left-sided tubes. A fiberscope is placed in the tracheal lumen through the open end of the tube or through a port in the connector specially designed for this purpose. As the fiberscope is advanced, the carina should come into view. The top surface of the blue bronchial cuff should be seen just below the carina in the left mainstem bronchus. The bronchial cuff should not herniate over the carina, nor should the carina be pushed to the right. An unobstructed view of the nonintubated right mainstem bronchus should be obtained.

The fiberscope should then be advanced through the bronchial lumen to check for narrowing of the lumen at the level of the cuff and an unobstructed view of the distal bronchial tree. Failure to check the bronchial lumen may result in problems (1073).

Right-sided tubes. Looking down the tracheal lumen, the upper surface of the bronchial cuff should be seen just below the carina in the right mainstem bronchus. The fiberscope is then placed in the bronchial lumen. The right middle-lower lobe bronchial carina should be seen below the end of the tube. The right upper lobe lumen should be located. The endoscopist should be able to look into the right upper lobe orifice by flexing the tip of the fiberscope superiorly. The mucosa should not be covering any part of the lumen.

Bronchospirometry

Pressure-volume and flow-volume loops are discussed in Chapter 19, "Airway Pressure, Volume, and Flow Measurements." Changes in compliance or resistance may mean that placement is not correct (1074–1081).

Monitoring Bronchial Cuff Pressure

Bronchial cuff pressure may decrease as the DLT is pulled out (1082).

Monitoring Exhaled Carbon Dioxide

Capnography can be used to check positioning of a DLT (1083). Capnometers attached to each lumen should show synchronous waveforms that are similar in shape and size. Variations from normal in the components of one of the capnograms such as altered base line, (angle, height, and slope of phase II slope of the alveolar plateau [phase III] may reflect lung problems (See Chapter 18, "Anesthesia Gas Monitoring") (1074). Capnography does not reliably indicate correct placement (1081).

Chest X-Ray

Confirmation of position by chest X-ray may be useful when a fiberscope is not available or cannot be used. However, it is less precise than the fiberoptic bronchoscopy, time-consuming, costly, and awkward to perform.

Stabilization of the Tube

Once it is confirmed that the tube is in the correct position, it should be secured in place. Special fixation methods have been recommended (909). The bronchial cuff should be kept deflated until the lung is isolated or collapsed to minimize damage to the bronchial mucosa.

Dislodgement during turning should be prevented by holding onto the tube at the level of the incisors and keeping the head immobile or in a neutral or slightly flexed position.

Intraoperative Manipulation (1084)

It may be possible for the surgeon to assist in correct placement once the chest is open. If it is determined that the tube is in the wrong bronchus, both cuffs are deflated and the tube withdrawn into the trachea. The surgeon then compresses the bronchus, and the anesthesia provider advances the tube into the correct side with surgical guidance. The cuffs are then reinflated. Similar manipulations can be performed if the tube is in the correct bronchus but not in the correct position.

Use of a Left-Sided Double-Lumen Tube for Left Lung Surgery

A left-sided DLT can be used for procedures below the tip of the tube. If a left pneumonectomy is to be performed, a left-sided DLT can be used until the left mainstem bronchus is to be clamped. At this point, both cuffs are deflated and the tube pulled back until the tip clears the left bronchus. The tracheal cuff is then reinflated, and the tube is used as a standard tracheal tube.

Replacement of a Double-Lumen Tube with a Single-Lumen Tube

If at the conclusion of a case in which a double-lumen bronchial tube was used it is necessary to have a tube in place for continued ventilation, it is usually desirable to replace the DLT with a standard tracheal tube. In most cases, the procedure is simply removing one tube and placing another. If the patient was difficult to intubate originally or circumstances make visualization of the larynx difficult, other techniques should be considered.

One would be to insert a flexible jet ventilation catheter before removal of the DLT, then advance a tracheal tube over the catheter (1085).

Another technique has been described (1086). At the conclusion of the case, both cuffs are deflated and the double-lumen tube withdrawn until the bronchial lumen is above the carina. The bronchial cuff is then inflated and the lungs ventilated through the bronchial lumen. The tracheal lumen adapter is clamped, and an opening created in the wall of the tracheal lumen. A single-lumen tube is then slipped over a fiberscope, and the fiberscope advanced through the hole in the tracheal lumen and inserted into the trachea. The opening in the DLT is extended, and the DLT slowly removed. The tracheal tube is then inserted into the trachea over the fiberscope, then the fiberscope removed.

Hazards Associated with Double-Lumen Tubes

Many of the hazards associated with conventional tracheal tubes can also occur with DLTs.

Difficulties with Insertion and Positioning

Insertion of a DLT is time consuming. When there is severe hemorrhage, this can be a major problem. Multiple insertions and repositionings increase the risk of trauma.

Tube Malposition (984, 1073, 1087)

Certain physical conditions may make it difficult or impossible for a DLT to be placed correctly (1035, 1088, 1089). Preoperative rigid or fiberoptic bronchoscopy may detect many of these problems. Even if a correct position is achieved during placement, movement of the head, a change in body positioning, or surgical manipulation may result in tube malposition.

Consequences

Unsatisfactory lung deflation (984, 1019, 1070). If the lung cannot be collapsed, operating time will be increased, and the surgical result may be compromised.

An obstruction in the unventilated lumen can prevent deflation of the unventilated lung (1090). Partial withdrawal of the tube or insertion of a

bronchial blocker through the bronchial lumen may remedy the situation (1091).

Obstruction to inflation. If the bronchial cuff is too deep, it may obstruct the upper lobe bronchus. If the bronchial cuff is not below the carina, the cuff may obstruct the trachea and right mainstem bronchus. With right-sided tubes, malalignment of the port for the right upper lobe can result in obstruction. If the right upper lobe bronchus originates from the trachea, it may be obstructed by the tracheal cuff (1092).

Gas trapping. Gas trapping, or obstruction to expiration, may be the result of a one-way valvular effect that allows inflation but not deflation. If unrecognized, it can result in cardiorespiratory embarrassment and/or lung parenchymal damage (1093).

Failure of lung separation. If the airway to a bronchopleural fistula cannot be isolated from that to the normal lung, tension pneumothorax may develop with positive pressure ventilation or the leak through the fistula may be so large that ventilation of the normal lung is compromised (1087).

With blood or infection in the non-dependent lung, an incompletely protected dependent lung may drown in blood or secretions. The need for lung isolation is even greater during bronchopulmonary lavage.

Possible Malpositions

Bronchial portion inserted into wrong mainstem bronchus. In some cases, the bronchial portion will enter the opposite lung. This should be easy to detect and correct.

Bronchial portion inserted too far into the appropriate bronchus (985, 1035, 1067, 1071, 1090, 1092, 1094–1096). A too-deep insertion may be the result of the use of too small a tube. It will result in obstruction of the upper lobe.

In a few patients a left-sided DLT placed so that the bronchial cuff is just distal to the carina still may cause left upper lobe obstruction (1017, 1097).

Bronchial segment not advanced sufficiently far into bronchus. If the tube is not sufficiently advanced into the bronchus, the bronchial cuff may protrude into the trachea. The need to inject more than 3 ml of air into the bronchial cuff to achieve a seal should alert the user that the tube may be misplaced. In many cases, no untoward sequelae will occur. However, there may be obstruction of gas flow to the other lung. The cuff may produce a valvular obstruction between itself and the tracheal wall, allowing the opposite lung to inflate but not deflate. Gas trapping may occur when both lumens are open or may occur only when the bronchial portion is clamped. The trapped gas can be released only by deflating the bronchial cuff. The bronchial segment may slip out of its bronchus, especially during positioning of the patient.

Tip of bronchial lumen above the carina. The tip of the bronchial lumen may be above the carina because of a tracheal lesion that prevents the tube from being advanced far enough (1087). With this malposition there will be unsatisfactory lung deflation and failure of lung separation.

Incorrect placement with respect to the upper lobe bronchus. Malposition with respect to the upper lobe bronchus is particularly a problem with right-sided tubes. The bronchial tip may be in the correct position, but the cuff occludes the lumen to the upper lobe. Even with left-sided tubes, it is possible to obstruct the upper lobe bronchus (1070, 1071, 1098). The result of such a misplacement is usually hypoxemia and, if the tube is on the operative side, failure of the upper lobe to deflate satisfactorily.

Asymmetrical bronchial cuff inflation. An inflated bronchial cuff can cause the tip of the bronchial lumen to face into the bronchial wall, producing one-way valvular obstruction that allows inflation but not deflation of the lung (984, 1099).

Hypoxemia

In many instances, hypoxemia during one-lung ventilation is at least partly the result of malpositioning of the DLT. For this reason, whenever hypoxia occurs, tube position should be reassessed and adjustment made if necessary. Even with correct positioning, hypoxemia can result from blood continuing to flow through the unventilated lung after one-lung ventilation is begun.

If hypoxemia is a problem, CPAP should be applied to the nonventilated lumen (1097). The reader is referred to Chapter 7, "Breathing Sys-

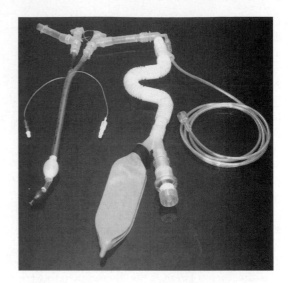

FIGURE 17.47. Device for applying continuous positive airway pressure (CPAP) to non-ventilated lung. The accordion tubing allows the bag and pressure valve to be remote from the patient. (Courtesy of Kendall Healthcare Products Co.)

tems II: Mapleson Systems" for a discussion of some devices used to deliver CPAP. Some double-lumen tube manufacturers include a CPAP device with each DLT (Fig 17.47 and 17.48).

Other measures to improve oxygenation include dependent lung PEEP, occasional ventilation of the nondependent lung (one breath every 5 to 10 min), and clamping of the pulmonary artery before excluding the lung from ventilation.

A change from two-lung to one-lung ventilation does not usually result in a significant increase in $PaCO_2$, provided minute volume is maintained at the same value. However, because the tidal volume is the same, more pressure must be applied during inspiration to overcome the increased resistance to higher flow through the single lumen of the DLT and the decreased compliance of the single lung.

Obstruction to Airflow

Many cases of obstruction are the result of malpositioning of the tube. In addition, overinflation of the bronchial cuff can cause narrowing of the lumen (1035, 1070).

In one reported case, the bronchial cuff was left

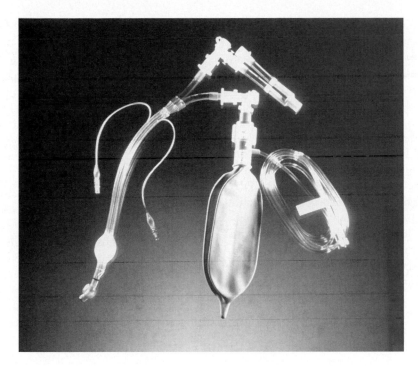

FIGURE 17.48.   Device for applying continuous positive airway pressure (CPAP) to non-ventilated lung. The adjustable valve applies pressures from 1 to 10 cm H_2O. (Courtesy of Mallinckrodt Medical Inc.)

deflated until one-lung ventilation was to begin (1100). A necrotic tumor migrated into the bronchus of the dependent lung, causing airway obstruction when one-lung ventilation was begun.

The bronchial lumen can become twisted (1073). This can result in partial obstruction to ventilation.

The bronchial cuff may cause the carina to be displaced laterally, producing obstruction of the other mainstem bronchus (1101).

In a DLT with a carinal hook, the hook may obstruct the tracheal lumen (1102).

Trauma

Trauma to the respiratory tract is a possibility whenever intubation with a DLT is performed. Rupture of a mainstem bronchus has been reported (1103–1109). The trachea may be perforated (1110, 1111). These complications may not be discovered until hours after the initial injury. An endobronchial inflammatory polyp consistent with the position of the bronchial cuff resulting in a fatal hemorrhage has been reported (1112).

Measures to reduce airway trauma include removing the stylet after the tip of the tube has passed the vocal cords, avoiding overinflating cuffs, deflating the tracheal and bronchial cuffs when repositioning the patient or the tube, and not advancing the tube when resistance is encountered. Using tubes with high-volume, low-pressure cuffs has been recommended but proof that high pressures cause airway damage during short-term intubation is lacking. Some bronchial cuffs can provide one-lung isolation with significantly lower bronchial pressures than others (1031). It has been recommended that the bronchial cuff be kept deflated until needed to minimize pressure on the bronchial mucosa (1108). This may not be prudent if there is a bronchial tumor, as necrotic tumor may migrate into the other lung (1100).

Tube Problems

Reported problems with DLTs include mislabeled lumens; distortion of the tracheal lumen such that a suction catheter would not pass; a slit in the septum that made it impossible to isolate the bronchus; a defect that made the bronchial lumen kink on itself; splitting of the tubing to the bronchial cuff so that it was impossible to keep the cuff inflated; and a protuberance of the wall of the tube that caused obstruction of the tracheal lumen (1091, 1113–1119).

Surgical Complications

The carinal hook may be clamped by the surgeon (1014). The bronchial cuff may be punctured. A suture may be placed through the DLT (897). The surgical procedure may result in a tight stenosis, which could entrap the bronchial segment (1120). If the bronchial segment is in the surgical side by mistake and this is not recognized, it is possible that when the bronchus is stapled and divided, the tip of the tube will be stapled and divided.

These possibilities should be considered when excessive resistance to extubation is encountered; reexploration of the chest may be warranted.

Circulatory Collapse

A mediastinal mass was compressed and displaced by a DLT in such a way that it compressed the great vessels from the heart (1121).

COAXIAL SYSTEMS FOR ONE-LUNG VENTILATION

Coaxial systems in which a bronchial tube is placed within a large-bore tracheal tube are available (1122–1125). The inner tube can be used as a bronchial blocker, or for suctioning, differential ventilation, or application of PEEP.

Tracheal and bronchial intubations are performed separately. The bronchial tube can be positioned blindly or with use of a rigid bronchoscope or a fiberscope (1122). Bronchial intubation can be performed without haste, while the patient is ventilated using the tracheal tube.

Advantages of this technique include not having to reintubate the patient at the end of the procedure. The bronchial tube can be positioned and removed many times, leaving the main tracheal tube in place.

A disadvantage is the necessity to use a large (at least 9 mm ID) tracheal tube. Another disadvantage is that this results in higher resistance than a DLT of a comparable external diameter (1126).

SINGLE-LUMEN BRONCHIAL TUBES

A single-lumen tube placed in the main bronchus of the nonoperative lung can be used to maintain ventilation while the other lung is blocked and isolated from the ventilated lung.

Indications

These tubes are used in situations where lung separation is desired and, when for some reason, a DLT cannot be used. They have been used frequently in pediatric patients whose airways are too small for double lumen tubes (987, 992, 995, 1127–1137). In patients with massive hemoptysis, bronchial intubation with a single-lumen tube is often the easiest and quickest method of separating the lungs. A bronchial tube may be used to treat atelectasis (1138). In patients with cystic fibrosis, use of a tracheal tube plus a bronchial blocker may result in better clearance of secretions than use of a DLT (1003).

Equipment

In the past, there were special tubes for bronchial intubation. Today bronchial intubation is usually carried out with a long small-diameter tracheal tube (583, 987, 1139). A long tube can be created by anastamosing two shorter tubes (1140, 1141) or may be obtained from a veterinary products supplier (1142). It is important that the tube have a narrow cuff and, beyond this, a short length of tube and short or absent bevel.

Techniques

Before insertion, the correct length for the tube can be estimated from a lateral chest X-ray by measuring the distance from the mouth to the carina and adding 1 cm (995).

The tube is placed before surgery and withdrawn into the trachea when the indication for one-lung ventilation is no longer present (992). It can be placed blindly but is more reliably placed using a fiberscope or rigid bronchoscope (1136, 1143). If placed blindly, the tube usually enters the right mainstem bronchus. The chance of intubating the left bronchus will be increased if the tube is rotated 180° from its usual position before advancing it beyond the carina and the head is turned to the right (583, 1041, 1042, 1144). A modification of this technique is to deliberately intubate a mainstem bronchus, advance the blocker through the tracheal tube, then withdraw the tube into the trachea (1145).

Another method is to insert a stylet into the chosen bronchus using a rigid bronchoscope (1146). The bronchoscope is then removed and an appropriate single-lumen tube inserted into position over the stylet.

Correct positioning can be confirmed by auscultation, X-rays, and/or fiberoptic bronchoscopy.

Disadvantages

With mainstem bronchial intubation, the upper lobe bronchus is easily obstructed, especially on the right (1129). It may be possible to rotate the tube so that the bevel faces the orifice of the upper lobe bronchus (1139). It is impossible to ventilate both lungs at the beginning of anesthesia, and the collapsed lung cannot be suctioned or re-expanded and ventilated until the tube is withdrawn into the trachea. Finally, use of a bronchial tube does not allow application of CPAP to the operative lung.

BRONCHIAL-BLOCKING DEVICES

With a bronchial blocker, the bronchus of a diseased lobe or lung is blocked while the balance of the lung is ventilated with a standard tracheal tube or bronchial intubation of the other lung can be performed.

Indications

Indications for bronchial blockers are similar to those for a double-lumen tube, with the exception of independent lung ventilation. They are often used in patients in whom use of a DLT is not possible or advisable (nasal intubation necessary, small patients, difficult intubation, anatomical problems) (1131, 1135, 1147–1155). One indication may be a patient on anticoagulants because insertion may cause less trauma than a DLT (1156). Another use is selective reinflation of a lung with lobar atelectasis (1157). Use of a blocker eliminates the need to change tubes at the conclusion of surgery if artificial ventilation is to be used postoperatively. An advantage over a DLT is the ability to block a segment of a lung rather than the entire lung (1158, 1159). Blockers may be helpful in controlling pulmonary bleeding (1160). They also can be used for short-term control of a leak from a bronchopleural fistula. One of the advantages is that the tube can be used for postoperative ventilation and this obviates the need to reintubate the trachea with a single-lumen tube following completion of surgery.

Use of a Univent tube as a means of providing high-frequency jet ventilation has been reported (1161).

Devices

A blocker typically consists of a central tube surrounded by an inflatable cuff. This allows suctioning, insufflation of oxygen, lavage, and ventilation.

Univent Bronchial-Blocking Tube (1162–1172)

The Univent tube is a single-lumen cuffed silicone tube with a small lumen along its concave side (Figs. 17.49 and 17.50). The small channel

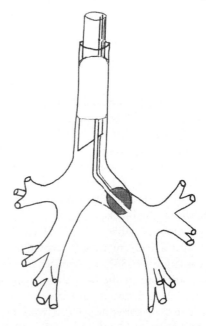

FIGURE 17.49. Univent bronchial blocker. The cuffed tracheal tube has a small lumen along its concave side, which contains a tubular cuffed bronchial blocker. The blocker can be advanced into a mainstem bronchus or smaller airway.

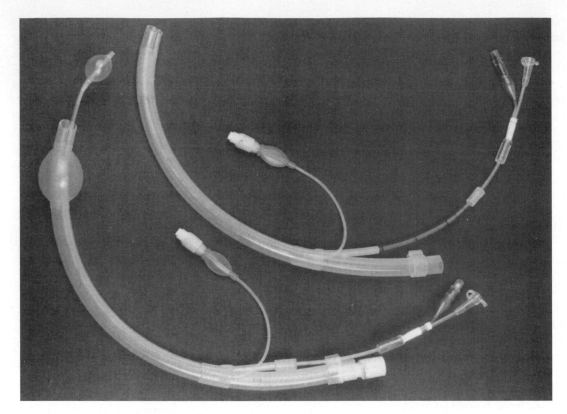

FIGURE 17.50.   Univent bronchial-blocking tubes. *Top,* the bronchial blocker is retracted. *Bottom,* the bronchial blocker is advanced and the cuff is inflated. (Courtesy of Vitaid.)

contains a tubular bronchial blocker that has a blue cuff. There are radiopaque rings at both ends of the cuff. The blocker can be advanced up to 8 cm beyond the main body of the tube and can block airways smaller than the mainstem bronchus. It has a slightly larger-than-usual external diameter for its internal diameter because of the space taken by the blocker.

All functions possible with a DLT can be performed with a Univent tube, except differential lung ventilation (1033). Intermittent re-expansion or suctioning of the lung during operation is accomplished without dislodgment of the blocker. Use of operative lung CPAP with the Univent tube has been described (1162).

The Univent tube may be easier to insert and position correctly than a double-lumen tube (1166, 1167). Its smaller external diameter compared to that of a DLT may make it useful in situa-

tions such as the patient with narrowing of the airway or a tracheostomy (1173, 1174).

One study found that in three of eight cases the Univent failed to occlude the bronchus, requiring replacement with a DLT (1156). This contrasts with satisfactory reports from other investigators (1166, 1167). It also offers a larger lumen for ventilation and pulmonary toilet of the unaffected lung. While one study found that the blocker cuff exerted high pressure (1175), another study found lower pressures (1176). Perforation of a bronchus by the blocker has been reported (1177).

Embolectomy Catheter

A balloon-tipped embolectomy catheter can be used as a bronchial blocker (1147–1149, 1157, 1178–1181). These come in a variety of sizes so that one can be used to block a second-order as well as a mainstem bronchus and can be used in both adults and children. It comes with a stylet in place so that it is possible to place a curvature in the distal tip. It can be passed through the glottis external to the tracheal tube.

Swan-Ganz Catheter

The Swan-Ganz catheter has been used in pediatric patients (1131, 1157). Its use allows delivery of oxygen to the involved lung.

Magill Blocker

The Magill bronchial blocker is a small catheter equipped with an inflatable cuff. It can be used in children.

Foley Catheter

A urinary catheter inserted down one lumen of a DLT has been used when there was a problem with the DLT (1091).

Techniques of Use (1178, 1179, 1182)

Univent Bronchial-Blocking Tube

Before intubation, both cuffs should be inflated and checked for leaks. After the cuffs have been deflated, the blocker is pushed back and forth to ensure free movement. The blocker is then fully retracted into the main body of the tube.

The Univent is inserted as a unit into the trachea. The cuff on the tracheal tube is inflated, and the patient ventilated. A fiberscope is inserted into the lumen of the tube while ventilation is maintained around it. The bronchial blocker is located by moving it in and out of its lumen, and the main tube rotated so that the blocker is directed toward the side to be occluded under direct vision and secured in place with its balloon deflated. The fiberscope is then withdrawn. A guidewire may be useful in directing the blocker into place (1158).

Blind insertion of the bronchial blocker is also possible. The whole tube is turned so that the concavity of the tube faces the side to be blocked. The blocker is advanced into the mainstem bronchus, and the cuff inflated. This method has not proved very successful in practice (1169).

Another method of placing the Univent blocker is to first insert the tube into the trachea.

A fiberscope is inserted into the bronchus to be blocked, and the tube is advanced into that bronchus. The blocker is then advanced into the bronchus, and the tube is withdrawn into the trachea, leaving the blocker in the bronchus.

Once the blocker is placed, its position should be checked using a fiberscope (1183), X-rays, or auscultation (1133, 1183).

Partially deflating the tracheal tube cuff and turning the patient's head to the side may aid in placement of the blocker (1184).

When the bronchus needs to be blocked, the lung is deflated with the blocker open to atmosphere, then suction applied to the lumen of the blocker until complete collapse is achieved. The bronchial blocker cuff should be inflated using the least amount of air that will provide a seal. This can be achieved by attaching a CO_2 analyzer to the proximal end of the blocker and noting when the waveform disappears (1185). When the need for the blocker is no longer present, the cuff is deflated and the blocker withdrawn into the main tube.

Other Bronchial Blockers

Before use, the cuff on the bronchial blocker should be tested for leaks, and the blocker fitted with a stylet. The blocker may be inserted into the trachea either before intubation with the tracheal tube or alongside it after intubation.

The blocker can be inserted using a bronchoscope or blindly (1186). Alternately the bronchoscope can be used to place a flexible stylet in the bronchus (1187). The blocker is inserted over the stylet, which is then removed.

The blocker also can be inserted beside the tracheal tube. A fiberscope is passed to the end of the single-lumen tube and the blocker visualized. The blocker is rotated until its distal tip is in the desired mainstem bronchus. It may be advanced into an intermediate bronchus if needed (1188).

Another technique of insertion employs two elbow connectors with self-sealing diaphragm ports in series (1189). The distal end of the connectors is connected to the single-lumen tracheal tube. The fiberscope is passed through the port, which offers a straight line down the tracheal tube. The blocker is placed through the other port.

Disadvantages (936, 1041)

With blockers other than the Univent, the blocker and tracheal tube are separate, and there may be difficulty maintaining or changing the position of the blocker (1166). Also, the obstructed lung segment cannot be suctioned or re-expanded until the blocker is removed.

A blocker may become dislodged (1156). If it slips into the trachea, separation of the lungs will be lost and the tracheal lumen distal to the tracheal tube will be obstructed. Pneumothorax has been reported with use of the Univent tube (1190). If the blocker is not withdrawn before the surgeon applies staples, it may become fixed (1191, 1192). Accidental inflation of the blocker's cuff instead of the cuff on the tube can occur, resulting in resistance to flow (1193). Part of the blocker may be lost (1183). The blocker balloon may be perforated by a surgical needle (1194).

The amount of air needed to inflate the bronchial cuff so that it blocks the bronchus may cause it to exert excessive pressure on the wall of the bronchus (1195).

In a comparison of the Univent with DLTs, the incidence of malposition was greater with the Univent (1065).

STYLETS AND BOUGIES
Stylets

A stylet (introducer, intubation guide) is designed to fit inside a tracheal tube so that the tube maintains a predetermined, fixed shape. It is most commonly used to facilitate insertion of the tube. It can also be used to check the patency of a tube.

Lighted intubation and optical stylets are discussed in Chapter 16, "Laryngoscopes."

Description (1196)

A variety of stylets is available (Figs. 17.51–17.54). Some have special nonfriction coverings (1197–1199). A stylet should have enough malleability so that its shape can be changed easily, yet enough rigidity to maintain its shape during insertion. It should be resistant to chipping and breaking. The distal end should be smooth to minimize trauma to soft tissues and the tube. It should be at least as long as the tube into which it is introduced.

There should be a means to limit the stylet's advancement into the tube (Figs. 17.51). If none is present, the stylet should be bent acutely at the proximal end (Fig. 17.52). The proximal end of the stylet may have an attachment that will fit firmly into the tracheal tube and prevent rotation of the tube on the stylet.

Some stylets allow the user to change their shape in situ (Figs. 17.53 and 17.54) (1200). These may be especially useful in the patient with a cervical spine injury (1201).

Techniques for Use

A stylet should always be immediately available when intubation is performed. Many anesthesia providers routinely use a stylet, while others reserve its use for difficult intubations. Some tracheal tubes require a stylet to give them sufficient rigidity for insertion.

Unless the stylet has a nonstick coating, a thin

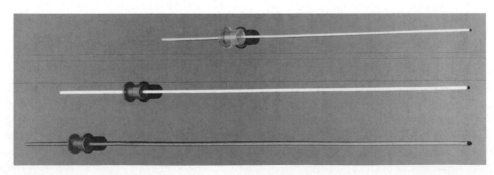

FIGURE 17.51.   Malleable stylets with adjustable stops. The stop fits into the tracheal tube and prevents the stylet from protruding beyond the distal tip of the tube. (Courtesy of Rusch Inc.)

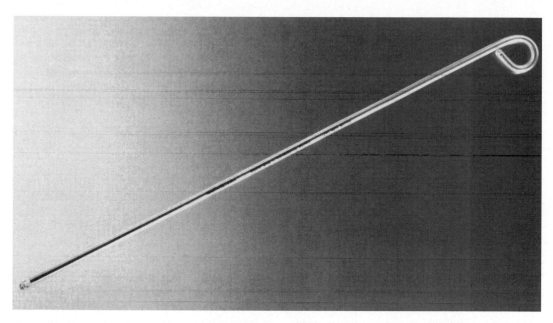

FIGURE 17.52. Malleable stylet. The proximal end must be bent to prevent it from protruding past the end of the tracheal tube. (Courtesy of Mallinckrodt Medical, Inc.)

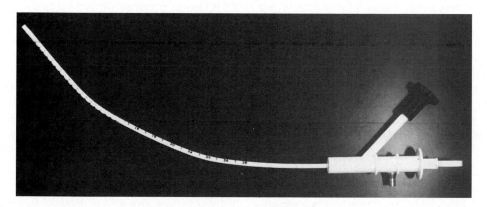

FIGURE 17.53. Flexguide. The distal tip can be flexed by means of the proximal grip handle. It has an attachment for a fiberoptic light source and a eyepiece. (Courtesy of Scientific Sales International, Inc.)

film of lubricant should be spread over its length before insertion. If this is not done, it may be difficult to remove the stylet after the tube is in place. Unless otherwise stated in the manufacturer's directions, the stylet should be inserted into the tube until the distal end is just inside the patient end of the tracheal tube and should be fixed so that the tip cannot advance. Removing the connector from the tube before inserting the stylet may make it easier to withdraw the stylet and decrease the likelihood of damage to the stylet (1197). The tube and stylet should then be bent to the desired shape. For routine intubations, a straight or slightly curved configuration is used. When an anterior larynx is encountered, a *J* or hockey stick configuration, with the distal end of the tube bent anteriorly to an angle of 70 to 80°, is most commonly used. Bending the midpoint of

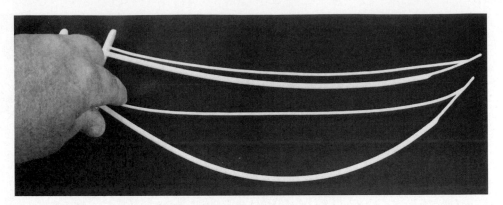

FIGURE **17.54.** Schroeder stylette. By pushing on the proximal part, the angle of the tube is increased.

the tube to the right or left at an angle of 70 to 80° to the first bend may result in a better view of the larynx (1202). The larynx is exposed in the usual manner, and the tracheal tube inserted. When the distal part of the tube is believed to have passed the vocal cords, the stylet is withdrawn from the tube.

A slightly different technique involves inserting the stylet into the tube and angling the distal portion anteriorly (336, 1203). The stylet is then removed from the tube. The tube is advanced to the vicinity of the larynx, and the stylet is then inserted. This technique may result in decreased trauma.

Problems with Stylets

Use of a stylet may result in trauma with serious consequences (425, 426, 428, 1204). Part of the stylet may be sheared off during removal (1205–1214). The inflation tube can become entangled in the stylet (1215). Finally, the stylet may damage the tracheal tube. Small pediatric tracheal tubes have been reported to kink at the distal tip of the Murphy eye. This was thought to have been the consequence of forceful intubation with a stylet (1216).

Bougies (1217, 1218)

A bougie (guide, intubation or tube guide, guiding catheter, director, stylet catheter, catheter guide, tracheal tube introducer, introducer, elastic stylet, tracheal tube replacement obturator, tube changer) (Figs. 17.55 and 17.56) can be used to aid intubation when the operator recognizes some anatomical landmarks but cannot direct the tip of the tracheal tube into the laryngeal inlet or when movement of the head and/or neck is undesirable (1219–1225). One study found that the bougie was superior to a stylet in a tracheal tube for difficult intubations (1222).

A bougie is also useful as a backup safety measure when changing tracheal or tracheostomy tubes or extubating a patient in whom manual ventilation and/or reintubation might be difficult (384, 385, 1226–1231). In addition, manipulation of the tube changer may be used to stimulate the cough reflex (1227). Placing the distal end of the changer in lidocaine jelly may help the patient tolerate it (1232). Because it is only a few millimeters in diameter, it represents a negligible obstruction to closure of the vocal cords. It can serve as a guide if reintubation is necessary. If the bougie is hollow, attachment of an adapter to the proximal end allows administration of oxygen or aspiration (384, 1233). Bag or jet ventilation through such a catheter can provide satisfactory gas exchange in most cases (1218, 1234).

Other uses include distinguishing esophageal from tracheobronchial intubation (483, 551), jet ventilation during microlaryngeal surgery (1235), and ventilating the patient during management of intraoperative tracheal injury (1236).

Description

Many intubating guides with different sizes, shapes, lengths, and materials have been devel-

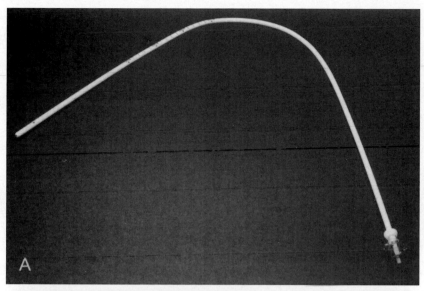

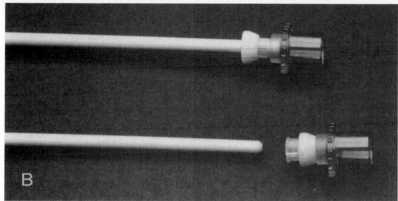

FIGURE 17.55. **A,** bougie. Note the marks showing the distance from the tip and the holes near the tip. **B,** the proximal connections allow administration of oxygen, jet ventilation, connection to a CO_2 analyzer, or suctioning. (Courtesy of Cook Critical Care, a division of Cook, Inc.)

oped (1237–1239). Other devices such as suction, embolectomy and urinary catheters, gastric tubes, and fiberscopes have been used (1240–1245). It should have marks to indicate the distance from the tip (see Fig. 17.55). The tip of the distal end may be angled (1246). The proximal end of the bougie may be adapted to allow administration of oxygen, suctioning, ventilation, or capnography (see Fig. 17.55).

Technique of Use

The bougie is advanced under direct vision to the area where the glottic opening is thought to be located. If the tip is held up at the anterior commissure, it should be rotated 180° then advanced (1247). If the bougie is solid when it enters the trachea, the stepwise advance of the distal end over the tracheal rings will produce a clicking sensation (1248). If it is hollow, the proximal end may be attached to a capnograph to confirm intratracheal placement (1233, 1249, 1250). However, CO_2 may not be detected if the openings are blocked by secretions (1251). A bougie may also be placed using a laryngeal mask or fiberscope (see chapter 15, "The Laryngeal Mask Airway," and Chapter 16, "Laryngoscopes").

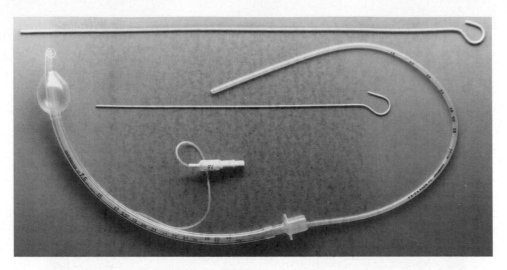

FIGURE **17.56.** Tube changer in place. (Picture courtesy of Kendall Healthcare Products, Inc.)

Once the bougie is believed to be in the trachea, the tracheal tube is advanced over it using a rotary motion. Sometimes after successful placement of a bougie in the trachea it is difficult or impossible to thread the tracheal tube over it (1252). Advancement of the tube may be enhanced by leaving the laryngoscope in the mouth and/or rotating the tracheal tube 90 or 180° (1253, 1254, 1247). Simultaneous bronchoscopy to visualize difficulties and the effects of interventions such as tracheal tube rotation may be helpful (1255). Another technique is to pass the bougie over a guide inserted translaryngeally and passed retrograde to the oropharynx (1210, 1256). The bougie is then withdrawn.

A bougie can be used as a tube exchanger (changer) (1085, 1235, 1257–1259). The tube changer is inserted into the tube and advanced to the tracheal tube's full length. Insertion farther than this may result in trauma (1234, 1260). Alternately, the bougie may be placed alongside the tube (1261). The bougie is held steady while the tracheal tube is removed. Care must be taken that the bougie is not pulled from the trachea. The replacement tracheal tube is slipped over the bougie and advanced into the trachea.

In a patient in whom reintubation or mask ventilation might be difficult is to be extubated, a bougie can be inserted into the trachea through the extant tracheal tube, which is then removed, leaving the bougie in place.

Perforation has been associated with use of a tube changer (1260, 1262, 1263). Use of jet ventilation with one may result in barotrauma (1218). The openings of a guide may be occluded by secretions incorrectly implying esophageal placement (1251). Bougies may be a source of contamination (1264, 1265). Part of one may be sheared off and aspirated (1266).

FORCEPS

A forceps can be used to direct a tracheal tube into the larynx or a gastric tube or other device into the esophagus. It also can be used to insert pharyngeal packing and retrieve foreign objects. Forceps should be readily available whenever an intubation is performed.

Description

A popular type is Magill's forceps (616). These are designed so that when the grasping ends are in the axis of the tracheal tube, the handle is to the right. Thus when the larynx is exposed, most of the forceps is out of the line of sight. Use of modifications of Magill's and other forceps have been described (1267–1276) as have other devices to manipulate the tube during intubation (1277–1280).

Problems with Forceps

Cuff damage may occur, especially when forceps are used with high-volume cuffs (1186). It is suggested that tubes be grasped at the tip, not the cuff. Another way to avoid cuff damage is to file the teeth from the end of the forceps (1268). The forceps may cause damage to the airway mucosa. Another problem is that one arm of the forceps may become lodged in a Murphy eye (28).

REFERENCES

1. Bolder PM, Healy TEJ, Bolder AR, et al. The extra work of breathing through adult endotracheal tubes. Anesth Analg 1986;65:853–859.
2. Brochard L, Rua F, Lorino H, et al. Inspiratory pressure support compensates for the additional work of breathing caused by the endotracheal tube. Anesthesiology 1991;75:739–745.
3. Le Souef PN, England SJ, Bryan AC. Total resistance of the respiratory system in preterm infants with and without an endotracheal tube. J Pediatr 1984;104:108–111.
4. Shapiro M, Wilson RK, Casar G, et al. Work of breathing through different sized endotracheal tubes. Crit Care Med 1986;14:1028–1031.
5. Wall MA. Infant endotracheal tube resistance: effects of changing length, diameter and gas density. Crit Care Med 1980;8:38–40.
6. Bersten AD, Rutten AJ, Vedig AE, et al. Additional work of breathing imposed by endotracheal tubes, breathing circuits, and intensive care ventilators. Crit Care Med 1989;17:671–677.
7. Brown ES, Hustead RF. Resistance of pediatric breathing systems. Anesth Analg 1969;48:842–848.
8. Bierman M, Blair L, Kreit J, et al. The contribution of in vivo endotracheal tube resistance to total airway resistance. Anesthesiology 1993;79:A241.
9. Blom H, Rytlander M, Wisborg T. Resistance of tracheal tubes 3.0 and 3.5 mm internal diameter. A comparison of four commonly used types. Anaesthesia 1985;40:885–888.
10. Baier H, Begin R, Sackner MA. Effect of airway diameter, suction catheters and the bronchofiberscope on airflow in endotracheal and tracheostomy tubes. Heart Lung 1976;5:235–238.
11. Heyer L, Louis B, Isabey D, et al. Noninvasive estimate of work of breathing due to the endotracheal tube. Anesthesiology 1996;85:1324–1333.
12. Hendricks HHL. Minimizing work of breathing through endotracheal tubes. Crit Care Med 1987;15:989–990.
13. Matthews JG, Ingenito E, Davison B, et al. Endotracheal tube resistance. The effects of tube curvature, tube interfaces, gas-liquid interaction and airflow direction. Anesthesiology 1992;77:A280.
14. Beatty PCW, Healy TEJ. The additional work of breathing through Portex Polar 'Blue-Line' preformed paediatric tracheal tubes. Eur J Anaesth 1992; 9:77–83.
15. Badenhorst CH. Changes in tracheal cuff pressure during respiratory support. Crit Care Med 1987;15:300–302.
16. Hatch DJ. Tracheal tubes and connectors used in neonates—dimensions and resistance to breathing. Br J Anaesth 1978;50:959–964.
17. Brown ES. Resistance factors in pediatric endotracheal tubes and connectors. Anesth Analg 1971;50:355–360.
18. Fleming BG, Nott MR. Resistance measurement and connectors. Anaesthesia 1988;43:1057.
19. Steen JA. Impact of tube design and materials on complications of tracheal intubation. Probl Anesth 1988;2:211–224.
20. Carroll RG, Kamen JM, Grenvick A, et al. Recommended performance specifications for cuffed endotracheal and tracheostomy tubes: a joint statement of investigators, inventors, and manufacturers. Crit Care Med 1973;1:155–156.
21. American Society for Testing and Materials. Standard specification for cuffed and uncuffed tracheal tubes (ASTM F1242-96). West Conshohocken, PA: ASTM, 1996.
22. Hirshman CA. Anaphylactic reactions to latex-containing medical devices. American Society of Anesthesiologists Newsletter 1992;56(8):21–22.
23. Klafta JM. Flexible tracheal tubes facilitate fiberoptic intubation. Anesth Analg 1994; 79:1211.
24. American Society for Testing and Materials. Standard test method for determining laser resistance of the shaft of tracheal tubes. (ASTM F246-94) West Conshohocken PA: ASTM, 1994.
25. Murphy FJ. Two improved intratracheal catheters. Anesth Analg 1941;20:102–105.
26. Baranowski AP. Unusual tracheal tube obstruction leading to an unusual bronchoscopic technique. Anaesthesia 1989;44:359–360.
27. Gregory GA. Pediatric Anesthesia. In: Miller RD, ed. Anesthesia. Vol. 2. San Francisco: Churchill Livingstone, 1981:1214.
28. Harrison JF. A problem with Murphy's eye. Anaesthesia 1986;41:445.
29. MacGillivray RG, Odell JA. Eye to eye with Murphy's law. Anaesthesia 1986;41:334.
30. Nichols KP, Zornow MH. A potential complication

of fiberoptic intubation. Anesthesiology 1989;70: 562–563.

31. Ovassapian A. Failure to withdraw flexible fiberoptic laryngoscope after nasotracheal intubation. Anesthesiology 1985;63:124–125.

32. Mackenzie CF, McDowell EM, Helrich M. Reduction of tracheal tube tip damage using a new tube. Crit Care Med 1984;12:259.

33. Pashayan AG, Gravenstein JS. Helium retards endotracheal tube fires from carbon dioxide lasers. Anesthesiology 1985;62:274–277.

34. Cole F. An endotracheal tube for babies. Anesthesiology 1945;6:627–628.

35. Brandstater B. Dilatation of the larynx with Cole tubes. Anesthesiology 1969;31:378–379.

36. Glauser EM, Cook CK, Bougas TP. Pressure-flow characteristics and dead spaces of endotracheal tubes used in infants. Anesthesiology 1961;22:339–341.

37. Mitchell MD, Bailey CM. Dangers of neonatal intubation with the Cole tube. Br Med J 1990;301: 602–603.

38. Ring WH, Adair JC, Elwyn RA. A new pediatric endotracheal tube. Anesth Analg 1975;54: 273–274.

39. Brunsoman JK, Altman VA, Johnson MA, et al. A new endotracheal tube for maxillofacial surgery. J Oral Surg 1980;38:847–848.

40. Olson KW, Culling DC. An alternative use for a nasotracheal tube. Can J Anaesth 1989;36: 252–253.

41. Chee WK. Orotracheal intubation with a nasal Ring-Adair-Elwyn tube provides an unobstructed view in otolaryngologic procedures. Anesthesiology 1995; 83:1369.

42. Alfery DD. Laryngeal mask airway and the ASA difficult airway algorithm: I. Anesthesiology 1996;85: 685.

43. Benumof JL. Laryngeal mask airway and the ASA difficult airway algorithm. In reply. Anesthesiology 1996;85:687–688.

44. Barker SWJ, Tremper KK. A new look at pressure loss through endotracheal tubes: RAE and CAT tubes. Anesth Analg 1986;65:S170.

45. Black AE, Mackersie AM. Accidental bronchial intubation with RAE tubes. Anaesthesia 1991;46: 42–43.

46. Shanahan EC. A nasotracheal tube for faciomaxillary surgery. Anaesthesia 1983;38:289–290.

47. McCoy EP, Russell WJ, Webb RK. Accidental bronchial intubation. Anaesthesia 1997; 52:24–31.

48. Mackersie AM. The length of RAE preformed tubes: a reply. Anaesthesia 1991;46:792.

49. Chung RA, Liban JB. Ludwig's angina and tracheal tube obstruction. Anaesthesia 1991;46:228–239.

50. Beckers HL. Use of a stabilized, armored endotracheal tube in maxillofacial surgery. Anesthesiology 1982;56:309–310.

51. Al-Kaisy AA, Kent AP, Watt JWH. Maintaining ventilation through the Montgomery t-tube. Can J Anaesth 1997; 44:340.

52. Steen JA, Lindhold C, Brdlik GC, et al. Tracheal tube forces on the posterior larynx: index of laryngeal loading. Crit Care Med 1982;10:186–189.

53. Calder I. When the endotracheal tube will not pass over the flexible fiberoptic bronchoscope. Anesthesiology 1992;77:398.

54. Brull SJ, Wiklund R, Ferris C, et al. Facilitation of fiberoptic orotracheal intubation with a flexible tracheal tube. Anesth Analg 1994;78:746–748.

55. Abramowitz MD, McNabb TG. A new complication of flexometallic endotracheal tubes. Br J Anaesth 1976;48:928.

56. Cohen DD, Dillon JB. Hazards of armored endotracheal tubes. Anesth Analg 1972;51:856–858.

57. Catane R, Davidson JT. A hazard of cuffed flexometallic endotracheal tubes. Br J Anaesth 1969;41: 1086.

58. Kohli MS, Manku RS. Reinforced endotracheal tube—diversion of air from cuff balloon producing obstruction. Anesthesiology 1966;27:513–514.

59. Lall NG. Airway obstruction with latex armoured endotracheal tube. Indian J Anaesth 1969;17:297.

60. Jacobson J. A hazard of armored endotracheal anesthesia. Anesth Analg 1969;48:37–41.

61. Mirakhur RK. Airway obstruction with cuffed armoured tracheal tubes. Can Anaesth Soc J 1974;21: 251–258.

62. Munson ES, Stevens DS, Redfern RE. Endotracheal tube obstruction by nitrous oxide. Anesthesiology 1980;52:275–276.

63. Ng TY, Krimili BI. Hazards in use of anode endotracheal tube: a case report and review. Anesth Analg 1975;54:710–714.

64. Ohn K, Wu W. Another complication of armored endotracheal tubes. Anesth Analg 1980;59: 215–216.

65. Ripoli I, Lindhold C, Carroll R, et al. Spontaneous dislocation of endotracheal tubes: a problem with too soft tube material. Crit Care Med 1978;6: 101–102.

66. Rendell–Baker L. A hazard alert: reinforced endotracheal tubes. Anesthesiology 1980;53:268–269.

67. Walton WJ. An invaginated tube. Br J Anaesth 1967;39:520.

68. Wright PJ, Mundy JVB. Tracheal tubes in neuroanesthesia. Nylon reinforced latex rubber tracheal tubes. Anaesthesia 1987;42:1012–1014.

69. Wright PJ, Mundy JVB, Mansfield CJ. Obstruction of armoured tracheal tubes: case report and discussion. Can J Anaesth 1988;35:195–197.

70. Brusco L, Weissman C. Pharyngeal obstruction of a reinforced orotracheal tube. Anesth Analg 1993; 76:653–654.

71. Singh B, Srivastava SK, Chhabra B. Reinforced orotracheal tube obstruction: Pharyngeal or oral? Anesth Analg 1994;79:193–194.

72. Gemma M, Ferrazza M. "Dental trauma" to oral airways. Can J Anaesth 1990;37:951.

73. Hoffmann CO, Swanson GA. Oral reinforced endotracheal tube crushed and perforated from biting. Anesth Analg 1989;69:552–553.

74. McTaggart RA, Shustack A, Noseworthy T, et al. Another cause of obstruction in an armored endotracheal tube. Anesthesiology 1983;59:164.

75. Martens P. Persistent narrowing of an armoured tube. Anaesthesia 1992;47:716–717.

76. Spiess BD, Rothenberg DM, Buckley S. Complete airway obstruction of armoured endotracheal tubes. Anesth Analg 1991;73:95–96.

77. Carden E, Crutchfield W. Anaesthesia for microsurgery of the larynx (a new method). Can Anaesth Soc J 1973;20:378–389.

78. Carden E, Ferguson GB, Crutchfield WM. A new silicone elastomer tube for use during microsurgery on the larynx. Ann Otol Rhinol Laryngol 1974;83:360–365.

79. Cooke JE, Hood JB, Thomas JD. A method for inserting the Carden tube. Anesth Analg 1976;55:882–883.

80. El-Naggar M, Keh E, Stemmers A, et al. Jet ventilation for micro laryngoscopic procedures: a further simplified technic. Anesth Analg 1974;53:797–804.

81. Edelman JD, Wingard W. Carden tube insertion. Anesthesiology 1978;49:220–221.

82. Singh A. A safe method of insertion of Carden's tube. Anaesthesia 1982;37:104–105.

83. Carden E. Carden tube. Can Anaesth Soc J 1980;27:512.

84. Soder CM, Haight J, Fredrickson JL, et al. Mechanical ventilation during laryngeal surgery. An evaluation of the Carden tube. Can Anaesth Soc J 1980;27:111–116.

86. Braverman I, Sichel J-Y, Halami P, et al. Complication of jet ventilation during microlaryngeal surgery. Ann Otol Rhinol Laryngol 1994;103:624–627.

87. Halimi P, Kadari A, Dayan M, et al. Gastric bleeding complicating esophageal intubation with a Carden's tube. J Clin Anesth 1994;6:168–169.

88. Dawson P, Rosewane F, Wells D. The Montando laryngectomy tube. Can J Anaesth 1989;36:486–487.

89. Riley RH, Mason SA, Barber CD. Obstruction of a preformed armoured tracheostomy tube. Can J Anaesth 1993;40:824.

90. Torres LE, Reynolds RC. Experiences with a new endotracheal tube for microlaryngeal surgery. Anesthesiology 1980;52:357–359.

91. Fry ENS. Difficult tracheal intubation. Anaesthesia 1985;40:206.

92. Asai T. Endotrol tube for blind nasotracheal intubation. Anaesthesia 1996;51:507.

93. Cook RT, Stene JK. The BAAM and endotrol endotracheal tube for blind oral intubation. J Clin Anesth 1993;5:431–432.

94. Cook RT, Stene JK, Marcolina B Jr. Use of a Beck airway airflow monitor and controllable-tip endotracheal tube in two cases of non-laryngoscopic oral intubation. Am J Emerg Med 1995;13:180–183.

95. Glinsman D, Pavlin EG. Airway obstruction after nasal-tracheal intubation. Anesthesiology 1982;56:229–230.

96. Miller BR. Problems associated with endotracheal tubes with monitoring lumens in pediatric patients. Anesthesiology 1987;67:1018–1019.

97. Green JM, Gonzalez RM, Sonbolian N, et al. The resistance to carbon dioxide laser ignition of a new endotracheal tube. Xomed Laser-Shield II. J Clin Anesth 1992;4:89–92.

98. Dillon F, Sosis M, Heller S. Evaluation of a new foil wrapped silicone endotracheal tube designed for laser airway surgery. Anesthesiology 1991;75:A392.

99. Sosis M, Pritikin J, Caldarelli D, et al. Effect of blood on the combustibility of laser resistant tracheal tubes. Anesthesiology 1992;77:A579.

100. Sosis MB Anesthesia for laser surgery. Clinical Updates. 1993;4(5):1–12.

101. Hawkins DB, Joseph MM. Avoiding a wrapped endotracheal tube in laser laryngeal surgery: experiences with apneic anesthesia and metal laser flex endotracheal tubes. Laryngoscope 1990; 100:1283–1287.

102. Garry B, Hivens HE. Laser safety in the operating room. Cancer Bull 1989;41:219–223.

103. Sosis MB. What is the safest endotracheal tube for Nd-YAG laser surgery?—A comparative study. Anesth Analg 1989;69:802–804.

104. Sosis MB. Which is the safest endotracheal tube for use with the CO_2 laser? A comparative study. J Clin Anaesth 1992;4:217–219.

105. Fried MP, Mallampati SR, Liu FC, et al. Laser resistant stainless steel endotracheal tube. Experimental and clinical evaluation. Lasers Surg Med 1991;11:301–306.

106. Anonymous. Laser-resistant endotracheal tubes and wraps. Health Devices 1990;19:109–139.

107. Sosis M, Dillon F. Reflection of CO_2 laser radiation from laser-resistant endotracheal tubes. Anesth Analg 1991;73:338–340.

108. Sprung J, Conley SF, Brown M. Unusual cause of difficult extubation. Anesthesiology 1991; 74:796.

109. Sosis MB. An analysis of the flow characteristics of pediatric laser resistant tracheal tubes. Anesth Analg 1995;80:S460.

110. Sosis M, Braverman V, Ivankovich AD. Evaluation of a new laser resistant fabric and copper foil wrapped endotracheal tube. Anesthesiology 1993; 79:A536.

111. Pashayan AG. Anesthesia for laser surgery. Atlanta: ASA Refresher Courses, 1995.

112. Norton ML, Vos P. New endotracheal tube for laser surgery of the larynx. Ann Otol Rhinol Laryngol 1978;87:554–557.

113. Sosis M. Large air leak during laser surgery with a Norton tube. Anesthesiol Rev 1989;16:39–41.

114. Skaredoff MN, Poppers PJ. Beware of sharp edges in metal endotracheal tubes. Anesthesiology 1983; 58:595.

115. Sosis MB. Hazards of laser surgery. Semin Anesth 1990;9:90–97.

116. Kamen JM, Wilkinson CJ. A new low-pressure cuff for endotracheal tubes. Anesthesiology 1971;34: 482–485.

117. Sosis M, Braverman B, Ivankovich AD. An evaluation of special tracheal tubes with the KTP laser. Anesth Analg 1991;72:S267.

118. Loeser EA, Machin R, Colley J, et al. Postoperative sore throat—importance of endotracheal tube conformity versus cuff design. Anesthesiology 1978;49: 430–432.

119. Wissler RN. The esophageal-tracheal Combitube. Anesth Rev 1993;20:147–152.

120. Baraka A, Salem R. The Combitube oesophageal-tracheal double lumen airway for difficult intubation. Can Anaesth Soc J 1993;40:1222–1223.

121. Butler BD, Little T, Drtil S. Combitube with a colorimetric carbon dioxide detector for emergency intubation/ventilation. Journal of Clinical Monitoring 1995;11:311–316.

122. Wafai Y, Salem MR, Joseph NJ, et al. Use of the self-inflating bulb with the esophageal tracheal Combitube. In response. Anesth Analg 1995;81: 1117–1118.

123. Maleck WH, Koetter KP. Esophageal-tracheal combitube, colorimetric carbon dioxide detection, and the esophageal detector device. Journal of Clinical Monitoring 1996;12:203.

124. Frass M, Rodler S, Frenzer R, et al. Esophageal tracheal combitube, endotracheal airway, and mask: comparison of ventilatory pressure curves. J Trauma 1989;29:1476-1479.

125. Frass M, Frenzer R, Zdrahal F, et al. The esophageal tracheal combitube: preliminary results with a new airway for CPR. Ann Emerg Med 1987;16: 768–772.

126. Frass M, Frenzer R, Rauscha F, et al. Evaluation of esophageal tracheal combitube in cardiopulmonary resuscitation. Crit Care Med 1987;15:609–611.

127. Frass M, Frenzer R, Rauscha F, et al. Ventilation with the esophageal tracheal combitube in cardiopulmonary resuscitation. Promptness and effectiveness. Chest 1988;93:781–784.

128. Staudinger T, Brugger S, Watschinger B, et al. Emergency intubation with the Combitube: comparison with the endotracheal airway. Ann Emerg Med 1993;22:1573–1575.

129. Forrest F. Millett S. Intermittent obstruction of tracheal tube revealed during pressure-supported ventilation. Anaesthesia 1991;46:799–800.

130. Frass M, Frenzer R, Zahler J, et al. Ventilation via the esophageal tracheal combitube in a case of difficult intubation. J Cardiothorac Anesth 1:1987: 565–568.

131. Atherton GL, Johnson JC. Ability of paramedics to use the Combitube in pre-hospital cardiac arrest. Ann Emerg Med 1993;22:1263–1268.

132. Banyai M, Falger S, Roggla M, et al. Emergency intubation with the Combitube in a grossly obese patient with bull neck. Resuscitation 1993;26: 271–276.

133. Bigenzahn W, Pesau B, Frass M. Emergency ventilation using the Combitube in cases of difficult intubation. Eur Arch Otorhinolaryngol 1991;248: 129–131.

134. Frass M, Frenzer R, Mayer G, et al. Mechanical ventilation with the esophageal tracheal Combitude (ETC) in the intensive care unit. Arch Emerg Med 1987;4:219–225.

135. Eichinger S, Schreiber W, Heinz T, et al. Airway management in a case of neck impalement: use of the oesophageal tracheal combitube airway. Br J Anaesth 1992;68:534–535.

136. Klauser R, Riggla G, Pidlich J, et al. Massive upper airway bleeding after thrombolytic therapy: successful airway management with the Combitube. Ann Emerg Med 1992;21:119.

137. Wiltschke C, Kment G, Swoboda H, et al. Ventilation with the Combitube during tracheotomy. Laryngoscope 1994;104:763–765.

138. Green K, KS, Beger TH. Proper use of the Combitube. Anesthesiology 1994;81:513.

139. Mest DR. Trauma applications of the Combitube. Anesthesiology News January 1995;13–30.

140. Bernhard WN, Yost L, Turndorf H, et al. Cuffed tracheal tubes: physical and behavioral characteristics. Anesth Analg 1982;61:36–41.

141. Cohen DD. Note on endotracheal tubes. Anesthesiology 1970;33:463.

142. Bernhard WN, Cottrell JE, Sivakumaran C, et al. Adjustment of intra-cuff pressure to prevent aspiration. Anesthesiology 1979;50:363–366.

143. Mehta S, Mickiewicz M. Pressure in large volume, low pressure cuffs. its significance, measurement and regulation. Intens Care Med 1985;11:267–272.

144. Seegobin RD, Van Hasselt GL. Endotracheal cuff pressure and tracheal mucosal blood flow: endoscopic study of effects of four large volume cuffs. Br Med J 1984;288:965–968.

145. Pavlin EG, Van Nimwegan D, Hornbein TF. Failure of a high-compliance low-pressure cuff to prevent aspiration. Anesthesiology 1975;42:216–219.

146. Guyton DC. Endotracheal and tracheotomy tube cuff design: influences on tracheal damage. Critical Care Updates 1990;1:10.

147. Mehta S. Safe lateral wall cuff pressure to prevent aspiration. Ann R Coll Surg Engl 1984;66:426–427.

148. Guyton DC, Barlow MR, Besseliebre TR. Influence of airway pressure on minimum occlusive endotracheal tube cuff pressure. Crit Care Med 1997; 25:91–94.

149. Bernhard WN, Yost LC, Turndorf H, et al. Physical characteristics of and rates of nitrous oxide diffusion into tracheal tube cuffs. Anesthesiology 1978;48:413–417.

150. Chandler M. Pressure in tracheal tube cuffs. Anaesthesia 1986;41:287–293.

151. Greene SJ, Cane RD, Shapiro BA. A foam cuff endotracheal tube T-piece system for use with nitrous oxide anesthesia. Anesth Analg 1986;65:1359–1360.

152. Mehta S. Effects of nitrous oxide and oxygen on tracheal tube cuff gas volumes. Br J Anaesth 1981;53:1227–1231.

153. Revenas R, Lindholm CE. Pressure and volume changes in tracheal tube cuffs during anaesthesia. Acta Anaesth Scand 1976;20:321–326.

154. Raeder JC, Borchgrevink PC, Sellevold OM. Tracheal tube cuff pressures. The effects of different gas mixtures. Anaesthesia 1985;40:444–447.

155. Stanley TH, Kawamura R, Graves C. Effects of nitrous oxide on volume and pressure of endotracheal tube cuffs. Anesthesiology 1974;41:256–262.

156. Stanley TH. Effects of anesthetic gases on endotracheal tube cuff gas volumes. Anesth Analg 1974;53:480–482.

157. Stanley TH. Nitrous oxide and pressures and volumes of high and low-pressure endotracheal-tube cuffs in intubated patients. Anesthesiology 1975;42:637–640.

158. Stevens WC, Crowley W. Tracheal wall pressure during nitrous oxide anesthesia and endotracheal intubation. Anesth Analg 1997;84:S271.

159. Latto IP. The cuff. In: Latto IP, Rosen M, eds. Difficulties in tracheal intubation. London: Baillière Tindall, 1985:48–74.

160. Lineberger CL, Johnson MD. A method for preventing endotracheal tube cuff overdistention caused by nitrous oxide diffusion. Anesth Analg 1991;72:843–844.

161. Morgan P. Prevention of nitrous oxide-induced increases in endotracheal tube cuff pressure. Anesth Analg 1991;73:232.

162. Fischer CG, Cook DR. Endotracheal tube cuff pressure in the use of nitrous oxide. Anesth Analg 1991; 73:99.

163. Brandt L. Nitrous oxide in oxygen and tracheal tube cuff volumes. Br J Anaesth 1982;54:1238–1239.

164. Ikeda D, Schweiss JF. Tracheal tube cuff volume changes during extracorporeal circulation. Can Anaesth Soc J 1980;27:453–457.

165. Partridge BL. Nitrous oxide and endotracheal tube cuff leaks. Anesthesiology 1988;68:167–168.

166. Patel RI, Oh TH, Epstein BS. Effects of nitrous oxide on pressure changes of tracheal tube cuffs following inflation with air and saline. Anaesthesia 1983;38:44–46.

167. Patel RI, Oh TH, Chandra R, et al. Tracheal tube cuff pressure. Changes during nitrous oxide anaesthesia following inflation of cuffs with air and saline. Anaesthesia 1984;39:862–864.

168. Sperry RJ, Johnson JO, Apfelbaum RI. Endotracheal tube cuff pressure increases significantly during anterior cervical fusion with the Caspar instrumentation system. Anesth Analg 1993;76:1318–1321.

169. Norman PH, Daley MD. Endotracheal tube cuff pressures in the absence of nitrous oxide. Anesth Analg 1994;78:S319.

170. Carroll R, Hedden M, Safar P. Intratracheal cuffs: performance characteristics. Anesthesiology 1969;31:275–281.

171. Dobrin P, Canfield T. Cuffed endotracheal tubes: mucosal pressures and tracheal wall blood flow. Am J Surg 1977;133:562–568.

172. Wu W, Lim I, Simpson FA, et al. Pressure dynamics

of endotracheal and tracheostomy cuffs. Crit Care Med 1973;1:197–202.

173. Cooper JD, Grillo HC. Analysis of problems related to cuffs on intratracheal tubes. Chest 1972;62: 21S–27S.

174. Jensen PJ, Hommelgaard P, Sondergaard P, et al. Sore throat after operation: influence of tracheal intubation, intracuff pressure and type of cuff. Br J Anaesth 1982;54:453–457.

175. Loeser EA, Orr DL, Bennett GM, et al. Endotracheal tube cuff design and postoperative sore throat. Anesthesiology 1976;45:684–687.

176. Loeser EA, Stanley TH, Jordan W, et al. Postoperative sore throat: influence of tracheal tube lubrication versus cuff design. Can Anaesth Soc J 1980; 27:156–158.

177. Jones R, Ueda I. Cuff bulk of tracheal tubes in adolescence. Can J Anaesth 1996;43:514–517.

178. Crawley BE, Cross DE. Tracheal cuffs. A review and dynamic pressure study. Anaesthesia 1975;30: 4–11.

179. Guyton D, Banner MJ, Kirby RR. High-volume, low-pressure cuffs. Are they always low pressure? Chest 1991;100:1076–1081.

180. Lewis FR, Schlobohm RM, Thomas AN. Prevention of complications from prolonged tracheal intubation. Am J Surg 1978;135:452–457.

181. Loeser EA, Bennett GM, Orr DL, et al. Reduction of postoperative sore throat with new endotracheal tube cuffs. Anesthesiology 1980;52:257–259.

182. Cross DE. Recent developments in tracheal cuffs. Resuscitation 1973;2:77–81.

183. Bernhard WN, Yost L, Joynes D, et al. Intracuff pressures in endotracheal and tracheostomy tubes. Related cuff physical characteristics. Chest 1985;87: 720–725.

184. Tonnesen AS, Vereen L, Arens JF. Endotracheal tube cuff residual volume and lateral wall pressure in a model trachea. Anesthesiology 1981;55: 680–683.

185. Wilder NA, Orr J, Westenskow D. Evaluation in animals of a system to estimate tracheal pressure from the endotracheal tube cuff. Journal of Clinical Monitoring 1996;12:11–16.

186. Mehta S. Performance of low-pressure cuffs. An experimental evaluation. Ann R Coll Surg Engl 1982; 64:54–56.

187. Nordin U. The trachea and cuff-induced tracheal injury. Acta Otolaryngol Suppl (Stockh) 1977;345: 1–74.

188. Stauffer JL, Olson DE, Petty TL. Complications and consequences of endotracheal intubation and tracheotomy. A prospective study of 150 critically ill adult patients. Am J Med 1981;70:65–76.

189. Jaeger JM, Wells NC, Blanch PB. Mechanical ventilation of a patient with decreased lung compliance and tracheal dilatation. J Clin Anesth 1992;4: 147–152.

190. Loeser EA, Hodges M, Gliedman J, et al. Tracheal pathology following short-term intubation with low- and high-pressure endotracheal tube cuffs. Anesth Analg 1978;57:577–579.

191. Bunegin L, Albin MS, Smith RB. Canine tracheal blood flow after endotracheal tube cuff inflation during normotension and hypotension. Anesth Analg 1993;76:1083–1090.

192. King K, Mandava B, Kamen JM. Tracheal tube cuffs and tracheal dilatation. Chest 1975;67:458–462.

193. Dinnick OP. Tracheal cuffs. Anaesthesia 1975;30: 553–554.

194. MacKenzie CF, Shin B, McAslan TC, et al. Severe stridor after prolonged endotracheal intubation using high-volume cuffs. Anesthesiology 1979;50: 235–239.

195. Pippin LK, Short DH, Bowes JB. Long-term tracheal intubation practice in the United Kingdom. Anaesthesia 1983;38:791–795.

196. Macrae W, Wallace P. Aspiration around high-volume, low-pressure endotracheal cuff. Br Med J 1981;283:1220.

197. Routh G, Hanning CD, Ledingham IM. Pressure on the tracheal mucosa from cuffed tubes. Br Med J 1979;1:1425.

198. Seegobin RD, van Hasselt GL. Aspiration beyond endotracheal cuffs. Can Anaesth Soc J 1986;33: 273–279.

199. Oikkonen M, Aromaa U. Leakage of fluid around low-pressure tracheal tube cuffs. Anaesthesia 1997; 52:567–569.

200. Young PJ, Rollinson M, Downward G, et al. Leakage of fluid past the tracheal tube cuff in a bench top model. Br J Anaesth 1997;78:557–562.

201. Sweatman AJ, Tomasello PA, Loughhead MO, et al. Misplacement of nasogastric tubes and oesophageal monitoring devices. Br J Anaesth 1978;50: 389–392.

202. Stark P. Inadvertent nasogastric tube insertion into the tracheobronchial tree. A hazard of new high-residual volume cuffs. Radiology 1982;142: 239–240.

203. Nakao MA, Killam D, Wilson R. Pneumothorax secondary to inadvertent nasotracheal placement of a nasoenteric tube past a cuffed endotracheal tube. Crit Care Med 1983;11:210–211.

204. Lee T, Schrader MW, Wright BD. Pseudo-failure of mechanical ventilator caused by accidental endobronchial nasogastric tube insertion. Respiratory Care 1980;25:851–853.

205. Carey TS, Holcombe BJ. Endotracheal intubation as a risk factor for complications of nasoenteric tube insertion. Crit Care Med 1991;19:427–429.

206. Dodd CM, Loken RG, Williams RT. Hazards associated with passage of nasogastric tubes. Can J Anaesth 1988;35:541–542.

207. Elder S, Meguid MM. Pneumothorax following attempted nasogastric intubation for nutritional support. J Parenter Enteral Nutr 1984;8:450–452.

208. Soroker D, Ezri T, Szmuk P. An unusual case of failure to ventilate the lungs. Anaesthesia 1994;49:1105.

209. Carroll RG, Grenvick A. Proper use of large diameter, large residual volume cuffs. Crit Care Med 1973;1:153–154.

210. Power KJ. Foam cuffed tracheal tubes. Clinical and laboratory assessment. Br J Anaesth 1990;65:433–437.

211. Kamen JM, Wilkinson C. Removal of an inflated endotracheal tube cuff. Anesthesiology 1977;46:308–309.

212. Wolman RL, Shapiro J, Kane F. Incidence of sore throat and hoarseness following cardiac surgery with foam versus air-filled cuff endotracheal tubes. Anesth Analg 1995;80:S557.

213. MacKenzie CF, Klose S, Browne DRG. A study of inflatable cuffs on endotracheal tubes. Br J Anaesth 1976;48:105–110.

214. Elliott CJR. Problems of cuff deflation. Anaesthesia 1973;28:535–537.

215. Tavakoli M, Corssen G. An unusual case of difficult extubation. Anesthesiology 1976;45:552–553.

216. Malone BT. A complication of Rusch armored endotracheal tubes. Anesth Analg 1975;54:756.

217. Dunn GL. Letter to the editor. Can Anaesth Soc J 1975;22:379–380.

218. Diaz JH. Continuous monitoring of intracuff pressures in endotracheal tubes. Anesthesiology 1988;68:813–818.

219. Morris JV, Latto IP. An electropneumatic instrument for measuring and controlling the pressures in the cuffs of tracheal tubes (the Cardiff cuff controller). J Med Eng Technol 1985;9:229–230.

220. Scott AA. Pressure monitoring device for low pressure cuffs on tracheostomy tubes. Can Anaesth Soc J 1974;21:120–122.

221. Cox PM, Schatz ME. Pressure measurements in endotracheal cuffs: a common error. Chest 1974;65:84–87.

222. Kosanin R, Maroff M. Continuous monitoring of endotracheal intracuff pressures in patients receiving general anesthesia utilizing nitrous oxide. Anesthesiol Rev 1981;8:29–32.

223. McGinnis GE, Shively JG, Patterson RL, et al. An engineering analysis of intratracheal tube cuffs. Anesth Analg 1971;50:557–564.

224. Magovern GJ, Shively JG, Fecht D, et al. The clinical and experimental evaluation of a controlled-pressure intratracheal cuff. J Thorac Cardiovasc Surg 1972;64:747–756.

225. Leigh JM, Maynard JP. Pressure on the tracheal mucosa from cuffed tubes. Br Med J 1979;1:1173–1174.

226. Carroll RG. Evaluation of tracheal tube cuff designs. Crit Care Med 1973;1:45–46.

227. Brandt L. Pressures on tracheal tube cuffs. Anaesthesia 1982;37:597–598.

228. Kumar CM, Scott G. Lanz valve—a method of circumventing a leaking valve. Anaesthesia 1986;41:772.

229. Burns SM, Shasby DM, Burke PA. Controlled pressure cuffed endotracheal tubes may not be controlled. Chest 1983;83:158–159.

230. Gravenstein N, Burwick N. Recoil of inflation syringe plunger limits excessive endotracheal tube cuff pressure. Anesthesiology 1988;69:A730.

231. Resnikoff E, Katz JA. A modified epidural syringe as an endotracheal tube cuff pressure-controlling device. Anesth Analg 1990;70:208–211.

232. Stanley TH, Foote JL, Lu WS. A simple pressure-relief valve to prevent increases in endotracheal tube cuff pressure and volume in intubated patients. Anesthesiology 1975;43:478–481.

233. Kay J, Fisher JA. Control of endotracheal tube cuff pressure using a simple device. Anesthesiology 1987;66:253.

234. Kim J. The tracheal tube cuff pressure stabilizer and its clinical evaluation. Anesth Analg 1980;59:291–296.

235. Joseph J, Epstein RH. Servoregulation of endotracheal tube cuff pressure in the presence of nitrous oxide. Anesth Analg 1994;78:S181.

236. Latto IP, Willis BA, Dyson A. The Cardiff cuff controller. Br J Anaesth 1987;59:651P–652P.

237. Willis BA, Latto IP, Dyson A. Tracheal tube cuff pressure. Clinical use of the Cardiff cuff controller. Anaesthesia 1988;43:312–314.

238. Willis BA, Latto IP. Profile-cuffed tracheal tubes and the Cardiff cuff controller. Anaesthesia 1989;44:524.

239. Lawler PG, Rayner RR. The limitations of the Shiley pressure relief adaptor. Anaesthesia 1982;37:865.

240. American Society for Testing and Materials. Standard specification for tracheal tube connectors (ASTM F1243-89) (Reapproved 1995). West Conshohocken, PA: ASTM, 1995.

241. Branson R, Lam AM. Increased resistance to breathing: a potentially lethal hazard across a coaxial circuit-connector coupling. Can J Anaesth 1987;34: S90–S91.

242. Villforth JC. FDA safety alert: breathing systems connectors. Rockville, MD: FDA, 1983.

243. Shupak RC. A new tracheal tube for head and neck surgery. Anesthesiology 1984;60:621–622.

244. Smith WDA. The effects of external resistance to respiration. Part II. Resistance to respiration due to anaesthetic apparatus. Br J Anaesth 1961;33: 610–627.

245. Galloon S. The resistance of endotracheal connectors. Br J Anaesth 1957;29:160–165.

246. Hayes SR, Johnson K, Munson ES. Removal of endotracheal tube connectors. Anesth Analg 1987;66: 1059–1060.

247. Scott RPF, Chapman I. A problem with the Argyll tracheal tube. Anaesthesia 1987;42:1123.

248. Sosis M, Dillon F. What is the safest foil tape for endotracheal tube protection during Nd-YAG laser surgery? A comparative study. Anesthesiology 1990; 72:553–555.

249. Sosis MB. Anesthesia for laser surgery. Int Anesthesiol Clin 1990;28:119–131.

250. Snow JC, Kripke J, Strong MS, et al. Anesthesia for carbon dioxide laser surgery on the larynx and trachea. Anesth Analg 1974;53:507–512.

251. Patel V, Stehling LC, Zauder HL. A modified endotracheal tube for laser microsurgery. Anesthesiology 1979;51:571.

252. Patil KF, Hicks JN. Prevention of fire hazards associated with use of carbon dioxide lasers. Anesth Analg 1981;60:885–888.

253. Vourc'h G, Tannieres ML, Freche G. Anaesthesia for microsurgery of the larynx using a carbon dioxide laser. Anaesthesia 1979;34:53–57.

254. Sosis MB. Evaluation of five metallic tapes for protection of endotracheal tubes during CO_2 laser surgery. Anesth Analg 1989;68:392–393.

255. Sosis M, Heller S. A comparison of five metallic tapes for protection of endotracheal tubes during CO_2 laser surgery. Can J Anaesth 1988;35:S63.

256. Munshi C, Connolly L. Comparison of laser-resistant wrappings of red rubber endotracheal tubes subjected to CO_2 and KTP laser. Anesth Analg 1993;76:S279.

257. Sosis MB. In response. Anesth Analg 1991;72: 415–416.

258. Williamson R. Why 70 watts to evaluate metal tapes for CO_2 laser surgery? Anesth Analg 1991;72: 414–415.

259. Sosis M, Dillon F. Prevention of CO_2 induced laser tracheal tube fires with Laser-Guard protective coating. Can J Anaesth 1989;36:S88–S89.

260. Gonzalez C, Smith M, Reinisch L. Endotracheal tube safety with the erbium:ytrium aluminum garnet laser. Ann Otol Rhinol Laryngol 1990;99: 553–555.

261. Burgess GE, LeJeune FE. Endotracheal tube ignition during laser surgery of the larynx. Arch Otolaryngol 1979;105:561–562.

262. Ngeow YK, Kashima H. More about protection of endotracheal tubes during laser microlaryngeal surgery. Anesthesiology 1981;55:714.

263. Fontenot R, Bailey BJ, Stiernberg CM, et al. Endotracheal tube safety during laser surgery. Laryngoscope 1987;97:919–921.

264. Brightwell AP. A complication of the use of the laser in ENT surgery. J Laryngol Otol 1983;97: 671–672.

265. Kaeder CS, Hirshman CA. Acute airway obstruction: a complication of aluminum tape wrapping of tracheal tubes in laser surgery. Can Anaesth Soc J 1979;26:138–139.

266. Hirshman CA, Leon D. Ignition of an endotracheal tube during laser microsurgery. Anesthesiology 1980;53:177.

267. Hirshman CA, Smith J. Indirect ignition of the endotracheal tube during carbon dioxide laser surgery. Arch Otolaryngol 1980;106:639–641.

268. Kalhan S, Regan AG. A further modification of endotracheal tubes for laser microsurgery. Anesthesiology 1980;53:81.

269. Malmros C, Fletcher R, Jonmarker C, et al. Cuffed endotracheal tubes for paediatric cardiac surgery cause a low incidence of post-operative airway problems. Anesthesiology 1991;75:A931.

270. Deakers TW, Reynolds H, Stretton M, et al. Cuffed endotracheal tubes in pediatric intensive care. J Pediatr 1994; 125:57–62.

271. Khine HH, Corddry DH, Kettrick RG, et al. Comparison of cuffed and uncuffed endotracheal tubes in young children during general anesthesia. Anesthesiology 1997;86:627–631.

272. Liu LMP, Li C-Y, Damiani–Rivera JA, et al. Can cuffed endotracheal tubes be used routinely in anesthetized children? Anesthesiology 1995;83:A1185.

273. Stenqvist O, Sonander H, Nilsson K. Small endotracheal tubes. Ventilator and intratracheal pressures during controlled ventilation. Br J Anaesth 1979; 51:375–381.

274. Zulliger JJ, Garvin JP, Schuller DE, et al. Assessment of intubation in croup and epiglottitis. Ann Otol Rhinol Laryngol 1982;91:403–406.

275. Downes JJ. Pediatric tracheal tube consideration. Paper presented at a workshop on tracheal tubes, Valley Forge, PA. April 30–May 1, 1981.

276. Board J. Endotracheal tube diameter. Anaesthesia and Intensive Care 1982;10:91–92.

277. Mackenzie CF, Shin B, Whitley N, et al. Human tracheal circumference as an indicator of correct cuff size. Anesthesiology 1980;53:S414.

278. Chandler M, Crawley BE. Rationalization of the selection of tracheal tubes. Br J Anaesth 1986;58:111–116.

279. Mackenzie CF, Shin B, Whitley N, et al. The relationship of human trachea size to body habitus. Anesthesiology 1979;51:S378.

280. Mackenzie CF, McAslan C, Shin B, et al. The shape of the human adult trachea. Anesthesiology 1978;49:48–50.

281. Mehta S, Myat HM. The cross-sectional shape and circumference of the human trachea. Ann R Coll Surg Engl 1984;66:356–358.

282. Bourne TM, Barker I. External diameters of paediatric tracheal tubes. Anaesthesia 1993;48:839.

283. DiCarlo JV, Sanders AI, Sweeney MF. Airway complications of endotracheal intubation in pediatric patients. Effect of endotracheal tube fit. Anesthesiology 1988;69:A775.

284. Finholt DA, Henry DB, Raphaely RC. Factors affecting leak around tracheal tubes in children. Can Anaesth Soc J 1985;32:326–329.

285. Finholt DA, Audenaert SM, Stirt JA, et al. Endotracheal tube leak pressure and tracheal lumen size in swine. Anesth Analg 1986;65:667–671.

286. Schwartz RE, Pasquariello CA. Tracheal tube leak test—is there inter-observer agreement? Can J Anaesth 1993; 40:1049–1052.

287. Sweeney MF, Egar M, Williams TA, et al. Total respiratory resistance in the intubated pediatric patient. Anesthesiology 1985;63:A477.

288. Lane GA, Pashley RT, Fishman RA. Tracheal and cricoid diameters in the premature infant. Anesthesiology 1980;53:S326.

289. Penlington GN. Endotracheal tube sizes for children. Anaesthesia 1974;29:494–495.

290. Anonymous. Standards for CPR and ECC. JAMA 1986;255:2972.

291. Luten RC, Wears RL, Broselow J, et al. Length-based endotracheal tube and emergency equipment in pediatrics. Ann Emerg Med 1992; 21:900–904.

292. Gregory GA. Respiratory care of the child. Crit Care Med 1980;8:582–587.

293. Fukuoka RH, Kelly JW, Franklin CM. Correlation between ETT size, distal digit diameter and the Penlington formula. Anesth Analg 1991;72:S85.

294. Fukuoka RH, Kelly JW, Franklin CM. Correlation between ETT size, distal digit diameter and the Penlington formulae. Anesth Analg 1991;72:S85.

295. van den Berg AA, Mphanza T. Choice of tracheal tube size for children: finger size or age-related formula? Anaesthesia 1997;52:695–703.

296. King BR, Baker MD, Braitman LE, et al. Endotracheal tube selection in children. Ann Emerg Med 1993;22:530–4.

297. Hinkle AJ. A rapid and reliable method of selecting endotracheal tube size in children. Anesth Analg 1988;67:S92.

298. McCoy E, Barnes S. A defect in a tracheal tube. Anaesthesia 1989;44:525.

299. McLean RF, McLean J, McKee D. Another cause of tracheal tube failure. Can J Anaesth 1989;36:733–734.

300. Smith MB, Watts JD. Splitting tubes. Anaesthesia 1992;47:363.

301. Heusner JE, Viscomi CM. Endotracheal tube cuff failure due to valve damage. Anesth Analg 1991;72:270.

302. Gold ML. Use of petroleum jelly. Anesthesiology 1985;63:339–340.

303. McMillan DD, Rademaker AW, Buchan KA, et al. Benefits of orotracheal and nasotracheal intubation in neonates requiring ventilatory assistance. Pediatrics 1986;77:39–44.

304. Fletcher R, Olsson K, Helbo–Hansen S, et al. Oral or nasal intubation after cardiac surgery? A comparison of effects on heart rate, blood pressure and sedation requirements. Anaesthesia 1984;39:376–378.

305. Donn SM, Blane CE. Endotracheal tube movement in the preterm neonate: oral versus nasal intubation. Ann Otol Rhinol Laryngol 1985;94:18–20.

306. Bach A, Boehrer H, Schmidt H, et al. Nosocomial sinusitis in ventilated patients. Anaesthesia 1992;47:335–339.

307. Coppolo DP, May JJ. Self-extubations in a 12-month experience. Chest 1990;98:165–169.

308. Berry FA, Blankenbaker WL, Ball CG. A comparison of bacteremia occurring with nasotracheal and orotracheal intubation. Anesth Analg 1973;52:873–876.

309. Dinner M, Tjeuw M, Artusio JF. Bacteremia as a complication of nasotracheal intubation. Anesth Analg 1987;66:460–462.

310. McShane AJ, Hone R. Prevention of bacterial endocarditis: does nasal intubation warrant prophylaxis? Br Med J 1986;292:26–27.

311. Rowse CW. Bacteraemia induced by endotracheal intubation. Br Dent J 1981;151:363.

312. Arens JF, LeJeune FE, Webre DR. Maxillary sinusitis: a complication of nasotracheal intubation. Anesthesiology 1974;40:415–416.

313. Aebert H, Hunefeld G, Regel G. Paranasal sinusitis and sepsis in ICU patients with nasotracheal intubation. Intens Care Med 1988;15:27–30.

314. Deutschman CS, Wilton PB, Sinow J, et al. Paranasal sinusitis. A common complication of nasotracheal intubation in neurosurgical patients. Neurosurgery 1985;17:296–299.

315. Deutschman CS, Wilton P, Sinow J, et al. Paranasal sinusitis associated with nasotracheal intubation. A frequently unrecognized and treatable source of sepsis. Crit Care Med 1986;14:111–114.

316. Fassoulaki A. Nasotracheal intubation, paranasal sinusitis and head injuries. Br J Anaesth 1989;62:236.

317. Fassoulaki A, Pamouktsoglou P. Prolonged nasotracheal intubation and its association with inflammation of paranasal sinuses. Anesth Analg 1989;69:50–52.

318. Hansen M, Poulsen MR, Bendixen DK, et al. Incidence of sinusitis in patients with nasotracheal intubation. Br J Anaesth 1988;61:231–232.

319. Halac E, Indiveri DR, Obregon RJ, et al. Complication of nasal endotracheal intubation. J Pediatr 1983;103:166.

320. Knodel AR, Beekman JF. Unexplained fevers in patients with nasotracheal intubation. JAMA 1982;248:868–870.

321. Linden BE, Aguilar EA, Allen SJ. Sinusitis in the nasotracheally intubated patient. Arch Otolaryngol Head Neck Surg 1988;114:860–861.

322. O'Reilly MJ, Reddick EJ, Black W, et al. Sepsis from sinusitis in nasotracheally intubated patients. A diagnostic dilemma. Am J Surg 1984;147:601–604.

323. Pope TL, Stelling CB, Leitner YB. Maxillary sinusitis after nasotracheal intubation. South Med J 1981;74:610–612.

324. Pedersen J, Schurizek BA, Melsen NC, et al. The effect of nasotracheal intubation on the paranasal sinuses. A prospective study of 434 intensive care patients. Acta Anaesthesiol Scand 1991;35:11–13.

325. Salord F, Gaussorgues P, Marti–Flich J, et al. Nosocomial maxillary sinusitis during mechanical ventilation: a prospective comparison of orotracheal versus the nasotracheal route for intubation. Intens Care Med 1990;16:390–393.

326. Willatts SM, Cochrane DF. Paranasal sinusitis. A complication of nasotracheal intubation. Br J Anaesth 1985;57:1026–1028.

327. Katkov WN, Ault MJ. Endotracheal intubation in massive hemoptysis. Advantages of the orotracheal route. Crit Care Med 1989;17:968.

328. Rhee KJ, Muntz CB, Donald PJ, et al. Does nasotracheal intubation increase complications in patients with skull base fractures? Ann Emerg Med 1993;22:1145–1147.

329. Conetta R, Nierman DM. Pneumocephalus following nasotracheal intubation. Ann Emerg Med 1992;21:100–102.

330. Quintin L, Ghignone M, Odelin P, et al. Decreasing the incidence of upper airway bleeding when using a large-size nasotracheal tube. Anesthesiology 1985;62:374.

331. Kay J, Bryan R, Hart HB, et al. Sequential dilatation. A useful adjunct in reducing blood loss from nasotracheal intubation. Anesthesiology 1985;63:A259.

332. Berger JM, Stirt JA. Aid to nasotracheal intubation. Anesthesiology 1983;58:105.

333. Moore DC. Bloodless turbinectomy following blind nasal intubation. Faulty technique. Anesthesiology 1990;73:1057.

334. Tahir AH. A simple manoeuvre to aid the passage of nasotracheal tube into the oropharynx. Br J Anaesth 1970;42:631–632.

335. Dryden GE. Use of a suction catheter to assist blind nasal intubation. Anesthesiology 1976;45:260.

336. Cohen PJ. An endotracheal-tube barb. Anesthesiology 1977;47:77.

337. Berry FA. The use of a stylet in blind nasotracheal intubation. Anesthesiology 1984;61:469–471.

338. Hamill M, Toung T. Blind nasotracheal intubations revisited. Anesth Analg 1994;79:390–391.

339. Liew RPC. A technique of naso-tracheal intubation with the soft Portex tube. Anaesthesia 1973;28:567–568.

340. Gorback MS. Inflation of the endotracheal tube cuff as an aid to blind nasal endotracheal intubation. Anesth Analg 1987;66:917–918.

341. Van Elstraete AC, Pennant JH, Gajraj NM, et al. Tracheal tube cuff inflation as an aid to blind nasotracheal intubation. Br J Anaesth 1993;70:691–693.

342. Szmuk P, Ezri T. Capnography and cuff inflation to aid blind tracheal intubation. Anaesthesia 1995;50:662.

343. Temperley AD, Walker PJ. Blind nasal intubation by monitoring capnography in a neonate with congenital microstomia. Anaesthesia and Intensive Care 1995;23:490–492.

344. Venditti RC. A novel application of the Nellcor Easy Cap end-tidal CO_2 detector. Anesth Analg 1994;78:1029–1030.

345. Bennett EJ, Grundy EM, Patel KP. Visual signs in blind nasal intubation. A new technique. Anesthesiol Rev 1978;5:18–20.

346. Barriot P, Riou B. Retrograde technique for tracheal intubation in trauma patients. Crit Care Med 1988; 16:712–713.

347. Mehta S. Intubation guide marks for correct tube placement. A clinical study. Anaesthesia 1991;46: 306–308.

348. Owen RL, Cheney FW. Endobronchial intubation: a preventable complication. Anesthesiology 1987; 67:255–257.

349. Spadafora MP, Roberts JR. Technique for determining proper depth of oral tracheal tube placement in the critically ill adult patient. Ann Emerg Med 1986;15:67.

350. Sosis MB, Harbut RE. A caution on the use of routine depth of insertion of endotracheal tubes. Anesthesiology 1991;74:961–962.

351. Eagle GCP. The relationship between a person's height and appropriate endotracheal tube length. Anaesthesia and Intensive Care 1992; 20:156–160.

352. Patel N, Mahajan RP, Ellis FR. Estimation of the correct length of tracheal tubes in adults. Anaesthesia 1993;48:74–75.

353. Yates AP, Harries AJ, Hatch DJ. Estimation of nasotracheal tube length in infants and children. Br J Anaesth 1987;59:524–526.

354. Soni AK, Paes ML. Getting the length right. Anaesthesia 1994;49:549.

355. Mamawadu BR, Miller R. Endotracheal cuff inflation. An improved technique. Anesthesiol Rev 1977;4:46–47.

356. Chandler S. Air volume in endotracheal tube cuffs. Anesthesiology 1980;53:437.

357. Mehta S. Aspiration around high-volume low-pressure endotracheal cuff. Br Med J 1982;284: 115–116.

358. Wedley JR, Mathias DB. Endotracheal cuffs. Anaesthesia 1976;31:114.

359. Doiron M, Stedman P. Are the endotracheal tube cuff pressures at our institution within the recommended range? Anesthesiology 1995;83:A500.

360. Fenje N, Steward DJ. A study of tape adhesive strength on endotracheal tubes. Can J Anaesth 1988;35:198–202.

361. Patel N, Smith CE, Pinchak AC, et al. Taping methods and tape types for securing oral endotracheal tubes. Can J Anaesth 1997;44:330–336.

362. Richards SD. A method for securing pediatric endotracheal tubes. Anesth Analg 1981;60:224–225.

363. Mikawa K, Maekawa N, Goto R, et al. Transparent dressing is useful for the secure fixation of the endotracheal tube. Anesthesiology 1991;75: 1123–1124.

364. Emmanual ER. Taping ETT connectors. Anaesthesia and Intensive Care 1993;21:380.

365. Benumof JL. Conventional (laryngoscopic) orotracheal and nasotracheal intubation (single-lumen type). In: Benumof JL, ed. Clinical procedures in anesthesia and intensive care. Philadelphia: JB Lippincott, 1992:115–148.

366. Shroff PK, Parton KR, Thomson JH, et al. A simple method of securing an endotracheal tube. J Am Assoc Nurse Anesth 1987;55:404.

367. Khorasani A, Bird DJ. Facial hair and securing the endotracheal tube: a new method. Anesth Analg 1996;83:886.

368. Dykes ER, Anderson R. Technic for fixation of endotracheal tubes. Anesth Analg 1964;43:238–240.

369. Klein DS. An endotracheal tube fixation device constructed from discarded oxygen tubing and umbilical tape. Anesthesiology 1984;60:76.

370. Steward DJ. Fixation of reinforced silicone tracheal tubes. Anesthesiology 1985;63:334.

371. Middleton H. Fixation of nasotracheal and nasogastric tubes. Anaesthesia 1991;46:600.

372. Jensen NF, Kealey GP. Securing an endotracheal tube in the presence of facial burns or instability. Anesth Analg 1992;75:641–642.

373. Garcia–Tornel S, Martin JM, Carits J, et al. Method of fixating tubes in infants and children. Respiratory Care 1978;22:58.

374. Molho M, Lieberman P. Safe fixation of oro- and nasotracheal tubes for prolonged intubation in neonates, infants and children. Crit Care Med 1975;3: 81–82.

375. Stubbing JF, Young JVI. Circumpalatal fixation of an orotracheal tube. Anaesthesia 1985;40:916–917.

376. Jobes DR, Nicolson S. An alternative method to secure an endotracheal tube in infants with midline facial defects. Anesthesiology 1986;64:643–644.

377. Birmingham PK, Horn B. An infant model to facilitate endotracheal tube fixation in the pediatric ICU patient. Anesthesiology 1989;70:163–164.

378. Kaplow R, Bookbinder M. A comparison of four endotracheal tube holders. Heart & Lung 1994; 23: 59–66.

379. Petros AJ. A new disposable system for tracheal tube fixation in children. Anaesthesia 1997;52:382–383.

380. Tasota F, Hoffman L, Zullo TG, et al. Evaluation of two methods used to stabilize oral endotracheal tubes. Heart Lung 1987;16:140–146.

381. Boyd GL, Funderburg BJ, Vasconez LO, et al. Long-distance anesthesia. Anesth Analg 1992;74: 477.

382. Gowdar K, Bull MJ, Schreiner RL, et al. Nasal de-

formities in neonates. Their occurrence in those treated with nasal continuous positive airway pressure and nasal endotracheal tubes. Am J Dis Child 1980;134:954–957.

383. Alfery DD. Changing an endotracheal tube. In: JL Benumof, ed. Clinical procedures in anesthesia and intensive care. Philadelphia: JB Lippincott, 1992: 177–194.

384. Bedger RC, Chang J. A jet-style endotracheal catheter for difficult airway management. Anesthesiology 1987;66:221–223.

385. Benumof JL. Additional safety measures when changing endotracheal tubes. Anesthesiology 1991; 75:921–922.

386. Desai SP, Fencl V. A safe technique for changing endotracheal tubes. Anesthesiology 1980;53:267.

387. Miller KA, Harkin CP, Bailey PL. Postoperative tracheal extubation. Anesth Analg 1995; 80:148–172.

388. Kong CS. A small child can bite through an armoured tracheal tube. Anaesthesia 1995;50:263.

389. Garla PGN, Skaredoff M. Tracheal extubation. Anesthesiology 1992;76:1058.

390. Benumof JF. Management of the difficult adult airway. Anesthesiology 1991;75:1087–1110.

391. Gillespie JA. Difficulty in extubation. Anaesthesia 1992;47:715.

392. Bourne TM, Tate K. Failed cuff deflation. Anaesthesia 1990;45:76.

393. Brock–Utne JG, Jaffe RA, Robins B, et al. Difficulty in extubation. A cause for concern. Anaesthesia 1992;47:229–230.

394. Singh B, Gupta B. Difficult extubation: A new management. Anesth Analg 1995;81:433.

395. Benumof JL. Management of the difficult airway. The ASA algorithm (ASA Refresher Course #134). New Orleans: ASA, 1992.

396. Kanefield JK, Munro JT, Eisele JH. Incidence of bleeding after oral endotracheal intubation. Anesth Rev 1990;17:43–45.

397. Gould DB, Banes CH. Iatrogenic disruptions of right temporomandibular joints during orotracheal intubation causing permanent closed lock of the jaw. Anesth Analg 1995;81:191–194.

398. Keane WM, Denneny JC, Rowe LD, et al. Complications of intubation. Ann Otol Rhinol Laryngol 1982;91:584–587.

399. Bembridge JL, Bembridge M. Pneumomediastinum during general anaesthesia: case report. Can J Anaesth 1989;36:75–77.

400. Dubost C, Kaswin D, Duranteau A, et al. Esophageal perforation during attempted endotracheal intubation. J Thorac Cardiovasc Surg 1979;78: 44–51.

401. de Espinosa H, de Paredes CG. Traumatic perforation of the pharynx in a newborn baby. J Ped Surg 1974;9:247–248.

402. Evron S, Beyth Y, Samueloff A, et al. Pulmonary complications following endotracheal intubation for anesthesia in breech extractions. Intensive Care Med 1985;11:223–225.

403. Eldor J, Ofek B, Abramowitz HB. Perforation of oesophagus by tracheal tube during resuscitation. Anaesthesia 1990;45:70–71.

404. Finer NN, Stewart AR, Ulan OA. Tracheal perforation in the neonate. Treatment with a cuffed endotracheal tube. J Pediatr 1976;89:510–512.

405. Hawkins DB, Seltzer DC, Barnett TE, et al. Endotracheal tube perforation of the hypopharynx. West J Med 1974;120:282–286.

406. Hirach M, Abramowitz HB, Shapira S, et al. Hypopharyngeal injury as a result of attempted endotracheal intubation. Radiology 1978;128:37–39.

407. Harmer M. Complications of tracheal intubation. In: Latto IP, Rosen M, eds. Difficulties in tracheal intubation. London: Baillière Tindall, 1985:36–47.

408. Johnson KG, Hood DD. Esophageal perforation associated with endotracheal intubation. Anesthesiology 1986;64:281–283.

409. Kanarek KS, David RF. Traumatic perforation of the esophagus in a newborn. J Fla Med Assoc 1979; 66:288–289.

410. Levine PA. Hypopharyngeal perforation. Arch Otolaryngol 1980;106:578–580.

411. Myers EM. Hypopharyngeal perforation: a complication of endotracheal intubation. Laryngoscope 1982;92:583–585.

412. McLeod BJ, Summer E. Neonatal tracheal perforation. Anaesthesia 1986;41:67–70.

413. Norman EA, Sosis M. Iatrogenic oesophageal perforation due to tracheal or nasogastric intubation. Can Anaesth Assoc J 1986;33:222–226.

414. Orta DA, Cousar JE, Yergin BM, et al. Tracheal laceration with massive subcutaneous emphysema: a rare complication of endotracheal intubation. Thorax 1979;34:665–669.

415. O'Neill JE, Giffin JP, Cottrell JE. Pharyngeal and esophageal perforation following endotracheal intubation. Anesthesiology 1984;60:487–488.

416. Stauffer JL, Petty TL. Accidental intubation of the pyriform sinus. A complication of "roadside" resuscitation. JAMA 1977;237:2324–2325.

417. Schild JP, Wuilloud A, Kollberg H. Tracheal perforation as a complication of nasotracheal intubation in a neonate. J Pediatr 1976;88:631–632.

418. Smith BAC, Hopkinson RB. Tracheal rupture during anaesthesia. Anaesthesia 1984;39:894–898.

419. Serlin SP, Daily WJR. Tracheal perforation in the neonate. A complication of endotracheal intubation. J Pediatr 1975;86:596–597.

420. Talbert JL, Rodgers B, Felman AH, et al. Traumatic perforation of the hypopharynx in infants. J Thorac Cardiovasc Surg 1977;74:152–156.

421. Touloukian RJ, Beardsley GP, Ablow RC, et al. Traumatic perforation of the pharynx in the newborn. Pediatrics 1977;59:1019–1022.

422. Tan CSH, Tashkin DP, Sassoon H. Pneumothorax and subcutaneous emphysema complicating endotracheal intubation. South Med J 1984;77:253–255.

423. Topsis J, Kinas HY, Kandall SR. Esophageal perforation—a complication of neonatal resuscitation. Anesth Analg 1989;69:532–534.

424. Wolff AP, Kuhn FA, Ogura JH. Pharyngeal-esophageal perforations associated with rapid oral endotracheal intubation. Ann Otol 1972;81:258–261.

425. Wengen DFA. Piriform fossa perforation during attempted tracheal intubation. Anaesthesia 1987;42:519–521.

426. Young PN, Robinson JM. Cellulitis as a complication of difficult tracheal intubation. Anaesthesia 1987;42:569.

427. Pembleton WE, Brooks JW. Esophageal perforation of unusual etiology. Anesthesiology 1976;45:680–681.

428. Majumdar B, Stevens RW, Obara LG. Retropharyngeal abscess following tracheal intubation. Anaesthesia 1982;37:67–70.

429. Ooi GC, Irwin MG, Lam LK, et al. An unusual complication of emergency tracheal intubation. Anaesthesia 1997;52:154–158.

430. Regragui IA, Fagan AM, Natrajan KM. Tracheal rupture after tracheal intubation. Br J Anaesth 1994;72:705–706.

431. Siler JN, Walton EW. Pyriform sinus intubation. A trainee complication of endotracheal intubation. Am J Anesth 1996;9:137–139.

432. Chortkoff BS, Perlman B, Cohen NH. Delayed pneumothorax following difficult tracheal intubation. Anesthesiology 1992;77:1225–1227.

433. Bowes WA, Johnson JO. Pneumomediastinum after planned retrograde fiberoptic intubation. Anesth Analg 1994;78:795–797.

434. Fisman DN, Ward ME. Intrapleural placement of a nasogastric tube: an unusual complication of nasotracheal intubation. Can J Anaesth 1996;43:1252–1256.

435. Horellou MF, Mathe D, Feiss P. A hazard of nasotracheal intubation. Anaesthesia 1978;33:73–74.

436. Jaffe BF. Postoperative hoarseness. Am J Surg 1972;123:432–437.

437. Kambic V, Radsel Z. Intubation lesions of the larynx. Br J Anaesth 1978;50:587–590.

438. Peppard SB, Dickens JH. Laryngeal injury following short-term intubation. Ann Otol Rhinol Laryngol 1984;92:327–330.

439. Stout DM, Bishop MJ. Perioperative laryngeal and tracheal complications of intubation. Probl Anesth 1988;2:225–234.

440. Prasertwanitch Y, Schwarz JJH, Vandam LD. Arytenoid cartilage dislocation following prolonged endotracheal intubation. Anesthesiology 1974;41:516–517.

441. Nicholls BJ, Packham RN. Arytenoid cartilage dislocation. Anaesthesia and Intensive Care 1986;14:196–198.

442. Gray B, Huggins NJ, Hirsch N. An unusual complication of tracheal intubation. Anaesthesia 1990;45:558–560.

443. Frink EJ, Pattison BD. Posterior arytenoid dislocation following uneventful endotracheal intubation and anesthesia. Anesthesiology 1989;70:358–360.

444. Quick CA, Merwin GE. Arytenoid dislocation. Arch Otolaryngol 1978;104:267–270.

445. Chatterji S, Gupta NR, Mishra TR. Valvular glottic obstruction following extubation. Anaesthesia 1984;39:246–247.

446. Castella X, Gilabert J, Perez C. Arytenoid dislocation after tracheal intubation. An unusual cause of acute respiratory failure? Anesthesiology 1991;74:613–615.

447. Dudley JP, Mancuso AA, Fonkalsrud EW. Arytenoid dislocation and computed tomography. Arch Otolaryngol 1984;110:483–484.

448. Roberts D, McQuinn T, Beckerman RC. Neonatal arytenoid dislocation. Pediatrics 1988;81:580–582.

449. Tolley NS, Cheesman TD, Morgan D, et al. Dislocated arytenoid: an intubation induced injury. Ann Roy Coll Surg Eng 1990;72:353–356.

450. Tintinalli JE, Claffey J. Complications of nasotracheal intubation. Ann Emerg Med 1981;10:142–144.

451. O'Connell JE, Stevenson DS, Stokes MA. Pathological changes associated with short-term nasal intubation. Anaesthesia 1996;51:347–350.

452. Binning R. A hazard of blind nasal intubation. Anaesthesia 1974;29:366–367.

453. Cooper R. Bloodless turbinectomy following blind nasal intubation. Anesthesiology 1989;71:469.

454. Kawamoto M, Shimidzu Y. A balloon catheter for nasal intubation. Anesthesiology 1983;59:484.

455. Knuth TE, Richards JR. Mainstem bronchial ob-

struction secondary to nasotracheal intubation. A case report and review of the literature. Anesth Analg 1991;73:487–489.

456. Mayumi T, Miyabe M. Complete endotracheal tube obstruction after nasotracheal intubation. Can Anaesth Soc J 1984;31:344–345.

457. Vitkun SA, Sidhu US, Lagade MRG, et al. Intranasal trauma caused by a sharp-edged laser-resistant (silicone) endotracheal tube. Anesthesiology 1985;62:834–835.

458. Rector FTR, DeNuccio DJ, Alden MA. Reducing the complications of routine nasotracheal intubations. J Am Assoc Nurse Anesth 1987;55:221–232.

459. Wilkinson JA, Mathis RD, Dire DJ. Turbinate destruction—A rare complication of nasotracheal intubation. J Emerg Med 1986;4:209–212.

460. Kras JF, Marchmont-Robinson H. Pharyngeal perforation during intubation in a patient with Crohn's disease. Am J Oral Maxillofac Surg 1989;47:405–407.

461. Daly WM. Unusual complication of nasal intubation. Anesthesiology 1953;14:96.

462. Hartley M, Vaughan RS. Problems associated with tracheal extubation. Br J Anaesth 1993;71:561–568.

463. Minkel DT, Kay J, Cheng EY, et al. Reducing blood loss from nasotracheal intubation by combining a warmed tube with vasoconstrictors. Anesth Analg 1987;66:S120.

464. Bhanumurthy S, McCaughey W. Gum elastic bougie for nasotracheal intubation. Anaesthesia 1994;49:824–825.

465. Munson ES, Lee R, Kushing LG. A new complication associated with the use of wire-reinforced endotracheal tubes. Anesth Analg 1979;58:152.

466. Short JA. An unusual cause of tracheal tube cuff damage. Anaesthesia 1997; 52:93–94.

467. Basagoitia JN, LaMastro M. Another complication of tracheal intubation. Anesth Analg 1990;70:460–461.

468. Bhanumurthy S, McCaughey W, Graham JL. Deflated tracheal tube cuff with inflated pilot balloon. Anaesthesia 1993;48:1109–1110.

469. McLintock TTC, Watson E. Failure to inflate the cuff of a tracheal tube. Anaesthesia 1989;44:1016.

470. Redahan CP, Young T. Failure to inflate the cuff of a tracheal tube. Anaesthesia 1989;44:1016.

471. Tahir AH, Adriani J. Failure to effect satisfactory seal after hyperinflation of endotracheal cuff. Anesth Analg 1971;50:540–543.

472. Herrema IH. Hazardous tracheal tube pilot balloons. Anaesthesia 1986;41:673.

473. Szekely SM, Webb RK, Williamson JA, et al. Problems related to the endotracheal tube: an analysis of 2000 incident reports. Anaesthesia and Intensive Care 1993;21:611–616.

474. Lim A. A leaking tracheal tube connector. Anaesthesia 1992;47:1106–1107.

475. Clyburn P, Rosen M. Accidental oesophageal intubation. Br J Anaesth 1994;73:55–63.

476. Holland R, Webb RK, Runciman WB. Oesophageal intubation: An analysis of 2000 incident reports. Anaesthesia and Intensive Care 1993;21:608–610.

477. Mackenzie CF, Martin P, Xiao Y. Video analysis of prolonged uncorrected esophageal intubation. Anesthesiology 1996;84:1494–1503.

478. Anonymous. Anesthetic "misintubation" alleged: 1.5 million malpractice suit filed. Biomedical Safety & Standards 1981;11:67.

479. Anonymous. Anesthesia allegedly incorrect in $520,000 settlement. Biomedical Safety & Standards 1983;13:79.

480. Anonymous. Anesthesia-related errors alleged in patient deaths & disabilities: suits filed. Biomedical Safety & Standards 1984;14:65.

481. Adriani J. Unrecognized esophageal placement of endotracheal tubes. South Med J 1986;79:1591–1592.

482. Ballester EE, Torres A, Rodriguez–Roisin R, et al. Pneumoperitoneum. An unusual manifestation of improper oral intubation. Crit Care Med 1985;13:138–139.

483. Birmingham PK, Cheney FW, Ward RJ. Esophageal intubation. A review of detection techniques. Anesth Analg 1986;65:886–891.

484. Vinen JD, Gaudry PL. Pneumoperitoneum complicating cardiopulmonary resuscitation. Anaesthesia and Intensive Care 1986;14:193–195.

485. Ford RWJ. Confirming tracheal intubation—a simple manoeuvre. Can Anaesth Soc J 1983;30:191–193.

486. Gentry WB, Shanks CA. Reevaluation of a maneuver to visualize the anterior larynx after intubation. Anesth Analg 1993;77:161–163.

487. Dhamee MS. Signs of endotracheal intubation. Anaesthesia 1981;36:328–329.

488. Howells TH, Riethmuller RJ. Signs of endotracheal intubation. Anaesthesia 1980;35:984–986.

489. Heiselman D, Potacek J, Snyder JV, et al. Detection of esophageal intubation in patients with intrathoracic stomach. Crit Care Med 1985;13:1069–1070.

490. Linko K, Paloheimo M, Tammisto T. Capnography for detection of accidental oesophageal intubation. Acta Anaesthesiol Scand 1983;27:199–202.

491. Pollard BJ, Junius F. Accidental intubation of the oesophagus. Anaesthesia and Intensive Care 1980;8:183–186.

492. Sharar SR, Bishop MJ. Complications of tracheal intubation. J Intensive Care Med 1992;7:12–23.

493. Baraka A, Tabakian H, Idriss A. Breathing bag refilling. Anaesthesia 1989;44:81–82.

494. Baraka A, Tabakian H, Idriss A. Breathing bag refilling. Anaesthesia 1989;44:81.

495. Stirt JA. Endotracheal tube misplacement. Anaesthesia and Intensive Care 1982;10:274–276.

496. Peterson AW, Jacker LM. Death following inadvertent esophageal intubation. A case report. Anesth Analg 1973;32:398–401.

497. Andersen KH, Hald A. Assessing the position of the tracheal tube. The reliability of different methods. Anaesthesia 1989;44:984–985.

498. Charters P. Normal chest expansion with oesophageal placement of a tracheal tube. Anaesthesia 1989;44:365.

499. Cundy J. Accidental intubation of oesophagus. Anaesthesia and Intensive Care 1981;9:76.

500. Ogden PN. Endotracheal tube misplacement. Anaesthesia and Intensive Care 1983;11:273–274.

501. Uejima T. Esophageal intubation. Anesth Analg 1987;66:481–482.

502. Howells TH. Oesophageal misplacement of a tracheal tube. Anaesthesia 1985;40:387.

503. Gillespie JH, Knight RG, Middaugh RE, et al. Efficacy of endotracheal tube cuff palpation and humidity in distinguishing endotracheal from esophageal intubation. Anesthesiology 1988;69:A265.

504. Haridas RP. Condensation on tracheal tubes is commonly seen with oesophageal intubation. Br J Anaesth 1995;75:115–116.

505. Warden JC. Accidental intubation of the oesophagus and preoxygenation. Anaesthesia and Intensive Care 1980;8:377.

506. Sosis MB, Sisamis J. Pulse oximetry in confirmation of correct tracheal tube placement. Anesth Analg 1990;71:309–310.

507. Hirsch NP. Confirmation of tracheal tube placement. Anaesthesia 1988;43:72.

508. Batra AK, Cohn MA. Uneventful prolonged misdiagnosis of esophageal intubation. Crit Care Med 1983;11:760–764.

509. Bagshaw O, Gillis J, Schell D. Delayed recognition of esophageal intubation in a neonate: role of radiologic diagnosis. Crit Care Med 1994;22:2020–2022.

510. Munro TN. Oesophageal misplacement of a tracheal tube. Anaesthesia 1985;40:919–920.

511. Horton WA, Ralston S. Cuff palpation does not differentiate oesophageal from tracheal placement of tubes. Anaesthesia 1988;43:803–804.

512. Cameron AE, Hyde RA, Sivalingam P, et al. Detection of accidental oesophageal intubation. Anaesthesia 1997;52:733–735.

513. Horton WA, Perera S, Charters P. Further developments in tactile tests to confirm laryngeal placement of tracheal tubes. Anaesthesia 1988;43:240–244.

514. Charters P, Wilkinson K. Tactile orotracheal tube placement test. A bimanual tactile examination of the positioned orotracheal tube to confirm laryngeal placement. Anaesthesia 1987;42:801–807.

515. Nunn JF. The oesophageal detector device. Anaesthesia 1988;43:804.

516. Wee MYK. The oesophageal detector device. Assessment of a new method to distinguish oesophageal from tracheal intubation. Anaesthesia 1988;43:27–29.

517. Wee MYK, Walker KY. The oesophageal detector device. Anaesthesia 1991;46:869–871.

518. Baraka A, Muallem M. Confirmation of correct tracheal intubation by a self-inflating bulb. MEJ Anesth 1991;11:193–196.

519. Morton NS, Stuart JC, Thomson MF, et al. The oesophageal detector device. successful use in children. Anaesthesia 1989;44:523–524.

520. O'Leary JJ, Pollard BJ, Ryan MJ. A method of detecting oesophageal intubation or confirming tracheal intubation. Anaesthesia and Intensive Care 1988;16:299–301.

521. Salem MR, Baraka A, Brennan AM, et al. Efficacy of the self-inflating bulb in detecting esophageal intubation in the presence of a nasogastric tube. Anesthesiology 1992;77:A1066.

522. Baraka A, Salem MR, Brennan AM, et al. Use of self-inflating bulb in detecting esophageal intubation following "esophageal ventilation." Anesthesiology 1992;77:A294.

523. Donahue PL. The oesophageal detector device. An assessment of accuracy and ease of use by paramedics. Anaesthesia 1994;49:863–865.

524. Foutch RG, Magelssen MD, MacMillan JG. The esophageal detector device: A rapid and accurate method for assessing tracheal versus esophageal intubation in a porcine model. Ann Emerg Med 1992;21:1073–1076.

525. Jenkins WA, Verdile VP, Paris PM, The syringe aspiration technique to verify endotracheal tube position. Am J Emerg Med 1994;12:413–416.

526. Oberly D, Stein S, Hess D, et al. An evaluation of the esophageal detector device using a cadaver model. Am J Emerg Med 1992;10:317–320

527. Kapsner CE, Seaberg DC, Stengel C, et al. The esophageal detector device: accuracy and reliability in difficult airway settings. Prehospital and Disaster Med 1996;11:60–62.

528. Stock MC. Tracheal tube position assessed by esophageal detector device. Crit Care Med 1993; 21:S189.

529. Williams KN, Nunn JF. The oesophageal detector device. A prospective trial on 100 patients. Anaesthesia 1989;44:412–414.

530. Zaleski L, Abello D, Gold MI. The esophageal detector device. Anesthesiology 1993; 79:244–247.

531. Wafai Y, Salem MR, Baraka A, et al. Effectiveness of the self-inflating bulb for verification of proper placement of the esophageal tracheal Combitube. Anesth Analg 1995;80:122–126.

532. Salem MR, Wafai Y, Joseph NJ, et al. Efficacy of the self-inflating bulb in detecting esophageal intubation. Anesthesiology 1994;80:42–48.

533. Salem MR, Baraka A, Brennan AM, et al. Efficacy of the self-inflating bulb in detecting esophageal intubation in the presence of a nasogastric tube. Anesthesiology 1992;77:A1066.

534. Salem MR, Wafai Y, Baraka A, et al. Use of the self-inflating bulb for detecting esophageal intubation after "esophageal ventilation." Anesth Analg 1993; 77:1227–1231.

535. Thean K, Webster S. Failure of test for tracheal intubation. Anaesthesia and Intensive Care 1989;17: 236–237.

536. Baraka A. The oesophageal detector device. Anaesthesia 1991;46:697.

537. Czinn EA, Wafal Y, Salem MR, et al. Efficacy of the self-inflating bulb for confirmation of emergency tracheal intubation in critically ill patients. Anesthesiology 1995;83:A266.

538. Baraka A, Choueiry P, Salem R. The esophageal detector device in the morbidly obese. Anesth Analg 1993;77:400.

539. Lang DJ, Wafai Y, Salem R, et al. Efficacy of the self-inflating bulb in confirming tracheal intubation in the morbidly obese. Anesthesiology 1996;85: 246–253.

540. Baraka A, Khoury PJ, Siddik SS, et al. Efficacy of the self-inflating bulb in differentiating esophageal from tracheal intubation in the parturient undergoing cesarean section. Anesth Analg 1997;84: 533–537.

541. Smith I. Confirmation of correct endotracheal tube placement. Anesth Analg 1991;72:263.

542. Wheeler S, Fontenot R, Gaughan S, et al. Use of the fiberoptic bronchoscope as a jet stylet. Anesth Rev 1993;20:16–17.

543. Calder I, Smith M, Newton M. The oesophageal detector device. Anaesthesia 1989;44:705.

544. Haynes SR, Morton NS. Use of the oesophageal

545. Murray D, Ward ME, Sear JW. SCOTI—a new device for identification of tracheal intubation. Anaesthesia 1995; 50:1062–1064.

546. Nandwani N, Caranza R, Lin ES, et al. Configuration of the SCOTI device with different tracheal tubes. Anaesthesia 1996;51:932–934,

547. Lockey DJ, Woodward W. SCOTI versus Wee. An assessment of two oesophageal intubation detection devices. Anaesthesia 1997;52:242–243.

548. Raphael DT, Conard FU. Ultrasound confirmation of endotracheal tube placement. J Clin Ultrasound 1987;15:459–462.

549. Lee ST. Partial lung ventilation test for differentiating esophageal and laryngeal intubation. Anesth Analg 1988;67:903–904.

550. Russell WJ. Tube in the trachea? Anaesthesia and Intensive Care 1992;20:536–537.

551. Kalpokas M, Russell WJ. A simple technique for diagnosing oesophageal intubation. Anaesthesia and Intensive Care 1989;17:39–43.

552. Birmingham PK, Cheney FW Jr. Incorrect tube placement. Prevention of a fatal complication. In: Bishop MJ, ed. Physiology and consequences of tracheal intubation. Vol. 2. No. 2. Problems in anesthesia. Philadelphia: JB Lippincott, 1988:278–279.

553. Mahdi M, Benyamin RM, Lang DJ, et al. Is the "old washboard-like" sign reliable in distinguishing tracheal from esophageal intubation? Anesthesiology 1995;83:A1090.

554. Stewart RD, Rosee A, Stoy A, et al. Use of a lighted stylet to confirm tube placement. Chest 1987;92: 900–903.

555. Owen RL, Cheney FW. Use of an apena monitor to verify endotracheal intubation. Respiratory Care 1985;30:974–976.

556. Deem S, Kasper C, Benson M. Confirmation of endotracheal tube placement after emergency intubation. Anesthesiology 1996;85:A232.

557. Zbinden S, Schupfer G. Detection of oesophageal intubation: the cola complication. Anaesthesia 1989;44:81.

558. Sum-Ping ST, Mehta MP, Anderton JM. A comparative study of methods of detection of esophageal intubation. Anesth Analg 1989;69:627–632.

559. Coaldrake LA. Capnography does not always indicate successful intubation. Anaesthesia and Intensive Care 1995;23:616–617.

560. Deluty S, Turndorf H. The failure of capnography to properly assess endotracheal tube location. Anesthesiology 1993;78:783–784.

561. Lababidi Z, Bland H, James E. Retrieval of an endo-

tracheal tube from the esophagus. J Pediat Rev 1978;93:1025.

562. Abrahams N, Goldacre M, Reynolds EOR. Removal of swallowed neonatal endotracheal tube. Lancet 1970;2:135–136.

563. Bowen A, III, Dominguez R. Swallowed neonatal endotracheal tube. Pediatr Radiol 1981;10: 178–179.

564. Dickson JAS, Fraser GC. "Swallowed" endotracheal tube: a new neonatal emergency. Br Med J 1967;1:811–812.

565. Flynn GJ, Lowe AK. Endotracheal tube swallowed by a neonate. Med J Aust 1973;1:62–63.

566. Finucane BT, Shanley V, Ricketts RR. "Disappearing" endotracheal tube following meconium aspiration. A possible solution to the problem. Anesthesiology 1989;71:469–470.

567. Hoffman S, Jedeikin R. Swallowed endotracheal tube in an adult. Anesth Analg 1984;63:457–459.

568. Kennedy S. Swallowed neonatal endotracheal tube. Lancet 1970;2:264.

569. Lee KW, Templeton JJ, Dougal RM. Tracheal tube size and post-intubation croup in children. Anesthesiology 1980;53:S325.

570. Mitchell SA, Shoults DL, Herren AL, et al. Deglutition of an endotracheal tube: case report. Anesth Analg 1978;57:590–591.

571. Mucklow ES. "Swallowed" endotracheal tube. Br Med J 1967;2:618.

572. Prinn MG. "Swallowed" endotracheal tube. Br Med J 1967;3:176.

573. Storch A, Calderwood GC. Endotracheal tube swallowed by neonate. J Pediatr 1970;77:123.

574. Stool SE, Johnson D, Rosenfeld PA. Unintentional esophageal intubation in the newborn. Pediatrics 1971;48:299–301.

575. Ezri T, Berry J, Ando K, et al. Unintentional left main bronchus intubation. Can J Anaesth 1994;41: 76–77.

576. Seto K, Goto H, Hacker DC, et al. Right upper lobe atelectasis after inadvertent right main bronchial intubation. Anesth Analg 1983;62:851–854.

577. Brunel W, Coleman DL, Schwartz DE, et al. Assessment of routine chest roentgenograms and the physical examination to confirm endotracheal tube position. Chest 1989;96:1043–1045.

578. Dronen S, Chadwick O, Nowak R. Endotracheal tip position in the arrested patient. Ann Emerg Med 1982;108:116–117.

579. Bednarek FJ, Kuhns LR. Endotracheal tube placement in infants determined by suprasternal palpation: a new technique. Pediatrics 1975;56: 224–229.

580. Kuhns LR, Poznanski AK. Endotracheal tube position in the infant. J Pediatr 1971;78:991–996.

581. Schwartz DE, Lieberman JA, Cohen NH. Women are at greater risk than men for malpositioning of the endotracheal tube after emergent intubation. Crit Care Med 1994;22:1127–1131.

582. Wells AL, Wells TR, Landing BH, et al. Short trachea, a hazard in tracheal intubation of neonates and infants. Syndromal associations. Anesthesiology 1989;71:367–373.

583. Baraka A, Akel S, Muallem M, et al. Bronchial intubation in children. Does the tube bevel determine the side of intubation. Anesthesiology 1987;67: 869–870.

584. Yamashita M. Endobronchial intubation by a non-beveled endotracheal tube in infants and small children. Anesthesiology 1993;79:1154.

585. Blatchley D. Signs of endotracheal intubation. Anaesthesia 1981;36:328.

586. Conrady PA, Goodman LR, Lainge F, et al. Alteration of endotracheal tube position. Crit Care Med 1976;4:8–12.

587. Donn SM, Kuhns LR. Mechanism of endotracheal tube movement with change of head position in the neonate. Pediatr Radiol 1980;9:37–40.

588. Lingenfelter AL, Guskiewicz RA, Munson ES. Displacement of right atrial and endobronchial catheters with neck flexion. Anesth Analg 1978;57: 371–373.

589. Roopchand R, Roopnarinesingh S, Ramsewak S. Instability of the tracheal tube in neonates. Anaesthesia 1989;44:107–109.

590. Todres ID, deBros F, Kramer SS. Endotracheal tube displacement in the newborn infant. J Pediatr 1976; 89:126–127.

591. Toung TJK, Grayson R, Saklad J, et al. Movement of the distal end of the endotracheal tube during flexion and extension. Anesth Analg 1985;64: 1030–1032.

592. Roopchand R, Roopnarinesingh S, Remsewak S. Instability of the tracheal tube in neonates. Anaesthesia 1989;44:107–109.

593. Rotschild A, Chitayat D, Puterman ML, et al. Optimal positioning of endotracheal tubes for ventilation of preterm infants. AJDC 1991;145: 1007–1012.

594. Hartrey R, Kestin IG. Movement of oral and nasal tracheal tubes as a result of changes in head and neck position. Anaesthesia 1995;50:682–687.

595. Sugiyama K, Mietani W, Hirota Y, et al. Displacement of the endotracheal tube caused by postural change: evaluation by fiberoptic observation. Anesth Pain Control Dent 1992;1:29–33.

596. Magaribuchi T, Hatano Y, Mori K. Movement of endotracheal tube tip during neck flexion or extension in children. Anesth Analg 1993;76:S234.

597. Lobato EB, Paige GB, Brown MM, et al. Pneumoperitoneum associated with laparoscopic gynecological procedures increases the risk of bronchial intubation. Anesth Analg 1997;84:S195.

598. Morimura N, Inoue K, Miwa T. Chest roentgenogram demonstrates cephalad movement of the carina during laparoscopic cholecystectomy. Anesthesiology 1994;8:1301–1302.

599. Brimacombe JR, Orland H, Graham D. Endobronchial intubation during upper abdominal laparoscopic surgery in the reverse Trendelenburg position. Anesth Analg 1994;78:607.

600. Chen PP, Chui PT. Endobronchial intubation during laparoscopic cholecystectomy. Anaesthesia and Intensive Care 1992;20:537–538.

601. Inada T, Uesugi F, Kawachi S, et al. Changes in tracheal tube position during laparoscopic cholecystectomy. Anaesthesia 1996;51:823–826.

602. Heinonen J, Takki S, Tammisto T. Effect of the Trendelenburg tilt and other procedures on the position of endotracheal tubes. Lancet 1969;1:850–853.

603. Birmingham PK, Cheney FW. Incorrect tube placement. Probl Anesthesia 1988;2:278–291.

604. Todres ID, deBros F, Kramer SS. Endotracheal tube displacement in the newborn. Papers presented at the American Society of Anesthesiologists meeting. 1975:27–28.

605. Goodman LR, Conrardy PA, Laing F, et al. Radiologic evaluation of endotracheal tube position. Am J Roentgenol 1976;127:433–434.

606. Freeman JA, Fredricks BJ, Best CJ. Evaluation of a new method for determining tracheal tube length in children. Anaesthesia 1995;50:1050–1052.

607. Bloch EC, Ossey K, Ginsberg B. Tracheal intubation in children. A new method for assuring correct depth of tube placement. Anesth Analg 1988;67:590–592.

608. Roberts J. Fundamentals of tracheal intubation. New York: Grune & Stratton, 1983.

609. Sosis M. Hazards of a new system for placement of endotracheal tubes. Anesthesiology 1988;68:299.

610. Pollard RJ, Lobato EB. Endotracheal tube location verified reliably by cuff palpation. Anesth Analg 1995;81:135–138.

611. Schellinger RR. The length of the airway to the bifurcation of the trachea. Anesthesiology 1964;25:169–172.

612. Aldrete JA, Wright AJ. Airway assessment systems. Anesthesiol News, July 12, 1992:12.

613. Morgan GAR, Steward DJ. Linear airway dimensions in children. including those with cleft palate. Can Anaesth Soc J 1982;29:1–8.

614. Tochen ML. Orotracheal intubation in the newborn infant: a method for determining depth of tube insertion. J Pediatr 1979;95:1050–1051.

615. Coldiron JS. Estimation of nasotracheal tube length in neonates. Pediatrics 1968;41:823–828.

616. Mattila MAK, Heikel PE, Suutarinen T, et al. Estimation of a suitable nasotracheal tube length for infants and children. Acta Anaesth Scand 1971;15:239–246.

617. Russell WJ, Smith JA. Endotracheal tube markings. Anaesthesia and Intensive Care 1985;13:210–211.

618. Mehta S. Endotracheal intubation: friend or foe? Br Med J 1986;292:694.

619. Loew A, Thiebeault DW. A new and safe method to control the depth of endotracheal intubation in neonates. Pediatrics 1974;54:506–508.

620. Wallace CT, Cooke JE. A new method for positioning endotracheal tubes. Anesthesiology 1976;44:272.

621. Dietrich KA, Strauss RH, Cabalka AK, et al. Use of flexible fiberoptic endoscopy for determination of endotracheal tube position in the pediatric patient. Crit Care Med 1988;16:884–887.

622. O'Brian D, Curran J, Conroy J, et al. Fibre-optic assessment of tracheal tube position. A comparison of tracheal tube position as estimated by fibre-optic bronchoscopy and by chest X-ray. Anaesthesia 1985;40:73–76.

623. Vigneswaran R, Whitfield JM. The use of a new ultra-thin fiberoptic bronchoscope to determine endotracheal tube position in the sick newborn infant. Chest 1981;80:174–177.

624. Sugiyama K, Yokoyama K. Reliability of auscultation of bilateral breath sounds in confirming endotracheal tube position. Anesthesiology 1995;83:1373.

625. Asai T, Barclay K, Eggers K. Confirmation of endotracheal tube position. Crit Care Med 1994;22:1306–1307.

626. Smith BL. Confirmation of the position of an endotracheal tube. Anaesthesia 1975;30:410.

627. Chander S, Feldman E. Correct placement of endotracheal tubes. NY State J Med 1979;79:1843–1844.

628. Imai M, Okuyama M, Okuyama A, et al. Cuff palpation technique in small children. Anesthesiology 1994;81:A1433.

629. Goldman JM, Armstrong JP. Tracheal tubes can be inserted to the correct depth using a cuff palpation technique. Anesthesiology 1994;81:A299.

630. Triner L. A simple maneuver to verify proper positioning of an endotracheal tube. Anesthesiology 1982;57:548–549.

631. Cullen DJ, Newbower RS, Gemer M. A new method for positioning endotracheal tubes. Anesthesiology 1975;43:596–599.

632. Kopman EA. A simple method for verifying endotracheal tube placement. Anesth Analg 1977;56: 121–124.

633. Hauser GJ, Muir E, Kline LM, et al. Prospective evaluation of a nonradiographic device for determination of endotracheal tube position in children. Crit Care Med 1990;18:760–763.

634. Zwass MS, Schriener MS, Raphealy RC. Noninvasive determination of tracheal tube position in infants and children. Anesthesiology 1988;69:A178.

635. Cote CJ, Szyfelbein SK, Liu LMP, et al. Intraoperative events diagnosed by expired carbon dioxide monitoring in children. Can Anaesth Soc J 1986; 33:315–320.

636. Gandhi SK, Munshi CA, Kampine JP. A sudden warning sign of an accidental endobronchial intubation. A sudden drop or sudden rise in $PaCO_2$? Anesthesiology 1986;65:114–115.

637. Riley RH, Marcy JH. Unsuspected endobronchial intubation—detection by continuous mass spectrometry. Anesthesiology 1985;63:203–204.

638. Riley RH, Finucane KE, Marcey JH. Early warning sign of an accidental endobronchial intubation. A sudden drop or sudden rise in $PaCO_2$? In reply. Anesthesiology 1986;65:115.

639. Stewart RD, LaRosee A, Kaplan RM, Ilkhanipour K. Correct positioning of an endotracheal tube using a flexible lighted stylet. Crit Care Med 1990;18: 97–99.

640. Watson CB, Clapham M. Transillumination for correct tube positioning. Use of a new fiberoptic endotracheal tube. Anesthesiology 1984;60:253.

641. Heller RM, Cotton RB. Early experience with illuminated endotracheal tubes in premature and term infants. Pediatrics 1985;75:664–666.

642. Barker SJ, Tremper KK. Detection of endobronchial intubation by noninvasive monitoring. Journal of Clinical Monitoring 1987;3:292–293.

643. Alberti J, Hanafee W, Wilson G, et al. Unsuspected pulmonary collapse during neuroradiologic procedures. Radiology 1967;89:316–320.

644. McCoy EP, Russell WJ. Endobronchial intubation: an analysis of 4000 incident reports. Anesthesiology 1996;85:A914.

645. Bernard SA, Jones BM. Endotracheal tube obstruction in a patient with status asthmaticus. Anaesthesia and Intensive Care 1991;19:121–123.

646. Seifert RD, Starsnic M, Zwillenberg D. Acute obstruction of the left mainstem bronchus following an attempted nasotracheal intubation. An unusual case report. Anesthesiology 1985;62:799–800.

647. Tahir AH. Endotracheal tube lost in the trachea. JAMA 1972;222:1061–1062.

648. Whyte MP. Aspiration of an endotracheal tube. JHEP 1977;6:332.

649. McGrath RB, Einterz RM. Aspiration of a nasotracheal tube. A complication of nasotracheal intubation and mechanism for retrieval. Chest 1987;91: 148–149.

650. Milstein J, Rabinovitz J, Goetzman B. A foreign body hazard in the neonate. Anesth Analg 1977; 56:726–727.

651. Harrington JF. An unusual cause of endotracheal tube obstruction. Anesthesiology 1984;61:116–117.

652. Chiu T, Meyers EF. Defective disposable endotracheal tube. Anesth Analg 1976;55:437.

653. Day C, Rankin N. Laceration of the cuff of an endotracheal tube during percutaneous dilatational tracheostomy. Chest 1994;105:644.

654. Yeung ML, Lett Z. An uncommon hazard of armoured endotracheal tubes. Anaesthesia 1974;29: 186–187.

655. Anonymous. Laser-resistant tracheal tube to be modified following recall. Biomedical Safety & Standards 1987;17:138.

656. Jackson S, Welch GW. Foreign body from a tube of anesthetic ointment. Anesthesiology 1987;67: 154–155.

657. Holley HS, Gildea JE. Vocal cord paralysis after tracheal intubation. JAMA 1971;215:281–284.

658. Kamhol SL, Rothman NI, Underwood PS. Fiberbronchoscopic retrieval of iatrogenically introduced endobronchial foreign body. Crit Care Med 1979; 7:346–348.

659. Liew PC. A hazard due to a commercially available topical spray. Anaesthesia 1973;28:346.

660. Yang LC, Jawan B, Lee JH. Iatrogenic foreign body after laryngoscopy. Br J Anaesth 1992;68:115.

661. Kearl RA, Hooper RG. Massive airway leaks: An analysis of the role of endotracheal tubes. Crit Care Med 1993;21:518–521.

662. Smotrilla MM, Nagel EL, Moya E. Failure of inflatable cuff resulting in foreign body in the trachea. Anesthesiology 1966;27:512–513.

663. Debnath SK, Waters DJ. Leaking cuffed endotracheal tubes: two case reports. Br J Anaesth 1968; 40:807.

664. Williamson R, Gorven AM. Cuff failure—a complication of tracheal intubation. Anaesthesia 1991;46: 593–594.

665. Jayasuriya KD, Watson WF. P.V.C. cuffs and ligno-caine-base aerosol. Br J Anaesth 1981;53:1368.

666. Reinders M, Gerber HR. Cuff failure of PVC tracheal tubes. Anaesthesia 1989;44:524–525.

667. Walmsley AJ, Burville LM, Davis TP. Cuff failure in polyvinyl chloride tracheal tubes sprayed with lignocaine. Anaesthesia 1988;43:399–401.

668. Blitt CD, Wright WA. An unusual complication of percutaneous internal jugular vein cannulation, puncture of an endotracheal tube cuff. Anesthesiology 1974;40:306–307.

669. Brown HI, Burnard RJ, Jensen M, et al. Puncture of endotracheal-tube cuffs during percutaneous subclavian-vein catheterization. Anesthesiology 1975;43:112–113.

670. Haddow GR, Tays R. Tracheal injury: A cause for unexplained endotracheal cuff leak during mediastinal dissection. Anesth Analg 1997;84:684–685.

671. Masterson GR, Smurthwaite GJ. A complication of percutaneous tracheostomy. Anaesthesia 1994;49:452–453.

672. Angelillo JC, Kosanin R, Fox WD. Damage to endotracheal tube during maxillofacial surgery. Anesthiol Rev 1986;13:17–20.

673. Bamforth BJ. Complications during endotracheal anesthesia. Anesth Analg 1963;42:727–733.

674. Fagraeus L, Angelillo JC, Dolan EA. A serious anesthetic hazard during orthognathic surgery. Anesth Analg 1980;59:150–152.

675. Job CA, Betcher AM, Pearson WT, et al. Intraoperative obstruction of endobronchial tubes. Anesthesiology 1979;51:550–553.

676. Ketzler JT, Landers DF. Management of a severed endotracheal tube during LeFort osteotomy. J Clin Anesth 1992;4:144–146.

677. Levack ID, Scott DHT. Conservative management of intra-operative cuff puncture in a bronchial tube. Anaesthesia 1985;40:1020–1021.

678. Mosby EL, Messer EJ, Nealis MF. Intraoperative damage to nasotracheal tubes during maxillary surgery: report of cases. J Oral Surg 1978;36:963–964.

679. Orr DL. Airway compromise during oral and maxillofacial surgery: case report and review of potential causes. Anesth Prog 1978;25:161–168.

680. Peskin RM, Sachs SA. Intraoperative management of a partially severed endotracheal tube during orthognathic surgery. Anesth Prog 1986;33:247–251.

681. Schwartz LB, Sordill WC, Liebers RM, et al. Difficulty in removal of accidentally cut endotracheal tube. J Oral Maxillofac Surg. 1982;40:518–519.

682. Tseuda K, Carey WJ, Gonty AA, et al. Hazards to anesthetic equipment during maxillary osteotomy: report of cases. J Oral Surg 1977;35:47.

683. Bevacqua BK, Cleary WF. An unusual case of endotracheal tube cuff dysfunction. J Clin Anesth 1993;5:237–239.

684. Wong RM. An unusual source of leakage from the cuff of an endotracheal tube. Anaesthesia and Intensive Care 1977;5:389.

685. Phillips B. Defect in a cuffed tube. Anaesthesia 1971;26:237.

686. Lacoste L, Thomas D. Unusual complication of tracheal intubation. Anesth Analg 1992;74:474–475.

687. Gonzales JG. Securing an endotracheal tube. Anesthesiology 1986;65:347.

688. Anonymous. Cuffed tracheal tubes may not inflate. Biomedical Safety & Standards 1993;23:126.

689. Chilvers R, Jenkins J. A hidden leak. Anaesthesia 1995;50:920.

690. Palmer JHM. Unexpected cause of tracheal cuff failure. Anaesthesia 1993;48:347–348.

691. Patel A, Smith M. Tracheal cuff failure. Anaesthesia 1995;50:568–569.

692. Hannington-Kiff JG. Faulty superset plastic catheter mounts. A cautionary tale applicable to other mass-produced disposable products. Anaesthesia 1991;46:671–672.

693. Nixon C. Endotracheal tube connector fracture—an avoidable hazard. Can Anaesth Soc J 1986;33:251.

694. Oyston J, Holtby H. Fracture of a RAE endotracheal tube connector. Can J Anaesth 1988;35:438–439.

695. Sun KO. A risk of using elastic adhesive bandage to secure the breathing circuit. Anaesthesia and Intensive Care 1993;21:125.

696. Spear RM, Sauder RA, Nichols DG. Endotracheal tube rupture, accidental extubation, and tracheal avulsion. Three airway catastrophes associated with significant decrease in leak pressure. Crit Care Med 1989;17:701–703.

697. McLean R, Houston P, Carmichael F, et al. Disruption of an armoured endotracheal tube caused by biting. Can Anaesth Soc J 1985;32:313.

698. Anonymous. Endotracheal tube severed by biting. Malpractice Reporter 1993;12:11.

699. O'Meara M, Buckley TA. Tracheal intubation of children in intensive care. Anaesthesia 1993;48:181.

700. Fisher MM. Repairing pilot balloon lines. Anaesthesia and Intensive Care 1988;16:500–501.

701. Sills J. An emergency cuff inflation technique. Respiratory Care 1986;31:199–201.

702. Stimmel S, Gutierrez CJ. Emergency cuff-inflation

technique revisited [Letter]. Respiratory Care 1986; 31:538.

703. Watson E, Harris MM. Leaking endotracheal tube. Chest 1989;95:709.

704. Sprung J, Bourke DL, Thomas P, et al. Clever cure for an endotracheal tube cuff leak. Anesthesiology 1994;81:790–791.

705. Schubert A, Kaenel WV, Ilyes L. A management option for leaking endotracheal tube cuffs. Use of lidocaine jelly. J Clin Anesth 1991;3:26–31.

706. Tinkoff G, Bakow ED, Smith RW. A continuous-flow apparatus for temporary inflation of damaged endotracheal tube cuffs. Respiratory Care 1991;35: 423–426.

707. Verborgh C, Camu F. Management of cuff incompetence in an endotracheal tube. Anesthesiology 1987;66:441.

708. Vitkun SA, Lagasse RS, Kyle KT, et al. Application of the Grieshaber air system to maintain endotracheal tube cuff pressure. J Clin Anaesth 1990;2: 45–47.

709. Wagner DL, Gammage GW, Wong M. Tracheal rupture following the insertion of a disposable double-lumen endotracheal tube. Anesthesiology 1985; 63:698–700.

710. Tornvall SS, Jackson KH, Oyanedel T. Tracheal rupture, complication of cuffed endotracheal tube. Chest 1971;59:237–239.

711. Kumar SM, Pandit SK, Cohen PJ. Tracheal laceration associated with endotracheal anesthesia. Anesthesiology 1977;47:298–299.

712. Gaukroger PB, Anderson G. Tracheal rupture in an intubated critically ill patient. Anaesthesia and Intensive Care 1986;14:199–201.

713. van Klarenbosch J, Meyer J, de Lange JJ. Tracheal rupture after tracheal intubation. Br J Anaesth 1994; 73:550–551.

714. Amodio JB, Berdon WE, Abramson SJ, et al. Retrocardiac pneumomediastinum in association with tracheal and esophageal perforations. Ped Radiol 1986;16:380–383.

715. Aziz EM, Suleiman KA. Tracheo-esophageal perforation in the newborn: A case report. Clin Pediatr 1983;22:584.

716. de Lange JJ, Booij LHDJ. Tracheal rupture. Anaesthesia 1985;40:211–212.

717. Kubota Y, Toyoda Y, Kubota H. A potential complication associated with a tracheal tube with Murphy eye. Anaesthesia 1989;44:866–867.

718. Van Der Spek AFL, Spargo PM, Norton ML. The physics of lasers and implications for their use during airway surgery. Br J Anaesth 1988;60:709–729.

719. Rampil IJ. Anesthetic considerations for laser surgery. Anesth Analg 1992;74:424–435.

720. Bargainnier DR, Hasnain JU, Matjasko MJ. How do you manage the patient requiring subglottic laser surgery? Surv Anesth 1993;37:53–55.

721. Sosis M, Dillon F. Hazards of a new, clear, unmarked polyvinyl chloride tracheal tube designed for use with the Nd-YAG laser. J Clin Anesth 1991; 3:358–360.

722. Casey KR, Fairfax WB, Smith SJ, et al. Intratracheal fire ignited by the Nd-YAG laser during treatment of tracheal stenosis. Chest 1983;84:295–296.

723. Denton RA, Dedhia HV, Abrons HL, et al. Long-term survival after endobronchial fire during treatment of severe malignant airway obstruction with the Nd-YAG laser. Chest 1988;94:1086–1088.

724. Krawtz S, Mehta AC, Wiedemann HP, et al. Nd-YAG laser-induced endobronchial burn. Management and long term follow-up. Chest 1989;95: 916–918.

725. McLaren ID, Bellman MH, Cooley J. Effects of the argon laser on anaesthetic gases and endotracheal tubes. Br J Anaesth 1983;55:1001–1004.

726. Green JM, Sonbolian N, Gonzalez RM, et al. CO_2 laser resistance of various ointments and tapes. Anesthesiology 1991;74:964–965.

727. Pashayan AG, Gravenstein JS, Cassisi NJ, et al. The helium protocol for laryngotracheal operations with CO_2 laser. A retrospective review of 523 cases. Anesthesiology 1988;68:801–804.

728. Sosis M. Nitrous oxide should not be used during laser endoscopic surgery. Anesth Analg 1987;66: 1054–1055.

729. Shapiro JD, El–Baz NM. N_2O has no place during oropharyngeal and laryngotracheal procedures. Anesthesiology 1987;66:447–448.

730. Byles PH, Kellman RM. The hazard of nitrous oxide during laser endoscopic surgery. Anesthesiology 1983;59:258.

731. Alhaddad S, Brenner J. Helium and lower oxygen concentrations do not prolong tracheal tube ignition time during potassium titanyl phosphate laser use. Anesthesiology 1994;80:936–938.

732. Wolf GL, Sidebotham GW, Aftel R, et al. Helium dilution increases flame spread velocity in endotracheal tubes. Anesthesiology 1996;85:A420.

733. Eisenkraft JB, Barker SJ. Helium and gas flow. Anesth Analg 1993;76:452–453.

734. Rampil IJ. Helium and gas flow. Anesth Analg 1993;76:S453.

735. Plost J, Campbell SC. The non-elastic work of breathing through endotracheal tubes of various sizes. American Review of Respiratory Disease 1984;129:A106.

736. Ohashi N, Asai M, Ueda S, et al. Hazard to endotracheal tubes by CO_2 laser beam. ORL J Otorhinolaryngol Relat Spec 1985;47:22–25.

737. Recommended practice on laser fire protection. Quincy MA: NFPA, 1996.

738. Sosis MB, Dillon FX. Saline-filled cuffs help prevent laser-induced polyvinyl chloride endotracheal tube fires. Anesth Analg 1991;72:187–189.

739. LeJeune FE, Guice C, LeTard F, et al. Heat sink protection against lasering endotracheal cuffs. Ann Otol Rhinol Laryngol 1982;92:606–607.

740. Sosis M, Dillon F. Saline filled cuffs help prevent polyvinyl chloride laser induced endotracheal tube fires. Can J Anaesth 1989;36:S142–S143.

741. Walsh M, Schubert A, Al Haddad S. The addition of lidocaine jelly to saline in the cuff of the endotracheal tube during laser surgery of the airway. Am J Anesth 1997;24:189–193.

742. Anonymous. Laser-resistant tracheal tubes. Technology for Anesthesia 1992;12(8):1–5.

743. Pashayan AG, SanGiovanni C, Davis LE. Positive end-expiratory pressure lowers the risk of laser-induced polyvinyl chloride tracheal-tube fires. Anesthesiology 1993;79:83–87.

744. Anonymous. Airway fires. Reducing the risk during laser surgery. Technology for Anesthesia 1990; 11(2):1–4.

745. Sosis MB, Braverman B. Advantage of rubber over plastic endotracheal tubes for rapid extubation in a laser fire. J Clin Laser Med & Surg 1996;14:93–95.

746. Sosis MB, Braverman B. Prevention of cautery-induced airway fires with special endotracheal tubes. Anesth Analg 1993;77:846–847.

747. Elton DR, Berkowitz GP. Endotracheal tube obstruction in neonates. Perinatol Neonatol 1981;5: 75–80.

748. Duffy BL. Delayed onset of respiratory obstruction during endotracheal anesthesia. S Afr Med J 1976; 50:1551–1552.

749. Johnson JT, Maloney RW, Cummings CW. Tracheostomy tube: cuff obstruction. JAMA 1977;238: 211.

750. Jago RH, Millar JM. Airway obstruction—an unusual presentation. Br J Anaesth 1985;57:541–542.

751. Kruczek ME, Hoff BH, Keszler BR, et al. Blood clot resulting in ball-valve obstruction in the airway. Crit Care Med 1982;10:122–123.

752. Flemming DC. Hazards of tracheal intubation. In: Orkin FK, Cooperman LH, eds. Complications in anesthesiology. Philadelphia: JB Lippincott, 1983: 165–172.

753. Dicpinigaitis PV, Mehta DC. Postoperative pulmonary edema induced by endotracheal tube occlusion. Intens Care Med 1995;21:1048–1050.

754. Gopalakrishnan M, Khoo ST, Tan PL. Pulmonary oedema associated with endotracheal tube occlusion. Anaesthesia and Intensive Care 1994;22:498.

755. Warner LO, Beach TP, Martino JD. Negative pressure pulmonary oedema secondary to airway obstruction in an intubated infant. Can J Anaesth 1988;35:507–510.

756. Russomanno JH, Brown LK. Pneumothorax due to ball-valve obstruction of an endotracheal tube in a mechanically ventilated patient. Chest 1992;101: 1444–1445.

757. de Soto H, Johnston JF. Pulmonary edema caused by endotracheal tube occlusion. Anesthesiol Rev 1987;14:39–40.

758. Hull JM. Occlusion of armoured tubes. Anaesthesia 1989;44:790.

759. Brock–Utne JG. Biting on ET tubes. Anaesthesia and Intensive Care 1997;25:309.

760. Webb CA. Hazard of reinforced tracheal tubes. Anaesthesia 1994;49:918–919.

761. Jayarajah MJ, Cole PJ. Hazard of reinforced tracheal tubes. Anaesthesia 1994;49:919.

762. King H-K, Lewis K. Guedel oropharyngeal airway does not prevent patient biting on the endotracheal tube. Anaesthesia and Intensive Care 1996;24: 729–730.

763. Harrison P, Bacon DR, Lema MJ. Perforation and partial obstruction of an armored endotracheal tube. J Neurosurg Anesth 1995;7:121–123.

764. Peck MJ, Needleman SM. Reinforced endotracheal tube obstruction. Anesth Analg 1994;79:193.

765. Vogel TM, Brock-Utne JG. A possible Solution to an occluded reinforced (armored) endotracheal tube. Am J Anesth 1997;24:58–61.

766. Stacey M, Asai T. Kinking of a tracheal tube in the nasal cavity. Anaesthesia 1995;50:917.

767. Roth DM, Benumof JL. Intubation through a laryngeal mask airway with a nasal RAE tube: stabilization of the proximal end of the tube. Anesthesiology 1996;85:1220.

768. Berwick EP, Chadd GD, Cox PN, et al. Armoured tracheal tubes for neuroanaesthesia. Anaesthesia 1986;41:775–776.

769. Kubota Y, Toyoda Y, Kubota H, et al. Armoured tubes are necessary for neuroanesthesia. Anaesthesia 1986;41:1064–1065.

770. Rao CC, Krishna G, Trueblood S. Stenting of the endotracheal tube to manage airway obstruction in the prone position. Anesth Analg 1980;59: 700–701.

771. Wilks DH, Tullock WC, Klain M. Airway obstruction caused by a kinked Hi-Lo jet endotracheal tube during high frequency jet ventilation. Anesth Analg 1989;69:116–118.

772. Shirley PJ, Kulkarni V, Frost N. A problem with the Boyle–Davis gag following difficult intubation. Anaesthesia 1994;49:551–552.

773. Graham D, Daddour HS. RAE tube obstruction during tonsil dissection. Br J Anaesth 1996;76:170–171.

774. Yamashita M, Motokawa K. A simple method for preventing kinking of 2.5-mm ID endotracheal tubes. Anesth Analg 1987;66:803–804.

775. Yamashita M, Motokawa K. Preventing kinking of disposable preformed endotracheal tubes. Can Anaesth Soc J 1987;34:103.

776. Arai T, Kuzume K. Endotracheal tube obstruction possibly due to structural fault. Anesthesiology 1983;59:480–481.

777. Singh B, Gombar KK, Chhabra B. Tracheal tube-kinking. Can J Anaesth 1993;40:682.

778. Callander CC. Intubation risk with patients with tracheostomy. Anaesthesia 1988;43:1061.

779. Batra AK. Complication following traumatic endotracheal intubation. Crit Care Med 1986;14:80.

780. Carter GL, Holcomb MC. An unusual cause of endotracheal tube obstruction. Anesthesiol Rev 1978;5:51–53.

781. Barat G, Ascorve A, Avello F. Unusual airway obstruction during pneumonectomy. Anaesthesia 1976;31:1290–1291.

782. Henzig D, Rosenblatt R. Thrombotic occlusion of a nasotracheal tube. Anesthesiology 1979;51:484–485.

783. Hitchen JE, Wiener AP. Unexpected obstruction of a nasotracheal tube: report of case. J Oral Surg 1973;31:722–724.

784. Robinson BC, Jarrett WJ. Postoperative complication after blind nasotracheal intubation for reduction of a fractured mandible: report of case. J Oral Surg 1971;29:340–343.

785. Hosking MP, Lennon RL, Warner M, et al. Endotracheal tube obstruction: recognition and management. Mil Med 1989;154:489–491.

786. Boysen K. An unusual case of nasotracheal tube occlusion. Anaesthesia 1985;40:1024.

787. Butt W. Unusual cause of endotracheal tube obstruction in a neonate. Anaesthesia and Intensive Care 1986;14:95.

788. Scamm FL, Babin RW. An unusual complication of nasotracheal intubation. Anesthesiology 1983;59:352–353.

789. Campbell WI, Hainsworth MA. Complications of nasal intubation . A report of two cases. Today's Anaesthetist 1988;3.

790. Biggerstaff MA, Starck TW, Hahn MB. A rare case of airway obstruction following nasotracheal intubation. Anesth Rev 1993;20:193–195.

791. Anderson CE, Savignac AC. Nasotracheal tube obstruction secondary to inferior turbinate impaction. J Am Assoc Nurse Anesth 1991;59:538–540.

792. Powell DR. Obstruction to endotracheal tubes. Br J Anaesth 1974;46:252.

793. Stark DCC. Endotracheal tube obstruction. Anesthesiology 1976;45:467–468.

794. Jenkins AV. Unexpected hazard of anaesthesia. Lancet 1959;1:761–762.

795. Haselhuhn DH. Occlusion of endotracheal tube with foreign body. Anesthesiology 1958;19:561–562.

796. Wittman FW. Airway obstruction due to a foreign body. Anaesthesia 1982;37:865–866.

797. Dutton CS. A bizarre cause of obstruction in an Oxford non-kink endotracheal tube. Anaesthesia 1962;17:395–396.

798. Stewart KA. Foreign body in endotracheal tube. Br Med J 1958;2:1226.

799. Rainer EH. Foreign body in endotracheal tube. Br Med J 1958;2:1357.

800. Goudsouzian NG, Ryan JF, Moench B. An unusual cause of endotracheal tube obstruction in a child. Anesthesiol Rev 1980;7:23–24.

801. Galley RL. Foreign body. Anaesthesia and Intensive Care 1987;15:471.

802. Peers B. Another intubation hazard. Anaesthesia 1975;30:827.

803. Ehrenpreis MB, Oliverio RM. Endotracheal tube obstruction secondary to oral preoperative medication. Anesth Analg 1984;63:867–868.

804. Singhal M, Gupta M, Singhal CK. Tube in tube. A case of acute airway obstruction. Br J Anaesth 1984;56:1317.

805. Galway JE. Airway obstruction. Anaesthesia 1972;27:102–103.

806. Singh CV. Bizarre airway obstruction. Anaesthesia 1977;32:812–813.

807. Mimpriss TJ. Respiratory obstruction due to a round worm. Br J Anaesth 1972;44:413.

808. Barst S, Yossefy Y Lebowitz P. An unusual cause of airway obstruction. Anesth Analg 1994;78:195.

809. Burlington DB. FDA Public Health Advisory. Occluded endotracheal tubes. Rockville, MD: Dept. Health and Human Services, 1994.

810. Robbie DS, Pearce DJ. Some dangers of armoured tubes. Anaesthesia 1959;14:379–385.

811. Ireland R. Potential hazard of Doughty tongue plate. Anaesthesia and Intensive Care 1986;14:209.

812. Palmieri AM, Scanni E, Spatola R, et al. Endotracheal tube obstruction. Anaesthesia and Intensive Care 1986;14:209.

813. Populaire C, Robarb S, Souron J. An armoured endotracheal tube obstruction in a child. Can J Anaesth 1989;36:331–332.

814. Bachand R, Fortin G. Airway obstruction with cuffed flexo metallic tracheal tubes. Can Anaesth Soc J 1976;23:330–333.

815. Guedj P, Eldor J. Endotracheal cuff herniation. Resuscitation 1991;21:293–294.

816. Davidson I, Zimmer S. Cuff herniation. Anaesthesia 1989;44:938–939.

817. Henderson MA. Airway obstruction with a cuffed single-use plastic endotracheal tube. Anaesthesia and Intensive Care 1993;21:370–372.

818. Brasch RC, Heldt GP, Hecht ST. Endotracheal tube orifice abutting the tracheal wall: a cause of infant airway obstruction. Radiology 1981;141:387–391.

819. Martin J, Hutchinson B. Tracheal tube obstruction by prominent aortic knuckle. Anaesthesia 1986;41:86–87.

820. Sapsford DJ, Snowdon SL. If in doubt, take it out. Obstruction of tracheal tube by prominent aortic knuckle. Anaesthesia 1985;40:552–554.

821. Stoen R, Smith–Erichsen N. Airway obstruction associated with an endotracheal tube. Intensive Care Med 1987;13:295–296.

822. Togashi H, Hirabayashi Y, Mitsuhata H, et al. The beveled tracheal tube orifice abutted on the tracheal wall in a patient with Forestier's disease. Anesthesiology 1993;79:1452–1453.

823. Sperry K, Smialek JE. The investigation of an unusual asphyxial death in a hospital. JAMA 1986;255:2472–2474.

824. Patterson KW, Keane P. Missed diagnosis of cuff herniation in a modern nasal endotracheal tube. Anesth Analg 1990;71:561–569.

825. Feinberg SE, Klein SL. Airway obstruction with the RAE endotracheal tube. J Maxillofac Surg 1983;41:260–262.

826. Bishop MJ. Endotracheal tube lumen compromise from cuff overinflation. Chest 1981;80:100–101.

827. Chan MCY. Collapse of endotracheal tubes. Anaesthesia and Intensive Care 1981;9:289–290.

828. Dunn HC. A defective endotracheal tube. N Z Med J 1988;101:460.

829. Famewo CE. A not so apparent cause of intraluminal tracheal tube obstruction. Anesthesiology 1983;58:593.

830. Hoffman S, Freedman M. Delayed lumen obstruction in endotracheal tubes. Br J Anaesth 1976;48:1025–1028.

831. Hebert RC, DeSessa PC. Compression of an endotracheal tube lumen by its cuff. A case report. Respiratory Care 1981;26:653–654.

832. Ketover AK, Feingold A. Collapse of a disposable endotracheal tube by its high-pressure cuff. Anesthesiology 1975;43:108–110.

833. Muir J, Davidson-Lamb R. Apparatus failure-cause for concern. Br J Anaesth 1980;52:705–706.

834. Perel A, Katzenelson R, Klein E, et al. Collapse of endotracheal tubes due to overinflation of high-compliance cuffs. Anesth Analg 1977;56:731–733.

835. Patel K, Teviotdale B, Dalal FY. Internal herniation of a Murphy endotracheal tube. Anesthesiol Rev 1978;5:60–61.

836. Roland P, Stovner J. Brain damage following collapse of a "polyvinyl" tube. Elasticity and permeability of the cuff. Acta Anaesth Scand 1975;19:303–309.

837. Priem L, Guntupalli K, Sladen A, et al. Inadvertent tracheal tube obstruction. Heart Lung 1982;11:285.

838. Hutchinson M, Himes TM, Davis LE. Preventing multiple body tube mix-ups. Nursing 1987;87:57.

839. Fergusson NV, Fang WB. Unusual problems of nasotracheal intubation. Anesthesiol Rev 1985;12:33–36.

840. Saade E. Unusual cause of endotracheal tube obstruction. Anesth Analg 1991;72:841–842.

841. Beaulieu P, Davies C. Airway obstruction during anaesthesia for anterior cervical cord decompression. Can J Anaesth 1994;41:874.

842. Bayes J, Slater EM, Hedberg PS, et al. Obstruction of a double-lumen endotracheal tube by a saber-sheath trachea. Anesth Analg 1994;79:186–188.

843. Mackenzie CF. Was it the trachea or inadequate tracheal cuff inflation? Anesth Analg 1995;80:427.

844. Lahay WD. Defective tracheal tube connector. Can Anaesth Soc J 1982;29:80–81.

845. McKinley AC. Occlusion of an endotracheal tube connector. Anesthesiology 1977;47:480.

846. Nott MR, Wainwright AC. Imperforate apparatus causing total airway obstruction. Anaesthesia 1977;32:77–78.

847. Osterud A. Dangerous fault in disposable connector for orotracheal tube. Br J Anaesth 1974;46:952.

848. Sansome AJ. Creasing of a paediatric tracheal tube connector. Anaesthesia 1990;45:343.

849. Zebrowski ME. Buckled adaptor. Anesthesiology 1979;51:276–277.

850. Gupta K, Harry R. Cutting paediatric tracheal

tubes-a potential cause of morbidity. Br J Anaesth 1997;78:627–628.

851. Nagan Kee WD. An unusual problem with an endotracheal tube. Anaesthesia and Intensive Care 1993; 21:247–248.

852. Emmanual ER. Kinking of tracheal tubes. Anaesthesia 1996;51:287.

853. Shimoda O, Nakayama R, Tashiro M, et al. A tracheal tube protector to prevent kinking. Br J Anaesth 1993;71:326.

854. Preis CA. Kinking of the proximal end of a nasal RAE tube after intubation via laryngeal mask airway: an alternative stabilization approach. Anesthesiology 1997;87:184–185.

855. Lieman BC, Hall ID, Stanley TH. Extirpation of endotracheal tube secretions with a Fogarty arterial embolectomy catheter. Anesthesiology 1985;62: 847.

856. Sizer J, Pierce JMT. Unblocking tracheal tubes. Anaesthesia 1992;47:278–279.

857. Smurthwaite GJ, Macdonald IJF. Another use of the Fogarty catheter. Anaesthesia 1995;50:86.

858. Elpern EH, Jacobs ER, Bone RC. Incidence of aspiration in tracheally intubated adults. Heart Lung 1987;16:527–531.

859. Petring OU, Adelhoj B, Jensen BN, et al. Prevention of silent aspiration due to leaks around cuffs of endotracheal tubes. Anesth Analg 1986;65: 777–780.

859A. Joseph JI, Torjman M, Lessin J, et al. Glottic incompetence and tracheal aspiration are common when using a double-lumen endotracheal tube. Anesth Analg 1993;76:S172.

860. Janson BA, Poulton TJ. Does PEEP reduce the incidence of aspiration around endotracheal tubes? Can Anaesth Soc J 1986;33:157–161.

861. Browning DH, Graves SA. Incidence of aspiration with endotracheal tubes in children. J Pediatr 1983; 102:582–584.

862. Goodwin S, Graves SA, Haberkern CM. Aspiration in intubated premature infants. Pediatrics 1985;75: 85–88.

863. Burgess GE, Cooper JR, Marino RJ, et al. Laryngeal competence after tracheal extubation. Anesthesiology 1979;51:73–77.

864. Healey J. Fine bore feeding tubes. Anaesthesia and Intensive Care 1983;11:81.

865. Hodgson CA, Mostafa SM. Riddle of the persistent leak. Anaesthesia 1991;46:799.

866. Adams AL. A complication following guided nasotracheal intubation. Anesthesiology 1983;58: 105–106.

867. Gravenstein N, Pashayan AG. More on eliminating

CT scan artifact due to endotracheal tubes. Anesthesiology 1988;68:823.

868. Tashiro C, Yagi M, Kinoshita H. Use of an endotracheal tube without radiopaque marker for cervical CT scans. Anesthesiology 1987;67:1022.

869. Brenn BR, Saldutti G. MRI image degradation from an endotracheal tube pilot balloon. Anesth Analg 1994;79:586–587.

870. Crofts S, Campbell A. A source of artefact during general anaesthesia for magnetic resonance imaging. Anaesthesia 1993;48:643.

871. Grady RE, Perkins WJ. An unexpected cause of magnetic resonance image distortion: the endotracheal tube pilot balloon. Anesthesiology 1997;86: 993–994.

872. Carroll M, Eljamel M, Cunningham AJ. Ferrous distortion during MRI. Br J Anaesth 1994;72: 727–728.

873. Black AE, Hatch DJ, Nauth-Misir N. Complications of nasotracheal intubation in neonates, infants and children. A review of 4 years' experience in a children's hospital. Br J Anaesth 1990;65:461–467.

874. Bosman YK, Foster PA. Endotracheal intubation and head posture in infants. S Afr Med J 1977;52: 71–73.

875. Dorsey M, Schwider L, Benumof JL. Unintentional endotracheal extubation by orogastric tube removal. Anesthesiol Rev 1988;15:30–33.

876. Mallampati SR, Ibrahim A. Orogastric intubation: near-strangulation of endotracheal tube. Anesth Analg 1993;76:671–672.

877. Grindlinger GA, Niehoff J, Hughes SL, et al. Acute paranasal sinusitis related to nasotracheal intubation of head-injured patients. Crit Care Med 1987;15: 214–217.

878. Bodin L, DoKhac T, Leguillou JL, et al. Retrospective incidence of maxillary and sphenoid bacterial sinusitis in critically ill patients. Br J Anaesth 1995; 74:115–116

879. Goldstein S, Wolf GL, Kim SJ, et al. Bacteraemia during laryngoscopy and endotracheal intubation: A study using a multiple culture, large volume technique. Anaesthesia and Intensive Care 1997;25: 239–244.

880. Holzapfel L, Chevret S, Madinier G, et al. Influence of long-term oro- or nasotracheal intubation on nosocomial maxillary sinusitis and pneumonia: Results of a prospective, randomized clinical trial. Crit Care Med 1993;21:1132–1138

881. Allison JM, Gunawardene WMS. Problems with cuffs on tracheal tubes. Anaesthesia 1984;39:191.

882. Heyman DM, Greeneld AL, Rogers JS, et al. Ability to deflate the distal cuff of the laser-flex tracheal

tube preventing extubation after laser surgery of the larynx. Anesthesiology 1994;80:236–237.

883. Virag R. Inability to deflate the distal cuff of the laser-Flex tracheal tube preventing extubation after laser surgery of the larynx. Anesthesiology 1994;80:237–238.

884. Hedden M, Smith RBF, Torpey DJ. A complication of metal spiral-imbedded latex endotracheal tubes. Anesth Analg 1972;51:859–862.

885. Sivaneswaran N, O'Leary J. Failure of endotracheal tube cuff deflation. Anaesthesia and Intensive Care 1984;12:88.

886. Tanski J, James RH. Difficult extubation due to a kinked pilot tube. Anaesthesia 1986;41:1060.

887. Sklar GS, Alfonso AE, King BD. An unusual problem in nasotracheal extubation. Anesth Analg 1976;55:302–303.

888. Fagraeus L. Difficult extubation following nasotracheal intubation. Anesthesiology 1978;49:43–44.

889. Grover VK. Difficulty in extubation. Anaesthesia 1985;40:198–199.

890. Khan RM, Khan TZ, Ali M, et al. Difficult extubation. Anaesthesia 1988;43:515.

891. Lall NG. Difficult extubation. A fold in the endotracheal cuff. Anaesthesia 1980;35:500–501.

892. Mishra P, Scott DL. Difficulty at extubation of the trachea. Anaesthesia 1983;38:811.

893. Ng TY, Datta TD. Difficult extubation of an endotracheal tube cuff. Anesth Analg 1976;55:876–877.

894. Pavlin EG, Nelson E, Pulliam J. Difficulty in removal of tracheostomy tubes. Anesthesiology 1976;44:69–70.

895. Asai T. Difficult tracheal extubation in a patient with an unsuspected congenital subglottic stenosis. Anaesthesia 1995;50:243–245.

896. Bhaskar PB, Scheffer RB, Drummond JN. Bilateral fixation of a nasotracheal tube by transfacial Kirschner wires. J Oral Maxillofac Surg 1987;45:805–807.

897. Dryden GE. Circulatory collapse after pneumonectomy (an unusual complication from the use of a Carlens catheter): case report. Anesth Analg 1977;56:451–452.

898. Hilley MD, Henderson RB, Giesecke AH. Difficult extubation of the trachea. Anesthesiology 1983;59:149–150.

899. Lee C, Schwartz S, Mok MS. Difficult extubation due to transfixation of a nasotracheal tube by Kirschner wire. Anesthesiology 1977;46:427.

900. Lang S, Johnson DH, Lanigan DT, et al. Difficult tracheal extubation. Can J Anaesth 1989;36:340–342.

901. Guntupalli KK, Bouchek CD. Cricothyroid punc-

ture of an undeflatable endotracheal tube cuff. Crit Care Med 1984;12:924.

902. Yau G, Jong W, Oh TE. Failure of endotracheal tube cuff deflation. Anaesthesia and Intensive Care 1990;18:425.

903. Tashayod M, Oskoui B. A case of difficult extubation. Anesthesiology 1973;39:337.

904. Gard MA, Cruickshank LFG. Factors influencing the incidence of sore throat following endotracheal intubation. Can Med Assoc J 1961;84:662–665.

905. Harding CJ, McVey FK. Interview method affects incidence of postoperative sore throat. Anaesthesia 1987;42:1104–1107.

906. Lund LO, Daos FG. Effects on postoperative sore throats of two analgesic agents and lubricants used with endotracheal tubes. Anesthesiology 1965;26:681–683.

907. Conway CM, Miller JS, Sugden FLH. Sore throat after anesthesia. Br J Anaesth 1960;32:219–223.

908. Alexopoulous C, Lindholm CE. Airway complaints and laryngeal pathology after intubation with an anatomically shaped endotracheal tube. Acta Anaesthesiol Scand 1983;27:339–344.

909. Cohen E, Koorn R. An easy way to safely tie a double-lumen tube. J Cardiothorac Anesth 1991;5:194–195.

910. Fink BR. Laryngeal complications of general anesthesia. In: Orkin FK, Cooperman LH, eds. Complications in anesthesiology. Philadelphia: JB Lippincott, 1983:144–151.

911. Saarnivaara L, Grahne B. Clinical study on an endotracheal tube with a high-residual volume, low-pressure cuff. Acta Anaesth Scand 1981;25:89–92.

912. Monroe MC, Gravenstein N, Saga–Rumley S. Postoperative sore throat: effect of oropharyngeal airway in orotracheally intubated patients. Anesth Analg 1990;70:512–516.

913. Stout D, Dwersteg J, Cullen BF, et al. Correlation of endotracheal tube size with sore throat and hoarseness. Anesth Analg 1986;65:S155.

914. Stout DM, Bishop MJ, Dwersteg JF, et al. Correlation of endotracheal tube size with sore throat and hoarseness following general anesthesia. Anesthesiology 1987;67:419–421.

915. Wilson JE, Ozinga DW, Baughaman VL. Sore throat—does endotracheal tube size really matter? Anesthesiology 1989;71:A458.

916. Hartsell CJ, Stephen CR. Incidence of sore throat following endotracheal intubation. Can Anaesth Soc J 1964;11:307–312.

917. Mandoe H, Nikolajsen L, Lintrup U, et al. Sore throat after endotracheal intubation. Anesth Analg 1992;74:897–900.

918. Jones MW, Catling S, Evans E, et al. Hoarseness after tracheal intubation. Anaesthesia 1992;47:213–216.

919. Loeser EA, Kaminsky A, Diaz A, et al. The influence of endotracheal tube cuff design and lubrication on postoperative sore throat. Anesthesiology 1981;55:A121.

920. Loeser EA, Kaminsky A, Diaz A, et al. The influence of endotracheal tube cuff design and cuff lubrication on postoperative sore throat. Anesthesiology 1983;58:376–379.

921. Stock MC, Downs JB. Lubrication of tracheal tubes to prevent sore throat from intubation. Anesthesiology 1982;57:418–420.

922. Stride PC. Postoperative sore throat. topical hydrocortisone. Anaesthesia 1990;45:968–971.

923. Winkel E, Knudsen J. Effect on the incidence of postoperative sore throat of 1% cinchocaine jelly for endotracheal intubation. Anesth Analg 1971;50:92–94.

924. Goldberg ME, Larijani G, Gratz I, et al. Emla use reduces the incidence of postoperative sore throat (post) with endotracheal intubation. Anesth Analg 1997;84:S295.

925. Stenqvist O, Nilsson K. Postoperative sore throat related to tracheal tube cuff design. Can Anaesth Soc J 1982;29:384–386.

926. Sprague NB, Archer PL. Magill versus Mallinckrodt tracheal tubes. A comparative study of postoperative sore throat. Anaesthesia 1987;42:306–311.

927. Navarro RM, Baughman VL. Lidocaine in the endotracheal tube cuff reduces postoperative sore throat. J Clin Anes 1997;9:394–397.

928. Jones GOM, Hale DE, Wasmuth CE, et al. A survey of acute complications associated with endotracheal intubation. Cleve Clin Q 1968;35:23–31.

929. Baron SH, Kohlmoos HW. Laryngeal sequelae of endotracheal anesthesia. Ann Otol Rhinol Laryngol 1951;60:767–792.

930. Jones MW, Catling S, Evans E, et al. Hoarseness after tracheal intubation. Anaesthesia 1992;47:213–216.

931. Ishida T, Yoshiya I, Morita Y, et al. Quantitative analysis of tracheal damage. Crit Care Med 1983;11:283–285.

932. Winter R, Munro M. Lingual and buccal nerve neuropathy in a patient in the prone position. A case report. Anesthesiology 1989;71:452–454.

933. Faithfull NS. Injury to terminal branches of the trigeminal nerve following tracheal intubation. Br J Anaesth 1985;57:535–537.

934. Brimacombe J. Bilateral lingual nerve injury following tracheal intubation. Anaesthesia and Intensive Care 1993;21:107–108.

935. Streppel M, Bachmann G, Stennert E. Hypoglossal nerve palsy as a complication of transoral intubation for general anesthesia. Anesthesiology 1997;86:1007.

936. Haselby KA, McNiece WL. Respiratory obstruction from uvular edema in a pediatric patient. Anesth Analg 1983;62:1127–1128.

937. Newman T, Franssen R. Uvular edema in pediatric patients. Anesth Analg 1984;63:701–702.

938. Ravindran R, Priddy S. Uvular edema, a rare complication of endotracheal intubation. Anesthesiology 1978;48:374.

939. Seigne TD, Felske A, DelGiudice PA. Uvular edema. Anesthesiology 1978;49:375–376.

940. McEwan AI, Cashman JN. Unexpected airway obstruction. Anaesthesia 1990;45:998.

941. Claxton AR, Philips J. A complication of tracheal intubation? Anaesthesia 1994;49:920–921.

942. Diaz JH. Is uvular edema a complication of endotracheal intubation? Anesth Analg 1993;76:1139–1141.

943. Hatanaka T, Yamashita T. Another cause of upper airway obstruction. Anesthesiology 1991;75:1117–1118.

944. Huehns TY, Yentis SM, Cumberworth V. Apparent massive tongue swelling. A complication of orotracheal intubation on the intensive care unit. Anaesthesia 1994;49:414–416.

945. Koka BV, Jeon IS, Andre JM, et al. Postintubation croup in children. Anesth Analg 1977;56:501–505.

946. Darmon J, Rauss A, Dreyfuss D, et al. Evaluation of risk factors for laryngeal edema after tracheal extubation in adults and its prevention by dexamethasone. A placebo controlled double blind, multicenter study. Anesthesiology 1992;77:245–251.

947. Litman RS, Keon TP. Postintubation croup in children. Anesthesiology 1991;75:1122–1123.

948. Brandwein M, Abramson AL, Shikowitz MJ. Bilateral vocal cord paralysis following endotracheal intubation. Arch Otolaryngol Head Neck Surg 1986;112:877–882.

949. Cavo JW. True vocal cord paralysis following intubation. Laryngoscope 1985;95:1352–1359.

950. Ellis PDM, Pallister WK. Recurrent laryngeal nerve palsy and endotracheal intubation. J Laryngol Otol 1975;89:823–826.

951. Gibbin KP, Egginton MJ. Bilateral vocal cord paralysis following endotracheal intubation. Br J Anaesth 1981;53:1091–1092.

952. Komorn RM, Smith CP, Erwin JA. Acute laryngeal injury with short-term endotracheal anesthesia. Laryngoscope 1973;83:683–690.

953. Kennedy RL. Questions and answers. Anesth Analg 1977;56:321–322.

954. Lim EK, Chia KS, Ng BK. Recurrent laryngeal nerve palsy following endotracheal intubation. Anaesthesia and Intensive Care 1987;15:342–345.

955. Mass L. Another post-endotracheal vocal cord paralysis of uncertain etiology. Anesthesiol Rev 1975; 2:28–30.

956. Minuck M. Unilateral vocal cord paralysis following endotracheal intubation. Anesthesiology 1976;45: 448–449.

957. Nuutinen J, Karja J. Bilateral vocal cord paralysis following general anesthesia. Laryngoscope 1981; 91:83–86.

958. Salem MR, Wong AY, Barangan, VC, et al. Postoperative vocal cord paralysis in paediatric patients. Br J Anaesth 1971;43:696–699.

959. Whited RE. Laryngeal dysfunction following prolonged intubation. Ann Otol 1979;88:474–478.

960. Cheong KF, Chan MYP, Sin–Fai–Lam KN. Bilateral vocal cord paralysis following endotracheal intubation. Anaesthesia and Intensive Care 1994;22: 206–208.

961. Ault ML, Kimovec MA, Keeley S, et al. Vocal cord dysfunction after neurosurgical procedures. Anesthesiology 1995;83:A187.

962. Cox RH, Welborn SG. Vocal cord paralysis after endotracheal anesthesia. South Med J 1981;74: 1258–1259.

963. Anonymous. Laryngeal paralysis after endotracheal intubation. Lancet 1986;1:536–537.

964. Colice GL, Stukel TA, Dain B. Laryngeal complications of prolonged intubation. Chest 1989;96: 877–884.

965. Dubick MN, Wright BD. Comparison of laryngeal pathology following long-term oral and nasal endotracheal intubations. Anesth Analg 1978;57: 663–668.

966. Burns HP, Dayal VS, Scott A, et al. Laryngotracheal trauma: observations on its pathogenesis and its prevention following prolonged orotracheal intubation in the adult. Laryngoscope 1979;89:1316–1325.

967. Weymuller EA, Bishop MJ, Fink BR, et al. Quantification of interlaryngeal pressure exerted by endotracheal tubes. Acta Otol Rhinol Laryngol 1983;92: 444–447.

968. Nordin U. The regeneration after cuff-induced tracheal injury. Acta Otolaryngol 1982;94:541–555.

969. Commins DJ, Whittet H, Okoli UC, et al. Postintubation uvular necrosis. Anaesthesia 1994;49: 457–458.

970. Clark GPM. Necrosis of the uvula. Anaesthesia 1994;49:925.

971. Krantz MA, Solomon DL, Polus JG. Uvular necrosis following endotracheal intubation. J Clin Anesth 1994;6:139–141.

972. Bergstrom J. Post-intubation granuloma of the larynx. Acta Otolaryngol 1964;57:113–118.

973. Etsten B, Mahler D. Subglottic membrane. A complication of endotracheal intubation. N Engl J Med 1951;245:957–960.

974. Lewis RN, Swerdlow M. Hazards of endotracheal anaesthesia. Br J Anaesth 1964;36:504–515.

975. Muir AP, Straton J. Membranous laryngo-tracheitis following endotracheal intubation. Anaesthesia 1954;9:105–113.

976. Tonkin JP, Harrison GA. The effect on the larynx of prolonged endotracheal intubation. Med J Aust 1966;2:581–587.

977. Young N, Steward S. Laryngeal lesions following endotracheal anaesthesia: a report of twelve adult cases. Br J Anaesth 1953;25:32–42.

978. Strome M, Ferguson CF. Multiple postintubation complications. Ann Otol 1974;83:432–438.

979. King EG. Aftermath of intubation. Emerg Med 1983;154:201–209.

980. Fine J, Finestone SC. An unusual complication of endotracheal intubation: report of a case. Anesth Analg 1973;52:204–206.

981. Barkin ME, Trieger N. An unusual complication of nasal-tracheal anesthesia. Anesth Prog 1976;23: 57–58.

982. Rennie T, Catania AF, Haanaes HR. Ulceration of the nasal ala and dorsum secondary to improper support of the nasoendotracheal tube. J Am Assoc Nurse Anesth 1978;46:282–285.

983. Yang KL. Tracheal stenosis after a brief intubation. Anesth Analg 1995;80:625–627.

984. Burton NA, Watson DC, Brodsky JB, et al. Advantages of a new polyvinyl chloride double-lumen tube in thoracic surgery. Ann Thorac Surg 1983;36: 78–84.

985. MacGillivray RG, Rocke DA, Mahomedy AE. Endobronchial tube placement in repair of ruptured bronchus. Anaesthesia and Intensive Care 1987;15: 459–462.

986. Brodsky JB, Welti RS, Mark JBD. Thoracoscopy for retrieval of intrathoracic foreign bodies. Anesthesiology 1981;54:91–92.

987. Tobias JD. Anesthetic implications of thoracoscopy in the pediatric patient. Anesth Rev 1994;21: 133–137.

988. Peden CJ, Prys–Roberts C. Capnothorax: implications for the anaesthetist. Anaesthesia 1993;48: 664–666.

989. Carron H, Hill S. Anesthetic management of lobec-

tomy for massive pulmonary hemorrhage. Anesthesiology 1972;37:658–659.

990. Morell RC, Prielipp RC, Foreman AS, et al. Intentional occlusion of the right upper lobe bronchial orifice to tamponade life-threatening hemoptysis. Anesthesiology 1995;82:1529–1531.

991. Shivaram U, Finch P, Nowak P. Plastic endobronchial tubes in the management of life-threatening hemoptysis. Chest 1987;92:1108–1110.

992. Baraka A, Dajani A, Maktabi M. Selective contralateral bronchial intubation in children with pneumothorax or bronchopleural fistula. Br J Anaesth 1983; 55:901–904.

993. Brown CR. Postpneumonectomy empyema and bronchopleural fistula—use of prolonged endobronchial intubation: a case report. Anesth Analg 1973;52:439–441.

994. Dennison PH, Lester ER. An anaesthetic technique for the repair of bronchopleural fistula. Br J Anaesth 1961;33:655–659.

995. Cullum AR, English ICW, Branthwaite MA. Endobronchial intubation in infancy. Anaesthesia 1973; 28:66–70.

996. McGuire GP. Lung ventilation and bronchopleural fistula. Can J Anaesth 1996;43:1275–1276.

997. Ratliff JL, Hill JD, Tucker H, et al. Endobronchial control of bronchopleural fistulae. Chest 1977;71: 98–99.

998. Bochenek KJ, Brown M, Skupin A. Use of a double-lumen endotracheal tube with independent lung ventilation for treatment of refractory atelectasis. Anesth Analg 1987;66:1014–1017.

999. Glass DD, Tonnesen AS, Gabel JC, et al. Therapy of unilateral pulmonary insufficiency with a double lumen endotracheal tube. Crit Care Med 1976;4: 323–326.

1000. Murray JF. Treatment of acute total atelectasis. Anaesthesia 1985;40:158–162.

1001. Mullelm M, Baraka A. A simple double lumen adapter for differential lung ventilation. Anaesthesia 1988;43:254–255.

1002. Venus B, Pratap KS, Tholt TO. Treatment of unilateral pulmonary insufficiency by selective administration of continuous positive airway pressure through a double-lumen tube. Anesthesiology 1980;53: 74–77.

1003. Kraenzler EJ, Kirby T, Hearn C, et al. Airway management of cystic fibrosis patients during double lung transplantation: single lumen endotracheal tubes are superior to double lumen endotracheal tubes. J Cardiothor Vasc Anesth 1994;8:157.

1004. Kubota Y, Toyoda Y, Nagata N, et al. Tracheobronchial angles in infants and children. Anesthesiology 1986;64:374–376.

1005. Sibai AN, Baraka A. A new double lumen tube adaptor. Anaesthesia 1986;41:628–630.

1006. Tanguturi S, Capan LM, Patel K, et al. A new double-lumen tube adapter. Anesth Analg 1980;59: 507–508.

1007. Worsley MH, Hawkins DJ, Scott DHT. Attachments to double-lumen bronchial tubes. Anaesthesia 1990;45:1001–1002.

1008. Hannallah MS, Benumof JL, Bachenheimer LC, et al. The resting volume and compliance characteristics of the bronchial cuff of left polyvinyl chloride double-lumen endobronchial tubes. Anesth Analg 1993;77:1222–1226.

1009. Hannallah MS, Benumof JL, Bachenheimer LC, et al. The resting volume and compliance characteristics of the bronchial cuff of left polyvinyl chloride double-lumen endobronchial tubes. Anesth Analg 1993;77:1222–1226.

1010. Benumof JL. Improving the design and function of double-lumen tubes. J Cardiothorac Anesth 1988; 2:729–733.

1011. Benumof JL, Partridge BL, Salvatierra C, et al. Margin of safety in positioning modern double-lumen endotracheal tubes. Anesthesiology 1987;67: 729–738.

1012. Edwards EM, Hatch DJ. Experiences with double-lumen tubes. Anaesthesia 1965;20:461–467.

1013. Butman BB. Experience with the Carlens double-lumen catheter for anesthesia in thoracic surgery. N Y State J Med 1954;54:2463–2466.

1014. Clarke AD. The White double lumen tube. A report on its use in fifty cases. Br J Anaesth 1962;34: 822–824.

1015. White GMJ. A new double lumen tube. Br J Anaesth 1960;32:232–234.

1016. McKenna MJ, Wilson RS, Botelho RJ. Right upper lobe obstruction with right-sided double-lumen endobronchial tubes. A comparison of two tube types. J Cardiothorac Anesth 1988;2:734–740.

1017. Keating JL, Benumof JL. An analysis of margin of safety in positioning double-lumen tubes. Anesthesiology 1985;63:A563.

1018. Robertshaw FL. Low resistance double-lumen endobronchial tubes. Br J Anaesth 1962;34:576–579.

1019. Read RC, Friday CD, Eason CN. Prospective study of the Robertshaw endobronchial catheter in thoracic surgery. Ann Thorac Surg 1977;24:156–161.

1020. Conacher ID, Herrema IH, Batchelor AM. Robertshaw double lumen tubes: a reappraisal thirty years on. Anaesthesia and Intensive Care 1994;22: 179–183.

1021. Benumof JL. Anesthesia for thoracic surgery. Philadelphia: WB Saunders, 1987.

1022. Bryce–Smith R. A double-lumen endobronchial tube. Br J Anaesth 1959;31:274–275.

1023. Brodsky JB, Macario A. Modified BronchoCath double-lumen tube. J Cardiothorac Vasc Anesth 1995;9:784–785.

1024. Alfery DD. Increasing the margin of safety in positioning left-sided double-lumen endotracheal tubes. Anesthesiology 1988;69:149–150.

1025. Desai FM, Rocke DA. Double-lumen tube design fault. Anesthesiology 1990;73:575–576.

1026. Virag RA. Double-lumen tube design fault. Anesthesiology 1990;73:576.

1027. Yahagi N, Furuya H, Matsui J, et al. Improvements of the left Broncho-Cath double-lumen tube. Anesthesiology 1994;81:781–782.

1028. Slinger P, Triolet W. A clinical comparison of three different designs of right-sided double-lumen endobronchial tubes. Can J Anaesth 1989;36:S59–S60.

1029. Hurford WE, Alfille PH. A quality improvement study of the placement and complications of double-lumen endobronchial tubes. J Cardiothorac Vasc Anesth 1993;7:517–520.

1030. Van Dyck MJ, Astiz I. Kinking of a right-sided double-lumen tube in the right upper lobe bronchus. Anesthesiology 1994;80:1410–1411.

1031. Slinger PD, Chripko D. A clinical comparison of bronchial cuff pressures in three different designs of left double-lumen tubes. Anesth Analg 1993;77:305–308.

1032. Benumof JL. Anesthesia for pulmonary surgery (ASA Refresher Course #225). New Orleans: ASA, 1991.

1033. Rocke DA, MacGillivray RG, Mahomedy AE. Positioning of double lumen tubes. Anaesthesia 1986;41:770–771.

1034. Burk WJ. Should a fiberoptic bronchoscope be routinely used to position a double-lumen tube? Anesthesiology 1988;68:826.

1035. Watson CB. Problems with endobronchial intubation. Anesthesiol Rev 1986;13:52–55.

1036. Aggarwal A, Bousamra M, Kotter G, et al. Obstruction of left double-lumen endotracheal tubes after left upper lobectomy. Anesth Analg 1996;82:SCA11.

1037. Habibi A, Mackey S, Brodsky JB. Selecting a double-lumen tube after lung transplantation. Anesth Analg 1997;84:940.

1038. Brodsky JB, Macario A, Mark JBD. Tracheal diameter predicts double-lumen tube size: a method for selecting left double-lumen tubes. Anesth Analg 1996;82:861–864.

1039. Hannallah MS, Benumof JL, Ruttimann UE. The relationship between left mainstem bronchial diameter and patient's size. Anesth Analg 1994;78:S150.

1040. Russell WJ. A blind guided technique for placing double-lumen endobronchial tubes. Anaesthesia and Intensive Care 1992;20:71–74.

1041. Neustein SM, Eisenkraft JB. Proper lateralization of left-sided double-lumen tubes. Anesthesiology 1989;71:996.

1042. Kubota H, Kubota Y, Toyoda Y, et al. Selective blind endobronchial intubation in children and adults. Anesthesiology 1987;67:587–589.

1043. Lieberman D, Littleford J, Horan T, et al. Placement of left double-lumen endobronchial tubes with or without a stylet. Can J Anaesth 1996;43:238–242.

1044. Panadero A, Iribarren MJ, Fernandoz–Liesa I, et al. A simple method to decrease malposition of Robertshaw-type tubes. Can J Anaesth 1996;43:984.

1045. El–Etr AA. Improved technic for insertion of the Carlens catheter. Anesth Analg 1969;48:738–740.

1046. Bjork VO, Carlens E, Friberg O. Endobronchial anesthesia. Anesthesiology 1953;14:60–72.

1047. Brodsky J, Benumof JL, Ehrenworth J, et al. Depth of placement of left double-lumen endobronchial tubes. Anesth Analg 1991;73:570–572.

1048. Matthew EB, Hirschmann RA. Placing double-lumen tubes with a fiberoptic bronchoscope. Anesthesiology 1986;65:118–119.

1049. Ross DG. Fiberoptic intubation and double-lumen tubes. Anaesthesia 1990;45:895.

1050. Shulman MS, Brodsky JB, Levesque PR. Fibreoptic bronchoscopy for tracheal and endobronchial intubation with a double-lumen tube. Can J Anaesth 1987;34:172–173.

1051. Shinnick JP, Freedman AP. Bronchofiberscopic placement of a double-lumen endotracheal tube. Crit Care Med 1982;10:544–545.

1052. Scanzillo MA, Shulman MS. Lighted stylet for placement of a double-lumen endobronchial tube. Anesth Analg 1995;81:205–206.

1053. Russell WJ. Further reflections on a blind guided technique for endobronchial intubation. Anaesthesia and Intensive Care 1996;24:123.

1054. Coe VL, Brodsky JB, Mark JBD. Double-lumen endotracheal tubes for patients with tracheostomies. Anesth Analg 1984;63:882.

1055. Simpson PM. Tracheal intubation with a Robertshaw tube via a tracheostomy. Br J Anaesth 1976;48:373–375.

1056. Seed RF, Wedley JR. Tracheal intubation with a Robertshaw tube via a tracheostomy. Br J Anaesth 1977;49:639.

1057. Brodsky JB, Tobler HG, Mark JBD. A double-lumen endobronchial tube for tracheostomies. Anesthesiology 1991;74:387–388.

1058. Hannallah MS, Benumof JL, McCarthy PO, et al. Comparison of three techniques to inflate the bronchial cuff of left polyvinyl chloride double-lumen tubes. Anesth Analg 1993;77:990–994.

1059. Riley RH, Marples FL. Relocation of a double-lumen tube during patient positioning. Anesth Analg 1992;75:1071.

1059. Cobley M, Kidd JF. Willis BA, et al. Endobronchial cuff pressures. Br J Anaesth 1993;70:576–578.

1060. Saito S, Dohi S, Naito H. Alteration of double-lumen endobronchial tube position by flexion and extension of the neck. Anesthesiology 1985;62:696–697.

1061. Alliaume B, Coddens J, Deloof T, Reliability of auscultation in positioning of double-lumen endobronchial tubes. Can J Anaesth 1992;39:687–690.

1062. Desiderio DP, Burt M, Kolker AC, et al. The effects of endobronchial cuff inflation on double lumen endotracheal tube movement after lateral decubitus positioning. Anesth Analg 1995;80:SCA43.

1063. Pescod DC, Fernandes JK. Inadvertent relocation of a double-lumen endotracheal tube by surgical traction. Anaesthesia and Intensive Care 1994;22:720–723.

1064. Yazigi A, Madi–Jebara S, Haddad F, et al. Relocation of a double-lumen tube during surgical dissection. Anesth Analg 1993;77:1303.

1065. Campos JH, Reasoner DK, Moyers JR. Comparison of a modified double-lumen endotracheal tube with a single-lumen tube with enclosed bronchial blocker. Anesth Analg 1996;83:1268–1272.

1066. Brodsky JB, Macario A, Cannon WB, et al. "Blind" placement of plastic left double-lumen tubes. Anaesthesia and Intensive Care 1995;23:583–586.

1067. Brodsky JB, Mark JBD. A simple technique for accurate placement of double-lumen endobronchial tubes. Anesthesiol Rev 1983;10:26–30.

1068. Zbinden S. Fibreoptic bronchoscopy and double-lumen endobronchial tubes. Can J Anaesth 1993;40:681.

1069. Slinger PD. Fiberoptic bronchoscopic positioning of double-lumen tubes. J Cardiothorac Anesth 1989;3:486–496.

1070. Smith GB, Hirsch NP, Ehrenwerth J. Placement of double-lumen endobronchial tubes. Br J Anaesth 1986;58:1317–1320.

1071. Hirsch NP, Smith GB. Malposition of left-sided double-lumen endobronchial tubes. Anesthesiology 1985;63:563.

1072. Benumof JL. Fiberoptic bronchoscopy and double-lumen tube position. Anesthesiology 1986;65:117–118.

1073. Asai T. Torsion of a double-lumen tube in the left bronchus. Anesthesiology 1992;76:1064–1065.

1074. Kumar AY, Shankar KB, Mosley HSL. Capnography does not reliably detect double-lumen endotracheal tube malplacement. Journal of Clinical Monitoring 1993;9:207.

1075. deVries JW, Haanschoten MC. Capnography does not reliably detect double-lumen endotracheal tube malplacement. Reply. Journal of Clinical Monitoring 1993;9:207–208.

1076. Bardoczky GI, deFrancquen P, Engelman E, et al. Continuous monitoring of pulmonary mechanics with the sidestream spirometer during lung transplantation. J Cardiothorac Vasc Anesth 1992;6:731–734.

1077. Bardoczky GI, Levarlet M, Engelman E, et al. Continuous spirometry for detection of double-lumen endobronchial tube displacement. Br J Anaesth 1993;70:499–502.

1078. Bardoczky GI, Engelman E, D'Hollander A. Continuous spirometry: an aid to monitoring ventilation during operation. Br J Anaesth 1993;71:747–751.

1079. Simon BA, Hurford WE, Alfille PH, et al. An aid in the diagnosis of malpositioned double-lumen tubes. Anesthesiology 1992;76:862–863.

1080. Iwasaka H, Itoh K, Miyakawa H, et al. Continuous monitoring of ventilatory mechanics during one-lung ventilation. Journal of Clinical Monitoring 1996;12:161–164.

1081. de Vries JW, Haanschoten MC. Capnography does not reliably detect double-lumen endotracheal tube malplacement. Journal of Clinical Monitoring 1992;8:236–237.

1082. Araki K, Nomura R, Urushibara R, et al. Displacement of the double-lumen endobronchial tube can be detected by bronchial cuff pressure changes. Anesth Analg 1997;84:1349–1353.

1083. Shafieha MJ, Sit J, Kartha R, et al. End-tidal CO_2 analyzers in proper positioning of the double-lumen tubes. Anesthesiology 1986;64:844–845.

1084. Cohen E, Kirschner PA, Goldofsky S. Intraoperative manipulation for positioning of double-lumen tubes. Anesthesiology 1988;68:170.

1085. Hannallah M. Evaluation of tracheal tube exchangers for replacement of double-lumen endobronchial tubes. Anesthesiology 1992;77:609–610.

1086. Gatell JA, Barst SM, Desiderio DP, et al. A new technique for replacing an endobronchial double-lumen tube with an endotracheal single-lumen tube. Anesthesiology 1990;73:340–341.

1087. Black AMS, Harrison GA. Difficulties with positioning Robertshaw double lumen tubes. Anaesthesia and Intensive Care 1975;3:299–311.

1088. Cohen JA, Denisco RA, Richards TS, et al. Hazardous placement of a Robertshaw-type endobronchial tube. Anesth Analg 1986;65:100–101.

1089. Saito S, Dohi S, Tajima K. Failure of double-lumen endobronchial tube placement. Congenital tracheal stenosis in an adult. Anesthesiology 1987;66: 83–85.

1090. Brodsky JB. Malposition of left-sided double-lumen endobronchial tubes. Anesthesiology 1985;62: 667–669.

1091. Conacher JD. The urinary catheter as a bronchial blocker. Anaesthesia 1983;38:475–477.

1092. Brodsky JB, Mark JBD. Bilateral upper lobe obstruction from a single double-lumen tube. Anesthesiology 1991;74:1163–1164.

1093. Brodsky JB. Complications of double-lumen tracheal tubes. Problems in Anesthesia 1988;2: 292–306.

1094. Cohen E, Goldofasky S, Neustein S, et al. Fiberoptic evaluation of endobronchial tube position: red rubber vs polyvinyl chloride. Anesth Analg 1989;68: S54.

1095. Greene ER, Gutierrez FA. Tip of polyvinyl chloride double-lumen endobronchial tube inadvertently wedged in left lower lobe bronchus. Anesthesiology 1986;64:406.

1096. Varma YS. An unusual complication with the Bryce–Smith double-lumen tube. A case report. 1969;41:551–552.

1097. Benumof JL. Anesthesia for pulmonary surgery (ASA Refresher Course #213). New Orleans: ASA, 1989.

1098. Gibbs N, Giles K. Malposition of left-sided double-lumen endobronchial tubes. Anaesthesia and Intensive Care 1986;14:92–93.

1099. Desai FM, Rocke DA. Double lumen tube design fault. Anesthesiology 1990;73:575–576.

1100. Maguire DP, Spiro AW. Bronchial obstruction and hypoxia during one-lung ventilation. Anesthesiology 1987;66:830–831.

1101. Sibell DM, Jaeger JM. Failure to ventilate through a double-lumen tube due to carinal shift during lung volume reduction surgery. Anesth Analg 1996;82: 881–882.

1102. Pollak Y, Kogan A, Grunwald Z. Double-lumen tube malfunction caused by the carinal hook. Anesthesiology 1995;83:639.

1103. Guernelli N, Bragaglia RB, Briccoli A, et al. Tracheobronchial ruptures due to cuffed Carlens tubes. Ann Thorac Cardiovasc Surg 1979;28:66–68.

1104. Heiser M, Steinberg JJ, MacVaugh H, et al. Bronchial rupture, a complication of the use of the Rob-

ertshaw double-lumen tube. Anesthesiology 1979; 51:88.

1105. Hannallah M, Gomes M. Bronchial rupture associated with the use of a double-lumen tube in a small adult. Anesthesiology 1989;71:457–459.

1106. Foster JMG, Alimo EB. Ruptured bronchus following endobronchial intubation. Br J Anaesth 1983; 55:687–688.

1107. Brodsky JB, Shulman MS, Mark JBD. Airway rupture with a disposable double-lumen tube. Anesthesiology 1986;64:415.

1108. Burton NA, Fall SM, Lyons T, et al. Rupture of the left main-stem bronchus with a polyvinyl chloride double-lumen tube. Chest 1983;83:928–929.

1109. Peden CJ, Galizia EJ, Smith RB. Bronchial trauma secondary to intubation with a PVC double-lumen tube. J Roy Soc Med 1992;85:705–706.

1110. Hasan A, Ganado AL, Norton R, et al. Tracheal rupture with disposable polyvinyl chloride double-lumen endotracheal tubes. J Cardiothorac Vasc Anesth 1992;6:208–211.

1111. Peden CJ, Galizia EJ, Smith RB. Bronchial trauma secondary to intubation with a PVC double-lumen tube. J Roy Soc Med 1992;85:705–706.

1112. Ikeda M, Ishida H, Tsujimoto S, et al. Endobronchial inflammatory polyp after thoracoabdominal aneurysm surgery: a late complication of use of a double-lumen endobronchial tube. Anesthesiology 1996;84:1234–1236.

1113. Bickford–Smith P, Evans CS. Error in labeling. Anaesthesia 1987;42:572.

1114. Jenkins V. Unusual difficulty with double-lumen endo-bronchial tube. Anaesthesia 1963;18: 236–237.

1115. Anonymous. Tracheal tube lumens may be distorted. Biomedical Safety & Standards 1989;19:68.

1116. Wyatt R, Garner S. A defect in Robertshaw double-lumen endotracheal tubes corrected. Anaesthesia 1981;36:830–831.

1117. Campbell C, Viswanathan S, Riopelle JM, et al. Manufacturing defect in a double-lumen tube. Anesth Analg 1991;73:825–826.

1118. Pritchard N. An incorrectly labeled Mallinckrodt double-lumen endobronchial tube. Anaesthesia 1994;49:744.

1119. Fikkers BG, Zandstra DF. Incorrectly labeled double-lumen tube. J Cardiothorac Vasc Anesth 1994; 8:605.

1120. Akers JA, Riley RH. Failed extubation due to "sutured" double-lumen tube. Anaesthesia and Intensive Care 1990;18:577.

1121. Wells DG, Zelcer J, Podolakin W, et al. Cardiac arrest from pulmonary outflow tract obstruction due to a double-lumen tube. Anesthesiology 1987;66: 422–423.

1122. Conacher ID. A coaxial technique for facilitating one-lung ventilation. Anaesthesia 1991;46: 400–403.

1123. Nazari S, Trazzi R, Moncalvo F, et al. Selective bronchial intubation for one-lung anaesthesia in thoracic surgery. Anaesthesia 1986;41:519–526.

1124. Nazari S, Trazzi R, Moncalvo F, et al. A new method for separate lung ventilation. Surv Anesth 1988;32: 355–356.

1125. Welsh BE. Selective bronchial intubation. Anaesthesia 1987;42:82.

1126. Chiaranda M, Rossi A, Manani G, et al. Measurement of the flow-resistive properties of double-lumen bronchial tubes in vitro. Anaesthesia 1989; 44:335–340.

1127. Baskoff JD, Stevenson RL. Endobronchial intubation in children. Anesthesiol Rev 1981;8:29–31.

1128. Brooks JG, Bustamante SA, Koops BL, et al. Selective bronchial intubation for the treatment of severe localized pulmonary interstitial emphysema in newborn infants. J Pediatr 1972;91:648–652.

1129. Baraka A, Slim M, Dajani A, et al. One-lung ventilation of children during surgical excision of hydatid cysts of the lung. Br J Anaesth 1982;54:523–528.

1130. Dickman GL, Short BL, Krauss DR. Selective bronchial intubation in the management of unilateral pulmonary interstitial emphysema. Am J Dis Child 1977;131:365.

1131. Dalens B, Labbe A, Haberer J. Selective endobronchial blocking versus selective intubation. Anesthesiology 1982;57:555–556.

1132. Fisk GC. Endobronchial anaesthesia in young children. Br J Anaesth 1966;38:157.

1133. Hogg CE, Lorhan PH. Pediatric bronchial blocking. Anesthesiology 1970;33:560–562.

1134. Mathew OP, Thach BT. Selective bronchial obstruction for treatment of bullous interstitial emphysema. J Ped 1980;96:475–477.

1135. Rao CC, Krishna G, Grosfeld JL, et al. One lung pediatric anesthesia. Anesth Analg 1981;60: 450–452.

1136. Watson CB, Bowe EA, Burk W. One-lung anesthesia for pediatric thoracic surgery. A new use for the fiberoptic bronchoscope. Anesthesiology 1982;56: 314–315.

1137. Yeh TF, Pildes RS, Salem MR. Treatment of persistent tension pneumothorax in a neonate by selective bronchial intubation. Anesthesiology 1978;49: 37–38.

1138. Sachdeva SP. Treatment of post-operative pulmonary atelectasis by active inflation of the atelectatic lobe(s) through an endobronchial tube. Acta Anaesthesiol Scand 1974;18:65–70.

1139. McLellan I. Endobronchial intubation in children. Anaesthesia 1974;29:757–758.

1140. Bragg CL, Vukelich GR. Endotracheal tube extension for endobronchial intubation. Anesth Analg 1989;69:548–549.

1141. Holzman RS. A tracheal tube extension for emergency tracheal reanastomosis. Anesthesiology 1989; 70:170–171.

1142. Riebold TW. Source of specialized endotracheal tubes. Anesthesiology 1989;71:322–323.

1143. Aps C, Towey RM. Experiences with fibre-optic bronchoscopic positioning of single-lumen endobronchial tubes. Anaesthesia 1981;36:415–418.

1144. Bloch EC. Tracheo-bronchial angles in infants and children. Anesthesiology 1986;65:236–237.

1145. Arndt GA, Kranner PW, Lorenz D. Co-axial placement of endobronchial blocker. Can J Anaesth 1994;41:1126–1127.

1146. Russell GN, Frazer S, Richardson JC. Difficult bronchial intubation. Anaesthesia 1987;42:82.

1147. Cant WF, Tinker JH, Tarhan S. Bronchial blockade in a child with a bronchopleural-cutaneous fistula using a balloon-tipped catheter. Anesth Analg 1976; 55:874–876.

1148. Vale R. Selective bronchial blocking in a small child. Br J Anaesth 1969;41:453–454.

1149. Welsh BE. Selective bronchial intubation. Anesthesiology 1987;42:82.

1150. Gozal Y, Lee W. Nasal intubation and one-lung ventilation. Anesthesiology 1996;84:477.

1151. Harvey SC, Alpert CC, Fishman RL. Independent placement of a bronchial blocker for single-lung ventilation: an alternative method for the difficult airway. Anesth Analg 1996;83:1330–1331.

1152. Hammer GB, Manos SJ, Smith BM, et al. Single-lung ventilation in pediatric patients. Anesthesiology 1996;84:1503–1506.

1153. Chen K-P, Chan H-C, Huang S-J. Foley catheter used as bronchial blocker for one lung ventilation in a patient with tracheostomy—a case report. Acta Anaesthesiol Sin 1995;31:41–44.

1154. Scheller MS, Kriett JM, Smith CM, et al. Airway management during anesthesia for double-lung transplantation using a single-lumen endotracheal tube with an enclosed bronchial blocker. J Cardiothorac Vasc Anesth 1992;6:204–207.

1155. Zilberstein M, Katz RI, Levy A, et al. An improved method for introducing an endobronchial blocker. J Cardiothorac Anesth 1990;4:481–483.

1156. Herenstein R, Russo JR, Mooka N, et al. Management of one-lung anesthesia in an anticoagulated patient. Anesth Analg 1988;67:1120–1122.

1157. Maewal HK, Kirk BW. Balloon catheter re-expansion of atelectatic lung. Crit Care Med 1976;4: 301–303.

1158. Cohen DJ. A unique use of the Univent tube. Anesthesiology 1995;83:229.

1159. Campos JH, Ledet V, Moyers JR. Improvement of arterial oxygen saturation with selective lobar bronchial block during hemorrhage in a patient with previous contralateral lobectomy. Anesth Analg 1995; 81:1095–1096.

1160. Brodsky JB. Complications of double-lumen tracheal tubes. In: Bishop, MJ ed. Physiology and consequences of tracheal intubation [Special Issue]. Probl Anesth 1988;2(2):292–306.

1161. Ransom E, Detterbeck F, Klein JI, et al. Univent tube provides a new technique for jet ventilation. Anesthesiology 1996;84:724–726.

1162. Benumof JL, Gaughan S, Ozaki GT. Operative lung constant positive airway pressure with the Univent bronchial blocker tube. Anesth Analg 1992;74: 406–410.

1163. Hultgren BL, Krishna PR, Kamaya H. A new tube for one lung ventilation. experience with Univent tube. Anesthesiology 1988;65:A481.

1164. Inoue H, Shohtsu A, Ogawa J, et al. New device for one-lung anesthesia. Endotracheal tube with moveable blocker. J Thorac Cardiovasc Med 1982; 83:940–941.

1165. Inoue H, Shohtsu A, Ogawa J, et al. Endotracheal tube with moveable blocker to prevent aspiration of intratracheal bleeding. Ann Thorac Surg 1984;37: 497–499.

1166. Inoue H. Endotracheal tube with movable blocker (Univent). Jpn J Med Inst 1989;59:241–244.

1167. Kamaya H, Krishna PR. New endobronchial tube (Univent tube) for selective blockade of one lung. Anesthesiology 1985;63:342–343.

1168. Karwande SV. A new tube for single lung ventilation. Chest 1987;92:761–763.

1169. MacGillivray RG. Evaluation of a new tracheal tube with a moveable bronchus blocker. Anaesthesia 1988;43:687–689.

1170. Inoue H, Suzuki I, Mwasaki M, et al. Selective exclusion of the injured lung. J Trauma 1993;34: 496–498.

1171. Slinger P. Con: The Univent tube is not the best method of providing one-lung ventilation. J Cardiothorac Vasc Anesth 1993;7:108–112.

1172. Gayes JM. The Univent tube is the best technique for providing one-lung ventilation. Pro: One-lung ventilation is best accomplished with the Univent endotracheal tube. J Cardiothorac Vasc Anesth 1993;7:103–107.

1173. Andros TG, Lennon PF. One-lung ventilation in a patient with a tracheostomy and severe tracheobronchial disease. Anesthesiology 1993;79: 1127–1128.

1174. Bellver J, Gardia–Aguado RG, De Andres J, et al. Selective bronchial intubation with a Univent system in patients with a tracheostomy. Anesthesiology 1993;79:1453–1454.

1175. Kelley JG, Gaba DM, Brodsky JB. Bronchial cuff pressures of two tubes used in thoracic surgery. J Cardiothorac Vasc Anesth 1992;6:190–192.

1176. Guyton DC, Delima L, Besselievre TR, et al. One lung ventilation: the effect of Univent cuff inflation technique on tracheal wall pressure. Anesth Analg 1995;80:S168.

1177. Schwartz DE, Yost CS, Larson MD. Pneumothorax complicating the case of a Univent endotracheal tube. Anesth Analg 1993;76:443–445.

1178. Lines V. Selective bronchial blocking in a small child. Br J Anaesth 1969;41:893.

1179. Ginsberg RJ. New technique for one-lung anesthesia using an endobronchial blocker. J Thorac Cardiovasc Surg 1981;82:542–546.

1180. Cay DL, Csenderits LE, Lines V, et al. Selective bronchial blocking in children. Anaesthesia and Intensive Care 1975;3:127–130.

1181. Ransom ES, Norfleet EA. Syringe cap prevents leaks during one-lung ventilation. Anesthesiology 1995; 82:1538.

1182. Oxorn D. Use of fiberoptic bronchoscope to assist placement of a Fogarty catheter as a bronchial blocker. Can J Anaesth 1987;34:427–428.

1183. Arai T, Hatano Y. Yet another reason to use a fiberoptic bronchoscope to properly site a double lumen tube. Anesthesiology 1987;66:581–582.

1184. Doyle DJ. A simple technique for placement of the Univent bronchial blocker. Anesthesiology 1993; 79:399.

1185. Essig K, Freeman JA. Alternative bronchial cuff inflation technique for the Univent tube. Anesthesiology 1992;76:478–479.

1186. Stark DCC. Anesthesia for thoracic surgery. Anesthesiol Rev 1980;7:14–19.

1187. Finucane BT, Kupshik HL. A flexible stilette for replacing damaged tracheal tubes. Can Anaesth Soc J 1978;25:153–154.

1188. Veit AM, Allen RB. Single-lung ventilation in a patient with a freshly placed percutaneous tracheostomy. Anesth Analg 1996;82:1292–1293.

1189. Larson CE, Gasior TA. A device for endobronchial blocker placement during one-lung anesthesia. Anesth Analg 1990;71:311–312.

1190. Schwartz DE, Yost CS, Larson MD. Pneumothorax

complicating the use of a Univent endotracheal tube. Anesth Analg 1993;76:443–445.

1191. Buchanan CCR, Vaughan RS, Verdi I. Right upper lobectomy in a patient with an iatrogenic tracheo-oesophageal fistula after laryngectomy. Br J Anaesth 1995;74:461–463.

1192. Thielmeier KA, Anwar M. Complication of the Univent tube. Anesthesiology 1996;84:491.

1193. Dougherty P, Hannallah M. A potentially serious complication that resulted from improper use of the Univent tube. Anesthesiology 1992;77:835–836.

1194. Gayes JM. Management of Univent bronchial blocking balloon perforation during one-lung ventilation. Anesth Analg 1994;79:1210.

1195. Hannallah M. The Univent tube. Bronchial cuff inflation. Anesthesiology 1991;75:165.

1196. Cobley M, Vaughn RS. Recognition and management of difficult airway problems. Br J Anaesth 1992;68:90–97.

1197. Linder GS. A new polyolefin-coated endotracheal tube stylet. Anesth Analg 1974;53:341–342.

1198. Linder GS. More on wire stylets. Anesth Analg 1977;56:325.

1199. Marshall J. Self-lubricated stylet for endotracheal tubes. Anesthesiology 1968;29:385.

1200. Swales H. Difficulty in using the Schroeder oral/nasal directional stylet. Anaesthesia and Intensive Care 1995;23:407–408.

1201. Salem MR, Nimmagadda UR, Salazar JL, et al. Evaluation of a new intubation guide in patients with cervical spine injuries. Crit Care Med 1990;18:S199.

1202. Smith M, Buist RJ, Mansour NY. A simple method to facilitate difficult intubation. Can J Anaesth 1990;37:144–145.

1203. Berry FA. Anesthesia for the child with a difficult airway. In: Berry FA, ed. Anesthetic management of difficult and routine pediatric patients. New York: Churchill Livingstone, 1990:167–198.

1204. Conacher ID. Instrumental bronchial tears. Anaesthesia 1992;47:589–590.

1205. Restall CJ. Plastic-covered wire stylet. Anesth Analg 1976;55:755.

1206. Martin P, Campbell AM. Tracheal intubation: a complication. Anaesthesia 1992;47:75.

1207. Larson CE, Gonzalez RM. A problem with metal endotracheal tubes and plastic-coated stylets. Anesthesiology 1989;70:883–884.

1208. Zmyslowski WP, Kam D, Simpson GT. An unusual cause of endotracheal tube obstruction. Anesthesiology 1989;70:883.

1209. Fishman RL. Reuse of a disposable stylet with life-threatening complications. Anesth Analg 1991;72:266–267.

1210. Kubota Y, Toyoda Y, Kubota H, et al. Shaping tracheal tubes. Anaesthesia 1987;42:896.

1211. Kubota Y, Toyoda Y, Kubota H. No more complications with stylets. Anaesthesia 1992;47:628.

1212. Sharma ML, Bhardwaj N, Chari P. Broken metal intubating stylet. Anaesthesia and Intensive Care 1994;22:624.

1213. Stevens DC, Merk PF, Fenton LJ, et al. Airway foreign body. Clin Ped 1982;21:510–511.

1214. Larson CE, Gonzalez RM. A problem with metal endotracheal tubes and plastic-coated stylets. Anesthesiology 1989;70:883–884.

1215. Kataria B, Starnes M. Another problem with a stylet in an endotracheal tube. Anesth Analg 1989;68:422.

1216. Gottschalk SK, Schuth CR, Quinby GE Jr. A complication of tracheal intubation: Distal kinking of the tube. J Pediatr 1978;92:161–162.

1217. Macintosh RR. An aid to oral intubation. Br Med J 1949;1:28.

1218. Cooper RM, Cohen DR. The use of an endotracheal ventilation catheter for jet ventilation during a difficult intubation. Can J Anaesth 1994;41:1196–1199.

1219. Nolan JP, Wilson ME. An aid to oral intubation in patients with potential cervical spine injuries. Anesth Analg 1992;75:153–154.

1220. Benson PF. The gum-elastic bougie: a life saver. Anesth Analg 1992;74:318.

1221. Hung OR, McNeil P. The use of an intubating guide (gum elastic bougie) for orotracheal intubation in patients with potential difficult airways. Anesthesiology 1996;85:A988.

1222. Gataure PS, Vaughan RS, Latto IP. Simulated difficult intubation. Comparison of the gum elastic bougie and the stylet. Anaesthesia 1996;51:935–938.

1223. Nolan JP, Wilson ME. An evaluation of the gum elastic bougie. Intubation times and incidence of sore throat. Anaesthesia 1992;47:878–881.

1224. Nolan JP, Wilson ME. Orotracheal intubation in patients with potential cervical spine injuries. An indication for the gum elastic bougie. Anaesthesia 1993;48:630–633.

1225. Morris GN. Orotracheal intubation in a patient with cervical spine injury. Anaesthesia 1994;49:258.

1226. Finucane BT, Kipshik HL. A flexible stilette for replacing damaged tracheal tubes. Can Anaesth Soc J 1978;25:153–154.

1227. Chipley PS, Castresana M, Bridges MT, et al. Prolonged use of an endotracheal tube changer in a pediatric patient with a potentially compromised airway. Chest 1994;105:961–962.

1228. Cooper RM. The use of an endotracheal ventilation

catheter in the management of difficult extubations. Can J Anaesth 1996;43:90–93.

1229. Hannallah M, Brager R, Ved S, et al. Jet stylets as an aid for replacement of tracheostomy tubes. Ann Otol Rhinol Laryngol 1995;104:695–697.

1230. Robles B, Hester J, Brock–Utne JG. Remember the gum-elastic bougie at extubation. J Clin Anesth 1993;5:329–331.

1231. Wright TM, Vinayakom K. Endotracheal tube replacement in patients with cervical spine injury. Anesthesiology 1995;82:1307–1308.

1232. Topf AI, Eclavea A. Extubation of the difficult airway. Anesthesiology 1996;85:1213–1214.

1233. Artru AA, Schultz AB, Bonneu JJ. Modification of an Eschmann introducer to permit measurement of end-tidal carbon dioxide. Anesth Analg 1989;68: 129–131.

1234. Gaughan SD, Benumof JL, Ozaki GT. Quantification of the jet function of a jet stylet. Anesth Analg 1992;74:580–585.

1235. Dhara SS. A multilumen catheter guide for difficult airway management. Its uses in anaesthesia and intensive care. Anaesthesia 1994;49:974–978.

1236. Montgomery PQ, Mochloulis G, Sid VS. A Cook airway exchange catheter in the management of intraoperative tracheal injury. Anaesthesia and Intensive Care 1996;24:617.

1237. Hung OR. Airway adjuncts and alternative techniques of endotracheal intubation. Can J Anaesth 1995;42:R31–R34.

1238. Manos SJ. Jaffe RA, Brock–Utne JG. An alternative to the gum elastic bougie and/or the jet stylet. Anesth Analg 1994;79:1017.

1239. Rosewarne FA. Teflon bougies to assist difficult intubations. Anaesthesia and Intensive Care 1993;21: 722–723.

1240. Coveler LA. More on management of the difficult airway. Anesthesiology 1987;67:154.

1241. Gormley MJ, Lee DS. Make a difficult intubation simple. Anesthesiology 1988;68:811–812.

1242. Suhasini T, Murthy NVVS, Rao SM. Nasogastric tube as a tracheal tube introducer. Anaesthesia 1995;50:270.

1243. Steinberg MJ, Chmiel RA. Use of a nasogastric tube as a guide for endotracheal reintubation. J Oral Maxillofac Surg 1989;47:1232–1233.

1244. Scott CJ. An alternative to the gum elastic bougie in infants. Anaesthesia 1997;52:185.

1245. Upton TE. A simple endotracheal tube guide. Anesth Analg 1994;79:1215.

1246. McCarroll SM, Lamont BJ, Buckland MR, Yates APB. The gum-elastic bougie: old but still useful. Anesthesiology 1988;68:643–644.

1247. Cossham PS. Nasotracheal tube placement over a bougie. Anaesthesia 1997;52:184–185.

1248. Kidd JF, Dyson A, Latto IP. Successful difficult intubation. Use of the gum elastic bougie. Anaesthesia 1988;43:437–438.

1249. Spencer RF, Rathmell JP, Viscomi CM. A new method for difficult endotracheal intubation: the use of a jet stylet introducer and capnography. Anesth Analg 1995;81:1079–1083.

1250. Takata M, Benumof JL, Ozaki GT. Confirmation of endotracheal intubation over a jet stylet: In vitro studies. Anesth Analg 1995;80:800–805.

1251. Haridas RP, Arsiradam NM. Failure of the Augustine stylet to detect tracheal intubation. Anesthesiology 1995;83:228–229.

1252. Boys JE. Failed intubation in obstetric anesthesia. Br J Anaesth 1983;55:187–188.

1253. Cossham PS. Difficult intubation. Br J Anaesth 1985;57:239.

1254. Dogra S, Falconer R, Latto IP. Successful difficult intubation. Tracheal tube placement over a gum-elastic bougie. Anaesthesia 1990;45:774–776.

1255. Schwartz D, Johnson C, Roberts J. A maneuver to facilitate flexible fiberoptic intubation. Anesthesiology 1989;71:470–471.

1256. Freund PR, Rooke A, Schwid H. Retrograde intubation with a modified Eschmann stylet. Anesth Analg 1988;67:605–606.

1257. Montgomery G, Dueringer J, Johnson C. Nasal endotracheal tube change with an intubating stylette after fiberoptic intubation. Anesth Analg 1991;72: 713.

1258. Millen JE, Glauser FL. A rapid simple technic for changing endotracheal tubes. Anesth Analg 1978; 57:735–736.

1259. Novella J. Intraoperative nasotracheal to orotracheal tube change in a patient with Klippel-Feil syndrome. Anaesthesia and Intensive Care 1995;23: 402–403.

1260. Seitz PA, Gravenstein N. Endobronchial rupture from endotracheal reintubation with an endotracheal tube guide. J Clin Anaesth 1989;1:214–217.

1261. Hambly PR, Field JM. An unusual case for reintubation. Anaesthesia 1995;50:568.

1262. Smith BL. Haemopneumothorax following bougie-assisted tracheal intubation. Anaesthesia 1994;49: 91.

1263. deLima LGR, Bishop MJ. Lung laceration after tracheal extubation over a plastic tube changer. Anesth Analg 1991;73:350–351.

1264. Letheren MJR. Sterilisation of gum elastic bougies. Anaesthesia 1994;49:921.

1265. Jerwood DC, Mortiboy D. Disinfection of gum elastic bougies. Anaesthesia 1995;50:376.

1266. Andrews BW, Targ AG. Fragmentation of tube exchanger. Anesth Analg 1995;80:638–639.

1267. Agosti L. Modification of Magill's intubating forceps. Anaesthesia 1976;31:574.

1268. Aun NC, Jawan B, Lee JH. A modification of Magill's forceps. Anesthesiology 1988;68:649.

1269. Burtles R. A new design of intubation forceps. Br J Anaesth 1987;59:1475–1477.

1270. Klaustermeyer WB. An oropharyngeal loop to guide nasotracheal intubation. American Review of Respiratory Disease 1970;102:978.

1271. Liberman H. A new intubating forceps. Anaesthesia and Intensive Care 1978;6:162–163.

1272. Pelimon A, Simunovic Z. Modified Magill forceps for difficult tracheal intubation. Anaesthesia 1987;42:83.

1273. Rees DF. A modification of Magill's forceps. Anaesthesia 1976;31:302–303.

1274. Vonwiller JB, Liberman H, Maver E. Modified Magill forceps for difficult tracheal intubation. Anaesthesia 1987;42:777.

1275. Zuck D. Magill intubating forceps. Br J Anaesth 1982;54:373.

1276. Vas L. Nasal packing forceps as a part of anaesthesia armamentarium. Anaesthesia 1996;51:514.

1277. Munson ES, Cullen SC. Endotracheal intubation in a patient with ankylosing spondylitis of the cervical spine. Anesthesiology 1965;26:365.

1278. Singh A. Blind nasal intubation. Anaesthesia 1966;21:400–402.

1279. Chester MH. Tracheal tube guide to facilitate nasotracheal intubation. Anesthesiology 1984;60:522–523.

1280. Berman AJ. Device for nasotracheal intubation. Anesthesiology 1962.23:130–131.

QUESTIONS

1. The best way to detect an esophageal intubation is
   A. Seeing the tube pass through the vocal cords
   B. Observing chest wall movement during inspiration and exhalation
   C. Hearing breath sounds during controlled ventilation
   D. Monitoring carbon dioxide in exhaled gases
   E. Drop in oxygen saturation as measured by pulse oximeter

Each question below contains four suggested answers of which one or more is correct.
Choose the answer:
A if 1, 2, and 3 are correct
B if 1 and 3 are correct
C if 2 and 4 are correct
D if 4 is correct
E if 1, 2, 3, and 4 are correct

2. Factors helping to determine the resistance to breathing resulting from use of a tracheal tube include
   1. Tube length
   2. Internal diameter
   3. Tube configuration
   4. Gas viscosity

3. Which statements about dead space are accurate?
   1. The dead space of the tube plus connector is greater than natural dead space in adults
   2. Using a shorter tracheal tube will decrease dead space
   3. Mechanical ventilation can overcome the effects of increased dead space
   4. Pediatric tubes and connectors can increase dead space above normal

4. Materials commonly used in tracheal tubes today include
   1. Polyvinyl chloride
   2. Rubber
   3. Silicone
   4. Polyethylene

5. Concerning the Murphy eye
   1. Its area is less than 80% of the cross-sectional area of the tube lumen
   2. Fiberoptic scopes may be trapped in it
   3. It may mask a right mainstem bronchial intubation
   4. Secretions may tend to accumulate there

6. Advantages of a spiral embedded tracheal tube include
   1. Ease of insertion over a fiberscope
   2. Resistance to kinking
   3. Flexible enough to be placed in tracheostomies
   4. Unlikely to be the cause of obstruction

7. With respect to tracheal tube size
   1. Pediatric tubes are sized by the outside diameter
   2. Tubes larger than size six must have the outside diameter marked on them
   3. The French scale is required to be marked on the tube
   4. Size is often displayed on the pilot balloon

8. With tracheal tube cuffs
   1. Cuff pressure should be kept between 25 and 34 cm H_2O
   2. Measuring the intracuff pressure in high-pressure cuffs gives an indication of the pressure applied to the tracheal wall
   3. Nitrous oxide can cause the cuff pressure to increase
   4. Intracuff pressure in low pressure cuffs does not vary during controlled ventilation

9. Advantages of the foam cuff tube include
   1. Measuring intracuff pressure is not necessary
   2. Even large cuffs do not present excessive pressure on the tracheal wall
   3. Diffusion of anesthetic agents will not affect cuff pressure

4. A seal sufficient to prevent aspiration will be achieved regardless of the relative size of the tube and trachea

10. Features of the Lanz pressure-regulating valve include
    1. It gives an indication of cuff inflation
    2. It has an external reservoir for cuff air
    3. It limits the pressure in the cuff
    4. Intracuff pressure is maintained at 26 to 33 torr

11. Products approved for use as a laser-resistant wrap for laser tracheal tubes include
    1. Copper foil
    2. Aluminum tape
    3. Aluminum foil
    4. Sponge and adhesive backed corrugated silver foil

12. Disadvantages of wrapping tracheal tubes include
    1. The outer diameter of the tube is increased
    2. A rough surface may be created
    3. A reflected beam could damage other tissues
    4. The airway could become obstructed

13. Problems associated with a tracheal tube cuff that is too large include
    1. Pressure on the tracheal wall will be increased
    2. Trauma to the vocal cords is more likely
    3. Intracuff pressure will be increased
    4. Aspiration is more likely to occur

14. In determining proper inflation of a low-pressure, high-volume cuff
    1. The volume of air just needed to abolish the air leak may not be enough to prevent aspiration
    2. The feel of the inflation balloon is a good indication of the cuff pressure
    3. Measurement of cuff pressure is needed to determine proper inflation
    4. Cuff pressure needs to be checked during the exhalation phase of ventilation

15. Possible complications of nasotracheal intubation include:
    A. Removal of segments of turbinates
    B. Mediastinitis
    C. Perforation of the nasal septum
    D. Perforation into the retropharyngeal space

16. Ways to minimize trauma when a nasal intubation is performed include
    A. Avoiding lubricants
    B. Warming the tracheal tube
    C. Vasodilating the nasal mucosa
    D. Using smaller tubes than would be used for oral intubation

17. If there is a leak around the tracheal tube that recurs in spite of added air
    1. The tube may be sliding in and out of a bronchus
    2. The cuff may be above the cords
    3. Gas may be diffusing out of the cuff
    4. There may be a leak in the cuff

18. Factors that tend to promote bronchial intubation include
    1. Trendelenburg position
    2. Neck flexion
    3. Placement of upper abdominal packs
    4. Use of RAE tubes

19. Methods unreliable in determining the presence of a bronchial intubation include
    1. Auscultation of the lungs
    2. Pulse oximetry
    3. Fiberscopic visualization through the tube
    4. End-tidal carbon dioxide monitoring

20. Ways to handle a cuff leak include
    1. Reintubation
    2. Packing the pharynx
    3. Attaching a mechanism for continuous air infusion to the cuff inflation system
    4. Do nothing

21. Precautions to minimize the risk of a tracheal tube fire from a laser include
    1. Filling the cuff with saline
    2. Minimizing the laser power density and duration

3. Using a laser-resistant tube
4. Using low oxygen concentrations in the inspired gas

22. Ways of preventing tracheal tube obstruction include
    1. Checking the cuff for even inflation
    2. Not withdrawing the tube with the cuff inflated
    3. Using an oral airway or bite block
    4. Putting traction on the tracheal tube

23. Factors increasing the incidence of aspiration of gastric contents include
    1. Head-up position
    2. Controlled ventilation
    3. Accumulation of fluid above the cuff
    4. High-pressure cuffs

24. Factors that increase the likelihood of accidental extubation include
    1. Secretions, skin oil, and prep solutions
    2. Use of antidisconnect devices
    3. Placement of a nasogastric tube
    4. Placement of tube at the carina

25. Possible causes of difficult extubation include
    1. Obstruction of the inflating mechanism
    2. Pulling the pilot balloon and inflation device from the inflating mechanism
    3. Surgical transfixion
    4. Swelling in the airway

26. Postoperative sore throat
    1. Is more common in males than females
    2. Is present in 10% to 22% of nonintubated patients
    3. Is related to both duration of anesthesia and age of the patient
    4. Is associated with use of larger tubes

27. Concerning hoarseness following intubation
    1. The incidence is decreased with the use of low pressure cuffs
    2. Lubrication of the tube with Xylocaine jelly does not decrease the incidence
    3. Smaller tubes are associated with a decreased incidence
    4. The incidence is not increased if the intubation was traumatic

28. Laryngeal edema
    1. May be caused by preexisting inflammation, bacterial contamination, or chemicals
    2. May be caused by inadequate muscle relaxation or too large a tube
    3. May be caused by an allergic reaction to the tube or lubricants
    4. Can occur anytime in the first 48 hours after extubation

29. Granulomas of the vocal cords
    1. Are found most commonly in males
    2. Are associated with head and neck surgery
    3. Most often occur on the anterior portion of the vocal cords
    4. May be symptomless

30. Indications for a double-lumen tube
    1. Patient with hemorrhage
    2. Patients with one-lung surgery
    3. Control of infection from one lung
    4. Patient with a lesion in the trachea

31. When placing a left-sided double-lumen tube
    1. The outermost acceptable position for the bronchial cuff is just below the carina
    2. If the tip of the bronchial segment is pulled out lung deflation will not be possible
    3. The tip of the bronchial lumen should be at the proximal edge of the left upper lobe bronchus
    4. The margin of safety is less than for right-sided tubes

32. Factors influencing the choice of a double-lumen tube include
    1. A left double-lumen tube should be used for right lung surgery
    2. A left double-lumen tube can be used for left pneumonectomy
    3. A right double-lumen tube must be used for left lung surgery if there is rupture of the left mainstem bronchus
    4. Manipulation and retraction during surgery are likely to alter the position of a tube in the contralateral bronchus

33. Which considerations apply to the insertion of the double-lumen bronchial tube?
    1. A stylet needs to be used for all intubations
    2. The tube should be inserted at a 90° angle from where it will eventually rest
    3. The stylet should be removed after passing the cords
    4. If the tube is to be placed in the left mainstem bronchus, the head and neck should be rotated to the right before rotating and advancing the tube

34. Techniques useful in confirming the position of a double-lumen bronchial tube include
    1. Auscultation of the chest with one lumen open to air
    2. Fiberoptic examination
    3. Chest X-Ray
    4. Capnography

35. Possible consequences of bronchial tube malposition include
    1. Unsatisfactory lung deflation
    2. Air trapping
    3. Airway obstruction
    4. Trauma and hemorrhage

36. Possible malpositions of a double-lumen bronchial tube include
    1. Obstruction of an upper lobe bronchus
    2. Bronchial tip above the carina
    3. Bronchial tip inadequately advanced into the bronchus
    4. Insertion into the wrong mainstem bronchus

37. Possible causes of obstruction to ventilation when a double-lumen tube is in use include
    1. Malposition of the tube

2. Foreign body migration into the dependent lung
3. Overinflation of the bronchial cuff
4. Surgical retraction

38. Possible consequences of trauma resulting from double-lumen tubes include
    1. Hemorrhage
    2. Rupture of a mainstem bronchus or the trachea
    3. Mediastinal emphysema
    4. Vocal cord paralysis

39. Uses of the bronchial-blocking devices include
    1. Patient on anticoagulants
    2. Bronchopleural fistula
    3. Pulmonary hemorrhage
    4. Differential lung ventilation

ANSWERS

1. D	21. E
2. A	22. A
3. C	23. B
4. A	24. A
5. E	25. E
6. A	26. C
7. D	27. C
8. B	28. E
9. B	29. C
10. A	30. A
11. D	31. A
12. E	32. A
13. D	33. C
14. B	34. E
15. E	35. A
16. C	36. E
17. C	37. E
18. E	38. A
19. C	39. A
20. E	

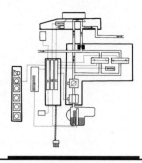

SECTION
IV

MONITORING DEVICES

CHAPTER 18

Gas Monitoring

I. **Definitions**
II. **Comparison of Nondiverting and Diverting Monitors**
  A. Nondiverting (Mainstream)
    1. Advantages
    2. Disadvantages
  B. Diverting
    1. Intubated Patients
    2. Face Mask in Use
    3. Laryngeal Mask
    4. Unintubated Patient Breathing Spontaneously
    5. Jet Ventilation
    6. Advantages
    7. Disadvantages
III. **Technology**
  A. Mass Spectrometry
    1. Components
      a. Sampling Tube
      b. Sample Pump
      c. Multiplexer
      d. Vacuum Pump
      e. Sample Inlet System
      f. Ion Source
      g. Analyzer
        (1) Magnetic Sector
        (2) Quadrupole Mass Filter
      h. Processing Circuit
        (1) Spectrum Overlap Eraser
        (2) Automatic Summing circuit
      i. Displays
    2. Shared System versus Stand-Alone Units
      a. Turn-Around Time
      b. Down-Time
      c. Special Installation Required
      d. Difficulties in Monitoring Remote Locations
      e. Decrease in Accuracy
    3. Advantages of Mass Spectrometers
      a. Multigas Capability
      b. Multiple Agent Detection

c. Fast Response Time
d. Convenience
e. Reliability
f. Low Cost
g. Measurement of Nitrogen
    4. Disadvantages
      a. Measurement of Only Preprogrammed Gases
      b. Necessity for Scavenging
      c. Warm-up Time
      d. Space
  B. Raman Light Scattering Gas Analysis
    1. Technology
    2. Advantages
      a. Multiple Gas Capability
      b. Multiple Agent Detection
      c. Fast Response Time
      d. Portability
      e. Fast Startup Time
      f. Convenience
      g. No Need for Scavenging Gases
      h. Accuracy
      i. No Artifacts with Propellants
    3. Disadvantages
      a. Size
      b. Nonanesthetic Gases Added to the Breathing System
      c. Not All Gases Can Be Measured
      d. Cost
      e. Inaccuracy with Fruit-Flavored Oils
      f. Artifacts with Nitric Oxide
  C. Infrared Analysis
    1. Technology
      a. Optical
        (1) Diverting (Sidestream)
        (2) Nondiverting (Mainstream)
      b. Photoacoustic
    2. Advantages
      a. Multigas Capability
      b. Volatile Agent Detection

c. No Need to Scavenge Gases
d. Portability
e. Quick Response Time
f. Short Warm-up Time
g. Convenience
h. Lack of Interference from Nitric Oxide or Argon
3. Disadvantages
  a. Oxygen and Nitrogen Are Not Measured
  b. Interference among Gases
  c. Inaccuracy with Alcohols, Acetone, Methane, and Propellants
  d. Interference from Water Vapor
  e. Slow Response Time
  f. Addition of Air to the Breathing System
  g. Interference from Radio Frequencies.
D. Paramagnetic Analysis
E. Electrochemical Analysis
  1. Technology
    a. Galvanic Cell
    b. Polarographic Electrode
  2. Use
    a. Calibration
    b. Checking the Alarms
    c. Placement in the Breathing System
    d. Setting Alarms Limits
  3. Advantages
    a. Ease of Use
    b. Cost
    c. Automatic Enabling
    d. Compact
    e. No Effect from Argon
  4. Disadvantages
    a. Maintenance
    b. Calibration
    c. User Enabling
    d. Difficulty Using Outside the Breathing System
    e. Inaccuracy
    f. Slow Response Time
F. Piezoelectric Analysis
  1. Technology
  2. Advantages
    a. Accuracy
    b. Fast Response Time
    c. No Need for Scavenging
    d. Short Warm-up Time
    e. Compactness
  3. Disadvantages
    a. Only One Gas Measured
    b. No Agent Detection
    c. Inaccuracy with Water Vapor

G. Chemical Carbon Dioxide Detection
  1. Technology
    a. Hygroscopic
    b. Hydrophobic
  2. Use
  3. Advantages
  4. Disadvantages
H. Refractometry
  1. Technology
  2. Advantages
  3. Disadvantages
IV. Gases
A. Oxygen
  1. Standard Requirements
  2. Technology
  3. Applications of Oxygen Analysis
    a. Detection of Hypoxic or Hyperoxic Mixtures
    b. Detection of Disconnections and Leaks
    c. Detection of Hypoventilation
    d. Other
B. Carbon Dioxide Analysis
  1. Terminology
  2. The Capnometer
    a. Standards Requirements
    b. Technology
    c. Water Vapor Considerations
    d. Atmospheric Pressure Considerations
      (1) Mass Spectrometer
      (2) Sidestream Infrared and Raman Analyzers
      (3) Mainstream Infrared Analyzers
  3. Clinical Significance of Capnometry
    a. Metabolism
    b. Circulation
    c. Respiration
    d. Equipment Function
  4. Correlation between Arterial and End-tidal Carbon Dioxide Levels
    a. Problems with Sampling
    b. Disturbances in the Ventilation: Perfusion Ratio
    c. Capnometer Inaccuracy
    d. Other
  5. Capnography
C. Volatile Anesthetic Agents
  1. Standard Requirements
  2. Measurement Techniques
  3. Usefulness of Anesthetic Agent Monitoring
    a. Vaporizer Function and Contents
    b. Inadvertent Administration
    c. Information on Uptake and Elimination
    d. Teaching Low-Flow Anesthesia

ONE STUDY SHOWED that nearly 60% of critical incidents during anesthesia involve either the patient's respiratory system or the gas delivery system (1). Adverse outcomes associated with respiratory events were the single largest class of injury in the American Society of Anesthesiologists closed claim project (2).

Reliable, affordable, and easy-to-use monitors of respiratory and anesthetic gas concentrations are now available. Some use more than one technology to measure different gases. Some combine gas analysis with other types of monitoring such as pulse oximetry and spirometry (Fig. 18.1).

DEFINITIONS (3–6)

1. Delay time (transit time, response time, transport delay, time delay, lag time) is the time to achieve 10% of a step change in reading at the gas monitor.
2. Response (rise) time is the time required for a rise from 10 to 90% of the change in a gas value with a step change at the sampling site.
3. The total system response time is the sum of the delay and rise times. A fast response time is essential to obtain accurate values and waveforms. Use of an instrument with a long response time may result in underestimation of end-tidal CO_2 during rapid ventilation (7, 8).
4. The sensor (measuring head or chamber) is the part of a respiratory gas monitor that is sensitive to the presence of the gas.
5. A nondiverting (mainstream, direct probe, flow through, in-line, on airway, nonsampling) monitor is one that measures the gas concentration at the sampling site. The sensor is usually connected by a cable to the display module.
6. A diverting (sidestream, withdrawal, sampling, aspirating, sniffer, sampled system) monitor is one that transports a portion of the gas being measured from the sampling site through a sampling tube to the sensor, which is remote from the sampling site.
7. The sampling (sensing) site is the location from which respiratory gases are diverted for measurement in a diverting monitor or the location of the sensor in a nondiverting monitor.
8. The sampling tube (inlet line, sample gas transport tube, sample capillary tube, sampling catheter or tube, transport tube, aspirating tube, sample line) is the conduit for transfer of gases from the sampling site to the sensor in a diverting gas monitor.
9. An alarm is a warning signal that is activated when the concentration(s) of the gas(es) being monitored reaches or exceeds the alarm limit. Alarms for gas monitors fall into three categories: (a) high priority, which requires immediate operator response; (b) medium priority, which requires prompt operator response; (c) low priority, which requires operator awareness.
10. An alarm set point is the setting of the adjustment control or display value that indicates the reading at or beyond which the alarm is intended to be activated.
11. An alarm system monitor consists of those parts that establish the alarm set point(s) and activate an alarm when the reading is less than or equal to the low alarm set point or is equal to or greater than the high alarm set point.
12. Useful life is the period of time during which the performance of a monitor or any of its components meets the requirements of the applicable standard.
13. Warmup time is the time necessary for the monitor to meet the accuracy specified by the manufacturer.
14. Accuracy is the ability of an instrument to

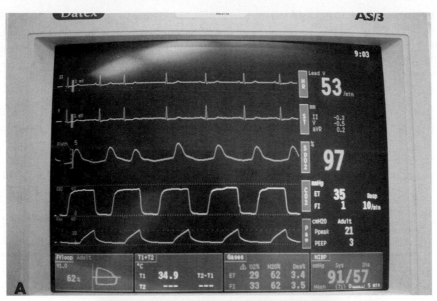

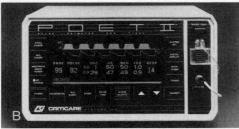

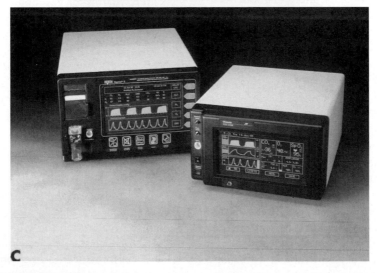

FIGURE **18.1.** Sidestream monitors. Note the water traps on **B** and **C**. (**A,** Courtesy of Datex; **B,** Courtesy of Criticare Systems, Inc.; **C,** Courtesy of Ohmeda, a division of BOC, Inc.)

indicate the actual concentration of the gas it is measuring.

15. Resolution is the ability of an instrument to distinguish between two measured values that are different.
16. Level is the concentration of a gas in a gaseous mixture. It may be expressed either as volumes percent or partial pressure.
17. The partial pressure of a gas is the pressure that that gas would exert in a gas mixture if it alone occupied the volume of the mixture at the same temperature.
18. The percent (%, V/V, volumes percent, vol %) of a gas is the level of that gas in a mixture, expressed as a percentage volume fraction.

COMPARISON OF NONDIVERTING AND DIVERTING MONITORS (9–11)
Nondiverting (Mainstream) (12)

A nondiverting or mainstream gas monitor is one which measures the gas directly in the breathing system. The sensor is connected to the monitor by a cable. Nondiverting monitors in common use measure oxygen (O_2) and carbon dioxide (CO_2).

In a nondiverting CO_2 monitor, the patient's respiratory gas stream passes through a wide-bore chamber (cuvette) with two windows. The cuvette (Fig. 18.2) is placed between the breathing system and the mask or tracheal tube, directly in the path of the patient's exhaled gases (Fig. 18.3A). The sensor, which houses both the light source and detector, fits over the cuvette (Figs. 18.2 and 18.3). The windows of the cuvette are usually made from sapphire, which is transparent to infrared (IR) light. IR light shines through the window on one side of the adaptor, and the sensor receives the light on the opposite side. To ensure that water vapor does not condense on the windows and obstruct the optical path, the sensor contains a heater that warms the adaptor to slightly above body temperature. Condensed water, secretions, or blood on the windows of the cuvette will interfere with light transmission. In one reported case, this caused a very high end-tidal CO_2 reading. Calibration is performed using sealed reference gas cells (Fig. 18.4).

This adaptor for the nondiverting CO_2 sensor adds from 5 to 17 ml for adult-size adapters and 0.6 to 2 ml for pediatric adapters (13, 14). However, studies show that end-tidal CO_2 values obtained using a mainstream IR analyzer with a pediatric adapter in healthy neonates and infants are close to arterial values (13).

The sensor may become dislodged from the

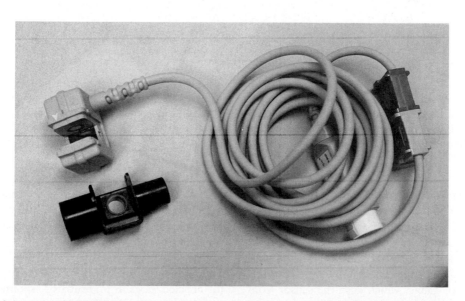

FIGURE 18.2.   Mainstream IR CO_2 analyzer. At lower left is the cuvette, which is placed between the breathing system and the patient. Above this is the sensor which houses the light source and detector.

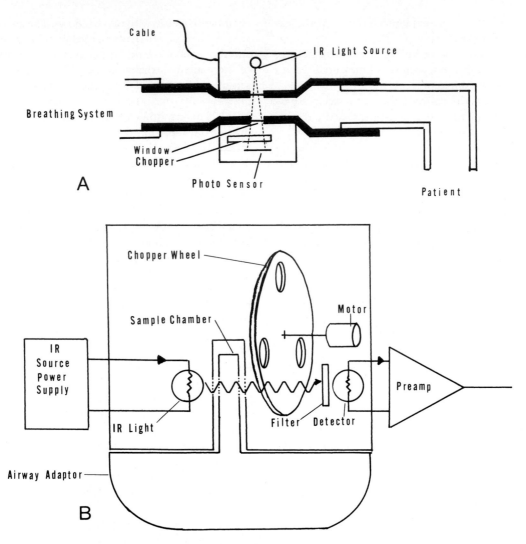

FIGURE 18.3. Mainstream infrared analyzer. **A,** side view. The light source and detector are housed in the sensor which fits over the cuvette. The infrared (IR) light shines through the windows of the cuvette and is detected by the photosensor. **B,** cross-sectional view. Gases pass through the airway adapter (cuvette). The infrared light that is transmitted through the windows is filtered and then detected by the photodetector in the sensor.

cuvette. If it is completely dislodged, no waveform will be seen. If it is slightly dislodged (Fig. 18.5), the reading may be incorrect although the waveform appears normal (15–17).

Thermal skin burns have been reported with use of a mainstream analyzer despite use of multiple layers of gauze, which kept the sensor from direct contact with the skin (18). To prevent this, it may be necessary to interpose a piece of alumi-

num foil between two pieces of soft material to reflect the radiant energy. Prolonged contact of the sensor assembly with the patient could cause pressure injury.

This type of monitor can be adapted to act as a diverting monitor so that it can be used to monitor exhaled gases in unintubated, spontaneously breathing patients (19, 20) or to find leaks in CO_2 insufflation equipment (21). Main-

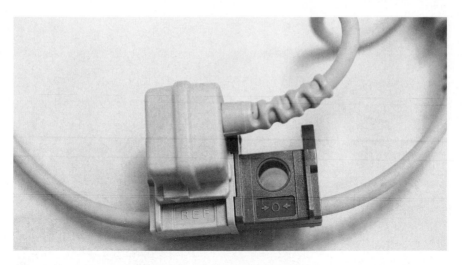

FIGURE 18.4. Calibration cells for mainstream infrared CO_2 analyzer. For convenience they are attached to the cable going to the sensor.

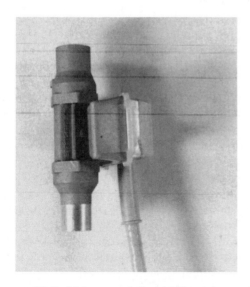

FIGURE 18.5. Mainstream infrared CO_2 analyzer with the sensor not completely covering the windows of the cuvette. This can result in falsely low CO_2 readings.

stream monitors with diverting capability are available (Fig. 18.6)

Advantages

1. Mainstream monitors have fast response times because there is no delay time. The gas waveform generated is of higher fidelity than one generated by a diverting monitor.

2. Because no gas is removed from the breathing system, it is not necessary to scavenge these devices or to increase the fresh gas flow to compensate for gas removed from the breathing system.
3. Water and secretions are seldom a problem with this type of analyzer, although secretions on the windows of the cuvette can cause erroneous readings.
4. Contamination of the sample by fresh gas flow is less likely than with a diverting monitor.
5. A standard gas is not required for calibration.
6. These monitors use fewer disposable items than diverting ones.

Disadvantages

1. To obtain accurate end-tidal values, the airway adapter and analysis module sensor must be placed near the patient. The sensor will add weight and may cause traction on the tracheal tube.
2. Use of an adapter between the patient and the breathing system will increase dead space.
3. Leaks, disconnections, and circuit obstructions can occur (22–25).
4. Condensed water, secretions, or blood on the windows of the cuvette will interfere with light transmission.

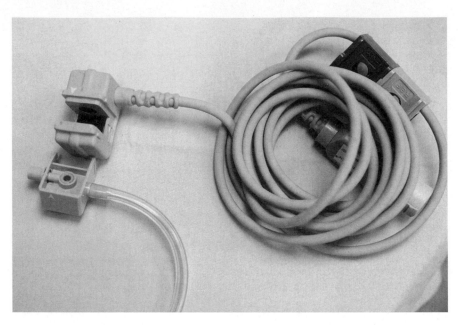

FIGURE **18.6.** Mainstream infrared CO_2 analyzer used as a diverting monitor. Gas is drawn through the cuvette by a pump.

5. The sensor may become dislodged from the cuvette. If it is completely dislodged, no waveform will be seen. If it is slightly dislodged (Fig. 18.5), the reading may be incorrect although the waveform appears normal (15–17).

6. The sensor is exposed to damage and may be expensive to repair or replace. Newer units are more resistant to mechanical trauma (11).

7. Warmup time is usually longer than with a diverting monitor.

8. At present, mainstream monitors can measure only O_2 and CO_2. They do not have the capability of measuring nitrogen, nitrous oxide, or anesthetic agents. The user must indicate the presence of nitrous oxide so a correction for this can be made.

9. A mainstream monitor is difficult to use with unintubated, spontaneously breathing patients.

10. The adapter must be cleaned and disinfected between uses. There is potential for cross-contamination between patients if this is not done properly.

11. Thermal skin burns have been reported with use of a mainstream analyzer despite use of multiple layers of gauze, which kept the sensor from direct contact with the skin (18). To prevent this, it may be necessary to interpose a piece of aluminum foil between two pieces of soft material to reflect the radiant energy. Prolonged contact of the sensor assembly with the patient could cause pressure injury.

12. Modules placed in the airway are subject to interference by condensed water, secretions and blood.

Diverting

In a diverting monitor the sensor is located in the main unit and a pump aspirates gas from the sampling site through a sampling tubing. Keeping the sampling tube as short as possible will decrease the delay time and result in more satisfactory waveforms.

To avoid contamination of the monitor by water or particulate matter, manufacturers have used traps (Figs. 18.1 and 18.7) (which must be emptied periodically), filters, hydrophobic membranes (which must be changed periodically), and

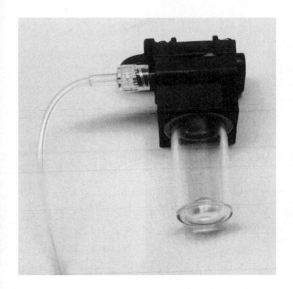

FIGURE **18.7.** Water trap. This should be emptied periodically to prevent water from entering the monitor.

nafion tubing (which allows water to diffuse though its walls) (26, 27).

Accuracy decreases with increasing respiratory rate, with changes in the I:E from 1:1 and with longer sampling lines (28, 29). Most diverting capnometers are accurate at the respiratory rates normally encountered (20 to 40 breaths per minute). Above 40 breaths per minute there is a slight decay in end-tidal accuracy and elevation of the capnographic baseline (30). When the I:E ratio is greater than 1:1, errors appear first in the end-tidal or expiratory values, and when it is less than 1:1, errors appear first in the inspiratory data. Other factors that may affect accuracy are the sampling flow rate and the composition of the sampling tube. On some monitors the flow rate can be varied.

The flow rate should be proportional to the size of each patient. However, it has been suggested that a sampling flow rate less than 150 ml/ min not be used because delay time and rise time are inversely proportional to the flow rate and a low sampling flow may result in an elevated baseline, erroneously low peak readings and absence of an end-tidal plateau (Fig 18.41), especially when the respiratory rate is high and tidal volume is small (31). A high flow rate will decrease the delay and rise times, but may cause fresh gas to

be entrained into the sample line. This will result in incorrect end-tidal readings and a capnogram with a decrease in CO_2 at the end of the expiratory plateau (Fig. 18.42) (32). These analyzers are usually zeroed using room air or automatically using electronics and calibrated against a gas of known composition.

The sampling site will vary, depending on the anesthetic technique being used.

Intubated Patients

In intubated patients the sensing site can be an adapter placed between components or a port in a component (Fig. 18.8). To measure both inspired and exhaled gases, the site must be between the patient and the breathing system. Many disposable breathing systems and heat and moisture exchangers have built-in sample ports. The sampling site should be away from the fresh gas port. When a Mapleson breathing system is used, continuous inflow of fresh gas close to the sampling site can cause erroneous readings and an abnormal waveform (Fig. 18.42).

Tracheal tubes that incorporate a sampling lumen that extends to the middle or distal end of the tube are available. Some are described in Chapter 17, "Tracheal Tubes." Tracheal tube connectors with a hole for inserting a sampling tube are available or can be created (33, 34). Various devices have been used for sampling (35–39). These may result in measurements that more closely approximate alveolar values, especially in small patients with breathing systems in which the fresh gas flow can mix with exhaled gases (40–45). However, they may be associated with increased airway resistance and the sampling tube may become obstructed by water or secretions.

Alternately, a hole that will accept a small tubing can be drilled into a component such as the elbow adaptor or tracheal tube connector (46, 47).

Face Mask in Use

A face mask has a relatively large dead space relative to tidal volume, making it difficult to obtain accurate end-tidal values if the sampling site is between the mask and breathing system. In this case, a sampling catheter can be attached to the upper lip or placed in the patient's nares or the

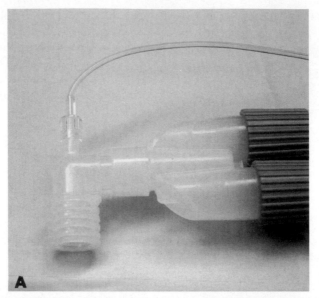

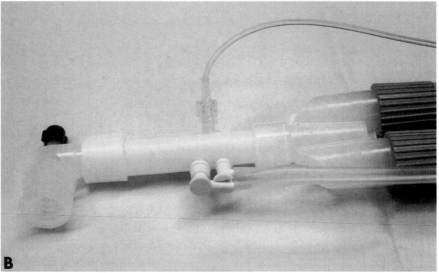

FIGURE 18.8. Ports for gas sampling in breathing system components.

lumen of an oral or nasopharyngeal airway under the mask (48, 49). Another method is to insert the sampling tube through the right-angle connector that attaches to the mask (50, 51).

Laryngeal Mask

With a laryngeal mask, a sampling tube can be inserted through the elbow connector (52, 53). The preferred sampling site is the distal end of the shaft (54) but in most patients sampling at the proximal connector will result in satisfactory readings (55–57).

Unintubated Patient Breathing Spontaneously

Plastic O_2 masks may be fitted with a sampling port (58). Alternatively, the sampling tube may be connected to the mask outlet (59), inserted through a vent hole (60–64) or slipped under the mask and attached near the nostrils (65).

Nasal cannulae may be fitted with a connection for the sampling tubing (62, 66–81). O_2 should not be delivered through the same port (82). They are available in several configurations (Fig. 18.9). The $PetCO_2$ measured by the two-prong nasal cannula is reported to provide a better estimate of $PaCO_2$ than that obtained by the four-prong nasal cannula (83).

A sampling catheter can be advanced into the nasopharynx (84, 85) or hypopharynx (86). A catheter can be left in the trachea after extubation and CO_2 monitored through it (87).

The end can be placed in front of or inside the patient's nostril (20, 88) or a nasopharyngeal airway (49). If the patient is a mouth breather, it can be placed in front of the mouth or in the posterior nasopharynx.

Optimal placement should be determined by the CO_2 waveform. Most of these devices are well tolerated by patients and do not interfere with administration of supplemental O_2. Mucosal irritation, blocking of the catheter, and mechanical interference by the surgeon are sometimes problems.

Jet Ventilation

For capnography during jet ventilation for laryngoscopy, a modified injector incorporating a sampling lumen may be used (89–91). However the end-tidal CO_2 values are significantly lower than arterial values (90).

Advantages

1. Sampling from patients who are not intubated is relatively easy.
2. Warmup is usually faster than with nondiverting devices.
3. Calibration and zeroing are usually automatic. Occasional calibration to a standard is necessary but is usually easily accomplished.
4. The patient interface is lightweight and inexpensive.
5. The added dead space is minimal.
6. The potential for cross-contamination between patients is low if the adapter and sample tube are changed between patients.
7. With some technologies several gases can be measured simultaneously. This allows auto-

matic correction for nitrous oxide and/or oxygen.
8. The sampling port can be used to administer bronchodilators (see Chapter 6, "Breathing Systems II: General Considerations") (92).
9. A diverting capnometer can be used to localize the site of leaks in CO_2 insufflation equipment (21), diagnose a tracheoesophageal or bronchoesophageal fistula (93, 94), or assist in placement of a feeding tube (95).
10. These devices can be used when the monitor must be remote from the patient (e.g., magnetic resonance imaging) (96–98).

Disadvantages (99)

1. Problems with the catheter sampling system can occur. Particulate matter, blood, secretions, or water can cause obstruction of the tubing (100–102). Some water traps may be overwhelmed so that water enters the measurement system (3). Leaks in the sampling system, obstruction of the sampling tube by kinking or external pressure, or failure of the aspirator pump can occur.
2. The gases aspirated must be either routed to the scavenging system (Fig. 12.3) or returned to the breathing system. If scavenging is employed, the fresh gas flow may need to be increased to compensate for the gas removed or negative pressure will be created in the breathing system (103).
3. In some diverting monitors room air or argon is added to the gas exiting the monitor. If this is returned to the breathing system this will create problems during closed circuit anesthesia.
4. Some delay time is inevitable.
5. A supply of calibration gas needs to be kept.
6. A number of disposable items (adapters and catheters) must be used.
7. When used with a Mapleson system, there may be deformation of the waveform and erroneously low CO_2 readings due to dilution by fresh gas.

TECHNOLOGY
Mass Spectrometry (104, 105)

The mass spectrometer can be used to measure inspired and end-tidal concentrations of O_2, ni-

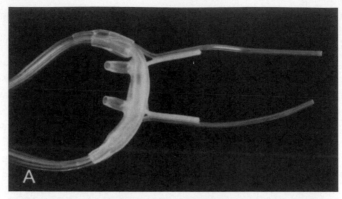

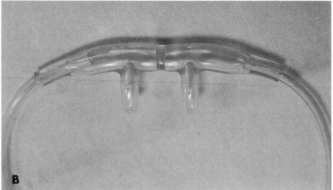

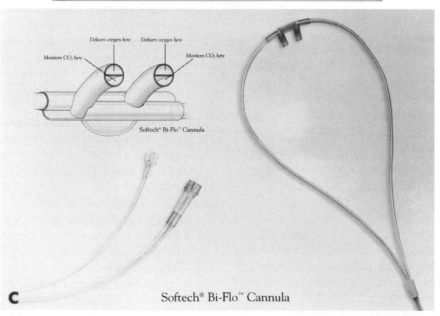

FIGURE **18.9.**   Devices for simultaneous administration of O₂ and gas sampling. **A,** This device is designed for patients who are predominantly mouth breathers. The longer oral sampling prongs can be cut and shaped to suit individual patients. (Courtesy of Bio-chem International, Inc.) **B,** One prong is used for administration of oxygen and one for gas sampling. There is a septum between the two prongs. **C,** With this device, the two prongs are divided so that oxygen is delivered and gas sampled through different prongs.

trogen, CO_2, nitrous oxide, and the volatile anesthetic agents. Argon and/or helium can be measured on some units.

The mass spectrometer spreads gases and vapors of differing molecular weights into a spectrum, according to their mass:charge ratios. By analyzing the spectrum, the composition and relative abundance of each component of a sample can be determined. The gas sample cannot be returned to the breathing system.

The mass spectrometer differs from most other measuring devices in that it measures concentrations in volumes percent, not partial pressure. This can cause inaccurate readings if a gas that the mass spectrometer cannot measure is present.

These units are calibrated with cylinders containing mixtures of the gases to be analyzed and room air.

Two basic types are available: shared (multiplexed) and dedicated (stand alone, single room, mini-mass spectrometer). With a shared system the mass spectrometer is located centrally, usually outside of the anesthetizing sites, but within the operating room suite. There are multiple stations from which gases are sampled and to which data are returned (Fig. 18.10). Tubings pass from each station through specially installed ductwork to a valve box (multiplexer) at the inlet of the mass spectrometer. The valve box sequentially directs the sample flows to the mass spectrometer, so that one station at a time is sampled. Information derived centrally is relayed to the individual stations and displayed. It may also be displayed centrally. Such an arrangement permits one central analyzer to serve up to 31 sampling locations on a time-shared basis.

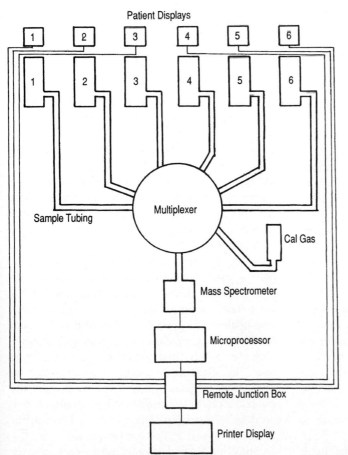

FIGURE 18.10. Shared mass spectrometer. The mass spectrometer is locally centrally. Long sample tubings pass from each sampling location through specially installed ductwork to the multiplexer, which sequentially directs sample flows to the mass spectrometer. Information derived centrally is relayed to the individual stations and displayed. The central display and printer are optional.

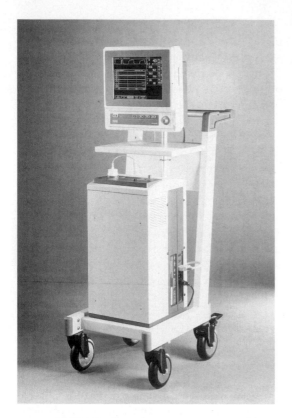

FIGURE **18.11.** Dedicated mass spectrometer. (Courtesy of Marquette Electronics.)

A dedicated mass spectrometer (Fig. 18.11). is used in only one location. It consists of two parts: the analyzer and the display/control unit, which are connected by a cable. A short tubing carries the gas sample from the sampling site to the analyzer. It uses a lower sampling flow rate than a shared mass spectrometer.

Components
Sampling Tube (99)

With a dedicated mass spectrometer, only a single short sampling tube is required. With a shared system, a tubing transports gas from the sampling site to a plate located in the wall or ceiling. This plate has two connections: one accepts the sampling tube and the other is an electrical connection that transmits information to and from a display unit. From the plate a longer catheter extends to the central mass spectrometer.

The tubing must be made of a material that is resistant to the gases being sampled and will not allow them to diffuse out or outside air to be drawn in. Of the various materials tried, nylon has proved most satisfactory (106, 107). Nafion, which is a braided nylon tubing that is permeable to water vapor and will allow most water to diffuse through its walls to atmosphere, is commonly used.

These lines should be as short as possible to keep the delay time to a minimum. Long sampling lines will cause smeared inspired and end-tidal peaks with erroneous readings, especially at high respiratory rates and high I:E ratios (28). Signal distortion can be lessened by increasing the sampling flow, but there is a limit to the amount of improvement that can be achieved (108).

Particulate matter and fluids may cause distorted waveforms, inaccurate measurements, and damage to the monitor. For these reasons a filter is commonly used. Despite this, fluid may be aspirated into the tube, causing malfunction (109).

Sample Pump

A pump is needed to withdraw the gas from the sampling site at flow rates up to 240 ml/min for shared units and 30 ml/min for dedicated units. A pressure drop from approximately 760 torr at the inlet to less than 50 torr at the mass spectrometer inlet is common (104). The gas profiles from several breaths can be stored in the sampling line without significant loss of information by continuously pulling gas through the lines going to stations not being monitored but at a slower rate than the mass spectrometer sampling rate. When the line is connected to the mass spectrometer, the flow rate is accelerated.

Multiplexer

A multiplexer (switching mechanism, multiplexing valve) is found in shared mass spectrometers. It serially samples from each station that has the remote monitor turned on for a specified period of time or a certain number of breaths, then sends the gas sample on to the mass spectrometer (Fig. 18.10). It then switches to a new sample line. The sequence of sampling is controlled by the central station computer. With some units, the sequence can be overridden if a particular station requests an immediate (stat) analysis. This will put that station next in line for sampling.

Some mass spectrometers use a rotary valve for

multiplexing. This sequentially directs gas samples to the mass spectrometer. Others use three-way solenoid valves on each sample gas tubing. Gas is continually sampled from all patient lines. The solenoid valves direct gas from one sampling line into the central unit at twice the original sampling rate and gas in the other lines to a scavenging system. This permits analysis of stored line data in less time. However, if the solenoid valve mechanism malfunctions, the entire system will be out of order. If the rotary valve malfunctions, only one station will be affected.

Vacuum Pump

The creation and manipulation of ions must be carried out in a vacuum to avoid interference by outside air and minimize random collisions between the ions and residual gases. The vacuum pump maintains a very low pressure, normally less than 10^{-5} mm Hg, within the ionization chamber. Achievement of a suitable vacuum may take up to 15 minutes.

Sample Inlet System

A small amount of the gas sampled enters the ionization chamber through the sample inlet (molecular leak inlet system, capillary inlet system, molecular leak, molecular inlet leak), a tiny hole, or a porous plug. The pressure falls and the flow changes from viscous to molecular. This means that the pressure and density are so low that the molecules rarely collide with one another and are only affected by collisions with the walls of the container (104).

Ion Source

Electrons are emitted by a heated wire filament, focused magnetically or electrically and directed into the ionization chamber. There they pass across the chamber and are collected by a positively charged plate on the opposite side. Neutral molecules of the sample gas enter the ionization chamber and are bombarded by the electrons. Some molecules are transformed into positively charged ions of the same mass as the molecule from which they were produced. Some molecules are split into fragments, one or more of which are positively charged. The positively charged ions then travel into the ion focal system, a set of electrodes that establishes an electrostatic field. The ions are accelerated, focused into a beam, and projected into the analyzer section.

Analyzer

The analyzer (ion filter) separates ions according to mass. There are several types, based on the method of separation (104). Two have been used for monitoring gases in anesthesia.

Magnetic sector (10, 105–110). The most common type of mass spectrometer is the magnetic sector (deflector) analyzer, so named because it uses a magnet to separate the ions (Fig. 18.12). Within the ionization chamber is a magnetic field at right angles to the ions' direction of travel. When a charged particle moves across a magnetic field, its path is deflected into an arc whose radius of curvature is determined by its mass:charge ratio. The degree of deflection is greater for lighter than for heavier ions, if they have equal charges. Thus a number of separate ion beams will exit the magnetic field.

The ion collectors (cathodes, detectors, detector plates, collector electrodes, ion counters, Faraday cups) are metal plates that receive the ions. These are placed at locations that correspond to the trajectories of the mass:charge ratios of the ion species for which the mass spectrometer has been programmed. The number of ions impacting on each plate during a fixed time interval is detected and an electric current that is proportional to the concentration of the gas in the original sample is produced.

A disadvantage of this type of analyzer is the need to specify the gases being monitored in advance of purchase (111). Most mass spectrometers use seven collectors. More can sometimes be added.

Quadrupole mass filter (110, 112). A quadrupole mass spectrometer works on the principle that a controlled oscillating electric field can prevent all but a narrow range of charged molecules from reaching a target (Fig. 18.13). Four parallel electrically conducting rods are arranged at the corners of a square. Opposite rods are electrically connected together. There is only one collector, which is at the end of the rods.

To the two pairs of rods are applied equal but opposite potentials, each of which has direct current and radio frequency voltage components. Gas molecules enter the unit and are ionized, and the ions are accelerated along the longitudinal axis of the four rods. To reach the collector the ions must

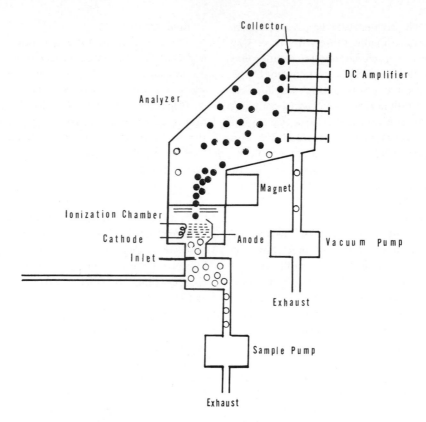

FIGURE 18.12. Magnetic sector mass spectrometer. The *open circles* represent un-ionized molecules; *the closed circles,* ions. A magnetic field acting on the ions does the same thing as a prism does with a light beam. It separates the different components, in this case according to their mass:charge ratios.

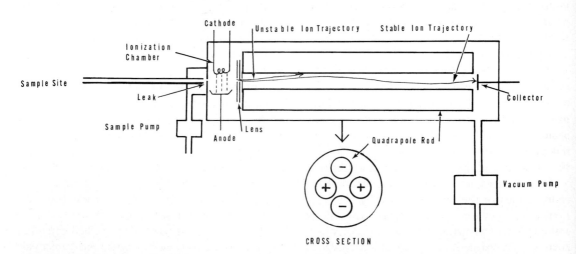

FIGURE 18.13. Quadrupole mass spectrometer. The name of this device comes from the four parallel electrically conducting rods arranged symmetrically. All electrons, except those of a selected mass:charge ratio, strike the sides of the quadrupole and are discharged. The number of hits on the collector for each mass:charge ratio is detected and is proportional to the partial pressure of the selected gas in the sample.

traverse this region without colliding with any of the rods. Radio frequency and direct current voltage generators are applied to the two pairs of rods so that the quadrupole's electrostatic charge changes in steps. For any given radio frequency to direct current voltage level, only ions of a specific mass:charge ratio avoid collision with one of the rods and reach the collector at the distal end of the chamber. All other ions collide with one of the rods and, because of the DC voltage, are discharged. The number of hits on the collector for each ion mass:charge ratio is detected and apportioned to indicate the concentration of the selected gas in the sample. This cycle of filtering out all but one mass:charge ratio and then measuring its abundance is repeated until each component of the mixture has been analyzed.

Compared with the magnetic sector, the quadrupole mass spectrometer is smaller, more lightweight, and has a lower sampling rate (104). This is the analyzer found in stand-alone mass spectrometers. The response time is almost identical. One advantage of a quadrupole system is that it may be adapted to measure new or additional gases by changes in software.

Processing Circuit

The measured currents from the collector(s) are entered into a computer that converts them into numbers representing the fractional components of the different constituents or partial pressures for each gas. Two special mechanisms are used for dealing with the data: a spectrum overlap eraser and an automatic summing circuit.

Spectrum overlap eraser (113, 114). A major problem in the use of mass spectrometry during anesthesia is the overlap in the spectra of several gases. Nitrous oxide and CO_2, which have the same atomic mass, are detected at the same mass:charge ratio. Likewise, isoflurane and enflurane have the same molecular weight.

Spectrum overlap erasing allows evaluation of individual gases or agents when more than one contribute to the signal at a specific mass:charge ratio. When compounds enter the analyzer, fragmentation (cracking), in which a molecule is split into smaller positively charged ions, occurs. This results in the production of a mass spectrogram (cracking pattern) rather than a discrete peak for each gas. Fortunately, gas molecules fragment in

a fixed proportion. One fragment is detected as the sole output of that gas at a particular mass number. The proportion of the parent substance in the original gas mixture as well as the contribution made by the parent substance to the outputs detected at the mass:charge ratios of the other gases present can then be determined.

Automatic summing circuit. Another problem with mass spectrometry is that the amount of charged material arriving at the collectors may vary with time. An automatic summing circuit (automatic stability control, automatic sensitivity control) electronically adds together all the measured concentrations of gases being monitored and adjusts the sensitivity to maintain the sum at 100%. Thus it corrects automatically for alterations in barometric pressure and water vapor and ignores gases for which the mass spectrometer has not been programmed. One problem is that if a gas for which the mass spectrometer is not programmed, e.g., helium, is used the gas will not be detected and the automatic summing circuit will show erroneously high concentrations of the other gases (115).

Algorithms use the maximum and minimum CO_2 levels to identify inspiration and end expiration. Other gases measured at these times are displayed as inspired and end-tidal values.

Displays

Data display is a function of software design and can be tailored to the needs of the user. Most units allow the operator to select the display format and alarm limits (Fig. 18.14). Typically, the screen will display a capnogram and one other waveform, inspired and expired gas concentrations in numerics or bar graphs, trend data, and alarm values. With shared systems, units may emit a beep when a new analysis is displayed.

Shared System versus Stand-Alone Units

The shared system offers advantages in initial and maintenance costs. Unfortunately there are a number of disadvantages.

Turn-Around Time

Shared systems have a small but finite turn-around time. The delay may be unacceptable for detection of sudden changes such as those seen with air embolism or for verifying placement of a

FIGURE **18.14.** Display unit for shared mass spectrometer. Inspired and end-tidal readings for the gases measured are displayed. To the right are trend data, and at the bottom is the CO_2 waveform display. Note the STAT control at the bottom. (Courtesy of Marquette Electronics.)

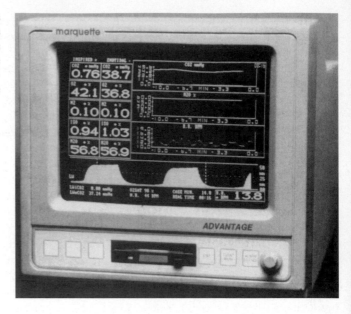

tracheal tube. Some systems can be programmed to sample certain locations more frequently than others to facilitate detection of certain events. Alternately, another type of monitoring than mass spectrometry may be used during such cases.

The frequency of sampling and time from sampling to display of results depends on four factors: (*a*) the distance from the mass spectrometer to the sampling location; (*b*) the number of stations on line at a particular time; (*c*) the number of breaths or time sampled (dwell time); and (*d*) priority settings (99). Priority settings enable the user to obtain a stat analysis (Fig. 18.14). Frequent use of this will delay the updating of information from other locations.

Down Time

If the system goes down, the entire operating room suite may be without gas monitoring. Two shared mass spectrometers can be linked to help solve this problem (116). Because O_2 and CO_2 monitoring are probably of greatest importance, manufacturers of shared systems offer optional continuous IR CO_2 detectors, which are placed in series between the patient sampling tube and the adapter at each sampling location. O_2 monitoring is standard on modern anesthesia machines.

To reduce down time, a spare mass spectrome-

ter may be purchased. If there is more than one mass spectrometer in close proximity, it may be possible to link them to provide continuous monitoring during system failure (116, 117).

Special Installation Required

With a shared system, the central unit requires a separate room, which may need independent air-conditioning. Special ductwork to each anesthetizing location must be installed.

Difficulties in Monitoring Remote Locations

With a shared mass spectrometer, there are limits to how far away from the central unit a sampling station can be located.

Movement of a dedicated unit requires a closedown and a startup time of 6 minutes or more. Special startup and closedown sequences must be followed.

Decrease in Accuracy

There may be a decrease in accuracy when gases are measured at remote locations. This is related to the accumulation of particulate materials in long transport tubes (118). In addition, when the respiratory rate is high as would be the case in pediatric patients, the signal from the patient may become unacceptably distorted during passage down long catheters.

Advantages of Mass Spectrometers

Multigas Capability

It can measure nearly every gas of importance to anesthesia.

Multiple Agent Detection

It can detect mixtures of volatile anesthetic agents (119). A variation of multiple agent detection is the indirect detection of carbon monoxide in the breathing circuit. This is a product of the chemical decomposition of difluoromethyl-ethyl ethers in dry CO_2 absorbents. On the mass spectrometer this will show up as a combination of isoflurane and enflurane if isoflurane or desflurane is being used. Carbon monoxide cannot be directly measured by the mass spectrometer. (120, 121)

Fast Response Time

The response time is fast enough to allow end-tidal measurements, although values may not be accurate at high respiratory frequencies. Mass spectrometer systems are adequate for the respiratory rates typically encountered in an adult population and some pediatric patients, if they are not too distant from the analyzer (28). A stand-alone mass spectrometer can accurately measure expired gas concentrations in subjects requiring tidal volumes as low as 3 to 4 ml and at respiratory rates up to 80 breaths/min (122).

Convenience

Mass spectrometers are easy to use, maintain, and calibrate. With a shared system, minimal space is needed. However, the stand-alone version requires several square feet of floor space.

Reliability

Most mass spectrometer systems function reliably for long periods with little down time.

Low Cost

Despite the large outlay needed to install and maintain a mass spectrometer, multipatient monitoring with a single, centrally located mass spectrometer results in relatively low cost per patient (117). A dedicated mass spectrometer is comparable in cost to the Raman spectrometer but more expensive than most IR monitors.

Measurement of Nitrogen

Since the mass spectrometer can measure nitrogen, it can detect leaks in the aspiration mechanism and increases in nitrogen in the breathing system which could result from an air embolus.

Disadvantages

Measurement of Only Preprogrammed Gases

With a mass spectrometer, the reliability of the readings presupposes that no gases other than those for which it is programmed are present in the gas sample. When an unmeasured gas is introduced into a mass spectrometer, the concentrations of the measured gases will be erroneously high and gases not present may be reported (115, 123–126).

Argon, which is found in increased concentration in gas mixtures generated by O_2 concentrators (see Chapter 3, "O_2 Concentrators") will not be detected correctly unless the mass spectrometer is programmed for it (127).

Carbon monoxide cannot be measured directly by the mass spectrometer but results in a small increase in nitrogen and CO_2 readings (120, 121, 128). When isoflurane or desflurane is broken down by contact with dry CO_2 absorbent, the mass spectrometer may incorrectly indicate enflurane (120, 121).

Mass spectrometers may give readings of multiple agents as a result of calibration error (129).

In mass spectrometers that are programmed for helium analysis, another problem may arise (130). Some spectrometers cannot evacuate the helium quickly from the high-vacuum chamber of the analyzer. After analyzing a gas mixture containing helium, the shared mass spectrometer may switch to the next station before all the helium has been evacuated from the chamber, and the partial pressure readings from the station not using helium will be erroneously low. Use of helium saturates the ion pump in the high-vacuum chamber more quickly, necessitating more frequent replacement of the pump (99).

Some substances, such as those found in propellants used in bronchodilators, may be read erroneously as anesthetic agents or CO_2 (131–134). There may be a decrease or increase in the CO_2 or anesthetic agent readings (135, 136). Fortunately, the effect of propellant gases is transient. If a shared unit is being used, the aerosol should be administered while the spectrometer is sampling other stations. If sampling is continuous, removing the sample port briefly from the circuit during administration of medication will prevent incorrect readings.

Necessity for Scavenging

The gas aspirated must be scavenged. It cannot be returned to the breathing system. The fresh gas flow may need to be increased to compensate for the gas removed. This is less of a problem with dedicated mass spectrometers which use lower sampling flow rates than shared units.

Warm-up Time

The dedicated mass spectrometer requires a fairly long warmup time to evacuate the analyzing chamber.

Space

The dedicated mass spectrometer takes up space in the operating room. A special room is needed for a shared system.

Raman Spectometry (105, 110, 137–141)

Technology

In Raman spectometry (light scattering gas analysis) a laser emits monochromatic light. When this light interacts with a gas molecule that has interatomic molecular bonds, some of its energy is converted into vibrational and rotational modes within the molecule. A fraction of the energy absorbed is reemitted at different wavelengths in a phenomenon called Raman scattering. The magnitude of this shift is characteristic for particular molecules, enabling their identification. This technology can be applied to all gases likely to be present in the respiratory gas mixture, including CO_2, O_2, nitrogen, nitrous oxide, and up to three anesthetic agents (3). These need to be selected in advance. Monoatomic gases such as helium, xenon, and argon do not exhibit Raman scattering and cannot be measured using this technology.

A Raman spectrometer is shown in Figure 18.1C. The gas mixture to be analyzed is drawn continuously through a water separator and particulate filter into the instrument.

The internal construction is shown in Figure 18.15. The measuring cell is a cylinder with a window at each end. The light is generated by a helium-neon laser. Two mirrors increase light intensity within the cell. The illumination is so powerful

that it could combust the anesthetic agents. To prevent this, room air is drawn into the cell close to the windows, creating an air dam across the windows. If the sample gas is returned to the breathing system increased nitrogen concentrations will appear (139).

There are port holes on the side of the sample cell. Each has a filter of narrow optical bandwidth tuned to a specific Raman scatter frequency. Transmitted light is detected by photo diodes. The number of photons at each wavelength is directly proportional to the concentration of the particular gas present. A pressure transducer downstream of the measuring cell monitors flow.

The Raman spectrometer periodically calibrates itself automatically, using an internal argon cylinder and room air. This takes about 8 seconds. It needs to be calibrated periodically with test gases.

Advantages (142)

Multiple Gas Capability

The Raman spectrometer can identify and measure inspired and expired partial pressures for most gases of interest in anesthesia, including CO_2, nitrous oxide, O_2, nitrogen, hydrogen, and the volatile anesthetic agents.

Multiple Agent Detection

Mixtures of volatile agents can be detected.

Fast Response Time

Although the response time is slower than that for mass spectrometry, it is adequate for breath-by-breath end-tidal monitoring in adults (142).

Portability

This monitor can be easily transported to remote locations.

Fast Startup Time

It has a very short startup time. This is especially advantageous if the monitor must be moved. It is recommended that the monitor be kept in a standby mode. If the analyzer must be turned off, the startup time is longer.

Convenience

The Raman spectrometer is easy to use and requires relatively little maintenance. The manufacturer recommends calibration at 30-day intervals. Without these calibrations, volatile agent quantification may drift significantly upward (141).

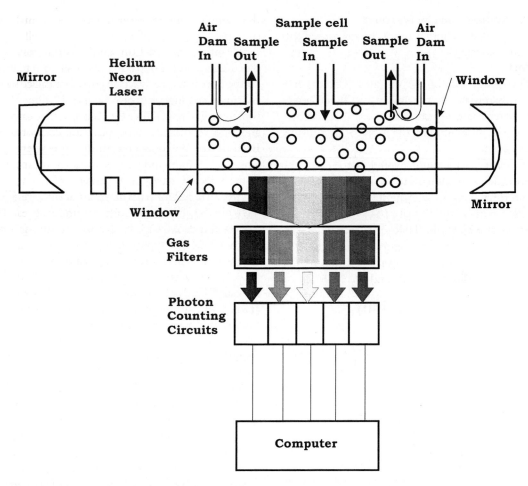

FIGURE 18.15.   Raman light scattering gas analyzer. The gas sample is drawn continuously into the sample cell. Light traversing this cell is scattered. The scattered light is directed through a series of filters that select particular wavelengths corresponding to the gases being analyzed.

No Need for Scavenging Gases

Because the aspirated gases undergo no change during analysis, they can be returned to the breathing system. The gases can also be vented to the scavenging system.

Accuracy

It has a high degree of accuracy (138).

No Artifacts with Propellants

Aerosol propellants that affect the readings of a mass spectrometer do not affect the accuracy of the Raman spectrometer (135). It also gives accurate readings in the presence of unknown or unusual gases such as helium, ethyl or isopropyl alcohol, or ethanol (139).

Disadvantages

Size

Although the later versions are smaller than the first models, the analyzer is still fairly large and heavy compared to IR monitors.

Nonanesthetic Gases Added to the Breathing System

If the sample gas is returned to the breathing system after passing through the sample chamber, air and argon will be added to the breathing system (143). Since more gas is added to the breathing system than has been withdrawn this will pose a problem with closed system anesthesia. This can be overcome by scavenging these gases.

Not All Gases Can be Measured

Argon and helium cannot be measured by Raman scattering.

Cost

The initial cost of the monitor is somewhat higher than with other technologies. If new anesthetic agents are introduced, there is a cost involved in reprogramming the monitor to measure these agents.

Inaccuracy with Fruit-Flavored Oils

Fruit-flavored oils used to scent face masks may be interpreted as an anesthetic ether or a nonspecific agent by the Rascal (144).

Artifacts with Nitric Oxide

Nitric oxide produces spurious nitrogen, nitrous oxide and isoflurane signals, but has no direct effect on those for CO_2 and O_2 (145).

IR Analysis (105, 146–150)

Technology

IR analyzers are based on the fact that gases that have two or more dissimilar atoms in the molecule (nitrous oxide, CO_2, and the halogenated agents) have specific and unique absorption spectra of IR light. Since the amount of light absorbed is proportional to the concentration of the absorbing molecules, the concentration can be determined by comparing the absorbance with that of a known standard. The nonpolar molecules of argon, nitrogen, helium, xenon, and O_2 do not absorb IR light and cannot be measured using this technology.

The analyzer selects the appropriate IR wavelength, using an individual filter or a filter wheel, to maximize absorption by the selected anesthetic at its peak wavelength and minimize its absorption by other gases and vapors that could interfere with the measurement of the desired component. Some IR units are equipped with a dial or switch to select and indicate the agent being measured, while others require a different filter and scale to measure each agent. After the transmitted IR energy is detected by the sensor, an electrical signal is produced and amplified, and the concentration is displayed in analog or digital form.

IR CO_2 analyzers may be diverting or nondiverting. Analyzers that measure anesthetic agents are diverting. Because the gases are not altered, the sample can be returned to the breathing system.

Monitors that identify and quantify halogenated agents use a separate chamber to measure absorption at several wavelengths. Typically, these are single channel, four-wavelength IR filter photometers. There is a filter for each anesthetic agent and one to provide a baseline for comparison. Each of the four filters transmits a specific wavelength of IR light and each gas absorbs differently in the selected wavelength bands (149).

Most IR instruments have an accuracy of ± 0.2% for CO_2 concentrations over the range of 0% to 10% and ± 2.0% for N_2O concentrations from 0% to 100%. For typical halogenated agents, the accuracy is ± 0.4% over a range of 0 to 5% (146). Most investigators believe that these monitors are sufficiently accurate for clinical purposes (151–158), although they tend to underestimate the inspired level and overestimate end-tidal values at high respiratory rates (159). With increasing respiratory rate, accuracy is diminished more for volatile anesthetic values than CO_2 (160).

Optical (10)

Diverting (sidestream). Figure 18.16 shows a sidestream IR analyzer. IR light is continuously focused on a spinning (chopper) wheel. The wheel has holes with filters specially selected for the gases to be measured. The gas to be measured is pumped continuously through a sample (measuring) chamber. The selectively filtered and pulsed light is passed through the sample chamber and also through a reference chamber with no absorption characteristics. The light is then focused on an IR light detector (photosensor). The amount of light absorbed by the sample gas is proportional to the partial pressures of gases whose IR light absorption patterns correspond to the wavelengths selected by the filters on the chopper wheel. The changing light levels on the photosensor produce changes in the electrical current that runs through it. Rotating the filter wheel thousands of times per minute provides hundreds of readings for each respiratory cycle. For practical purposes, the waveform on the display is continuous.

Monochromatic sidestream optical IR analyzers use one wavelength to measure potent inhalational agents and are unable to distinguish be-

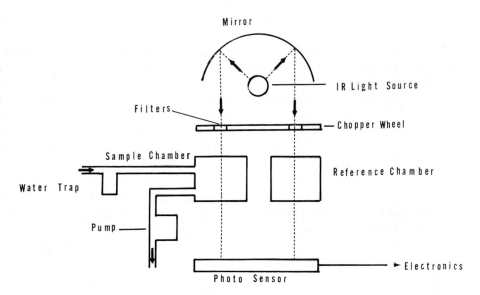

FIGURE 18.16. Sidestream optical infrared analyzer. A beam of infrared (IR) light is at one end and a photo detection device is at the other. The chopper wheel contains several filters, which are divided into sections that will allow passage of only the frequencies most readily absorbed by the gases to be measured. The filtered and pulsatile IR light is directed through both the sample chamber and a reference chamber with no absorption qualities. The amount of IR light absorbed at each frequency depends on the levels of gases in the sample chamber.

tween agents or to detect a mixture of agents (161). When such an analyzer is used, the clinician must select which agent is to be monitored. If an incorrect agent is selected, incorrect values will be reported (162–166). Polychromatic IR analyzers use multiple wavelengths to both identify and quantify the various agents (167–170). This eliminates the need for the user to select the agent to be monitored and allows detection of a mixture of agents.

When a new anesthetic agent is introduced, new monitors capable or measuring this agent may be required, or existing equipment may be updated (e.g., with new filters and software) if possible.

Most sidestream analyzers have fixed sampling rates (usually 150 ml/min), although some permit selection of other rates. The measuring cell is calibrated to zero using gas free of the gases of interest (usually room air) and to a standard level using a calibration gas mixture. Some optical sidestream IR monitors are shown in Figure 18.1.

Nondiverting (mainstream) . With a nondiverting CO_2 monitor the patient's respiratory gas stream passes through a chamber (cuvette) with two windows (Fig. 18.2). The windows are usually made from sapphire, which is transparent to IR light. The cuvette is placed between the breathing system and the patient (Fig. 18.3A). The sensor, which houses both the light source and detector, fits over the cuvette. To prevent condensation of water, the sensor is heated slightly above body temperature. IR light shines through the window on one side of the adapter, and the sensor receives the light on the opposite side. After passing through the sample chamber, the light goes through three ports in a rotating wheel, which contains (a) a sealed cell with a known high CO_2 concentration, (b) a chamber vented to the sensor's internal atmosphere, and (c) a sealed cell containing only nitrogen (Fig. 18.3B). The radiation then passes through a filter that screens the light to the correct wavelength to isolate CO_2 information from interfering gases and onto a photo detector. The signal is amplified and sent to the display module.

A mainstream monitor with diverting capability is shown in Figure 18.6. Gas is aspirated through a special cuvette and is analyzed by the sensor.

Calibration is performed using two sealed cells in a plastic unit that attaches to the control unit (Fig. 18.4). It is shaped so that the sensor can clip over either cell. The low calibration cell contains 100% nitrogen while the high cell contains a known partial pressure of CO_2. The actual value is printed on the unit and must be programmed into the control unit. Correction factors for nitrous oxide and/or O_2 must be made manually.

The adapter adds from 5 to 17 ml for adult-size adapters and 0.6 to 2 ml for pediatric adapters (13, 14). End-tidal CO_2 values obtained using a mainstream IR analyzer with a pediatric adapter are close to arterial values in healthy neonates and infants (13).

The sensor may become dislodged from the cuvette. If it is completely dislodged, no waveform will be seen. If it is slightly dislodged (Fig. 18.5), the reading may be incorrect although the waveform appears normal (15–17). Condensed water, secretions, or blood on the windows of the cuvette will interfere with light transmission and may cause erroneous readings (171).

Photoacoustic (10, 105, 149, 172, 173)

Photoacoustic spectroscopy (PAS) is based on the fact that absorption of IR light by molecules causes them to expand and thereby increases the pressure of the gas. If the light is delivered in pulses, the pressure increase will be intermittent. If the frequency of pulsation is in the audible range, the changes in pressure will create an acoustic signal that can be detected by a microphone. The amplitude of the signal caused by the pressure fluctuation is directly proportional to the partial pressure of gas present.

A photoacoustic gas analyzer is shown in Figure 18.17. Broad-band IR radiation is used to produce the increase in pressure, but to differentiate between the signals for each measured gas, it is necessary to divide the emitted beam into three different sections. For this, a chopper disk with three concentric bands of holes is employed. This causes the emitted radiation to be modulated at three different frequencies. The divided light beam then passes through three different optical filters, which form one wall of the measurement chamber. Each of these filters allows only IR radia-

tion of a specific wavelength to pass through so that the wavelengths of the emitted light are matched to the absorption spectra of the gases to be measured. The filters on the measuring cell are positioned to match the radiation pulses emerging from the chopper wheel. The frequency at which the light is turned on and off is selected to get the maximum acoustic response.

The PAS system has better long-term stability than traditional IR instruments because it measures IR absorption directly rather than indirectly (172). Accuracy is similar to that of the mass spectrometer (174) and greater than other IR technologies (166).

Anesthetic agent identification is not possible with PAS. However, because photoacoustic monitors use a different wavelength from optical infrared monitors, the errors in the readings when an incorrect agent is selected are less (165, 172, 175).

Advantages

Multigas Capability

IR analyzers are capable of measuring CO_2, nitrous oxide, and all of the commonly used potent volatile agents.

Volatile Agent Detection

Although the monochromatic analyzers are unable to identify anesthetic agents and mixtures of agents, most newer models provide agent detection and can detect and quantify mixtures. Analyzers handle a mixture of agents in different ways. They may give a display saying that there is a mixture of agents, or may compensate for the additional agent.

No Need to Scavenge Gases

After measurement, the gases can be returned to the breathing system if desired.

Portability

The units are small, compact, and lightweight.

Quick Response Time

The response time is fast enough to measure both inspired and exhaled concentrations. Response times for anesthetic agents and nitrous oxide are longer than for CO_2 (146).

Short Warm-up Time

The warm-up time is short. The instruments do not need to be kept in a standby mode.

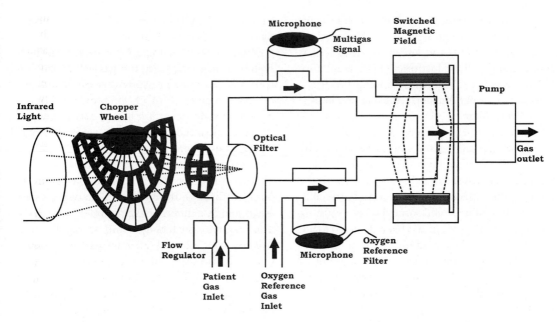

FIGURE 18.17. Photoacoustic infrared analyzer. The gas sample is drawn into the measurement chamber through a flow regulator. This makes the sample flow rate independent of changes in the patient's airway pressure. Light from an infrared source is aimed toward a window in the measurement chamber. Before the light enters the chamber, it passes through a spinning chopper wheel that causes it to pulsate. To differentiate between the three signals caused by carbon dioxide (CO_2), nitrous oxide, and anesthetic agents, the chopper has three concentric bands of holes. This causes the light to pulsate at three different frequencies. Each light beam then passes through an optical filter that only allows light of a specific wavelength to pass through. Thus the frequencies and wavelengths of the incident light are matched to the infrared (IR) absorption spectra of the three gases to be measured. In the measurement chamber, each beam excites one of the gases, causing it to expand and contract at a frequency equal to the pulsation frequency of the appropriate infrared beam. The periodic expansion and contraction of the gas sample produce a fluctuation of audible frequency that can be detected by a microphone. In this monitor an alternating magnetic field is applied to a separate sample of gas. Because oxygen has paramagnetic properties, this will produce a sound wave. The amplitude of this wave will be proportional to the concentration of O_2 present.

Convenience

Although early units required a complicated calibration with test gases with each use, with newer units periodic calibration with a standardized gas mixture is sufficient.

Lack of Interference from Nitric Oxide or Argon

Argon or low concentrations of nitric oxide do not interfere with monitoring of volatile agents by IR analyzers (127, 176).

Disadvantages

Oxygen and Nitrogen Not Measured

O_2 and nitrogen cannot be measured by IR technology.

Interference among Gases

While O_2 is not absorbed by IR light it causes broadening of the CO_2 absorption spectra, which results in lower CO_2 readings (3, 146). In a typical IR CO_2 analyzer, 95% O_2 causes a 0.5% decline in measured CO_2 (99). Some units have a user-actuated electronic offset for O_2 (177).

There is some overlap of the CO_2 and nitrous oxide IR absorption peaks so that nitrous oxide can cause falsely high CO_2 readings, with an increase of 0.1 to 1.4 torr per 10% nitrous oxide (3). Most IR analyzers that measure both CO_2 and nitrous oxide automatically correct for nitrous oxide's effect on the CO_2 reading. Some require the user to indicate when nitrous oxide is present.

If the analyzer is set to measure a volatile agent different from that present in the gas mixture being analyzed, CO_2 and nitrous oxide as well as agent readings will be incorrect (178). A mixture of agents can cause erroneous readings (179).

Inaccuracy from Alcohols, Acetone, Methane, and Propellants

Ethanol, methanol, isopropanol, methane, or acetone in sampled gases can cause spuriously high volatile agent readings (151, 166, 180–189). The magnitude of the interference varies with the monitor. Polychromatic and photoacoustic analyzers are less affected and some display a warning that the interfering agent has been detected (158, 168, 173, 190). Nafion tubing allows some alcohol to escape and this decreases the amount of interference (191). Some analyzers detect halogenated propellants as anesthetic gases (134, 135, 192–194).

Interference from Water Vapor (195)

Water vapor absorbs IR light at many wavelengths and will cause increased CO_2 and volatile agent readings (146). Monitors use nafion tubing, water traps, filters, and/or hydrophobic membranes to minimize this. Water that gets into the monitor can cause expensive or irreversible damage (196).

Slow Response Time

With rapid respiratory rates, the response time may be too slow to measure inspired and end-tidal levels of volatile agents accurately (154, 197).

Addition of Air to the Breathing System

If the sample gas from the agent monitor is returned to the breathing system, unexpectedly high levels of nitrogen may be seen due to air added to the sample gas after it had passed through the analyzing chamber (143). Because more gas is returned to the breathing system than was removed, closed circuit anesthesia is difficult (143).

Interference from Radio Frequencies

Hand-held radios used near an IR analyzer may cause the CO_2 readings to be increased (198).

Paramagnetic Analysis (149, 150, 173, 199–201)

When introduced into a magnetic field, some substances locate themselves in the strongest portion of the field. These substances are termed paramagnetic. Of the gases of interest in anesthesia, only O_2 is paramagnetic.

When a gas containing O_2 is passed through a switched magnetic field, the gas will expand and contract, causing a pressure wave proportional to the partial pressure of O_2 present. To obtain a high degree of accuracy it is necessary to compare the pressure in the gas sample to a reference signal obtained using air.

A paramagnetic O_2 analyzer is shown in Figure 18.18. Reference (air) and sample gases are pumped through the analyzer. The two gas paths are joined by a differential pressure or flow sensor. The magnet is switched on and off rapidly. If the streams of sample and reference gas have different O_2 partial pressures, the magnet will cause their pressures to differ. This difference is detected by the transducer and converted into an electrical signal that is displayed as O_2 partial pressure (or converted to volumes percent). The short rise time of this technique allows measurement of inspired and end-tidal O_2 levels at high respiratory rates. The paramagnetic analyzer is strongly temperature dependent; therefore accurate temperature compensation is needed.

Some monitors combine photoacoustic infrared analysis of CO_2, anesthetic agents, and nitrous oxide with paramagnetic O_2 analysis (Fig. 18.17). Switching the magnet on and off at a certain frequency generates a pressure wave that can be detected in the acoustic spectrum. This is known as magnetoacoustics.

One problem with these instruments is that if the gas from the analyzer is returned to the breathing system, the air that is used as a reference will dilute the other gases and cause an increase in nitrogen (99).

These analyzers are not affected by argon (127).

Electrochemical Analysis

An electrochemical O_2 analyzer consists of a sensor, which is exposed to the gas to be sampled, and the analyzer box, which contains the electric circuitry, display, and alarms (Fig. 18.19). The sensor contains a cathode and an anode surrounded by electrolyte gel. The gel is held in place by a membrane that is nonpermeable to ions, proteins, or other such materials, yet permeable to gases such

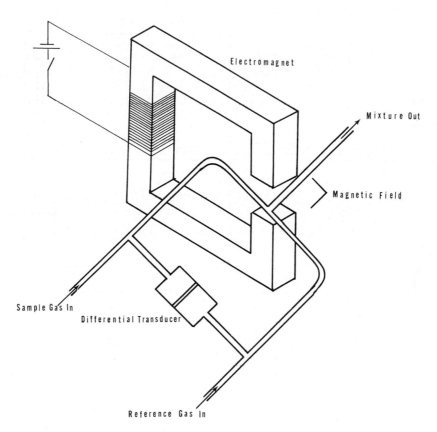

Electromagnet

Mixture Out

Magnetic Field

Sample Gas In

Differential Transducer

Reference Gas In

FIGURE **18.18.** Paramagnetic O_2 analyzer. A reference gas of known or no O_2 content and the gas whose O_2 level is to be measured are pumped through the analyzer and converge into a tube at the outlet. The two gas paths are joined at their midpoints by a differential pressure or flow sensor. The magnet is switched on and off at a rapid rate. Because the reference and sample gases have different O_2 levels, the pressures in the paths will differ. The pressure difference is detected by the sensor.

as O_2. The membrane prevents evaporation of the electrolyte. It should not be touched because dirt and grease reduce its usable area.

O_2 diffuses through the membrane and electrolyte to the cathode, where it is reduced, causing a current to flow between the electrodes. The rate at which O_2 enters the cell and generates current is proportional to the partial pressure of O_2 in the gas outside the membrane. For convenience, however, the display scale is usually marked in percent O_2. A gain control allows the analyzer to be calibrated with gas containing a known partial pressure of O_2.

These analyzers respond slowly to changes in O_2 pressure, so that they cannot be used to measure end-tidal concentrations.

There are two basic types of sensors: galvanic cell and polarographic electrode.

Technology
Galvanic Cell (149, 150)

A galvanic cell (fuel cell, microfuel cell) sensor is shown in Figure 18.20. It consists of a lead anode and a gold cathode surrounded by potassium hydroxide electrolyte (202, 203). The cathode acts as the sensing electrode and is not consumed. The hydroxyl ions formed there react with the lead anode, forming lead oxide. The lead anode is gradually consumed (worn out).

$$\text{Cathode: } O_2 + 2H_2O + 4e^- \rightarrow 4OH^-$$
$$\text{Anode: } 4OH^- + 2Pb \rightarrow 2PbO + 2H_2O + 4e^-$$

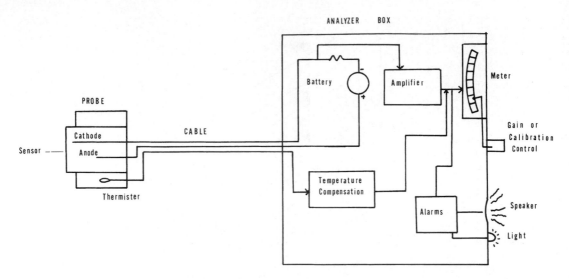

ANALYZER   BOX

Meter

Battery   Amplifier

PROBE

Gain or
Calibration
Control

Cathode   CABLE

Sensor   Anode

Temperature
Compensation

Thermister

Alarms

Speaker

Light

FIGURE 18.19. Electrochemical O_2 analyzer. The sensor is connected by a cable to the analyzer box, which contains the meter, alarms, and controls. A thermistor compensates for changes in O_2 diffusion caused by temperature. An amplifier is present in the polarographic analyzer. Those monitors with manual calibration require adjustment of a gain control until the correct reading is obtained for a standard O_2 concentration. Those with automatic calibration simply require a button to be pressed in the presence of a gas of standard concentration (usually air). This puts the monitor into calibration mode, and it returns to normal readings automatically when calibration is complete.

FIGURE 18.20. Galvanic cell sensor. The membrane is permeable to gases but not to liquids. At the cathode, oxygen molecules are reduced to hydroxide ions. At the anode, hydroxide ions give up electrons. An electron flow between the anode and cathode, which is directly proportional to the partial pressure of O_2 in the sample gas, is generated. (Courtesy of Biomarine Industries, Inc.)

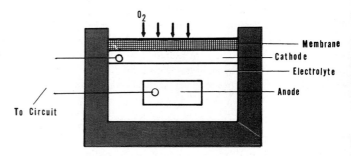

O_2

Membrane
Cathode
Electrolyte

To Circuit

Anode

Because the current is strong enough to operate the meter, a separate power source is not required to operate the analyzer. A power source (either battery or wall current) is required for alarms.

The sensor comes packaged in a sealed container from which O_2 has been removed. Its lifespan begins when the package is opened (202, 204). Its useful life is cited in percent hours, which is the product of hours of exposure and O_2 percentage. If it is left in areas of high O_2 concentration, its life expectancy will be decreased. Sensor life can be prolonged by leaving it exposed to air when not in use (Fig. 18. 21). Galvanic sensors require no membrane or electrolyte replacement. The entire sensor must be replaced when it becomes exhausted (Fig. 18.22).

Polarographic Electrode

A polarographic (Clark electrode) sensor is shown in Figure 18.23. It consists of a silver anode, a platinum or gold cathode, electrolyte, and a gas-permeable membrane (202, 204–206). There is a power source (battery or AC line) for inducing a potential between the anode and the cathode.

O_2 molecules diffuse through the membrane

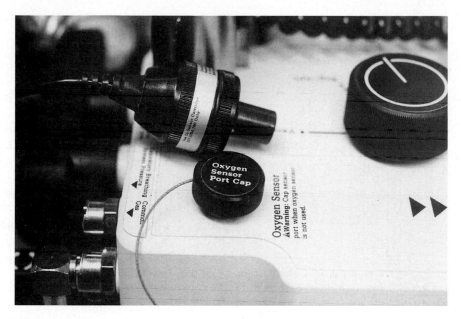

FIGURE 18.21. The life of a galvanic (fuel cell) electrochemical O_2 analyzer can be prolonged by leaving it exposed to room air when not in use.

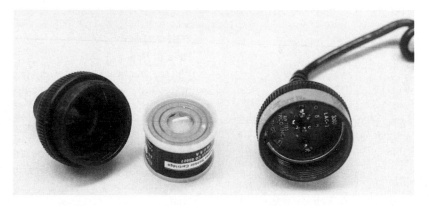

FIGURE 18.22. Galvanic cell sensor. The entire sensor must be replaced when it becomes exhausted.

and the electrolyte. When a polarizing voltage is applied to the cathode, electrons combine with the O_2 molecules and reduce them to hydroxide ions:

$$\text{Cathode: } O_2 + 2H_2O + 4e^- \rightarrow 4OH^-$$
$$\text{Anode: } 4Ag + 4Cl^- \rightarrow 4AgCl + 4e^-$$

A current that is proportional to the partial pressure of O_2 in the sample flows between the anode and cathode.

Polarographic sensors may be either preassem-

bled, disposable cartridges or units that can be disassembled and reused by changing the membrane and/or electrolyte (207). The sensor remains unconsumed when not turned on, so the analyzer should be kept on standby when not in use.

Use

Calibration

Calibration should be performed daily before use and at least every 8 hours after that. Some instruments remind the user when calibration is

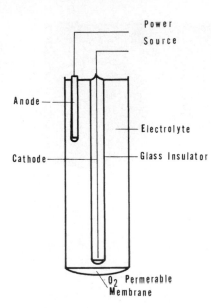

Power
Source

Anode —

Electrolyte

Cathode —

Glass Insulator

O₂ Permerable
Membrane

FIGURE **18.23.** Polarographic sensor. O_2 diffuses through the membrane and electrolyte to the cathode. When a polarizing voltage is applied to the cathode, the oxygen molecules are reduced to hydroxide ions. The current flow between cathode and anode will be proportional to the partial pressure of O_2. (Courtesy of Bageant RA. Oxygen analyzers. Respir Care 1976;21:415.)

due and will not give a reading unless calibration is performed. The calibration can be checked quickly by exposing the sensor to room air and verifying that it indicates approximately 21% O_2 (Fig. 18.21 and 18.24).

Checking the Alarms

In some polarographic O_2 analyzers, there are three batteries: two for operating the sensor and one for the alarms (208). Checking the battery-test function may not check the battery for the alarms.

The sensor should be put in room air and the low O_2 alarm set above 21%. The visual signal should flash and the audible alarm sound. If the unit has a high O_2 alarm, the setting for that should be moved below 21%. The visual and audible signals should be activated. If the lamp(s) fails to light or the audible alarm is weak, the batteries should be replaced and the alarms rechecked. If this fails to remedy the situation, the unit should

be returned to the manufacturer for servicing or replacement.

Placement in the Breathing System

Sites for placement in breathing systems are discussed in Chapter 7, "Breathing Systems II: Mapleson Systems," and Chapter 8, "Breathing Systems III: Circle System." High pressure will cause the fuel cell to read a higher O_2 percentage than is actually present (209). The service life of the sensors of some galvanic cell analyzers is reduced by exposure to CO_2, so locating the sensor on the inspiratory side of the system may be preferable.

The junction between the cable and the sensor should not be under strain. The sensor should be upright or tilted slightly to prevent moisture from accumulating on the membrane.

Setting Alarms Limits

The low O_2 alarm should be set a little below the minimum and the high O_2 level alarm a little above the maximum acceptable concentrations. There should be places on the anesthesia record for recording the alarm set points and O_2 percentages.

Advantages

Ease of Use

Electrochemical O_2 analyzers are dependable, accurate, and user friendly. Galvanic analyzers appear capable of delivering more reliable service than polarographic ones (210). The warmup time is short. The polarographic analyzer has a faster response time than the galvanic (207, 211, 212). This is probably not clinically significant but does facilitate calibration.

Cost

These instruments cost less than other means of O_2 analysis. Galvanic cell analyzers are less costly to purchase and maintain than polarographic ones (210).

Automatic Enabling

O_2 analyzers that are a component part of the anesthesia machine are automatically enabled when the machine is turned on. Thus the possibility of the user forgetting to turn it on is eliminated.

Compact

Compared with other technologies for measuring O_2, the electrochemical analyzer takes up little space.

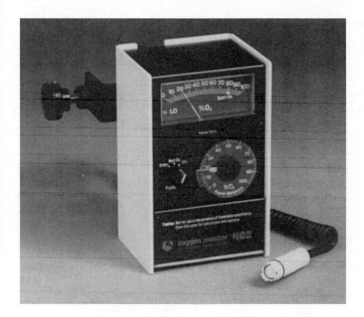

FIGURE 18.24. The electrochemical O_2 analyzer is calibrated by exposing the sensor to room air.

No Effect from Argon

Argon does not affect galvanic cell monitoring (127).

Disadvantages

Maintenance

While maintenance on the newer models has been simplified, some instruments need frequent membrane and electrolyte changes. Polarographic monitors require more maintenance than the galvanic cell ones (210).

Calibration

These instruments need to be calibrated before use each day and at least every 8 hours.

User Enabling

Instruments that are not an integral part of anesthesia machines need to be turned on by the user.

Difficulty Using Outside the Breathing System

With spontaneously breathing patients who are not connected to a breathing system and receiving O_2 via mask or nasal cannulae, it is difficult to monitor the inspired O_2 concentration using these instruments.

Inaccuracy

A study found that electrochemical analyzers had a high percentage of errors, most commonly caused by humidity (213).

Slow Response Time

These analyzers cannot be used to measure end-tidal O_2.

Piezoelectric Analysis (149, 150, 214, 215)

Technology

The piezoelectric method uses vibrating crystals coated with a layer of lipid (Fig. 18.25). When exposed to a volatile anesthetic agent, the vapor is adsorbed into the lipid. The resulting change in the mass of the lipid alters the vibration frequency. By use of an electronic system consisting of two oscillating circuits, one of which has an uncoated (reference) crystal and the other a coated (detector) crystal, an electric signal which is proportional to the vapor concentration is generated. The reference crystal and microprocessor compensate for the effects of temperature and atmospheric pressure variations.

The first device using this technology was a mainstream device, which had many problems associated with its use. Newer models are sampling devices (Fig. 18.26) and have a superior performance compared with earlier models (215). Some piezoelectric-based units have a separate non-dispersive IR sensor that differentiates inspiration and expiration.

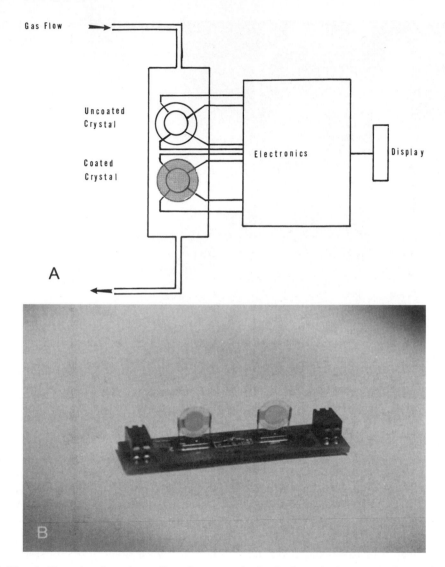

FIGURE 18.25. A, Piezoelectric analyzer. One vibrating crystal is coated with lipid, and the other is uncoated. By comparing the vibration frequencies of the crystals, the level of anesthetic agent in the gas being analyzed can be measured. **B,** Piezoelectric crystals. (Courtesy of Biochemical International, Inc.)

Advantages

Accuracy

Investigations show an accuracy of better than 0.1% (214–216). Water vapor and nitrous oxide affect the reading, but the worst case interference is less than 0.1%. The analyzer does not give artifactual results in the presence of aerosol propellants used to administer bronchodilators (135). Although alcohol adheres to the surface of a coated crystal it has a minimal effect on readings (183).

Fast Response Time

Newer models can measure inspired and expired levels of halogenated agents.

No Need for Scavenging

Because the agents are not altered, the gas removed can be returned to the breathing system.

Short Warmup Time

The warmup period is shorter than with an infrared analyzer or mass spectrometer (214).

Compactness

These units are small.

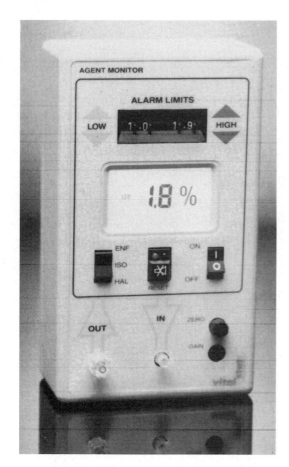

FIGURE 18.26.   Piezoelectric anesthetic agent monitor. The agent to be measured must be selected. (Courtesy of Vital Signs, Inc.)

Disadvantages

Only One Gas Measured

This analyzer cannot measure O_2, CO_2, nitrogen, or nitrous oxide.

No Agent Discrimination

This device cannot discriminate between agents. If the wrong agent is selected the reading can be in error by as much as 118% (214). With a mixture of agents, the reading may be close to the sum of the delivered percents of the agents (217).

Inaccuracy with Water Vapor

Water will cause errors with the piezoelectric monitor (166). In one case the pipes to the pump were reversed so that water vapor was removed after its passage rather than before (218).

Chemical Carbon Dioxide Detection (219–223)

Chemical (colorimetric) chemical indicator devices consist of a pH-sensitive chemical indicator whose pH is just above the level where the dye chosen is expected to change its color enclosed in a disposable housing. When the detector is exposed to CO_2, it becomes more acidic and changes color. During inspiration, the color returns to its resting state unless it is used with a breathing system that allows rebreathing.

The inlet and outlet ports are 15 mm, so the device can fit between patient and the breathing system or resuscitation bag. With Mapleson systems it may be possible to place the detector elsewhere in the breathing system (224).

Technology

Hygroscopic

The hygroscopic CO_2 detector contains hygroscopic filter paper impregnated with a colorless liquid base and an indicator (metacresol purple) that changes color as a function of the pH.

The device is shown in Figure 18.27. The filter paper is visible through a clear window. The color chart on the dome was designed to be read under fluorescent light. An auxiliary color chart included in each package should be consulted if other lighting is encountered. A (purple, mauve) for low levels of CO_2 (0.5%) ; B (beige) for moderate levels of CO_2 (.5 to 2%); and yellow for high levels (>2%) of CO_2 (225, 226). The mean minimum concentration of CO_2 needed to produce a color change is 0.54% with a range from 0.25 to 0.60% (222).

Its useful life may last from a few minutes up to several hours, depending on the humidity of the gas monitored (227). Reducing the relative humidity of exhaled gases by insertion of a heat and moisture exchanger to trap moisture before it reaches the device markedly prolongs the useful life of this device (228). Use with an active humidifier will shorten its workable life (229). Exposure to ambient room air conditions should be avoided prior to use. It has a shelf life of only 15 months (230).

Hydrophobic (227)

Another device using a hydrophobic indicator has been developed. This allows this indicator to work in a relative humidity range of 15 to 85%. On exposure to CO_2 the color changes from blue

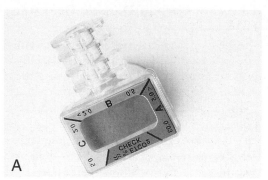

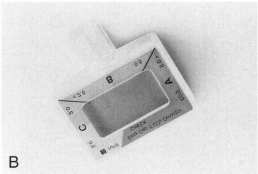

FIGURE **18.27.** Colorometric carbon dioxide (CO_2) detector. A color code around the outside provides a reference. **A,** Adult size. **B,** Pediatric version. (Pictures courtesy of Nellcor, a division of Mallinkrodt Medical Inc.)

to green to yellow. Liquids will cause the device not to function but if allowed to dry out it will recover its activity.

It has a faster response time that the hygroscopic model and performs better at high respiratory frequencies (227). It is only slightly affected by exposure to humidity. It has been shown to function for 24 hours in the ICU and for more than 9 hours during low flow anesthesia (231).

Use

The chemical CO_2 detector is used primarily for confirming successful tracheal intubation. It may be useful in determining the position of the Combitube (see Chapter 17, "Tracheal Tubes") (232). It can be used during an intubation in a hyperbaric chamber (233).

A minimum of six breaths should be performed before a determination is made to avoid errors caused by CO_2 forced into the stomach during mask ventilation or by antacids or cola in the stomach. Usually, the color change can be seen long before this.

A pediatric version has been developed (Fig. 18.27). While it has been found to be more accurate than the adult version in pediatrics, the sensitivity is decreased during rapid respiration (234).

Advantages

1. The device is easy to use.
2. Its performance is not affected by nitrous oxide or anesthetic vapors.

3. Its small size allows it to be used in locations where access to a CO_2 monitor is not possible. It may be useful for intubations performed at remote locations and during transport of patients where space is limited, as in an ambulance or helicopter (235–237).
4. It is portable and requires no power source.
5. Compared with other methods of CO_2 analysis the cost is low.
6. Studies show the device to be very accurate in diagnosing esophageal intubation, even in small children (219, 221, 224, 236, 238–246).
7. The device can serve to indicate the effectiveness of resuscitation or as a prognostic indicator of successful short-term resuscitation, after the tracheal tube has been correctly positioned (240, 247, 248). A negative test result may indicate either esophageal intubation or airway intubation with poor or absent pulmonary blood flow (242, 249).
8. It offers minimal resistance to flow.
9. The device is always ready for use, does not require sterilization, and limits the risk of transmission of infection.

Disadvantages

1. It may take several breaths before conclusions can be drawn about the location of the tracheal tube.
2. False-negative results may be seen with very low tidal volumes and low end-tidal CO_2 con-

centrations (250, 251). It may not indicate CO_2 in cases of compromised lung perfusion (227, 245, 252–254). During CPR, a positive test correctly indicates that the tracheal tube is in the airway, but a negative result (suggesting esophageal placement) requires an alternate method of confirming tracheal tube position (239). Best results are in patients with spontaneous circulation (255). Failure to inflate the tracheal tube cuff may cause equivocal color change (220).

3. Contamination of this device with drugs instilled in the trachea or gastric contents can cause irreversible damage (230, 254, 256, 257).

Both hygroscopic and hydrophobic devices fail to function when liquid water covers the active surface area. Chemicals may leach out from a hygroscopic unit, causing permanent damage, while the hydrophobic unit will recover on drying (227).

4. False-positives can occur if there is CO_2 in the stomach (from ingestion of carbonated beverages, administration of antacids, or mask ventilation) (258–262). The display may initially turn color, and only slowly revert to its original color. A false positive result may occur if the tip of the tube is in the pharynx (245).

5. Difficulty in distinguishing color changes has been reported (259). It may be difficult to determine whether a subtle color change is due to the patient's low end-tidal CO_2 or to misplacement of the tracheal tube (256).

6. These devices are not suited for continuous monitoring. There is no alarm or waveform.

7. This device may not be cost effective for routine use when compared to a capnometer (230). Its cost effectiveness may be greater with a small number of applications (263).

8. Airflow obstruction resulting from a manufacturing defect has been reported (264).

Refractometry (265–267)
Technology

In an optical interference refractometer (interferometer), one portion of a split light beam passes through a chamber into which the sample gas has been aspirated, while the other portion passes through an identical chamber containing air. Because vapor slows the velocity of light, the portion passing through the vapor chamber is delayed. The beams are then recombined to form an interference pattern consisting of dark and light bands. The position of these bands yields the vapor concentration.

Advantages

This technology is commonly used to calibrate monitors and vaporizers. Interactions between agents is not a problem (267).

Disadvantages

Nitrous oxide interferes with the readings, making it unsatisfactory for clinical monitoring (148).

GASES
Oxygen

The standards for basic intraoperative monitoring during administration of general anesthesia of the American Society of Anesthesiologists and American Association of Nurse Anesthetists include measurement of the level of O_2 in the breathing system. The anesthesia machine standard requires that the anesthesia machine be equipped with an O_2 analyzer with a high-priority alarm that is activated when the measured O_2 level is below the user-set alarm threshold (268).

Standard Requirements

An international standard on O_2 analyzers was published in 1997 (269). A U.S. standard was published in 1993 (4). The following requirements are in the U.S. standard.

1. O_2 readings shall be within ± 3% of the actual level. This accuracy shall be maintained for at least 8 hr of continuous use.

2. Humidity up to 100%, concentrations of nitrous oxide up to 80%, CO_2 up to 5%, halothane up to 4%, enflurane up to 5%, and isoflurane up to 5% shall not cause the O_2 readings to vary from actual level by more than 5%.

3. The low O_2 alarm limit shall not be adjustable or preset below 15%. There must be a visual indication to the user when the low alarm limit is below 21%. If a manual control is provided to override the low-O_2-level alarm, it shall only

override the auditory signal and shall automatically cancel after not more than 120 seconds following its most recent activation.

Technology

O_2 levels may be measured using mass spectrometry, Raman scattering, electrochemical, magnetoacoustics, or paramagnetic technology. Electrochemical analysis can measure only mean concentrations. The other four methods have sufficiently rapid response times that inspired and end-tidal levels can be measured if the sensing site is located between the patient and the breathing system. It may be desirable to measure the inspired O_2 with nonintubated spontaneously breathing patients. This is possible with a diverting device such as the mass spectrometer, Raman spectrometer, acoustomagnetic or paramagnetic analyzer but not with an electrochemical monitor. O_2 analysis can be used during jet ventilation (270).

Using more than one device to monitor oxygen is desirable, especially if a shared system mass spectrometer is in use.

If helium is to be used, an electrochemical analyzer should be used to supplement the mass spectrometer, which may display erroneously high oxygen readings (115).

Applications of Oxygen Analysis

Detection of Hypoxic or Hyperoxic Mixtures

The first line of defense against hypoxemia is avoidance of a hypoxic inspired gas mixture. Low O_2 levels provide an earlier warning of inadequate O_2 than pulse oximetry (154). In a study of 2000 critical incidents, 1% were first detected by the O_2 monitor (271).

O_2 analysis can also help to prevent problems resulting from hyperoxygenation such as awareness, damage to the lungs and eyes, and airway fires with laser use (272).

Detection of Disconnections and Leaks

Disconnection of the tubing to an O_2 mask may be detected using a diverting O_2 analyzer (273).

An O_2 monitor can detect disconnections in the breathing system (154, 274–276). However, it cannot be depended on for this purpose (277–280). Whether or not the O_2 level falls at the point being monitored depends on several factors, including the type of breathing system in use, the position of the sensor in the system, the site of disconnection, the alarm set points, whether the patient is breathing spontaneously or ventilation is controlled and the type of ventilator in use (277).

With a sidestream analyzer a decrease in inspired and expired O_2 may result from a leak in the sampling system (281).

Detection of Hypoventilation

Normally the difference between inspired and expired O_2 is 4 to 5%. A difference of more than 5% after a steady state has been reached is a sensitive indicator of acute hypoventilation (282, 283).

Other

End-tidal O_2 has been used as an indication of the adequacy of preoxygenation (284–288).

Knowledge of expired O_2 concentration allows estimates of the patient's O_2 consumption and cardiac output and can aid in the diagnosis of malignant hyperthermia. O_2 consumption can be estimated from the difference between the inspired and exhaled O_2 concentrations (289, 290). This can be useful in determining the prognosis with resuscitation.

The concentration of nitrous oxide can be estimated from the concentration of O_2.

End-tidal O_2 has been used to detect air embolism. When a significant amount of air enters the vascular bed, there is an increase in end-tidal O_2 and a decrease in the $F_{(I-e)}O_2$ (291–293).

Carbon Dioxide Analysis

The ASA and AANA practice guidelines for basic intraoperative monitoring include end-tidal CO_2 monitoring for verification of tracheal intubation (294). A court case has held that a reasonably prudent health care facility would supply a CO_2 monitor to a patient undergoing general anesthesia (295). Some states have mandated use of CO_2 monitors (150).

CO_2 analysis provides a means for assessing ventilation and can detect many equipment- and patient-related problems that other monitors may either fail to detect or detect so slowly that patient safety may be compromised (296). A closed claims analysis found that capnography plus pulse oximetry was potentially preventative in 93% of avoidable anesthetic mishaps (297). In one study, 10% of intraoperative problems were initially diagnosed by CO_2 monitoring (298). In another, end-tidal CO_2 was useful in confirming the occurrence of 58% of already suspected anesthesia-related critical incidents and was the initial detector of 27% (299). In still another study it was estimated that a capnometer used on its own would have detected 55% of critical incidents had they been allowed to evolve and 43% would have been detected before any potential organ damage (300).

The respiratory cycle (i.e., inspiration versus expiration) is defined in terms of CO_2 measurement so determination of end-tidal values for other gases depends on measurement of CO_2.

Terminology

Capnometry is the measurement and numerical display of CO_2 concentrations during the respiratory cycle. A capnometer is the device that performs the measurement and displays the readings. Capnography is the graphic record of CO_2 concentration on a screen or paper. A capnograph is the machine that generates a waveform, and the capnogram is the actual waveform (301). It may be possible to connect a capnometer to a patient monitor and/or recorder and generate a waveform.

The Capnometer

Standards Requirements

A U.S. standard on capnometers was published in 1992 (5). It contains the following specifications.

1. The CO_2 reading shall be within $\pm$ 12% of the actual value or $\pm$ 4 mm Hg (0.53 kPa), whichever is greater, over the full range of the capnometer.
2. The manufacturer must disclose any interference caused by O_2, nitrous oxide, halothane, enflurane, isoflurane, ethanol, acetone, or chlorodifluromethane.
3. Alarms.
   a. The capnometer shall have a high CO_2 alarm for both inspired and exhaled CO_2. When the capnometer is switched on, the high CO_2 alarm shall be at least medium priority.

   b. It should have a low CO_2 reading alarm for exhaled CO_2. If a low CO_2 reading alarm is provided it shall be medium priority.
   c. The audible components of the alarms should allow silencing until the capnometer is placed in use (i.e., connected to the patient) to reduce nuisance alarms.

Technology

Methods to measure CO_2 levels include mass spectrometry, Raman scattering, IR, and chemical colorimetric analysis. IR CO_2 analyzers may be diverting or nondiverting.

A wide variety of display formats is available on CO_2 monitors (Fig. 18.1). The CO_2 level may be reported as either partial pressure or volumes percent and may be displayed continuously or as peak (normally end-tidal) value. The minimum inspired level may also be shown. Many capnometers have more than one speed. Slower speeds are used for trending and faster ones for waveform observation. Some have optional recorders. Other parameters such as respiratory rate and I:E ratio may be displayed. Portable, battery-operated CO_2 monitoring devices that are suitable for emergency medicine (e.g., pre-hospital use, emergency rooms, crash carts) and patient transport are available (302–305). MRI-compatible IR CO_2 monitors that measure CO_2 without interfering with the MR image and do not produce heating (because all sample lines and patient attachments are nonconductive) are available.

Many capnometers are part of multipurpose monitors with other parameters such as blood pressure, pulse oximetry, and analysis of other gases. The CO_2 waveform may be one of several on a display.

Water Vapor Considerations (105, 195, 306)

Water vapor dilutes the CO_2 in a gas sample. Because most sampling catheter materials are permeable to water, with a diverting capnometer, gas entering the sample cell will have the water vapor concentration of room air, even though the gas being measured may have a higher water vapor pressure. The capnometer will calculate the CO_2 partial pressure using the following formula:

$$PetCO_2 = FetCO_2 \times Pb$$

where Pb is atmospheric pressure. With 5% CO_2 and an atmospheric pressure of 760 torr

$$PetCO_2 = 0.05 \times 760$$
$$PetCO_2 = 38 \text{ mm Hg}$$

To calculate the correct end-tidal CO_2 level, the formula should be

$$PetCO_2 = FetCO_2 \times (Pb - 47)$$

Using the same figures as above,

$$PetCO_2 = 0.05 \times (760 - 47)$$
$$PetCO_2 = 35.65 \text{ mm Hg.}$$

Atmospheric Pressure Considerations (3, 105, 147, 307, 308)

Atmospheric pressure can influence CO_2 readings. Some instruments incorporate a barometer to compensate for changes in atmospheric pressure. Others require the user to enter the atmospheric pressure manually. Still others do not correct for atmospheric pressure.

The 1992 capnometer standard (5) states that if automatic compensation for barometric pressure is not provided, the accompanying documents of a capnometer shall contain an explanation that the readings are correct only at the pressure at which the capnometer is calibrated.

Mass spectrometer. A mass spectrometer measures gases in volumes percent. If the reading is converted to partial pressure, the atmospheric pressure must be known to obtain a correct reading. Furthermore, because the mass spectrometer does not measure water vapor, a correction needs to be made for this.

$PetCO_2 = FetCO_2$ 100

$\times$ (atmospheric pressure $-$ water vapor pressure)

At 760 mm Hg atmospheric pressure and a $FetCO_2$ of 5%

$$PetCO_2 = 0.05 \times (760 - 47) \text{ mm Hg} = 36 \text{ mm Hg}$$

If atmospheric pressure is reduced to 500 mm Hg,

$$PetCO_2 = 0.05 \times (500 - 47) \text{ mm Hg} = 23 \text{ mm Hg}$$

Sidestream Infrared and Raman analyzers. Sidestream IR and Raman analyzers measure partial pressure. Calibration is usually accomplished using a tank whose contents are known in volumes percent. If the atmospheric pressure at the time of calibration is known, the analyzer can compute

the partial pressure of the calibration gas. Readings will reflect the partial pressure of the gas being measured, regardless of changes in atmospheric pressure.

When a sidestream IR or Raman analyzer reports results in volumes percent, the atmospheric pressure at the time of measurement time must be known to compute the value correctly.

$FetCO_2$ = partial pressure

$\times$ (atmospheric pressure $-$ water vapor pressure) $\times$ 100

At 760 mm Hg atmospheric pressure and a CO_2 level of 38 mm Hg,

$$FetCO_2 = 38 (760 - 47) \times 100 = 5\%$$

If the atmospheric pressure is reduced to 500 mm Hg,

$$FetCO_2 = 38 (500 - 47) \times 100 = 8\%$$

If a correction for atmospheric pressure is not made, the capnometer will show erroneously low concentrations at increased altitude (308).

Mainstream Infrared analyzers. Mainstream IR instruments are calibrated from sealed gas cells of known partial pressure. These instruments will always correctly report measurements in units of partial pressure (3). If such an analyzer reports results in volumes percent, the atmospheric pressure at measurement time must be known. Corrections are similar to those for mainstream IR and Raman analyzers.

Clinical Significance of Capnometry

CO_2 is produced in the body by cellular metabolism, conveyed by the circulatory system to the lungs, excreted by the lungs and transported by the breathing system. Therefore, changes in respired CO_2 may reflect alterations in metabolism, circulation, respiration, the airway, or breathing system. Tables 18.1 to 18.4 list some sources of changes in CO_2 levels.

Metabolism

Monitoring CO_2 elimination gives an indication of the patient's metabolic rate. Table 18.1 lists some metabolic causes of increased or decreased CO_2 excretion. An increase in end-tidal CO_2 is a reliable indicator of increased metabolism only in mechanically ventilated subjects. In spon-

TABLE 18.1. **Capnography and Capnometry with Altered Carbon Dioxide Production**[a]

	Waveform on Capnograph	End-Tidal CO_2	Inspiratory CO_2	End-Tidal to Arterial Gradient
Absorption of CO_2 from peritoneal cavity	Normal	↑	0	Normal
Injection of sodium bicarbonate	Normal	↑	0	Normal
Pain, anxiety, shivering	Normal	↑	0	Normal
Increased muscle tone (as from muscle relaxant reversal)	Normal	↑	0	Normal
Convulsions	Normal	↑	0	Normal
Hyperthermia	Normal	↑	0	Normal
Hypothermia	Normal	↓	0	Normal
Increased depth of anesthesia (in relation to surgical stimulus)	Normal	↓	0	Normal
Use of muscle relaxants	May see curare cleft	↓	0	Normal
Increased transport of CO_2 to the lungs (restoration of peripheral circulation after it has been impaired, e.g., after release of a tourniquet)	Normal	↑	0	Normal

[a] Normal end-tidal CO_2 is 38 torr (5%). Inspired CO_2 is normally 0. The arterial to end-tidal gradient is normally less than 5 torr.

TABLE 18.2. **Capnographic and Capnometric Alterations as a Result of Circulatory Changes**

	Waveform on Capnograph	End-Tidal CO_2	Inspiratory CO_2	End-Tidal to Arterial Gradient
Decreased transport of CO_2 to the lungs (impaired peripheral circulation)	Normal	↓	0	Normal
Decreased transport of CO_2 through the lungs (pulmonary embolus, either air or thrombus; surgical manipulations)	Normal	↓	0	Elevated
Right-to-left shunt	Normal	↑	0	Elevated
Increased patient dead space	Normal	↓	0	Elevated

TABLE 18.3. **Capnometry and Capnography with Respiratory Problems**

	Waveform on Capnograph	End-Tidal CO_2	Inspiratory CO_2	End-Tidal to Alveolar Gradient
Disconnection	Absent		0	
Apneic patient, stopped ventilator	Absent		0	
Hyperventilation	Normal	↓	0	Normal
Hypoventilation, mild to moderate	Normal	↑	0	Normal
Upper airway obstruction	Abnormal[a]	↑	0	Elevated
Rebreathing, e.g., (under drapes)	Baseline elevated	↑	↑	Normal
Esophageal intubation	Absent		0	

[a] See Figure 18.34.

TABLE 18.4. **Capnographic and Capnometric Alterations with Equipment**

Problem	Waveform on Capnograph	End-Tidal CO_2	Inspiratory CO_2	End-Tidal to Arterial Gradient
Increased apparatus dead space	Baseline Elevated	↑	↑	Normal
Rebreathing with circle system: faulty or exhausted absorbent, bypassed absorber (may be masked by high fresh gas flow)	Baseline Elevated See Figure 18.35	↑	↑	Normal
Rebreathing with Mapleson system (inadequate fresh gas flow, misassembly, problem with inner tube of Bain system)	Baseline Elevated See Figure 18.35	↑	↑	Decreased
Rebreathing due to malfunctioning non-rebreathing valve	Baseline Elevated See Figure 18.35	↑	↑	Decreased
Obstruction to expiration in the breathing system	See Figure 18.34	↑	0	Decreased
Blockage of sampling line	Absent	0	0	
Leakage in sampling line	See Figure 18.39	↓	0	Increased
Low sampling rate with diverting device	See Figure 18.41	↓	↑	Increased
Too high a sampling rate with diverting device	See Figure 18.42	↓	0	Increased
Inadequate seal around tracheal tube	See Figure 18.44	↓	0	Increased

taneously breathing patients, PetCO$_2$ may not increase as a result of hyperventilation (309, 310).

Metabolic causes of increases in expired CO_2 include increased temperature (311), shivering, convulsions, excessive production of catecholamines, administration of blood or bicarbonate (312, 313), release of an arterial clamp or tourniquet (314–319), glucose in the intravenous fluid (320), parenteral hyperalimentation (321), and CO_2 used to inflate the peritoneal cavity during laparoscopy (322–325), the pleural cavity during thorascopy (326) or a joint during arthroscopy (327). Extraperitoneal or subcutaneous insufflation of CO_2 increases end-tidal CO_2 more than intraperitoneal insufflation (328, 329).

Malignant hyperthermia is a hypermetabolic state with a massive increase in CO_2 production. The increase occurs early, before the rise in temperature. Early detection of this syndrome is one of the most important reasons for routinely monitoring CO_2 (298, 330–336). Capnometry can be used to monitor the effectiveness of treatment.

CO_2 production falls with decreased temperature, increased muscle relaxation, and increased depth of anesthesia (337).

Circulation

Table 18.2 lists some of the circulatory causes of changes in exhaled CO_2. A decrease in end-tidal CO_2 is seen with a decrease in cardiac output if ventilation remains constant (338–341).

In addition to reduced cardiac output, reduced blood flow to the lungs can result from surgical manipulations of the heart or thoracic vessels (342, 343), wedging of a pulmonary artery catheter, and pulmonary embolism (thrombus, tumor, gas, fat, marrow, or amniotic fluid) (344–350). If the embolized gas is CO_2, the end-tidal CO_2 may increase or decrease (351–355). Although not as sensitive as the Doppler for detecting air embolism, CO_2 monitoring is less subjective, is unaffected by electrosurgery apparatus, and can be used in major ear, nose, and throat cases for which the Doppler method is not applicable. Capnometry may not be sufficiently sensitive to detect fat and marrow microemboli (356).

During resuscitation, exhaled CO_2 is a better guide to the presence of circulation than the electrocardiogram (ECG), pulse, or blood pressure. The effectiveness of resuscitation measures can be gauged by capnometry (247, 357–368). The capnometer is not susceptible to the mechanical artifacts associated with chest compression, and chest compressions do not have to be interrupted to assess circulation. However, if high-dose epinephrine or bicarbonate is used, end-tidal CO_2 is not a good indicator of resuscitation measures (369–375).

End-tidal CO_2 levels may be of value in predicting the outcome of resuscitation (240, 358, 362–364, 376–382). A sudden increase in end-tidal CO_2 is an early clue that spontaneous cardiac output has been restored (367).

Exhaled CO_2 concentrations are helpful in determining which patients are likely to be successfully resuscitated. The patient is more likely to be resuscitated if the concentration of exhaled CO_2 is greater than 10 to 15 mm Hg (240, 377, 383, 384). With a colorimetric CO_2 detector, no color change despite correct tracheal intubation indicates that successful resuscitation is unlikely (248).

Epinephrine injected subcutaneously has been shown to increase the end-tidal CO_2. One possible explanation is that cardiac output may be increased with additional CO_2 being transported to the lungs. Peripheral vasoconstriction might increase central blood volume and pulmonary blood flow (385).

Respiration

CO_2 monitoring gives information about the rate, frequency, and depth of respiration. For patients breathing spontaneously, exhaled CO_2 levels can provide an estimate of the depth of anesthesia. CO_2 monitoring can be used to evaluate the patient's ability to breathe spontaneously as well as the effects of bronchodilator or nitric oxide treatment or changing ventilation parameters. It allows control of ventilation with fewer blood gas determinations. End-tidal analysis is noninvasive, available on a breath-by-breath basis and not affected by hyperventilation induced by drawing an arterial blood sample.

Table 18.3 lists some respiratory causes of increased and decreased end-tidal CO_2. A capnometer can warn of esophageal intubation, apnea, extubation, disconnection, ventilator malfunction, a change in compliance or resistance, partial obstruction of a tracheal tube, airway obstruction, poor mask fit, or a leaking tracheal tube cuff.

A dependable means to determine when a tracheal tube has been correctly positioned in the airway is obviously of great value. Placement of the tracheal tube in the esophagus has been a leading cause of death or cerebral damage in the past (386). A discussion of ways to detect inadvertent esophageal placement is found in Chapter 17, "Tracheal Tubes." CO_2 monitoring is usually considered the best method (387–389).

CO_2 detection of esophageal placement has some drawbacks and limitations. Bronchospasm, equipment malfunction, application of PEEP, or cricoid pressure occluding the tip of the tube can result in failure to detect CO_2 (390–393). The analyzer may be in a calibration mode when the tube is placed or a shared mass spectrometer system may be sampling another location.

If no effective pulmonary circulation is present during cardiopulmonary resuscitation, sufficient CO_2 may not be present in the lung to generate a waveform. This can result in confusion about the placement of the tracheal tube.

With esophageal intubation, small waveforms may be transiently seen as a result of CO_2 that has entered the stomach during mask ventilation or from carbonated beverages or medications (258–260, 394, 395). This could give the impression that the tube is correctly placed in the trachea. However, rapidly diminishing concentrations and abnormal waveforms will usually differentiate esophageal from tracheal intubation (388, 394, 396, 397).

While placement of the tube in the esophagus will most likely be detected using end-tidal CO_2, there is no guaranty that the tube is in the trachea. CO_2 could be sensed from a tracheal tube positioned above the vocal cords (398).

End-tidal CO_2 can aid in performing a blind oral or nasal intubation (399–405, 420). A capnograph is attached to the tracheal tube as it is being inserted into a spontaneously breathing patient and the CO_2 waveform and/or peak CO_2 level used as a guide. As the tube approaches the larynx, the CO_2 increases and decreases as it moves away.

As the tube is advanced and the tip passes between the vocal cords, a normal capnogram is observed.

Capnography can be used in conjunction with a jet stylet introducer in cases where the glottic opening cannot be visualized (406).

Capnography can be used to identify needle placement during transtracheal cricothyrotomy (407).

A CO_2 monitor can be used to monitor respiratory rate and exhaled CO_2 in unintubated patients breathing spontaneously (19, 20, 49, 60, 65, 76–81, 88, 408–410). Apnea and/or airway obstruction can be detected. If ventilation of the breathing space is inadequate, rebreathing will occur and can be detected by a rising inspired carbon dioxide level (78, 410). Although some studies have shown a poor correlation between the peak expired and arterial CO_2 using this method of monitoring (49, 411–414), others have yielded good results (20, 75, 78, 79, 415, 416). Peak CO_2 values correlate more closely with $PaCO_2$ values than average end-tidal levels (417). Poor correlation is associated with partial airway obstruction and high respiratory rates (417). Results may be improved by isolating insufflated O_2 from exhaled gases, observing the waveform for normal configuration, and decreasing the O_2 flow rate (79, 416, 418). In mouth breathers, the cannula may be realigned over the mouth or the mouth may be closed (419).

Capnometry has been used to help in determining proper position and detecting dislodgment of a double-lumen bronchial tube (421, 422). Correct placement can be checked by examining the waveform from each lung during clamping and unclamping procedures. However, it is somewhat less reliable than other methodologies used for this purpose (423–425).

CO_2 monitoring can serve as a warning of accidental bronchial intubation. This may result in a transient fall or rise in end-tidal CO_2 (426–428).

CO_2 monitoring can be used to aid in weaning patients from artificial ventilation (429–432). In pediatric seizure patients it provides an assessment of pulmonary status that can assist with the decision of whether to provide ventilatory support (433).

Patients who are partially paralyzed with muscle relaxants may make respiratory efforts. This can alert the anesthesia provider that the muscle relaxant is wearing off. It may occur anywhere in the respiratory cycle (Fig. 18.32). If the patient is spontaneously breathing and the depression occurs in the later third of the waveform it is referred to as a curare cleft (Fig. 18.31) (434).

Equipment Function

A problem with the breathing system can cause an inspired CO_2 level greater than zero. Examples of such problems are listed in Table 18.4 and include a leak, faulty or exhausted absorbent, channeling, a bypassed absorber, increased dead space, inadequate fresh gas flow to a Mapleson system, a defect in the inner tube of a Bain system, accidental administration of CO_2, and a defective nonrebreathing valve (435–442). With an expiratory valve leak, the inspired CO_2 level is inversely related to inspiratory flow, because as inspiratory flow increases, a smaller portion of each breath passes through the incompetent valve (436, 443, 444).

If the sample line is plugged, there will be a loss of waveform and no CO_2 detected (445). Misassembly of the capnometer can cause erroneous readings (446).

Correlation Between Arterial and End-Tidal Carbon Dioxide Levels

The relationship between arterial and end-tidal CO_2 tensions is affected by many factors. There may be a constant relationship or one which varies, sometimes in different directions both within and between patients (447). Although there is usually a linear relationship between end-tidal and arterial CO_2 levels, the gradient may be unexpectedly large, or even negative (448–452).

Numerous studies have shown that the correlation between arterial and end-tidal CO_2 tensions in children and adults without cardiorespiratory dysfunction is good enough to warrant routine monitoring (13, 453–463). End-tidal CO_2 is usually lower than $PaCO_2$ by 2 to 5 torr (464). The gradient may be less in pregnant patients and small children than in adults (13, 40, 457, 458, 465–467) and is reduced with rebreathing (468). Tables 18.1 through 18.4 show some conditions with altered gradients.

Problems with Sampling

The correlation between arterial and end-tidal CO_2 tensions is better during use of a laryngeal mask than face mask ventilation (469).

Accurate measurement of end-tidal CO_2 is especially difficult with high ventilatory frequencies and sidestream monitors (30). In small patients, distal sampling from the tracheal tube results in a closer approximation to arterial CO_2 than proximal sampling (40–44). Mainstream capnometers, while adding dead space and bulkiness, do not suffer from the problems associated with sampling and may yield end-tidal CO_2 values more closely approximating $PaCO_2$ in infants (13, 30, 44, 470, 471).

One possible source of sampling error is a leak at the interface of the patient and the equipment. Poor mask fit, use of an uncuffed tracheal tube or a tube with a defective cuff, or a loose connection or crack in the sampling catheter may cause an erroneously low end-tidal CO_2 reading.

Hypoventilation may result in a diminished expiratory flow rate. If the expiratory flow rate of the patient decreases below the rate of sampling, CO_2-free gases will be aspirated into the capnometer. This can result in erroneously low values of $PetCO_2$, particularly if the sampling flow rate is high. Use of lower sampling flows may produce more accurate end-tidal CO_2 readings.

While placing the gas sampling line on the patient side of a heat-moisture exchanger (HME) may avoid contamination and waterlogging of the sample, this may result in erroneous values (472).

With unintubated, spontaneously breathing patients most studies have shown good correlation between end-tidal and arterial CO_2, (20, 71, 75, 78, 79, 86, 416, 417, 473), although some have not (49, 410, 470, 474). Poor correlation is associated with partial airway obstruction, high respiratory rates, low tidal volumes, O_2 delivery through the ipsilateral nasal cannula and mouth breathing (82, 86, 417).

When a sidestream capnometer is used with a Mapleson system, dilution of exhaled gas by fresh gas can occur during the latter portion of expiration if the expiratory flow rate is less than the sampling flow rate of the capnometer. This will cause the measured end-tidal CO_2 level to be lowered even if the alveolar phase of the capnogram is flat or has a small positive slope (45, 465, 475). The magnitude of the lowering will depend on several factors, including whether spontaneous or controlled ventilation is used, the type of ventilator and breathing circuit, the fresh gas flow, the sampling rate and the expiratory flow rate (40, 42, 43, 45, 465–477). This is especially a problem in infants, because of their low expiratory flow rates. Studies show that the most proximal and acceptable site to sample CO_2 in infants is at the point of narrowing of the tracheal tube connector with the tracheal tube (478). In critically ill neonates, distal sampling may be necessary (44).

Maneuvers to obtain a $PetCO_2$ reading that is closer to the $PaCO_2$ with Mapleson systems include using lower fresh gas flows, extending the time of expiratory flow, adding dead space between the breathing system and gas sampling point, and using a circuit that automatically interrupts the fresh gas flow after inspiration or prevents mixing of exhaled and fresh gases (465, 479, 480). A quick method of checking to see whether the $PetCO_2$ is artifactually low is to temporarily disconnect the fresh gas supply (481). If there is an abrupt rise in $PetCO_2$ when the diluting effect of the fresh gas flow is removed, then the first breaths that follow will give a measure of the true $PetCO_2$.

Even with a circle system, dilution of exhaled gas may occur if the sampling site is far from the patient (45). If there is a break in the sample line or its connections, air will be added to the sample and the end-tidal CO_2 reading will be lower than the actual value (482, 483). An internal leak can result in artifactually high peak values (484).

If the rise time of the analyzer is prolonged, the end-tidal CO_2 reading may be falsely low with high respiratory rates (7). Rise time will be longer with lower sampling flow rates. For this reason, it has been recommended that a sampling flow rate less than 150 ml/min not be used (31). Kinking of the sampling catheter can cause the sampling flow rate to be decreased.

During high-frequency ventilation $PetCO_2$ is a poor index of $PaCO_2$ (485–487). For this reason, it is necessary to measure $PetCO_2$ by single tidal volume breaths during ventilation lapses (486, 488–490).

If a patient has not fully exhaled before the

next breath, the end-tidal value will be falsely low (14). In this situation, a gentle squeeze of the patient's chest or abdomen will often produce a sample of alveolar gas.

Disturbances in the Ventilation:Perfusion Ratio (268, 491)

In the lung, ideally a normally ventilated alveolus is adjacent to a normally perfused capillary. When there is ventilation-perfusion mismatching, the relationship between end-tidal and arterial tensions of CO_2 is disturbed.

Clinical conditions that can alter the volume and/or distribution of pulmonary blood flow include pulmonary embolism, stenosis or occlusion of the pulmonary artery, reduced cardiac output, pulmonary hypotension, and various heart lesions (342, 464, 492–496).

The end-tidal to arterial CO_2 gradient increases as venous admixture (right-to-left shunt) occurs (464). This can be caused by atelectasis, bronchial intubation, or certain heart conditions. The effect is less dramatic than that caused by an increase in dead space, but when the venous admixture is large (as in cyanotic congenital heart disease) its contribution can be considerable (453, 493, 495).

Changes in body position such as placement in the lateral decubitus position may cause an increase in the $Pa/PetCO_2$ gradient (497).

Patients with pulmonary disease have an uneven distribution of ventilation and, to a lesser extent, blood flow. This leads to an increased gradient (464, 459, 498–502). While the gradient can be decreased by using lower ventilatory rates and larger tidal volumes, these maneuvers do not improve estimation of arterial CO_2 from end-tidal CO_2 (503, 504).

After bilateral lung transplantation, there is marked alveolar deadspace ventilation which improves in the first hours after reperfusion. End-tidal CO_2 is not a reliable guide to $PaCO_2$ during this time (505).

PEEP can affect the gradient (506). It has been suggested that the gradient be used to titrate PEEP.

Capnometer Inaccuracy (3)

Factors related to the capnometer that may result in an inaccurate $PetCO_2$ reading include lack of display resolution, sampling system resistance, instability, changes in atmospheric pressure, temperature dependence, improper calibration, drift, noise, selectivity, pressure effects from the sampling system or patient environment, water vapor, and foreign substances (3). With some analyzers, the gas used for zeroing is obtained from room air. If CO_2-containing gas enters the zeroing sample, there will be a shift in the baseline and falsely low CO_2 readings with normal-looking waveforms (507).

Other

A significant discrepancy between $PaCO_2$ and $PetCO_2$ may occur in patients taking acetazolamide, which delays the conversion of HCO_3^- to CO_2, causing a decrease in end-tidal CO_2 (508).

End-tidal CO_2 is occasionally higher than arterial CO_2 (20, 417, 465, 477, 509–512). Causes include errors in calibration, rebreathing, and inadvertent addition of CO_2 to the inspired gas (195, 513–515). $PetCO_2$ may exceed $PaCO_2$ if functional residual capacity is reduced, as in pregnant or obese patients or during laparoscopy (457, 458, 467, 516).

Capnography (14, 105, 480, 517)

Most CO_2 monitors include a waveform. Many older capnometers have an analog output that can be connected to an oscilloscopic display for a low-cost capnograph (518). Most capnograms are calibrated so that values for end-tidal CO_2 can be estimated. Waveforms can be displayed on an oscilloscope or printed on paper. Slow speeds can be used to show trends. Faster speeds are used for examination of individual waveforms. Some capnographs have the ability to analyze waveforms and alert the viewer when they should be checked (519, 520).

Examination of the waveform will often explain readings that appear inaccurate. If the capnometer reads several peaks per breath (as can be seen with certain artifacts) or does not note breaths that do not have a plateau, the respiratory rate and peak CO_2 readings will be inaccurate. Misassembly or a leak in the capnometer can often be detected by examining the capnogram (446, 484).

The waveform should be examined systematically for height, frequency, rhythm, baseline, and shape. Height depends on the end-tidal level of CO_2. Frequency depends on the respiratory rate.

The baseline should be zero (unless CO_2 is deliberately added to the inspired gases or there is deliberate rebreathing without CO_2 absorption).

The volume of CO_2 in each breath is equal to the area under the curve of the capnogram. Adding individual breath volumes allows CO_2 production to be calculated.

Elevation of the baseline (Fig. 18.35) can result from deliberate administration of CO_2, rebreathing or artifact. One cause is parabolic distortion of CO_2 plugs traversing long sampling catheters (521). Elevations of the baseline are associated with exhausted absorbent or an incompetent expiratory unidirectional valve. The baseline may or may not be elevated with an incompetent inspiratory unidirectional valve, depending on the relationship between the volume of the inspiratory breathing hose and the tidal volume setting on the ventilator (11). A sudden elevation in both the baseline and end-tidal CO_2 usually indicates contamination of the sample cell with water, mucus, or dirt (105).

The shape of the normal waveform is illustrated in Figure 18.28. Only one shape (top hat or sine wave) is considered normal. Phase I begins at E. The CO_2 is zero.

Phase II begins at B and continues to C. As gas from alveoli begins to be exhaled, the level of CO_2 rises rapidly (BC). With airway obstruction, phase II will become slanted and shortened and may continue into Phase III.

Phase III begins at C and continues to just before D. As gas coming almost entirely from alveoli is exhaled, a plateau (CD), is seen. It includes expiratory flow and the expiratory pause. The very last portion of Phase III, identified by point D, is

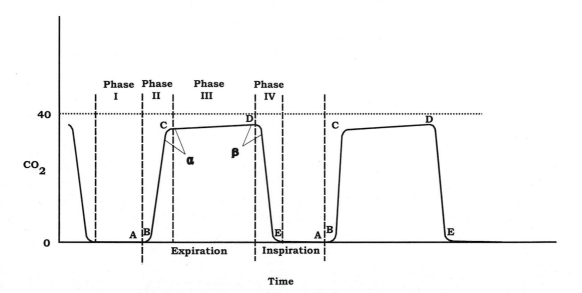

FIGURE 18.28.   Normal CO_2 waveform. **EA,** (Phase I) is the latter part of inspiration, during which the CO_2 level remains at zero. **BC,** (Phase II) represents the emptying of connecting airways and the beginning of the emptying of alveoli. As exhalation continues, gas from alveoli in regions with relatively short conducting airways appears and mixes with dead space gas from regions with relatively long conducting airways, resulting in an increasing CO_2 level. **CD,** (Phase III) shows the alveolar plateau. Because of uneven emptying of alveoli, the slope continues to rise gently. Point **D,** shows the best approximation of alveolar CO_2 (end of expiration, beginning of inspiration). In **DE,** (Phase IV) as the patient inhales, CO_2-free gas enters the patient's airway and the CO_2 level abruptly falls to zero. Characteristics of the normal capnogram include (1) rapid increase from **B** to **C**, (2) nearly horizontal plateau between **C**, and **D**, (3) rapid decrease from **D** to **E** to zero, and (4) a zero baseline (**EA, AB**). A good alveolar plateau greatly increases the chances that the end-tidal reading is a reliable estimate of the alveolar level.

termed the end-tidal point. The CO_2 level here is at its maximum. In normal individuals this is 5 to 5.5%, or 35 to 40 torr.

The angle between Phases II and III is called the α angle. Normally it is between 100 and 110°. It increases as the slope of Phase III increases. The slope of Phase III depends on the ventilation/perfusion status of the lung. Airway obstruction causes an increased slope and a larger angle (301, 461, 522). Other factors that affect the angle are the response time of the capnometer, sweep speed, and the respiratory cycle time (301).

The angle between the end of Phase III and the descending limb of the capnogram is called the β angle. It is normally approximately 90°. This angle is used to assess the extent of rebreathing. If there is rebreathing, the angle will be increased. Another possible cause of an increased β angle is a prolonged response time compared to the respiratory cycle time of the patient, particularly in children (301).

In Phase IV the patient inhales, and the level of CO_2 falls abruptly to zero and remains at zero until the next exhalation.

Examination of the waveform will reveal whether or not an alveolar plateau is present. If it is not, the maximum value obtained may not be equivalent to the end-tidal level and the correlation between arterial and end-tidal CO_2 is not likely to be good.

Loss or absence of a CO_2 waveform has a number of possible implications. It could mean that the gas being sampled does not contain CO_2 as would be the case if the tracheal tube was not in the trachea. It could mean that there was no circulation to the lung. It could mean that there was a disconnection or obstruction in the sample line (523). Another possible cause is a fault with the monitor or an automatic recalibration.

A number of special situations can be demonstrated by waveform analysis. Some special waveforms are shown in Figures 18.29–18.47.

Volatile Anesthetic Agents

The measurement of concentrations of volatile anesthetic gases is becoming common practice. In some countries (but not the United States at the time of writing) it is a standard of care (166).

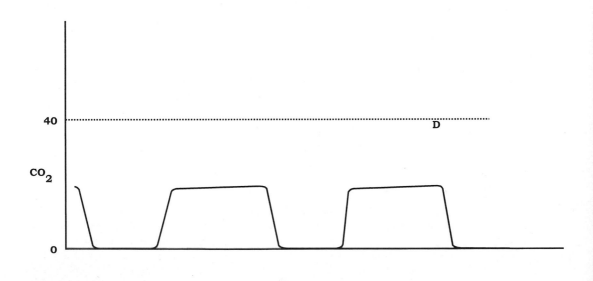

FIGURE 18.29. Low end-tidal carbon dioxide (CO_2) with a good alveolar plateau may be the result of hyperventilation or an increase in dead space ventilation. Comparison of $PetCO_2$ with partial pressure of carbon dioxide in arterial gas ($PaCO_2$) is necessary to distinguish these two conditions.

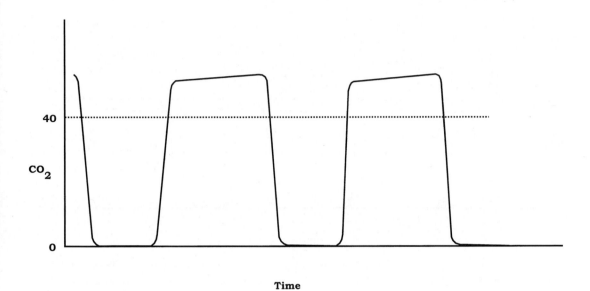

FIGURE 18.30. Elevated end-tidal carbon dioxide (CO_2) with good alveolar plateau may be caused by hypoventilation or increased CO_2 delivery to the lungs.

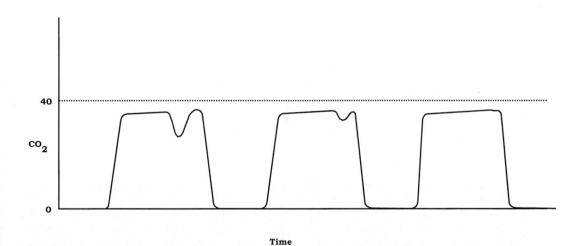

FIGURE 18.31. Curare cleft or notch, which is seen during spontaneous ventilation. The capnogram on the *left* shows the notch. As the muscle relaxant is reversed the curve becomes normal in shape. The cleft is in the last third of the plateau and is caused by a lack of synchronous action between the intercostal muscles and the diaphragm most commonly caused by inadequate muscle relaxant reversal. The depth of the cleft is proportional to the degree of muscle paralysis. The notch also is seen in patients with cervical transverse lesions, flail chest, hiccups, and pneumothorax and when a patient tries to breathe during mechanical ventilation.

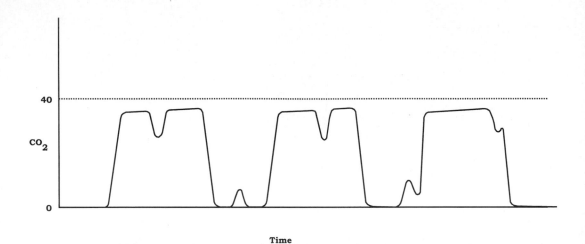

FIGURE **18.32.** Spontaneous respiratory efforts during mechanical ventilation. The capnogram shows small breaths at various places during expiration and inspiration. Causes include improper ventilator settings, inadequate muscle paralysis, severe hypoxia, or the patient waking up. The end-tidal carbon dioxide (CO_2) may rise slightly because of increasing metabolism of the contracting respiratory muscles. This pattern may also be caused by pressure on the patient's chest or ventilator malfunction (323).

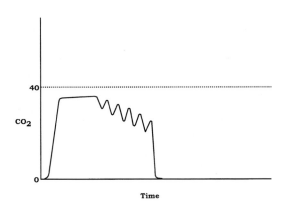

FIGURE **18.33.** Cardiogenic oscillations appear as small, regular, tooth-like humps at the end of the expiratory phase. They may be single or multiple and the heights may vary considerably. They are believed to be due to the contraction and relaxation of the heart and intrathoracic great vessels on the lungs, forcing air in and out. The rate of oscillation matches that of a simultaneously recorded heart rate on the electrocardiogram (ECG). A number of factors contribute to the appearance of cardiogenic oscillations, including negative intrathoracic pressure, a low respiratory rate, diminution in the vital capacity:heart size ratio, a low inspiratory: expiratory ratio, low tidal volumes, and muscular relaxation (324, 325, 519). In many cases, adjustment of the ventilator rate, flow, or tidal volume will remove this pattern from the screen. Other times, however, it cannot be corrected. Cardiogenic oscillations are the rule rather than the exception in pediatric patients because of the relative size of the infant's heart and thorax (326). Capnograms from patients with severe emphysema tend not to register cardiogenic oscillations. Less sophisticated capnometers may count each oscillation as a breath, displaying an artificially high respiratory rate.

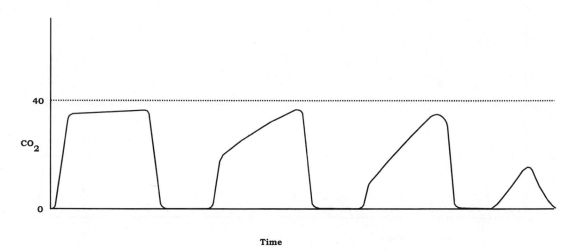

FIGURE 18.34. Prolonged expiratory upstroke. At the *left* is a normal waveform. The other three curves show progressive slanting and prolongation of the expiratory upstroke. As expiration is progressively prolonged, inspiration may start before expiration is complete so that the end-tidal CO_2 reading is decreased. This is indicative of obstruction to gas flow caused by a partially obstructed tracheal tube or obstruction in the patient's airways (chronic obstructive lung disease, bronchospasm, or upper-airway obstruction).

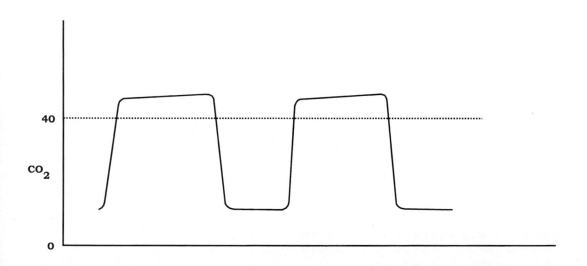

FIGURE 18.35. The baseline is elevated, and the waveform is normal in shape. This may be caused by an incompetent expiratory valve or exhausted absorbent in the circle system, insufficient fresh gas flow to a Mapleson system, problems with the inner tube of a Bain system, deliberate addition of CO_2 to the fresh gas, or in some cases, an incompetent inspiratory valve. It may also be the result of rebreathing under drapes in a spontaneous breathing patient who is not intubated (238, 327).

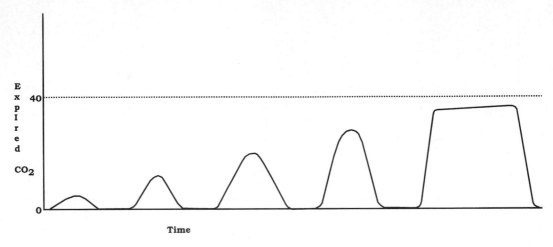

FIGURE 18.36. Return to spontaneous ventilation. The first breath is typically of small volume. Subsequent breaths show progressively higher peaks with gradual resumption of a normal waveform.

FIGURE 18.37. Incompetent inspiratory unidirectional valve. The waveform shows a prolonged plateau and a slanting inspiratory downstroke. The inspiratory phase is shortened, and the baseline may or may not reach zero, depending on the fresh gas flow (261, 264, 328). A similar pattern may be seen with suction applied to a chest tube (329).

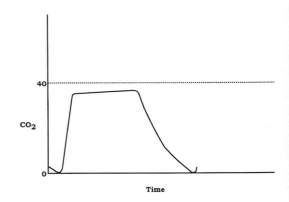

FIGURE 18.38. Irregular plateau and/or baseline may result from displacement of the tracheal tube into the upper larynx or lower pharynx with intermittent ventilation of the stomach and lungs or from pressure on the chest which causes small volumes of gas to move in and out of the lungs.

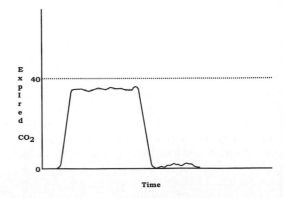

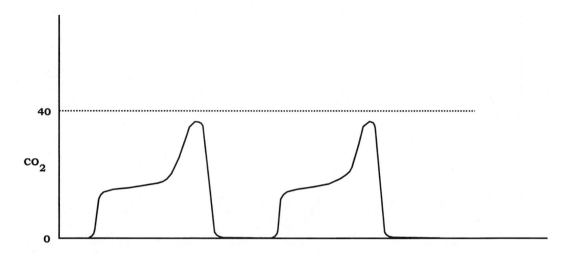

FIGURE 18.39.   A leak in the sampling line during positive pressure ventilation will result in an upswing at the end of phase III (59, 172, 330, 541). A plateau of long duration is followed by a peak of brief duration. The height of the plateau is inversely proportional to the size of the leak. The brief peak is caused by the next inspiration when positive pressure transiently pushes undiluted end-tidal gas through the sampling line. If nitrogen is being monitored, an increase will be noted. This pattern is not seen if the patient is breathing spontaneously. A falsely low end-tidal CO_2 reading can be obtained owing to air entrainment, but no terminal hump is seen. An upswing at the end of phase III may also be seen in obese and pregnant patients (301).

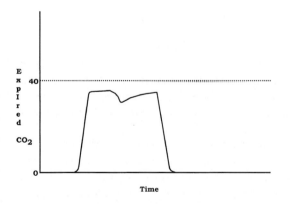

FIGURE 18.40.   If the compliance, airway resistance, or ventilation-perfusion ratios in one lung differ substantially from the other lung, a biphasic expiratory plateaus may be seen (542). This type of capnogram has been reported in a patient with severe kyphoscoliosis (543) and following single lung transplantation (544).

Standard Requirements

A U.S. standard for anesthetic gas monitors is available (6). The following are provisions of that document.

1. For halogenated anesthetic gases, the difference between the mean anesthetic gas reading and the anesthetic gas level shall be within ± (0.15% vol % + 15% of the anesthetic gas level). In addition, six standard deviations (SD) of the anesthetic gas readings shall be less than or equal to 0.6 vol %. This means that greater than 68% of all readings occur within 0.1 vol % of the mean reading, over 95% of all readings occur within 0.2 vol % of the mean reading, and more than 99% of all readings occur within 0.3 vol % of the mean reading.

2. High concentration alarms are mandatory. Low concentration alarms are optional. The alarm set point for both high and low concen-

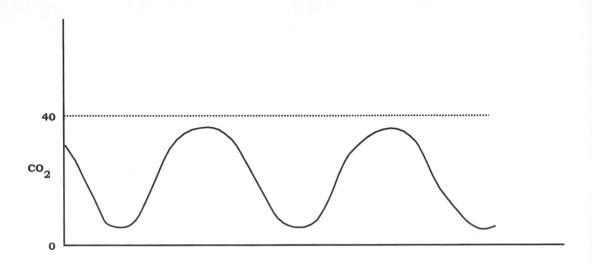

FIGURE 18.41. Too low a sampling rate with a side-stream capnometer will result in a low peak and, often, elevation of the baseline. Erroneous values for both inspired and end-tidal carbon dioxide will be reported.

tration alarms must be operator adjustable. The high gas reading alarm(s) shall be medium priority. If low concentrations alarm(s) are provided, they must be low priority.

Measurement Techniques

Volatile anesthetic agents can be measured using mass spectrometry, Raman analysis, IR analysis, refractometry (266) or oscillating crystal technology. Response times for volatile agent monitors vary (524). Factors that decrease the response time include decreasing the length or internal diameter of the sample tube and increasing the sampling flow. The composition of the sample line is important; the partition coefficient of the halogenated agent in the material of a tube correlates with the response time (524).

Usefulness of Anesthetic Agent Monitoring (525)

Vaporizer Function and Contents

An advantage of monitoring potent agents is the ability to assess the output of a vaporizer. Agent-specific analyzers can detect an incorrect agent, and non-agent-specific analyzers will usually exhibit unusual readings when an agent error is made. They also allow determination of the concentration of agent when a setting below the lowest calibration on a vaporizer is dialed or when the vaporizer is used with gas flows outside those for which it is calibrated. Finally, anesthetic agent monitoring will alert the user when a vaporizer has become empty or is turned off.

Inadvertent Administration

Anesthetic agent monitors can detect a vaporizer inadvertently left in the on position. They can also detect when a vaporizer not in use is allowing significant amounts of vapor to leak into the fresh gas line.

Information on Uptake and Elimination

Monitoring volatile anesthetic agents provides information on uptake and elimination. The difference between inspired and expired levels provides a measure of patient saturation.

Teaching Low-Flow Anesthesia

Anesthetic agent monitoring can be used to demonstrate the relationship between levels in the fresh gas line and those in the breathing system. This makes them useful in teaching low-flow anesthesia.

Information on Anesthetic Depth

Knowledge of volatile agent concentrations may provide evidence that the patient who is paralyzed is neither awake nor grossly overdosed, per-

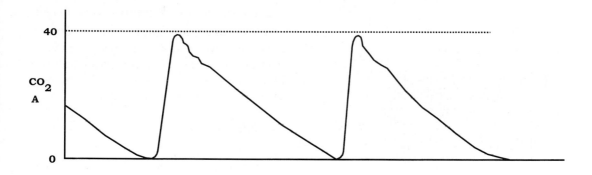

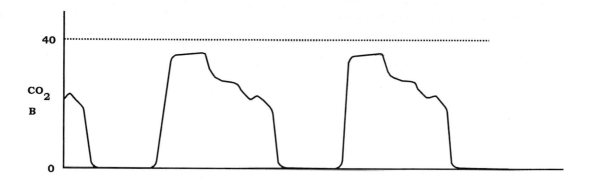

Time

FIGURE 18.42.   Contamination of expired sample by fresh gas or ambient air may be caused by placing the sampling site too near the fresh gas inlet, a leak, or too high a sampling flow rate. **A,** A large leak is indicated by the progressive decrease in the plateau. **B,** Here, the contamination is of lesser magnitude and a drop occurs at the end of the plateau.

mit more rapid awakening of the patient, and aid in the diagnosis of delayed emergence. Awareness due to a low concentration of inhalational agent may be avoided (526).

Studies show that volatile anesthetic agents are involved in up to one-third of cardiac arrests in anesthesia (525, 527). End-tidal concentrations of volatile anesthetic agents can be used as a measure of anesthetic depth.

However, caution should be exercised. A study on anesthetized patients found that prediction of arterial levels from end-tidal concentrations was difficult (528). Improvement in intraoperative hemodynamic stability or early recovery with either high or low total gas flows has not been found with agent monitoring (529–531). Anesthetic

agent monitoring should not be regarded as a replacement for other means of measuring depth, but as an additional source of information.

Detection of Contaminants

Contaminants in the nitrous oxide supply were detected with an agent monitor that indicated the presence of a volatile agent when no vaporizer was turned on (532).

Nitrous Oxide
Technology

Nitrous oxide can be measured by IR, mass spectrometry, or Raman scattering technology.

Standard Requirements

The standard for anesthetic gas monitors (6) requires that the difference between the mean

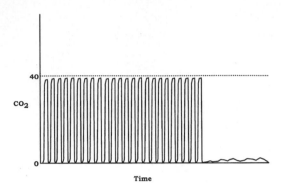

FIGURE **18.43.** A sudden drop of end-tidal carbon dioxide (CO_2) to zero is usually caused by an acute event relating to the airway, such as extubation, esophageal intubation, complete breathing system disconnection, ventilator malfunction, or a totally obstructed tracheal tube. It may also be the result of a plugged gas sampling tube.

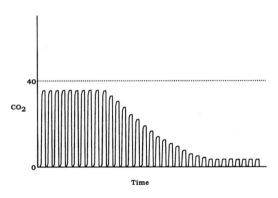

FIGURE **18.44.** The causes of a sudden drop of end-tidal carbon dioxide (CO_2) to a low but nonzero value include a poorly fitting tracheal tube or mask, a leak or partial disconnection in the breathing system, and a partial obstruction of the tracheal tube.

reading and the actual nitrous oxide level be within ($\pm$ 2.0 vol % + 8%) of the nitrous oxide level. In addition, 6 standard deviations (SD) of the nitrous oxide reading (for a given level) shall be less than or equal to 10.0 vol %. This means that more than 68% of all readings occur within 1.7 vol % of the mean reading, over 95% of all readings occur within 3.3 vol % of the mean reading, and more than 99% of all readings occur within 5.0 vol % of the mean reading.

Significance of Nitrous Oxide Levels

Analysis of nitrous oxide will show whether the flowmeters are functioning properly. At the end of a case, the washout of nitrous oxide will avoid diffusion hypoxia. A decrease may be caused by entrainment of room air (281, 533).

Nitrogen (525)
Technology

Nitrogen can be measured only by mass spectrometry or Raman scattering. Intermittent monitoring with a shared mass spectrometer could miss a sudden increase in nitrogen (534).

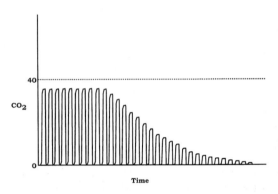

FIGURE **18.45.** Events that cause an exponential decrease in end-tidal carbon dioxide (CO_2) include sudden hypotension owing to massive blood loss or obstruction of a major blood vessel, circulatory arrest with continued pulmonary ventilation, and pulmonary embolism (air, clot, thrombus, or marrow).

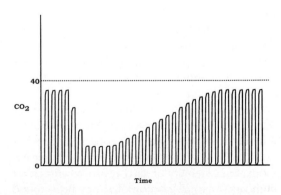

FIGURE **18.46.** Small air embolus with resolution.

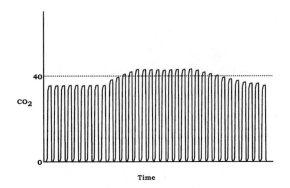

FIGURE **18.47.** Release of a tourniquet or unclamping of a major vessel may result in a sudden increase in end-tidal carbon dioxide (CO_2) that gradually returns to normal.

Significance

Verifying Adequate Denitrogenation

An important use of nitrogen monitoring is to ensure adequate denitrogenation before induction. This is especially a concern with pediatric patients, patients with lung disease, and patients with a reduced functional residual capacity (e.g., obesity or pregnancy) as well as during a rapid sequence induction.

Detection of Venous Air Emboli (535, 536)

A rise in exhaled nitrogen may indicate that air from some source has entered the breathing system. During certain surgical procedures, this is most likely the result of air entering a venous sinus or open vein, provided that the breathing system is tight enough that no air can be entrained. Used in connection with CO_2 monitoring, nitrogen monitoring can provide information helpful in distinguishing between air emboli from other events that cause reduced CO_2 elimination.

Monitoring Breathing System Integrity

Normally, during general anesthesia the level of nitrogen in the breathing system drops rapidly at first then more slowly. A slow drop or a rise may be caused by room air entering through a leak, disconnection, poorly fitting mask, an uncuffed tracheal tube, or breathing out of synchrony with a ventilator (533, 537).

A leak in the sampling system can cause nitrogen to be detected (100, 538). To determine if this is occurring, pure O_2 from the anesthesia ma-chine should be sampled. If the monitor continues to show nitrogen, air is leaking into the sampling line.

Detecting Nitrogen Accumulation

In spite of high initial gas flows, excreted nitrogen can build up in the breathing system during low-flow anesthesia. Nitrogen levels as high as 15% have been reported (539). Such a level can cause a significant decrease in the levels of O_2, nitrous oxide, and volatile agents.

Carbon Monoxide

No operating monitor is available for carbon monoxide but detection of mixed agents with isoflurane or desflurane anesthesia and a small increase in nitrogen and CO_2 may be seen with the mass spectrometer. (120, 121, 128). Infrared analyzers were less effective at detection and may not give any indication (540).

REFERENCES

1. Cooper JB, Newbower RS, Kitz RJ. An analysis of major errors and equipment failure in anesthesia management. Considerations for prevention and detection. Anesthesiology 1984;60:34–42.
2. Caplan RA, Posner KL, Ward RJ, et al. Adverse respiratory events in anesthesia: A closed claims analysis. Anesthesiology 1990;72:828–833.
3. Raemer DB, Calalang I. Accuracy of end-tidal carbon dioxide tension analyzers. Journal of Clinical Monitoring 1991;7:195–208.
4. American Society for Testing and Materials. Specification for oxygen monitors (F-1462-93). West Conshohocken, PA: ASTM, 1993.
5. American Society for Testing and Materials. Specification for capnometers (F-1456-92). West Conshohocken, PA: ASTM, 1992.
6. American Society for Testing and Materials. Specification for the minimum performance and safety requirements for components and systems of anesthetic gas monitors (F-1452-92). West Conshohocken, PA: ASTM, 1992.
7. Brunner JX, Westinskow DR. How the rise time of carbon dioxide analyzers influences the accuracy of carbon dioxide measurements. Br J Anaesth 1988; 61:628–638.
8. Breen PH, Mazumdar B, Skinner SC. Capnometer transport delay: measurement and clinical implications. Anesth Analg 1994;78:584–586.
9. Block FE, McDonald JS. Sidestream versus mainstream carbon dioxide analyzers. Journal of Clinical Monitoring 1992;8:139–141.

10. Deluty SH. Capnography: how does it work and what can we learn from it? Progress in Anesthesiology 1990;4:273–288.

11. Good ML. Principles and practice of capnography (ASA Refresher Course #226). New Orleans: ASA, 1996.

12. Kinsella SM. Assessment of the Hewlett-Packard HP47210A capnometer. Br J Anaesth 1985;57: 919–923.

13. Badgwell JM, Heavner JE. End-tidal carbon dioxide pressure in neonates and infants measured by aspiration and flow-through capnography. Journal of Clinical Monitoring 1991;7:285–288.

14. Swedlow DB. Capnometry and capnography. The anesthesia disaster early warning system. Semin Anesth 1986;5:194–205.

15. Quarmby R, Schmitt L. A simple, inexpensive device to prevent airway disconnection when using remote capnometry. Anesth Analg 1989;69:414–415.

16. Hurley MR, Paull JD. A spuriously low end-tidal carbon dioxide. Anaesthesia and Intensive Care 1991; 19:615–616.

17. Ornstein E. False-positive abrupt decrease in EtCO$_2$ during craniotomy in the sitting position. Anesthesiology 1985;62:542.

18. Reder RF, Brown EG, DeAsla RA, et al. Thermal skin burns from a carbon dioxide analyzer in children. Ann Thoracic Surg 1983;35:329–330.

19. Marks LF. Monitoring of tidal carbon dioxide in spontaneously breathing patients using a mainstream analyzing monitor. Anaesthesia 1991;46:154–155.

20. Lenz G, Heipertz W, Epple E. Capnometry for continuous postoperative monitoring of nonintubated, spontaneously breathing patients. Journal of Clinical Monitoring 1991;7:245–248.

21. Pesonen P, Luukonen P. Use of a capnometer to detect leak of carbon dioxide during laparoscopic surgery. Anesthesiology 1992;76:661.

22. Lenoir RJ. Hewlett-Packard HP4720A capnometer. Br J Anaesth 1986;58:1204.

23. Anonymous. Hewlett-Packard Model 47210A Capnometers. Technology for Anesthesia 1987;8(2): 4–5.

24. Russell WJ, Webb RK, van der Walt JH, et al. Problems with ventilation: an analysis of 2000 incident reports. Anaesthesia and Intensive Care 1993;21: 617–620.

25. Webb RK, Russell WJ, Klepper I, et al. Equipment failure: analysis of 2000 incident reports. Anaesthesia and Intensive Care 1993;21:673–677.

26. Shankar KB, Kannan S. Prevention of occlusion of sampling tubes in side-stream capnographs. Can J Anaesth 1997;44:453.

27. Sprung J, Cheng EY. Modification to an anesthesia breathing circuit to prolong monitoring of gases during the use of humidifiers. Anesth Analg 1991;72: 264–265.

28. Paulsen AW. Factors influencing the relative accuracy of long-line time-shared mass spectrometry. Biomed Instrum Technol 1989;23:476–480.

29. Scamman FL. Accuracy of a central mass spectrometer system at high respiratory frequencies. Journal of Clinical Monitoring 1988;4:227–229.

30. From RP, Scamman FL. Ventilatory frequency influences accuracy of end-tidal CO$_2$ measurements. Anesth Analg 1988;67:884–886.

31. Gravenstein N. Capnometry in infants should not be done at lower sampling flow rates. Journal of Clinical Monitoring 1989;5:63–64.

32. Epstein RA, Reznik AM, Epstein MAF. Determinants of distortions in CO$_2$ catheter sampling systems. A mathematical model. Respir Physiol 1980; 41:127–136.

33. Beaumont AC, Diamond JG. CO$_2$ measurement and the Minilink system. Anaesthesia 1989;44:535.

34. Friederich JA, Brooker RF. A pediatric end-tidal carbon dioxide sampling port. Anesth Analg 1994;79: 198.

35. Reid MF, Matthews A. A simple arrangement to sample expired gas in small children. Anaesthesia 1988; 43:902–903.

36. Levytam S, Kavanagh BP, Cooper RM, et al. Distal tracheal capnography following general anesthesia. Anesth Analg 1993;76:S223.

37. Duthie GM. Measurement of end-tidal carbon dioxide tension in adults. Anaesthesia 1984;39:605.

38. Levytam S, Kavanagh BP, Cooper RM, et al. Distal tracheal capnography following general anesthesia. Anesth Analg 1993;76:S223.

39. Mather SJ. Capnography in babies and small children. Anaesthesia 1994;49:1096–1097.

40. Badgwell JM, McLeod ME, Lerman J, et al. End-tidal PCO$_2$ measurements sampled at the distal and proximal ends of the endotracheal tube in infants and children. Anesth Analg 1987;66:959–964.

41. Hillier SC, Badgwell JM, McLeod E, et al. Accuracy of end-tidal PCO$_2$ measurements using a sidestream capnometer in infants and children ventilated with the Sechrist infant ventilator. Can J Anaesth 1990; 37:318–321.

42. McEvedy BAB, McLeod ME, Mulera M, et al. End-tidal, transcutaneous, and arterial PCO$_2$ measurements in critically ill neonates. A comparative study. Anesthesiology 1988;69:112–116.

43. Rich GF, Sullivan MP, Adams JM. Is distal sampling of end-tidal CO$_2$ necessary in small subjects. Anesthesiology 1990;73:265–268.

44. McEvedy BAB, McLeod ME, Kirpalani H, et al. End-tidal carbon dioxide measurements in critically ill neonates: a comparison of sidestream and mainstream capnometers. Can J Anaesth 1990;37:322–326.

45. Schieber RA, Namnoum A, Sugden A, et al. Accuracy of expiratory carbon dioxide measurements in small subjects. Journal of Clinical Monitoring 1985;1:149–155.

46. Beaumont AC, Diamond JG. CO_2 measurement and the Minilink system. Anaesthesia 1989;44:535.

47. Machin JR, MacNeil A. Gas sampling from a face mask for capnography. Anaesthesia 1986;41:971.

48. Bredas P, Bardoczky I, Wathieu M. Simple capnometry during inhalational anesthesia with mask ventilation. Journal of Clinical Monitoring 1991;7:108–109.

49. Norman EA, Zeig NJ, Ahmad I. Better designs for mass spectrometer monitoring of the awake patient. Anesthesiology 1986;64:664.

50. Machin JR, MacNeil A. Gas sampling from a face mask for capnography. Anaesthesia 1986;41:971.

51. Campbell FA, Bissonnette B. End-tidal carbon dioxide measurement in infants and children during and after general anaesthesia. Can J Anaesth 1994;41:107–110,

52. Ball AJ. Pediatric capnography. Anaesthesia 1995;50:833–834.

53. Newell S, Brimacombe J. A modified tracheal tube mount for sampling gases from the distal shaft of the laryngeal mask airway. J Clin Anesth 1995;7:444–445.

54. Spahr–Schopfer IA, Bissonnette B, Hartley EJ. Capnometry and the paediatric laryngeal mask airway. Can J Anaesth 1993;40:1038–1043.

55. Chhibber AK, Kolano JW, Roberts WA. Relationship between end-tidal and arterial carbon dioxide with laryngeal mask airways and endotracheal tubes in children. Anesth Analg 1996;82:247–250.

56. Chhibber AK, Fickling K, Kolano JW, et al. Comparison of end-tidal and arterial carbon dioxide in infants using laryngeal mask airway and endotracheal tube. Anesth Analg 1997;84:51–53.

57. Hicks IR, Soni NC, Shephard JN. Comparison of end-tidal and arterial carbon dioxide measurements during anaesthesia with the laryngeal mask airway. Br J Anaesth 1993;71:734–735.

58. Evans D. New oxygen mask for clinical practice. Reg Anes 1995;20:80–81.

59. Frankell R, Karram T, Simon K. Monitoring during sedation. Anaesthesia 1990;45:786–787.

60. Pressman MA. A simple method of measuring $ETCO_2$ during MAC and major regional anesthesia. Anesth Analg 1988;67:905–906.

61. Asai T. Fixation of capnograph sampling tube to a Hudson mask. Anaesthesia 1994;49:745.

62. Risdall JE, Geraghty IF. Respiratory monitoring in patients undergoing regional anaesthesia. Anaesthesia 1994;49:179.

63. Skjellerup N. Respiratory monitoring for regional anaesthesia. Anaesthesia 1994;49:1097.

64. Lee G, Shankleton E, Bodlander FMS. Monitoring respiration in sedated patients. Anaesthesia and Intensive Care 1994;22:497.

65. Inomata S, Nishikawa T. Early detection of airway obstruction with a capnographic probe attached to an oxygen mask. Can J Anaesth 1992;39:744.

66. Ackerman WE, Phero JC, Reaume D. End-tidal carbon dioxide and respiratory rate measurement during conscious sedation through a nasal cannula. Anesth Prog 1990;37:199–200.

67. Herrera A, Suan C, Perez–Torres MC, et al. Capnography and oxigraphy monitoring in non-intubated patients. Br J Anaesth 1997;78:20.

68. Reah G. Nasal cannulae and capnography for all. Anaesthesia 1995;50:95–96.

69. Shah MG, Epstein L. Measurement of carbon dioxide at both nares and mouth using standard nasal cannula. Anesthesiology 1994;81:779–780.

70. Tobias JD, Flanagan J, Garrett J, et al. End-tidal CO_2 monitoring via nasal cannulae in spontaneously breathing children. Crit Care Med 1994;22:A146.

71. Tobias JD, Flanagan JFK, Wheeler TJ, et al. Noninvasive monitoring of end-tidal CO_2 via nasal cannulas in spontaneously breathing children during the perioperative period. Crit Care Med 1994;22:1805–1808.

72. Hunter JA. A cost-free, simple method for monitoring end-tidal carbon dioxide through nasal cannulae. Anesth Prog 1990;37:301–303.

73. Tsui BCH. A simple method with no additional cost for monitoring $ETCO_2$ using a standard nasal cannulae. Can J Anaesth 1997;44:787–788.

74. Derrick SJ, Waters H, Kang SW, et al. Evaluation of a nasal/oral discriminate sampling system for capnographic respiratory monitoring. J Am Assoc Nurse Anesth 1993;61:509–520.

75. Bowe EA, Boysen PG, Broome JA, et al. Accurate determination of end-tidal carbon dioxide during administration of oxygen by nasal cannulae. Journal of Clinical Monitoring 1989;5:105–110.

76. Desmarattes R, Kennedy R, Davis DR. Inexpensive capnography during monitored anesthesia care. Anesth Analg 1990;71:100–101.

77. Goldman JM. A simple, easy, and inexpensive method for monitoring $ETCO_2$ through nasal cannulae. Anesthesiology 1987;67:606.

78. Gallacher BP. The measurement of end-tidal carbon dioxide concentrations using modified nasal prongs in ophthalmologic patients under regional anesthesia. Reg Anesth 1991;16:189.

79. Roy J, McNulty SE, Torjman MC. An improved nasal prong apparatus for end-tidal carbon dioxide monitoring in awake sedated patients. Journal of Clinical Monitoring 1991;7:249-252.

80. Turner KE, Sandler AN, Vosu HA. End-tidal CO_2 monitoring in spontaneously breathing adults. Can J Anaesth 1989;36:248–249.

81. Zimmerman D, Loken RG. Modified nasal cannula to monitor $ETCO_2$. Can J Anaesth 1992;39:1119.

82. Friesen RH, Alswang M. End-tidal PCO_2 monitoring via nasal cannulae in pediatric patients: accuracy and sources of error. Journal of Clinical Monitoring 1996;12:155–159.

83. Roth JV, Barth LJ, Womack LH, et al. Evaluation of two commercially available carbon dioxide sampling nasal cannulae. Journal of Clinical Monitoring 1994; 10:237–243.

84. Jones D, Rushmer J, McIntyre A, et al. Airway monitoring in the post anaesthetic recovery room. Anaesthesia and Intensive Care 1996;24:115–116.

85. Lenz G, Heipertz W, Epple E. Capnometry for continuous postoperative monitoring of nonintubated, spontaneously breathing patients. Journal of Clinical Monitoring 1991;7:245–248.

86. Oberg B, Waldau T, Larsen VH. The effect of nasal oxygen flow and catheter position on the accuracy of end-tidal carbon dioxide measurements by a pharyngeal catheter in unintubated, spontaneously breathing patients. Anaesthesia 1995;50:695–698.

87. Athayde J, Cooper RM, Sandler AN. Use of endotracheal ventilation catheter in monitoring end-tidal CO_2 in postoperative cardiac patients after "early extubation." Anesth Analg 1994;78:S13.

88. Bonsu AK, Tamilarasan A, Bromage PR. A nasal catheter for monitoring tidal carbon dioxide in spontaneously breathing patients. Anesthesiology 1989;71: 318.

89. Gottschalk A, Edwards MW. A simple device to enable capnography during jet ventilation for laryngoscopy. Anesthesiology 1993;79:620–621.

90. Gottschalk A, Mirza N, Weinstein GS, et al. Capnography during jet ventilation for laryngoscopy. Anesth Analg 1997;85:155–159.

91. Ward KR, Menegazzi JJ, Yealy DM, et al. Trans laryngeal jet ventilation and end-tidal pCO_2 monitoring during varying degrees of upper airway obstruction. Ann Emerg Med 1991;20:1193–1197.

92. Craen RA, Hickman JA. Use of end-tidal CO_2 sampling connector to administer bronchodilators into the anaesthetic circuit. Anaesthesia and Intensive Care 1991;19:299–300.

93. Fazlollah TM, Tosone SR. End-tidal carbon dioxide monitoring may help diagnosis of H-type tracheoesophageal fistula. Anesthesiology 1995;83:878–879.

94. Read MS, John G. Capnography and broncho-esophageal fistula. Anaesthesia 1992;47:1102.

95. Asai T, Stacey M: Confirmation of feeding tube position; how about capnography? Anaesthesia 1994;49: 451.

96. Patteson SK, Chesney JT. Anesthetic management for magnetic resonance imaging: problems and solutions. Anesth Analg 1992;74:121–128.

97. Peden CJ, Menon DK, Hall AS, et al. Magnetic resonance for the anaesthetist. Part II. Anaesthesia and monitoring in MR units. Anaesthesia 1992;47: 508–517.

98. Shellock FG. Monitoring sedated pediatric patients during MR imaging. Radiology 1990;177:586–587.

99. Eisenkraft JB, Raemer DB. Monitoring gases in the anesthesia delivery system. In: Ehrenwerth J, Eisenkraft JB, eds. Anesthesia equipment. Principles and applications. New York: CV Mosby, 1993:201–220.

100. Skeehan TM, Biebuyck JF. Erroneous mass spectrometer data caused by a faulty patient sampling tube: case report and laboratory study. Journal of Clinical Monitoring 1991;7:313–319.

101. Raynond RN, Tolley PM. Water damage to capnography equipment. Anaesthesia and Intensive Care 1992;20:249.

102. Carlon GC, Miodownik S, Ray C, et al. An automated mechanism for protection of mass spectrometry sampling tubing. Journal of Clinical Monitoring 1988; 4:264–266.

103. Mushlin PS, Mark JB, Elliott WR, et al. Inadvertent development of subatmospheric airway pressure during cardiopulmonary bypass. Anesthesiology 1989; 71:459–462.

104. Sodol IE, Clark JS, Swanson GD. Mass spectrometers in medical monitoring. In: Webster, JG, ed. Encyclopedia of medical devices and instrumentation. New York: Wiley, 1988:1848–1859.

105. Bhavani–Shankar K, Moseley H, Kumar AY, et al. Capnometry and anaesthesia. Can J Anaesth 1992; 39:617–632.

106. Scamman FL, Fishbaugh JK. Frequency response of long mass-spectrometer sampling catheters. Anesthesiology 1986;65:422–425.

107. Lerou JGC, van Egmond J, Kolmer HHB. Evaluation of long sampling tubes for remote monitoring by mass spectrometry. Journal of Clinical Monitoring 1990;6:39–52.

108. Cramers CA, Leclercq PA, Lerou JG, et al. Mass spec-

trometry in monitoring anaesthetic gas mixtures using long sampling tubes. Band broadening in capillary tubes caused by flow and diffusion. In: Vickers MD, Crul J, eds. Mass spectrometry in anesthesiology. New York: Springer–Verlag, 1981:120–130.

109. Munshi CA, Bardeen–Henschel A. Mass spectrometer failure: an unusual cause. Journal of Clinical Monitoring 1987;3:288–290.

110. Ilsley AH, Lillie PE. In-circuit analyzers. Anaesthesia and Intensive Care 1994;22:415–418.

111. Buckingham JD, Holme AE. Mass spectrometry for respiratory gas analysis. Br J Clin Equip 1977;2: 142–148.

112. Beatty PCW. The Spectralab-M quadrupole medical mass spectrometer. J Med Eng Technol 1988;12: 265–272.

113. Beatty PCW. Potential inaccuracies in mass spectrometers with spectrum overlap erasure units used during anaesthesia. Clin Phys Physiol Meas 1984;5: 93–104.

114. Davis WOM, Spence AA. A modification of the MGA 200 mass spectrometer to enable measurement of anaesthetic gas mixtures. Br J Anaesth 1979;51: 987–988.

115. Williams EL, Benson DM. Helium-induced errors in clinical mass spectrometry. Anesth Analg 1988;67: 83–85.

116. Steinbrook RA, Elliott WR, Goldman DB, et al. Linking mass spectrometers to provide continuing monitoring during system failure. Journal of Clinical Monitoring 1991;7:271–273.

117. Frazier WT, Odom SH. Efficiency and expense of time-shared mass spectrometer systems. Biomed Instrum Technol 1989;23:481–484.

118. Carlon GC, Kopec IC, Miodownik S, et al. Frequency response of the peripheral sampling sites of a clinical mass spectrometer. Anesthesiology 1990;72: 187–190.

119. Munshi C, Dhamee S, Bardeen–Henschel A, et al. Recognition of mixed anesthetic agents by mass spectrometer during anesthesia. Journal of Clinical Monitoring 1986;2:121–124.

120. Woehick HJ, Dunning III M, Gandhi S, et al. Indirect detection of intraoperative carbon monoxide exposure by mass spectrometry during isoflurane anesthesia. Anesthesiology 1995;83:213–217.

121. Woehick HJ, Dunning M, Nithipatikom K, et al. Mass spectrometry provides warning of carbon monoxide exposure via trifluoro methane. Anesthesiology 1996;84:1489–1493.

122. Perkins WJ, Marsh BT. Continuous and accurate end-tidal CO_2 and anesthetic concentration measurements at high respiratory frequencies. Anesthesiology 1991;75:A486.

123. McCleary U. Potential effects of an unknown gas on mass spectrometer readings. Anesthesiology 1985; 63:724–725.

124. Siegel M, Gravenstein N. Evaluation of helium interference with mass spectrometry. Anesth Analg 1988; 67:887–889.

125. Abel M Eisenkraft JB. Erroneous mass spectrometer readings caused by desflurane and sevoflurane. Journal of Clinical Monitoring 1995;11:152–158.

126. Bennett JA, Seitman D. Desflurane and the unmodified mass spectrometer. Anesth Analg 1995;80:853.

127. Friesen RM. Oxygen concentrators and the practice of anaesthesia. Can J Anaesth 1992;39:R80–R84.

128. Breen PH. Detection of carbon monoxide with mass spectroscopy during anesthesia. Anesthesiology 1995;83:1383.

129. Dhruva SA, Dhamee MS, Hensler T. Mass spectrometer artifact: simultaneous detection of two volatile anesthetics. Journal of Clinical Monitoring 1988;4: 122–124.

130. Gravenstein JS, Gravenstein N, van der Aa JJ, et al. Pitfalls with mass spectrometry in clinical anesthesia. Int J Clin Monit Comp 1984;1:27–34.

131. Gravenstein N, Theisen GJ, Knudsen AK. Misleading mass spectrometer reading caused by an aerosol propellant. Anesthesiology 1985;62:70–72.

132. Kharasch ED, Sivarajan M. Aerosol propellant interference with clinical mass spectrometers. Journal of Clinical Monitoring 1991;7:172–174.

133. Theisen GJ, Gravenstein N, Knudsen AL, et al. More on mass spectrometers and aerosol propellants. Anesthesiology 1985;63:568–569.

134. Bickler PE, Sohn YJ. Mass spectrometers and infrared gas analyzers interpret bronchodilator propellants as anesthetic gases. Anesth Analg 1992;75:142–143.

135. Elliott WR, Raemer DB, Goldman DB, et al. The effects of bronchodilator-inhaler aerosol propellants on respiratory gas monitors. Journal of Clinical Monitoring 1991;7:175–180.

136. Paulsen AW. Spare mass spectrometer vs linking systems in the event of a single system failure. Journal of Clinical Monitoring 1992;8:319–320.

137. Van Wagenen RA, Westinskow DR, Benner RE, et al. Dedicated monitoring of anesthetic and respiratory gases by Raman scattering. Journal of Clinical Monitoring 1986;2:215–222.

138. Westenskow DR, Smith KW, Coleman DL, et al. Clinical evaluation of a Raman scattering multiple gas analyzer for the operating room. Anesthesiology 1989;70:350–355.

139. Lockwood GG, Landon MJ, Chakrabarti, et al. The Ohmeda Rascal II. A new gas analyser for anesthetic use. Anaesthesia 1991;49:44–53.

140. Westenskow DR, Coleman DL. Raman scattering for respiratory gas monitoring in the operating room: advantages, specifications and future advances. Biomed Instrum Technol 1989;23:485–489.

141. Lawson D, Samanta S, Magee PT, et al. Stability and long-term durability of Raman spectroscopy. Journal of Clinical Monitoring 1993;9:241–251.

142. Westenskow DR, Coleman DL. Can the Raman scattering analyzer compete with mass spectrometers. An affirmative reply. Journal of Clinical Monitoring 1989;5:34–36.

143. Stevens WC, Nash JA, Bunney R. A source of nitrogen in the breathing circuit during closed system anesthesia.. Anesthesiology 1996;85:1492–1493.

144. Niedfeldt JW, Hoffman GM, Farber NE. Fruit flavored oils are falsely detected by Raman spectrometers as anesthetic agents. Anesthesiology 1996;85: A433.

145. Firestone L, Mitchell J, Carrera J, et al. Nitric oxide-induced measurement artifacts with the Rascal I gas monitor. Anesth Analg 1994;78:S111.

146. Walker SD. Respiratory gas measurements by infrared technology. Biomed Instrum Technol 1989;23: 466–469.

147. Mogue LR, Rantala B. Capnometers. Journal of Clinical Monitoring 1988;4:115–121.

148. Anonymous. An overview of halogenated anesthetics analyzers. Technology for Anesthesia 1995;15(8): 1–3.

149. Anonymous. An overview of multiple medical gas monitors. Technology for Anesthesia 1996;16(7): 1–4.

150. Anonymous. Gas monitoring and the standard of care in the OR. Health Devices 1990;19:207–241.

151. Colquhoun AD, Gray WM, Asbury AJ. An evaluation of the Datex Normac anaesthetic agent monitor. Anaesthesia 1986;41:198–204.

152. Ilsey AH, Plummer JL, Runciman WB, et al. An evaluation of three volatile anaesthetic agent monitors. Anaesthesia and Intensive Care 1986;14:437–442.

153. Jameson LC, Springman SR. Laboratory performance of two commercially available infrared anesthetic monitors and a mass spectrometer. Anesthesiology 1988;69:A301.

154. Luff NP, White DC. Evaluation of the Datex "Normac" anaesthetic agent monitor. Anaesthesia 1985; 40:555–559.

155. Schulte GT, Block FE. Infrared-paramagnetic versus mass spectrometer measurement of anesthetic and respiratory gas values. Anesthesiology 1988;69:A225.

156. Springman SR, Jameson LC. A comparison of two infrared gas monitors and a multiplexed mass spectrometer with a stand-alone mass spectrometer in adult patients. Anesthesiology 1988;69:A302.

157. Zbinden AM, Westenskow D, Thomson DA, et al. A laboratory investigation of two new portable gas analyzers. Int J Clin Monit Comp 1986;2:151–161.

158. Nielsen J, Kann T, Moller JT. Evaluation of three transportable multigas anesthetic monitors: the Bruel and Kajer anesthetic gas monitor 1304, the Datex Capnomac Usltima, and the Nellcor N-2500. Journal of Clinical Monitoring 1993;9:91–98.

159. Synott A, Wren WS. Accuracy of the Datex Normac anaesthetic vapour analyser. Anaesthesia 1986;41: 322.

160. Jameson LC, Popic PM. Adverse effect of respiratory rate on volatile anesthetic reporting in three infrared anesthetic monitors. Anesthesiology 1991;75:A418.

161. McPeak H, Palayiwa E, Madgwick R, et al. Evaluation of a multigas anaesthetic monitor. The Datex Capnomac. Anaesthesia 1988;43:1035–1041.

162. Bjoraker DG. The Ohmeda 5250 respiratory gas monitor. Anesthesiol Rev 1990;17:44–48.

163. Deriaz H, Baras E, Benmosbah L, et al. Misfilled vaporizer: can it be detected with a monochromatic infrared analyzer? Anesthesiology 1989;71:A364.

164. Gravenstein N, Guyton D. Infrared analysis of anesthetic gases: impact of selector switch setting, anesthetic mixtures, and alcohol. Journal of Clinical Monitoring 1989;5:292.

165. Nielsen J, Kann T, Moller JT. Evaluation of two newly developed anesthetic agent monitors: Bruel & Kjaer anesthetic agent monitor 1304 (BK1304) and Datex Capnomac Ultima (Ultima). Anesthesiology 1990;73:A538.

166. Walder B, Lauber R, Zbinden AM. Accuracy and cross-sensitivity of 10 different anesthetic gas monitors. Journal of Clinical Monitoring 1993;9: 364–373.

167. Jameson LC. Detection and quantification of mixed volatile anesthetics by Poet II and a mass spectrometer. Anesthesiology 1990;73:A440.

168. Lai NC. Multiple-filter infrared system as an alternative to mass spectrometer. Journal of Clinical Monitoring 1991;7:87–89.

169. Munshi CA, Brennan S. Evaluation of Poet II (Criticare) multigas infrared analyzer. Anesthesiology 1990;73:A478.

170. Sosis MB, Braverman B, Ivankovich AD. Evaluation of a new three wavelength infrared anesthetic agent monitor. Anesth Analg 1993;76:S408.

171. Honan D, Synnott A. Capnometry error. Anaesthesia 1996;51:289–290.

172. Mollgaard K. Acoustic gas—measurement. Biomed Inst Technol 1989;23:495–497.

173. McPeak HB, Palayiwa E, Robinson GC, et al. An evaluation of the Bruel and Kjaer monitor 1304. Anaesthesia 1992;47:41–47.

174. Abenstein JP, Welna JO. Clinical evaluation of a photoacoustic gas analyzer. Anesthesiology 1991;75: A463.

175. Guyton DC, Shomaker TS. Effect of incorrect agent setting or alcohol on a photoacoustic gas monitor. Journal of Clinical Monitoring 1991;7:120.

176. Gerard J-L, Hanouz J-L, Flais F, et al. Does nitric oxide interfere with monitoring of volatile anesthetic agents? Anesthesiology 1994;81:A558.

177. Anonymous. Carbon dioxide monitors. Health Devices 1986;15:255–272.

178. Wilkes AR, Mapleson WW. Interference of volatile anaesthetics with infrared analysis of carbon dioxide and nitrous oxide tested in the Drager Cicero EM using sevoflurane. Br J Anaesth 1996;76:737–739.

179. Morrison JE, McDonald C. Erroneous data from an infrared anesthetic gas analyzer. Journal of Clinical Monitoring 1993;9:293–294.

180. Yamashita M, Tsuneto S. "Normac" falsely recognizes "fruit extract" as an anesthetic agent. Anesthesiology 1987;66:97–98.

181. Doyle DJ. Factitious readings from anaesthetic agent monitors. Can J Anaesth 1988;35:667.

182. Foley MA, Wood PR, Peel WJ, et al. The effect of exhaled alcohol on the performance of the Datex Capnomac. Anaesthesia 1990;45:232–234.

183. Crawford MW, Volgyesi GA, Carmichael FJ, et al. The effect of ethanol vapor on the detection of inhalational anesthetics using infrared and piezoelectric monitors. Anesthesiology 1990;73:A522.

184. Yamashita M, Tsuneto S. Alcohol vapour and the Normac analyser. Anaesthesia 1987;42:209.

185. Veyckemans F, Muller G, Pelsser MO, et al. The "ozone-friendly" lidocaine spray affects the monitoring of volatile anesthetics. Anesthesiology 1994;80: 480–481.

186. Gloss S. The "ozone-friendly" lidocaine spray affects the monitoring of volatile anesthetics. In reply. Anesthesiology 1994;80:481.

187. Rolly G, Versichelen LF, Mortier E. Methane accumulation during closed-circuit anesthesia. Anesth Analg 1994;79:545–547.

188. Rolly G, Mortier E, Versichelen L, et al. Laboratory analysis of influence of methane on infrared read-out of volatile anaesthetics. Br J Anaesth 1997;78:22.

189. Rolly G, Versichelen L. Laboratory analysis of influence of methane on the infrared readout of volatile anesthetics. Anesthesiology 1996;85:A445.

190. Strachan AN, Richmond MN. Ether in an isoflurane vaporizer and the use of vapour analyzers in safe anaesthesia. Br J Anaesth 1997;78:107–108.

191. Volgyesi GA, Crawford MW. The effect of alcohols and acetone on the 3.3 nm infrared anesthetic agent monitors. Anesthesiology 1991;75:A488.

192. Hoskin RW, Dallen LT Bronchodilator aerosol propellant interferes with an infrared photoacoustic spectrophotometer respiratory gas analyzer. Journal of Clinical Monitoring 1993;9:65–66.

193. Yamashita M. Freon affects infrared gas monitors. Anaesthesia 1992;47:816.

194. Parslow M. Freon affects infrared gas monitors. Reply. Anaesthesia 1992;47:816–817.

195. Severinghaus JW. Water vapor calibration errors in some capnometers. Respiratory conventions misunderstood by manufacturers? Anesthesiology 1989;70: 996–998.

196. Raymond RN, Tolley PM. Water damage to capnography equipment. Anaesthesia and Intensive Care 1992;20:249.

197. Synnott A, Wren WS. Accuracy of the Datex Normac anaesthetic vapour analyser. Anaesthesia 1986;41: 322.

198. Sprung J, Siker D, Koch R, et al. Disruption of an infrared capnograph by hand-held radio transceivers. Anesthesiology 1995;83:1352–1354.

199. Kocache R. Oxygen analyzers. In: Webster JG, ed. Encyclopedia of medical devices and instrumentation. New York: Wiley, 1988;2154-2161.

200. Merilainen PT. A fast differential paramagnetic O_2-sensor. Int J Clin Monit Comput 1988;5:187–195.

201. Merilainen PT. A differential paramagnetic sensor for breath-by-breath oximetry. Journal of Clinical Monitoring 1990;6:65–73.

202. Figallo EM, Smith RB, Pautler S, et al. Continuous oxygen analyzers in clinical anesthesia. Anesthesiol Rev 1978;5:25–31.

203. Roe PG, Tyler CKG, Tennant R, et al. Oxygen analyzers. An evaluation of five fuel cell models. Anaesthesia 1987;42:175–181.

204. Bageant RA. Oxygen analyzers. Respiratory Care 1976;21:410–616.

205. Smith AC, Hahn CEW. Electrodes for the measurement of oxygen and carbon dioxide tensions. Br J Anaesth 1969;41:731–741.

206. Wilson RS, Laver MB. Oxygen analysis: advances in methodology. Anesthesiology 1972;37:112–116.

207. Anonymous. Oxygen analyzers for breathing circuits. Health Devices 1983;12:183–197.

208. Mazze N, Wald A. Failure of battery-operated alarms. Anesthesiology 1980;53:246–248.

209. Wilson AM. Location of oxygen sensor. Anaesthesia 1990;45:697.

210. Meyer RM. Oxygen analyzers: failure rates and life spans of galvanic cells. Journal of Clinical Monitoring 1990;6:196–202.

211. Erdmann K, Jantzen JAH, Etz C, et al. Evaluation of two oxygen analyzers by computerized data acqui-

sition and processing. Journal of Clinical Monitoring 1986;2:105–113.

212. Ilsey AH, Runciman WB. An evaluation of fourteen oxygen analyzers for use in patient breathing circuits. Anaesthesia and Intensive Care 1986;14:431–436.

213. Bengtson JP, Sonander H, Stenqvist O. Oxygen analyzers in anaesthesia. Performance in a simulated clinical environment. Acta Anaesthesiol Scand 1986;30: 656–659.

214. Westenskow DR, Silva FH. Laboratory evaluation of the vital signs (ICOR) piezoelectric anesthetic agent analyzer. Journal of Clinical Monitoring 1991;7: 189–194.

215. Humphrey SJE, Luff NP, White DC. Evaluation of the Lamtec anaesthetic agent monitor. Anaesthesia 1991;46:478–481.

216. Westenskow DR, Silva FH. Evaluation of the vital stat (ICOR) anesthetic agent analyzer. Anesthesiology 1989;71:A358.

217. Schulte GT, Block FE. What really happens when the wrong agent is poured into a vaporizer? Anesthesiology 1991;75:S420.

218. Pollock CH. Reliability of monitoring. Anaesthesia 1996;51:612.

219. Denman WT, Hayes M, Higgins D, et al. The Fenem CO_2 detector device. Anaesthesia 1990;45:465–467.

220. Goldberg JS, Rawle PR, Zehnder JL, et al. Colorimetric end-tidal carbon dioxide monitoring for tracheal intubation. Anesth Analg 1990;70:191–194.

221. O'Flaherty D, Adams AP. The end-tidal carbon dioxide detector. Anaesthesia 1990;45:653–655.

222. Jones BR, Dorsey MJ. Sensitivity of a disposable end-tidal carbon dioxide detector. Journal of Clinical Monitoring 1991;7:268–270.

223. Heller MB, Yealy DM, Seaberg DC, et al. End-tidal CO_2 detection. Ann Emerg Med 1989;18:1375.

224. Higgins D. Confirmation of tracheal intubation in a neonate using the Fenem CO_2 detector. Anaesthesia 1990;45:591–592.

225. Sanders KC, Clum WB III, Nguyen SS, et al. End-tidal carbon dioxide detection in emergency intubation in four groups of patients. J Emerg Med 1994; 12:771–777.

226. Wilkinson DJ, Hayes M, Denman WP, et al. The Fenem FEF CO_2 detector. Anaesthesia 1990;45:694.

227. Gedeon A, Krill P, Mebius C. A new colorimetric breath indicator (Colibri). Anaesthesia 1994;49: 798–803.

228. Ponitz AL, Gravenstein N, Banner MJ. Humidity affecting a chemically based monitor of exhaled carbon dioxide. Anesthesiology 1990;73:A515.

229. Feinstein R, White PF, Westerfield SZ III. Intraoperative evaluation of a disposable end-tidal CO_2 monitor. Anesthesiology 1989;71:A460.

230. Muir JD, Randalls PB, Smith GB, et al. Disposable carbon dioxide detectors. Anaesthesia 1991;46:323.

231. Gedeon A, Krill P, Mebius C. A new colorimetric CO_2 indicator. Anesthesiology 1994;81:A583.

232. Butler BD, Little T, Drtil S. Combined use of the esophageal-tracheal combitube with a colorimetric carbon dioxide detector for emergency intubation/ ventilation. Journal of Clinical Monitoring 1995;11: 311–316.

233. Larson SR, Sutton T, Koch S, et al. Use of a disposable carbon dioxide detector with emergency intubation in a hyperbaric chamber. Aviation, Space and Environmental Med 1993;64:1133–1134.

234. Freid EB, Brink L, Farrington G, et al. Accuracy of the pedi-cap, a new disposable pediatric end-tidal CO_2 detector. Anesth Analg 1995;80:S132.

235. Campbell RC, Boyd CR, Shields RO, et al. Evaluation of an end-tidal carbon dioxide detector in the aeromedical setting. J Air Med Transport 1990;9: 13–15.

236. Bhende MS, Thompson AE, Orr RA. Utility of an end-tidal carbon dioxide detector during stabilization and transport of critically ill children. Pediatrics 1992; 89:1042–1044.

237. Rosenberg M, Block CS. A simple, disposable end-tidal carbon dioxide detector. Anesth Prog 1991;38: 24–26.

238. Bhende MS, Thompson AE, Howland DF. Validity of a disposable end-tidal carbon dioxide detector in verifying endotracheal tube position in piglets. Crit Care Med 1991;19:566–568.

239. Bhende MS, Thompson AE, Cook DR, et al. Validity of a disposable end-tidal CO_2 detector in verifying endotracheal tube placement in infants and children. Ann Emerg Med 1992;21:142–145.

240. Varon AJ, Morrina J, Civetta JM. Clinical utility of a colorimetric end-tidal CO_2 detector in cardiopulmonary resuscitation and emergency intubation. Journal of Clinical Monitoring 1991;7:289–293.

241. Anton WR, Gordon RW, Jordan TM, et al. A disposable end-tidal CO_2 detector to verify endotracheal intubation. Ann Emerg Med 1991;20:271–275.

242. Bhende MS, Thompson AE. Evaluation of an end-tidal CO_2 detector during pediatric cardiopulmonary resuscitation. Pediatrics 1995;95:395–399.

243. Kelly JS, Wilhoit RD, Brown RE, et al. Efficacy of the FEF colorimetric end-tidal carbon dioxide detector in children. Anesth Analg 1992;75:45–50.

244. Higgins D, Forrest ETS, Lloyd–Thomas A. Colorimetric end-tidal carbon dioxide monitoring during transfer of intubated children. Intens Care Med 1991;17:63–64.

245. MacLeod BA, Heller MB, Gerard J, et al. Verification

of endotracheal tube placement with colorimetric end-tidal CO_2 detection. Ann Emerg Med 1991;20:267–270.

246. Sanders JC, Lynn AM. Accuracy of the easy cap colorimetric end-tidal carbon dioxide detector in children with cyanotic heart disease and in infants aged 1 day to 6 months. Journal of Clinical Monitoring 1994;10:287–288.

247. Higgins D, Hayes M, Denman W, et al. Effectiveness of using end-tidal carbon dioxide concentration to monitor cardiopulmonary resuscitation. Br Med J 1990;300:581.

248. Varon AJ, Morrina J, Civetta JM. Use of colorimetric end-tidal carbon dioxide monitoring to prognosticate immediate resuscitation from cardiac arrest. Anesthesiology 1990;73:A412.

249. Varon AJ, Morrina J, Civetta JM. Clinical utility of a colorimetric end-tidal CO_2 detector in cardiopulmonary resuscitation and emergency intubation. Journal of Clinical Monitoring 1991;7:289–293.

250. Freid EB, Good ML, Bonett S, et al. Disposable end-tidal CO_2 detector. Tidal volume threshold. Anesthesiology 1990;73:A464.

251. Mehta MP, Symreng T, Sum Ping JST. Reliability of FEF end-tidal CO_2 detector during CPR. Anesthesiology 1990;73:A473.

252. Varon AJ, Morrina J, Civetta JM. Clinical utility of a colorimetric end-tidal carbon dioxide detector in emergency intubation. Anesthesiology 1990;73:A413.

253. Menegazzi JJ, Heller MB. Endotracheal tube confirmation with colorimetric CO_2 detectors. Anesth Analg 1990;71:441–442.

254. Muir JD, Randalls PB, Smith GB. End-tidal carbon dioxide detector for monitoring cardiopulmonary resuscitation. Br Med J 1990;301:41–42.

255. Ornato JP, Shipley JB, Racht EM, et al. Multicenter study of a portable, hand-size, colorimetric end-tidal carbon dioxide detection device. Ann Emerg Med. 1992;21:518–523.

256. Anonymous. End-tidal CO_2 detector questions arise. JEMS 1991;1616:22–23.

257. Bhende MS, Thompson AE. Gastric juice, drugs, and end-tidal carbon dioxide detectors. Pediatrics 1992;90:1005.

258. Petrioanu G, Widjaja B, Bergler WF. Detection of esophageal intubation: can the "cola complication" be potentially lethal? Anaesthesia 1992.47:70–71.

259. Sum Ping ST, Mehta MP, Symreng T. Accuracy of the FEF CO_2 detector in the assessment of endotracheal tube placement. Anesth Analg 1992;74:415–419.

260. Sum Ping ST, Mehta MP, Symreng T. Reliability of capnography in identifying esophageal intubation with carbonated beverage or antacid in the stomach. Anesth Analg 1991;73:333–337.

261. O'Flaherty D, Adams AP. False-positives with the end-tidal carbon dioxide detector. Anesth Analg 1992;74:467–468.

262. Petrioanu G, Widjaja B, Bergler WF. Detection of oesophageal intubation: can the cola complication' be potentially lethal? Anaesthesia 1992;47:70–71.

263. Anonymous. Issues in using and purchasing $ETCO_2$ monitoring devices. Health Devices 1991;20:51–54.

264. Anonymous. End-tidal CO_2 detector obstructed by plastic caps. Biomedical Safety & Standards 1995;25:11–12.

265. Wallroth CF, Gippert K-L, Ryschka M, et al. Refractive indices for volatile anesthetic gases: equipment and method for calibrating vaporizers and monitors. Journal of Clinical Monitoring 1995;11:168–174.

266. Allison JM, Gregory RS, Birch KP, et al. Determination of anaesthetic agent concentration by refractometry. Br J Anaesth 1995;74:85–88.

267. Cheam EWS, Lockwood GG. The use of a portable refractometer to measure desflurane. Anaesthesia 1995;50:607–610.

268. American Society for Testing and Materials. Standard specification for minimum performance and safety requirements for components and systems of anesthesia gas machines (F-1161-88). West Conshohocken, PA: ASTM, 1988.

269. International Organization for Standardization. Oxygen monitors for monitoring patient breathing mixtures—safety requirements (ISO 7767:1997). Geneva, Switzerland: ISO, 1997.

270. Baer GA, Paloheimo M, Rahnasto J, et al. End-tidal oxygen concentration and pulse oximetry for monitoring oxygenation during intratracheal jet ventilation. Journal of Clinical Monitoring 1995;11:373–380.

271. Barker L, Webb RK, Runciman WB, et al. The oxygen analyser: applications and limitations—An analysis of 2000 incident reports. Anaesthesia and Intensive Care 1993;21:570–574.

272. Ransom M, Burk N, Benumof J. Avoiding airway fires with laser use: change in $FetO_2$ after a step change in FIO_2. Anesthesiology 1989;71:A1121.

273. Hanowell LH, Kanefield J. Case report. The importance of monitoring inspired oxygen concentrations during regional anesthesia. Reg Anesth 1988;13:126–127.

274. Knaack–Steinegger R, Thomson DA. The measurement of expiratory oxygen as disconnection alarm. Anesthesiology 1989;70:343–344.

275. Meyer RM. A case for monitoring oxygen in the expi-

ratory limb of the circle. Anesthesiology 1984;61:347.

276. Ritchie PA. Another use for an oxygen analyser. Anaesthesia 1984;39:1038–1039.

277. Marks MM, Wrigley FRH. Oxygen analyzers as disconnection alarms. Can Anaesth Soc J 1981;28:611.

278. Spooner RB. Oxygen analyzers unreliable as disconnection alarms. Anesth Analg 1984;63:962.

279. Spooner RB. The measurement of expired oxygen as disconnection alarm. Anesthesiology 1989;71:994.

280. Vreede E, Liban JB. Disconnection and inspired oxygen alarms—a hazard. Anaesthesia 1993;48:739–740.

281. Zupan J, Martin M, Benumof JL. End-tidal CO_2 excretion waveform and error with gas sampling line leak. Anesth Analg 1988;67:579–581.

282. Linko K, Paloheimo M. Inspired end-tidal oxygen content difference. A sensitive indicator of hypoventilation. Crit Care Med 1989;17:345–348.

283. Gronstand M, Paloheimo M. End-tidal oxygen for routine monitoring. Journal of Clinical Monitoring 1989;5:292–293.

284. Berry CB, Myles PS. Preoxygenation in healthy volunteers: a graph of oxygen "washin" using end-tidal oxygraphy. Br J Anaesth 1994;72:116–118.

285. Bhatia PK, Bhandari SC, Tulsiani KL, et al. End-tidal oxygraphy and safe duration of apnoea in young adults and elderly patients. Anaesthesia 1997;52:175–178.

286. Butler PJ, Munro HM, Kenny MB. Preoxygenation in children using expired oxygraphy. Br J Anaesth 1996;77:333–334.

287. Machlin HA, Myles PS, Berry CB, et al. End-tidal oxygen measurement compared with patient assessment for determining preoxygenation time. Anaesthesia and Intensive Care 1993;21:409–413.

288. Sultana A, Lucas J, Roberts N. End-tidal oxygraphy is a reliable monitor of preoxygenation in the parturient. Anaesthesia and Intensive Care 1995;23:244.

289. Barnard JPM, Sleigh JW. Breath-by-breath analysis of oxygen uptake using the Datex Ultima. Br J Anaesth 1995;74:155–158.

290. Watanabe S, Kimura T, Asakura N. End-tidal O_2 and CO_2 after resuscitation. Can J Anaesth 1994;41:354–355.

291. Mallick A, Moss E. Venous air embolism: is end-tidal oxygen monitoring more informative than end-tidal carbon dioxide? Br J Anaesth 1996;76:475.

292. Kytta J, Randell T, Tanskanen P, et al. Monitoring lung compliance and end-tidal oxygen content for the detection of venous air embolism. Br J Anaesth 1995;75:447–451.

293. Russell GB, Graybeal J. Oxygram analysis for venous air embolism detection: a new clinical application for the inspired to expired oxygen difference. Anesthesiology 1993;79:A507.

294. Cheney FW. ASA closed claims project progress report. The effect of pulse oximetry and end-tidal CO_2 monitoring on adverse respiratory events. American Society of Anesthesiologists Newsletter 1992;56(6):6–10.

295. Anonymous. From the literature. Standards of care and capnography. Anesthesia Patient Safety Foundation Newsletter 1991;6:20–21.

296. Lillie PE, Roberts JG. Carbon dioxide monitoring. Anaesthesia and Intensive Care 1988;16:41–44.

297. Tinker JH, Dull DL, Caplan RA, et al. Role of monitoring devices in prevention of anesthetic mishaps. A closed claims analysis. Anesthesiology 1989;71:541–546.

298. Cote CJ, Liu LMP, Szyfelbein SK, et al. Intraoperative events diagnosed by expired carbon dioxide monitoring in children. Can Anaesth Soc J 1986;33:315–320.

299. Brown ML. End-tidal carbon dioxide monitoring in the detection of anesthesia-related critical incidents. JAANA 1992;60:33–40.

300. Williamson JA, Webb RK, Cockings J, et al. The capnograph: Applications and limitations—An analysis of 2000 incident reports. Anaesthesia and Intensive Care 1993;21:551–557.

301. Bhavani–Shankar K, Kumar AY, Moseley HSL, et al. Terminology and the current limitations of time capnography: a brief review. Journal of Clinical Monitoring 1995;11:175–182.

303. Junker H, Petroianu GA, Maleck WH. Capnometers for out-of-hospital' use. Anaesthesia 1996;51:91–92.

304. Vukmir RB, Heller MB, Stein KL. Confirmation of endotracheal tube placement: a miniaturized infrared qualitative CO_2 detector. Ann Emerg Med 1991;20:726–729.

305. McLeod GA, Inglis MD. The MiniCAP® III CO_2 detector: assessment of a device to distinguish oesophageal from tracheal intubation. Arch Emerg Med 1992;9:373–376.

306. Lauber R, Seeberger B, Zbinden AM. Carbon dioxide analyzers: accuracy, alarm limits and effects of interfering gases. Can J Anaesth 1995;42:643–656.

307. Hilberman M. Capnometer readings at high altitude. Anesthesiology 1990;73:354–355.

308. James MF, White JF. Anesthetic considerations at moderate altitude. Anesth Analg 1984;63:1097–1105.

309. Alas VD, Geddes LA, Voorhees WD, et al. End-tidal CO_2, CO_2 production, and O_2 consumption as early indicators of approaching hyperthermia. Biomed Instrum Technol 1990;24:440–444.

310. de las Alas V, Voorhees WD, Geddes LA, et al. End-tidal carbon dioxide concentration, carbon dioxide production, heart rate and blood pressure as indicators of induced hyperthermia. Journal of Clinical Monitoring 1990;6:183–185.

311. Donati F, Maille J, Blain R, et al. End-tidal carbon dioxide tension and temperature changes after coronary artery bypass surgery. Can Anaesth Soc J 1985; 32:272–277.

312. Okamoto H, Hoka S, Kawasaki T. Changes in end-tidal CO_2 following sodium bicarbonate administration reflect cardiac output and hemoglobin levels. Anesthesiology 1992;77:A247.

313. Deriaz H, Verillon M, Delva E, et al. Influence of blood transfusion on cardiac index and end-tidal carbon dioxide tension relationship in anesthetized patients: Br J Anaesth,1994;72(Suppl 1):23.

314. Dickson M, White H, Kinney W, et al. Extremity tourniquet deflation increases end-tidal PCO_2. Anesth Analg 1990;70:457–458.

315. Giuffrida JG. Extremity tourniquet deflation increases end-tidal PCO_2. Anesth Analg 1990;71:568.

316. Patel AJ, Choi C, Giuffrida JG. Changes in end-tidal CO_2 and arterial blood gas levels after release of tourniquet. South Med J 1987;80:213–216.

317. Akata T, Tominaga M, Sagiyama M, et al. Changes in end-tidal CO_2 level following tourniquet deflation during orthopedic surgery. J Anesth 1992;6:9–16.

318. Bourke DL, Sllberberg MS, Ortega R, et al. Respiratory responses associated with release of intraoperative tourniquets. Anesth Analg 1989;69:541–544.

319. Takahashi S, Mizutani T, Sato S, et al. Changes in oxygen consumption and carbon dioxide elimination after release of tourniquet. Anesth Analg 1994;78: S427.

320. Hagerdal M, Caldwell CB, Gross JB. Intraoperative fluid management influences carbon dioxide production and respiratory quotient. Anesthesiology 1983; 59:48–50.

321. Salem MR. Hypercapnia, hypocapnia, hypoxemia. Semin Anesth 1987;6:202–215.

322. Khan RM, Maroof M, Bhatti TH, et al. Correlation of end-tidal CO_2 and hemodynamic variation following CO_2 insufflation during laparoscopic cholecystectomy. Anesthesiology 1992;77:A464.

323. Baraka A, Jabbour S, Hammoud R, et al. End-tidal carbon dioxide tension during laparoscopic cholecystectomy. Anaesthesia 1994;49:304–306.

324. Bongard FS, Pianim NA, Leighton TA, et al. Helium insufflation for laparoscopic operation. Surg Gynecol Obstet 1993;177:140–146.

325. Kazama T, Ikeda K, Kato T, et al. Carbon dioxide output in laparoscopic cholecystectomy. Br J Anaesth 1996;76:530–535.

326. Biles DT, Carroll GJ, Smith MV, et al. Elevated end-tidal carbon dioxide during thoracoscopy: An unusual cause. Anesthesiology 1994;80:953–955.

327. Goode JG, Gumnit RY, Carel WD, et al. Hypercapnia during laser arthroscopy of the knee. Anesthesiology 1990;73:551–553.

328. Sha M, Katagiri J, Ohmura A, et al. A greater increase in $PetCO_2$ during endoscopic inguinal herniorrhaphy by extraperitoneal approach. Anesthesiology 1995; 83:A467.

329. Hall D, Goldstein A, Tynan E, et al. Profound hypercarbia late in the course of laparoscopic cholecystectomy: Detection by continuous capnometry. Anesthesiology 1993;79:173–174.

330. Baudendistel L, Goudsouzian N, Cote C, et al. End-tidal CO_2 monitoring. Its use in the diagnosis and management of malignant hyperthermia. Anaesthesia 1984;39:1000–1003.

331. Dunn CM, Maltry DE, Eggers GWN. Value of mass spectrometry in early diagnosis of malignant hyperthermia. Anesthesiology 1985;63:333.

332. Holzman RS. Mass spectrometry for early diagnosis and monitoring of malignant hyperthermia crisis. Anesthesiol Rev 1988;15:31–34.

333. Neubauer KR, Kaufman RD. Another use for mass spectrometry. Detection and monitoring of malignant hyperthermia. Anesth Analg 1985;64:837–839.

334. Triner L, Sherman J. Potential value of expiratory carbon dioxide measurement in patients considered to be susceptible to malignant hyperthermia. Anesthesiology 1981;55:482.

335. Knill RL. Practical CO_2 monitoring in anaesthesia. Can J Anaesth 1993;40:R40–R44.

336. Karan SM, Crowl F, Muldoon SM. Malignant hyperthermia masked by capnographic monitoring. Anesth Analg 1994;78:590–592.

337. Jordan WS, Jordan RB, Westenskow DR, et al. CO_2 production (VCO_2) related to anesthetic depth. Anesthesiology 1984;61:A173.

338. Isserles SA, Breen PH. Can changes in end-tidal PCO_2 measure changes in cardiac output. Anesth Analg 1991;73:808–814.

339. Ornato JP, Garnett AR, Glauser FL. Relationship between cardiac output and the end-tidal carbon dioxide tension. Ann Emerg Med 1990;19:1104–1106.

340. Shibutani K, Muraoka M, Shirasaki S, et al. Do changes in end-tidal PCO_2 quantitatively reflect changes in cardiac output? Anesth Analg 1994;79: 829–833.

341. Wahba RWM, Tessler MJ, Beique F, et al. Changes in PCO_2 with acute changes in cardiac index. Can J Anaesth 1996;43:243–245.

342. Schuller JL, Bovill JG, Nijveld A. End-tidal carbon

dioxide concentration as an indicator of pulmonary blood flow during closed heart surgery in children. A report of two cases. Br J Anaesth 1985;57: 1257–1259.

343. Schuller JL, Bovill JG. Severe reduction in end-tidal PCO$_2$ following unilateral pulmonary artery occlusion in a child with pulmonary hypertension. Evidence for reflex pulmonary vasoconstriction. Anesth Analg 1989;68:792–794.

344. Symons NLP, Leaver HK. Air embolism during craniotomy in the seated position: a comparison of methods for detection. Can Anaesth Soc J 1985;32: 174–177.

345. Hurter D, Sebel PS. Detection of venous air embolism. A clinical report using end-tidal carbon dioxide monitoring during neurosurgery. Anaesthesia 1979; 34:578–582.

346. Drummond JC, Prutow RJ, Scheller MS. A comparison of sensitivity of pulmonary artery pressure, end-tidal carbon dioxide, and end-tidal nitrogen in the detection of venous air embolism in the dog. Anesth Analg 1985;64:688–692.

347. Carroll GC. Capnographic trend curve monitoring can detect 1-ml pulmonary emboli in humans. Journal of Clinical Monitoring 1992;8:101–106.

348. Byrick RJ, Forbes D, Waddell JP. A monitored cardiovascular collapse during cemented total knee replacement. Anesthesiology 1986;65:213–216.

349. Clarke RCN, Daly JG, Morrow B. Unusually low PaCO$_2$ as a sign of pulmonary embolism in acute severe asthma? Anaesthesia and Intensive Care 1996; 24:617–618.

350. Gibby GL. Real-time automated computerized detection of venous air emboli in dogs. Journal of Clinical Monitoring 1993;9:354–363.

351. Shulman D, Aronson HB. Capnography in the early diagnosis of carbon dioxide embolism during laparoscopy. Can Anaesth Soc J 1984;31:455–459.

352. Diakun TA. Carbon dioxide embolism: successful resuscitation with cardiopulmonary bypass. Anesthesiology 1991;74:1151–1153.

353. Couture P, Boudreault D, Derouin M, et al. Venous carbon dioxide embolism in pigs: An evaluation of end-tidal carbon dioxide, transesophageal echocardiography, pulmonary pressure and precordial auscultation as monitoring modalities. Anesth Analg 1994; 79:867–873.

354. Shulman D, Aronson HB. Capnography in the early diagnosis of carbon dioxide embolism during laparoscopy. Can Anaesth Soc J 1984;31:455–459.

355. Beck DH, McQuillan PJ. Fatal carbon dioxide embolism and severe haemorrhage during laparoscopic salpingectomy. Br J Anaesth 1994;72:243–245.

356. Byrick RJ, Kay JC, Mullen JB. Capnography is not as sensitive as pulmonary artery pressure monitoring in detecting marrow micro embolism. Anesth Analg 1989;68:94–100.

357. Falk JL, Rackow EC, Weil MH. End-tidal carbon dioxide concentration during cardiopulmonary resuscitation. N Engl J Med 1988;318:607–611.

358. Gudipati CV, Weil MH, Bisera J, et al. Expired carbon dioxide: a noninvasive monitor of cardiopulmonary resuscitation. Circulation 1988;77:234–239.

359. Barton C, Callaham M. Lack of correlation between end-tidal carbon dioxide concentrations and PaCO$_2$ in cardiac arrest. Crit Care Med 1991;19:108–110.

360. Kalenda Z. The capnogram as a guide to the efficacy of cardiac massage. Resuscitation 1976;6:259–263.

361. Lepilin MG, Vasilyev AV, Bildinov OA, et al. End-tidal carbon dioxide as a noninvasive monitor of circulatory status during cardiopulmonary resuscitation. A preliminary clinical study. Crit Care Med 1987;15: 958–959.

362. Sanders AB, Atlas M, Ewy GA, et al. Expired PCO$_2$ as an index of coronary perfusion pressure. Am J Emerg Med 1985;3:147–149.

363. Sanders AB, Ewy GA, Bragg S, et al. Expired PCO$_2$ as a prognostic indicator of successful resuscitation from cardiac arrest. Ann Emerg Med 1985;12: 948–952.

364. Von Planta M, von Planta I, Weil MH, et al. End-tidal carbon dioxide as an haemodynamic determinant of cardiopulmonary resuscitation in the rat. Cardiovasc Res 1989;23:364–368.

365. Gueugniaud P-Y, Muchada R, Bertin–Maghit M, et al. Non-invasive continuous haemodynamic and PetCO$_2$ monitoring during preoperative cardiac arrest. Can J Anaesth 1995;42:910–913.

366. Gudipati CV, Weil MH, Bisera J, et al. Expired carbon dioxide: a noninvasive monitor of cardiopulmonary resuscitation. Circulation 1988;77:234–239.

367. Steedman DJ, Robertson CE. Measurement of end-tidal carbon dioxide concentration during cardiopulmonary resuscitation. Arch Emerg Med 1990;7: 129–134.

368. Ward KR, Menegazzi JJ, Zelenak RR, et al. A comparison of chest compressions between mechanical and manual CPR by monitoring end-tidal PCO$_2$ during human cardiac arrest. Ann Emerg Med 1993;22: 669–674.

369. Paradis NA, Martin GB, Rivers EP, et al. End-tidal CO$_2$ and high dose epinephrine during cardiac arrest in humans [Abstract]. Crit Care Med 1990;18:S276.

370. Cantineau JP, Merckx P, Lambert Y, et al. Effect of epinephrine on end-tidal carbon dioxide pressure during prehospital cardiopulmonary resuscitation. Am J Emerg Med 1994;12:267–270.

371. Callaham M, Barton C, Matthay M. Effect of epinephrine on the ability of end-tidal carbon dioxide readings to predict initial resuscitation from cardiac arrest. Crit Care Med 1992;20:337–343.

372. Merckx P, Lambert Y, Cantineau JP, et al. Effect of bicarbonate on end-tidal CO_2 during prehospital CPR. Anesthesiology 1992;77:A236.

373. Martin GB, Gentile NT, Paradis NA, et al. Effect of epinephrine on end-tidal carbon dioxide monitoring during CPR. Ann Emerg Med 1990;19:396–398.

374. Okamoto H, Hoka S, Kawasaki T. Changes in end-tidal CO_2 following sodium bicarbonate administration reflect cardiac output and hemoglobin levels. Anesthesiology 1992;77:A247.

375. Angelos MG, DeBehnke DJ. Epinephrine-mediated changes in carbon dioxide tension during reperfusion of ventricular fibrillation in a canine model. Crit Care Med 1995;23:925–930.

376. Barton CW, Callaham ML. Successful prediction by capnometry of resuscitation from cardiac arrest. Ann Emerg Med 1988;17:393.

377. Callaham M, Barton C. Prediction of outcome of cardiopulmonary resuscitation from end-tidal carbon dioxide concentration. Crit Care Med 1990;18:358–362.

378. Gazmuri RJ, von Planta M, Weil MH, et al. Arterial PCO_2 as an indicator of systemic perfusion during cardiopulmonary resuscitation. Crit Care Med 1989;17:237–240.

379. Kern KB, Sanders AB, Voorhees WD, et al. Changes in expired end-tidal carbon dioxide during cardiopulmonary resuscitation in dogs: a prognostic guide for resuscitation efforts. J Am Coll Cardiol 1989;13:1184–1189.

380. Sanders AB, Kern KB, Otto CW, et al. End-tidal carbon dioxide monitoring during cardiopulmonary resuscitation. JAMA 1989;262:1347–1351.

381. Domsky M, Wilson RF, Heins J. Intraoperative end-tidal carbon dioxide values and derived calculations correlated with outcome: prognosis and capnography. Crit Care Med 1995;23:1497–1503.

382. Kern KB, Sanders AB, Voorhees WD, et al. Changes in expired end-tidal carbon dioxide during cardiopulmonary resuscitation in dogs: A prognostic guide for resuscitation efforts. J Am Coll Cardiol 1989;13:1184–1189.

383. Coates NE. End-tidal carbon dioxide ($EtCO_2$) predicts the emergency department survival of traumatically injured, intubated patients. Crit Care Med 1994;22:A137.

384. Cantineau JP, Lambert Y, Merckx P, et al. End-tidal carbon dioxide during cardiopulmonary resuscitation in humans presenting mostly with asystole: a predictor of outcome. Crit Care Med 1996;24:791–796.

385. Brunner JX, Westenkow DR. How carbon dioxide analyzer rise time affects the accuracy of carbon dioxide measurements. Journal of Clinical Monitoring 1988;4:344.

386. Utting JE, Gray TC, Shelley FC. Human misadventures in anaesthesia. Can Anaesth Soc J 1979;26:472–478.

387. Guggenberger H, Lenz G, Federle R. Early detection of inadvertent oesophageal intubation: pulse oximetry vs. capnography. Acta Anesthesiol Scand 1989;33:112–115.

388. Linko K, Paloheimo M, Tammisto T. Capnography for detection of accidental oesophageal intubation. Acta Anaesthesiol Scand 1983;27:199–202.

389. Vaghadia H, Jenkins LC, Ford RW. Comparison of end-tidal carbon dioxide, oxygen saturation and clinical signs for the detection of oesophageal intubation. Can J Anaesth 1989;36:560–564.

390. Dunn SM, Mushlin PS, Lind LJ, et al. Tracheal intubation is not invariably confirmed by capnography. Anesthesiology 1990;73:1285–1287.

391. Markovitz BP, Silverberg M, Godinez RI. Unusual cause of an absent capnogram. Anesthesiology 1989;71:992–993.

392. Bowie JR, Smith RA, Downs JB. Absence of a capnogram after positive end-expiratory pressure. Journal of Clinical Monitoring 1993;9:78–80.

393. Tang TKK, Davies JM. Absence of a capnograph trace after confirmed tracheal intubation. Can J Anaesth 1993;40:581.

394. Garnett AR, Gervin CA, Gervin AS. Capnographic waveforms in esophageal intubation: effect of carbonated beverages. Ann Emerg Med 1989;18:387–390.

395. Zbinden S, Schupfer G. Detection of oesophageal intubation: the cola complication. Anaesthesia 1989;44:81.

396. Good ML, Modell JH, Rush W. Differentiating oesophageal from tracheal capnograms. Anesthesiology 1988;69:A266.

397. Sum Ping ST. Esophageal intubation. Anesth Analg 1987;66:483.

398. Deluty S, Turndorf H. The failure of capnography to properly assess endotracheal tube location. Anesthesiology 1993;78:783–784.

399. Schmidt SI, Latham J. Blind oral intubation directed by capnography. J Clin Anesth 1991;3:81.

400. King H-K, Wooten DJ. Blind nasal intubation by monitoring end-tidal CO_2. Anesth Analg 1989;69:412–413.

401. Dohi S, Inomata S, Tanaka M, et al. End-tidal carbon dioxide monitoring during awake blind nasotracheal intubation. J Clin Anesth 1990;2:415–419.

402. Omoigui S, Glass P, Martel DLJ, et al. Blind nasal

intubation with audio-capnometry. Anesth Analg 1991;72:392–393.

403. Szmuk P, Ezri T. Capnography and cuff inflation to aid blind tracheal intubation. Anaesthesia 1995;50:662.

404. Temperley AD, Walker PJ. Blind nasal intubation by monitoring capnography in a neonate with congenital microstomia. Anaesthesia and Intensive Care 1995;23:490–492.

405. Venditti RC. A novel application of the Nellcor (Easy Cap) end-tidal CO_2 detector. Anesth Analg 1994;78:1029–1030.

406. Spencer RF, Rathmell JP, Viscomi CM. A new method for difficult endotracheal intubation: The use of a jet stylet introducer and capnography. Anesth Analg 1995;81:1079–1083.

407. Tobias JD, Higgins M. Capnography during transtracheal needle cricothyrotomy. Anesth Analg 1995;81:1077–1078.

408. Ibarra E, Lees DE. Error in measurement of oxygen uptake due to anesthetic gases when using a mass spectrometer. Anesthesiology 1985;63:572.

409. Huntington CT, King H. A simpler design for mass spectrometer monitoring of the awake patient. Anesthesiology 1986;65:565–566.

410. Zeitlin GL, Hobin K, Platt J, et al. Accumulation of carbon dioxide during eye surgery. J Clin Anesth 1989;1:262–267.

411. Dunphy JA. Accuracy of expired carbon dioxide partial pressure sampled from a nasal cannula II. Anesthesiology 1988;68:960–961.

412. Urmey WF. Accuracy of expired carbon dioxide partial pressure sampled from nasal cannula. I. Anesthesiology 1988;68:959–960.

413. Louwsma DL, Silverman DG. Reproducibility of end-tidal CO_2 measurements in sedated patients receiving supplemental O_2 by nasal cannula. Anesthesiology 1988;69:A268.

414. Dunphy JA. Accuracy of expired carbon dioxide partial pressure sampled from a nasal cannula. II. Anesthesiology 1988;68:960–961.

415. McNulty SE, Torjman M, Toy J, et al. Correlation between arterial carbon dioxide and end-tidal carbon dioxide using a nasal sampling port. Anesthesiology 1989;71:A354.

416. Mogue LR, Rantala B. Reply. Journal of Clinical Monitoring 1989;5:63–64.

417. McNulty SE, Roy J, Torjman M, et al. Relationship between arterial carbon dioxide and end-tidal carbon dioxide when a nasal sampling port is used. Journal of Clinical Monitoring 1990;6:93–98.

418. Roth JV, Wiener LB, Barth LJ, et al. A new CO_2 sampling nasal cannula for oxygenation and capnography. Anesthesiology 1991;75:A481.

419. Witkowski TA, McNulty SE, Epstein RH. A comparison of three techniques for monitoring end-tidal CO_2 in awake sedated patients. Journal of Clinical Monitoring 1991;7:92.

420. Dinner M, Steuer M. Capnography as an aid to blind nasal intubation (BNI). Anesthesiology 1992;77:A469.

421. Shafieha MJ, Sit J, Kartha R, et al. End-tidal CO_2 analyzers in proper positioning of the double-lumen tube. Anesthesiology 1986;64:844–845.

422. Shankar KB, Moseley HSL, Kumar AY. Dual end-tidal CO_2 monitoring and double-lumen tubes. Can J Anaesth 1992;39:100.

423. De Vries JW, Haanschoten MC. Capnography does not reliably detect double-lumen endotracheal tube malplacement. Journal of Clinical Monitoring 1992;8:236–237.

424. Kumar AY, Shankar KB, Moseley HSL. Capnography does not reliably detect double-lumen tube malplacement. Journal of Clinical Monitoring 1993;9:207.

425. De Vries JW, Haanschoten MC. Capnography does not reliably detect double-lumen endotracheal tube malplacement. Reply. Journal of Clinical Monitoring 1993;9:207–208.

426. Gandhi SK, Munshi CA, Kampine JP. Early warning sign of an accidental endobronchial intubation. A sudden drop or sudden rise in $PACO_2$. Anesthesiology 1986;65:114–115.

427. Gandhi SK, Munshi CA, Coon R, et al. Capnography for detection of endobronchial migration of an endotracheal tube. Journal of Clinical Monitoring 1991;7:35–38.

428. Johnson DH, Chang PC, Hurst TS, et al. Changes in $PetCO_2$ and pulmonary blood flow after bronchial occlusion in dogs. Can J Anaesth 1992;29:184–191.

429. Thrush DN, Mentis SW, Downs JB. Weaning with end-tidal CO_2 and pulse oximetry. J Clin Anesth 1991;3:456–460.

430. Morley TF, Giaimo J, Maroszan E, et al. Use of capnography for assessment of the adequacy of alveolar ventilation during weaning from mechanical ventilation. American Review of Respiratory Disease 1993;148:339–344.

431. Niehoff J, DelGuercio C, LaMorte W, et al. Efficacy of pulse oximetry and capnometry in postoperative ventilatory weaning. Crit Care Med 1988;16:701–705.

432. Smith RA, Novak RA, Venus B. End-tidal CO_2 monitoring utility during weaning from mechanical ventilation. Respiratory Care 1989;34:972–975.

433. Abramo TJ, Wiebe RA, Scott S, et al. Noninvasive capnometry monitoring for respiratory status during pediatric seizures. Crit Care Med 1997;25:1242–1246.

434. Bissinger U, Lenz G. Capnographic detection of diaphragm movements ("curare clefts") during complete vecuronium neuromuscular block of the adductor pollicis muscle. Anesth Analg 1993;77: 1303–1304.

435. Martin DG. Leak detection with a capnograph. Anaesthesia 1987;42:1025.

436. Berman LS, Pyles ST. Capnographic detection of anaesthesia circle valve malfunctions. Can J Anaesth 1988;35:473–475.

437. Carlon GC, Ray C, Miodownik S, et al. Capnography in mechanically ventilated patients. Crit Care Med 1988;1616;550–556.

438. Kumar AY, Bhavani–Shankar K, Moseley HS, et al. Inspiratory valve malfunction in a circle system: pitfalls in capnography. Can J Anaesth 1992;39: 997–999.

439. Pyles ST, Berman LS, Modell JH. Expiratory valve dysfunction in a semiclosed circle anesthesia circuit—verification by analysis of carbon dioxide waveform. Anesth Analg 1984;63:536–537.

440. Parry TM, Jewkes DA, Smith M. A sticking flutter valve. Anaesthesia 1991;46:229.

441. van Genderingen HR, Gravenstein N, van der Aa JJ, et al. Computer-assisted capnogram analysis. Journal of Clinical Monitoring 1987;3:194–200.

442. Riley RH, Harris LA, Hale AP, et al. Detection of faulty CO_2 absorber by capnography. Anaesthesia and Intensive Care 1992;20:246.

443. Goldman JM. Inspiratory flow rate affects inspired CO_2 concentration in the presence of a circle circuit expiratory valve leak. Journal of Clinical Monitoring 1992;8:176–177.

444. Anlognini J. Capnograph questioned. Anesthesia Patient Safety Foundation Newsletter 1990;5:21.

445. Hussain S, Raphael DT. Analysis of a straight-line capnographic waveform. Anesth Analg 1997;85:465.

446. Hall AC, Llewellyn R. Inaccurate capnograph waveform. Journal of Clinical Monitoring 1993;9: 309–310.

447. Wahba RWM, Tesler MJ. Misleading end-tidal CO_2 tensions. Can J Anaesth 1996;43:862–866.

448. Isert P. Control of carbon dioxide levels during neuroanaesthesia: Current practice and an appraisal of our reliance upon capnography. Anaesthesia and Intensive Care 1994;22:435–441.

449. Russell Gb, Graybeal JM. Reliability of the arterial to end-tidal carbon dioxide gradient in mechanically ventilated patients with multisystem trauma. J Trauma 1994;36:317–322.

450. Russell GB, Graybeal JM. End-tidal carbon dioxide as an indicator of arterial carbon dioxide in neurointensive care patients. J Neurosurg Anesth 1992;4: 245–249.

451. Russell GB, Graybeal JM. The arterial to end-tidal carbon dioxide difference in neurosurgical patients during craniotomy. Anesth Analg 1995;81: 806–810.

452. Kerr ME, Zempsky J, Sereika S, et al. Relationship between arterial carbon dioxide and end-tidal carbon dioxide in mechanically ventilated adults with severe head trauma. Crit Care Med 1996;24:785–790.

453. Lindahl SGE, Yates AP, Hatch DJ. Relationship between invasive and noninvasive measurements of gas exchange in anesthetized infants and children. Anesthesiology 1987;66:168–175.

454. Fletcher R, Jonson B. Dead space and the single breath test for carbon dioxide during anaesthesia and artificial ventilation. Br J Anaesth 1984;56:109–119.

455. Phan CQ, Tremper KK, Lee SE, et al. Noninvasive monitoring of carbon dioxide. A comparison of the partial pressure of transcutaneous and end-tidal carbon dioxide with the partial pressure of arterial carbon dioxide. Journal of Clinical Monitoring 1987;3: 149–154.

456. Reid CW, Martineau RJ, Miller DR, et al. A comparison of transcutaneous, end-tidal and arterial measurements of carbon dioxide during general anesthesia. Can J Anaesth 1992;39:31–36.

457. Shankar KB, Moseley H, Kumar Y, et al. Arterial to end-tidal carbon dioxide tension difference during Caesarean section anaesthesia. Anaesthesia 1986;41: 698–702.

458. Shankar KB, Moseley H, Vemula V, et al. Arterial to end-tidal carbon dioxide tension difference during anaesthesia in early pregnancy. Can J Anaesth 1989; 36:124–127.

459. Whitesell R, Asiddao C, Gollman D, et al. Relationship between arterial and peak expired carbon dioxide pressure during anesthesia and factors influencing the difference. Anesth Analg 1981;60:508–512.

460. Engoren M. Evaluation of capnography to predict arterial pCO_2 in neurosurgical patients. J Neurosurg Anesth 1992;4:241–244.

461. Nyarwaya J-B, Mazoit J-X, Samii K. Are pulse oximetry and end-tidal carbon dioxide tension monitoring reliable during laparoscopic surgery? Anaesthesia 1994;49:775–778.

462. Reid CW, Miller DR, Hull KA, et al. A comparison of transcutaneous, end-tidal, and arterial measurements of carbon dioxide during general anaesthesia. Can J Anaesth 1992;39:31–36.

463. Sharma SK, McGuire GP, Cruise CJE. Stability of the arterial to end-tidal carbon dioxide difference during anaesthesia for prolonged neurosurgical procedures. Can J Anaesth 1995;42:498–503.

464. Fletcher R. The arterial-end-tidal CO_2 difference

during cardiothoracic surgery. J Cardiothorac Anesth 1990;4:105–117.

465. Badgwell JM, Heavner JE, May WS, et al. End-tidal PCO_2 monitoring in infants and children ventilated with either a partial-rebreathing or non-rebreathing circuit. Anesthesiology 1987;66:405–410.

466. Rich GF, Sullivan MP, Adams JM. Is distal sampling of end-tidal CO_2 necessary in small subjects? Anesthesiology 1989;71:A1005.

467. Shankar KB, Moseley H, Kumar Y, et al. Arterial to end-tidal carbon dioxide tension difference during anaesthesia for tubal ligation. Anaesthesia 1987;42:482–486.

468. Bowie JR, Knox P, Downs JB, et al. Rebreathing improves accuracy of ventilatory monitoring. Journal of Clinical Monitoring 1995;11:354–357.

469. Ivens D, Verborgh C, Phan Thi H, et al. The quality of breathing and capnography during laryngeal mask and face mask ventilation. Anaesthesia 1995;50:858–862.

470. Bissonnette B, Lerman. Single breath end-tidal CO_2 estimates of arterial PCO_2 in infants and children. Can J Anaesth 1989;36:110–112.

471. Pascucci RC, Schena JA, Thompson JE. Comparison of a sidestream and mainstream capnometer in infants. Crit Care Med 1989;17:560–562.

472. Hardman JG, Mahajam RP, Curran J. End-tidal CO_2 measurement in children: the effect of breathing system filters. Br J Anaesth 1997;78:102.

473. Barton CW, Wang ESJ. Correlation of end-tidal CO_2 measurements to arterial $PaCO_2$ in nonintubated patients. Ann Emerg Med 1994;23:560–563.

474. Kavanagh BP, Sandler AN, Turner KE, et al. Use of end-tidal PCO_2 and transcutaneous PCO_2 as noninvasive measurement of arterial PCO_2 in extubated patients recovering from general anesthesia. Journal of Clinical Monitoring 1992;8:226–230.

475. Kaplan RF, Paulus DA. Error in sampling of exhaled gases. Anesth Analg 1983;62:955–956.

476. Gravenstein N, Lampotang S, Beneken JEW. Factors influencing capnography in the Bain circuit. Journal of Clinical Monitoring 1985;1:6–10.

477. Rich GF, Sconzo JM. Continuous end-tidal CO_2 sampling within the proximal endotracheal tube estimates arterial CO_2 tension in infants. Can J Anaesth 1991;38:201–203.

478. Halpern L. The most proximal and accurate site for sampling end-tidal CO_2 in infants. Can J Anaesth 1994;41:984–990.

479. Bissonnette B, Lerman J. Single breath end-tidal CO_2 estimates of arterial PCO_2 in infants and children. Can J Anaesth 1989;36:110–112.

480. Halpern L, Bissonnette B. A new endotracheal tube connector for sampling end-tidal CO_2 in infants. Anesthesiology 1991;75:A930.

481. Hardwick M, Hutton P. Capnography: fundamentals of current clinical practice. Current Anaesthesia and Critical Care 1990;3:176–180.

482. Barton FL: Monitoring line failure. Anaesthesia 1994;49:457.

483. Fletcher JE, Foster JMT, Heard CMB. Carbon dioxide sampling error due to leaking O-ring? Can J Anaesth 1996;43:880.

484. Healzer JM, Spiegelman WG, Jaffe RA. Internal gas analyzer leak resulting in an abnormal capnogram and incorrect calibration. Anesth Analg, 1995;81:202–203.

485. Capan LM, Ramanathan S, Sinha K, et al. Arterial to end-tidal CO_2 gradients during spontaneous breathing, intermittent positive-pressure ventilation and jet ventilation. Crit Care Med 1985;13:810–813.

486. Mortimer AJ, Cannon DP, Sykes MK. Estimation of arterial pCO_2 during high frequency jet ventilation. Br J Anaesth 1987;59:240–246.

487. D'Haese J, Noppen M, Claeys MA, et al. Arterial to end-tidal CO_2 gradients during intermittent positive-pressure ventilation and high frequency jet ventilation delivered with a Hi-Lo jet endotracheal tube. Br J Anaesth 1997;78:50.

488. Mihm FG, Feeley TW, Rodarte A. Monitoring end-tidal carbon dioxide tensions with high-frequency jet ventilation in dogs with normal lungs. Crit Care Med 1984;12:180–182.

489. Mason CJ. Single breath end-tidal PCO_2 measurement during high frequency jet ventilation in critical care patients. Anaesthesia 1986;41:1251–1254.

490. Algora–Weber A, Rubio JJ, De Villota ED, et al. Simple and accurate monitoring of end-tidal carbon dioxide tensions during high-frequency jet ventilation. Crit Care Med 1986;14:895–897.

491. Paulus DA. Capnography. Int Anesthesiol Clin 1989;27:167–175.

492. Puri GD, Venkatraman R, Singh H. End-tidal CO_2 monitoring in mitral stenosis patients undergoing closed mitral commissurotomy. Anaesthesia 1991;46:494–496.

493. Burrows FA. Physiologic dead space, venous admixture, and the arterial to end-tidal carbon dioxide difference in infants and children undergoing cardiac surgery. Anesthesiology 1989;70:219–225.

494. Fletcher R. The relationship between the arterial to end-tidal PCO_2 difference and hemoglobin saturation in patients with congenital heart disease. Anesthesiology 1991;75:210–216.

495. Lazzell VA, Burrows FA. Stability of the intraoperative arterial to end-tidal carbon dioxide partial pres-

sure difference in children with congenital heart disease. Can J Anaesth 1991;38:859–865.

496. Ip–Yam PC, Innes PA, Jackson M, et al. Variation in the arterial to end-tidal PCO_2 difference during one-lung thoracic anaesthesia. Br J Anaesth 1994;72:21–24.

497. Pansard JL, Cholley B, Devilliers C, et al. Variation in arterial to end-tidal CO_2 tension differences during anesthesia in the "kidney rest" lateral decubitus position. Anesth Analg 1992;75:506–510.

498. Hatle L, Rokseth R. The arterial to end-expiratory carbon dioxide tension gradient in acute pulmonary embolism and other cardiopulmonary diseases. Chest 1974;66:352–357.

499. Fletcher R. Smoking, age and the arterial-end-tidal PCO_2 difference during anaesthesia and controlled ventilation. Acta Anaesthesiol Scand 1987;31:355–356.

500. Yamanaka MK, Sue DY. Comparison of arterial-end-tidal PCO_2 difference and dead space/tidal volume ratio in respiratory failure. Chest 1987;92:832–835.

501. Watkins AMC, Weindling AM. Monitoring of end-tidal CO_2 in neonatal intensive care. Arch Dis Child 1987;62:837–839.

502. Helm M, Haurer J, Sauermuller G, et al. Arterial to end-tidal carbon dioxide gradient and Horbitz quotient of value in diagnostic blunt chest trauma. Br J Anaesth 1995;74:127.

503. Ip–Yam PC: Can one predict PCO_2 from end-tidal PCO_2? Br J Anaesth 1994;72:495.

504. Tavernier B, Rey D, Thevenin D, et al. Can prolonged expiration manoeuvers improve the prediction of arterial PCO_2 from end-tidal PCO_2? Br J Anaesth 1997;78:536–540.

505. Jellinek H, Hiesmayr M, Simon P, et al. Arterial to end-tidal CO_2 tension difference after bilateral lung transplantation. Crit Care Med 1993;21:1035–1040.

506. Blanch L, Fernandez R, Benito S, et al. Effect of PEEP on the arterial minus end-tidal carbon dioxide gradient. Chest 1987;92:451–454.

507. Hruby J, Marvulli T. A carbon dioxide calibration error during automatic correction of measurements in the N1000 Nellcor pulse oximeter/capnometer. Journal of Clinical Monitoring 1990;6:339.

508. Lee T-S. End-tidal partial pressure of carbon dioxide does not accurately reflect $PaCO_2$ in rabbits treated with acetazolamide during anaesthesia. Br J Anaesth 1994;73:225–226.

509. Raemer DB, Francis D, Philip JH, et al. Variation in PCO_2 between arterial blood and peak expired gas during anesthesia. Anesth Analg 1983;62:1065–1069.

510. Moorthy SS, Losasso AM, Wilcox J. End-tidal PCO_2 greater than $PaCO_2$. Crit Care Med 1984;12:534–535.

511. Russell GB, Graybeal JM, Strout JC. Stability of arterial to end-tidal carbon dioxide gradients during postoperative cardiorespiratory support. Can J Anaesth 1990;37:560–566.

512. Rampton AJ, Mallaiah S, Garrett CPO. Increased ventilation requirements during obstetric general anaesthesia. Br J Anaesth 1988;61:730–737.

513. Gibbs MN, Braunegg PW, Hensley FA, et al. Hazard associated with CO_2 as the cooling gas during endobronchial Nd:YAG laser therapy. Anesthesiology 1988;68:966–967.

514. Bowie JR, Knox P, Downs JB. Rebreathing reduces arterial to end-tidal CO_2 gradient. Anesthesiology 1992;77:A4710.

515. Steinbrook RA, Fencl V, Gabel RA, et al. Reversal of arterial-to-expired CO_2 partial pressure differences during rebreathing in goats. J Appl Physiol 1983;55:736–741.

516. Brampton WJ, Watson RJ. Arterial to end-tidal carbon dioxide tension difference during laparoscopy. Anaesthesia 1990;45:210–214.

517. Ward SA. The capnogram: scope and limitations. Semin Anesth 1987;6:216–228.

518. Block FE. A carbon dioxide monitor that does not show the waveform is worthless. Journal of Clinical Monitoring 1988;4:213–214.

519. Smith TC, Green A, Hutton P. Recognition of cardiogenic artifact in pediatric capnograms. Journal of Clinical Monitoring 1994;10:270–275.

520. Patil C, Stokes M, Clutton–Block T, et al. Automated analysis of th capnogram and its derived parameters. Br J Anaesth 1989;63:634P–635P.

521. Badgwell JM, Kleinman SE, Heavner JE. Respiratory frequency and artifact affect the capnographic baseline in infants. Anesth Analg 1993;77:708–712.

522. Watson R, Benumof J, Clausen J, et al. Expiratory CO plateau slope predicts airway resistance. Anesthesiology 1989;71:A1072.

523. Lyew MA. Another cause of an absent capnogram. Anesth Analg 1994;79:389–390.

524. Frei FJ, Zbinden AM, Wecker H, et al. Parameters influencing the response time of volatile anesthetics monitors. Int Journal Clin Monitor Comput 1989;6:21–30.

525. Jameson LC. Are end-tidal anesthetic concentrations clinically useful? (ASA Refresher Course #422). New Orleans: ASA, 1988.

526. Osborne GA, Webb RK, Runciman WB. The Australian Incident Monitoring Study. Patient awareness during anaesthesia: an analysis of 2000 incident reports. Anaesthesia and Intensive Care 1993;21:653

527. Keenan RL, Boyan CP. Cardiac arrest due to anesthesia. JAMA 1985;253:2373–2377.

528. Frei FJ, Zbinden AM, Thomson DA, et al. Is the end-tidal partial pressure of isoflurane a good predictor of its arterial partial pressure? Br J Anaesth 1991;66: 331–339.

529. Klein KW, Wang JK, Liu J, et al. Anesthetic gas monitoring does not improve hemodynamic stability or recovery times. Anesthesiology 1993;79:A449.

530. Liu J, Klein KW, Griffin JD, et al. Does monitoring end-tidal isoflurane concentration improve titration during general anesthesia. J Clin Anesth 1995;7: 186–191.

531. Wang J, Liu J, White PF, et al. Effects of end-tidal gas monitoring and flow rates on hemodynamic stability and recovery profiles. Anesth Analg 1994;79: 538–544.

532. Johnson EB. Detection of contaminated nitrous oxide. Anesthesiology 1987;66:257.

533. Martin M, Zupan J. Unusual end-tidal CO_2 waveform. Anesthesiology 1987;66:712–713.

534. Matjasko J, Daffern G, Marquis B, et al. End-tidal nitrogen and venous air embolism in dogs breathing N_2O. Anesthesiology 1985;63:A390.

535. Matjasko J, Petrozza P, Mackenzie CF. Sensitivity of end-tidal nitrogen in venous air embolism detection in dogs. Anesthesiology 1985;63:418–423.

536. Russell GB, Graybeal JM. The sensitivity of Raman spectrometry for detection of air embolism in dogs. Anesth Analg 1994;78:S372.

537. Lanier WL. Intraoperative air entrainment with Ohio Modulus anesthesia machine. Anesthesiology 1986; 64:266–268.

538. Komatsu T, Nishiwakii K, Shimada Y. A system for automated spectral analysis of arterial blood pressure oscillation. Anesthesiol Rev 1988;15:46–49.

539. Barton F, Nunn JF. Totally closed circuit nitrous oxide/oxygen anesthesia. Br J Anaesth 1975;47: 350–357.

540. Dunning III M, Woehick H, Nithipatikom K. Comparison of clinical gas monitors to detect breakdown of isoflurane or desflurane to carbon monoxide. Anesthesiology 1995;83:A1079.

541. Sims C. An unusual capnogram. Anaesthesia and Intensive Care 1990;18:272.

542. Good ML. Capnography—Principles and Practice. ASA Annual Refresher Courses. New Orleans, October 20, 1996.

543. Nichols KP, Benumof JL. Biphasic carbon dioxide excretion wave form from a patient with severe kyphoscoliosis. Anesthesiology 1989;71:986–987.

544. Williams EL, Jellish WS, Modica PA, et al. Capnography in a patient after single lung transplantation. Anesthesiology 1991;74:621–622.

QUESTIONS

1. Which method of analysis requires molecules with interatomic bonds to analyze agents?
   A. Infrared
   B. Mass spectroscopy
   C. Paramagnetic
   D. Raman light scattering
   E. Piezoelectric

2. Which technology is based on the fact that molecules with two or more dissimilar atoms have specific and unique absorption spectra?
   A. Raman spectroscopy
   B. Paramagnetic
   C. Infrared
   D. Vibrating crystal
   E. Mass spectrometer

Each question below contains four suggested answers of which one or more is correct. Choose the answer:
A if 1, 2, and 3 are correct
B if 1 and 3 are correct
C if 2 and 4 are correct
D if 4 is correct
E if 1, 2, 3, and 4 are correct

3. Resolution is:
   1. The ability to indicate the actual concentration of the gas being monitored
   2. The ability to read values as displayed on a monitor screen
   3. The ability to quickly indicate changes in concentration as the concentration of measured gas varies
   4. The ability of the instrument to distinguish between two measured values

4. Advantages of a nondiverting monitor include
   1. Quick response time
   2. Water is less likely to cause problems
   3. Scavenging of gases is not necessary
   4. A standard calibrating gas can be used

5. Disadvantages of a nondiverting monitor include
   1. Only carbon dioxide and oxygen can be measured by this method
   2. Blood in the system will cause inaccuracy problems
   3. The sensor can be damaged by mishandling
   4. It cannot be used on patients who do not have a tracheal tube in place

6. Possible sampling sites for a diverting monitor include
   1. A heat and moisture exchanger
   2. The base or inside of the nose
   3. An elbow adapter
   4. The distal end of a tracheal tube

7. If the sampling flow rate of a diverting monitor is too low
   1. The delay time and rise time will be decreased
   2. The peak readings on the capnogram will be lowered
   3. The base line on the capnogram will be depressed
   4. The plateau on the capnogram will be absent

8. Advantages of a diverting gas monitor include
   1. Calibration and zero are usually automatic
   2. The patient connection is usually disposable and therefore does not need to be cleaned and sterilized
   3. Remote monitoring is possible in the MRI suite
   4. Fast warmup time

9. Disadvantages of a diverting gas monitor include
   1. Need for daily calibration
   2. Gases from the monitor must be returned to the breathing system or scavenged
   3. Warmup is usually prolonged
   4. The delay time is prolonged

10. Gases that can be monitored with the mass spectrometer include
    1. Carbon dioxide
    2. Argon
    3. Nitrous oxide
    4. Helium

11. In a magnetic sector mass spectrometer
    1. The ion source breaks molecules into charged ions
    2. The electrical charge of ions striking the collector is proportional to the concentration of a gas
    3. Collectors are placed at points where certain ions are expected to contact
    4. A magnetic field causes the ions to be deflected with the degree of deflection being less for lighter ions

12. The purposes for the high subatmospheric pressure in a mass spectrometer include
    1. The mode of gas flow becomes molecular rather than viscous
    2. Separation of one gas species from another is hindered
    3. The molecules rarely collide at this pressure
    4. Gas is drawn into the ionization chamber

13. Advantages of the mass spectrometer include
    1. Fast response time
    2. Nitrogen can be measured
    3. These instruments are easy to calibrate
    4. Mixtures of agents can be detected

14. Disadvantages of the mass spectrometer include
    1. Gases cannot be returned to the breathing system after analysis
    2. Only programmed gases can be analyzed
    3. Long warmup time
    4. Erroneous high readings will be reported if an unknown gas is present

15. Advantages of Raman spectrometry include
    1. Multiple gas detection
    2. Fast response time
    3. Fast startup
    4. High degree of accuracy

16. Disadvantages of Raman spectrometry include
    1. Artifacts when propellants are used
    2. Artifacts with nitric oxide
    3. Gases must be scavenged rather than added to the breathing system
    4. Large size of the instrument

17. Technology(ies) that can measure nitrogen include(s)
    1. Infrared
    2. Raman light scattering
    3. Oscillating crystal
    4. Mass spectrometer

18. Technology(ies) that can measure oxygen include(s)
    1. Raman light scattering
    2. Paramagnetic
    3. Mass spectrometry
    4. Infrared

19. Technologies that can measure nitrous oxide include
    1. Mass spectrometry
    2. Infrared
    3. Raman light scattering
    4. Vibrating crystal

20. Technologies that measure volatile agents include
    1. Infrared
    2. Vibrating crystal
    3. Raman light scattering
    4. Paramagnetic

21. Which technology(ies) can be used with mainstream (nondiverting) analyzers?
    1. Raman spectroscopy
    2. Vibrating crystal
    3. Mass spectrometer
    4. Infrared

22. Technology(ies) that can detect mixtures of volatile agents include
    1. Mass spectrometer
    2. Infrared
    3. Raman spectrometry
    4. Vibrating crystal

23. Advantages of infrared monitors include
1. They do not need to be kept on standby
2. Response time is fast enough to measure both inspiratory and end-tidal values
3. Units are small and lightweight
4. Periodic calibration with a standard gas is sufficient

24. Disadvantages of infrared gas analysis include
1. Gases must be scavenged after analysis and cannot be added to the breathing system
2. Alcohols and acetone will cause inaccuracy
3. Aerosols will cause artifacts
4. Water vapor will cause interference

25. Method(s) for measuring inspired and end-tidal oxygen include
1. Mass spectrometry
2. Paramagnetic analysis
3. Raman spectroscopy
4. Electrochemical monitors

ANSWERS

1. D		**14.** E	
2. C		**15.** E	
3. D		**16.** C	
4. A		**17.** C	
5. A		**18.** A	
6. E		**19.** A	
7. C		**20.** A	
8. E		**21.** D	
9. C		**22.** A	
10. E		**23.** E	
11. B		**24.** A	
12. B		**25.** A	
13. E			

Airway Pressures, Volumes, and Flows

2. Controlled Ventilation with PEEP
3. Controlled Ventilation with an Inspiratory Pause
4. Spontaneous Respiration without PEEP
5. Spontaneous Respiration with PEEP
6. Mask Ventilation
7. Spontaneous Breath during Controlled Ventilation
8. Ventilator with Descending Bellows
9. Open Loop
10. Overshoot Loop
11. Tubing Misconnection
12. Disconnection Proximal to the Sensor
13. Leak between Sensor and Breathing System
14. Disconnection Distal to Sensor
15. Changes in Compliance
16. Changes in Resistance
17. Severe Chronic Obstructive Lung Disease
18. Tracheal or Upper Airway Obstruction
19. Restrictive Disease
20. Inadvertent Bronchial Intubation
21. Double Lumen Bronchial Tube Problems
22. Esophageal Intubation

MONITORING OF AIRWAY pressures, flow, and volumes is helpful in assessing the mechanics of the respiratory system and selecting and verifying appropriate ventilator settings. Frequently these monitors will give duplicate information. This redundancy should be regarded as desirable. A single signal may be artifactual. Two signals delivering consistent information increase the likelihood that each is authentic.

DEFINITIONS
Tidal Volume

The tidal volume is the volume of gas entering or leaving the patient during the inspiratory or expiratory phase time, respectively.

Ventilatory (Respiratory) Rate or Frequency

The number of respiratory cycles per unit time, usually per minute, is the ventilatory rate or frequency.

Minute Volume

The minute volume is the sum of all tidal volumes within 1 minute.

Inspiratory Flow Time

The period between the beginning and end of inspiratory flow is the inspiratory flow time (Fig. 19.1).

Inspiratory Pause Time (T_{IP})

The inspiratory pause (inspiratory hold, inflation hold, inspiratory plateau) is that portion of the inspiratory phase time during which the lungs are held inflated at a fixed pressure or volume (i.e., the time during the inspiratory phase time when the flow is zero) (see Fig. 19.1).

Inspiratory Phase Time (T_I)

The inspiratory phase time is the time between the start of inspiratory flow and the beginning of expiratory flow (see Fig. 19.1). It is the sum of the inspiratory flow and inspiratory pause times. The inspiratory pause time:inspiratory phase time (T_{IP}:T_I) may be expressed as a percentage.

Expiratory Flow Time

The time between the beginning and end of expiratory flow is the expiratory flow time (see Fig. 19.1).

Expiratory Pause Time

The expiratory pause time is the time from the end of expiratory flow to the start of inspiratory flow (see Fig. 19.1).

Expiratory Phase Time

The time between the start of expiratory flow and the start of inspiratory flow is the expiratory phase time. It is the sum of the expiratory flow and expiratory pause times (see Fig. 19.1).

Inspiratory: Expiratory I:E Phase Time, T_I:T_E Ratio

The I:E ratio is the ratio of the inspiratory phase time to the expiratory phase time. It is commonly expressed by assigning the inspiratory portion of the ratio a value of one. For example, an I:E ratio of 1:2 means that the inspiratory phase time is one third of the ventilatory cycle time.

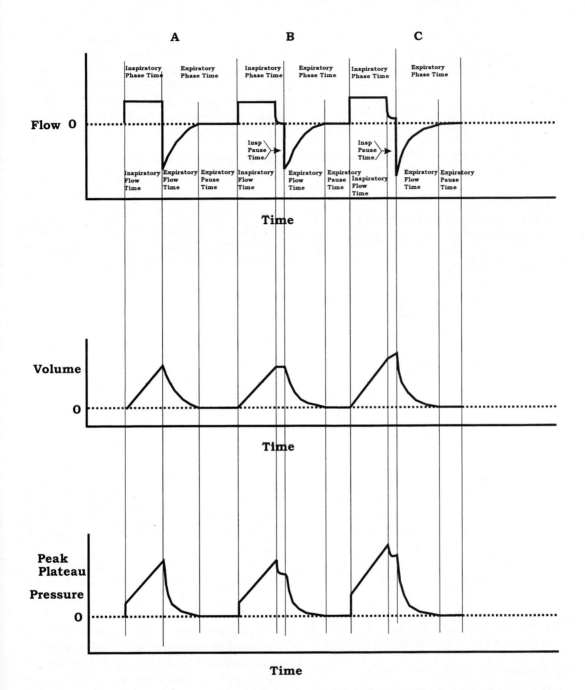

FIGURE 19.1.   Flow, volume, and pressure curves from a ventilator that produces a rectangular inspiratory flow wave. **A,** this represent controlled ventilation with no inspiratory pause. The end-inspiratory pressure will equal the peak pressure. **B,** with an inspiratory pause there is a decrease from peak pressure to a lower plateau pressure. **C,** this illustrates the effect of continuing fresh gas flow during inspiration. The inspired volume increases and the peak pressure falls, then rises.

Inspiratory Flow Rate

The inspiratory flow rate is the rate at which gas flows into the patient expressed as volume per unit of time.

Expiratory Flow Rate

The expiratory flow rate is the rate at which gas is exhaled by the patient expressed as volume per unit of time.

Peak Pressure

The peak pressure is the maximum pressure during the inspiratory phase time (see Fig. 19.1).

Plateau Pressure

The plateau pressure is the resting pressure during the inspiratory pause. There is usually a lowering of airway pressure from peak pressure when there is an inspiratory pause (see Fig. 19.1).

Positive End–Expiratory Pressure (PEEP)

Positive end–expiratory pressure (PEEP) is positive pressure in the airway at the end of exhalation.

Compliance

Compliance is the ratio of a change in volume to a change in pressure. It is a measure of distensibility and is usually expressed in milliliters per centimeter of water (ml/cm H_2O). Most commonly compliance is used in reference to the lungs and chest wall. Breathing system components, especially breathing tubes and the reservoir bags, also have compliance (1).

Elastance

Elastance is the reciprocal of compliance.

Resistance

Resistance, the property that opposes gas flow, is the ratio of the change in driving pressure to the change in flow rate. It is commonly expressed as centimeters of water per liter per second (cm $H_2O/l/sec$).

Timed Expiratory Flow

The timed expiratory flow (V.1) is the percentage of the expired volume exhaled in 1 second. It is similar to the FEV_1 (forced expiratory volume in 1 second) determined in routine spirometry. The FEV_1 requires that the patient make a maximal effort at expiration. For the V.1 the patient is passively exhaling. A V.1 value of 70% is normal. A lower value indicates increased resistance or decreased compliance.

Work of Breathing (2)

The work of breathing is the energy expended by the patient and/or ventilator to move gas in and out of the lungs. It is expressed as the ratio of work to volume moved, commonly as joules per liter. It includes both the work needed to overcome the elastic and flow-resistive forces of the respiratory system and work required to overcome the forces added by apparatus.

Loops

A loop shows the dynamic relationship between two variables on a graph.

GENERAL CONSIDERATIONS
Ventilatory (Respiratory) Cycle

Airway pressure with controlled ventilation is shown in Figure 19.1. There is a rise in pressure with no preceding negative pressure. A fast rise to peak pressure suggests too high a flow setting. The peak pressure will increase if tidal volume, inspiratory flow rate, or resistance increases or compliance decreases. A decrease in peak pressure may result from a leak or a spontaneous inspiratory effort by the patient.

Figure 19.1B shows the respiratory cycle with an inspiratory pause. The presence or absence of an inspiratory pause will depend on the characteristics and settings of the ventilator in use. If the pause is long enough, a plateau pressure will occur at the end of inspiration. The plateau pressure is usually preceded by a higher peak pressure. Plateau pressure depends upon tidal volume and the patient's total static compliance but is independent of resistance (1).

Compliance and Resistance

Measurement of compliance and resistance during anesthesia has traditionally been difficult, involving bulky apparatus. They can now be measured accurately on a real-time basis with relatively compact equipment.

Compliance

Compliance measurement may be dynamic or static. Dynamic compliance is calculated by dividing the difference in volume by the difference in pressure at two points during the ventilatory cycle.

$$Dynamic\ Compliance = \frac{Tidal\ Volume}{Peak\ Pressure - PEEP}$$

This is not a true measure of total compliance because peak airway pressure includes the pressure needed to overcome resistance.

Static compliance is calculated using the end-inspiratory occlusion pressure (3) (see Fig. 19.22). Conditions of zero gas flow are achieved by employing an inspiratory hold or occluding the expiratory port long enough to allow airway pressure to reach a constant value. This pressure, commonly termed "plateau pressure", represents the static elastic recoil pressure of the total respiratory system at end-inflation volume.

$$Static\ Compliance = \frac{Tidal\ Column}{Plateau\ Pressure - PEEP}$$

In adults, normal total static compliance is 35 to 100 ml/cm H_2O. In children, normal static compliance is greater than 15 ml/cm H_2O (4).

Total compliance values reflect the elastic properties of the lungs, thorax, and abdomen and are influenced by such factors as muscular tension, interstitial lung water, pulmonary fibrosis, lung inflation, and the alveolar surface tension. A low compliance value reflects a stiff chest wall or lungs or increased abdominal pressure. Muscle relaxants will cause the compliance of the chest wall to increase but will not affect the compliance of the lungs so that in paralyzed patients, changes in compliance reflect mainly alterations in lung compliance or abdominal pressure.

Resistance

When gas flows through a tube, energy is lost. This is reflected in a decrease in pressure. The pressure drop can be expressed as the product of resistance and flow rate. For a given tidal volume, a high resistance may be overcome by using a lower flow for a longer time or a higher driving pressure. During controlled ventilation, if there is an increase in airway resistance, the pressure needed to deliver a given volume will increase. This can usually be supplied by the ventilator or the person squeezing the reservoir bag so that inspiratory flow is not affected. Because exhalation is passive during anesthesia, expiratory flow depends on the elastic and resistive forces of the patient's lungs and the resistance in the expiratory limb of the breathing system.

Total resistance, which may differ during inspiration and expiration, is determined predominantly by the resistance of the patient's airway, the tracheal tube, and the breathing system. Decreased airway caliber from bronchoconstriction, secretions, tumor, swelling, foreign body, or airway closure is associated with increased resistance. Tracheal tube resistance depends primarily upon its internal diameter, but partial obstruction of the tube by secretions, kinking, or dislodgment will cause an increase in resistance. Breathing system resistance is affected by the length and internal diameter of its components and is increased by sharp bends and constrictions.

Total airway resistance can be estimated using the difference between peak and plateau pressures, which is normally 2 to 5 cm H_2O. If there is an increase in resistance, a higher peak pressure will be necessary to produce the same flow. Plateau pressure, however, depends only on compliance and will not be affected by resistance. Therefore, if the inspiratory flow and the tidal volume remain essentially constant but resistance increases, there will be a greater difference between peak and plateau pressure.

RESPIRATORY VOLUME AND FLOW MEASUREMENTS

A respirometer (spirometer, ventilation or respiratory meter or monitor, ventilometer, volume measuring device, flow monitor, respiratory flowmeter) is a device that measures the volume of gas passing through a location in a flow pathway over a period of time and displays volumetric measurements such as tidal and minute volumes.

Monitoring respiratory volumes and flows can aid in detecting obstructions, disconnections, apnea, leaks, ventilator failure, and high tidal and minute volumes in spontaneously breathing patients as well as those ventilated mechanically. Some monitors can detect reversed flow, an indication of an incompetent unidirectional valve or a leak. A discrepancy between expired and inspired tidal volume should suggest a leak around the tracheal tube or mask. A decrease in tidal volume associated with migration of a tracheal tube into a bronchus may be detected (5). Although there are other ways of detecting these problems, such as observation of chest wall movements, monitoring breath sounds, capnometry, and airway pressure monitoring, use of a volume monitor provides additional protection. One study found that for detecting and classifying breathing system faults, a volume monitor was better than an airway pressure or CO_2 monitor (6).

Respiratory volume monitoring may fail to detect some problems. With occlusion of the airway there may be enough flow during expiration due to compression of gas within the breathing system during inspiration that the alarm may not be activated. During spontaneous breathing, a disconnection may go undetected. Also flow does not guarantee gas exchange. It is possible to have fairly normal flow in the breathing system with esophageal intubation. A ventilator with a descending bellows may draw in room air.

Older respirometers were strictly mechanical devices. On most newer devices, flow is converted into an electronic signal that is processed. Most purely mechanical devices are not equipped with alarms and do not display respiratory rate. Electronic processing permits display of respiratory frequency, detection of reverse flow, and alarm capability.

On monitors with alarm capability, the alarm should be set as close as possible to the displayed tidal or minute volume without producing an unacceptable incidence of false alarms (7).

Equipment

Ventilator Bellows Scale

Ventilators used in anesthesia are described in Chapter 11, "Anesthesia Ventilators." They often have a scale on the bellows housing. This can provide a rough estimate of the tidal volume delivered by the bellows into the breathing system but is not an accurate estimate of the volume delivered to the patient.

Wright Respirometer (8, 9, 10)

Description

Typical Wright respirometers are shown in Figure 19.2. They are supplied with adaptors to facilitate connection to a mask, tracheal tube, or breathing system. There is an ON-OFF control in the form of a sliding stud and a spring-loaded reset button to set the hands of the scales to zero.

An infant version that can measure volumes down to 15 ml is available (11) (Fig. 19.3). Its dead space is 15 ml. An electronic version is available (7).

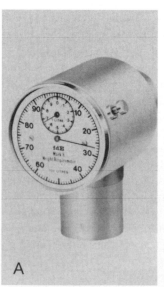
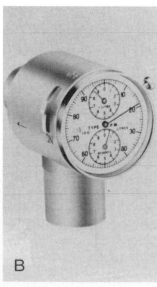

A   B

FIGURE **19.2.** Wright respirometers. **A,** this small instrument can be hand held or inserted into the breathing system. It has two dials: a large peripheral one and a smaller one on the upper part of the main dial. The small dial indicates volumes up to 1 liter and the large dial, up to 100 liters. Note the reset button on the side. **B,** this version has three dials. The top small dial reads up to 1 liter, the large dial indicates volumes up to 100 liters, and the bottom small dial reads up to 10,000 liters. Note the on-off control and the directional flow arrow. This is a larger version which is designed to be mounted into a breathing system. The long hand indicates volumes up to 1 liter on the inner scale and the small hand indicates volumes up to 100 liters on the concentric outer scale. Note the directional arrow at the bottom, the reset button, and the on-off control. (Courtesy of Ferraris Medical, Inc.)

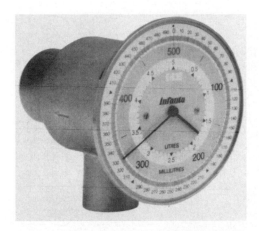

FIGURE 19.3. Infant version of Wright respirometer. The outer scale goes up to 500 ml and the inner scale goes up to 5 liters. (Courtesy of Ferraris Medical, Inc.)

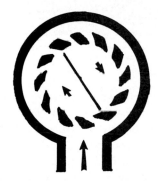

FIGURE 19.4. Internal construction of Wright respirometer. Gas entering the casing is directed through a series of tangential slots and strikes the vane in the center, causing it to rotate.

The internal construction is shown in Figure 19.4. Gas entering through the outer casing is directed through a series of tangential slots enclosed in a cylindrical housing and strikes a vane, causing it to rotate. The vane is connected by a mechanical gear system to the hands on the dial so that a reading corresponding to the volume of gas passing through the device is registered.

Evaluation

Most studies have found that the Wright respirometer over reads at high flows and under reads with low flows (8–15), although one investigation found it consistently under read (16). Pulsatile

flows can cause additional over reading. It will give slightly higher readings with mixtures of nitrous oxide and oxygen than for air (9).

Advantages of the Wright respirometer include small size and light weight, which make it quite portable. Another advantage is its low dead space, which makes it suitable for use between the patient and the breathing system.

The main disadvantage is that it has no alarms. It is somewhat difficult to read and does not give respiratory rate. Determination of minute volume requires a watch. Maintenance can be expensive. Many instruments in use are inaccurate because of poor mechanical condition (8). Its portability can result in inaccuracy due to pocket dirt and a high incidence of damage from dropping. Guards designed to reduce damage from physical abuse are available. Another disadvantage is that it measures flow in only one direction.

Drager Volumeter and Minute Volumeter

Description

The Drager minute volumeter is a large instrument, which is usually permanently mounted on the anesthesia machine and incorporated into the circle system. It is also sold as a separate component.

The instrument is shown in Figure 19.5. Gas flow is from top to bottom. There are two control buttons at the top. When the left button is depressed, a black dot appears on the left side of the

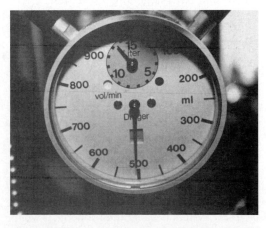

FIGURE 19.5. Drager volumeter (see text for details).

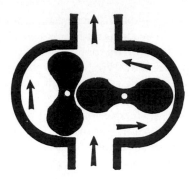

FIGURE **19.6.** Internal construction of Drager minute volumeter. Gas flow along the sides of the case causes the rotors to turn.

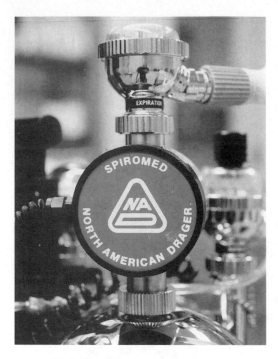

FIGURE **19.7.** Spiromed in place in breathing system.

face and a timer begins to run. After 1 minute, the hands stop and a black disc fills the space under the pointer. The minute volume is then displayed. When the right button is depressed, a black dot appears in the right-hand window and the tidal volume is measured. To stop the pointer, the right-hand button is depressed halfway; depressing it fully starts it again.

The internal construction is shown in Figure 19.6. There are two hourglass-shaped rotors, which mesh as they spin. Gas flow actuates the rotors. The rotation is transmitted by means of a cog-wheel mechanism to the pointer on the gauge.

Evaluation

The Volumeter tends to give erroneously low readings at low flows and high readings with high flows (10, 16). It is easy to read, but rather cumbersome and has a large internal volume.

Spiromed

Description

The Spiromed is an electronic respirometer designed for use with North American Drager breathing systems. It employs a displacement rotating-lobe impeller that generates electronic pulses in response to flow. The sensor in the breathing system is shown in Figure 19.7 and the display is shown in Figure 19.8. Tidal volume, minute volume, and respiratory rate are displayed digitally. An indicator on the left side of the panel will flash red and green if the electronic system fails. If the system is operating properly, it will be green.

Various alarms are built into the device. If no exhaled volume is detected for 15 seconds, *LO* is shown on the breaths-per-minute display accompanied by an intermittent repeating tone. If apnea persists for 30 seconds, the *LO* on the breaths-per-minute display is augmented by a repeating tone, and both tidal- and minute-volume displays are blanked. If the minute volume falls below 1 l/min, *LO* is displayed on the minute-volume display and an intermittently repeating tone is generated. If the measured respiratory rate exceeds 60 breaths/min, *HI* is shown on the breaths-per-minute display. If reversed flow during inspiration is detected, a reversed flow indicator appears on the left side of the front panel, accompanied by a brief audible tone. An alarm silence button is located on the side of the anesthesia machine (Fig. 19.9).

Evaluation

This instrument is programmed to measure tidal volumes equal to or greater than 0.15 liter. If the tidal volume is less than 0.15 liter, the instrument will automatically add two or more consecutive tidal volumes and reduce the frequency accordingly. The minute-volume reading remains

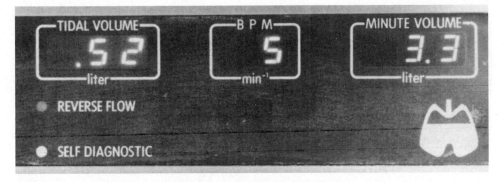

FIGURE **19.8.** Drager Spiromed.

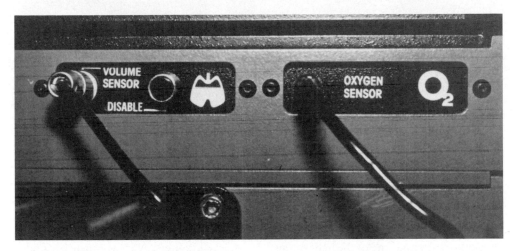

FIGURE **19.9.** Drager Spiromed alarm silence button on the side of an anesthesia machine.

correct. The accuracy of tidal volume measurement is reported as ± 0.04 liter, minute volume as ± 10% of reading or 0.1 liter, and respiratory rate as ± 8% of reading or 1 breath/min.

Ohmeda 5400 Series Volume Monitors
Description
The Ohmeda 5400 volume monitors are available in two configurations. It may be an integral part of an anesthesia machine or ventilator. With this arrangement the monitor obtains power from the anesthesia machine and has an internal rechargeable back-up battery pack. The other configuration is a stand-alone unit that can operate off either a remote charger or a battery pack. When the monitor is operating from the battery pack, the heater in the sensor (see below) is turned off to conserve power. The instrument can operate for up to 8 hours on battery power.

The monitor consists of a sensor that fits into the breathing system, a display unit, and a coiled electrical cord connecting the two.

Sensor
The sensor portion (Fig. 19.10) consists of two parts: a cartridge, which is placed in the breathing system, and a clip-on optical coupler, which fits over the cartridge. The clip is marked with arrows to indicate the correct direction of flow and contains a small heater to help prevent condensation. The cartridge has an internal volume of 6 to 10 ml. As gas passes through the cartridge, it strikes

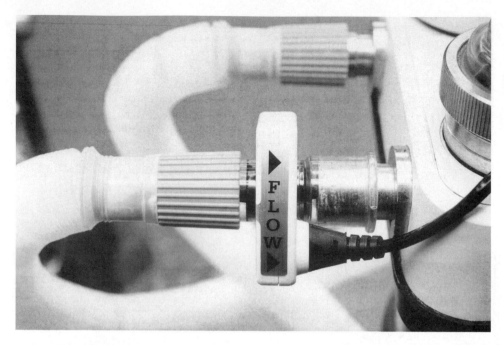

FIGURE **19.10.** Flow sensor for the Ohmeda 5420 volume monitor. Note the flow directional arrow.

the vanes of a rotor, causing it to spin. The coupler contains two light beam sources and an optical sensor. As the rotor spins, it interrupts the light beams shining through the cartridge. The sensor generates a pulse each time one of the light beams is blocked. The number of pulses is proportional to the volume of gas flowing through the sensor. A computer in the monitor counts these pulses and calculates tidal volume, minute volume, and respiratory rate. Calculations for respiratory rate and minute volume are performed at the end of each detected breath or at 10-second intervals and averaged over the last six breaths. Averaging helps reduce the effect of artifacts such as coughing. The computer can detect reverse flow by determining the order in which the light beams are blocked. If the light beams are blocked by condensate or other contaminants, the sensor may not work and the cartridge must be cleaned or replaced.

Display

The liquid crystal display unit is shown in Figure 19.11. An ON-OFF switch is located at the lower right. The unit will display respiratory rate and either tidal or minute volume. Respiratory rate is shown by two small digits to the left of the larger volume display. Tidal volume may be displayed in milliliters or liters. Minute volume is displayed in liters. A 15-segment bar graft shows the tidal volume with each breath. Each bar segment represents approximately 50 ml. If the volume exceeds 750 ml, an arrow will be displayed. Other displays are possible.

Control and Power Mechanism

A switch on the left of the independent unit allows the operator to select either tidal volume or minute volume. An alarm silence switch, which will suppress all audible tones for 30 seconds, is located between these two switches. An alarm light is located just above the alarm silence switch. It will be illuminated during alarm conditions, whether the alarm silence switch is activated or not. At the top are thumb-wheel switches, which allow the operator to select the alarm thresholds for low and high minute volumes. The upper minute volume alarm limits can be adjusted to between 1 and 99 liters and the low between 0.0 and 9.9 liters.

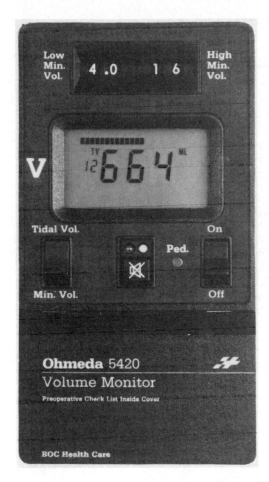

FIGURE **19.11.** Display unit for the Ohmeda 5420 volume monitor. (Courtesy of Ohmeda, a division of BOC Health Care, Inc.)

Inside the door at the bottom are two switches. One is for changing the source of power (line or battery). The switch to battery is not automatic on built-in units. When the line power source fails, the monitor is turned off. It is important to switch back to line power when it is restored to avoid running down the batteries. The other switch is to activate the reverse flow detector. A *REV OFF* message appears on the display when this switch is in the *OFF* position. When the switch is in the *ON* position, reverse flow volumes greater than 50 ml are indicated by an audio tone. This should not be used when the sensor is located where gas

flow will be bidirectional, such as between the breathing system and the patient.

Alarm Functions

An alarm will be triggered if the monitor malfunctions or the batteries are low. This is indicated by a continuous high tone with a blank display and the alarm light staying on. The apnea alarm will be triggered if at least a 150-ml breath is not sensed within 30 seconds. An apnea message will appear on the screen and the light will flash. If the condition persists, there will be a single tone after 30 seconds, two tones after 60 seconds, three tones after 90 seconds, and a continuous tone after 120 seconds. Low- and high-minute-volume alarms are activated if the volume falls below or rises above the selected limits. A low- or high-minute-volume message will appear on the screen. An intermittent low tone signifies a low minute volume and an intermittent high tone a high minute volume. If the reverse flow detection switch is in the ON position, a reverse flow volume greater than 50 ml will be indicated by a *REV FLOW* message and an audible alarm with a continuous low tone.

Evaluation

The unit is intended for use on patients over 20 kg. It is not intended for tidal volumes less than 150 ml. The manufacturer specifies an accuracy of either $\pm$ 8% or $\pm$ 40 ml, whichever is greater. Respiratory rate is stated to be accurate to within 1 breath/min.

One evaluation found it accurate to within 10% when measuring flows between 23 and 44 l/min, provided the respiratory rate did not exceed 30 breaths per minute (17). At lower flows, the instrument recorded falsely high values and at higher flows, falsely low values were recorded. The device was inaccurate with respiratory rates over 30 breaths per minute. The monitor tended to give falsely low values with accelerating waveforms. Values recorded with 100% oxygen and 66% nitrous oxide in oxygen were 20 to 30% higher than those recorded with air. Halothane, isoflurane, and enflurane in clinically-used concentrations did not affect the accuracy of the device. Another study found that it gave low readings at low minute volumes and when used with saturated water vapor or nitrous oxide (15).

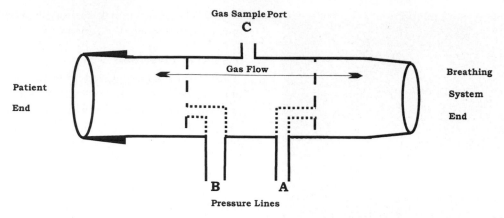

FIGURE 19.12. D-Lite flow sensor and gas sampler The patient end has a 15-mm internal and 22-mm outside diameter connector to fit a mask or tracheal tube connector. The other end has a 15-mm outside diameter connector. Because the pressure tubes point in opposite directions, gas flows can be measured during both inspiration and exhalation. Note that one pressure tube is larger than the other to avoid misconnection of the tubings. There is a gas sampling port on the opposite site of the sensor.

One problem reported with this monitor is that when the operating room light was focused on the transducer, it interfered with the photosensitive detector (18). The monitor alarmed and indicated incorrect volumes.

D-Lite Gas Sampler and Flow Sensor (19–23)

Description

The flow sensor (Fig. 19.12) is a modified Fleisch Pneumotach with a two-sided Pitot tube. The Fleisch pneumotach measures flow by putting a flow resistor (capillary tube) in a flow tube and measuring the pressure difference across the resistor. The Pitot tube uses two tubes to make a differential pressure measurement. One tube faces the direction of flow (total pressure) and the other faces the opposite direction to measure the static pressure (23). The difference in pressure between the total pressure and static pressure is the dynamic pressure, which is proportional to the square of gas flow.

The sensor (Fig. 19.13) consists of a straight tube with a combined 15-mm female/22-mm male connector on the patient end and a 15-mm male connector on the machine end. Two small hollow pressure tubes perforate the side of the tube and extend into the lumen. Each makes a 90° turn inside the lumen so that the end of one tube faces the breathing system and the end of the other, the patient.

The sensor is placed between the breathing system and the patient, preferably as close to the patient as possible. A filter or heat and moisture exchanger may be placed on either side of the sensor. If placed between the patient and the sensor, mucus and humidity will be prevented from entering the gas sampling tube.

During inspiration, gas moves from the breathing system toward the patient. The pressure in the hollow tube facing the breathing system and the pressure in the tube that faces away from the direction of gas flow are measured. Since the pressure tubings face in both directions, similar measurements can be made during exhalation, when the gas flow is reversed.

In the monitor concentrations of CO_2, oxygen and anesthetic agents are determined. The monitor then compensates for the effects of different gas compositions on the measured volumes. Pressure differences between the two pressure ports together with gas concentration information is used to calculate flows. From the derived flows (flow rate, peak flow) and measured pressures (end-expiratory, plateau, minimum, and maximum), the inspiratory and expiratory tidal and minute volumes, and compliance and resistance

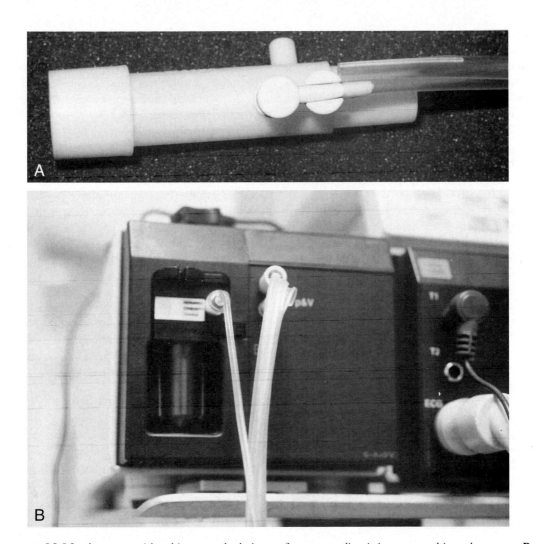

FIGURE 19.13. **A,** sensor with tubings attached. A port for gas sampling is incorporated into the sensor. **B,** attachment of tubings to the monitor.

are calculated and displayed. From these values, flow-volume and pressure-volume loops are drawn. Inspired and expired gas concentrations are also displayed.

Alarms include a high PEEP alarm with a default value of 10 cm H_2O. High pressure and low inspiratory pressure alarms have default settings of 40 and 0 cm H_2O. There are high and low expiratory minute volume alarms and messages for leak, disconnection, and obstruction.

Sensor Calibration (24)

The sensor needs to be calibrated at least every 6 months. One indication that calibration needs

to be performed is an open or overshoot loop. The operations manual should be consulted for the complete procedure. It should be performed with the equipment in the configuration that will be used with the next patient. Accessories such as heat and moisture exchangers placed proximal to the sensor will not affect calibration. However, if the clinician wishes to place an accessory on the distal end of the sensor, then the unit should be calibrated with this in place. A different sized tracheal tube or the omission of the connector could affect the calibration value and result in incorrect volume measurements.

Evaluation

The D-lite is used to measure flows in ranges common for adults and children down to 3 kg. Resistance to flow is 0.5 cm H_2O at 30 l/min. Its dead space is 9.5 ml. One study found that flow measurements were within ± 10% accuracy (25). Tidal volumes of 250 to 2000 ml and minute volumes of 2.5 to 30 l/minute can be measured. The range of measurement for airway pressure is −20 to +80 cm water. The range of flow rates is −100 to +100 l/min.

Regular visual inspection and removal of water are required for trouble-free performance. If used for extended periods with heavy humidification, condensed water in the pressure sensing or gas sampling tubes may cause occlusion.

The D-Lite sensor has a number of advantages. It has a simple and robust construction, light weight, low dead space, and no moving parts. It is not position dependent and allows bidi-

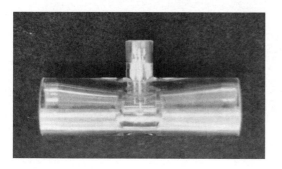

FIGURE **19.14.** Heated wire anemometer. One wire is for measuring flow and one for determining the effect of various gases during no flow.

rectional measurement of gas flow. Small amounts of mucus and water droplets do not affect the measurements. Only one adapter is needed for respirometry and gas sampling. It can be used with both circle and Mapleson systems. Another important advantage is the ability to monitor flow-volume and pressure-volume loops.

Heated Wire Anemometer

In this sensor (Figs. 19.14 and 19.15), the gas flows around a thin wire heated to a constant temperature in a measuring tube. Heat is dissipated when gas flows past this wire. The greater the volume of gas flowing past per unit time, the more heat will be dissipated so the current required to keep the wire at a constant temperature is an indicator of gas flow.

The effect of the various types of gases is compensated for using a second heated wire. The heat dissipated by the second wire is determined when there is no gas flow (e.g., during inhalation in the exhalation side of the breathing system).

Variable Orifice Flow Sensor

The variable orifice flow sensor (VOS) is used with the Ohmeda 7900 Ventilator and the circle system. Sensors at the connections to the carbon dioxide absorber are used to measure inspiratory and expiratory flows.

Construction

Each sensor (Fig. 19.16) uses the principle of pressure drop across an orifice. A Milar flap is placed across the direction of gas flow. Flow causes the flap to bend, creating an orifice with a pressure drop across it. Tubes on either side of

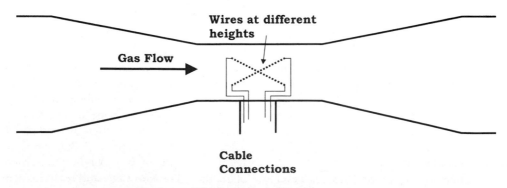

FIGURE **19.15.** Heated wire anemometer.

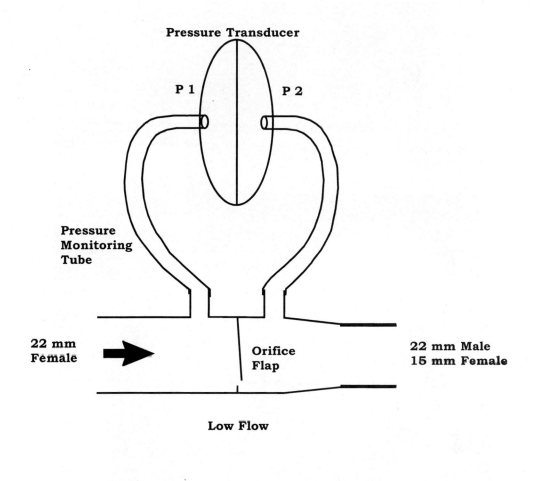

Pressure Transducer

P 1   P 2

**Pressure
Monitoring
Tube**

**22 mm
Female**

**Orifice
Flap**

**22 mm Male
15 mm Female**

Low Flow

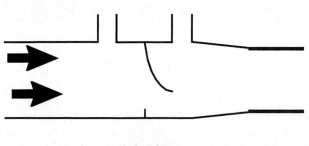

High Flow

FIGURE **19.16.** Variable orifice sensor (VOS). Gas flow causes the Milar flap to bend. There is a pressure drop across the flap. A transducer inside the ventilator converts the pressure drop into a flow.

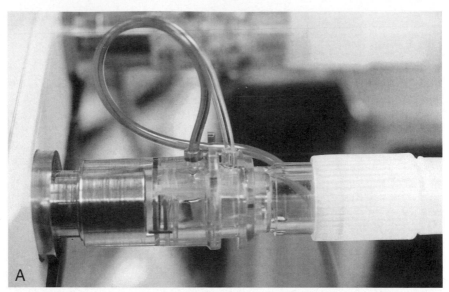

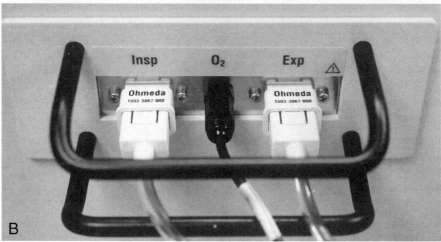

FIGURE **19.17.** **A,** Variable orifice sensor (VOS) sensor. Tubings are attached on either side of the flap. **B,** tubings from the sensors attached to the anesthesia machine. It is important that they be attached to the proper connection.

the orifice are connected to a differential pressure transducer inside the anesthesia machine (Fig. 19.17). A memory chip in the tubing connector contains the calibration curve for each sensor so that flow can be measured accurately. The sensor used on the inspiratory side is also connected to a pressure sensor so that breathing system pressure is measured.

Use

The length of the tubes affects the response time of the sensor and its accuracy in measuring volumes. Before use, the tubes should be checked to make sure they are clear, pointed up, and do not have kinks, cracks, or other problems. Use of filters is recommended to protect the sensors from contamination.

Calibration on a weekly basis is recommended. It is performed using a menu on the ventilator. The sensor tubing must be disconnected during the calibration.

Accuracy

The sensor can measure flows from 1 to 120 l/min. There are no respiratory rate limits. The instruments will read high by 0.95 for each 1%

of anesthetic agent. Effects of nitrous oxide and air are inconsequential.

Since both inspiratory and exhaled volumes are measured, the ventilator can make adjustments so that changes in fresh gas flow do not affect the delivered volumes. However, since the sensors are located at the absorber, they cannot compensate for gas compression or expansion of the breathing tubes. This is a small error unless very compliant breathing tubes are used.

Advantages and Disadvantages

The main advantage of this device is that it allows the ventilator to automatically compensate for changes in fresh gas flow.

Disadvantages include the need for two sensors and filters.

Respirometer Position in the Breathing System

Figure 19.18 shows a possible location for a respirometer with the circle system. From the standpoint of accuracy, the most desirable location is between the breathing system and the patient (position C), so that the volume of gas measured is that actually exhaled or inhaled. In this location, breathing system leaks and compliance and gas compression do not affect the readings. Comparison of these measurements with the set tidal volumes can help to detect a breathing system leak or disconnection. Both inspired and expired volumes can be measured. A large discrepancy between these might indicate a leaking tracheal tube cuff. Placing the sensor at this site will increase the dead space. Condensation of water may be a significant problem. This position may result in increased likelihood of damage, a disconnection, or tracheal tube kinking.

A common practice is to locate the respirometer in the exhalation limb of the circle just upstream of the unidirectional valve (positions A and B). An advantage of these positions is that if the respirometer can sense reverse flow, a malfunc-

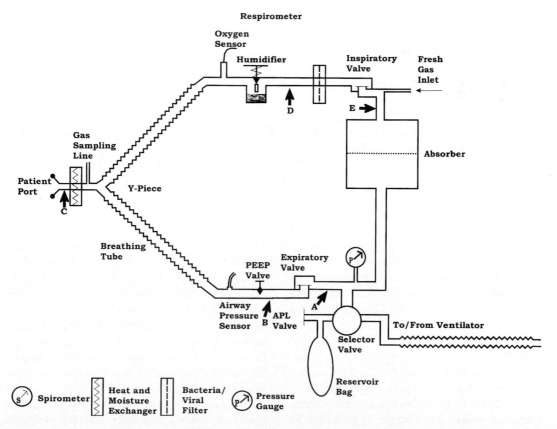

FIGURE 19.18. Possible sites for a respirometer in the circle system. See text for details.

tioning unidirectional valve can be detected. A respirometer in this location will usually read accurately during spontaneous respiration, but during controlled respiration, it will usually give inaccurately high readings (26, 27). If a ventilator with a hanging bellows is used, a respirometer in this position may still indicate flow when a disconnection occurs (28).

If the respirometer is located downstream of the absorber (position E), the volume of gas measured will be decreased by the absorption of carbon dioxide.

Another possible location is on the inspiratory side of the system (position D). In this location, the respirometer will display erroneously high readings since gas that does not inflate the patient's lungs may pass the respirometer (as with a leak or disconnection). During controlled ventilation, a disconnection may not be detected.

When these devices are used in Mapleson systems, placement between the patient connection port and the patient will result in the most accurate readings (7)

AIRWAY PRESSURE MONITORING

Airway pressure monitors (ventilator or respiratory monitors or alarms; pressure alarms; pressure alarm systems; anesthesia, patient, or breathing circuit monitors; ventilator monitoring alarms; breathing gas interruption monitors; disconnect monitors; breathing pressure monitors) warn of abnormal pressure conditions in the breathing system.

Excessive or inadequate pressure in the breathing system has been a major cause of anesthesia mortality and morbidity (29–33). Therefore use of a device that responds to pressure changes within the breathing system and provides warning of a problem is strongly recommended (34). Other parameters such as exhaled carbon dioxide and exhaled volumes may remain relatively normal in the presence of dangerously abnormal airway pressures.

Equipment

Airway pressure monitors may be freestanding or incorporated into a ventilator or an anesthesia machine. Most of these devices are inexpensive, robust, easy to use, and reliable. They should be

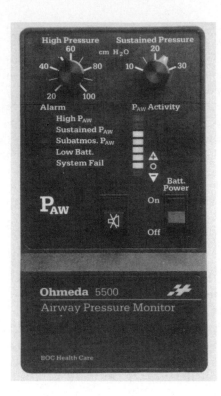

FIGURE 19.19. Airway pressure monitor. The high and sustained elevated pressure alarm limits are user adjustable. This monitor can be run on main power (with the batteries for back up) or on batteries. Note the low battery indicator and the mute button.

powered either from the main electrical system with battery backup or by a battery with battery test capability (Fig. 19.19).

Airway pressure monitors can be purely mechanical or have electromechanical or solid-state transducers. Mechanical gauges were discussed in Chapter 6, "Breathing Systems I: General Considerations." All circle breathing systems have a manometer that displays the pressure at the absorber. This does not allow electronic recording or the data to be integrated with other parameters such as in compliance calculations. Also the device must be continually scanned, which is tedious. Therefore automatic devices with transducers are now widely employed

Most pressure alarms have a delay (reset, mute, silencing) control that when activated will delay the audible signal for some or all functions (Fig. 19.19). Such muting should not prevent the visual indicator from functioning. Some units' audible alarms can be completely turned off (35). Other features on some devices include automatic activation when a pressure pulse is detected, the ability to detect impending battery failure, and protection from accidental inactivation or power failure (34, 36). Some airway pressure monitors have the ability to display pressure waveforms. This is useful for detecting deviations from normal.

Low Peak Inspiratory Pressure

Basic monitoring standards adopted by the American Society of Anesthesiologists and the American Association of Nurse Anesthetists state that when ventilation is controlled by a mechanical ventilator, there shall be a means of detecting disconnection of components of the breathing system in continuous use. The device must give an audible signal when its alarm threshold is exceeded (37). Such an alarm has been recommended by several other responsible bodies around the world (38).

A low peak inspiratory pressure (minimum airway pressure, low airway pressure, ventilation failure, apnea, cycling, pressure failure, disconnect, ventilator disconnect, minimum ventilatory, ventilation pressure, threshold pressure, low-pressure, peak airway, fail-to-cycle, low pressure, low circuit pressure) alarm is activated if the pressure detected does not exceed a preset minimum threshold within a fixed time.

On some of these devices, the pressure is preset by the manufacturer, either at a fixed value or by a value that varies according to the ventilator setting. Others allow the user to select the threshold. These may have discrete values (Fig. 19.20) or allow continuous variation. The time span should be long enough that the peak pressure must fall below the set point for several successive breaths so that a single low-pressure breath will not cause an alarm. This will avoid false alarms due to short-term disturbances. Most of these alarms are enabled when the ventilator is turned on. However, older systems that must be turned on by the user are still in use.

Conditions that can cause a minimum pressure monitor to alarm include a disconnection or major leak in the breathing system, failure of the fresh

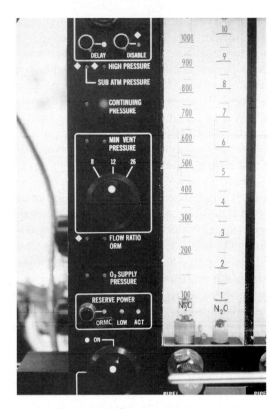

FIGURE 19.20. Airway pressure monitor. The user has a choice of three low pressures: 8, 12, and 26 cm H_2O. The sustained elevated (continuing), subambient, and high-pressure alarm levels are not adjustable. The delay button is at the top.

gas flow, a leaking tracheal tube cuff, extubation, failure of the ventilator to cycle, an unconnected ventilator, incorrect ventilator settings, a malfunctioning scavenging system, failure of the gas supply to the ventilator, increased compliance, and reduced resistance. Most of these are accompanied by a reduced or absent signal from the capnograph and the respirometer. Low pressure monitors are of little or no use during spontaneous breathing when the pressure in the system does not rise and fall appreciably (39).

The alarm threshold should be set just below the minimum peak pressure expected during inspiration (34, 35, 40, 41). This peak pressure will vary not only from patient to patient but also during a given case. Often the threshold is set lower in an attempt to prevent false alarms. If the threshold value is too low, the alarm may be fooled (42–47).

It has been suggested that a pressure threshold of less than 8 to 10 cm H_2O is unacceptable (48). On most modern delivery systems, the circuit pressure waveform and the low pressure alarm threshold are displayed to make it easy for the user to adjust the threshold properly. On some, an advisory signal will be activated if the threshold is set a certain amount below the peak pressure. Some units automatically set the threshold based on the pressure sensed during previous breaths.

Problems with these monitors have been reported. A disconnection or leak may not be detected if the alarm is not switched on (49) or the threshold is set too low. The alarm can be fooled during use of PEEP if the end-expiratory pressure is above the threshold pressure (50, 51). Other conditions that may produce a pressure large enough to exceed the threshold when a disconnection occurs include the breathing system connector's becoming obstructed by a pillow, sheet, or surgical drape; high resistance components such as a heat and moisture exchanger, capnometer cuvette, or humidifier; entrainment of air into the breathing system (especially with a ventilator bellows descending during expiration); partial extubation; compression of an empty ventilator bellows; a Mapleson system with a high flow resistance; and separation of the tracheal tube from its adaptor (52–58). Oscillation of a water 'plug' can falsely silence an alarm; conversely, droplets in the tube can attenuate the sensed airway pressure, leading to a false alarm (35, 59, 60, 62). Positioning the alarm unit above the breathing system and watching for buildup of condensate may help prevent these problems (35, 59). Those operating on batteries will not alarm if the batteries fail (63, 64). It is essential that the alarm be checked before use by making a disconnection at the patient connector while the ventilator is cycling (42). Unfortunately, studies show that this test is not performed routinely or correctly (40). It is important that another means of detecting a disconnection (such as a capnograph or volume or flow monitor) be used.

Sustained Elevated Pressure

A sustained elevated (continuous, continuing, continuing elevated) pressure monitor measures airway pressure and alarms if the pressure does not fall below a certain level during part of the respiratory cycle. The pressure threshold may be fixed or user adjustable (see Figs. 19.19 and 19.20). These alarms have lower threshold values and shorter delays than low peak inspiratory pressure alarms (34). Most are always functional. Some incorporate a valve that opens to relieve the pressure after a certain time (53).

Several mechanisms can produce a sustained elevated pressure: accidental activation of the oxygen flush valve; occlusion or obstruction of the expiratory limb; an improperly adjusted adjustable pressure limiting (APL) valve; occlusion of the scavenging system; a malfunctioning ventilator; or a malfunctioning or incorrectly set PEEP valve (34, 36, 54, 65, 66).

High Pressure

A high pressure alarm is activated immediately if the pressure exceeds a certain limit. On some devices, the threshold is fixed (usually 50 to 80 cm water); on others it is adjustable (35, 63, 67) (see Fig 19.19). On some, the alarm is automatically set at a value above the expected peak inspiratory pressure. This is calculated as the average peak pressure for several previous breaths. Most of these alarms are always functional. Some anesthesia delivery systems are fitted with pressure-limiting valves that vent gas out of the breathing system and activate an audible alarm when high pressure is detected (35).

Possible causes of high pressure include airway obstruction, reduced compliance, increased resistance, a kinked or occluded tracheal tube or breathing system, operation of the oxygen flush during the inspiratory phase, a punctured ventilator bellows, occlusion or obstruction of the expiratory limb of the breathing system, scavenger malfunction, or the patient's coughing or straining (30, 34, 68). However, even in the presence of complete obstruction, this alarm will not be activated if the peak inspiratory pressure does not reach the set limit (41). High compliance, low resistance, leaks, low inspiratory flow rates, high respiratory rates, low I:E ratios, low tidal volumes, and low fresh gas flows can all decrease the peak inspiratory pressure so that there is no alarm (1, 67).

Subambient Pressure

A subambient (subatmospheric) pressure alarm is activated by pressures that fall below atmospheric pressure by a predetermined amount. Subatmospheric pressure can be generated by a patient attempting to inhale against a collapsed reservoir bag or increased resistance, a blocked inspiratory limb (during the ventilator's expiratory phase), malfunctioning of an active scavenging system, suction applied to a nasogastric tube placed in the tracheobronchial tree or to the working channel of a fiberscope passed into the airway, or a sidestream sampling gas analyzer or the refilling of a ventilator with a hanging bellows with a low fresh gas flow (34, 41, 64, 69–71).

Other

With some monitors, an alarm is activated if PEEP is above a certain level or warn if PEEP is active (35, 41).

Monitoring Site

The location where pressure is sensed will affect its usefulness. Figure 19.21 shows possible sites. Ideally, the site should be close to the patient's airway (position *C*). Many disposable breathing

systems have a small port at the Y-piece that can serve as the connection site for tubing that transmits the pressure changes to a separate pressure-monitoring device (58).

The more distant the site of measurement is from the patient, the less useful it is as an estimate of airway pressure (1, 72). Breathing system resistance and compliance, leaks, obstructions, and other mechanical factors may cause the measured pressure to be very different from the pressure in the patient's airway (73).

While placement between the patient and the breathing system is best from this standpoint, in practice it may present problems with dead space, disconnections, tracheal tube kinking, contamination, and water buildup in the pilot line. Also it is necessary to connect the line for every case.

Frequently the site is in the breathing system (Positions *A, B,* and *D*). An occlusion in the breathing system will cause a low-pressure state

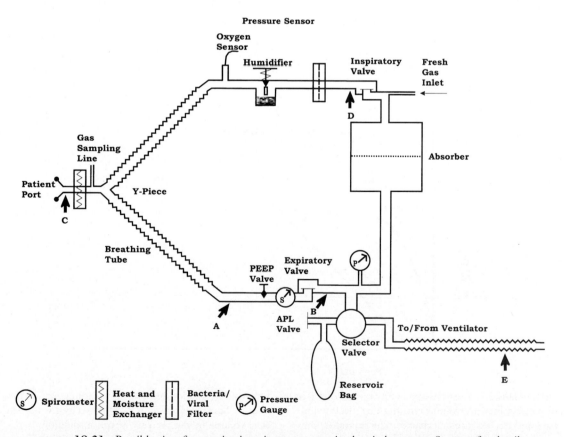

FIGURE **19.21.** Possible sites for monitoring airway pressure in the circle system. See text for details.

distal to the obstruction and a high-pressure state proximal to it, so the alarm may miss certain types of problems (58).

In the past, the sensor was sometimes located in the ventilator (Position *E*). This is unsatisfactory because under certain circumstances, sufficient back pressure to inhibit the minimum pressure alarm may be generated at the bellows even when there is a disconnection (54, 55, 60). Placing the sensing point in the ventilator may also result in failure to detect an incorrectly set bag/ventilator selector valve (57).

SPIROMETRY LOOPS AND WAVE FORMS (4, 21, 22)

The value of loops is that certain patterns are easily recognizable and changes in these patterns signify alterations in equipment or patient conditions. For this reason, it is desirable to save a baseline loop for comparison with later ones. Compliance, resistance, and timed expiratory flow should also be compared with earlier values. Deviations from baseline can signify a problem, although the exact site and nature of the problem cannot always be determined from the loop configuration or changes in resistance and/or compliance.

The Pressure-Volume (Compliance) Loop

The pressure-volume loop shows volume on the vertical axis and pressure on the horizontal axis (Fig. 19.22). The direction of the inspiratory half of the loop will depend on whether the pressure during inspiration is negative (spontaneous ventilation) or positive (controlled ventilation). The tidal volume is the point on the vertical axis that corresponds to the highest point on the loop. The portion of the loop representing expiration starts at the point of highest volume and moves downward toward zero. The area inside the loop is related to the work of breathing (2).

The Flow-Volume (Resistance) Loop

The flow-volume loop (Fig. 19.23) has volume on the horizontal axis and flow on the vertical axis. The zero point for volume is to the right on the horizontal axis. This corresponds to the functional residual capacity. During inspiration, flow rate increases (plotted downward) rapidly, is sustained as the volume increases (moves to the left) and drops to zero as inspiration ends. The tidal volume is reached at the point where flow crosses the horizontal axis. Exhalation is represented by the part

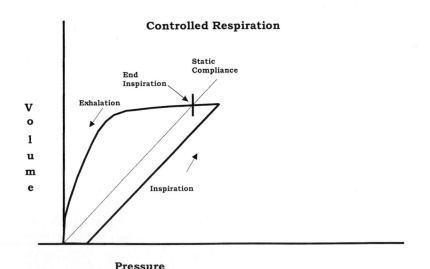

FIGURE **19.22.**   Illustrative pressure-volume loop. The inspiratory pressure-volume relationship reflects pulmonary and tracheal tube mechanics. The expiratory pressure-volume relationship reflects breathing system mechanics. Static compliance is determined by dividing the tidal volume by the pressure at end inspiration.

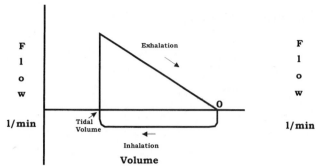 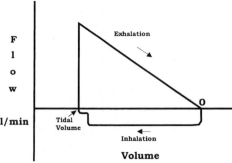

FIGURE 19.23. Illustrative flow-volume loops. Left, controlled ventilation without continuing fresh gas flow. Right, with continuing fresh gas flow.

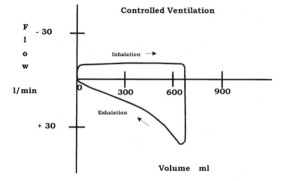

FIGURE 19.24. Alternative method of displaying flow-volume loops. See text for details.

of the loop above the horizontal axis. The shape of this portion of the loop is determined by the rate of passive lung deflation, which is in turn determined by elastic recoil of the lung and chest wall and by the total flow resistance offered by the bronchial tree, tracheal tube, expiratory limb of the breathing system, and any additional equipment. With a normal loop, the flow rate during exhalation increases rapidly at the beginning and quickly reaches a peak, then slows and gradually returns to zero.

Figure 19.24 shows another way of illustrating a flow-volume loop, which is used by some manufacturers. The zero point is at the junction with the vertical axis. Inhalation is above the horizontal axis and exhalation is below. Flow-volume loops illustrated in this chapter use the representation used by pulmonologists.

Representative Loops (24)

Loops illustrated in this chapter are stylized, but taken from actual loops whenever possible. The reader should not expect to see an exact reproduction when monitoring a patient. Clinical conditions are rarely straightforward. A patient may have a number of conditions, each of which will contribute to the configuration of the loop that is displayed.

Controlled Ventilation with No Inspiratory Pause

The normal pressure-volume loop for controlled ventilation with no inspiratory pause is shown in Figure 19.25. The shape of the loop is double convex. It begins at zero volume and near-zero pressure. During inspiration, both pressure and volume increase so the loop moves counterclockwise. The slope from the beginning of inspiration to the end of inspiration depicts compliance. At the end of inspiration, both peak pressure and volume are attained. If there is no inspiratory pause, the transition point between inspiration and expiration will be sharp.

The flow-volume loop seen with controlled ventilation is shown in Figure 19.26. It has a smoothly curved, rectangular inspiratory limb below the horizontal axis and an upper, triangular expiratory portion whose apex represents peak expiratory flow. Through most of inspiration, the flow is relatively steady and will depend on the characteristics and settings of the ventilator rather than the patient. Toward the end of inspiration, the flow drops rapidly to zero, as the tidal volume

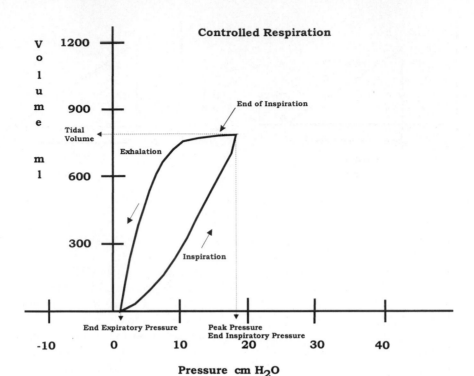

FIGURE 19.25. This is a pressure-volume loop drawn during use of a ventilator with no inspiratory pause. Tidal volume is approximately 775 ml. Peak pressure is 18 cm water. It is normal for there to be a small amount of positive end–expiratory pressure (PEEP) when a ventilator with a standing bellows is used.

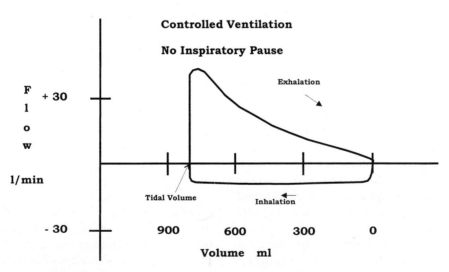

FIGURE 19.26. This is a flow-volume loop drawn during a complete respiratory cycle with constant inspiratory flow provided by an anesthesia ventilator. It has a smoothly curved slightly rectangular inspiratory limb influenced largely by the flow of the ventilator and a triangular expiratory limb, with the apex of the triangle representing peak expiratory flow, followed by a concave descending limb, joining the volume axis at the zero flow-volume point. The tidal volume is approximately 750 ml.

is reached. As exhalation begins, the flow is positive on the vertical axis and there is a rapid ascent to a peak. As flow decreases, the loop falls smoothly toward zero flow and volume. The angle at the top of the loop is narrow. The slope of the descending portion of the expiratory flow curve reflects the resistance and recoil pressure of the entire ventilatory system. The height of the curve reflects the peak flow rate of gas leaving the lungs and correlates with the V1.0% value.

Controlled Ventilation with (PEEP)

Addition of PEEP causes the pressure-volume loop to shift to the right so that it begins at the PEEP value (Fig. 19.27). PEEP may cause an increase in compliance (see Fig. 19.56), so that peak pressure is decreased. One of the advantages of displaying loops is that inadvertent PEEP may be detected. This could result from a PEEP valve being inadvertently turned on, a partial obstruction in the breathing system, a malfunctioning exhalation unidirectional valve or scavenging inter-

face, or an incorrectly set APL valve. During mechanical ventilation, patients with airflow obstruction may develop inadvertent PEEP (auto-PEEP, occult or intrinsic PEEP, dynamic hyperinflation) if there is not enough time for complete exhalation (74, 75).

Patients with obstructive airways disease may not complete full exhalation prior to the start of the next inhalation, resulting in persistent positive pressure.

The flow-volume loop with PEEP is shown in Figure 19.28. In normal patients, application of PEEP will decrease the expiratory driving pressure, producing lower flows during expiration (3).

Controlled Ventilation with an Inspiratory Pause

Figure 19.29 shows the pressure-volume loop with an inspiratory pause. After the peak pressure is reached, there is a pause during which the pressure drops to a plateau level, usually 2 to 5 cm water lower than peak pressure. The inspired vol-

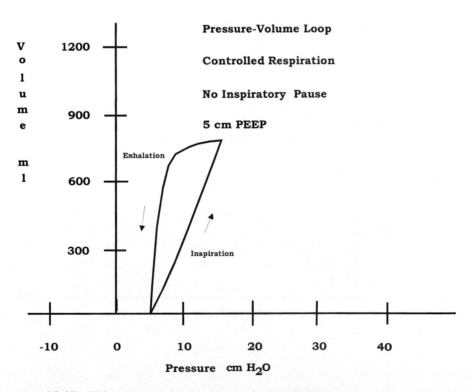

FIGURE 19.27. With positive end–expiratory pressure (PEEP) the loop is shifted to the right.

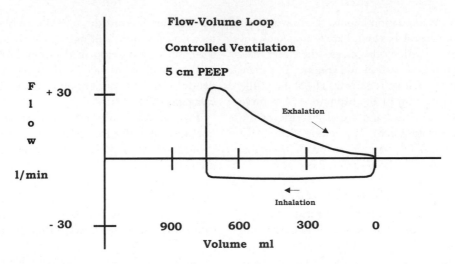

FIGURE 19.28. Positive end–expiratory pressure (PEEP) produces a decrease in expiratory flow.

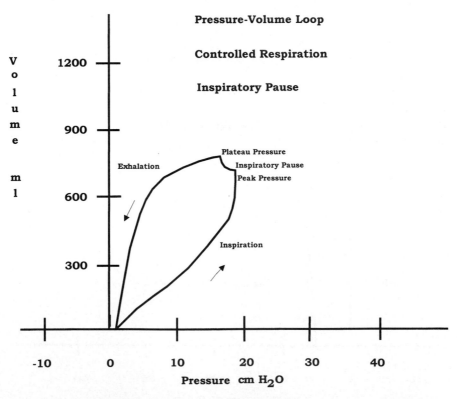

FIGURE 19.29. During an inspiratory pause, it is common for the airway pressure to decline 2 to 5 cm H_2O. The lower pressure is called the plateau pressure.

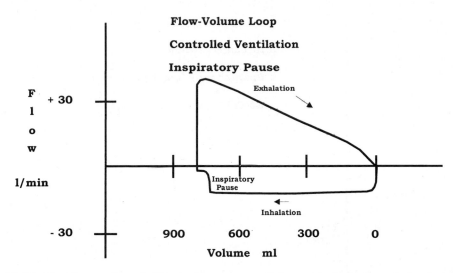

FIGURE 19.30.   The blip near the end of inspiration represents the increase in tidal volume during the inspiratory pause due to fresh gas continuing to flow into the breathing system.

ume will increase during the inspiratory pause because of the fresh gas flowing into the breathing system from the anesthesia machine. These factors make the portion of the loop corresponding to the plateau more rounded. During exhalation, the pressure and volume will drop in the expected manner.

The flow-volume loop seen with an inspiratory pause is shown in Figure 19.30. There is a drop in flow near the end of inspiration with a small increase in tidal volume due to fresh gas flowing into the breathing system during the pause. This pattern should not be confused with a spontaneous breath during mechanical ventilation (see Fig. 19.38). The increase in volume resulting from fresh gas flow is steady and close to the zero flow line. With a spontaneous breath, the inspiratory flow rate will be more variable.

Spontaneous Respiration without PEEP

With spontaneous respiration and no PEEP, the pressure-volume loop (Fig. 19.31) starts at zero. During inspiration, airway pressure is negative, so the loop moves clockwise. At the end of inspiration, the pressure returns to zero. During exhalation, airway pressure is positive so the loop moves to the right. At the same time, the volume drops. At the end of exhalation, the pressure and

volume have returned to zero. The shape of the loop is still double convex, but its slope is quite different from that seen with controlled ventilation. Compliance cannot be calculated because the inspiratory pressure is negative. The area of the loop represents the work of breathing.

The corresponding flow-volume loop is shown in Figure 19.32. The flow rate during inspiration varies more than with mechanical ventilation. Flow increases to a peak midway through inspiration and then decreases. A sawtooth pattern on a flow-volume loop during spontaneous breathing suggests the presence of secretions (3).

Spontaneous Respiration with PEEP

If PEEP is applied during spontaneous ventilation, the pressure-volume loop will start out at the PEEP value and move to the left (Fig. 19.33). During exhalation the loop moves toward the right and downward to the point of origin. The loop has a rectangular shape. The corresponding flow-volume loop is shown in Figure 19.34. The exhalation portion is more rounded than when there is no PEEP.

Mask Ventilation

When the upper airway is not bypassed by a tracheal tube, the pressures during inspiration and expiration are dispersed through the mask, nose,

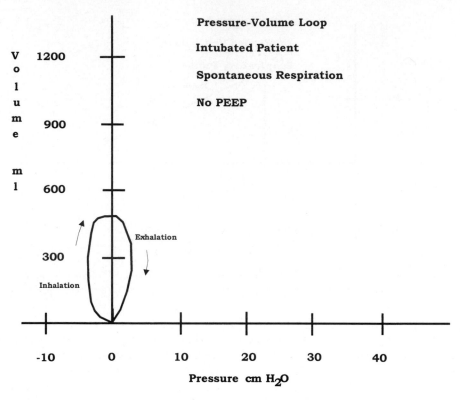

FIGURE 19.31. With spontaneous ventilation the shape of the loop is double convex, but the slope is different from that seen with controlled ventilation.

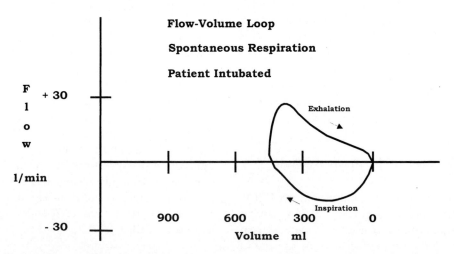

FIGURE 19.32. With spontaneous ventilation the flow rate during inspiration varies more than with mechanical ventilation. Inspiration and exhalation tend to mirror each other. Tidal volume during spontaneous ventilation is usually lower than with controlled ventilation.

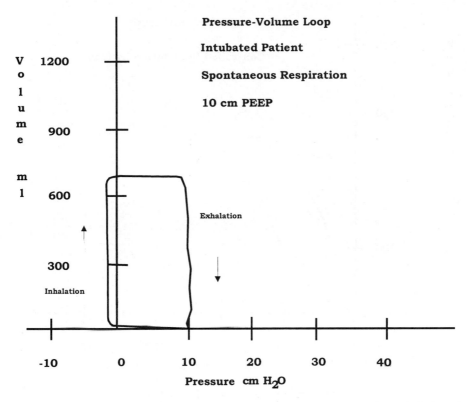

FIGURE 19.33. With spontaneous ventilation and positive end–expiratory pressure (PEEP) the loop is shifted leftward and becomes rectangular.

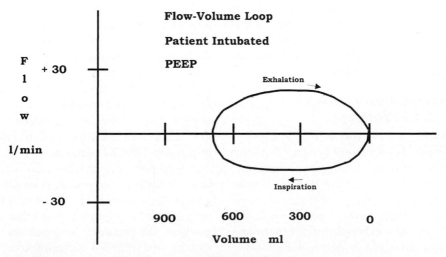

FIGURE 19.34. Positive end–expiratory pressure (PEEP) during spontaneous respiration results in lower flows during both inspiration and exhalation.

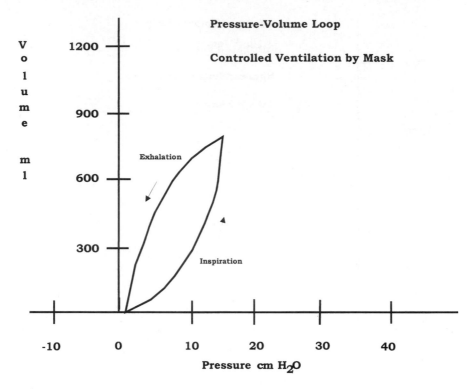

FIGURE **19.35.**   With mask ventilation, the pressure rises more slowly during inspiration. During expiration, the absence of the tracheal tube decreases resistance to flow and volume and pressure drops rapidly.

mouth, pharynx, and esophagus as well as the trachea and lungs. The basic shape of the pressure-volume loop is still double convex (Fig. 19.35). The inspiratory portion of the loop is more rounded. If there is a significant leak around the mask, an open loop may be seen. The flow-volume loop during mask ventilation (Fig. 19.36) is more rounded during both inspiration and exhalation than that seen with intubation.

Spontaneous Breath during Controlled Ventilation

It is possible for a non-paralyzed patient to initiate a spontaneous breath during controlled ventilation. This can occur at any time during the respiratory cycle. Usually, the spontaneous breath has a lower inspiratory flow than the mechanical breath. Figure 19.37 shows a pressure-volume loop with a spontaneous breath during exhalation. As the spontaneous breath occurs, the pressure drops below the expected level while the volume rises above the usual curve. As the spontaneous breath is exhaled, the pressure increases briefly, and the volume drops. The remainder of the loop follows the expected shape.

Figure 19.38 depicts a flow-volume loop with a spontaneous breath near the end of inspiration. There is a sudden increase in the inspiratory flow and volume. As the breath is exhaled the flow and volume again move toward zero.

Figure 19.39 shows a series of pressure-volume loops with the solid line (loop 1) representing the normal loop produced with mechanical ventilation. Loop 2 shows a spontaneous effort during inspiration. The loop moves towards the right (pressure increase) with a decrease in the tidal volume. In loop 3, the patient is clearly breathing against the ventilator. The loop moves to the negative side of the pressure axis and then changes to positive. The pressures generated are quite high and the tidal volume is decreased since the patient is exhaling during inspiration.

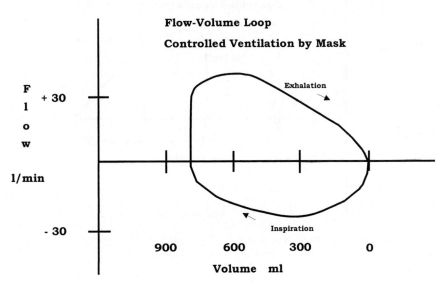

FIGURE 19.36. Mask ventilation. The inspiratory flow is more variable when ventilation is manually controlled than when a ventilator is used. During exhalation the lower resistance due to the absence of a tracheal tube results in higher flows.

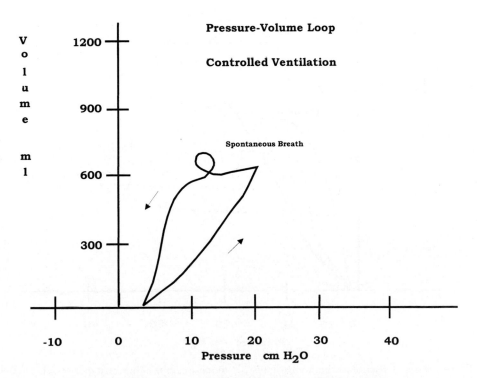

FIGURE 19.37. This spontaneous breath occurs during expiration.

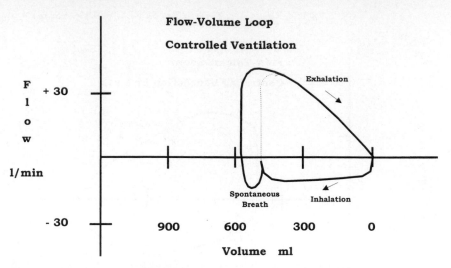

FIGURE 19.38. The spontaneous breath occurs near the end of inspiration. The dotted line represents the normal loop. Instead of returning to zero at the end of inspiration, the flow increases. There is a small increase in volume as well.

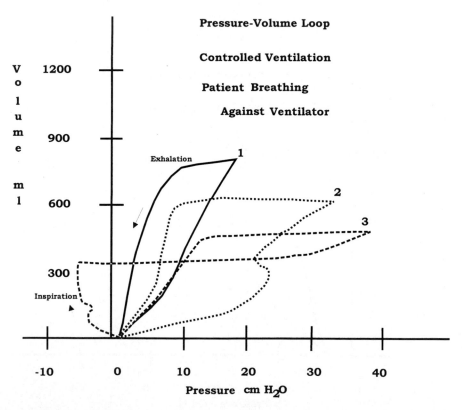

FIGURE 19.39. Loop 1 represents the normal loop. Loop 2 shows a spontaneous breath during inspiration. The pressure drops and the volume increases briefly. There is a decrease in compliance caused by an increase in tension in the chest wall muscles. In Loop 3 the patient inhales at the beginning of the respiratory cycle, so the loop moves to the left of the vertical axis. There is a further decrease in compliance.

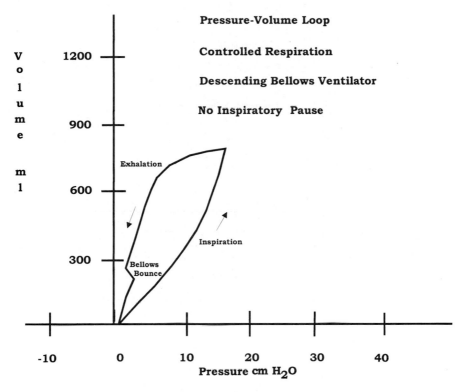

FIGURE 19.40. Expansion of the bellows is halted abruptly when it reaches its set limit. This causes a disruption (bounce) in the expiratory limb.

Ventilator with Descending Bellows

While most anesthesia ventilators in use today have bellows that ascend during expiration, there are some in which the bellows expands downward. The loops associated with these ventilators have special characteristics. The pressure-volume loop is shown in Figure 19.40. As the bellows expands during exhalation, there is a slight bounce as it reaches a stop. At that point, there is a slight increase in pressure, which is manifested in a small blip to the right. The corresponding flow-volume loop (Fig. 19.41) has a small step near the end of exhalation.

Open Loop

A loop should return to its starting point at the end of the respiratory cycle. An open loop (Figs. 19.42 and 19.43) has a gap between the end and starting points, indicating that the exhaled volume is significantly less than the inhaled volume. The greater the difference in the two volumes, the more open the loop will appear.

There are several possible causes for an open loop. An open loop is normal with an uncuffed tracheal tube or an LMA (76). Incorrect calibration has been previously discussed and should be considered. Another possibility is a leak distal to the sensor. This could be due to a partial disconnection, a tracheal tube cuff leak, or partial extubation. Tension pneumothorax should also be considered. In this case, it is likely that the loop would also show a decrease in compliance.

Gas exchange imbalance is another possible cause of an open loop. The volume of oxygen consumed is normally somewhat higher than the volume of carbon dioxide produced. This makes the exhaled volume smaller than the inhaled volume, but this alone is not enough to open a loop. If nitrous oxide and volatile agents are used, the uptake of these agents, especially during induction, may be sufficient to produce an open loop.

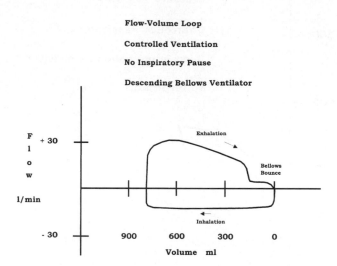

FIGURE 19.41. The step at the end of exhalation is caused by the descending bellows reaching its set limit.

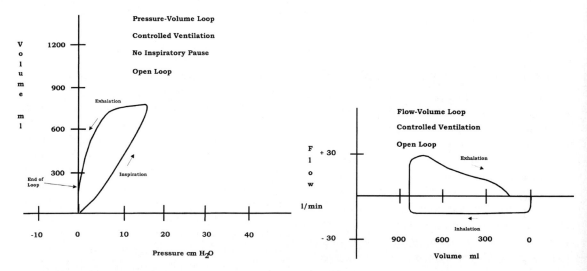

FIGURE 19.42 and FIGURE 19.43. There is a leak, so that exhaled volume is approximately 150 ml less than the inhaled volume. This produces open pressure-volume (PV) and flow-volume (FV) loops.

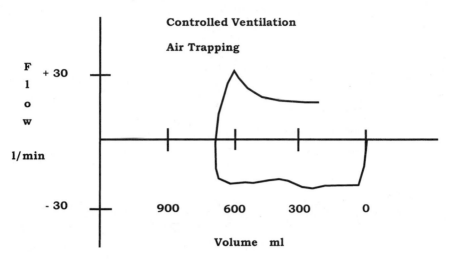

FIGURE 19.44. The gap in the flow-volume loop indicates that there was still expiratory flow when the next respiration commenced.

If exhalation is not completed before the next inhalation begins, the exhaled volume will be substantially less than the inspired volume (Fig. 19.44). This will be indicated by the absence of a period of zero flow before the next inhalation. This may occur in patients with chronic airway obstruction or increased expiratory resistance due to an equipment problem. A retractor compressing the lung can cause this problem (19). Another possible cause is a flap-valve obstruction in a large airway (77). A double-lumen bronchial tube may impose sufficient resistance to result in incomplete emptying of the lungs even in patients with normal airways (20).

Overshoot Loop

An overshoot loop (Figs. 19.45 and 19.46) indicates that the exhaled volume is greater than the inspired volume. This usually indicates the need for recalibration. It can also result if there is pressure on the thorax causing some of the functional residual volume to be added to the tidal volume.

Tubing Misconnection

Older sensors had a long and a short nipple that are designed to connect to the short and long lumens of the pressure tubing respectively. It was possible to connect the tubings long to long and short to short. If this is done, the monitor senses exhalation as inhalation and vice versa. The loops will be drawn backwards and upside down (Figs. 19.47 and 19.48). In addition, it will take two respiratory cycles to produce a full loop. The monitor will be unable to compute the compliance. Extremely high PEEP pressures will be recorded. Newer sensors with male and female connections make tubing misconnections less likely.

Disconnection Proximal to the Sensor

If there is a disconnection between the breathing system and the spirometry sensor, there will be no flow through the sensor during mechanical ventilation and a loop will not be generated (Figs. 19.49 and 19.50). If the patient begins to breathe spontaneously, loops similar to those seen with spontaneous respiration will be generated.

Leak Between Sensor and Breathing System

If there is a leak or partial disconnection between the sensor and the breathing system, some gas will be lost. The pressure-volume loop (Fig. 19.51, solid line) will be normal in shape but will show a decrease in tidal volume and a decrease in peak airway pressure. The flow-volume loop (Fig. 19.52, solid line) also will show a decreased tidal volume and a decrease in peak expiratory flow.

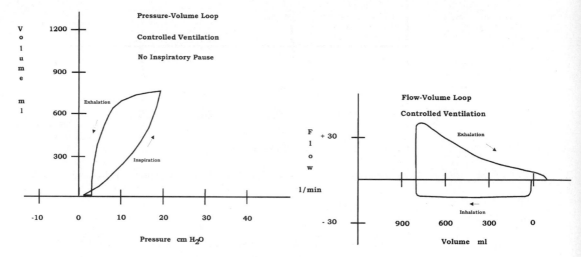

FIGURE 19.45 and **FIGURE 19.46.** The exhaled volume exceeds the inhaled volume, producing an overshoot loop.

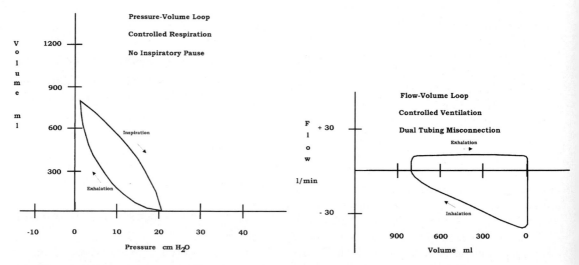

FIGURE 19.47 and **FIGURE 19.48.** Misconnection of the tubings will cause the loop to be drawn backwards and upside down.

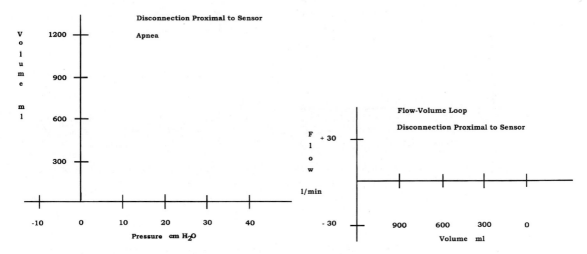

FIGURE 19.49 and **FIGURE 19.50.** A disconnection between the breathing system and the sensor will result in no flow through the sensor.

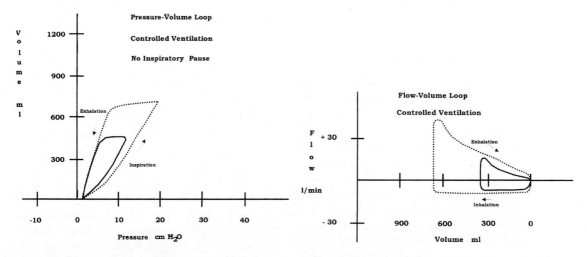

FIGURE 19.51 and **FIGURE 19.52.** With a leak between the breathing system and the sensor, the loop will have a normal shape but the tidal volume, peak pressure, and expiratory flows will be decreased. The dotted line represents the normal loop and the solid line the loop with a leak.

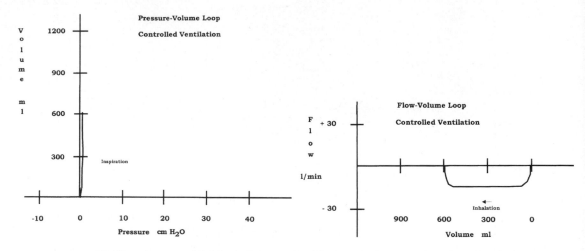

FIGURE 19.53 and **FIGURE 19.54.** A disconnection distal to the sensor will result in flow during inspiration, but none during exhalation.

The loops will not be open because the same volume that the patient inhales will be exhaled.

Disconnection Distal to Sensor

With a disconnection distal to the sensor, during controlled ventilation, there will be flow during inspiration but not exhalation (Figs. 19.53 and 19.54).

Changes in Compliance

A major advantage of pressure-volume loops is the ability to detect changes in compliance. If the lungs or chest wall become stiffer, the pressure necessary to deliver the tidal volume increases. This causes the pressure-volume loop to be displaced clockwise (Fig. 19.55). Increased compliance will cause it to be displaced counterclockwise. Since changes in compliance often occur gradually, they may not be recognized unless the change is large. It is useful, therefore, to store a loop from the beginning of the case for comparison.

Decreases in compliance can result from inadequate muscle relaxation; air embolism; diseases and tumors that invade large areas of the lung or alter its distensibility; narcotics; bronchial intubation; bronchoconstriction; pneumothorax; reduction pneumoplasty; lateral decubitus, lithotomy, or Trendelenburg position; external pressure on the chest or abdomen; abdominal retractors or packing; abdominal enlargement; curvature of the spine; obesity; prone position; or pressurization of the peritoneal cavity for laparoscopic surgery (4, 22, 78–89).

PEEP may cause an increase in compliance (Fig. 19.56, solid line). Loops may help to determine when the maximum benefit of PEEP has been reached.

Decreases in compliance will affect the flow-volume loop (Fig. 19.57, dotted line). Flow will be increased during exhalation, with a higher peak and a steeper slope.

Changes in Resistance

In intubated patients, an increase in resistance distal to the sensor may be caused by obstruction of the tracheal tube (kinking, dislodgment, secretions), bronchoconstriction, collapse of airways from loss of elastic recoil, or obstruction in a large airway caused by secretions, blood, foreign body, neoplasm, or inflammation. This pattern may also be seen when using a tracheal tube that is too small. Non-intubated patients may have obstruction in the upper airway as well. Changes in the loops toward normal indicate the effectiveness of treatment.

During controlled ventilation, increased resistance causes higher inspiratory pressures to be required to deliver a given flow. Tidal volume may be reduced. As shown in Figure 19.58 (solid line)

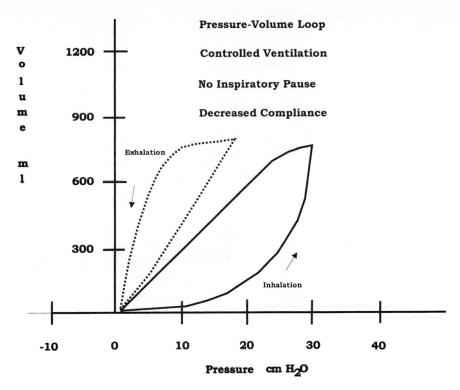

FIGURE 19.55. Low compliance causes the loop to be moved closer to the horizontal axis. High compliance causes the loop to move closer to the vertical axis. The dotted line represents normal compliance; the solid line represents decreased compliance.

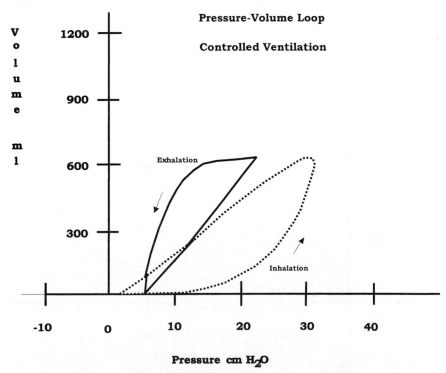

FIGURE 19.56. The dotted line represents decreased compliance. The addition of positive end–expiratory pressure (PEEP) results in a more normal-looking loop.

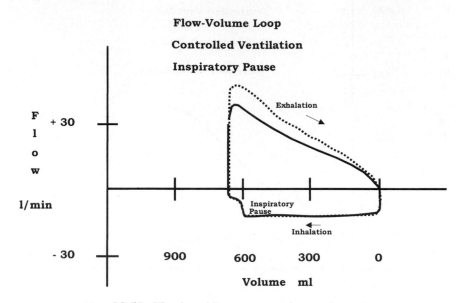

FIGURE **19.57.** The dotted line represents decreased compliance.

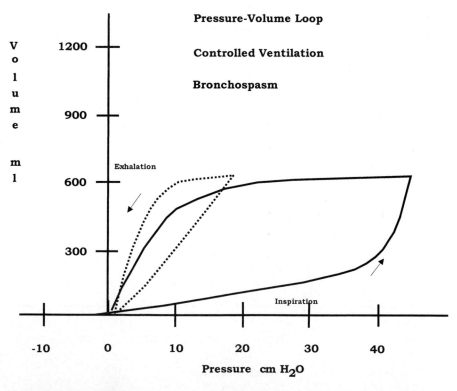

FIGURE **19.58.** With an increase in resistance, a higher pressure is needed to deliver the same volume (solid curve). Tidal volume may be reduced.

the pressure-volume loop is shifted to the right and downward with a large internal area. The pressure falls rapidly after inspiration is complete. There may be a negative pressure as the ventilator bellows tries to expand (19). The loop may be open if there is air trapping. With spontaneous ventilation, the inspiratory limb is displaced leftward (Fig. 19.59, solid line).

If resistance is increased, the flow-volume loop will show decreased peak expiratory flow and decreased flow throughout exhalation (Fig. 19.60, solid line) (3, 19, 21). While mild bronchospasm causes only slight changes in the flow-volume loop, as it increases, there will be changes in both the inspiratory and exhalation portions, as seen in Figure 19.61 (solid line). With severe expiratory resistance, expiratory flow may stop abruptly before the next mechanical inflation.

Severe Chronic Obstructive Lung Disease

Emphysema is characterized by a progressive loss of elastic tissue in the lung. These patients have no problem with inflating the lungs but must do work to exhale. The pressure-volume (PV) loop seen with this condition is shown in Figure 19.62. During exhalation the pressure drops with little change in volume until the end of exhalation. The corresponding flow-volume loop is shown in Figure 19.63. During expiration, there is a severe reduction in flow. These loops may be open if the patient does not have sufficient time to exhale completely.

Tracheal or Upper Airway Obstruction (90)

Flow-volume curves may be helpful in identifying tracheal or upper airway obstruction (91).

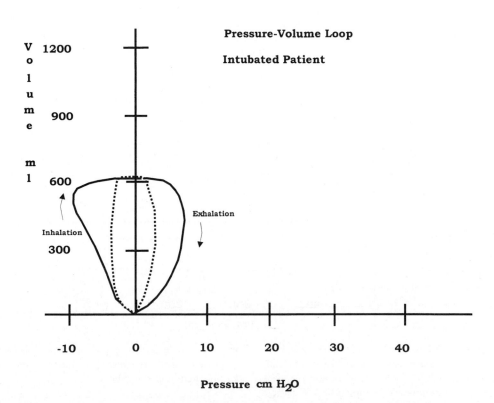

FIGURE 19.59. Spontaneous respiration with increased resistance. The normal loop is shown with dotted lines. With increased resistance greater pressure (more negative during inspiration, more positive during exhalation) will be needed to move the same volume of gas.

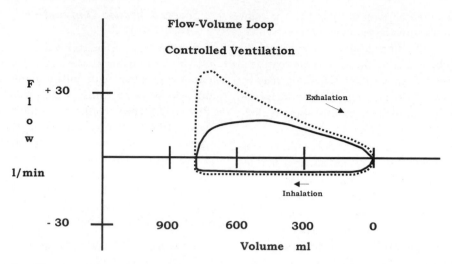

FIGURE 19.60. The dotted line represents the curve with normal resistance. With increased resistance there is diminished expiratory flow. The convex configuration of the expiratory limb reflects uneven lung emptying.

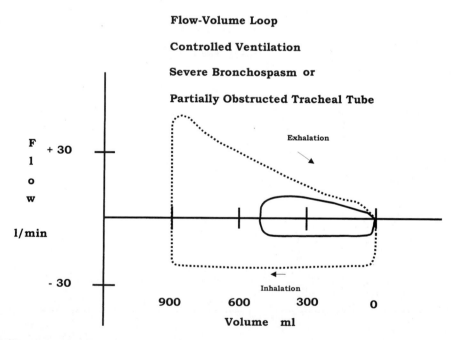

FIGURE 19.61. A kinked tracheal tube results in both inspiratory and expiratory obstruction. With a severe increase in resistance, the ventilator cannot fully compensate and inspiratory flow will be diminished. Tidal volume may be decreased. Expiratory flow is also severely decreased. The dotted line represents the curve without an obstruction in the tube.

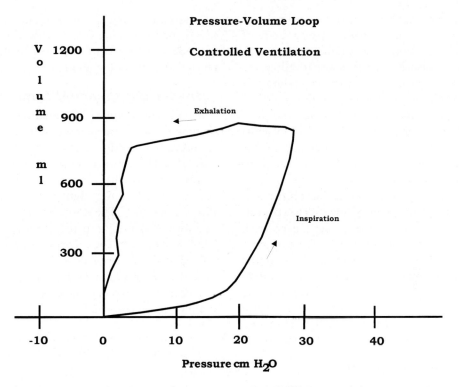

FIGURE 19.62. With severe chronic obstructive pulmonary disease (COPD), resistance during expiration is greatly increased. The patient may have difficulty exhaling completely before the next inspiration, producing an open loop.

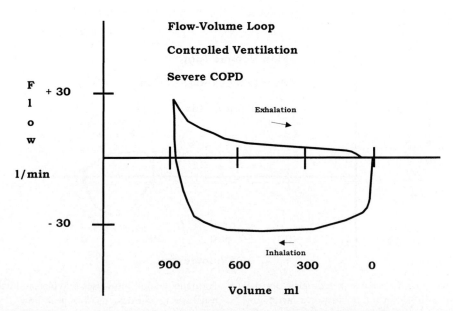

FIGURE 19.63. With severe chronic obstructive pulmonary disease (COPD) expiratory flow is severely reduced.

When the cross-sectional area of the airway is decreased to a critical level, characteristic patterns of flow occur with spontaneous ventilation. Typically the flow rate will plateau. The value of the flow rate at this plateau is proportional to the minimum area of the flow-limiting segment of the airway.

With a fixed obstruction and spontaneous ventilation, both the inspiratory and expiratory limbs of the flow-volume curve are flattened. If there is a variable obstruction, only one limb is flattened, depending on whether the obstruction is intra- or extrathoracic. When there is a variable obstruction within the thorax, expiratory flow rises to a plateau instead of the usual rise to, and descent from, peak flow (Fig. 19.64, solid line) (92). Conversely, a variable obstruction located outside the thorax will cause decreased flow during inspiration (92) (Fig. 19.65, solid line). A lesion located at the thoracic outlet will not be affected by pressures above or below the lesion since flow is limited equally during both inhalation and exhalation.

Restrictive Disease (90)

The increase in elastic recoil in restrictive defects increases the force driving expiratory flow. Thus, even before lung volumes are decreased, the flow-volume loop usually shows a high expiratory flow associated with a steep descending limb. As the process becomes more severe, lung volumes are decreased and the flow-volume loop becomes tall and narrow (Fig. 19.66, solid line). With severe reduction of lung volumes, the flow-volume loop may have a relatively normal shape, but be smaller than normal in all dimensions.

Inadvertent Bronchial Intubation

Inadvertent bronchial intubation can occur anytime a tracheal tube is inserted. If this happens, the pressure needed to deliver a set tidal volume rises (19). The pressure-volume loop will show a decrease in compliance with a rightward and downward shift and a high peak pressure (Fig. 19.67, solid line). The flow-volume loop associated with bronchial intubation is shown in Figure 19.68 (solid line). The increase in peak pressure will increase the peak flow during exhalation. After the tracheal tube has been properly repositioned, there should be a decrease in peak pressure and increase in compliance.

Double-Lumen Bronchial Tube Problems (4, 19, 20, 88, 93, 94)

Double-lumen bronchial tubes are often placed incorrectly or may be displaced during patient positioning or surgery. Continuous spirometric monitoring can help in detecting a problem. Baseline flow-volume and flow-pressure loops should be established for each patient in the supine position during two-lung ventilation to allow comparison with later ones.

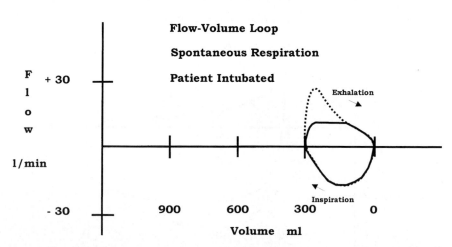

FIGURE **19.64.** With a variable intrathoracic obstruction (such as a tumor in the trachea or a mediastinal mass), inspiratory flow may be relatively normal, but during expiration, flow rises to a plateau instead of the usual rise to and descent from peak flow.

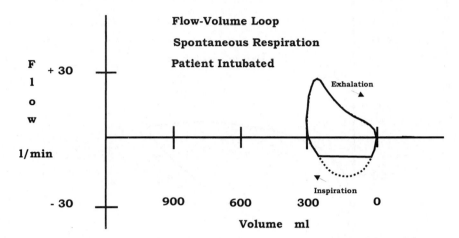

FIGURE 19.65. A variable obstruction located outside the thorax will cause a plateau during inspiration. The expiratory portion of the curve is close to normal.

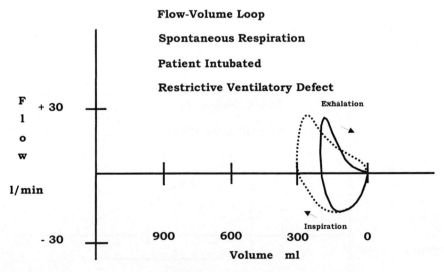

FIGURE 19.66. With a restrictive defect the increase in elastic recoil is associated with higher expiratory flows. As the process becomes more severe and lung volumes are decreased, the flow-volume curve becomes tall and narrow.

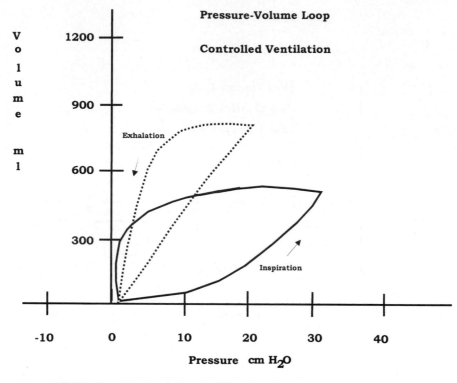

FIGURE **19.67.** Bronchial intubation (solid loop) will result in a decrease in compliance.

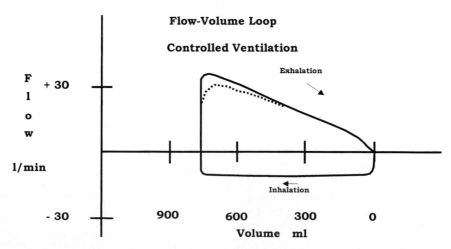

FIGURE **19.68.** Bronchial intubation. The solid loop shows an increase in expiratory flow, especially during the early part of expiration.

When one-lung ventilation is begun, the pressure-volume loop should show a slight shift of the slope to the right, reflecting decreased compliance, if the double-lumen tube is positioned correctly (88, 93, 94). The flow-volume loop will show a slightly decreased expiratory flow rate. With surgical handling of the non-dependent lung, compliance may decrease further (88).

If a double-lumen tube is placed too deeply, there will be a decrease in compliance (Fig. 19.69, solid line). The flow-volume loop will show diminished inspiratory and expiratory flows. Tidal volumes may be decreased. Incomplete emptying of the lung with production of an open loop may occur (20).

The loops shown in Figure 19.70 resulted from the tip of the bronchial lumen's impinging on the wall of the bronchus. Loop 1 (solid line) is the normal loop. In loop 3 (dotted line), the tube tip has impinged on the wall of the bronchus. Pressure rises rapidly with little increase in volume until sufficient pressure has been exerted to move the tip away from the wall. At this point the volume rises rapidly. There will be an increase in peak pressure and/or a decrease in compliance. If there is a ball-valve action, during exhalation, the pressure will decrease rapidly with little change in volume until the pressure in the bronchial tube has fallen sufficiently to allow exhalation. Adjusting the depth of the tube will cause a change in the

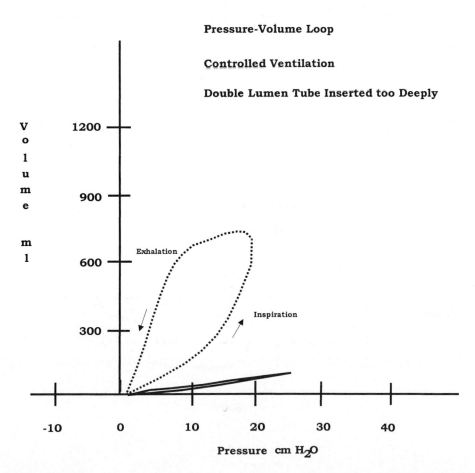

FIGURE 19.69.   The dotted line represents the loop when the double-lumen tube is correctly positioned. If the bronchial lumen is inserted too deeply, a severe reduction in compliance and tidal volume will be seen.

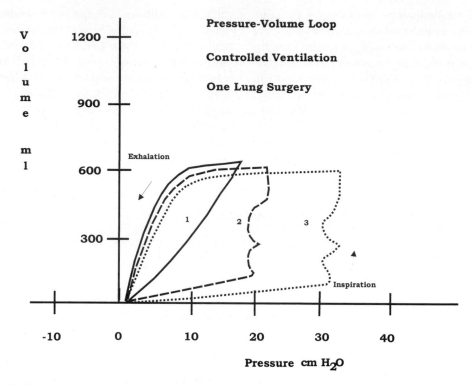

FIGURE 19.70. Impingement of the end of the tube on the bronchial wall has created a ball-valve obstruction. The pressure rises rapidly with little increase in volume until the pressure is sufficient to overcome the obstruction. The volume then increases and the pressure drops. If the pressure drops low enough, there will again be obstruction to flow, creating another notch on the upswing of the loop.

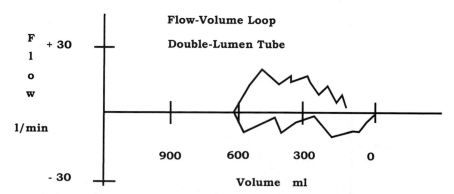

FIGURE 19.71. The loop represents repeated ball-valve obstruction to flow during both inspiration and expiration.

pressure-volume loop (Loop 2 dashed line). Figure 19.71 is the corresponding flow-volume curve. In addition to the irregular shape, there is incomplete expiration, as shown by the open loop.

The flow-volume loop that would be generated if there were a disconnection of one limb of a double-lumen tube or a leaking bronchial cuff is shown in Figure 19.72 (solid line). The inspiratory portion is normal. Because much of the inspired tidal volume is lost through the leak, the loop is open. In addition, there would be decreased flow during exhalation.

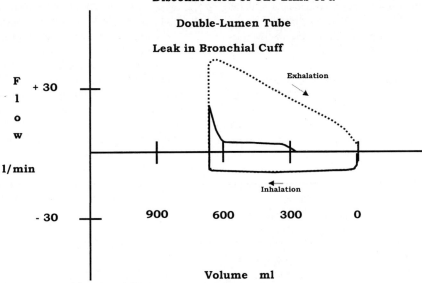

Flow-Volume Loop

Controlled Ventilation

Disconnection of One Limb of a

Double-Lumen Tube

Leak in Bronchial Cuff

FIGURE **19.72.** With a leak in the bronchial cuff or a disconnection of one limb (solid loop), there will be an open loop, with the inhaled volume exceeding the exhaled volume. Exhaled flows will be decreased.

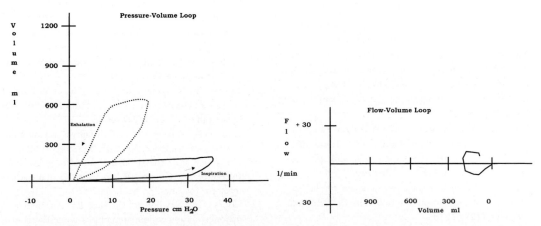

FIGURE **19.73** and FIGURE **19.74.** The loops associated with esophageal intubation may vary greatly. Compliance may be increased, decreased, or normal.

Esophageal Intubation (19)

With esophageal intubation, the pressure-volume loop will usually show a decrease in compliance (Fig. 19.73, solid line), although compliance may be increased or normal. In addition, the loop may be open. The flow-volume loop will be distorted and show small inspiratory and expiratory volumes, often with an open loop (Fig. 19.74).

REFERENCES

1. Elliott WR, Topulas GP. The influence of the mechanics of anesthesia breathing circuits on respiratory monitoring. Biomed Inst Tech 1990;24: 260–265.
2. Banner MJ. Respiratory muscle loading and the work of breathing. J Cardiothorac Vasc Anesth 1995;9: 192–204.
3. Tobin MJ. Monitoring of pressure, flow and volume during mechanical ventilation. Respiratory Care 1992; 37:1081–1096.
4. Bardoczky G, de Vries J, Merilainen P, et al. Side stream spirometry. Monitoring patient ventilation during anaesthesia. Datex Division Instrumentation Corp, Helsinki, Finland
5. Wilson S, Frerk C. A paediatric airway monitor for use with the T-piece. Anaesthesia 1997;52:185.
6. Orr JA, Westenskow DR, Farrell RM. Information content of three breathing circuit monitors: a neural network analysis. Anesthesiology 1992;77:A517.
7. Hatch DJ, Jackson EA. A new critical incident monitor for use with the paediatric T-piece. Anaesthesia 1996; 51:839–842.
8. Wright BM. A respiratory anemometer. J Physiol 1955;127:25.
9. Nunn JF, Ezi–Ashi TI. The accuracy of the respirometer and ventigrator. Br J Anaesth 1962;34:422–432.
10. Byles PH. Observations on some continuously-acting spirometers. Br J Anaesth 1960;32:470–475.
11. Meeke R, Wren W, Davenport J, et al. The measurement of tidal volumes in spontaneously breathing children during general anaesthesia using a Haloscale infant Wright respirometer. Acta Anaesthesiol Scand 1984;28:696–699.
12. Bushman JA. Effect of different flow patterns on the Wright respirometer. Br J Anaesth 1979;51:895–898.
13. Hall KD, Reeser FH. Calibration of Wright spirometer. Anesthesiology 1962;23:126–129.
14. Lunn JN, Hillard EK. The effect of repairs on the performance of the Wright respirometer. Br J Anaesth 1970;42:1127–1130.
15. Ilsley AH, Hart JD, Withers RT, et al. Evaluation of five small turbine-type respirometers used in adult an-

esthesia. Journal of Clinical Monitoring 1993;9: 196–201.
16. Kittredge P. Accuracy of clinical ventilation meters. Respiratory Care 1972;17:181–187.
17. Synnott AJ, Wren WS. Assessment of the Ohio 5400 volume monitor Ohmeda SE302 spirometer and the flow meters of the Servo 900C ventilator. Acta Anaesthesiol Scand 1988;32:30–32.
18. Cotter TP, Bush GL. Volume monitor malfunction caused by an overhead operating room light. Anesthesiology 1989;70:1022.
19. Bardoczky GI, Engelman E, D'Hollander A. Continuous spirometry: an aid to monitoring ventilation during operation. Br J Anaesth 1993;71:747–751.
20. Bardoczky GI, deFrancquen P, Engelman E, et al. Continuous monitoring of pulmonary mechanics with the sidestream spirometer during lung transplantation. J Cardiothorac Vasc Anesth 1992;6:731–734.
21. Huffman LM. AANA journal course: new technologies in anesthesia: update for nurse anesthetists—monitoring ventilation and compliance with Side Stream Spirometry. J Am Assoc Nurse Anesth 1991;59:249–258.
22. Huffman LM. Monitoring compliance: a sensitive indicator of change. J Am Assoc Nurse Anesth 1992;60: 217–220.
23. Merilainen P, Hanninen H, Tuomaala L. A novel sensor for routine continuous spirometry of intubated patients. Journal of Clinical Monitoring 1993;9: 374–380.
24. Anonymous. An Atlas of Spirometry, Datex Corporation.
25. Filmyer W, Weissman C, Sardar A. In-vitro evaluation of an instrument designed to measure ventilation during anesthesia. Anesthesiology 1994;81:A524.
26. Purnell RJ. The position of the Wright anemometer in the circle absorber system. Br J Anaesth 1968;40: 917–918.
27. Feldman JM, Muller J. Tidal volume measurement errors—the impact of lung compliance and a circuit humidifier. Anesthesiology 1990;73:A468.
28. Thorpe CM. Ventilators, circle systems and respirometers. Anaesthesia 1992;47:913.
29. Cooper JB, Newbower RS, Long CD, et al. Preventable anesthesia mishaps. A study of human factors. Anesthesiology 1978;49:399–406.
30. Newton NI, Adams AP. Excessive airway pressure during anaesthesia. Anaesthesia 1978;33:689–699.
31. Holland R. Anesthesia-related mortality in Australia. In: Pierce EC, Cooper JB, eds. Analysis of anesthetic mishaps. Int Anesth Clin 1984;22:61–71.
32. Cooper JB, Newbower RS, Kitz RJ. An analysis of major errors and equipment failures in anesthesia management. Considerations for prevention and detection. Anesthesiology 1984;60:34–42.

33. Keenan RL, Boyan P. Cardiac arrest due to anesthesia. A study of incidence and causes. JAMA 1985;253:2373–2377.

34. Myerson KR, Ilsley AH, Runciman WB. An evaluation of ventilator monitoring alarms. Anaesthesia and Intensive Care 1986;14:174–185.

35. Anonymous. An overview of airway pressure alarms. Technology for Anesthesia 1995;16(3):1–4.

36. Mimpriss T, Spivey A. A simple disconnect alarm. J Med Eng Technol 1989;13:222–224.

37. Anonymous. Standards for basic intra-operative monitoring. American Society of Anesthesiologists Newsletter 1986;50:12–13.

38. Winter A, Spence AA. An international consensus on monitoring [Editorial]. Br J Anaesth 1990;64:263–266.

39. Epstein RA. The elusive "disconnect alarm" examined. Anesthesia Patient Safety Foundation Newsletter 1988;3:39.

40. Campbell RM, Sheikh A, Crosse MM. A study of the incorrect use of ventilator disconnection alarms. Anaesthesia 1996;51:369–370.

41. Eisenkraft JB. Complications of anesthesia delivery systems. ASA Annual Refresher Courses, 1996, No. 255.

42. Pryn SJ, Crosse MM. Ventilator disconnexion alarm failures. Anaesthesia 1989;44:978–981.

43. Picard UM, Hancock DE, Pinchak AC. Pressure transients in anesthesia ventilators—failure of disconnect alarm system. Anesthesiology 1987;67:A189.

44. Reynolds AC. Disconnect alarm failure. Anesthesiology 1983;58:488.

45. Schreiber PJ. Corrections concerning alleged disconnect alarm failure. Anesthesiology 1983;59:601.

46. Bourke AE, Snowdon SL, Ryan TDR. Failure of a ventilator alarm to detect patient disconnection. J Med Eng Technol 1987;11:65–67.

47. Murphy PJ, Rabey FG. The Humphrey ADE breathing system and ventilator alarm. Anaesthesia 1991;46:1000.

48. Lawrence JC. Breathing system gas pressure monitoring and venting, ventilator monitors and alarms. Anaesthesia and Intensive Care 1988;16:38–40.

49. Russell WJ, Webb RK, Van der Walt JH, et al. Problems with ventilation: an analysis of 2000 incident reports. Anaesthesia and Intensive Care 1993;21:617–620.

50. Anonymous. Alert. Breathing circuit alarms. Health Devices 1980;9:1.

51. Anonymous. Canadian government issues alert on Monagahan/Hospital 703 ventilator alarm. Biomedical Safety & Standards 1980;10:135.

52. Hommelgaard P, Nissen T. A water-insensitive ventilator alarm. Anaesthesia 1979;34:1048–1051.

53. Seed RF. Alarms for lung ventilators. Br J Clin Equip 1978;4:114–121.

54. McEwen JA, Small CF, Jenkins LC. Detection of interruptions in the breathing gas of ventilated anaesthetized patients. Can J Anaesth 1988;35:549–561.

55. Sinclair A, VanBergen J. Flow resistance of coaxial breathing systems: investigation of a circuit disconnect. Can J Anaesth 1992;39:90–94.

56. Sarnquist FH, Demas K. The silent ventilator. Anesth Analg 1982;61:713–714.

57. Schreiber P. Safety guidelines for anesthesia systems. Boston: Merchants, 1984.

58. Raphael DT. An algorithmic response for the breathing system low-pressure alarm condition. Progress in Anesthesiology 1997;11:219–244.

59. Anonymous. Airway pressure monitor. Biomedical Safety & Standards 1982;12:123.

60. Anonymous. Evaluation of ventilator alarms. J Med Eng Technol 1984;8:270–276.

63. Schreiber PJ. Anesthesia ventilators should have adjustable high-pressure alarms: a reply. Anesthesiology 1985;63:232–233.

64. Spielman FJ, Sprague DH. Another benefit of the subatmospheric alarm. Anesthesiology 1981;54:526–527.

65. Anonymous. Ventilation alarms. Health Devices 1981;10:204–220.

66. Rendell–Baker L, Meyer JA. Accidental disconnection and pulmonary barotrauma. Anesthesiology 1983;58:286.

67. Bashein G, MacEvoy B. Anesthesia ventilators should have adjustable high-pressure alarms. Anesthesiology 1985;63:231–232.

68. Anonymous. Heat/moisture exchange humidifiers. Technology for Anesthesia 1991;11(8):5.

69. Stirt JA, Lewenstein LN. Circle system failure induced by gastric suction. Anaesthesia and Intensive Care 1981;9:161–162.

70. Hodgson CA, Mostafa SM. Riddle of the persistent leak. Anaesthesia 1991;46:799.

71. Walker T. Another problem with a circle system. Anaesthesia 1996;51:89.

72. Sola A, Farina D, Rodriguez S, et al. Lack of relationship between the true airway pressure and the pressure displayed with an infant ventilator. Crit Care Med 1992;20:778–781.

73. Sinclair A, Van Bergen J. Flow resistance of coaxial breathing system: investigation of a circuit disconnect. Can J Anaesth 1992;39:90–94.

74. Bardoczky G, d'Hollander A, Yernault J-C, et al. On-line expiratory flow-volume curves during thoracic surgery: occurrence of auto-PEEP. Br J Anaesth 1994;72:25–28.

75. Patel H, Yang KL. Variability of intrinsic positive end-expiratory pressure in patients receiving mechanical ventilation. Crit Care Med 1995;23:1074–1079.

76. Darling JR, D'Arcy JT, Murray JM. Split laryngeal mask airway is an aid to fiberoptic intubation. Anaesthesia 1993;48:79–80.

77. Breen PH, Serina ER, Barker SJ. Exhaled flow monitoring can detect bronchial flap-valve obstruction in a mechanical lung model. Anesth Analg 1995;81:292–296.

78. Oikkonen M, Tallgren M. Changes in respiratory compliance at laparoscopy: measurement using side stream spirometry. Can J Anaesth 1995;42:495–497.

79. Bardoczky GI, Engelman E, Levarlet M, et al. Ventilatory effects of pneumoperitoneum monitored with continuous spirometry. Anaesthesia 1993;48:309–311.

80. Bennett JA, Abrams JT, VanRiper DF, et al. Difficult ventilation after opioid induction is caused by laryngospasm. Anesthesiology 1995;83:A74.

81. Chassard D, Berrada K, Tournadre J-P, et al. The effects of neuromuscular block on peak airway pressure and abdominal elastance during pneumoperitoneum. Anesth Analg 1996;82:525–527.

82. Fahy B, Barnas G, Flowers J, et al. Effects of increased abdominal pressure on lung and chest wall mechanics during laparoscopy. Anesthesiology 1995;83:A1223.

83. Makinen M-T, Yli-Hankala A. The effect of laparoscopic cholecystectomy on respiratory compliance as determined by continuous spirometry. J Clin Anesth 1996;8:119–122.

84. Kytta J, Randell T, Tanskanen P, et al. Monitoring lung compliance and end-tidal oxygen content for the detection of venous air embolism. Br J Anaesth 1995;75:447–451.

85. Makinen M-T, Yli-Hankala A, Kansanaho M. Early detection of CO_2 pneumothorax with continuous spirometry during laparoscopic fundoplication. Acta Anaesthesiol Scand 1995;39:411–413.

86. Fahy BG, Barnas GM, Nagle SE, et al. Effects of Trendelenburg and reverse Trendelenburg postures on lung and chest wall mechanics. J Clin Anesth 1996;8:236–244.

87. Dash HH, Bithal PK, Joshi S, et al. Airway pressure monitoring as an aid in the diagnosis of air embolism. J Neurosurg Anesth 1993;5:159–163.

88. Iwasaka H, Itah K, Miyakawa H, et al. Continuous monitoring of ventilatory mechanics during one-lung ventilation. Journal of Clinical Monitoring 1996;12:161–164.

89. Dueck R, Cooper S, Kapelanski D, et al. Intraoperative spirometry during reduction pneumoplasty for emphysema. Anesthesiology 1996;85:A1109.

90. Murray JF, Nadel JA. Textbook of respiratory medicine. Philadelphia: WB Saunders, 1994:804–823.

91. Weissman C. Flow-volume relationship between spontaneous breathing through endotracheal tubes. Crit Care Med 1992;20:615–620.

92. Dahlberg CGW, Hales CA. Pulmonary function tests to evaluate the airway. In: Roberts JT, ed. Clinical management of the airway. Philadelphia: WB Saunders, 1994:56–62.

93. Simon BA, Hurford WE, Alfille PH, et al. An aid in the diagnosis of malpositioned double-lumen tubes. Anesthesiology 1992;76:862–863.

94. Bardoczky GI, Levarlet M, Engelman E, et al. Continuous spirometry for detection of double-lumen endobronchial tube displacement. Br J Anaesth 1993;70:499–502.

QUESTIONS

1. Normal static compliance in adult is
   A. 15 ml/cm H_2O
   B. 35 to 100 ml/cm H_2O
   C. 20 to 35 ml/cm H_2O
   D. 35 to 50 ml/cm H_2O
   E. 75 to 125 ml/cm H_2O_2

2. For greatest accuracy the gas flow sensor should be placed
   A. In the inspiratory limb at the canister
   B. Between the inspiratory limb and the Y-piece
   C. Between the Y-piece and the patient
   D. Between the Y-piece and the expiratory limb
   E. On the canister on the exhalation side

3. The preferred site for monitoring airway pressure is
   A. At the ventilator
   B. In the inspiratory limb at the canister
   C. At the connection between the Y-piece and the breathing system
   D. On the expiratory limb at the canister
   E. At the bag mount connection

Each question below contains four suggested answers of which one or more is correct. Choose the answer:
A if 1, 2, and 3 are correct
B if 1 and 3 are correct
C if 2 and 4 are correct
D if 4 is correct
E if 1, 2, 3, and 4 are correct

4. Plateau pressure
   1. Is seen when there is an expiratory pause
   2. Depends on the resistance
   3. Is independent of system compliance
   4. Is normally 2 to 5 cm H_2O less than peak pressure

5. Use of muscle relaxants
   1. May cause the compliance of the lungs to increase
   2. May cause the compliance of the chest wall to increase
   3. May cause a decrease in resistance
   4. May result in a decrease in plateau pressure

6. A rise in peak airway pressure may occur as a result of
   1. An increase in tidal volume
   2. An increase in inspiratory flow rate
   3. An increase in resistance
   4. An increase in compliance

7. Factors which influence compliance include
   1. Interstitial lung water
   2. Alveolar surface tension
   3. Pulmonary fibrosis
   4. Muscle tension

8. Increased resistance to breathing during controlled respiration can be overcome by
   1. Adding or increasing PEEP
   2. Increasing the driving pressure
   3. Increasing the inspired oxygen
   4. Decreasing inspiratory flow

9. Total resistance during inspiration and expiration is influenced by
   1. The patient's airway
   2. The exhalation portion of the breathing system
   3. The size and characteristics of the tracheal tube
   4. The amount of PEEP added to the breathing system

10. Technologies useful for detecting a leak around a tracheal tube include
    1. Airway pressure monitors
    2. Respiratory breath sound monitoring
    3. Respiratory volume measurement
    4. Capnography

11. Respiratory volume monitoring may fail to detect
    1. Occlusion of the airway
    2. A disconnection during spontaneous breathing
    3. Apnea
    4. Esophageal intubation

12. During controlled ventilation the delivered volume may differ from that set on the ventilator due to
    1. Expansion of breathing system components
    2. Fresh gas flow into the breathing system
    3. Gas compression in the breathing system
    4. Leaks

13. Conditions that can be detected using a minimum pressure alarm include
    1. An unconnected ventilator
    2. A major leak in the breathing system
    3. A malfunctioning scavenging system
    4. An increase in resistance

14. The minimum airway pressure alarm should be set
    1. At the lowest setting
    2. At different settings during a case
    3. Greater than 10 cm H_2O
    4. Slightly less than the peak pressure during inspiration

15. Conditions that may prevent activation of the minimum pressure alarm with a disconnection include
    1. PEEP
    2. Partial extubation
    3. High resistance of components of the breathing system
    4. Water in the tubing between the breathing system and the alarm

16. A sustained pressure may be caused by
    1. Occlusion of the inspiratory limb of the breathing system
    2. Occlusion of the scavenging system
    3. Activation of the oxygen flush valve
    4. Improper adjustment of the APL valve

17. An excessively high pressure in the breathing system may be caused by
    1. Patient coughing or straining
    2. Use of the oxygen flush during the inspiratory phase of the ventilator cycle
    3. A punctured ventilator bellows
    4. Increased compliance

18. Subambient pressure in the breathing system may be caused by
    1. A nasogastric tube placed in the trachea and attached to suction
    2. A blocked expiratory limb
    3. Inspiration with an empty reservoir bag
    4. Refilling of a ventilator with a standing bellows with low fresh gas flows

19. On a pressure-volume loop
    1. The furthest point to the right on the horizontal axis represents the tidal volume
    2. The slope of the inspiratory portion is determined by the resistance
    3. The highest point on the curve represents the peak pressure
    4. The curve can slope to the right or left during inspiration

20. On the flow-volume loop
    1. The portion below the horizontal line represents inspiration
    2. The portion above the horizontal line represents the passive deflation as determined by the elastic recoil of the lungs and chest wall
    3. The tidal volume is that point where the loop crosses the horizontal line
    4. This loop is known as a compliance loop

21. Effects of PEEP on the pressure-volume loop include
    1. The loop is moved upward
    2. The point of the loop is flattened
    3. The loop is widened
    4. The beginning point of the loop is moved to the right

22. Possible causes of inadvertent PEEP include
    1. Partial obstruction of the breathing system
    2. Malfunctioning scavenging device
    3. Patients with obstructive airway disease
    4. Patients with airflow obstruction

23. Possible causes of an open loop include
    1. Improper calibration of the monitor
    2. An uncuffed tube

3. A leak distal to the sensor
4. Tension pneumothorax

24. Decreases in compliance may be caused by
1. Inadequate muscle relaxation
2. Prone position
3. Obesity
4. Reverse Trendelenburg position

25. With restrictive lung disease
1. The peak expiratory flow will be increased
2. The flow-volume loop may become tall and narrow
3. The flow-volume loop may have a relatively normal shape but appear smaller in all dimensions
4. Resistance is increased

26. With inadvertent bronchial intubation
1. There will be a decrease in compliance
2. The pressure-volume loop will be shifted to the right and downward
3. The peak pressure will be increased
4. The flow-volume loop will show an increase in peak expiratory flow.

27. If a double-lumen tube is placed too deeply
1. The pressure-volume loop will be shifted to the right and downward
2. There will be a decrease in compliance
3. Resistance will increase
4. An overshoot loop may result

ANSWERS

1. B		**15.** E	
2. C		**16.** C	
3. C		**17.** A	
4. D		**18.** B	
5. C		**19.** D	
6. A		**20.** A	
7. E		**21.** D	
8. C		**22.** E	
9. A		**23.** E	
10. E		**24.** B	
11. E		**25.** A	
12. E		**26.** A	
13. A		**27.** A	
14. C			

Pulse Oximetry

8. Anemia
9. Skin Pigmentation
10. Dyes
11. Optical Interference
12. Nail Polish and Coverings
13. Loss of Accuracy at Low Values
14. Electrical Interference
15. Motion Artifacts
16. Pressure on the Sensor
17. Hyperemia
G. False Alarms
H. Failure to Detect Absence of Circulation
I. Discrepancies in Readings from Different Monitors
J. Failure to Detect Hypoventilation
K. Problems with Sound Recognition
L. Lack of User Knowledge
M. Interference with Other Monitors
XI. Patient Complications
A. Corneal Abrasions
B. Pressure and Ischemic Injuries
C. Burns
D. Electric Shock

INTRODUCTION

PULSE OXIMETRY IS a non-invasive method of measuring oxygen saturation (SpO_2) from a light signal transmitted through tissue, taking into account the pulsatile volume changes that occur.

A reliable, continuous non-invasive method of measuring oxygen delivery was a goal of researchers for many years. Until the 1980s, non-invasive oximeters, known as ear oximeters, were large, expensive, and cumbersome. They required "arterialization" by heat or chemical treatment, and their utility was limited by technical difficulties in differentiating light absorbance of arterial blood from that of venous blood and tissues.

Technical advances, including light-emitting diodes (LEDs), miniaturized photo detectors, and microprocessors, allowed the creation of a new generation of oximeters, which are smaller, less expensive, and easier to use than the earlier models. These differentiate the absorption of incident light by the pulsatile arterial component from the static components. Hence they are called pulse oximeters. Many pulse oximeters are combined with other monitors, such as electrocardiographic

(ECG) monitors and capnometers, into one instrument and may be incorporated into an anesthesia machine.

The American Society of Anesthesiologists has made pulse oximetry a standard for monitoring intraoperatively and in the postanesthesia care unit. International standards for safe practice endorsed by the World Federation of Societies of Anesthesiologists highly recommend continuous use of a quantitative monitor of oxygenation such as pulse oximetry (1). In some states, its use is mandatory. A study of closed claims of anesthetic-related malpractice cases determined that a combination of pulse oximetry and capnography could have prevented 93% of avoidable mishaps (2). A retrospective study in Australia of 2000 incident reports determined that pulse oximetry provided the first warning of an incident in 27% of situations (3). One study found that the number of unanticipated intensive care unit admissions decreased after the introduction of pulse oximetry (4).

PRINCIPLES OF OPERATION (5–11)

The pulse oximeter estimates SpO_2 by measuring pulsatile signals across perfused tissue at two discrete wavelengths, using the constant component of absorption (caused by everything except arterial blood) at each wavelength to normalize the signals (12). It then computes the ratio between these two normalized signals and relates this ratio to the arterial oxygen saturation, using an empirical algorithm. Most pulse oximeters base their calculations on calibration curves derived from studies in healthy volunteers (7).

The two wavelengths allow differentiation of reduced hemoglobin and oxyhemoglobin. Reduced hemoglobin absorbs more light in the red band than does oxyhemoglobin (Fig. 20.1). Oxyhemoglobin absorbs more light in the infrared band. Fractional oxygen saturation (% HbO_2) is the ratio of oxyhemoglobin to the sum of all hemoglobin species present, whether available for reversible binding to oxygen or not (13). Functional oxygen saturation (SaO_2) is defined as the ratio of oxyhemoglobin to all functional hemoglobins. These must be determined using an in vitro oximeter. For patients with low dyshemoglobin levels, the difference between fractional and functional saturation is very small. However, when the dyshemoglobin levels are elevated, the two values

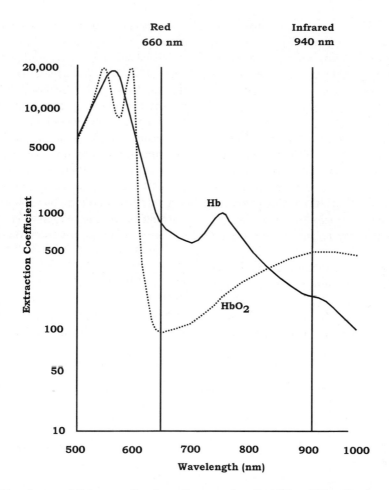

Red
660 nm

Infrared
940 nm

FIGURE **20.1.**   Absorbance of light as a function of wavelength. The extinction coefficient is a measure of the tendency of a substance to absorb light. At the red wavelengths (650 to 750 nm) reduced hemoglobin absorbs more light than does oxyhemoglobin. In the infrared region (900 to 1000 nm) the reverse is true.

can vary greatly and pulse oximeter readings are unlikely to agree with either the true fractional or functional saturation values (12).

The principal barrier to the clinical use of oximetry was the difficulty in separating the absorption of light by arterial blood from that of venous blood and tissues. Modern pulse oximeters discriminate between arterial blood and other components by considering only the change in transmitted light caused by the flow of arterial blood. The transmitted light signal during diastole serves as a reference. The oximeter pulses the red and infrared LEDs on and off several hundred times per second. The rapid sampling rate allows recognition of the times of the peak and trough of each

pulse wave. Absorbance data from both peaks and troughs are saved and used in calculations. At the trough, the vascular bed contains arterial, capillary, and venous blood as well as intervening tissue. At the peak, it contains all this plus a quantity of arterial blood. The presence of this additional arterial blood changes the amount of transmitted light in both the red and infrared bands. Most oximeters have a phase with both LEDs off to allow detection of and compensation for extraneous light. Readings during the off period are subtracted from the next sequence. Data from several sequences are used to calculate the oxygen saturation.

A microcomputer in the pulse oximeter monitors and controls signal levels, coordinates the functional elements, performs the calculations, implements signal validity schemes, activates alarms and messages, and monitors its own circuitry to warn of malfunctions.

PHYSIOLOGY

Efficient oxygen transport relies on the ability of hemoglobin to reversibly load and unload oxygen. The relationship between oxygen tension and oxygen binding is shown in the oxyhemoglobin dissociation curve (Fig. 20.2), which plots the oxygen saturation of hemoglobin against the oxygen tension. The sigmoid shape is essential for physiological transport. As oxygen is taken up in the lungs, the blood is nearly fully saturated over a wide range of tensions. During passage through the systemic capillaries, a large amount of oxygen is released with a relatively small drop in tension. This allows oxygen to be released at sufficiently high concentrations to provide an adequate gradient for diffusion into the cells.

The shape of the oxyhemoglobin dissociation curve (Fig. 20.2) limits the degree of desaturation that can be tolerated. Between 90 and 100% saturation, the partial pressure of arterial oxygen (PaO_2) will be 60 torr or above. Below 90% saturation, the curve becomes steeper and small drops in saturation correspond to large drops in the partial pressure. Thus there is a narrow range of saturation that can be considered the safety zone and if a problem develops there may not be much warning before the oxygen level reaches dangerous levels. Normal saturation will decrease as altitude above sea level increases (14).

EQUIPMENT
Sensors

The sensor (probe) is the part intended to come in contact with the patient. It contains two

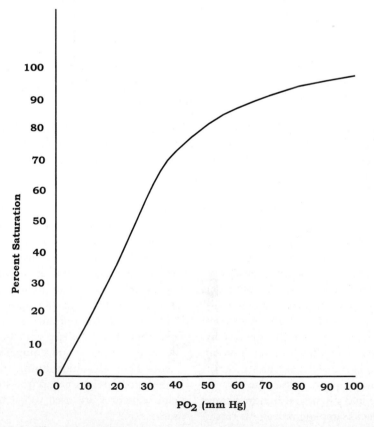

FIGURE 20.2. The oxyhemoglobin dissociation curve. Hemoglobin saturation is plotted as a function of oxygen tension.

or more LEDs (photo diodes) that emit light at specific wavelengths and a photodetector (photocell, transducer). These are mounted in a probe that supports them and maintains them in contact with the pulsatile tissue.

The LEDs provide monochromatic light. This means they emit a constant wavelength throughout their life, so that once calibrated they never need recalibration. The exact wavelengths used vary somewhat with different models. LEDs cause little heating. Thus, the sensor can be left in place for long periods of time without thermal injury. LEDs are so inexpensive they may be used in a disposable probe. The light, partially absorbed and modulated as it passes through the tissue sample, is converted into an electronic signal by the photodetector, which transmits it to the console.

Sensors may be reusable or disposable. A disposable sensor may be attached using an adhesive.

Reusable sensors either clip on or are attached using adhesive. Disposable sensors may be preferable when cross-contamination is a concern. They are sometimes easier to use, but reusable sensors are more economical (15, 16). Tape-on (band) probes are less susceptible to motion artifact and less likely to come off if the patient moves. However, they are usually not as well shielded from ambient light as slide-on probes. Probes lined with soft material may be associated with fewer motion artifacts (17).

Figures 20.3 through 20.9 show several types of available probes. A circumferential design may preclude use in people with extremely large fingers. A metal nose clip from a disposable face mask may be useful in fitting a nasal or flexible probe. Some probes are available in different sizes. If a probe is too large for the patient, some of the output of the LED can reach the photocell without passing through tissue and falsely high SpO_2

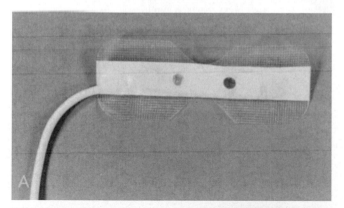

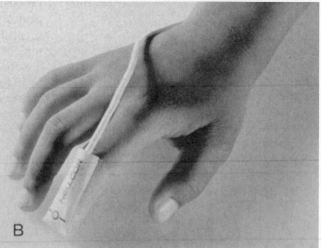

FIGURE **20.3. A,** This disposable probe is most commonly used on the finger, as shown in **B.** Other sites where it has been used include the ear, cheek, tongue, toe, penis, hypothenar or thenar eminence, palm, forefoot, and wrist. (Courtesy of Nellcor, Inc.)

FIGURE 20.4. A, Disposable probe designed for use on the nose. It may come with a means for degreating the skin. **B,** The disposable nasal probe in place. (Courtesy of Nellcor, Inc.)

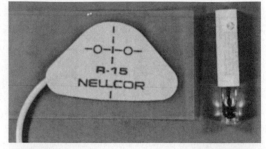

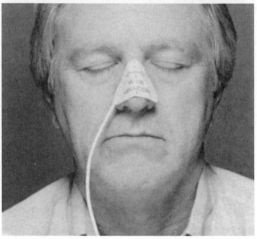

FIGURE 20.5. Reusable probe designed for use on the ear. This may also be used on various other locations, including the cheek.

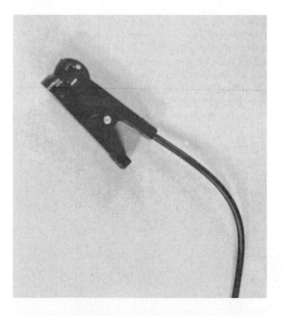

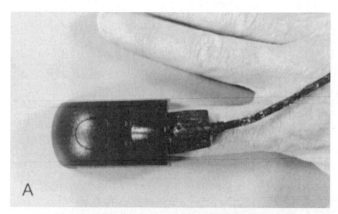

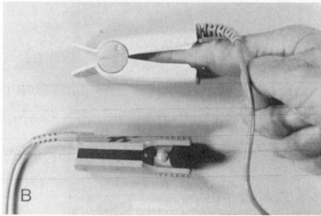

FIGURE **20.6.** Reusable probes for use on fingers or toes in adults and children. In infants, this type of probe can be placed on part of the hand, including some fingers, or part of the foot, including some toes. These probes offer better shielding from ambient light than some other probes.

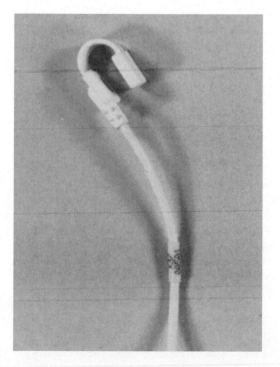

FIGURE **20.7.** Reusable probe for use on finger or toe of pediatric patient. It may also be used on the thenar or hypothenar eminence, the wings of the nostrils, or the nasal septum. The probe should be taped in place.

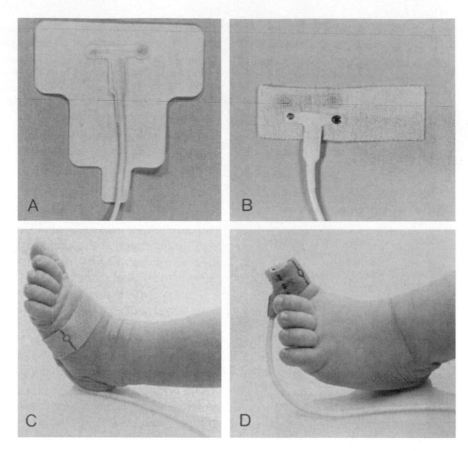

FIGURE **20.8.**   Reusable flexible probes. **A,** This probe is attached to the patient using a disposable adhesive backing. **B,** This probe is attached to an elastic bandage for attachment to the patient. **C** and **D,** The probe is wrapped around the finger, palm, foot, or toe in a manner similar to a common bandage. These probes offer some shielding from ambient light.

readings will be produced (18). Probes specially designed for use during magnetic resonance imaging (MRI) are available (19, 20). Aluminum foil and other materials may be used to shield the probe (19, 21).

Various methods have been devised to hold probes in place. It should be determined that these do not affect the accuracy of the device before use. Making it difficult to separate a reusable sensor from the cable will reduce loss of reusable sensors (16). Attaching the probe to the oximeter case when not in use will reduce damage and make it easy to find (22).

Cable

The probe is connected to the console by an electrical cable. Cables from different manufacturers should not be used interchangeably.

Console

Many different consoles are available. Most are line operated but will work on batteries, making them suitable for use during transport. Most units have a bright display, allowing them to be seen in a darkened room. The front panel usually displays percent saturation, pulse rate, and alarm limits. A variety of messages may be provided to inform the operator of its functional status (8). Pulse amplitude may be represented using a lighted vertical post whose height rises with an increase in pulse amplitude, by a bar graph on a dot matrix display, or as a plethysmograph waveform.

The displayed values for SpO_2 and pulse rate are usually weighted averages. This provides a value with lower sensitivity to motion and other "noise." Some oximeters allow the averaging period to be adjusted. A mode that averages over a

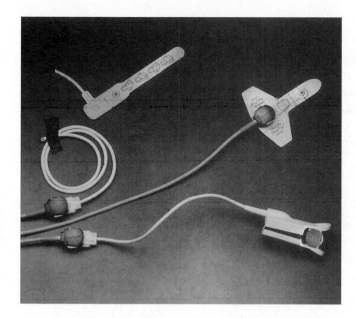

FIGURE **20.9.** Three types of probes. At top is a disposable infant probe that can be wrapped around different vascular beds. The middle is an adult disposable finger probe. The cable snaps onto the probe. The lower probe is an adult reusable probe. (Courtesy of Ohmeda, a division of BOC Healthcare Inc.)

longer period of time is better if there is much probe motion (23). However, changes in pulse rate or saturation will be reflected more rapidly in a mode that averages over a shorter period of time. Most instruments provide an audible tone whose pitch changes with the saturation with each pulse. In this way, the operator can be made aware of changes in SpO$_2$ without looking at the oximeter. There may be a means to control the volume of the beep. Alarms are commonly provided for low and high pulse rates and low and high saturations. Most units generate an alarm when the sensor is not properly applied to the patient or for some other reason the signal is inadequate.

Many pulse oximeters offer trend data (24). Interfaces for hard copy recording and data management systems are sometimes available.

OXIMETER STANDARDS

A U.S. standard (25) and an international standard (26) were published in 1992. Among the provisions are the following:

1. Manufacturers must disclose the accuracy and range of hemoglobin saturation over which the accuracy is claimed; whether the calibration was to functional or fractional saturation; the accuracy and range for the pulse rate if this is provided and the range over which this accuracy is claimed.

2. If intended for continuous monitoring, the pulse oximeter must have a low SpO$_2$ alarm, whose default limit is 80% or greater.
3. Visual indication of signal adequacy should be provided.
4. If a pulse waveform is displayed, a visual display of pulse strength shall also be provided.
5. If a variable pitch audible annunciation is provided for the pulse signal, the change in pitch or amplitude should parallel the reading.
6. If the pulse oximeter is provided with user-adjustable controls to compensate for dysfunctional hemoglobin, there shall be a clear indication that these controls have been adjusted.
7. If intended for continuous monitoring, a probe fault alarm shall be provided.

USE
Sites

The sensor is attached to a pulsatile vascular bed. Such a bed may include the fingertip; hypothenar or thenar eminence; cheek; penis; toe; earlobe; nose; or in infants, the palm, forefoot, or wrist. It is essential that an assortment of probes be available. If the signal is unsatisfactory, the sensor site should be changed.

Finger

The probe is most commonly attached over the fingertip (see Figs. 20.3*B* and 20.6). The failure rate is less when the probe is placed on the finger than on the earlobe (27, 28).

Under conditions of poor perfusion, finger probes perform better than ear probes (29). If there is poor circulation, a finger block or intraarterial vasodilators may restore circulation and oximeter detection (30–32). Vigorously rubbing the fingertip may temporarily improve circulation to the area (33).

A disadvantage of probes placed on an extremity is that desaturation and resaturation are detected less rapidly than when probes are placed more centrally (34–40). Response time may be quicker when the sensor is placed on the thumb (39). In neonates, SpO_2 obtained from the hand is a better index of oxygenation than that obtained from the foot (41).

The finger with the strongest pulsatile signal can be located using the pulse signal strength. Motion artifacts are less frequent when the sensor is placed on one of the larger fingers (17). The little finger may be useful if the patient is particularly large.

In general, the arm opposite from that on which the blood pressure cuff is applied or in which an arterial catheter has been inserted should be used. Insertion of a radial artery catheter is commonly followed by a transient decrease in blood flow and loss of an adequate signal for a pulse oximeter whose probe is placed on a finger of that hand (42). With some monitors, the pulse oximeter is integrated with the non-invasive blood pressure monitor so that the pulse oximeter will not alarm during the inflation cycle. Occasionally, poor function may occur with probe attachment to the same extremity as the intravenous infusion, due to local hypothermia and vasoconstriction. When one limb is above the other, the pulse amplitude and SpO_2 will be greater in the upper than the dependent hand (43).

If there is dark fingernail polish or synthetic fingernails, the probe should be oriented so that it transmits light from one side of the finger to the other (44). Some types of clear acrylic nails do not affect pulse oximeter readings (45).

The pulse oximeter may be placed over a finger with a second degree burn and massive exudation (46).

Toe

The toe is an alternate site when the finger is not available or the signal from the finger is unsatisfactory. Detection of desaturation or resaturation will not be as rapid as with more centrally placed sensors (40). However, in patients who have had an epidural block the toe may provide a more reliable signal (47). An increase in pulse amplitude from the toe may aid in early detection of a successful block.

Nose

The nose is usually a convenient location. The bridge of the nose (see Fig. 20.4B), the wings of the nostrils, and the nasal septum have been used (48). The nose clip from a disposable oxygen face mask can be attached to the outer surface of a flexible sensor to make it fit snugly (49). The nose has been recommended for conditions such as hypothermia, hypotension, and infusion of vasoconstrictor drugs (50). The evidence on this is conflicting. One study found that nasal probes often give grossly erroneous results and had a higher failure rate than other sites under conditions of poor perfusion (29). However, another study found that in hypothermic patients the nasal septum was a more reliable site than the finger. Another study found that nasal probes were associated with a higher failure rate than finger probes (51).

Nasal pulse oximeter SpO_2 readings are higher than those with finger probes (48, 52) and may be more accurate (48). Nasal probes respond more rapidly to desaturation than probes placed on extremities. If the patient is placed in the Trendelenburg position, venous congestion may occur around the nose, causing the pulse oximeter to read low (53).

Ear

The ear probe is useful when the hand is not accessible or significant finger motion is expected. It may be held in place by a plastic semicircular device hung around the ear. Stabilizing devices such as headbands or around-the-ear loops may be useful. The nose clip from a disposable oxygen face mask can be used to hold the sensor in place (49).

The earlobe should be massaged for 30 to 45

seconds with alcohol or vasodilator cream before sensor application to increase perfusion and improve oximeter performance. Response time is faster with an ear probe than with a finger probe (35, 36, 39, 54), but ear probes are associated with a higher failure rate (51). Under conditions of poor perfusion, some ear probes perform well compared with finger probes (29). Ear probes may give more erroneous readings than finger probes in patients with tricuspid incompetence (55). A probe in this location will not produce a consistently good signal during cardiopulmonary resuscitation (56).

Tongue

A tongue probe can be fashioned by placing a malleable aluminum strip behind the sensor to allow it to bend around the tongue (57, 58). A disposable probe wrapped around the tip of the tongue in the sagittal plane may also be used (59). The mouth should be closed.

A lingual probe is somewhat difficult to maintain in place during emergencies but is more resistant to signal interference from electrosurgery than peripheral sites (57, 58). Glossal pulse oximetry has been shown to be accurate (59).

The major causes of lingual probe failure are malposition and tongue movement, especially if the patient is lightly anesthetized. Tongue quivering may mimic tachycardia. Other causes are venous congestion from the Trendelenburg position and excess oral secretions. The probe must be positioned after tracheal intubation and can be dislodged easily.

This site may be especially useful in patients with burns over a large percentage of their body surface (58, 59). Desaturation and resaturation are detected by a sensor at the tongue quicker than one on the finger or toe (40).

Cheek

A probe with a metal strip backing can be used to hold a disposable probe around the cheek or lips (60, 61). A clip-on probe can also be used (62–64).

Buccal pulse oximetry is more accurate than finger pulse oximetry (61, 65, 66). Sensors at this location have been shown to react to increases and decreases in saturation quicker than at the finger

or toe (40). Buccal oximetry has been found to be effective during hypothermia, decreased cardiac output, increased systemic vascular resistance and other low pulse pressure states. Disadvantages include difficult placement, poor acceptance by awake patients and artifacts during airway maneuvers. This site is useful in patients with burns (67).

Other

In infants, flexible probes may work through the palm, foot, penis, ankle, lower calf, or even arm (68–70) (see Fig. 20.8C). Adhesive tape or wrap can be used to attach a flexible probe to the vascular bed. The probe should be snug against the skin but not so tight as to cause vasoconstriction. Circulation distal to the sensor location should be checked frequently. Clip-on reusable probes can be used in infants by placing the probe on the palm, finger, foot, or toe (69).

Fixation

Proper probe placement is crucial for good performance. Care needs to be taken to align the LEDs and the sensor and the site to be sensed between them. A malpositioned probe can result in false-positive and false-negative alarms (71). Probes can be totally or partially dislodged without this being noticed, especially if the probe is under drapes. Adhesive probes may stay on better than clip-on probes. It may be beneficial to tape probes in place when they will be inaccessible during surgery, but it is important to avoid compression of the finger or other part. Wrapping the limb with gauze may help to fix the probe in position. Another method is to slip the cut finger of a glove over the probe (72). The sensor should be protected from bright light.

Stabilization

The pulse search that occurs when a probe is initially applied (or dislodged) includes sequential trials of various intensities of light in an effort to find a pulse strong enough to transmit through the tissue but not so strong that the detection system is saturated (7). Once a pulse is found, there is generally a delay of a few more seconds while SpO_2 values for several pulses are averaged.

Appearance of a satisfactory waveform is a good indication that the readings are reliable. Comparison of the pulse rate shown by the oximeter and that by an ECG monitor is a good indication that saturation readings are accurate (73). A discrepancy between the rates is frequently an indication of malposition or malfunction of the probe.

Reuse of Probes

Because disposable sensors are costly, many institutions reuse them (74–82). Although concerns about this have been raised (83, 84), several studies show that the failure rate of recycled probes is equal to or less than that of new probes and the accuracy is not affected (80–82).

TESTING

One of the drawbacks of pulse oximetry is the inability of the user to check the calibration. There are now devices on the market that can be used to test pulse oximeters (85–88). Some allow the user to set plethysmographic waveforms of different amplitude and test the accuracy of the heart rate as well as SpO_2.

APPLICATIONS
Monitoring Oxygenation

The main purpose of pulse oximetry is to provide warning of hypoxemia, the final common pathway for many life-threatening events, so that treatment can be initiated before irreversible changes occur. Body stores of oxygen are small so changes in oxygenation occur rapidly. The magnitude and speed of a decrease in SpO_2 will depend on the initial SpO_2 and the cause of the decrease. Saturation will fall more quickly with obstructive than central apnea (89).

Anesthetizing Areas

Oxygen desaturation can occur anytime during anesthesia, regardless of the skill and experience of the anesthesia provider. Desaturation greater than 10% occurs in up to 53% of anesthetized patients (90–94). Pediatric patients are especially at risk for hypoxemia (68, 95–99). Most severe desaturations occur during induction or emergence. During maintenance, desaturations are milder but more frequent (100). Studies have shown that a reduction in the number of hypoxemic events occurred when pulse oximetry was used (96, 101).

The incidence of myocardial ischemia is also decreased (102).

Pulse oximetry may help to detect inadvertent bronchial intubation (3, 103–105); however, it is not reliable for this, especially with elevated FIO_2 (7, 106, 107). Also, the absence of desaturation does not rule out bronchial intubation (108).

Oximetry is useful in managing one-lung anesthesia (109, 110). It can help to assess the effectiveness of measures taken to increase the oxygen saturation.

Oximetry is useful for patients undergoing conduction anesthesia and monitored anesthesia care (111, 112). Often the signs of hypoxia are confused with restlessness from an inadequate block and instead of supplying oxygen and assisting respiration, additional sedation is provided, which compounds the problem. With oximetry, the patient's oxygenation status can be assessed and adjustments made to provide the best SpO_2.

Pulse oximetry may be useful to confirm correct tracheal tube placement when a carbon dioxide monitor is not available or nonfunctional (113). If oxygen saturation rises after intubation, correct tube placement is likely. However, it should not be relied on for this purpose since preoxygenation may delay the onset of desaturation beyond the time when esophageal placement of the tube would be considered a possibility.

Other problems that can be manifested by desaturation include fat embolism, amniotic fluid embolism, pulmonary edema, breathing system disconnections and leaks, aspiration, tracheal tube obstruction, hypoxic gas mixture, failure of oxygen delivery, hypoventilation, anaphylaxis, bronchospasm, pneumothorax, malignant hyperthermia, and pulmonary embolism (3, 114–122).

Postanesthesia Care Unit

The recovery room is another situation where desaturation is common (93, 123–134). Routine administration of oxygen to recovering patients may not be necessary if patients are monitored with pulse oximetry (135). Pulse oximetry has been found to increase the patient's safety in the postoperative period when being treated with opiates (136). Before leaving the recovery room, a trial of room air while monitoring oxygen saturation may provide an indication of the need to continue oxygen (137).

Transport

Unrecognized oxygen desaturation may occur during transportation between the operating room and the postanesthesia care unit and between this unit and other areas (138–148). Battery-operated pulse oximeters should be used. Pulse oximetry is included on many transport monitors.

Other Intrahospital Uses

Patients frequently experience hypoxic episodes in the postoperative period (149–154). Pulse oximetry can detect these and aid in deciding when therapy should be discontinued.

It is also useful for monitoring patients in the intensive care unit (155). It may be helpful during weaning from artificial ventilation (156, 157).

It has been used during cardiopulmonary resuscitation (56, 158–160). However, because of artifacts and lag times, it is more useful in primary respiratory arrest than in cardiac arrest. It is useful in assessing oxygenation during newborn resuscitation (161).

Another area where it may prove useful is the emergency department (162–164).

Out-of-Hospital Use

Pulse oximetry may be useful in the prehospital setting, including during transport of patients by helicopter or ambulance (165–175).

Other Uses

Pulse oximetry may be useful in identifying which patients with tonic-clonic seizures are at risk of hypoxic cerebral brain damage (176).

Controlling Oxygen Administration

Pulse oximetry allows administration of the lowest concentration and flow of oxygen compatible with safe levels of arterial oxygenation (177).

Oximetry is useful in situations in which as low an inspired oxygen concentration as possible is desired. These include laser procedures in the airway, during which keeping the oxygen concentration low will diminish the potential for a fire (178).

Monitoring Circulation

Pulse oximetry can be used to detect positions that compromise circulation (179–180). If the pulse oximeter is unable to detect a pulse, the position should be altered. Monitoring oxygen saturation during shoulder arthroscopy has been recommended as a test for brachial artery compression (181). However, an adequate pulse signal may be present with brachial plexus compression (182).

Patients with limb fractures, especially supracondylar fractures of the humerus, may have compromised circulation distal to the fracture (183). Pulse oximetry may serve as a useful guide to blood flow to that area (184).

Pulse oximetry may be used to evaluate the effect of a sympathetic block as indicated by an increase in peripheral blood flow (185).

Pulse oximetry has been used to monitor reimplanted or revascularized digits (186–188). Continuous saturation monitoring can provide warning of decreased perfusion.

Pulse oximetry may be used to determine the best site of amputation or arterial bypass surgery (189). It is a more sensitive index of peripheral perfusion than transcutaneous oxygen or Doppler pressure. It has proved useful in evaluation of the painful hand after creation of an arteriovenous fistula (190).

Pulse oximetry can be used to measure palmar collateral circulation (191–200). However, its usefulness for this has been disputed (201–203). There is a case report of radial artery occlusion which was detected by loss of the pulse oximetry signal (204). A similar examination of the dorsalis pedis and posterior tibial collateral arteries may be performed (192).

Determining Systolic Blood Pressure

A pulse oximeter can be used to determine the systolic blood pressure (205–211). The blood pressure cuff is applied to the same arm as the pulse oximeter. The cuff is inflated slowly and the pressure at the point at which the waveform is lost is noted. It also can be determined by inflating the cuff well past the systolic pressure and looking for the onset of a signal as the cuff is deflated. One study found that the best agreement with Korotkoff sounds and non-invasive blood pressure equipment occurred when the average of blood pressures estimated at the disappearance and reappearance of the waveforms was taken as the systolic pressure (205).

In pediatrics, blood pressure by this method was found to be more accurate than that determined by an automatic non-invasive blood pressure monitor (212).

Pulse oximetry may be used in patients with pulseless diseases of the extremities to monitor saturation and systolic blood pressure (213).

Locating Vessels

When the axillary artery cannot be palpated, it may be located by placing a pulse oximeter on a finger on that side and pressing in the axilla until the pulse wave disappears (214, 215).

The dorsalis pedis artery can be localized by placing the oximeter probe on the second toe and occluding the posterior tibial artery behind the medial malleolus (216). Pulse oximetry has been used to locate the femoral artery when obesity prevented palpation of a pulse (217).

Avoidance of Hyperoxemia

In premature neonates, administration of oxygen is sometimes associated with retrolental fibroplasia. Pulse oximetry can aid in titrating inspired oxygen by detecting hypoxemia (218–221). However, the range of saturation to protect against hyperoxia must be established for each brand or model of oximeter. It is generally agreed that pulse oximetry is not adequate for evaluating hyperoxia in this setting (198).

Monitoring Vascular Volume

If the pulse oximeter begins skipping beats or performing intermittently, the cause could be hypovolemia (222). A correlation between pulse waveform amplitude variation during positive pressure ventilation and hypovolemia has been seen (223, 224). The diagnosis may sometimes be confirmed by interruption of ventilation for 15 seconds. If this causes the pulse waveform to return to normal or more constant function, a trial of fluid therapy may be warranted.

Other Uses

Other situations in which oximetry may be useful include high-frequency jet ventilation (225)

and determining the effectiveness of therapeutic bronchoscopy. It can be combined with measurement of mixed venous oxyhemoglobin saturation to estimate oxygen consumption (226, 227).

Pulse oximetry has been used to gauge pulmonary blood flow in infants and children with cyanotic congenital heart lesions (228, 229).

ADVANTAGES
Accuracy

The instrument is accurate, and accuracy does not change with time. Numerous studies have shown the difference between saturation determined by pulse oximetry and arterial blood gas analysis to be clinically insignificant above an SpO_2 of 70% (8, 34, 37, 50, 68, 73, 110, 220, 230–262). Most manufacturers claim that errors are less than $\pm 3\%$ at saturations above 70% (198). This accuracy should be sufficiently precise for most clinical purposes, except possibly neonatal hyperoxia. Changes in accuracy are negligible over the temperatures encountered in clinical use (263).

Pulse oximetry is accurate in patients with dysrhythmias, provided the SpO_2 is stable and the plethysmogram is noise free and has reasonable amplitude (264). The SpO_2 may be correct even if the pulse rate is not. Pulse oximeters may be less accurate at lower saturations (35, 231, 241, 253, 265–268).

Independence from Gases and Vapors

Pulse oximetry readings are not affected by anesthetic gases or vapors.

Dependability

The instruments are dependable. Studies have found the failure rate to be less than 2% (269–271). Performance is unaffected if pulse oximeter readings are made on the arm in which an arterial cannula is present (272). The failure rate is increased with ear and nose sensors (51).

Fast Response Time

Pulse oximetry has a fast response time, especially compared with transcutaneous measurements (110). This allows rapid determination of changes.

Non-Invasiveness

It is non-invasive, which allows it to be used as a routine monitor. It is readily accepted by awake patients, so it can be applied before induction. The bleeding, arterial insufficiency, embolization, and infection sometimes seen after arterial puncture are avoided. Temporary elevation of the PaO_2 induced by pain and apprehension is avoided.

Continuous Measurement

Monitoring is continuous. Developing trends can be detected and remedial action taken before severe hypoxia ensues.

Continuous Pulse Rate

Pulse oximetry provides a continuous pulse rate. Many monitors allow the pulse to be taken either from the ECG or the pulse oximeter. A discrepancy between these may alert the clinician to arrhythmias which are affecting cardiac output. Pulse discrepancy may also be an indication of optical interference with the probe or electrical interference.

Provision of Separate Respiratory and Circulatory Variables (273)

Perfusion is indicated by the pulse strength signal and oxygenation by saturation. Unlike transcutaneous monitoring, the values displayed do not require interpretation. Most oximeters will signal if the flow is not adequate to provide a saturation value. This is helpful in determining a truly low saturation value as opposed to one due to low flow.

Monitoring of Peripheral Blood Flow

There is continuous beat-to-beat monitoring of the quality of the peripheral pulse. This may be helpful in determining whether a hypotensive patient has good cardiac output. If blood pressure is low and pulse signal strength is high, the patient is probably vasodilated but perfusing adequately. If, however, both blood pressure and pulse strength are low, perfusion may be inadequate.

Easy Sensor Application

Application of the sensor is simple and fast. No skill is required.

Convenience

No calibration or changing of electrolyte or membrane is required.

Minimal Site Preparation

Site preparation is minimal. "Arterialization" of the skin is not necessary, except when the earlobe is the monitoring site (273).

Fast Start Time

There is minimal delay in starting. Readout occurs within a few beats after application of the sensor. This is a distinct advantage over transcutaneous monitoring, which requires a prolonged warmup time.

Verification of Proper Operation

By providing an arterial pulse wave, it gives immediate verification of proper sensor operation.

Tone Modulation

Changes in pulse tone with varying saturation allow the user to be continuously updated on pulse rate and SpO_2 without taking his or her eyes off the patient.

User Friendliness

Most instruments are user friendly. Minimal training is required to learn to operate the instrument.

Light Weight and Compactness

The console can be made compact and lightweight. This facilitates use during transport.

Rugged Sensors

The sensors are rugged.

Variety of Sensor Configurations

The wide variety of sensor configurations confers broad clinical applicability to all types of patients, including preterm infants (73). The ability to use various vascular beds offers advantages from the standpoint of access during surgery and avoiding the surgical field.

No Heating Required

No heating of the skin is required. The sensor can be left in place for extended periods without risk of thermal injury.

Battery Operated

Most stand-alone units and those incorporated into transport monitors can be operated on batteries.

Economical

Use of pulse oximetry can save money by allowing oxygen administration only when needed and decreasing the number of blood gas analyses (154, 274–276).

LIMITATIONS AND DISADVANTAGES

Failure

There is a small but definite incidence of failure with pulse oximetry (269, 277–280). Factors reported to contribute to higher failure rates include American Society of Anesthesiologists (ASA) physical status 3, 4, or 5; young and elderly patients; orthopedic, vascular and cardiac surgery; use of electrocautery; hypothermia; hypotension; hypertension; duration of intraoperative procedure; chronic renal failure; low hematocrit; and pigmented skin (269, 277–279, 281–283). The actual failure rate varies with the individual monitor (284). Monitors that can analyze the signal and reject artifacts have fewer episodes of failure. The failure rate is increased with ear and nose sensors (51).

Poor Function with Poor Perfusion

Pulse oximeters require adequate pulsations to distinguish arterial blood light absorption from venous blood and tissue light absorption (285). Readings may be unreliable or unavailable if there is loss or diminution of the peripheral pulse (proximal blood pressure cuff inflation, leaning on an extremity, improper positioning, hypotension, hypothermia, cardiopulmonary bypass, low cardiac output, hypovolemia, peripheral vascular disease, or infusion of vasoactive drugs) (29, 50, 208, 285–291). A Valsalva maneuver, such as is seen in laboring patients, will cause a decrease in pulse amplitude, which adversely affects the oximeter's ability to provide useful data (292). Cold alone may not impair the functioning of the pulse oximeter unless the patient has Raynaud's phenomenon (293). Under these conditions, some pulse oximeters blank the display or give a message such as *Low Quality Signal* or *Inadequate Signal*. Others freeze the display when they are unable to detect a consistent pulse wave. The presence of a functioning pulse oximeter should not be construed as evidence of adequate tissue oxygenation or oxygen delivery to vital organs (198, 208, 294).

Methods to improve the signal include application of vasodilating cream, digital nerve blocks, administration of intraarterial vasodilators, or placing a glove filled with warm water in the patient's hand (30–32, 295–297). Warming cool extremities may increase the pulse amplitude, provided the cardiac output is not depressed (297, 298). Some studies indicate the finger probe performs best under conditions of poor perfusion (29). Placing a probe on the cheek or tongue may also work (58). Pulse oximeters with signal extraction technology may perform better during low perfusion (299, 300).

Difficulty in Detecting High Oxygen Partial Pressures

At high saturations, small changes in saturation are associated with relatively large changes in PaO_2. Thus it has limited ability to distinguish high but safe levels of arterial oxygen from excessively elevated levels (301).

Delayed Detection of Hypoxic Events

While the response time of the pulse oximeter is generally fast, there may be a significant delay between a change in alveolar oxygen tension and a change in the oximeter reading. It is possible for arterial oxygen to reach dangerous levels before the pulse oximeter alarm is activated (302).

Delay in response is related to sensor location (39, 54, 303). Desaturation is detected earlier when the sensor is placed more centrally. Lag time will be increased with poor perfusion and decreased if blood flow to the site is increased (208, 304). Performance of a neural block may cause the lag time to decrease (305, 306). Venous obstruction, peripheral vasoconstriction, cold, and motion artifacts delay detection of hypoxemia (17, 287, 289). Increasing the time over which the pulse signals are averaged also increases the delay time.

Erratic Performance with Irregular Rhythms

Irregular heart rhythms can cause erratic performance. During aortic balloon pulsation, the augmentation of diastolic pressure exceeds that of systolic pressure. This leads to a double- or triple-peaked arterial pressure waveform that confuses the pulse oximeter so that it may not provide a reading (307). However, pulse oximetry works in patients who have had an aortomyoplasty (308).

Inaccuracy

While accuracy is one of the advantages of pulse oximetry, there are many sources of error.

Different Hemoglobins

Whole blood contains not only reduced hemoglobin and oxyhemoglobin but, frequently, other moieties such as carboxyhemoglobin (HbCO) and methemoglobin. In vitro cooximetry can measure the percentages of other moieties by using more than two wavelengths.

Dyshemoglobins are important because they do not carry oxygen. This disturbs the absorbance ratio of the wavelengths that are used to determine oxygen saturation (309).

Methemoglobin (310, 311)

Normally less than 1% of the total hemoglobin, methemoglobin (metHb) is an oxidation product of hemoglobin that forms a reversible complex with oxygen and impairs the unloading of oxygen to tissues. Methemoglobinemia can be congenital (312) or acquired. Causes of acquired methemoglobinemia include nitrobenzene (313), benzocaine (314, 315), prilocaine (316, 317) and dapsone (311, 318, 319).

Methemoglobin absorbs light equally at the red and infrared wavelengths used by pulse oximeters. All two-wavelength pulse oximeters will overread compared with fractional saturation when metHb is present (12). When compared with functional saturation, pulse oximeters give falsely low readings for saturations above 85% and falsely high values for saturations below 85%. As methemoglobin increases, SpO$_2$ seeks the 80 to 85% range and stays there once methemoglobin is above 40% (310, 320–324). The discrepancy between SpO$_2$ and functional saturation increases as the level of metHb increases and functional hemoglobin saturation decreases (310). With treatment of the methemoglobinemia, the SpO$_2$ readings become more accurate (316, 317, 319, 323). If there are conflicting results between the pulse oximeter and arterial blood gas analysis, methemoglobinemia should be suspected and the diagnosis should be confirmed by multiwavelength cooximetry, because standard blood gas analysis is not capable of detecting and measuring metHb (325).

Carboxyhemoglobin

HbCO exists in varying degrees as a consequence of smoking and urban pollution, but may occur in very high concentrations as a result of smoke inhalation (12). An increase in HbCO occurs during laser surgery of the airway, but the levels are not high enough to keep pulse oximetry from reliably estimating saturation (326). HbCO has an absorption spectrum similar to oxyhemoglobin so most pulse oximeters will overread by the percentage of HbCO present (327–330). Pulse oximeters that differentiate between oxyhemoglobin and HbCO are available.

Fetal Hemoglobin

Although the presence of fetal hemoglobin (Hb F) does not appear to affect the accuracy of pulse oximetry to a clinically important degree (73, 231, 232, 331–335), very high levels will cause some inaccuracy (336).

Hemoglobin S

The accuracy of pulse oximetry in the patient with sickle cell disease is controversial. Several studies have found that saturation measured by pulse oximetry was not an adequate predictor of arterial oxygen saturation in patients with sickle cell anemia (337–340), although a few small studies found good correlation (341, 342).

Other Hemoglobinopathies

Hemoglobin Koln is associated with an artifactually low oxygen saturation as measured by the pulse oximeter (343, 344). Hemoglobin Hammersmith has been shown to cause the pulse oximeter to read so low that it is not useful in patients with this hemoglobinopathy (345). Hemoglobin-H disease will cause the pulse oximeter to indicate a higher saturation than is actually present (346). A patient with hemoglobin Constant Springs and

α-thalassemia 2 in which pulse oximetry readings were consistently low has been reported (347).

Bilirubinemia

Severe hyperbilirubinemia can cause an artifactual elevation of methemoglobin and HbCO using in vitro oximetry, but does not affect pulse oximetry readings (231, 232, 331, 348–351).

Low Saturations

Pulse oximetry may become less accurate at lower saturations (5, 34–36, 38, 231, 235, 237, 241, 242, 248, 253, 257, 265–268, 352–356). It should be used with caution in children with cyanotic congenital heart disease (357–359).

Malpositioned Sensor

Oximeters with sensors that are not well applied vary greatly in their behavior, depending on both the actual SpO_2 and the manufacturer and model (43, 360–364). There are marked differences in the forces required to displace various probes (365). Use of too large a probe may result in inaccurate readings (18, 366). Long fingernails can cause inaccurate positioning (286). In one reported case, the sensor was completely unattached but continued to provide apparently accurate readings (368). Closer examination of the waveform revealed an unusual pattern.

To avoid these problems, sensor position should be checked frequently and inaccessible locations avoided whenever possible.

Poor Peripheral Pulsation

Because pulse oximeters rely on adequate arterial pulsation, a significant decrease in pulsation—such as with hypotension, vasoconstriction, hypothermia, cardiopulmonary bypass, or cardiac arrest—can produce a signal too small to be processed reliably (289, 369, 370). In patients with low peripheral vascular resistance, underreading of the saturation may occur (371).

Venous Pulsations

Pulse oximeter design assumes that the pulsatile component of light absorbance is due to arterial blood. Prominent pulsations of venous blood may lead to underestimation of the SpO_2 (43, 372–375). Pulse rate determination may be correct. The error may be worse when ear probes are used (55) but less when the probe is placed on the distal part of the finger (376). High airway pressures during artificial ventilation may cause phasic venous congestion, which may be interpreted by the oximeter as a pulse wave (377). In some cases, it may be necessary to turn off the ventilator to obtain a correct reading.

Mixing of Sensors

SpO_2 measurements may not be accurate if a sensor from a different manufacturer is used on a particular monitor (378, 379).

Anemia

The pulse oximeter tends to overestimate SpO_2 at low saturations in patients with anemia (380–385).

Skin Pigmentation

Studies show that pulse oximeter readings are erroneously high in patients with dark skin color (236, 386–389). The effect is more pronounced at low saturations (390, 391).

Dyes

Certain dyes including methylene blue, indocyanine green, and indigo carmine when injected intravenously or into the uterine cavity can cause large transient decreases in SpO_2 readings without actual decreases in saturation (392–398). In vitro oximetry is also affected by dyes (318, 399). The reaction of the pulse oximeter to exogenous dyes has been advocated as a means of confirming intravascular catheter placement. The dye is injected into the catheter and the pulse oximeter observed (400). The pulse oximeter may be useful to estimate cardiac output by the dye dilution method (401). Intradermal patent blue dye used for mapping of the lymphatic drainage may be associated with a false decrease in saturation as determined by the pulse oximeter (402). Fingerprinting ink will cause a low saturation reading (403). Henna, a stain used by some Middle Eastern women on the fingers and toes, can cause a low saturation reading (404). Children who have been fingerpainting with blue paints may exhibit low SpO_2 readings (405).

Optical Interference

Stray light or light flickering at frequencies similar to the frequencies of the LEDs, including sunlight, operating room lights, infrared heating lamps, light sources for various scopes, xenon lamps, and bilirubin lights, can enter the photodetector, resulting in inaccurate or erratic readings (9, 406–415). Although excessive ambient light usually prevents the oximeter from tracking the pulse, in some instances it can result in apparently normal but inaccurate measurements (413). Oximeters vary significantly in their susceptibility to optical interference (288, 409). Sensitivity to light sources may be increased with reduced pulse amplitude. One clue that this is occurring is inconsistency between the pulse oximeter generated pulse and that on other monitors such as the ECG (309). If the sensor seems to be malfunctioning, it should be shielded from ambient light to determine whether this is the problem.

Several ways exist of minimizing the effects of external optical interference. These include selection of the correct sensor for the patient and use, applying the sensor so the detector is across from the LEDs, making certain the sensor remains properly positioned, and shielding the sensor from bright light and other nearby sensors. It is usually sufficient to cover the probe with an opaque material such as a surgical towel, gauze, finger cot, blanket, alcohol wipe packet, or other foil shield (75, 416–418). This may also help to stabilize the sensor. However, some light may not be adequately shielded by a simple covering (406, 413).

Some manufacturers try to minimize the effect of stray light by taking intermittent background readings when both of the LEDs in the sensor are turned off and subtracting these readings from measurements taken by the photodetector when either LED is turned on.

Nail Polish and Coverings

Some shades of black, blue, and green (but not red or purple) nail polish may cause significantly lower saturation readings (419–421). Synthetic nails may interfere with pulse oximetry readings (273). One way to overcome this problem (besides removing the polish or the fingernail) is to orient the probe so it transmits light from one side of the finger to the other side (44, 422). The presence of onychomycosis, a yellowish gray color caused by fungus, can cause falsely low SpO_2 readings (423). Dirt under the nail can also cause difficulty in obtaining reliable readings (423). Although there is one report of dried blood on a finger causing erroneous low saturation readings (424), other authors have found that dried blood does not affect the accuracy of the pulse oximeter (425, 426).

Loss of Accuracy at Low Values

Measurement of SpO_2 is less accurate at low values (34, 36, 38, 231, 235, 237, 241, 242, 248, 253, 257, 266–268, 353–355).

Electrical Interference

Electrical interference from an electrosurgical unit can cause the oximeter to give an incorrect pulse count (usually by counting extra beats) or to falsely register a decrease in oxygen saturation (427). This problem may be increased in patients with weak pulse signals (8). The effect is transient and limited to the duration of the cauterization. Manufacturers have made significant progress in reducing their instruments' sensitivity to electrical interference (8, 198, 288). Some monitors display a notice when significant interference is present. Steps to minimize electrical interference include locating the electrosurgery grounding plate as close to, and the oximeter sensor as far from, the surgical field as possible; routing the cable from the sensor to the oximeter away from the electrosurgery apparatus; keeping the pulse oximeter sensor and console as far as possible from the surgical site and the electrosurgery grounding plate and table; raising the high pulse rate alarm; and operating the unit in a rapid response mode. The electrosurgical apparatus and pulse oximeter should not be plugged into the same power source (427).

Motion Artifacts

Motion of the sensor relative to the skin can cause an artifact that the pulse oximeter is unable to differentiate from normal arterial pulsations. Motion may produce a prolongation in the detection time for hypoxemia without giving a warning (17). Motion is usually not a problem during general anesthesia, but if the patient is shivering, moving about or being transported it can be significant

(428, 429). Evoked potential monitors and nerve stimulators can produce motion artifacts if the pulse oximeter sensor is on the same extremity (430–432). Evoked potential monitoring and nerve stimulators can also produce motion artifacts. Motion artifacts have been noted in patients under regional anesthesia who tapped their fingers to music (433).

The ability of an oximeter to deal with motion artifacts depends on the correlation with the onset of the motion and the start of monitoring. If the motion precedes the onset of monitoring there is a greater decrement in performance (434). Motion artifacts can usually be recognized by false or erratic pulse rate displays or distorted plethysmographic waveforms. Increased pulse amplitude is an indicator of movement but not necessarily of artifactual SpO$_2$ readings (435, 436). Artifacts caused by motion can be decreased by careful sensor positioning. Whenever possible, the pulse oximetry sensor should be located on a different extremity from that being stimulated. Ear, cheek, and nose probes may be more useful than finger probes in restless patients. Flexible probes that are taped in place are less susceptible to motion artifacts than clip-on probes (8). Probes lined with soft material may be associated with fewer motion artifacts (17). Smaller fingers are more susceptible to motion artifact (17).

Pulse oximeters vary in their ability to identify readings associated with movement (437). Lengthening the averaging mode will increase the likelihood that enough true pulses will be detected to reject motion artifacts (10, 438). Use of longer averaging times reduces motion artifacts. Some manufacturers use the R-wave of the patient's ECG to synchronize the optical measurements. Oximeters with signal extraction technology which uses mathematical manipulation of the oximeter's light signals to measure and subtract the noise components associated with motion will have fewer artifacts (434, 439).

Pressure on the Sensor

Pressure on the sensor may result in inaccurate SpO$_2$ readings without affecting pulse rate determination (375).

Hyperemia

If a limb is hyperemic, the flow of capillary and venous blood becomes pulsatile. In this situation, the absorption of light from these sources will be included in the saturation computations with resulting decrease in accuracy of the oxygen saturation measured by pulse oximetry (440). A pulse oximeter placed near the site of blood transfusion may show transient decreases in oxygen saturation with rapid infusion of the blood (441).

False Alarms

A high percentage of pulse oximetry alarms are spurious or trivial (428, 442–449). False alarms are most commonly caused by motion artifact but also are associated with poor signal quality, sensor displacement, and electrosurgical interference. Some false alarms can be avoided by simple measures such as putting the probe on an extremity without the automated blood pressure cuff or in a location where it will not be affected by external pressure (443). Delaying the time between detection of low SpO$_2$ and alarm activation and setting the low SpO$_2$ alarm limit lower can reduce the number of false alarms (446, 450–452). On some pulse oximeters, turning off the low pulse rate alarm prevents alarming when a blood pressure cuff is inflated (8). Some pulse oximeters have sophisticated methods to reject noise and motion artifacts. Frequent running averages of saturation throughout a pulse pressure wave are carefully weighted to avoid showing sudden changes, and many factors are taken into account to determine when to indicate no reading if the signal quality is poor (453). Use of neural networks may reduce false alarms (454).

Synchronizing the pulse oximeter with the ECG monitor is another way to lessen motion artifacts (17, 23). However, the oximeter may synchronize with ECG artifacts generated by motion or shivering, resulting in erroneous readings (8). Furthermore, with this system, the pulse rate displayed by the oximeter will necessarily be equal to the pulse rate shown by the ECG monitor so that equality of the pulse rates cannot be used as an indication that the displayed saturation data are valid. Another method for decreasing false alarms is signal extraction technology (439, 455–458). This uses mathematical manipulation of the oximeter's light signals to measure and subtract the noise components associated with motion and low perfusion.

Analyzing the shape of the arterial waveform can reduce false alarms (284). The arterial pulse wave is characterized by a rapid rise and slow decay, whereas artifactual pulsations caused by motion are characterized by equally fast rise and decay. By rejecting these, motion artifacts are filtered out. Pulse oximeters that display the plethysmographic waveform have an advantage over those that display only the amplitude of the signal, because this allows the operator to assess the quality of the signal and to observe noise such as motion artifacts that may alter its accuracy (459).

Failure to Detect Absence of Circulation

A pulse oximeter signal and a normal reading do not necessarily imply adequacy of tissue perfusion. Some pulse oximeters show pulses despite inadequate tissue perfusion (208, 289) or even when no pulse is present (159, 460–462). Ambient light may produce a false signal (414). Pulse oximetry does not appear to be reliable in the diagnosis of impaired perfusion with increased intracompartmental pressures (463, 464).

Discrepancies in Readings from Different Monitors

A discrepancy in readings between different brands of oximeters on the same patient at the same time is not uncommon (13, 465–468). One reason for this is differences in methods of calibration. There is variation in the time it takes various monitors to detect resaturation (469).

Failure to Detect Hypoventilation

Hypoventilation and hypercarbia may occur without a decrease in hemoglobin oxygen saturation, especially if the patient is receiving supplemental oxygen (470). Pulse oximetry should not be relied upon to assess the adequacy of ventilation (471), or to detect disconnections (472) or esophageal intubation (473).

Problems with Sound Recognition

Some clinicians have trouble detecting changes in the pitch of the sound emitted by pulse oximeters as the saturation changes (474).

Lack of User Knowledge

Pulse oximetry is often used by personnel whose knowledge of it is limited. Physicians, nurses, and others using the instrument often do not know the basic principles and make serious errors in interpretation of readings (309, 475, 476).

Interference with Other Monitors

Electromagnetic interference from the power supply of a pulse oximeter may cause artifacts and false readings on certain thoracic impedance monitors (477).

PATIENT COMPLICATIONS
Corneal Abrasions

Patients recovering from general anesthesia frequently rub their eyes. If a pulse oximeter is on the index finger, a corneal abrasion may result (478, 479). It is suggested that a finger other than the index finger may be more appropriate for the sensor (480).

Pressure and Ischemic Injuries

Persistent numbness of a finger on which a probe was placed has been reported (481–483). Ischemic injuries associated with reusable finger probes have also been reported (484–487).

These risks may be increased by prolonged probe application, compromised perfusion of the extremity, or tight application of tape. Frequent examination of the site and moving the sensor to different sites will reduce the likelihood of injury (484, 488).

Burns

Injuries ranging from tan areas to third-degree burns under pulse oximeter probes have been reported (486, 489–498). Burns can result from incompatibility between the sensor from one manufacturer with the pulse oximeter of another (494, 499). A number of pulse oximeter sensors has compatible connectors but incompatible probes. Use of a damaged probe can result in a burn (489, 500, 501). Burns associated with pulse oximetry during MRI as a result of induced skin current beneath looped cables have been reported (502–504). A second degree burn has been reported when a pulse oximeter was used with photodynamic therapy (505).

To avoid these injuries, frequent inspection of probe sites and site rotation are recommended. When a probe is placed on a finger or toe, the light source should be placed on the nail rather than the pulp (506). A glove can be placed on the hand to protect from thermal injury without affecting the accuracy of the instrument (507). Any freezing of the pulse oximeter display should be investigated. Only the probes recommended by the oximeter manufacturer should be used (494). During MRI, the danger of burns can be reduced by the following measures:

1. All potential conductors should be checked before use to ensure absence of frayed insulation, exposed wires, and other hazards.
2. All unnecessary conductive materials such as unused surface coils should be removed from the bore of the MRI system before initiation of patient monitoring.
3. The sensor should be placed as far from the imaging site as possible.
4. All cables, leads, or wires from monitoring devices should be positioned so that no loops are formed. A braid should be made of the slack portion of wires.
5. If possible, no potential conductors should touch the patient's body at more than one location.
6. A thick layer of thermal insulation should be placed between any wires or cables and the patient's skin.
7. Monitoring devices that do not appear to be operating properly should be removed from the patient immediately.

Electric Shock

An electrical shock related to diathermy has been reported (508). In this case there were bare wires in the pulse oximeter probe.

REFERENCES

1. Gravenstein JS. International standards for safe practice endorsed by WFSA. APSF Newslett 1992;7:29–31.
2. Tinker JH, Dull DL, Caplan RA, et al. Role of monitoring devices in prevention of anesthetic mishaps. A closed claims analysis. Anesthesiology 1989;71:541–546.
3. Runciman WB, Webb RK, Barker L, et al. The pulse oximeter: Applications and limitations—An analysis of 2000 incident reports. Anaesthesia and Intensive Care 1993;21:543–550.
4. Scuderi PE, Bowton DL, Anderson RL, et al. Pulse oximetry: would further technical alterations improve patient outcome? Anesth Analg 1992;74:177–180.
5. Tremper KK, Barker SJ. Pulse oximetry. Anesthesiology 1989;70:98–108.
6. Wukitsch MW, Petterson MT, Tobler DR, et al. Pulse oximetry. Analysis of theory, technology, and practice. Journal of Clinical Monitoring 1988;4:290–300.
7. Kelleher JF. Pulse oximetry. Journal of Clinical Monitoring 1989;5:37–62.
8. Alexander CM, Teller LE, Gross JB. Principles of pulse oximetry. Theoretical and practical considerations. Anesth Analg 1989;68:368–376.
9. Anonymous. Pulse Oximeters. Health Devices 1989;18:185–230.
10. Hamlin MD. A guide to pulse oximetry monitoring and troubleshooting. J Clin Eng 1995;20:476–483.
11. Schnapp LM, Cohen NH. Pulse oximetry. Uses and abuses. Chest 1990;98:1244–1250.
12. Reynolds KJ, Palayiwa E, Moyle JTB, et al. The effect of dyshemoglobins on pulse oximetry. Part I: theoretical approach. Part II: experimental results using an in vitro test system. Journal of Clinical Monitoring 1993;9:81–90.
13. Pologe JA. Functional saturation versus fractional saturation. What does pulse oximetry read. Journal of Clinical Monitoring 1989;5:298–299.
14. Thilo EH, Park–Moore B, Berman ER, et al. Oxygen saturation by pulse oximetry in healthy infants at an altitude of 1610 m (5280 ft). AJDC 1991;145:1137–1140.
15. Anonymous. Hospitals look for savings in pulse oximetry sensors. Technology for Anesthesia 1992;13(5):1–2.
16. Maruschak GF, Johnson RM. Pulse oximeter cost per use—securing savings. Anesthesiology 1989;71:167–168.
17. Langton JA, Hanning CD. Effect of motion artefact on pulse oximeters. Evaluation of four instruments and finger probes. Br J Anaesth 1990;65:564–570.
18. Zahka KG, Dean MJ. Failure of pulse oximetry to detect severe hypoxia: importance of sensor selection. Clin Pediatr 1988;27:403–404.
19. Peden CJ, Menon DK, Hall AS, et al. Magnetic resonance for the anaesthetist. Part II. Anaesthesia and monitoring in MR units. Anaesthesia 1992;47:508–517.

20. Shellock FG, Myers SM, Kimble KJ. Monitoring heart rate and oxygen saturation with a fiber-optic pulse oximeter during MR imaging. AJR 1992;15(8): 663–664.

21. Wagle WA. Technique for RF isolation of a pulse oximeter in a 1.5-T MR unit. Am J Neuroradiol 1989;10:208.

22. Yoder RD. Preservation of pulse oximetry sensors. Anesthesiology 1988;68:308.

23. Barrington KJ, Finer NN, Ryan CA. Evaluation of pulse oximetry as a continuous monitoring technique in the neonatal intensive care unit. Crit Care Med 1988;16:1147–1153.

24. Pasterkamp H, Daien D. The use of a personal computer for trend data analysis with the Ohmeda 3700 pulse oximeter. Journal of Clinical Monitoring 1988; 4:215–222.

25. American Society for Testing and Materials. Specification for pulse oximeters (F1415-92). West Conshohocken, PA: ASTM, 1992.

26. International Organization for Standardization. Pulse oximeters for medical use—requirements (ISO 9919-1992). Geneva: ISO, 1992.

27. Barker SJ, Lee N, Hyatt J. Failure rates of transmission and reflectance pulse oximetry for various sensor sites. Journal of Clinical Monitoring 1991;7: 102–103.

28. Swedlow DB, Running V, Feaster SJ. Ambient light affects pulse oximeters: a reply. Anesthesiology 1987; 67:865.

29. Clayton DG, Webb RK, Ralston AC, et al. Pulse oximetry probes. A comparison between finger, nose, ear and forehead under conditions of poor perfusion. Anaesthesia 1991;46:260–265.

30. Bourke DL, Grayson RF. Digital nerve blocks can restore pulse oximeter signal detection. Anesth Analg 1991;73:815–817.

31. Gentili ME, Chevaleraud E, Viel E, Digital block of the flexor tendon sheath can restore pulse oximeter signal detection. Reg Anesth 1995;20:82–83.

32. Holroyd K, Lui M, Beattie C. Intraarterial vasodilator administration to restore pulse oximeter function. Anesthesiology 1993;79:388–390.

33. Eastwood DW. Digital nerve blocks and pulse oximeter signal detection. Anesth Analg 1992;74:931.

34. Kagle DM, Alexander CM, Berko RS, et al. Evaluation of the Ohmeda 3700 pulse oximeter: steady-state and transient response characteristics. Anesthesiology 1987;66:376–380.

35. Severinghaus JW, Naifeh KH. Accuracy of response of six pulse oximeters to profound hypoxia. Anesthesiology 1987;67:551–558.

36. Severinghaus JW, Naifeh KH, Koh SO. Errors in 14 pulse oximeters during profound hypoxia. Journal of Clinical Monitoring 1989;5:72–81.

37. Warley ARH, Mitchell JH, Stradling JR. Evaluation of the Ohmeda 3700 pulse oximeter. Thorax 1988; 42:892–896.

38. Webb RK, Ralston AC, Runciman WB. Potential errors in pulse oximetry. Part II. Effects of changes in saturation and signal quality. Anaesthesia 1991;46: 207–212.

39. Young D, Jewkes C, Spittal M, et al. Response time of pulse oximeters assessed using acute decompression. Anesth Analg 1992;74:189–195.

40. Reynolds LM, Nicolson SC, Steven JM, et al. Influence of sensor site location on pulse oximetry kinetics in children. Anesth Analg 1993;76:751–754.

41. Dimich I, Singh PP, Adell A, et al. Evaluation of oxygenation monitoring by pulse oximetry in neonates in the delivery system. Can J Anaesth 1991;38: 985–988.

42. Kurki TS, Sanford TJ, Smith NT, et al. Effects of radial artery cannulation on the function of finger blood pressure and pulse oximeter monitors. Anesthesiology 1988;69:778–782.

43. Kim J-M, Arakawa K, Benson KT, et al. Pulse oximetry and circulatory kinetics associated with pulse volume amplitude measured by photoelectric plethysmography. Anesth Analg 1986;65:1333–1339.

44. White PF, Boyle WA. Nail polish and oximetry. Anesth Analg 1989;68:546–547.

45. Edelist G. Acrylic nails and pulse oximetry. Anesth Analg 1995;81:884.

46. Imaizumi H, Ujike Y, Sumita S, et al. Pulse oximetry in an extensively burned patient. Journal of Clinical Monitoring 1995;11:80.

47. Peduto VA, Tani R, Pani S. Pulse oximetry during lumbar epidural anesthesia: Reliability of values measured at the hand and the foot. Anesth Analg 1994; 78:921–924.

48. Ezri T, Lurie S, Konichezky S, et al. Pulse oximetry from the nasal septum. J Clin Anesth 1991;3: 447–450.

49. Segstro R. Nasal sensor attachment. Can J Anaesth 1989;36:365–366.

50. Yelderman M, New W. Evaluation of pulse oximetry. Anesthesiology 1983;59:349–352.

51. Barker SJ, Hyatt J, Rumack WA. Pulse oximeter failure rates. Effects of manufacturer, sensor site, and patient. Anesth Analg 1992;74:S15.

52. Rosenberg J, Pedersen MH. Nasal pulse oximetry overestimates oxygen saturation. Anaesthesia 1990; 45:1070–1071.

53. Stoddart AP, Anaes FC, Kao Y, et al. Trendelenburg position affects the accuracy of pulse oximetry on dif-

ferent probe sites: A quantitative analysis. Anesthesiology 1993;79:A528.

54. Broome IJ, Harris RW, Reilly CS. The response times during anaesthesia of pulse oximeters measuring oxygen saturations during hypoxemic events. Anaesthesia 1992;47:17–19.

55. Skacel M, O'Hare E, Harrison D. Invalid information from the ear probe of a pulse oximeter in tricuspid incompetence. Anaesthesia and Intensive Care 1990; 18:270.

56. Spittal MJ. Evaluation of pulse oximetry during cardiopulmonary resuscitation. Anaesthesia 1993;48: 701–703.

57. Jobes DR, Nicolson SC. Monitoring of arterial hemoglobin oxygen saturation using a tongue sensor. Anesth Analg 1988;67:186–188.

58. Cote CJ, Daniels AL, Connolly M, et al. Tongue oximetry in children with extensive thermal injury. Comparison with peripheral oximetry. Can J Anaesth 1992;39:454–457.

59. Hickerson W, Morrell M, Cicala RS. Glossal pulse oximetry. Anesth Analg 1989;69:73–74.

60. Gunter JB. A buccal sensor for measuring arterial oxygen saturation. Anesth Analg 1989;69:417–418.

61. O'Leary RJ, Landon M, Benumof JL. Buccal pulse oximeter is more accurate than finger pulse oximeter in measuring oxygen saturation. Anesth Analg 1992; 75:495–498.

62. Sosis MB, Coleman N. Use of an Ohmeda ear oximetry probe for "buccal" ' oximetry. Can J Anaesth 1990;37:489–490.

63. Lema GE. Oral pulse oximetry in small children. Anesth Analg 1991;72:414.

64. Groudine SB, Cost-effective buccal oximetry. Anesthesiology 1996;84:484.

65. Landon M, Benumof JL, O'Leary RJ. Buccal pulse oximetry: an accurate alternative to the finger probe. Anesthesiology 1992;77:A526.

66. Langdon M. Buccal pulse oximetry: an accurate alternative to finger oximetry. Anesthesiology 1992;77: A526.

67. Cook TM, Gaylord D, Wood F. Another site for the pulse oximeter probe. Anaesthesia 1995;50: 1096–1097.

68. Miyasaka K, Katayama M, Kusakawa I, et al. Use of pulse oximetry in neonatal anesthesia. J Perinatol 1987;7:343–345.

69. Mikawa K, Maekawa N. A simple alternate technique for the application of the pulse oximeter probe to infants. Anaesthesia 1992;47:400.

70. Robertson RE, Kaplan RF. Another site for the pulse oximeter probe. Anesthesiology 1991;74:198.

71. Barker SJ, Hyatt J, Shah NK. The accuracy of malpositioned pulse oximeters during hypoxemia. Anesthesiology 1992;77:A496.

72. Prasad MK, Puri GD, Chari P. Glove finger for fixing pulse oximeter probe. Anaesthesia 1994;49:831.

73. Deckardt R, Steward DJ. Non-invasive arterial hemoglobin oxygen saturation versus transcutaneous oxygen tension monitoring in the preterm infant. Crit Care Med 1984;12:935–939.

74. Foltz BD. Another technique for extending the life of oximetry monitoring probes. Anesth Analg 1987; 66:367–374.

75. Alpert CC, Cooke JE. Extending the life of oximetry monitoring probes. Anesth Analg 1986;65: 826–827.

76. Shlamowitz M, Miguel R. Prolonging the lifespan of disposable Nellcor pulse oxisensors. Journal of Clinical Monitoring 1990;6:160.

77. Tharp AJ. A cost-saving method of modifying the Nellcor pulse oximeter finger probe. Anesthesiology 1986;65:446–447.

78. Anonymous. Pulse oximetry sensor recycling cuts Utah hospital's costs. Technology for Anesthesia 1994;14(11):11–12.

79. Mangar D, Samuels DJ, Rasanen J. Cost saving with reusable pulse oximeter probes. Anesth Analg 1993; 77:638–646.

80. Salyer JW, Burton K, Lynch J, et al. Adventures in recycling: the reuse of "disposable" pulse oximeter probes. Resp Care 1993;38:1072–1076.

81. Gerber DR, Santarelli RJ, Scott WE, et al. Evaluation of a protective sheath for disposable pulse oximetry probes. Resp Care 1996;41:197–201.

82. Russell GB, Graybeal JM. Accuracy of laminated disposable pulse-oximeter sensors. Resp Care 1995;40: 728–733.

83. Racys V, Nahrwold ML. Reusing the Nellcor pulse oximeter probe. Is it worth the savings? Anesthesiology 1987;66:713.

84. Swedlow DB, Larson LH. Prolonging the Lifespan disposable Nellcor pulse oxisensors. Journal of Clinical Monitoring 1991;7:211.

85. Anonymous. Pulse oximeters. Technology for Anesthesia 1996;17(1):8.

86. Volsko TA, Chatburn RL, Kallstrom TJ. Evaluation of a commercial standard for checking pulse oximeter performance. Resp Care 1996;41:100–104.

87. Reynolds KJ, Moyle JTB, Gale OB, et al. In vitro performance test system for pulse oximeters. Med Biol Eng Comput 1992;30:629–635.

88. Fisher JA, Volgyesi GA. Evaluation of a new pulse oximeter testing device. Can J Anaesth 1996;43: 179–183.

89. Hanning CD. Oximetry and anaesthetic practice

(preoperative, intraoperative, postoperative and critical care). Leicester, UK: BOC Healthcare Group, 1985.

90. Raemer DB, Warren DL, Morris R, et al. Hypoxemia during ambulatory gynecologic surgery as evaluated by the pulse oximeter. Journal of Clinical Monitoring 1987;3:244–248.

91. Moller JT, Joannessen NW, Berg H, et al. Hypoxemia during anaesthesia. An observer study. Br J Anaesth 1991;66:437–444.

92. Walsh JF. Training for day-case dental anaesthesia. Oxygen saturation during general anaesthesia administered by dental undergraduates. Anaesthesia 1984; 39:1124–1127.

93. Hempenstall PD, de Plater RMH. Oxygen saturation during general anaesthesia and recovery for outpatient oral surgical procedures. Anaesthesia and Intensive Care 1990;18:517–521.

94. McCormick ASM, Saunders DA. Oxygen saturation of patients recovering from electroconvulsive therapy. Anaesthesia 1996;51:702–704.

95. Bone ME, Galler D, Flynn PJ. Arterial oxygen saturation during general anesthesia for paediatric dental extraction. Anaesthesia 1987;42:879–882.

96. Cote CJ, Goldstein EA, Cote MA, et al. A single-blind study of pulse oximetry in children. Anesthesiology 1988;68:184–188.

97. Cote CJ, Rolf N, Liu LMP, et al. A single-blind study of combined pulse oximetry and capnography in children. Anesthesiology 1991;74:980–987.

98. Laycock GJA, McNicol LR. Hypoxemia during induction of anaesthesia—an audit of children who underwent general anaesthesia for routine elective surgery. Anaesthesia 1988;43:981–984.

99. Moorthy SS, Dierdorf SF, Krishna G. Transient hypoxemia during emergence from anesthesia in children. Anesthesiol Rev 1988;15:20–23.

100. McKay WPS, Noble WH. Critical incidents detected by pulse oximeter during anaesthesia. Can J Anaesth 1988;35:265–269.

101. Moller JT, Jensen PF, Johannessen NW, et al. Hypoxemia is reduced by pulse oximetry monitoring in the operating theatre and in the recovery room. Br J Anaesth 1992;68:146–150.

102. Moller JT, Johannessen NW, Espersen K, et al. Randomized evaluation of pulse oximetry in 20,802 patients: II. Perioperative events and postoperative complications. Anesthesiology 1993;78:445–453.

103. Riley R. Detection of unsuspected endobronchial intubation by pulse oximetry. Anaesthesia and Intensive Care 1989;17:381–382.

104. Burton A, Steinbrook RA. Precipitous decrease in oxygen saturation during laparoscopic surgery. Anesth Analg 1993;76:1177–1178.

105. Baraka A, Jabbour S, Rizkallah P. Left bronchial intubation by the laryngectomy tube. Anesthesiology 1993;78:995,

106. Barker SJ, Tremper KK, Hyatt J, et al. Pulse oximetry may not detect endobronchial intubation. Anesthesiology 1987;67:A170.

107. Barker SJ, Tremper KK, Hyatt J, et al. Comparison of three oxygen monitors in detecting endobronchial intubation. Journal of Clinical Monitoring 1988;4: 240–243.

108. Barker JS, Tremper KK. Detection of endobronchial intubation by non-invasive monitoring. Journal of Clinical Monitoring 1987;3:292–293.

109. Brodsky JB, Shulman MS, Swan M, et al. Pulse oximetry during one-lung ventilation. Anesthesiology 1985;63:212–214.

110. Viitanen A, Salmenpera M, Heinonen J. Non-invasive monitoring of oxygenation during one-lung ventilation: a comparison of transcutaneous oxygen tension measurement and pulse oximetry. Journal of Clinical Monitoring 1987;3:90–95.

111. Davies MJ, Scott DA, Cook PT. Continuous monitoring of arterial oxygen saturation with pulse oximetry during spinal anesthesia. Reg Anesth 1987;12: 63–70.

112. Council of Scientific Affairs, American Medical Association. The use of pulse oximetry during conscious sedation. JAMA 1993;270:1463–1468.

113. Sosis MB, Sisamis J. Pulse oximetry in confirmation of correct tracheal tube placement. Anesth Analg 1990;71:309–310.

114. Michael S, Fraser RB, Reilly CS. Intra-operative pulmonary embolism. Detection by pulse oximetry. Anaesthesia 1990;45:225–226.

115. Byrick RJ, Forbes D, Waddell JP. A monitored cardiovascular collapse during cemented total knee replacement. Anesthesiology 1986;65:213–216.

116. Quance D. Amniotic fluid embolism: detection by pulse oximetry. Anesthesiology 1988;68:951–952.

117. Mason RA. The pulse oximeter—an early warning device? Anaesthesia 1987;42:784–785.

118. Allberry RAW, Westbrook D. Pulse oximetry. Anaesthesia and Intensive Care 1991;19:130.

119. Laishley RS, Aps C. Tension pneumothorax and pulse oximetry. Br J Anaesth 1991;66:250–252.

120. Bacon AK. Pulse oximetry in malignant hyperthermia. Anaesthesia and Intensive Care 1989;17: 208–210.

121. Breathwaite CEM, O'Malley KF, Ross SE, et al. Continuous pulse oximetry and the diagnosis of pulmonary embolism in critically ill trauma patients. J Trauma 1992;33:528–531.

122. Anonymous. Pulse oximetry—not just in the O.R. and PACU. ASA Newslett 1995;59(5):33.

123. Moller JT, Wittrup M, Johansen SH. Hypoxemia in the postanesthesia care unit. An observer study. Anesthesiology 1990;73:890–895.

124. Canet J, Ricos M, Vidal F, Early postoperative arterial desaturation. Determining factors and response to oxygen therapy. Anesth Analg 1989;69:207–212.

125. Smith DC, Canning JJ, Crul JF. Pulse oximetry in the recovery room. Anaesthesia 1989;44:345–348.

126. Tomkins DP, Gaukroger P. Oxygen saturation in children following general anaesthesia. Anaesthesia and Intensive Care 1987;15:111.

127. Bach A. Pulse oximetry in the recovery room. Anaesthesia 1989;44:1007.

128. Brown LT, Purcell GJ, Traugott FM. Hypoxemia during postoperative recovery using continuous pulse oximetry. Anaesthesia and Intensive Care 1990;18:509–516.

129. Motoyama EK, Glazener CH. Hypoxemia after general anesthesia in children. Anesth Analg 1986;65:267–272.

130. Mertzlufft FO, Jansen U, Dick W. Continuous monitoring of arterial oxygenation in the recovery room using pulse oximetry. Eur J Anaesth 1987;4:64–65.

131. McDonald J, Keneally J. Oxygen saturation in children during transit from operating theatre to recovery. Anaesthesia and Intensive Care 1987;15:360–361.

132. Morris RW, Bushman A, Warren DL, et al. The prevalence of hypoxemia detected by pulse oximetry during recovery from anesthesia. Journal of Clinical Monitoring 1988;4:16–20.

133. Fiechter FK. Results of a quality assurance study on the use of pulse oximetry in the postanesthesia care unit. J Post Anesth Nurs 1991;6:342–346.

134. Serpell Mgm, Padgham N, McQueen F, et al. The influence of nasal obstruction and its relief on oxygen saturation during sleep and the early postoperative period. Anaesthesia 1994;49:538–540.

135. DiBenedetto RJ, Graves SA, Gravenstein N, et al. Pulse oximetry monitoring can change routine oxygen supplementation practices in the postanesthesia care unit. Anesth Analg 1994;78:365–368.

136. Chrubasik J, Geller E, Graf R, et al. Evaluation of continuous pulse oximetry and capnometry during postoperative pain treatment with opioids. Anesth Analg 1994;78:S61.

137. Kimovec MA, Grutsch JF, Nacpil JA. Incidence of postoperative hypoxia prior to recovery room discharge. Anesthesiology 1989;71:A373.

138. Blair I, Holland R, Lau W, et al. Oxygen saturation during transfer from operating room to recovery after anaesthesia. Anaesthesia and Intensive Care 1987;15:147–150.

139. Chripko D, Bevan JC, Archer DP, et al. Decreases in arterial oxygen saturation in paediatric outpatients during transfer to the post-anesthetic recovery room. Can J Anaesth 1989;36:128–132.

140. Katarina BK, Harnik EV, Mitchard R, et al. Postoperative arterial oxygen saturation in the pediatric population during transportation. Anesth Analg 1988;67:280–282.

141. Meiklejohn BH, Smith G, Elling AE, et al. Arterial oxygen desaturation during postoperative transportation: the influence of operation site. Anaesthesia 1987;42:1313–1315.

142. Pullerits J, Burrows RA, Roy WL. Arterial desaturation in healthy children during transfer to the recovery room. Can J Anaesth 1987;34:470–473.

143. Patel R, Norden J, Hannallah RS. Oxygen administration prevents hypoxia during post-anesthetic transport in children. Anesthesiology 1988;69:616–618.

144. Riley RH, Davis NJ, Finucane KE, et al. Arterial oxygen saturation in anaesthetized patients during transfer from induction room to operating room. Anaesthesia and Intensive Care 1988;16:182–186.

145. Smith DC, Crul JF. Early postoperative hypoxia during transport. Br J Anaesth 1988;61:625–627.

146. Tyler IL, Tantisira B, Winter PM, et al. Continuous monitoring of arterial oxygen saturation with pulse oximetry during transfer to the recovery room. Anesth Analg 1985;64:1108–1112.

147. Tompkins DP, Gaukroger PB, Bentley MW. Hypoxia in children following general anesthesia. Anaesthesia and Intensive Care 1988;16:177–181.

148. Tait AR, Kyff JV, Crider B, et al. Changes in arterial oxygen saturation in cigarette smokers following general anesthesia. Can J Anaesth 1990;37:423–428.

149. Lampe GH, Wauk LZ, Whitendale P, et al. Postoperative hypoxemia after non-abdominal surgery. A frequent event not caused by nitrous oxide. Anesth Analg 1990;71:597–601.

150. Choi HJ, Little MS, Garber SZ, et al. Pulse oximetry for monitoring during ward analgesia. Epidural morphine versus parenteral narcotics. Journal of Clinical Monitoring 1989;5:87–89.

151. McKenzie AJ. Perioperative hypoxemia detected by intermittent pulse oximetry. Anaesthesia and Intensive Care 1989;17:412–417.

152. Choi HJ, Little MS, Garber SZ, et al. Pulse oximetry for monitoring during ward analgesia: epidural morphine versus parenteral narcotics. Journal of Clinical Monitoring 1989;5:87–89.

153. Pan PH, James CE. Anesthetic-postoperative morphine regimens for Cesarean section and postoperative oxygen saturation monitored by a telemetric pulse oximetry network for 24 continuous hours. J Clin Anesth 1994;6:124–128.

154. Bierman MI, Stein KL, Snyder JV. Pulse oximetry in the postoperative care of cardiac surgical patients: A randomized controlled trial. Chest 1992;102:1367–1370.

155. Klaas MA, Cheng EY. Early response to pulse oximetry alarms with telemetry. Journal of Clinical Monitoring 1994;10:178–180.

156. Withington DE, Ramsay JG, Saoud AT, et al. Weaning from ventilation after cardiopulmonary bypass. Evaluation of a non-invasive technique. Can J Anaesth 1991;38:15–19.

157. Neihoff J, DelGuercio C, LaMorte W, et al. Efficacy of pulse oximetry and capnometry in postoperative ventilatory weaning. Crit Care Med 1988;16:701–705.

158. Narang VPS. Utility of the pulse oximeter during cardiopulmonary resuscitation. Anesthesiology 1986;65:239–240.

159. Moorthy SS, Dierdorf SF, Schmidt SI. Erroneous pulse oximetry data during CPR. Anesth Analg 1990;70:339.

160. Griffin M, Cooney C. Pulse oximetry during cardiopulmonary resuscitation. Anaesthesia 1995;50:1008.

161. Sendak MJ, Harris AP, Donham RT. Use of pulse oximetry to assess arterial oxygen saturation during newborn resuscitation. Crit Care Med 1986;14:739–740.

162. Galdun JP, Paris PM, Stewart RD. Pulse oximetry in the emergency department. Am J Emerg Med 1989;7:422–425.

163. Jones J, Heiselman D, Cannon L, et al. Continuous emergency department monitoring of arterial saturation in adult patients with respiratory distress. Ann Emerg Med 1988;17:463–468.

164. Kellerman AL, Cofer CA, Joseph S, et al. Ann Emerg Med 1991;20:130–134.

165. Aughey K, Hess D, Eitel D, et al. An evaluation of pulse oximetry in pre-hospital care. Ann Emerg Med 1991;20:887–891.

166. Short L, Hecker RB, Middaugh RE, et al. A comparison of pulse oximeters during helicopter flight. J Emerg Med 1989;7:639–643.

167. Hankins CT. The use of pulse oximetry during infant transport from outside facilities. J Perinatol 1987;7:346.

168. Puttick NP, Lawler PGP. Pulse oximetry in mountain rescue and helicopter evacuation. Anaesthesia 1989;44:867.

169. Runcie CJ, Reeve W. Pulse oximetry during transport of the critically ill. Journal of Clinical Monitoring 1991;7:348–349.

170. Talke P, Nichols RJ, Traber DL. Monitoring patients during helicopter flight. Journal of Clinical Monitoring 1990;6:139–140.

171. Morley AP. Pre-hospital monitoring of trauma patients: experience of a helicopter emergency medical service. Br J Anaesth 1996;76:726–730.

172. Short L, Hecker RB, Middaugh RE, et al. A comparison of pulse oximeters during helicopter flight. J Emerg Med 1989;7:639–643.

173. Aughey K, Hess D, Eitel D, et al. An evaluation of pulse oximetry in pre-hospital care. Ann Emerg Med 1991;20:887–891.

174. McGuire TJ, Pointer JE. Evaluation of a pulse oximeter in the pre-hospital setting. Ann Emerg Med 1988;17:1058–1062.

175. Talke PO, Nichols RJ, Traber DL. Monitoring patients during helicopter flight. Journal of Clinical Monitoring 1990;6:139.

176. James MR, Mardhall H, Carew–McCollo M. Pulse oximetry during apparent tonic-clonic seizures. Lancet 1991;337:394–395.

177. Brodsky JB, Shulman MS. Oxygen monitoring of bleomycin-treated patients. Can Anaesth Soc J 1984;31:488.

178. Lennon RL, Hosking MP, Warner MA, et al. Monitoring and analysis of oxygenation and ventilation during rigid bronchoscopic neodymium-YAG laser resection of airway tumors. Surv Anesth 1988;32:100.

179. Skeehan TM, Hensley FA Jr. Axillary artery compression and the prone position. Anesth Analg 1986;65:518–519.

180. Hovagim AR, Backus WW, et al. Pulse oximetry and patient positioning. A report of eight cases. Anesthesiology 1989;71:454–456.

181. Herschman ZJ, Frost EAM, Goldiner PL. Pulse oximetry during shoulder arthroscopy. Anesthesiology 1986;65:565.

182. Gibbs N, Handal J, Nentwig MK. Pulse oximetry during shoulder arthroscopy. Anesthesiology 1987;67:150–151.

183. Ray SA, Ivory JP, Beavis JP. Use of pulse oximetry during manipulation of supracondylar fractures of the humerus. Injury 1991;21:103–104.

184. David HG. Pulse oximetry in closed limb fractures. Ann Roy Coll Surg Eng 1991;73:283–284.

185. Vegfors M, Tryggvason B, Sjoberg F, et al. Assessment of peripheral blood flow using a pulse oximeter. Journal of Clinical Monitoring 1990;6:1–4.

186. Graham B, Paulus DA, Caffee HH. Pulse oximetry for vascular monitoring in upper extremity replantation surgery. J Hand Surg 1986;11:687–692.

187. Skeen JT, Bacus WW, Hovagim AR, et al. Intraoperative pulse oximetry in peripheral revascularization in an infant. Journal of Clinical Monitoring 1988;4:272–273.

188. Reference deleted.

189. Joyce WP, Walsh K, Gough DB, et al. Pulse oximetry: a new non-invasive assessment of peripheral arterial occlusive disease. Br J Surg 1990;77:1115–1117.

190. Halevy A, Halpern Z, Negri M, et al. Pulse oximetry in the evaluation of painful hand after arteriovenous fistula creation. J Vasc Surg 1991;14:537–539.

191. Matsuki A. A modified Allen's test using a pulse oximeter. Anaesthesia and Intensive Care 1988;16:126–127.

192. Nowak GS, Moorthy SS, McNiece WL. Use of pulse oximetry for assessment of collateral arterial flow. Anesthesiology 1986;64:527.

193. Cheng EY, Lauer, KK, Stommel KA, et al. Evaluation of the palmar circulation by pulse oximetry. Journal of Clinical Monitoring 1989;5:1–3.

194. Pillow K, Herrick IA. Pulse oximetry compared with Doppler ultrasound for assessment of collateral blood flow to the hand. Anaesthesia 1991;46:388–390.

195. Persson E. The pulse oximeter and Allen's test. Anaesthesia 1992;47:451.

196. Raju R. The pulse oximeter and the collateral circulation. Anaesthesia 1986;41:783–784.

197. Rozenberg B, Rosenberg M, Birkhan J. Allen's test performed by pulse oximetry. Anaesthesia 1988;43:515–516.

198. Severinghaus JW, Kelleher JF. Recent developments in pulse oximetry. Anesthesiology 1992;76:1018–1038.

199. Hovagim AR, Katz RI, Poppers PJ. Pulse oximetry for evaluation of radial and ulnar blood flow. J Cardiothorac Anesth 1989;3:27–30.

200. Persson E. The pulse oximeter and Allen's test. Anaesthesia 1992;47:451.

201. Glavin RJ. Pulse oximeter and Allen's test. Anaesthesia 1992;47:917.

202. Lovinsohn DG, Gordon L, Sessler DI. The Allen's test. Analysis of four methods. J Hand Surg 1991;16A:279–282.

203. Glavin RJ, Jones HM. Assessing collateral circulation in the hand. Four methods compared. Anaesthesia 1989;44:594–595.

204. Munro FJ, Broome I. Radial artery occlusion detected by pulse oximetry. Anaesthesia 1994;49:1102.

205. Chawla R, Kumarvel V, Girdhar KK, et al. Can pulse oximetry be used to measure systolic blood pressure? Anesth Analg 1992;74:196–200.

206. Greenblott GB, Gerschultz S, Tremper KK. Blood flow limits and signal detection comparing five different models of pulse oximeters. Anesthesiology 1989;70:367–368.

207. Korbon GA, Wills MH, D'Lauro F, et al. Systolic blood pressure measurement. Doppler versus pulse oximeter. Anesthesiology 1987;67:A188.

208. Severinghaus JW, Spellman MJ. Pulse oximeter failure thresholds in hypotension and vasoconstriction. Anesthesiology 1990;73:532–537.

209. Talke P, Nichols RJ, Traber DL. Does measurement of systolic blood pressure with a pulse oximeter correlate with conventional methods? Journal of Clinical Monitoring 1990;6:5–9.

210. Wallace CT, Baker JD, Alpert CC, et al. Comparison of blood pressure measurement by Doppler and by pulse oximetry techniques. Anesth Analg 1987;66:1018–1019.

211. Talke PO. Measurement of systolic blood pressure using pulse oximetry during helicopter flight. Crit Care Med 1991;19:934–937.

212. Langbaum M, Eyal FG. A practical and reliable method of measuring blood pressure in the neonate by pulse oximetry. J Pediar 1994;125:591–595.

213. Chawla R, Kumarvel V, Girdhar KK, et al. Oximetry in pulseless disease. Anaesthesia 1990;45:992–993.

214. Sullivan MJ, Cooke JE, Baker JD III, et al. Axillary block utilizing the pulse oximeter. Anesthesiology 1989;71:166–167.

215. Okuda Y, Kitajima T, Asai T. Use of a pulse oximeter during performance of an axillary plexus block. Anaesthesia 1997;52:717.

216. Katz Y, Lee ME. Pulse oximetry for localization of the dorsalis pedis artery. Anaesthesia and Intensive Care 1989;17:114.

217. Introna RPS, Silverstein PI. A new use for the pulse oximeter. Anesthesiology 1986;65:342.

218. Blanchette T, Dziodzio J, Harris K. Pulse oximetry and normoxemia in neonatal intensive care. Respiratory Care 1991;36:25–32.

219. Bucher HU, Fanconi S, Baechert P, et al. Hyperoxemia in newborn infants: detection by pulse oximetry. Pediatrics 1989;84:226–230.

220. Southall DP, Bingall S, Stebbens VA, et al. Pulse oximeter and transcutaneous arterial oxygen measurements in neonatal and paediatric intensive care. Arch Dis Child 1987;62:882–888.

221. Poets CF, Wilken M, Seldenberg J, et al. Reliability of a pulse oximeter in the detection of hyperoxemia. J Pediatr 1993;122:87–89.

222. James DJ, Brown RE. Vascular volume monitoring with pulse oximetry during paediatric anaesthesia. Can J Anaesth 1990;37:266–267.

223. Partridge BL. Use of pulse oximetry as a non-invasive indicator of intravascular volume status. Journal of Clinical Monitoring 1987;3:263–268.

224. Bowes WA III, Haryadi DG, Westenskow DR. Positive pressure induced changes in pulse oximeter waveforms correlate with volume replacement after hemorrhage in mechanically ventilated dogs. Journal of Clinical Monitoring 1996;12:462–463.

225. Carlson CA, Gravenstein JS, Banner MJ, et al. Monitoring techniques during anesthesia and HFJV for extracorporeal shock-wave lithotripsy. Anesthesiology 1985;63:A178.

226. Rasanen J, Downs JB, Hodges MR. Continuous monitoring of gas exchange and oxygen use with dual oximetry. J Clin Anesth 1988;1:3–8.

227. Rasanen J, Downs JB, Malec DJ, et al. Oxygen tensions and oxyhemoglobin saturations in the assessment of pulmonary gas exchange. Crit Care Med 1987;15:1058–1061.

228. Stemp LI. Another use for pulse oximetry. Anesthesiology 1992;77:1236.

229. Casthely PA, Redko V, Dluzneski J, et al. Pulse oximetry during pulmonary artery banding. J Cardiothoracic Vasc Anesth 1987;1:297–299.

230. Anonymous. Pulse oximeters. Health Devices 1989; 18:185–230.

231. Fanconi S, Doherty P, Edmonds JF, et al. Pulse oximetry in pediatric intensive care. Comparison with measured saturations and transcutaneous oxygen tension. J Pediatr 1985;107:362–366.

231a. Boxer RA, Gottesfeld I, Singh S, et al. Non-invasive pulse oximetry in children with cyanotic congenital heart disease. Crit Care Med 1987;15:1062–1064.

232. Chapman KR, D'Urzo A, Rebuck AS. The accuracy and response characteristics of a simplified ear oximeter. Chest 1983;83:860–864.

232a. Ramanathan R, Durand M, Larrazabal C. Pulse oximetry in very low birth weight infants with acute and chronic lung disease. Pediatrics 1989;79: 612–617.

233. Cecil WT, Petterson MT, Lamoonpun S, et al. Clinical evaluation of the Biox IIA ear oximeter in the critical care environment. Respiratory Care 1985;30: 179–183.

234. Cecil WT, Morrison LS, Lampoonpun S. Clinical evaluation of the Ohmeda Biox III pulse oximeter. A comparison of finger and ear cuvettes. Respiratory Care 1985;30:840–845.

235. Chapman KR, Liu FLW, Watson RM, et al. Range of accuracy of two-wavelength oximetry. Chest 1986; 89:540–542.

236. Cecil WT, Thorpe KJ, Fibuch EE, et al. A clinical evaluation of the accuracy of the Nellcor N-100 and Ohmeda 3700 pulse oximeters. Journal of Clinical Monitoring 1988;4:31–36.

237. Chapman KR, Liu FLW, Watson RM, et al. Range of accuracy of two wavelength oximetry. Chest 1986; 89:540–542.

238. Fait CD, Wetzel RC, Dean JM, et al. Pulse oximetry in critically ill children. Journal of Clinical Monitoring 1985;1:232–235.

239. Hess D, Kochansky M, Hassett L, et al. An evaluation of the Nellcor N-10 portable pulse oximeter. Respiratory Care 1986;31:796–802.

240. Gabrielczyk MR, Buist RJ. Pulse oximetry and postoperative hypothermia. Anaesthesia 1988;43: 402–404.

241. Knill RL, Clement JL, Kieraszewicz HT, et al. Assessment of two non-invasive monitors of arterial oxygenation in anesthetized man. Anesth Analg 1982; 61:582–586.

242. Lynn AM, Bosenberg A. Pulse oximetry during cardiac catheterization in children with congenital heart disease. Journal of Clinical Monitoring 1986;2: 230–233.

243. Kim SK, Baidwan BS, Petty TL. Clinical evaluation of a new finger oximeter. Crit Care Med 1984;12: 910–912.

244. Mihm FG, Halperin BD. Non-invasive detection of profound arterial desaturations using a pulse oximetry device. Anesthesiology 1985;62:85–87.

245. Mackenzie N. Comparison of a pulse oximeter with an ear oximeter and an in-vitro oximeter. Journal of Clinical Monitoring 1985;1:156–160.

246. Mendelson Y, Kent JC, Shahnarian A, et al. Evaluation of the Datascope Accusat pulse oximeter in healthy adults. Journal of Clinical Monitoring 1988; 4:59–63.

247. Macnab AJ, Baker–Brown G, Anderson EE. Oximetry in children recovering from deep hypothermia for cardiac surgery. Crit Care Med 1990;18:1066–1069.

248. Nickerson BG, Sarkisian C, Tremper K. Bias and precision of pulse oximeters and arterial oximeters. Chest 1988;93:515–517.

249. Russell RIR, Helms PJ. Comparative accuracy of pulse oximetry and transcutaneous oxygen in assessing arterial saturation in pediatric intensive care. Crit Care Med 1990;18:725–727.

250. Rebuck AS, Chapman KR, D'Urzo A. The accuracy and response characteristics of a simplified ear oximeter. Chest 1983;83:860–864.

251. Ries AL, Farrow JT, Clausen JL. Accuracy of two ear oximeters at rest and during exercise in pulmonary patients. Am Rev Respir Dis 1985;132:685–689.

252. Shippy MB, Petterson MT, Whitman RA, et al. A clinical evaluation of the BTI Biox II ear oximeter. Respiratory Care 1984;29:730–735.

253. Sidi A, Rush W, Gravenstein N, et al. Pulse oximetry fails to accurately detect low levels of arterial hemoglobin oxygen saturation in dogs. Journal of Clinical Monitoring 1987;3:257–262.

254. Tytler JA, Seeley HF. The Nellcor N-100 pulse oximeter. A clinical evaluation in anaesthesia and intensive care. Anaesthesia 1986;41:302–305.

255. Tweeddale PM, Douglas NJ. Evaluation of Biox IIA ear oximeter. Thorax 1985;40:825–827.

256. Taylor MB, Whitwam JG. The accuracy of pulse oximeters. Anaesthesia 1988;43:229–232.

257. Sendak MJ, Harris AP, Donham RT. Accuracy of pulse oximetry during oxyhemoglobin desaturation in dogs. Anesthesiology 1988;68:111–114.

258. Hay WW, Brockway JM, Eyzaguirre M. Neonatal pulse oximetry: accuracy and reliability. Pediatrics 1989;83:717–722.

259. Hay WW. Physiology of oxygenation and its relation to pulse oximetry in neonates. J Perinatology 1987;7:309–319.

260. Haessler R, Brandl F, Zeller M, et al. Continuous intra-arterial oximetry, pulse oximetry, and co-oximetry during cardiac surgery. J Cardiothorac Vasc Anesth 1992;6:668–673.

261. Hannhart B, Haberer J-P, Saunier C, et al. Accuracy and precision of fourteen pulse oximeters. Eur Respir J 1991;4:115–119.

262. Hannhart B, Michalski H, Delorme N, et al. Reliability of six pulse oximeters in chronic obstructive pulmonary disease. Chest 1991;99:842–846.

263. Reynolds KJ, DeKock JP, Tarassenko L, et al. Temperature dependence of LED and its theoretical effect on pulse oximetry. Br J Anaesth 1991;67:638–643.

264. Wong DH, Tremper KK, Davidson J, et al. Pulse oximetry is accurate in patients with dysrhythmias and a pulse deficit. Anesthesiology 1989;70:1024–1025.

265. Thrush D, Hodges M. The accuracy of pulse oximetry during hypoxemia. Anesthesiology 1992;77:A537.

266. Ridley SA. A comparison of two pulse oximeters. Anaesthesia 1988;43:136–140.

267. Reynolds KJ, Moyle JTB, Sykes MK, et al. Response of 10 pulse oximeters to an in vitro test system. Br J Anaesth 1992;68:365–369.

268. Fanconi S. Reliability of pulse oximetry in hypoxic infants. J Pediatr 1988;112:424–427.

269. Freund PR, Overand PT, Cooper J, et al. A prospective study of intraoperative pulse oximetry failure. Journal of Clinical Monitoring 1991;7:253–258.

270. Gillies BSA, Overand PT, Bosse S, et al. Failure rate of pulse oximetry in the post anesthesia care unit. Anesthesiology 1990;73:A1009.

271. Overand PT, Freund PR, Cooper JO, et al. Failure rate of pulse oximetry in clinical practice. Anesth Analg 1990;70:S289.

272. Morris RW, Nairn M, Beaudoin M. Does the radial arterial line degrade the performance of a pulse oximeter? Anaesthesia and Intensive Care 1990;18:107–109.

273. New WJ. Pulse oximetry. Journal of Clinical Monitoring 1985;1:126–129.

274. King T, Simon RH. Pulse oximetry for tapering supplemental oxygen in hospitalized patients. Chest 1987;92:713–716.

275. Dib H, Gerber D, Dubois J, et al. Impact of routine pulse oximetry on arterial blood gas use in mechanically ventilated patients. Crit Care Med 1994;22:A30.

276. Roizen MF, Schreider B, Austin W, et al. Pulse oximetry, capnography, and blood gas measurements: reducing cost and improving the quality of care with technology. Journal of Clinical Monitoring 1993;9:237–240.

277. Gillies BS, Posner K, Freund P, et al. Failure of pulse oximetry in the postanesthesia care unit. Journal of Clinical Monitoring 1993;9:326–329.

278. Reich DL, Timcenko A, Bodian CA, et al. Predictors of pulse oximetry data failure. Anesthesiology 1996;84:859–864.

279. Moller JT, Pedersen T, Rasmussen LS, et al. Randomized evaluation of pulse oximetry in 20,802 patients: I. Design, demography, pulse oximetry failure rate, and overall complication rate. Anesthesiology 1993;78:436–444.

280. Trivedi NS, Barker SJ, Hyatt J, et al. Pulse oximeter failure during general anesthesia. Anesthesiology 1995;83:A473.

281. Armstrong N, Perrin LS. Pulse oximeter overload. Anesthesiology 1992;76:148.

282. Trivedi NS, Barker SJ, Shah NK, et al. Pulse oximeter failure during electrocautery use under general anesthesia. Anesthesiology 1995;83:A451.

283. Sipe S, Boyd G, Battito M, et al. High "failure" rate for pulse oximetry in patients with chronic renal failure. Crit Care Med 1992;20:S21.

284. Lie C, Kehlet H, Rosenberg J. Comparison of the Nellcor N-200 and N-3000 pulse oximeters during simulated postoperative activities. Anaesthesia 1997;52:450–452.

285. Clayton DG, Webb RK, Ralston AC, et al. A comparison of the performance of twenty pulse oximeters under conditions of poor perfusion. Anaesthesia 1991;46:3–10.

286. Falconer RJ, Robinson BJ. Comparison of pulse oximeters: accuracy at low arterial pressure in volunteers. Br J Anaesth 1990;65:552–557.

287. Langton JA, Lassey D, Hanning CD. Comparison of four pulse oximeters. Effects of venous occlusion and cold-induced peripheral vasoconstriction. Br J Anaesth 1990;65:245–247.

288. Morris RW, Nairn M, Torda TA. A comparison of fifteen pulse oximeters. Part I: a clinical comparison. Part II: a test of performance under conditions of poor perfusion. Anaesthesia and Intensive Care 1989;17:62–73.

289. Wilkins CJ, Moores M, Hanning CD. Comparison of pulse oximeters. Effects of vasoconstriction and venous engorgement. Br J Anaesth 1989;62: 439–444.

290. Ibanez J, Velasco J, Raurich JM. The accuracy of the Biox 2700 pulse oximeter in patients receiving vasoactive therapy. Intens Care Med 1991;17:484–486.

291. Palve H, Vuori A. Minimum pulse pressure and peripheral temperature needed for pulse oximetry during cardiac surgery with cardiopulmonary bypass. J Cardiothorac Vasc Anesth 1991;5:327–330.

292. Woods AM, Queen JS, Lawson D. Valsalva maneuver in obstetrics: the influence of peripheral circulatory changes on function of the pulse oximeter. Anesth Analg 1991;73:765–771.

293. Kurki TSO, Piirainen HI, Kurki PT. Effects of cold exposure on the function of finger blood pressure and pulse oximeter monitors. Anesthesiology 1989;71: A409.

294. Lawson D, Norley I, Korbon G, et al. Blood flow limits and pulse oximeter signal detection. Anesthesiology 1987;67:599–603.

295. Freund PR, Bowdle TA, Neuenfeldt T, et al. Reversal of intraoperative pulse oximetry failure by digital nerve block. Anesth Analg 1991;72:S81.

296. Palve H, Vuori A. Pulse oximetry during low cardiac output and hypothermia states immediately after open heart surgery. Crit Care Med 1989;17:66–69.

297. Gupta A, Vegfors M. A simple solution. Anaesthesia 1992;47:822.

298. Paulus DA, Monroe MC. Cool fingers and pulse oximetry. Anesthesiology 1989;71:168–169.

299. Shah NK, Trivedi NS, Alkire MT, et al. Impact of low perfusion on the performance of a new pulse oximeter. Anesth Analg 1995;80:S426.

300. Weber W, Elfadel IM, Barker SJ. Low-perfusion resistant pulse oximetry. Journal of Clinical Monitoring 1995;11:282.

301. Barker SJ, Tremper KK, Gamel DM. A clinical comparison of transcutaneous PO$_2$ and pulse oximetry in the operating room. Anesth Analg 1986;65: 805–808.

302. Verhoeff F, Sykes MK. Delayed detection of hypoxic events by pulse oximeters. Computer simulations. Anaesthesia 1990;45:103–109.

303. Reynolds LM, Jobes DR, Nicholson SC, et al. Changes in oxygen saturation in children are detected earlier by centrally placed pulse oximeter sensors. Anesthesiology 1992;77:A1178.

304. Ding Z, Shibata K, Yamamoto K, et al. Decreased circulation time in the upper limb reduces the lag time of the finger pulse oximeter response. Can J Anesth 1992;39:87–89.

305. Reference deleted.

306. Xue FS, Liao X, Tong SY, et al. Effect of epidural block on the lag time of pulse oximeter response. Anaesthesia 1996;51:1102–1105.

307. Smith TC. Intra-aortic balloon pumps and the pulse oximeter. Anaesthesia 1992;47:1010–1011.

308. Pandit JJ. Accuracy of pulse oximetry in aortomyoplasty and balloon counterpulsation. Anaesthesia 1997;52:87–88.

309. Smith J. Understanding pulse oximetry. Anaesthesia and Intensive Care 1992;20: 255–256.

310. Barker SJ, Tremper KK, Hyatt J. Effects of methemoglobinemia on pulse oximetry and mixed venous oximetry. Anesthesiology 1989;70:112–117.

311. Sprung J, Bourke DL, Mackenzie CF, et al. Chronic methemoglobinemia: improving hemoglobin saturation monitoring during anesthesia. Journal of Clinical Monitoring 1994;10:267–269.

312. Chisholm DG, Stuart H. Congenital methaemoglobinemia detected by pulse oximetry. Can J Anaesth 1994;41:519–522.

313. Kumar A, Chawla R, Ahuja S, et al. Nitrobenzene poisoning and spurious pulse oximetry. Anaesthesia 1990;45:949–951.

314. Severinghaus JW, Xu Fa-Di, Spellman MJ. Benzocaine and methemoglobin. Recommended actions. Anesthesiology 1991;74:385–386.

315. Anderson ST, Hajduczek J, Barker SJ. Benzocaine-induced methemoglobinemia in an adult: accuracy of pulse oximetry with methemoglobinemia. Anesth Analg 1988;67:1099–1101.

316. Marks LF, Desgrand D. Prilocaine associated methaemoglobinemia and the pulse oximeter. Anaesthesia 1991;46:703.

317. Bardoczky GI, Wathieu M, D'Hollander A. Prilocaine-induced methemoglobinemia evidenced by pulse oximetry. Acta Anaesthesiol Scand 1990;34: 162–164.

318. Eisenkraft JB. Pulse oximeter desaturation due to methemoglobinemia. Anesthesiology 1988;68: 278–282.

319. Trillo PA, Aukburg S. Dapsone-induced methemoglobinemia and pulse oximetry. Anesthesiology 1992;77:594–596.

320. Delwood L, O'Flaherty D, Prejean EJ, et al. Methaemoglobinemia and pulse oximetry. Anaesthesia 1992; 47:80.

321. Delwood L, O'Flaherty D, Prejean EJ, et al. Methemoglobinemia and its effect on pulse oximetry. Crit Care Med 1991;19:988.

322. Rieder HU, Frei FJ, Zbinden AM, et al. Pulse oximetry in methemoglobinemia. Anaesthesia 1989;44: 326–327.

323. Schweitzer SA. Spurious pulse oximeter desaturation due to methaemoglobinemia. Anesthesia and Intensive Care 1991;19:269–271.

324. Watcha MF, Connor MT, Hing AV. Pulse oximetry in methemoglobinemia. Am J Dis Child 1989;143:845–847.

325. Varpm AK. Methemoglobinemia and pulse oximetry. Crit Care Med 1992;20:1363–1364.

326. Goldhill DR, Hill AJ, Whitburn RH, et al. Carboxyhaemoglobin concentrations, pulse oximetry, and arterial blood-gas tensions during jet ventilation for Nd-YAG laser bronchoscopy. Br J Anaesth 1990;65:749–753.

327. Vegfors M, Lennmarken C. Carboxyhemoglobinaemia and pulse oximetry. Br J Anaesth 1991;66:625–626.

328. Gonzalez A, Gomez–Arnay J, Pensado A. Carboxyhemoglobin and pulse oximetry. Anesthesiology 1990;73:573.

329. Barker SJ, Tremper KT. The effect of carbon monoxide inhalation on pulse oximetry and transcutaneous pO_2. Anesthesiology 1987;66:677–679.

330. Tashiro C, Koo YH, Fukumitsu K, et al. Effects of carboxyhemoglobin on pulse oximetry in humans. J Anesth 1988;2:36–40.

331. Anderson JV. The accuracy of pulse oximetry in neonates: effects of fetal hemoglobin and bilirubin. J Perinatol 1987;7:323.

331a. Harris AP, Sendak MJ, Donham RT, et al. Absorption characteristics of human fetal hemoglobin at wavelengths used in pulse oximetry. Journal of Clinical Monitoring 1988;4:175–177.

332. Pologe JA, Raley DM. Effects of fetal hemoglobin on pulse oximetry. J Perinatol 1987;7:324–326.

333. Praud J-P, Carofilis A, Bridey F, et al. Accuracy of two wavelength pulse oximetry in neonates and infants. Pediatr Pulmonol 1989;6:180–182.

334. House JT, Schultetus RR, Gravenstein N. Continuous neonatal evaluation in the delivery room by pulse oximetry. Journal of Clinical Monitoring 1987;3:96–100.

335. Rajadurai VS, Walker AM, Yu VYH, et al. Effect of fetal haemoglobin on the accuracy of pulse oximetry in preterm infants. J Paediatr Child Health 1992;28:3–6.

336. Jennis MS, Peabody JL. Pulse oximetry. An alternative method for the assessment of oxygenation in newborn infants. Pediatrics 1988;79:524–528.

337. Craft JA, Alessandrini E, Kenney LB, et al. Comparison of oxygenation measurements in pediatric patients during sickle cell crises. J Ped 1994;124:93–95.

338. Goepp J, Murray C, Walker A, et al. Oxygen saturation measurement by pulse oximetry in patients with sickle cell anemia: lack of correlation with arterial blood gas measurement. Pediatr Emerg Care 1991;7:387.

339. McMahon B, Bell C, Moscovitz H. Accuracy of pulse oximetry during sickle cell vaso-occlusive crisis. Journal of Clinical Monitoring 1995;11:269.

340. Pianosi P, Charge TD, Esseltine DW, et al. Pulse oximetry in sickle cell disease. Arch Dis Child 1993;68:735–738.

341. Weston Smith SG, Glass UH, Acharya FJ, et al. Pulse oximetry in sickle cell disease. Clin Lab Haemat 1989;11:185–188.

342. Rackoff WR, Kunkel N, Silber JH, et al. Pulse oximetry and factors associated with hemoglobin oxygen desaturation in children with sickle cell disease. Blood 1993;81:3422–3427.

343. Gottschalk A, Silverberg M. An unexpected finding with pulse oximetry in a patient with hemoglobin Koln. Anesthesiology 1994;80:474–476.

344. Katoh R, Miyake T, Arai T. Unexpectedly low pulse oximeter readings in a boy with unstable hemoglobin Koln. Anesthesiology 1994;80:472–474.

345. Lang SA, Chang PC, Laxdal VA, et al. Haemoglobin Hammersmith precludes monitoring with conventional pulse oximetry. Can J Anaesth 1994;41:965–968.

346. Jay GD, Renzi FP. Evaluation of pulse oximetry in anemia from hemoglobin-H disease. Ann Emerg Med 1992;21:572–574.

347. Corkeron MA, Pavy TJG. Pulse oximetry in mixed haemoglobinopathy. Anaesthesia and Intensive Care 1996;24:619–620.

348. Beall SN, Moorthy SS. Jaundice, oximetry, and spurious hemoglobin desaturation. Anesth Analg 1989;68:806–807.

349. Chelluri L, Snyder JV, Bird JR. Accuracy of pulse oximetry in patients with hyperbilirubinemia. Respiratory Care 1991;36:1383–386.

350. Veyckemans F, Baele P, Guillaume JE, et al. Hyperbilirubinemia does not interfere with hemoglobin saturation measured by pulse oximetry. Anesthesiology 1989;70:118–122.

351. Veyckemans F, Baele PL. More about jaundice and oximetry. Anesth Analg 1990;70:335–336.

352. Thrush D, Hodges MR. Accuracy of pulse oximetry during hypoxemia. South Med J 1994;87:518–521.

353. Mendelson Y, Kent JC, Shahnarian A, et al. Simultaneous comparison of three non-invasive oximeters in healthy volunteers. Medical Instrum 1987;21:183–188.

354. Sendak MJ, Harris AP, Donham RT. Accuracy of pulse oximetry during severe arterial oxygen desaturation. Anesthesiology 1986;65:A133.

355. Sarnquist FH, Todd C, Whitcher C. Accuracy of a new non-invasive oxygen saturation monitor. Anesthesiology 1980;53:S163.

356. Inman KJ, Rutledge FS, Cunningham DG, et al. A visual method of comparing saturations obtained by pulse oximetry and the arterial blood gas. Crit Care Med 1993;21:S215.

357. Schmitt HJ, Schuetz WH, Proeschel PA, et al. Accuracy of pulse oximetry in children with cyanotic congenital heart disease. J Cardiothorac Vasc Anes 1993; 7:61–65.

358. Lebecue P, Shango P, Stijns M, et al. Pulse oximetry versus measured arterial oxygen saturation: A comparison of the Nellcor N100 and the Biox III. Pediatric Pulmonol 1991;10:132–135.

359. Gidding SS. Pulse oximetry in cyanotic congenital heart disease. Am J Cardiology 1992;70:391–392.

360. Barker SJ, Hyatt J, Shah NK, et al. The effect of sensor malpositioning on pulse oximeter accuracy during hypoxemia. Anesthesiology 1993;79:248–254.

361. Kelleher JF, Ruff RH. The penumbra effect. Vasomotion-dependent pulse oximeter artifact due to probe malposition. Anesthesiology 1989;71:787–791.

362. Serpell MG. Children's fingers and spurious pulse oximetry. Anaesthesia 1991;46:702–703.

363. Ordman AJ, Samra GS. Pulse oximetry: incorrect use leading to failure to fail safe. Anaesthesia 1994;49:927.

364. Southall DP, Samuels M. Inappropriate sensor application in pulse oximetry. Lancet 1992;340:481–482.

365. Langton JA, Hanning CD. Effect of motion artefact on pulse oximeters. Evaluation of four instruments and finger probes. Br J Anaesth 1990;65:564–570.

366. Anonymous. Oximeter probes. Technol for Anesth 1994;15(6):14.

367. Tweedie IE. Pulse oximeters and fingernails. Anaesthesia 1989;44:268.

368. Poets CF, Seidenberg J, van der Hardt H. Failure of pulse oximeter to detect sensor detachment. Lancet 1993;341:244.

369. Al Khudhairi D, Prabhu R, El Sharkawy M, et al. Evaluation of a pulse oximeter during profound hypothermia. An assessment of the Biox 3700 during induction of hypothermia before cardiac surgery in paediatric patients. Int J Clin Monit Comput 1990;7:217–222.

370. Vegfors M, Lindberg L-G, Lennmarken C. The influence of changes in blood flow on the accuracy of pulse oximetry in humans. Acta Anaesthesiol Scand 1992; 36:346–349.

371. Secker C, Spiers P. Accuracy of pulse oximetry in patients with low systemic vascular resistance. Anaesthesia 1997;52:127–130.

372. Mark JB. Systolic venous waves cause spurious signs of arterial hemoglobin desaturation. Anesthesiology 1989;71:158–160.

373. Sami HM, Kleinman BS, Lonchyna VA. Central venous pulsations associated with a falsely low oxygen saturation measured by pulse oximeter. Journal of Clinical Monitoring 1991;7:309–312.

374. Stewart KG, Rowbottom SJ. Inaccuracy of pulse oximetry in patients with severe tricuspid regurgitation. Anaesthesia 1991;46:668–670.

375. Bucher HU, Keel M, Wolf M, et al. Artifactual pulse-oximetry estimation in neonates. Lancet 1994;343:1135–1136.

376. Kao YJ, Norton RG. A quantitative study of venous congestion on pulse oximetry. Can J Anaesth 1991;38:A154.

377. Scheller J, Loeb R. Respiratory artifact during pulse oximetry in critically ill patients. Anesthesiology 1988;69:602–60.

378. Anonymous. Pulse oximeters. Technology for Anesthesia 1992;13(1):6–7.

379. Anonymous. Pulse oximeters. Technology for Anesthesia 1994;14(1):6.

380. Severinghaus JW, Koh SO. Effect of anemia on pulse oximeter accuracy at low saturation. Journal of Clinical Monitoring 1990;6:85–88.

381. Lee S, Tremper KK, Barker SJ. Effects of anemia on pulse oximetry and continuous mixed venous hemoglobin saturation monitoring in dogs. Anesthesiology 1991;75:118–122.

382. Tamsing TH, Rosenberg J. Pulse oximetry in severe anaemia. Intens Care Med 1992;18:125–126.

383. Vegfors M, Lindberg LG, Oberg PA, et al. The accuracy of pulse oximetry at two haematocrit levels. Acta Anaesthesiol Scand 1992;36:454–459.

384. Jay GD, Hughes L, Renzi FP. Pulse oximetry is accurate in acute anemia from hemorrhage. Ann Emerg Med 1994;24:32–35.

385. Kolesar R, Volgyesi G, Lerman J. Effect of hemoglobin concentration on the accuracy of pulse oximetry. Can J Anaesth 1990;37:588.

386. Cahan C, Decker MJ, Hoekje PL, et al. Agreement between non-invasive oximetric values for oxygen saturation. Chest 1989;97:814–819.

387. Emery JR. Skin pigmentation as an influence on the accuracy of pulse oximetry. J Perinatol 1987;7:329–330.

388. Ries AL, Prewitt LM, Johnson JJ. Skin color and ear oximetry. Chest 1989;96:287–290.

389. Jubran Am, Tobin MJ. Reliability of pulse oximeter in titrating supplemental oxygen therapy in ventilator-dependent patients. Chest 1990;97:1420–1425.

390. Volgyesi GA, Eng P, Spahr–Schopfer I. Does skin

pigmentation affect the accuracy of pulse oximetry? Anesthesiology 1991;75:A406.

391. Zeballos RJ, Weisman IM. Reliability of non-invasive oximetry in black subjects during exercise and hypoxia. Am Rev Respir Dis 1991;144:1240–1244.

392. Scheller MS, Unger RJ, Kelner MJ. Effects of intravenously administered dyes on pulse oximetry readings. Anesthesiology 1986;65:550–552.

393. Sidi A, Paulus DA, Rush W, et al. Methylene blue and indocyanine green artifactually lower pulse oximetry readings of oxygen saturation. Studies in dogs. Journal of Clinical Monitoring 1987;3:249–256.

394. Kessler MR, Eide T, Humayun B, et al. Spurious pulse oximeter desaturation with methylene blue injection. Anesthesiology 1986;65:435–436.

395. Gorman ES, Shnider MR. Effect of methylene blue on the absorbance of solutions of haemoglobin. Br J Anaesth 1988;60:439–444.

396. Robinson DN, McFadzean WA. Pulse oximetry and methylene blue. Anaesthesia 1990;45:884–885.

397. Scott DM, Cooper MG. Spurious pulse oximetry with intrauterine methylene blue injection. Anaesthesia and Intensive Care 1991;19:267–268.

398. Kumar A, Chawla R, Ahuja S, et al. Nitrobenzene poisoning and spurious pulse oximetry. Anaesthesia 1990;45:949–951.

399. Eisenkraft JB. Methylene blue and pulse oximetry readings: spuriouser and spuriouser! Anesthesiology 1988;68:171.

400. Bohrer H, Schmidt H, Bach A. Confirmation of intravascular catheter placement by pulse oximetry following indocyanine green injection. Anaesthesia 1993; 48:647–648.

401. Volgyesi GA, Eng P, Reimer H. Can pulse oximeter sensors be used to estimate cardiac output by dye dilution? Anesthesiology 1992;77:A475.

402. Morell RC, Heynecker T, Kasbtan HJ, et al. False desaturation due to intradermal patent blue dye. Anesthesiology 1993;78:363–343.

403. Battito MF. The effect of fingerprinting ink on pulse oximetry. Anesth Analg 1989;69:256.

404. Goucke R. Hazards of henna. Anesth Analg 1989; 69:416–417.

405. Sneyd JR. "Finger-painting" and the pulse oximeter. Anaesthesia 1991;46:420–421.

406. Anonymous. Ambient light interference with pulse oximeters. Technology for Anesthesia 1988;8(7): 3–4.

407. Amar D, Neidzwski J, Wald A, et al. Fluorescent light interferes with pulse oximetry. Journal of Clinical Monitoring 1989;5:135–136.

408. Anonymous. Pulse oximeter interference from surgical lighting. Health Devices 1987;16:50–51.

409. Anonymous. Pulse oximeter interference from surgical lighting. Technology for Anesthesia 1987;7(10): 8–9.

410. Anonymous. Ambient light interference with pulse oximeters. Health Devices 1987;16:346–347.

411. Brooks TD, Paulus DA, Winkle WE. Infrared heat lamps interfere with pulse oximeters. Anesthesiology 1984;61:630.

412. Block FE. Interference in a pulse oximeter from a fiberoptic light source. Journal of Clinical Monitoring 1987;3:210–211.

413. Costarino AT, Davis DA, Keon TP. Falsely normal saturation reading with the pulse oximeter. Anesthesiology 1987;67:830–831.

414. Hanowell L, Eisele JH, Downs D. Ambient light affects pulse oximeters. Anesthesiology 1987;67: 864–865.

415. Swedlow DB, Ronning V, Feaster SJ. In reply. Anesthesiology 1987;67:865

416. Siegel MN, Gravenstein N. Preventing ambient light from affecting pulse oximetry. Anesthesiology 1987; 67:280.

417. Zablocki AD, Rasch DK. A simple method to prevent interference with pulse oximetry by infrared heating lamps. Anesth Analg 1987;66:915.

418. Samuels SI, Shochat SJ. A new technique for stabilizing the oxygen saturation monitor probe in infants and children. Anesth Analg 1986;65:213.

419. Kataria BK, Lampkins R. Nail polish does not affect pulse oximeter saturation. Anesth Analg 1986;65: 824.

420. Cote CJ, Goldstein EA, Fuchsman WH, et al. The effect of nail polish on pulse oximetry. Anesth Analg 1988;67:683–6.

421. Rubin AS. Nail polish color can affect pulse oximeter saturation. Anesthesiology 1988;68:825.

422. Bignell S, Brimacombe J. A twist in your oximetry. Anaesthesia and Intensive Care 1994;22:738–746.

423. Ezri T, Szmuk P. Pulse oximeters and onychomycosis. Anesthesiology 1992;76:153.

424. Hopkins PM. An erroneous pulse oximeter reading. Anaesthesia 1989;44:868.

425. Rosewarne FA, Reynolds KJ. Dried blood does not affect pulse oximetry. Anaesthesia 1991;46: 886–887.

426. Oyston J, Ordman A. Erroneous explanation for an erroneous pulse oximeter reading. Anaesthesia 1990; 45:258.

427. Block FE, Detko GJ. Minimizing interference and false alarms from electrocautery in the Nellcor N-100 pulse oximeter. Journal of Clinical Monitoring 1986; 2:203–205.

428. Wilson S. Conscious sedation and pulse oximetry: false alarms? Pediatric Dentistry 1990;12:228–232.

429. Langton JA. Shivering and pulse oximeter function. Anaesthesia 1992;47:711.

430. Marks LF, Heath PJ. An unusual pulse oximeter artifact. Anaesthesia 1990;45:501.

431. Block RE, Stahl D. Interference in a pulse oximeter from a nerve stimulator. Journal of Clinical Monitoring 1995;11:392–393.

432. Gardner MW, Ashley EMC. Another pitfall of pulse oximetry. Anaesthesia 1996;51:991.

433. Cone AM, Sansome AJ. An unusual cause of motion artifact during pulse oximetry. Anaesthesia 1992;47:917.

434. Barker SJ, Shah NK. Effects of motion on the performance of pulse oximeters in volunteers. Anesthesiology 1997;86:101–108.

435. Ilsley AH, Zakaria Z, Plummer L, et al. Pulse oximeters outside the operating theatre: effect of movement on saturation readings. Anaesthesia and Intensive Care 1994;22:107–108.

436. Plummer JL, Zakaria AZ, Ilsley AH, et al. Evaluation of the influence of movement on saturation readings from pulse oximeters. Anaesthesia 1995;50:423–426.

437. Ilsley AH, Fronsko RRL, Owen H, et al. Susceptibility to movement artefact of the Nellcor N-200 and N-3000 pulse oximeters. Anaesthesia and Intensive Care 1997;25:190–191.

438. Ralston AC, Webb RK, Runciman WB. Potential errors in pulse oximetry. Anaesthesia 1991;46:291–295.

439. Dumas C, Wahr JA, Tremper KK. Clinical evaluation of a prototype motion artifact resistant pulse oximeter in the recovery room. Anesth Analg 1996;83:269–272.

440. Broome IJ, Mills GH, Spiers P, et al. An evaluation of the effect of vasodilatation on oxygen saturations measured by pulse oximetry and venous blood gas analysis. Anaesthesia 1993;48:415–416.

441. Nachman JA, Schwartz RE. Erroneous measurement of arterial oxygen saturation. J Paediatr Child Health 1993;29:396–397.

442. Wilson S. Conscious sedation and pulse oximetry. False alarms? Pediatr Dent 1990;12:228–232.

443. Rolf N, Cote CJ. Incidence of real and false positive capnography and pulse oximetry alarms during pediatric anesthesia. Anesthesiology 1991;75:A476.

444. Wiklund L, Hok B, Jordeby–Jonsson A, et al. Postanesthesia monitoring. More than 75% of pulse oximeter alarms are trivial. Anesthesiology 1992;77:A582.

445. Anonymous. Delay circuit may reduce pulse oximetry false alarms. Biomedical Safety & Standards 1992;22:162–163.

446. Pan PH, James CF. Effects of default alarm limit settings on alarm distribution in telemetric pulse oximetry network in ward setting. Anesthesiology 1991;75:A405.

447. Jones RDM, Lawson AD, Gunawardene WMS, et al. An evaluation of prolonged oximetric data acquisition. Anesthesia and Intensive Care 1992;20:303–307.

448. Lawless ST. Crying wolf: False alarms in a pediatric intensive care unit. Crit Care Med 1994;22:981–985.

449. Wiklund L, Jordeby–Jonsson A, Stahl K. Postanesthesia monitoring: More than 75% of pulse oximeter alarms are false. Acta Anaesthesiol Scand 1993;37:46.

450. Pan PH. False alarms distribution in intraoperative pulse oximetry. Anesthesiology 1992;77:A494.

451. Pan PH Gravenstein N. Intraoperative pulse oximetry: Frequency and distribution of discrepant data. J Clin Anesth 1994;6:491–495.

452. Leyssius ATR, Kalkman CJ. Influence of pulse oximeter lower alarm limits on the incidence of hypoxemia in the post anesthesia care unit. Anesthesiology 1994;81:A502.

453. Ralston AC, Webb RK, Runciman WB. Potential errors in pulse oximetry. Part I. Pulse oximeter evaluation. Anaesthesia 1991;46:202–206.

454. Egbert TP, Westenskow DR. Detection of artifact in pulse oximetry signals using a neural network. Anesthesiology 1992;77:A521.

455. Elfadel IM, Weber W, Baker SJ. Motion-resistant pulse oximetry. Journal of Clinical Monitoring 1995;11:262.

456. Pollard V, Prough DS. Signal extraction technology: A better mousetrap. Anesth Analg 1996;83:213–214.

457. Shah N, Barker S, Hyatt J, et al. Comparison of alarm conditions between new pulse oximeters during motion at normal and lower oxygen saturations. Anesthesiology 1995;83:A1067.

458. Trivedi NS, Shah NK, Jacobsen BP, et al. New pulse oximeter: resistant to motion artifacts. Anesth Analg 1995;80:S510.

459. Taylor MB. Erroneous actuation of the pulse oximeter. A reply. Anaesthesia 1987;42:1116.

460. Munley AJ, Sik MJ. An unpredictable and possibly dangerous artefact affecting a pulse oximeter. Anaesthesia 1988;43:334.

461. Norley I. Erroneous actuation of the pulse oximeter. Anesthesiology 1987;42:1116.

462. Dawalibi L, Rozario C, van den Bergh AA. Pulse oximetry in pulseless patients. Anaesthesia 1991;46:990–991.

463. Mars M, Hadley GP. Pulse oximetry in the assessment of limb perfusion. SAMJ 1992;82:486.

464. Mars M, Hadley GP. Failure of pulse oximetry in the assessment of raised limb intracompartmental pressure. Injury 1994;25:379–381.

465. Choe H, Tashiro C, Fukumitsu K, et al. Comparison of recorded values from six pulse oximeters. Crit Care Med 1989;17:678–681.

466. Goldstein S, Owusu, Dean D, et al. Comparison of simultaneous oxygen saturation values using Nellcor N-100 and Marquette Tramscope 12 oximetry. Journal of Clinical Monitoring 1995;11:265.

467. Poets CF, Southall DP. Non-invasive monitoring of oxygenation in infants and children: practical considerations and areas of concern. Pediatrics 1994;93: 737–746.

468. Thilo EH, Andersen D, Wasserstein ML, et al. Saturation by pulse oximetry: Comparison of the results obtained by instruments of different brands. J Pediatr 1993;122:620–626.

469. Shah NK, Trivedi NS, Hyatt J, et al. Response time of different pulse oximeters during resaturation. Anesthesiology 1994;81:A501.

470. Hutton P, Clutton–Brock T. The benefits and pitfalls of pulse oximetry. Br Med J 1993;307:457–458.

471. Davidson JAH, Hosie HE. Limitations of pulse oximetry: respiratory insufficiency—a failure of detection. Br Med J 1993;307:372–373.

472. Videira RLR, Mossqsuera MS, Junqueira PCM, et al. Pulse oximetry versus capnography for diagnosis of fresh gas flow disconnection in spontaneously breathing children. Anesthesiology 1993;79:A1180.

473. McShane AJ, Martin JL. Preoxygenation and pulse oximetry may delay detection of esophageal intubation. J Nat Med Assoc 1987;79:987, 991–992.

474. Schulte GT, Block FE. Can people hear the pitch change on a variable-pitch pulse oximeter? Journal of Clinical Monitoring 1992;8:198–200.

475. Kruger PS, Longden PJ. A study of a hospital staff's knowledge of pulse oximetry. Anaesthesia and Intensive Care 1997;25:38–41.

476. Stoneham MD, Saville GM, Wilson IH. Knowledge about pulse oximetry among medical and nursing staff. Lancet 1994;344:1339–1342.

477. Anonymous. Pulse oximeters. Technology for Anesthesia 1993;14(6):6–7.

478. Brock–Utne JG, Botz G, Jaffe RA. Perioperative corneal abrasions. Anesthesiology 1992;77:221.

479. Ball DR. A pulse oximetry probe hazard. Anesth Analg 1995;80:1251.

480. Metz S. Avoid rubber fingers. Anesth Analg 1996; 82:217.

481. Clark M, Lavies NG. Sensory loss of the distal phalanx caused by pulse oximeter probe. Anaesthesia 1997; 52:508–509.

482. Donahue PJ, Emery S. Digital sensory loss without pulse oximeter malfunction. Anesth Analg 1995;81: 1312.

483. Gates RE, Kinsella SB, Moorthy SS. Sensory loss of the distal phalanx and pulse oximeter probe. Anesth Analg 1995;80:855.

484. Rubin MM, Ford HC, Sadoff RS. Digital injury from a pulse oximeter probe. J Oral Maxillofac Surg 1991; 49:301–302.

485. Berge KH, Lanier WL, Scanlon PD. Ischemic digital skin necrosis. A complication of the reusable Nellcor pulse oximeter probe. Anesth Analg 1988;67: 712–713.

486. Bannister J, Scott DHT. Thermal injury associated with pulse oximetry. Anaesthesia 1988;43:424–425.

487. Chemello PD, Nelson SR, Wolford LM. Finger injury resulting from pulse oximeter probe during orthognathic surgery. Oral Surg Oral Med Oral Pathol 1990;69:161–163.

488. Stogner SW, Owens MW, Bethge BA. Cutaneous necrosis and pulse oximetry. Cutis 1991;48:235–238.

489. Sloan TB. Finger injury by an oxygen saturation monitor probe. Anesthesiology 1988;68:936–938.

490. Polar SM. Cutaneous injuries associated with pulse oximeters. Journal of Clinical Monitoring 1992;8: 185.

491. Alexander R, Levison A. Burns from a pulse oximeter [Letter]. Clin Intens Care 1991;2:188.

492. Miyasaka K, Ohata J. Burn, erosion, and "sun" tan with the use of pulse oximetry in infants. Anesthesiology 1987;67:1008–1009.

493. Poler SM, Walker SS, Kibelbek MJ, et al. Cutaneous injuries associated with pulse oximeters. Journal of Clinical Monitoring 1992;8:185–186.

494. Anonymous. Mismatched pulse oximeter probes. Tech for Anes 1996;16(11):1–2.

495. Sobel DB. Burning of a neonate due to a pulse oximeter: arterial saturation monitoring. Pediatrics 1992;89:489–498.

496. Murphy KG, Secunda JA, Rockoff MA. Severe burns from a pulse oximeter. Anesthesiology 1990;73: 350–352.

497. Pettersen B, Kongsgaard U, Aune H. Skin injury in an infant with pulse oximetry. Br J Anaesth 1992;69: 204–205.

498. Mills GH, Ralph SJ. Burns due to pulse oximetry. Anaesthesia 1992;47:276–277.

499. Murphy KG, Secunda JA, Rockoff MA. Severe burns from a pulse oximeter. Anesthesiology 1990;73: 350–352.

500. Reference deleted.

501. Anonymous. Oximeters, ear. Technology for Anesthesia 1985;6(3):10.

502. Bashein G, Syrovy G. Burns associated with pulse oximetry during magnetic resonance imaging. Anesthesiology 1991;75:382–383.

503. Shellock FG, Slimp GL. Severe burn of the finger caused by using a pulse oximeter during MR imaging. AJR Am J Roentgenol 1989;153:1105.

504. Kanal E, Shellock FG. Burns associated with clinical MR examinations. Radiology 1990;175:585.

505. Faber NE, McNeely J, Rosner D. Skin burn associ-ated with pulse oximetry during perioperative photo-dynamic therapy. Anesthesiology 1996;84:983–985.

506. Pettersen B, Kongsgaard U, Aune H. Skin injury in an infant with pulse oximetry. Br J Anaesth 1992;69:204–205.

507. Ackerman WE, Juneja MM, Baumann RC, et al. The use of a vinyl glove does not affect pulse oximeter monitoring. Anesthesiology 1989;70:558–559.

508. Wakeling HG. Diathermy frequency shock from faulty pulse oximeter probe. Anaesthesia 1995;50:749.

QUESTIONS

1. In which wavelength does reduced hemoglobin absorb more light?
   A. The purple band
   B. The red band
   C. The infrared band
   D. The near infrared band
   E. The blue band

Each question below contains four suggested answers of which one or more is correct. Choose the answer:
A if 1, 2, and 3 are correct
B if 1 and 3 are correct
C if 2 and 4 are correct
D if 4 is correct
E if 1, 2, 3, and 4 are correct

2. In operation of the pulse oximeter,
   1. Component absorption is measured at the site of measurement
   2. Calculation of the oxygen saturation is based on calibration curves determined from healthy volunteers
   3. Different wavelengths of infrared light are used
   4. Light transmitted during systole serves as a reference

3. Fractional oxygen saturation is
   1. The ratio of oxyhemoglobin to all the functional hemoglobins
   2. Close to functional oxygen saturation (SaO_2) in patients with low levels of dyshemoglobins
   3. Determined by in vitro oximetry
   4. The ratio of oxyhemoglobin to the sum of all the hemoglobin present

4. Effects on pulse oximeter readings of a methemoglobin level higher than 1% include
   1. Readings may be falsely low if the saturation is below 85%
   2. At high methemoglobin levels the SpO_2 reading will be 80 to 85%
   3. Readings may be falsely low if the saturation is above 85%
   4. Since methemoglobin has the same absorption coefficient in the red and infrared bands there will be no difference in the pulse oximeter readings

5. Which of the following do not affect pulse oximeter readings?
   1. Hyperbilirubinemia
   2. Hemoglobin S
   3. Hemoglobin F
   4. Severe anemia

6. When using a finger probe
   1. Response time is quicker if the probe is placed on the thumb
   2. Insertion of a radial artery catheter improves pulsation
   3. The probe can be placed sideways to avoid dark fingernail polish
   4. Smaller fingers cause fewer motion artifacts

7. Pulse oximetry can be used to
   1. Detect brachial artery compression during shoulder arthroscopy
   2. Monitor circulation to reimplanted or revascularized digits
   3. Determine the best site for arterial bypass surgery
   4. Evaluate a sympathetic block

8. Factors reported to contribute to higher familure rates with pulse oximetry include
   1. Physical status 3, 4, or 5, young and elderly patients
   2. Orthopedic, vascular, and cardiac surgery
   3. Hypertension
   4. Low hematocrit

9. Measures to improve the peripheral pulsation include
   1. Application of vasodilating cream
   2. Digital nerve blocks
   3. Administration of intraarterial vasodilators
   4. Sympathetic block

ANSWERS

1. B	6. B
2. A	7. E
3. C	8. E
4. A	9. E
5. B	

Neuromuscular Transmission Monitoring

INTRODUCTION

MUSCLE RELAXANTS ARE employed in anesthesia for muscular relaxation and/or abolition of patient movement. Monitoring of the degree of neuromuscular block (NMB) is accomplished by delivering an electrical stimulus near a peripheral motor nerve and evaluating the evoked response of the muscle(s) innervated by that nerve.

ADVANTAGES OF ROUTINE USE OF NEUROMUSCULAR STIMULATORS (1)

Use of neuromuscular (nerve) stimulators allows determination of the state of relaxation on a minute-to-minute basis. Numerous studies have documented enormous variation in patients' responses to muscle relaxants. Disease states and perioperative medications can also modify the responses.

During induction, the stimulator helps to determine the onset time of NMB and can be used to diagnose unusual sensitivity to relaxants. It can be used as a guide to whether the patient is sufficiently relaxed for tracheal intubation to be performed.

During maintenance, the stimulator can be used to titrate the relaxant dosage to the needs of the operative procedure so that both underdosage and overdosage are avoided. Too deep a NMB may result in intraoperative awareness or postoperative respiratory complications and may necessitate artificial support of ventilation in the postoperative period. Underdosage may result in inadequate relaxation or undesirable patient movement. In a study on closed claims against anesthesiologists, eye injuries constituted 3% of claims (2). Patient movement during anesthesia was the mechanism of injury in 30% of those cases. Peripheral nerve stimulators were not used in any of the claims for movement under anesthesia.

At the end of a procedure, use of a stimulator allows determination of whether the block is reversible and adjustment of the dose of reversal agent, if required, to the patient's requirements. It also can be used to assess the adequacy of recovery from NMB. Studies have shown that some patients entering the postanesthesia care unit have an unacceptable level of NMB (3–18). Use of a nerve stimulator may prevent residual NMB, which could lead to life-threatening impairment of ventilation (17, 19).

If a patient is not breathing adequately, use of a stimulator can help to tell whether residual relaxant effect is contributing to the problem.

Routine monitoring of NMB in the intensive care unit has been advocated to avoid overdosage (20–27).

Peripheral nerve stimulators have been used for locating nerves for regional block (28, 29). However, the current needed for stimulation of peripheral nerves is far below that needed for monitoring NMB. Stimulators with controls for both functions are available (30).

An unusual use for a stimulator was therapeutic suppression of a ventricular pacemaker (31).

EQUIPMENT

The equipment used for estimating NMB is inexpensive, easy to use, noninvasive (unless needle electrodes are used), and permits evaluation of the state of relaxation regardless of the patient's level of consciousness or cooperation.

The Stimulator

Several types of stimulators are shown in Figure 21.1. Desirable features include compactness, lightness, and simplicity. A battery-operated stimulator with a means to check the status of the battery is preferred. Mounting brackets for securing the device are desirable.

Current

Current, not voltage, is the determining factor in nerve stimulation. Because skin resistance may change, only stimulators that automatically adjust their output to maintain a constant direct current can ensure unchanging stimulation with changes in skin resistance. The force of muscle contraction is proportional to the number of activated muscle fibers. If a motor nerve is stimulated with sufficient current, all the muscle fibers supplied by that nerve will contract and the maximum force of contraction will be obtained. The current required for this is called the maximal current.

In the clinical setting, stimuli of greater than maximal (supramaximal) intensity are often used to ensure that maximal stimulation is still delivered if skin resistance increases. Supramaximal stimulation can be ensured if the current is 2.75 times that which first produces an identifiable response, with a minimum of 20 mA (32).

A submaximal current may be better in patients recovering from anesthesia because patient discomfort increases with the intensity of the stimulating current (33–37). Also use of a submaximal current may result in more reliable detection of residual NMB using visual or tactile monitoring (38). Stimulators are calibrated in milliamperes (mA) and deliver whatever voltage is required to achieve the set current. Currents suitable for stimulating nerves usually lie between 20 and 60 mA for stick-on skin electrodes and between 5 and 8 mA for needle electrodes (39, 40). It is recommended that stimulators be capable of delivering at least 70 mA and that adult patients be stimulated with at least 20 mA if surface electrodes are used (32, 41).

Display of the current is useful in alerting the

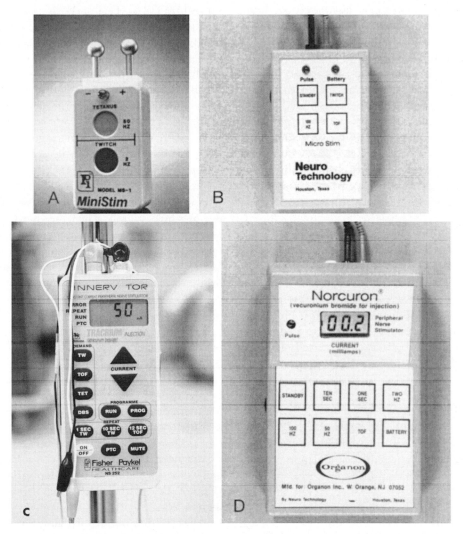

FIGURE 21.1. Neuromuscular stimulators. **A,** This simple device has only two patterns of stimulation: tetanus and single twitch. The delivered current cannot be varied and is not displayed. Note the metal ball electrodes. Reprinted with permission from Professional Instruments, a subsidiary of Life Tech, Inc. **B,** This unit has three modes of stimulation: single stimulus (twitch), tetanus, and train-of-four (TOF). The current is varied using a rheostat at the side, but there is no display of the current being delivered. **C,** This unit has four patterns of stimulation: single twitch (available at 0.1 and 1 Hz), TOF (which can be repeated automatically every 12 seconds), 50-Hz tetanus, and double burst stimulation (DBS). It also is capable of delivering the stimulus pattern for obtaining a post-tetanic count (PPC). The selected current is displayed in the window. Failure to deliver this current will cause a mark to be displayed to the right of the word *error*. Note that the connections for the lead wires are of different colors. **D,** This unit has three modes of stimulation: single stimulus (which can be delivered at 0.1, 1, or 2 Hz), tetanus (which is available at a frequency of 50 to 100 Hz), and TOF. Stimulus current is varied using a rheostat at the side. The delivered current is displayed in a window, to the left of which is an indicator that lights when a stimulus is being delivered. A battery status check button is present.

user to the possibility of a disconnection, lead breakage, weak battery, or poorly conducting electrodes, as the current will then be reduced. Some stimulators have an alarm to warn when the selected current is not delivered.

Although most modern stimulators are claimed by their manufacturers to deliver a constant current, the majority does so only within a certain range of impedances (42, 43). Some deliver a lower current as impedance increases. This could produce less than supramaximal stimulation and a decreased muscular response, leading to overestimation of NMB.

Frequency

The frequency of stimuli is usually expressed in Hertz (Hz), which is 1 cycle/sec; 0.1 Hz is equal to 1 stimulus every 10 seconds; and 10 Hz is 10 stimuli every sec. Commonly used rates of stimulation vary from 0.1 to 100 Hz. Frequent stimulation promotes fatigue and can lead to an increase in local blood flow, which will result in more rapid delivery of relaxant to the stimulated muscle.

Waveform

Ideally, the stimulus waveform should be rectangular (square wave) and monophasic. Biphasic waves may produce repetitive stimulation, which can lead to underestimation of the degree of NMB present (44).

Duration

The duration should be as short, 0.2 milliseconds or less (44). If the duration of the pulse is over 0.5 milliseconds, a second action potential may be triggered (45).

Patterns

Single Twitch

Single-twitch stimuli are usually delivered at a frequency of 0.1 or 1 Hz. Delivery more frequently than every 10 seconds is associated with a progressively diminished response and could result in overestimation of NMB (46). The strength of a (control) response is noted (Fig. 21.2A). The strengths of subsequent twitches are then compared with the control and expressed as a percentage of the control (single-pulse or -twitch depres-

sion, $T_1\%$, $T1\%$, $T_1:T_c$). With both a nondepolarizing and a depolarizing block, there will be progressive depression of the response as the block develops. A decrease in temperature will also cause a reduction in twitch response (47–50).

The single stimulus is useful in establishing a supramaximal stimulus and for identifying when conditions satisfactory for intubation have been achieved. It can be used (in conjunction with a tetanic stimulus) to monitor deep levels of NMB (the *post-tetanic* (twitch) count (PTC), discussed below).

There are several disadvantages associated with use of single stimuli. There needs to be a prerelaxant control twitch. It cannot distinguish between a depolarizing and nondepolarizing block. Most importantly, the presence of full-twitch height does not guarantee that full recovery from NMB has occurred (51).

Train of Four (52)

Train-of-four (TOF, T_4) consists of four single pulses of equal intensity delivered at intervals of 0.5 seconds over a period of 2 seconds (2 Hz) (Fig. 21.2B). TOF should not be repeated more frequently than every 10 to 12 seconds (46). Many modern stimulators do not allow it to be repeated more often. In the control response (before any relaxant has been given) all four responses are the same. The pattern seen with a depolarizing block differs from that of a nondepolarizing block (Fig. 21.2B). With a partial depolarizing block, there is equal depression of height with all four twitches. With a nondepolarizing block, there is progressive depression of height with each twitch (fade). As the block is deepened, the fourth twitch will be eliminated first, then the third, and so on (Fig. 21.3). Thus counting the number of twitches (train-of-four count or TOFC) permits quantitative assessment of a nondepolarizing block (53). With recovery or reversal of a nondepolarizing block, the TOF count increases, then fade decreases. The train-of-four ratio (T_r, T_4 ratio, $T_4:T_1$, TR%, TOF ratio, TOFR) is the ratio of the amplitude of the fourth response to that of the first. It may be expressed as a percentage or a fraction. It provides an estimation of the degree of nondepolarizing NMB. In the absence of nondepolarizing block, the TOFR is approximately 1.0 (100%). The deeper the block, the lower the

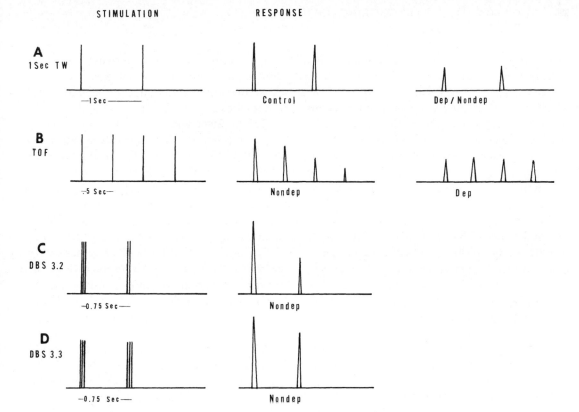

STIMULATION   RESPONSE

A 1 Sec TW

—1 Sec—

Control

Dep/Nondep

B TOF

—.5 Sec—

Nondep

Dep

C DBS 3.2

—0.75 Sec—

Nondep

D DBS 3.3

—0.75 Sec—

Nondep

FIGURE 21.2. Patterns of stimulation and response. **A,** Single stimulus stimulation at 1 Hz (1 stimulus/sec). The height of the control twitches is noted. With either a depolarizing or a nondepolarizing block, twitch height is decreased. **B,** Train-of-four (TOF) stimulation. Four successive single stimuli are delivered with 0.5-second intervals. With a nondepolarizing block, there will be progressive depression of the response with each stimulus (fade). With a depolarizing block, the responses will be depressed equally. **C** and **D,** Double-burst stimulation. Three stimuli are delivered at 50 Hz, followed 0.75 seconds later by two or three similar stimuli. There will be depression of the response to the second burst with a nondepolarizing block. Note the increased height of the response to the first burst compared with that seen with TOF stimulation.

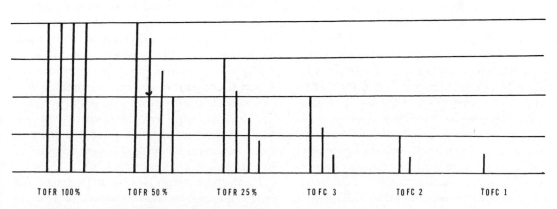

TOFR 100%   TOFR 50%   TOFR 25%   TOFC 3   TOFC 2   TOFC 1

FIGURE 21.3. Onset and progressive deepening of nondepolarizing block using train-of-four stimulation. When there is no neuromuscular block (NMB) present, all four responses are equal. With onset of the block, there is progressive depression of twitch height with each twitch (fade). As the block progresses, the last twitch is lost and the train-of-four count is less than four.

TOFR (Fig. 21.3). Because TOFR requires that four twitches be present, it cannot be used to monitor deep NMB. Accurate assessment of the TOFR may not require a supramaximal stimulus (6, 33). Testing at 10 mA above the lowest current at which four responses can be elicited may provide values that are consistent with those of supramaximal testing (54). Cooling of the monitoring site should be avoided since this will result in changes in TOF (50).

TOF has several advantages. It is a more sensitive indicator of residual NMB than the single twitch (55). Establishment of a control is not necessary. It can distinguish between a depolarizing and a nondepolarizing block and has proved of value in detecting and following the development of a phase II block following succinylcholine administration.

The main disadvantage of TOF is that it is not possible to detect fade reliably using visual or tactile methods (56–62).

Double-Burst Stimulation (DBS)

Double-burst stimulation (mini-tetanus) consists of two short trains of 50-Hz tetanic stimuli separated by 750 milliseconds. Although different combinations of stimuli have been used, the two most common are $DBS_{3,3}$ and $DBS_{3,2}$. $DBS_{3,3}$ consists of a burst of three 0.2-milliseconds impulses at 50 Hz, followed 750 milliseconds later by an identical burst (Fig. 21.2C). $DBS_{3,2}$ is a burst of three impulses followed by two such impulses 750 milliseconds later (Fig. 21.2D). $DBS_{3,3}$ and TOF maintain a close relationship over a wide range of NMB. Changes in $DBS_{3,2}$ correlate with, but are not identical to, changes in TOF (63).

The primary use of DBS has been to detect residual NMB. Numerous studies show that fade is more readily detected with DBS than TOF using visual or tactile monitoring (38, 56–67). It also has been used for intraoperative assessment of NMB (68). Another potential use of DBS is during assessment of deep block, since the first twitch in double burst can be detected at slightly deeper levels of block than the first twitch in TOF (69).

DBS causes more discomfort than TOF stimulation, but less than tetanic stimulation (34). It should not be repeated at intervals of less than 12 seconds (58).

Caution should be used in switching between double-burst and TOF stimulation (70). Up to 92 seconds may be required for stabilization of the responses.

Tetanic Stimulation

Tetanus is a rapidly repeated (e.g., 50, 100 or even 200 Hz) single stimulus. In the absence of NMB, this causes sustained contraction of the stimulated muscles. With a depolarizing block, the response will be depressed in amplitude but sustained. With a nondepolarizing block, the response is depressed in amplitude and the contraction is not sustained (fade or decrement). With profound NMB there is no response. Fade after tetanic stimulation is a more sensitive index of NMB than single twitch, but not sufficiently sensitive to be used for assessing the adequacy of recovery (71).

The most commonly used frequency is 50 Hz, because it stresses the neuromuscular junction to the same extent as a maximal voluntary effort. At lower frequencies, fade may not be seen when significant nondepolarizing block is present. As the frequency increases, the block appears to be more pronounced. This can lead to overestimation of the NMB present (72, 73). It may be better to use 100 Hz than 50 Hz when assessing residual NMB (74).

The duration of the tetanic stimulus is important, because it affects fade. A duration of 5 seconds is standard. With a nondepolarizing block, fade is seen after only 1 or 2 seconds. Tetanic stimulation should not be repeated more often than every 2 minutes (75). Some newer stimulators limit how frequently it can be used. Post-tetanic facilitation (potentiation, PTF or PTP) refers to a temporary increase in response to stimulation following a tetanic stimulus. It is seen with a nondepolarizing, but not a depolarizing, block and is greater with deeper NMB (76, 77). It is maximal in about 3 seconds and lasts up to 2 minutes following a tetanic stimulus of 50 Hz applied for 5 seconds (76).

In situations where NMB is so profound that there is no response to single twitch or TOF, it may be possible to estimate NMB by using the PTC (78). This is performed by administering a tetanic stimulus of 50 Hz for 5 seconds. After a

3-seconds pause, single-twitch stimuli are applied at 1 Hz and the number of (post-tetanic) responses counted. The number of twitches elicited increases as the depth of NMB decreases. The time to appearance of the first twitch in a pre-tetanic TOF is inversely related to the number of post-tetanic twitches present (78–82). The actual time varies among the different relaxants, being longer with longer-acting drugs. Even deeper block can be monitored by counting the number of responses following 100-Hz tetanus (83).

A significant disadvantage of tetanic stimulation is that it is very painful. Therefore, it should be avoided in the conscious patient.

Electrodes

Stimulation is achieved by placing two electrodes along a nerve and passing a current through them. Stimulation can be carried out either transcutaneously using surface electrodes or percutaneously with needle electrodes.

Types
Surface

Surface (gel, patch, pad) electrodes have adhesive surrounding a gelled foam pad in contact with a metal disc with a knob for attachment to the electrical lead. They are readily available, easily applied, disposable, self-adhering, and comfortable. The electrode-skin resistance decreases with a large conducting area, as do skin burns and pain. However, a large conducting area may make it difficult to obtain supramaximal stimulation and may cause stimulation of multiple nerves, so it may be better to use pediatric electrodes (84).

Electrodes specially designed for peripheral nerve stimulation are available. These have a different thickness than electrocardiographic (ECG) electrodes and chemical buffers to maintain skin surface pH. They are available in a dual-element configuration.

Metal

Some stimulators are supplied with two metal balls or plates spaced about 1 inch apart, which attach directly to the stimulator (Fig. 21.1*A*) These are convenient to use, but they may not make good contact. Burns have been reported with their use (85).

Needle Electrodes

In most cases, surface electrodes produce satisfactory stimulation. Needle electrodes may be useful when supramaximal stimulation cannot be achieved using surface electrodes. This usually occurs when the skin is thickened, cold, or edematous and in obese, hypothyroid, or renal-failure patients (86, 87). Additional complications (broken needles, infection, burns, and nerve damage) are associated with their use. Needle electrodes carry a greater risk of direct muscle stimulation than surface electrodes (88).

Polarity (89, 90)

Stimulators produce a direct current by using one negative and one positive electrode. Maximal effect is achieved when the negative electrode is placed close to the nerve being stimulated (39, 89). The positive electrode should be placed at a site where it would not induce depolarization of another nerve or direct muscle stimulation (41). The polarity of the outlet sockets should be indicated on the stimulator. If the polarity is unknown, the connections can be reversed to determine which arrangement evokes the greater response.

METHODS OF EVALUATING EVOKED RESPONSES
Visual

For visual assessment, the observer should be at an angle of 90° to the motion (91). Visual assessment can be used to count the number of responses present with a train-of-four stimulus, to determine the PTC, or to detect the presence of fade with TOF or DBS or PTF with tetanic stimulation. However, studies have shown that it is difficult to determine accurately the TOFR or to compare a single-twitch height with its control visually (56, 61). Visual recognition of fade with TOF stimulation may be more accurate with submaximal currents (56, 92).

Tactile (93)

Tactile monitoring is accomplished by placing the evaluator's fingertips lightly over the muscle to be stimulated so that there is a slight preload

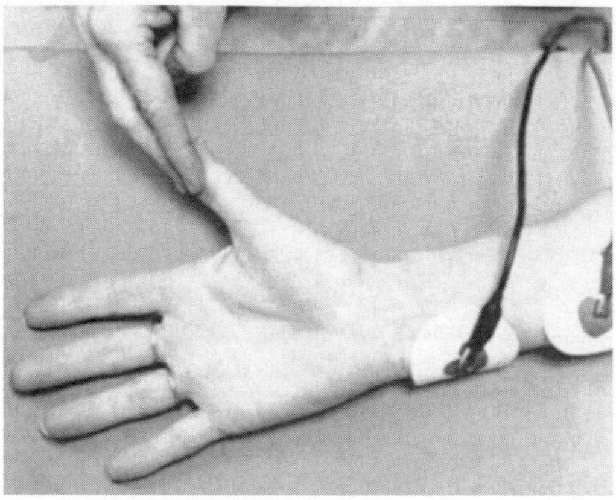

FIGURE 21.4. For tactile evaluation of thumb adduction, the hand is supine and a slight preload is applied.

and feeling the strength of contraction (Fig. 21.4). It is more sensitive than visual monitoring for assessing NMB using TOF (60). It can be used to evaluate the presence or absence of responses and/or fade with TOF, DBS, and tetanic stimulation. The PTC can be determined (94). If there is a response to all four stimuli with TOF stimulation, the T_4 ratio can be estimated. However, it is difficult for even trained observers to detect fade unless the TOF ratio is below 40% (56–61, 92). Determination of single-twitch depression also is not accurate using tactile monitoring. Using the index finger rather than the thumb will result in better detection of fade using tactile means (95).

Mechanomyogram (MMG)

The MMG uses a force-displacement transducer, such as a strain gauge, attached to a finger or other part of the body that will move when stimulated to quantitate the response to nerve stimulation. The transducer converts the contractile force into an electrical signal, which is amplified and displayed on a monitor screen or recorded on a chart. Single-twitch height, response to tetanic stimulation, and the T4 ratio can be accurately measured using a MMG. Use of the MMG entails a number of difficulties. The devices are cumbersome and difficult to set up for stable and accurate measurements. Proper transducer orien-

tation, isometric conditions and application of a constant preload are required (96).

Accelerography (ACG) (9, 97)

With ACG a thin piezoelectric transducer or a small aluminum rod with electrodes on both sides is fixed to the moving part (Fig. 21.5). When the part moves, an electrical signal proportional to the acceleration of the moving part is produced. This method requires less fixation than the MMG and does not require that a preload be applied. It can be used to assess MMB at the hand with the patient's arm tucked at the side.

Most studies show a fairly close relationship between TOF ratios measured by ACG and the MMG (9, 54, 97–107) or electromyography (EMG) (101, 108).

Electromyography (109–112)

When a motor nerve is stimulated, a biphasic action potential is generated in each of the muscle cells it supplies, unless some degree of NMB exists. The sum of a number of these action potentials can be sensed using electrodes placed over the muscle being stimulated. Two stimulating electrodes are placed over the nerve to be stimulated. Three electrodes, two receiving (sensing, recording) and one grounding, are used for recording. The best signal is usually obtained by placing the active receiving electrode over the belly of the muscle with the indifferent (reference) electrode over the tendon insertion site. The ground electrode, whose function is to decrease stimulation artifacts, is placed between the stimulating and recording electrodes. Best results will be seen when the electrodes have been in contact with the skin for at least 15 minutes before calibration (cure time). Movement artifact can be minimized by fixation or applying a constant pretension to the muscle being recorded (110, 113).

The evoked EMG signal is filtered, rectified, amplified, and then displayed and/or recorded at a much slower speed. Measurements may be made of peak amplitude of the major deflection from the isoelectric line, the sum of the amplitudes of

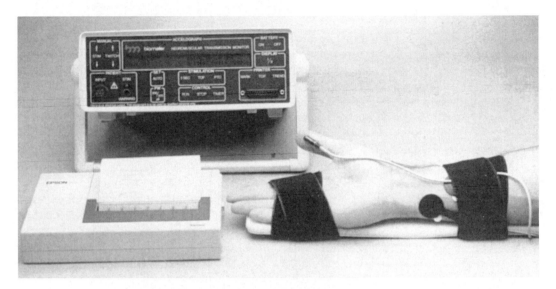

FIGURE 21.5.   Accelerography (ACG). The piezoelectric wafer is attached to the moving part, in this case the thumb. When the thumb moves, an electrical signal proportional to the acceleration is produced. The monitor allows determination of single twitch depression, train-of-four count or ratio and/or the post-tetanic count (PTC). Responses can be displayed using the printer. (Reprinted with permission from Biometer International A/S.)

the major positive and negative deflections, or the area under the curve (114). Changes in latency, duration of the action potential, and the power density spectrum have also been studied (115, 116).

EMG machines (Fig. 21.6) automatically determine the supramaximal stimulus, establish a control response, stimulate at a preselected interval, measure the response, and compare it to the control. Available features include an alarm to warn when the single pulse response exceeds a chosen value and a printer to provide a permanent record. Most have alarms to warn of errors in functioning, loose connections, increased skin resistance, absence of supramaximal stimulation, etc. Most show the EMG waveform and automatically adjust the gain so that it occupies the full scale.

With a nondepolarizing NMB, the amplitude of the action potential is decreased and there is fade with TOF. Frequently, the amplitude does not return to 100% of control with recovery, although TOFR will equal approximately 100%. Different hand positions may affect the results (117, 118). A number of studies comparing

EMG and MMG have been published (101, 119–139). With a nondepolarizing block, a correlation is usually seen, although the two techniques do not give identical information. With a depolarizing block, the relationship is more complex and studies show contradictory results (122, 125, 131, 133, 134). The EMG TOFR may be less affected by changes in temperature than the MMG (138).

EMG has several advantages over mechanical monitoring. Less immobilization is required. It does not require bulky apparatus near the muscle being monitored. The electrodes can be applied before the patient enters the operating room. It can be measured from muscles that are not accessible for mechanical recording to anesthesia personnel. It can be used to monitor intense NMB when the response to TOF is below the threshold of detection (140).

There are disadvantages to the EMG. It is sensitive to electrical interference. The response may vary according to the muscle used (125). The equipment takes some time and effort to set up. Skin preparation and placement of the electrodes must be done especially carefully.

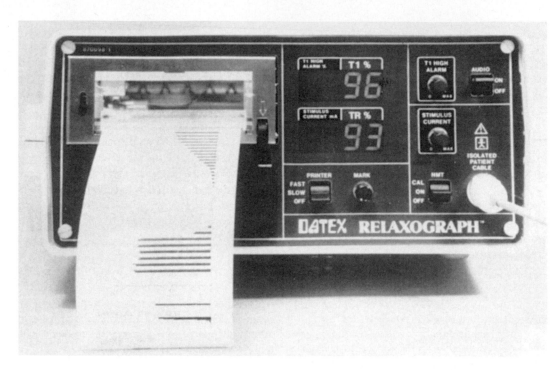

FIGURE 21.6. Electromyographic (EMG) monitor. The T_1%, train-of-four (TOF) ratio, and TOF count can be measured and are displayed in the boxes to the right of the printer. Responses can be recorded using the printer. A T_1% high alarm is present. TOF stimulation is performed automatically every 20 seconds. (Reprinted with permission from Datex Medical Instrumentation, Inc.)

Piezoelectric Film (103)

This method uses a disposable piezoelectric film (Fig. 21.7). This is placed so that it spans a movable joint (141). Muscle movement from evoked stimulation bends the film and generates a voltage which is proportional to the amount of bending. It has been used on the thumb, fifth digit, and the great toe (141–142). It can be used with patients' hands tucked at their sides (143).

This method is not as accurate as mechanomyography or EMG but may predict recovery of the TOFR better than visual or tactile evaluation (103, 144).

CHOICE OF MONITORING SITE (145)

The site of stimulation should be away from the surgical field. If visual or tactile monitoring is to be used, the location must be accessible to the anesthesia provider. If a muscle in an arm or leg is used, the blood pressure should be measured on a different extremity. If the patient has an upper-motor-neuron lesion, a nerve in an affected (paretic) extremity should not be used as it may falsely show resistance to nondepolarizing drugs (146, 147).

Ulnar Nerve

The ulnar nerve is most commonly used because of its accessibility during most surgical procedures and because of the anatomy of the muscles involved. The adductor pollicis (thumb) muscle is most commonly monitored. Because this muscle is on the side of the arm opposite to the site of stimulation, there is little direct muscle stimulation, which could lead to underestimation of the NMB. However, one study has shown that residual NMB may be easier to detect using the index finger (95). For EMG monitoring, use of the first dorsal interosseous or abductor digiti quinti muscle may be preferable (148).

The nerve can be stimulated at the wrist or

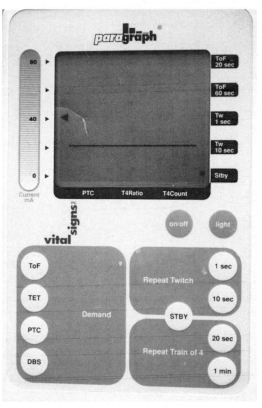

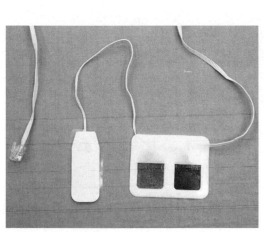

FIGURE 21.7. **A,** Piezoelectric film. This is placed so that it spans a movable joint. Muscle movement causes the film to bend, generating a signal. **B,** The unit itself has a scale at left to indicate the current delivered. Twitch amplitudes are shown on the screen.

elbow (Fig. 21.8 and 21.9). Responses are greater when the negative electrode is distal (37). Stimulation at the wrist will produce thumb adduction and flexion of the fingers. Stimulation at the elbow produces hand adduction as well. For tactile assessment, the thumb should be held in abduction and the observer's fingertips should be placed over the distal phalanx in the direction of movement (41) (Fig. 21.4). If a MMG or EMG is used for measuring the response, the stimulating electrodes should be placed at the wrist to limit motion of the hand. Placing the electrodes at the elbow may be preferable in children to avoid direct muscle stimulation artifact.

At the wrist, the two electrodes are usually placed along the medial aspect of the distal forearm, approximately 2 cm proximal to the junction of the hand and wrist (Fig. 21.8A). There the

ulnar nerve is superficial. Alternately, the positive electrode may be placed on the dorsal side of the wrist (Fig. 21.9). At the elbow, the electrodes should be placed over the sulcus of the medial epicondyle of the humerus (see Fig. 21.8B). Caution must be exercised to ensure that the electrodes do not cause ulnar nerve compression as this can cause a palsy (149).

When EMG monitoring is used, the recording electrodes can be placed over the abductor digiti quinti (hypothenar), the adductor pollicis brevis (thenar), or the first dorsal interosseous muscle. The electrical resistance of the palm skin may vary because of the production of sweat and may be increased in manual workers (150). The dorsum of the hand is less affected than the palm in both respects, so that use of the dorsal interosseous muscle may be preferred (151).

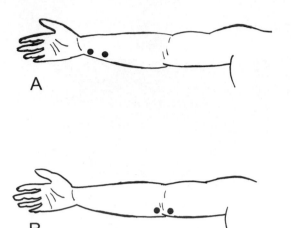

A

B

FIGURE 21.8. Placement of electrodes for ulnar nerve stimulation. **A,** The electrodes are placed along the ulnar aspect of the distal forearm. **B,** The electrodes are placed over the sulcus of the medial epicondyle of the humerus.

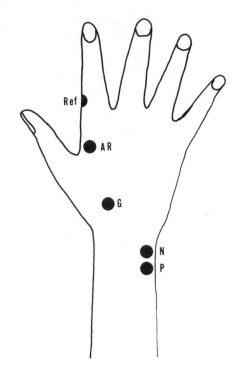

FIGURE 21.10. Sites for electrodes for electromyographic (EMG) monitoring with ulnar nerve stimulation and recording from the dorsal interosseous muscle. The active receiving electrode is placed in the web between the index finger and the thumb and the reference electrode, at the base of the second finger. *Ref,* reference electrode; *AR,* active receiving electrode; *G,* grounding electrode; *N,* negative-stimulating electrode; *P,* positive-stimulating electrode.

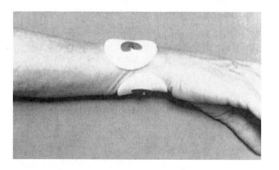

FIGURE 21.9. Alternate placement of electrodes for ulnar nerve stimulation. The negative electrode is placed along the ulnar aspect of the ventral side of the wrist. The positive electrode is placed on the dorsal side.

To record the reaction of the dorsal interosseous muscle, the active receiving electrode is placed in the web between the index finger and the thumb, and the other electrode at the base of the second finger (Fig. 21.10). Surface electrodes are simple to fix here, easy to maintain in position, and seldom disturbed by hand movements (151).

For the hypothenar EMG, both electrodes are placed on the palmar side over the hypothenar eminence or the active electrode is placed on the hypothenar eminence and the other below the

second line on the ring finger or at the base of the dorsum of the fifth finger (Fig. 21.11) (152). If the thenar muscle's EMG is recorded, electrodes are placed on the thenar eminence and the proximal phalanx of the middle or index finger (153) or the lateral side of the base of the thumb's (Fig. 21.12). Abduction of the thumb with a constant pretension will bring the muscles closer to the skin and minimize movement (39, 113).

Median Nerve (90)

The median nerve is larger than the ulnar, but less superficial. It can be stimulated at the wrist, by placing the electrodes medial to where the electrodes would be placed for ulnar nerve stimulation or at the elbow adjacent to the brachial artery.

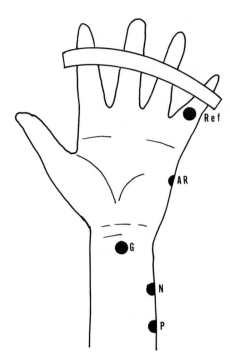

FIGURE 21.11. Placement of electrodes for electromyographic (EMG) monitoring from the hypothenar eminence. The active electrode is placed over the hypothenar eminence. The reference electrode may be placed more distally on the hypothenar eminence, below the second line on the ring finger or at the base of the fifth finger as shown. *Ref,* reference electrode; *AR,* active receiving electrode; *G,* grounding electrode; *N,* negative-stimulating electrode; *P,* positive-stimulating electrode.

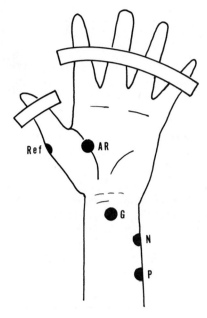

FIGURE 21.12. Placement of electrodes for monitoring the electromyographic (EMG) from the thenar eminence. The active receiving electrode is placed over the thenar eminence. The reference electrode may be placed as shown here or at the proximal phalanx of the middle or index finger. *Ref,* reference electrode; *AR,* active receiving electrode; *G,* grounding electrode; *N,* negative-stimulating electrode; *P,* positive-stimulating electrode.

This results in thumb adduction. The EMG signal can be monitored from the thenar muscles.

Posterior Tibial Nerve (154–156)

To stimulate the posterior tibial nerve, electrodes are placed behind the medial malleolus of the tibia and anterior to the Achilles tendon (Fig. 21.13). Stimulation causes plantar flexion of the foot and big toe. If EMG monitoring is used, the receiving electrodes are placed on the flexor hallucis brevis on the plantar surface of the foot or on the intermetatarsal muscles with the reference electrode on the big toe (Fig. 21.14). ACG can be used at this site (157, 158).

This site offers many advantages. It is especially useful in children, when it is difficult to find room

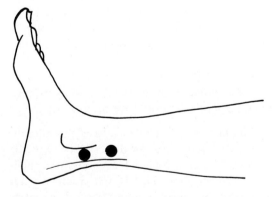

FIGURE 21.13. Placement of electrodes for stimulating the posterior tibial nerve. The negative electrode is placed behind the medial malleolus, anterior to the Achilles tendon. The positive electrode is placed just proximal to the negative electrode. Stimulation causes plantar flexion of the great toe.

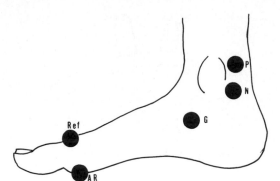

FIGURE **21.14.** Electromyographic (EMG) monitoring using the posterior tibial nerve. The active receiving electrode is placed over the flexor hallucis brevis and the reference electrode, on the big toe. *Ref,* reference electrode; *AR,* active receiving electrode; *G,* grounding electrode; *N,* negative-stimulating electrode; *P,* positive-stimulating electrode.

on the arm because of other monitors or invasive lines, and when the hand is inaccessible or for other reasons (amputation, burns, or infection) cannot be used. However, patients with peripheral vascular disease, metabolic neuropathies, or foot deformities may have reduced or absent evoked responses (159).

Peroneal Nerve

To stimulate the peroneal (lateral popliteal) nerve, electrodes are placed on the lateral aspect of the knee (Fig. 21.15). It may be necessary to try different positions to achieve the best response (160). Stimulation causes dorsiflexion of the foot.

Facial Nerve

For stimulation of the facial nerve, three configurations of electrodes have been used.

1. The negative electrode is placed just anterior to the inferior part of the ear lobe, and the other electrode is placed just posterior or inferior to the lobe (Fig. 21.16). Stimulation at this site will make it more likely that muscle contractions are the result of stimulation of the nerve rather than direct muscle stimulation.
2. The negative electrode is placed just anterior to the earlobe, and the positive electrode is placed over the lateral margin of the contralat-

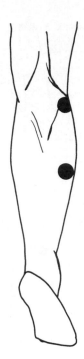

FIGURE **21.15.** Electrode placement for stimulating the peroneal (lateral popliteal) nerve. The electrodes are placed lateral to the neck of the fibula. Stimulation causes dorsiflexion of the foot.

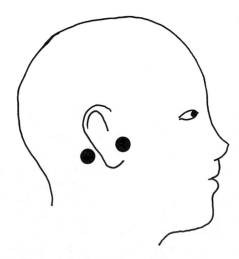

FIGURE **21.16.** Electrode placement for stimulating the facial nerve. The negative electrode is placed anterior to the earlobe. The positive electrode is placed posterior or inferior to the earlobe.

eral eyebrow (161). This results in direct muscle stimulation on the contralateral side and nerve stimulation on the ipsilateral side.

3. One electrode is placed lateral to and below the lateral canthus of the eye, and the other electrode is placed anterior to the earlobe (162, 163) or 2 cm lateral to and above the lateral canthus (164). This placement may result in direct muscle stimulation.

The orbicularis oculi and orbicularis oris muscles are observed. EMG monitoring is difficult to use with the facial nerve but ACG can be used (165, 166).

The facial nerve may be useful for monitoring NMB when the arms and legs are not accessible. However, the facial muscles, like the diaphragm, are relatively resistant to NMB drugs (162, 163, 165, 167). Therefore, managing NMB by stimulation of the facial nerve will result in relaxation greater than that from stimulating a limb nerve if equivalent responses are used. Great caution should be used when using facial nerve stimulation to assess recovery from NMB. The responses may show complete recovery while significant NMB is still present (162, 168–170).

Stimulating the facial nerve is useful in detecting the onset of relaxation in the muscles of the jaw, larynx, and diaphragm.

Mandibular Nerve (171)

The mandibular nerve, a branch of the trigeminal, supplies the masseter muscle. It can be stimulated by placing the negative electrode anterior and inferior to the zygomatic arch and by placing the positive electrode on the forehead. Stimulation causes closure of the jaw. The onset of NMB in this muscle is faster than in hand muscles (171–173). In adults, this muscle is more sensitive to both depolarizing and nondepolarizing drugs than the muscles of the hand (172, 174). In children, the sensitivity may be equal (173).

Spinal Accessory Nerve (175)

The spinal accessory nerve can be stimulated by placing the electrodes over the depression between the ramus of the mandible and the mastoid process/sternocleidomastoid muscle. Stimulation causes stimulation of the sternomastoid and trape-

zius muscles. This can cause movement of the shoulder and thorax and be transmitted to the abdomen (176).

USE
Before Induction

Prior to induction of anesthesia, the stimulator unit should be connected to electrodes positioned over the nerve selected. If EMG monitoring is to be used, the receiving electrodes should be placed at least 15 minutes before induction.

Electrode sites should be dry and free of excessive hair or scar tissue or other types of lesions. Proper preparation of the skin will decrease resistance. It should be thoroughly cleansed using a solvent such as alcohol, then dried and rubbed briskly with a dry gauze pad until a slight redness is visible (177).

The electrodes should be checked to verify that the gel is moist. It is important to avoid spreading of the gel or overlap of adhesive while placing the electrodes on the skin. A gel bridge between the electrodes can short circuit them and lead to poor stimulation (39). After the lead is attached to the electrode, a piece of tape should be placed over the leads to prevent movement. It is good practice to create a loop to prevent displacement (Fig. 21.17).

Induction

After induction and before administering any muscle relaxants, the stimulator should be turned on, and the clinician should feel or observe the response, as a final check on the functional integrity of the system. The stimulator should be adjusted to provide supramaximal stimulation by applying single-twitch stimuli at 0.1 Hz, and the output of the stimulator increased until the response shows no increase with an increase in current, then increased 10 to 20%. Applying stimulation more frequently will make it appear as if the time of onset of NMB were shorter (178–180). The same result will occur with use of train-of-four stimulation.

If maximal stimulation is not achieved with a current of 50 to 70 mA, the electrodes should be checked for proper placement, polarity, and drying. The wire connections should be checked.

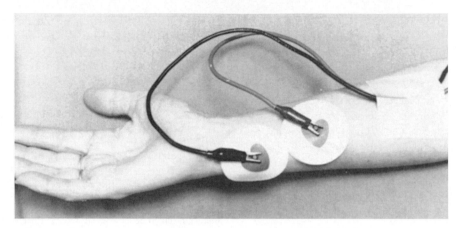

FIGURE 21.17. Electrodes in place. Creating loops and securing the wires with tape will decrease the likelihood that the wires will be pulled off the electrodes.

If maximal stimulation still cannot be achieved, needle electrodes should be used.

Special needle electrodes for nerve stimulators are available commercially, but ordinary injection needles can be used. They should be short and thin. The needles should be placed subcutaneously. Inserting them deeper may produce direct muscle excitation and/or cause damage to the nerve. The angle of insertion should be parallel to the nerve. There should be a few centimeters between the needles. They should be held in place with tape as movement of the tips may influence monitoring. The lead should be attached to the shaft of the needle unless the needle has a metal hub.

Correct EMG electrode placement should be verified by observing the quality of the evoked waveform, which should approximate a sine wave. The gain control should be adjusted so that the waveform occupies the full scale (181).

Intubation

The onset of NMB will be faster in centrally located muscles such as the diaphragm, facial, laryngeal, and jaw muscles than in peripheral muscles such as the adductor pollicis (171, 172, 182–185) The diaphragm, orbicular oculi, and most laryngeal muscles are more resistant to nondepolarizing relaxants than peripheral muscles (186, 187). The diaphragm is resistant to succinylcholine though the laryngeal muscles are quite sensitive to it. The masseter muscle is relatively sensitive to both nondepolarizing and depolarizing relaxants (174, 188).

Monitoring the response of the facial muscles will reflect the time of onset and the level of NMB at the airway musculature more closely than monitoring of peripheral muscles, which will underestimate the rate of onset of NMB in the airway musculature and may overestimate the degree of block (99, 162, 163, 165, 183, 189–196).

If the facial nerve cannot be used, a peripheral nerve will suffice in most cases. In the majority of patients, disappearance of an adductor pollicis response provides good to excellent intubating conditions. If the electromyographic responses are being monitored, monitoring at the hypothenar eminence may be preferable (151).

Whatever nerve is used, it is recommended that single twitch at 0.1 Hz be used and that the clinician wait until a response is barely perceptible before attempting laryngoscopy and intubation. Rapid stimulation may accelerate the onset of block at the stimulated site (197, 198). It should be kept in mind that the response to intubation is a function of both neuromuscular block and the level of anesthesia. It is possible to intubate a patient with less-than-complete paralysis if a sufficient depth of anesthesia is present.

The response to stimulation will usually disappear for a variable period of time, then appear and increase progressively to full recovery. Additional relaxants should not be given until there is evidence of some recovery to make sure the patient does not have an abnormal response. However, it is not necessary to wait for complete recovery.

Electroconvulsive Therapy

A common error in the practice of electroconvulsive therapy is premature delivery of the electrical stimulus (199). It is recommended that a single stimulus be applied at 1 Hz to the posterior tibial nerve (200). When there is complete abolition of response, the stimulus for the electroconvulsive therapy should be applied.

Maintenance

During a surgical procedure the aim is usually to produce the optimal paralysis compatible with quick recovery. The degree of NMB required depends on many factors, including the type of surgery, the anesthetic technique, and the depth of anesthesia. It is important to prevent cooling of the monitoring site to avoid impairment of nerve conduction or increased skin resistance, which may result in overestimation of the degree of NMB (201, 202).

It is important to correlate the reaction to nerve stimulation with the clinical condition of the patient, as there may be a discrepancy between the degree of relaxation of the monitored muscles and that of the muscles at the site of surgery. If the surgeon believes that relaxation is inadequate, the anesthesia provider should confirm that the depth of anesthesia is sufficient as the degree of NMB block necessary to produce adequate muscle relaxation is affected by the depth of anesthesia (203). It should also be confirmed that the stimulator is working properly. If it does not display the delivered current, electrodes may be placed on the user's arm and a low current used to confirm proper functioning.

TOF is commonly regarded as the most useful pattern for monitoring NMB during maintenance. Use of supramaximal currents is traditional. Use of submaximal current has been suggested but this is controversial (37, 38, 204–208). The goal for most cases in which abdominal muscle relaxation is required should be to maintain at least one response to TOF stimulation in a peripheral nerve (209, 210). If no response is present,

further administration of relaxants is not indicated. If two responses are present, abdominal relaxation should be adequate, using balanced anesthesia (211). Presence of three twitches is usually associated with adequate relaxation if a volatile agent is used. Deeper levels of NMB may be required for upper abdominal or chest surgery or if diaphragmatic paralysis is needed. If the facial muscles are used, at least one twitch should be added to the above recommendations.

Muscle relaxants are sometimes administered in cases such as eye surgery or laser surgery of the vocal cords to guarantee that movement does not occur. To ensure total diaphragmatic paralysis, the NMB should be so intense that there is no response to post-tetanic stimulation (i.e., the post-tetanic count is zero) (212). One approach is to give a bolus of a short-acting muscle relaxant when the post-tetanic count is one (213). Alternatively the twitch response at a resistant muscle such as the orbicularis oculi may be monitored and a dose of relaxant given as soon as there is any response. The type of anesthesia may influence the likelihood of reflex movement even with a PTC of zero (214).

Recovery and Reversal (215)

When relaxation is no longer required, administration of neuromuscular blocking drugs should be discontinued. As recovery progresses, the responses to TOF will progressively appear, then fade will disappear. The ease of reversal of a nondepolarizing block is inversely related to the degree of block at the time of reversal. Adequate reversal may not be possible if there is only one or no response to TOF stimulation.

Recovery of neuromuscular function is governed by the sensitivity of the muscle and rate of disappearance of the drug from the plasma. The diaphragm, laryngeal muscles and orbicularis oculi recover first, followed by more sensitive muscles, such as the masseter and muscles of the hand or foot (184, 185). It is best to use a peripheral muscle to monitor recovery, because its complete recovery would indicate that residual weakness of the muscles contributing to airway patency or respiration is unlikely (170, 174, 183, 216–218). The probability of detecting fade using the index finger is greater than if the thumb or great toe is used (95, 219). The facial muscles should not be used to determine the adequacy of recovery, as their resistance to NMB may cause overestimation of the degree of recovery.

A considerable body of evidence exists to show that a TOFR of 70% or greater in a limb muscle on MMG is associated with adequate mechanical respiratory response at rest (55, 220–224). A normal response to hypoxemia, protection from aspiration and absence of heaviness of the eyelids, diplopia, difficulty in swallowing or patient anxiety may require a higher TOFR (225–229).

Detection of residual blockade can be reliably accomplished using acceleromyography (108). If EMG monitoring is being used, residual anesthetic effects usually prevent the return of T_1% to preanesthetic reference levels (230). However, the TOFR should exceed 90% (126).

If visual and/or tactile monitoring is being used, residual NMB cannot be reliably detected using TOF (38, 60, 61, 108). Double-burst stimulation is more reliable and should be used if available (38, 56, 57, 65). Both may be more reliable at detecting fade at lower currents (38). If all four responses to TOF or both responses to DBS appear equal, a 50-Hz tetanic stimulus followed by TOF may be applied (93). A sustained response and absence of PTF provide additional indications of the absence of significant residual NMB. However it must be emphasized visual or tactile evaluation of responses is often inadequate to reliably exclude significant residual NMB (230).

Irrespective of the method used to assess the adequacy of recovery from NMB, the clinician should use clinical criteria to ascertain whether the return of muscle strength is adequate (231). The criteria used depend on whether the patient can respond to commands. Clinical criteria in an awake patient include the ability to (*a*) open the eyes for 5 seconds and not experience diplopia (*b*) sustain protrusion of the tongue, (*c*) sustain head lift for at least 5 seconds, (*d*) sustain hand grip, (*e*) sustain leg lifting in children and (*f*) cough effectively. Clinical criteria in an asleep patient include an adequate tidal volume and an inspiratory force of at least 25 cm H_2O negative pressure.

Postoperative Period

Even if a nerve stimulator has not been used during an operation, it can be of diagnostic value postoperatively. If the patient is not fully anesthetized, it is preferable to use less than supramaximal stimulation (33, 54, 232). This decreases the discomfort associated with stimulation and may improve the accuracy of visual assessment (56). Fade with TOFR or DBS and/or fade or PTF with tetanic stimulation suggests residual paralysis.

HAZARDS
Burns

Burns have been reported using a stimulator with metal ball electrodes, tetanic stimulation, and the stimulator set to deliver maximal stimulation (85, 233). With surface electrodes, erythema at the site may be seen (177, 234). Electrodes should not overlap, as gel could diffuse between them and this could result in burns. A high current in association with needle electrodes may result in burns. If the stimulator is electrically grounded while the indifferent electrode of the electrosurgery unit has a defective ground wire, the electrode of the nerve stimulator can become the ground and a burn can result (91).

Paresthesias

The pressure of an electrode on a nerve can result in a palsy (149). Thumb paresthesias were reported in nine patients whose muscular function was monitored using a MMG (235).

Complications Associated with Needle Electrodes

When needle electrodes are used, possible complications include infection, bleeding, pain, and damage to the nerve or other tissues.

Pain

Patient discomfort will be reduced by using lower currents and avoiding tetanic or double-burst stimulation when the patient is awake (34, 37).

Electrical Interference

Use of a nerve stimulator may cause changes in the ECG tracing that appear similar to non-captured pacing spikes (236) or suppression of an implanted pacemaker (31, 237).

Incorrect Information

With some stimulators when the batteries are low, only three pulses are generated during train-of-four stimulation (238). This could lead to incorrect interpretation of the degree of NMB.

REFERENCES

1. Viby-Mogensen J. Monitoring of neuromuscular blockade: technology and clinical methods in muscle relaxants. Agoston S, Bowman WC, eds. New York: Elsevier, 1990:141–162.
2. Gild WM, Posner KL, Caplan RA, et al. Eye injuries associated with anesthesia. Anesthesiology 1992;76: 204–208.
3. Andersen BN, Madsen JV, Schurizek BA, et al. Residual curarisation. A comparative study of atracurium and pancuronium. Acta Anaesthesiol Scand 1988;32: 79–81.
4. Bevan DR, Smith CE, Donati F. Postoperative neuromuscular blockage. A comparison between atracurium, vecuronium, and pancuronium. Anesthesiology 1988;69:272–276.
5. Beemer GH, Rozental P. Postoperative neuromuscular function. Anaesthesia and Intensive Care 1986; 14:41–45.
6. Brull SJ, Ehrenwerth J, Connelly NR, et al. Assessment of residual curarization using low-current stimulation. Can J Anaesth 1991;38:164–168.
7. Howardy-Hansen P, Rasmussen JA, Jensen BN. Residual curarization in the recovery room: atracurium versus gallamine. Acta Anaesthesiol Scand 1989;33: 167–169.
8. Hartmannsgruber M, Gravenstein N. Routine use of nerve stimulator reduces incidence of postoperative muscle weakness. Journal of Clinical Monitoring 1992;8:185–186.
9. Lennmarken C, Lofstrom JB. Partial curarization in the postoperative period. Acta Anaesthesiol Scand 1984;28:260–262.
10. Pedersen T, Viby-Mogensen J, Bang U, et al. Does perioperative tactile evaluation of the train-of-four response influence the frequency of postoperative residual neuromuscular blockade? Anesthesiology 1990; 73:835–839.
11. Shorten GD, Ali H, Merk H. Perioperative neuromuscular monitoring and residual curarization. Br J Anaesth 1992;68:438P–439P.
12. Viby-Mogensen J, Jorgensen BC, Ording H. Residual curarization in the recovery room. Anesthesiology 1979;50:539–541.
13. Baillard C, Gehan G, Reboul-Marty J, et al. Residual curarization in the recovery room. Br J Anaesth 1996; 76:12.
14. Fawcett WJ, Dash A, Francis GA, et al. Recovery from neuromuscular blockade: residual curarisation following atracurium and vecuronium by bolus dosing or infusions. Acta Anaesthesiol Scand 1995; 39: 288–293.
15. McEwin L, Merrick PM, Bevan DR. Residual neuromuscular blockade after cardiac surgery: pancuronium versus rocuronium. Can J Anaesth 1997;44: 891–895.
16. Bevan DR, Kahwaji R, Ansermino JM, et al. Residual block after mivacurium with or without edrophonium reversal in adults and children. Anesthesiology 1996;84:362–367.
17. Mortensen CR, Berg H, El-Mahdy A, et al. Perioperative monitoring of neuromuscular transmission using acceleromyography prevents residual neuromuscular block following pancuronium. Acta Anaesthesiol Scand 1995;39:797–801.
18. Kopman AF, Ng J, Zank LM, et al. Residual postoperative paralysis. Pancuronium versus mivacurium, does it matter? Anesthesiology 1996;85:1253–1259.
19. Shorten GD, Merk H, Sieber T. Perioperative train-of-four monitoring and residual curarization. Can J Anaesth 1995;42:711–715.
20. Dulin PG, Gilliard L, Williams C. To the editor. Crit Care Med 1992; 20:1623–1624.
21. Hodges UM. Vecuronium infusion requirements in paediatric patients in intensive care units: the use of acceleromyography. Br J Anaesth 1996;76:23–28.
22. Hansen-Flaschen J, Cowen J, Raps EC. Neuromuscular blockade in the intensive care unit: more than we bargained for. American Review of Respiratory Disease 1993;147:234–236.
23. Rudis MI, Sikora CA, Angus E, et al. A prospective, randomized, controlled evaluation of peripheral nerve stimulation versus standard clinical dosing of neuromuscular blocking agents in critically ill patients. Crit Care Med 1997; 25:575–583.
24. Watling SM, Dasta JF. Prolonged paralysis in intensive care unit patients after the use of neuromuscular blocking agents; a review of the literature. Crit Care Med 1994;22:884–893.
25. Sharpe MD. The use of muscle relaxants in the intensive care unit. Can J Anaesth 1992;39:949–962.
26. Sladen RN. Neuromuscular blocking agents in the intensive care unit: a two-edged sword. Crit Care Med 1995;23:423–428.
27. Viby-Mogensen J. Monitoring neuromuscular function in the intensive care unit. Intens Care Med 1993; 19:S74–S79.
28. Nielsen CH, Arnold DE. Performance of peripheral

nerve stimulators for regional anesthesia. Anesthesiology 1989;71:A464.

29. Raj PP, Rosenblatt R, Montgomery SJ. Use of the nerve stimulator for peripheral blocks. Regional Anesth 1980;5:14–21.

30. Sansome AJ, de Courcy JG. A new dual function nerve stimulator. Anaesthesia 1989;44:494–497.

31. Ducey JP, Fincher CW, Baysinger CL. Therapeutic suppression of a permanent ventricular pacemaker using a peripheral nerve stimulator. Anesthesiology 1991;75:533–536.

32. Kopman AF, Lawson D. Milliamperage requirements for supramaximal stimulation of the ulnar nerve with surface electrodes. Anesthesiology 1984;61:83–85.

33. Brull SJ, Ehrenwerth J, Silverman DG. Stimulation with submaximal current for train-of-four monitoring. Anesthesiology 1990;72:629–632.

34. Connelly NR, Silverman DG, O'Conner TZ, et al. Subjective responses to train-of-four and double burst stimulation in awake patients. Anesth Analg 1990;70:650–653.

35. Saitoh Y, Toyooka H. Optimal stimulating current for train-of-four stimulation in conscious subjects. Can J Anaesth 1995;42:992–995.

36. Satioh Y, Tanaka Y. Double burst stimulation$_{2,3}$ at submaximal current. Can J Anaesth 1997;44:570.

37. Brull SJ, Silverman DG. Pulse width, stimulus intensity, electrode placement, and polarity during assessment of neuromuscular block. Anesthesiology 1995;83:702–709.

38. Brull SJ, Silverman DG. Visual and tactile assessment of neuromuscular fade. Anesth Analg 1993;77:352–355.

39. Edmonds HL Jr, Paloheimo M, Wauquier A. Computerized EMG monitoring in anesthesia and intensive care. Schoutlaan, The Netherlands: Instrumentarium Science Foundation, 1988.

40. Mehta MP, Choi WW. Monitoring of neuromuscular blockade. In: Webster JA, ed. Encyclopedia of medical devices and instrumentation. New York: Wiley, 1988:2034–2041.

41. Brull SJ. Muscle relaxants, what should I monitor and what does it tell me? ASA Annual Refresher Courses, New Orleans, October 20, 1996.

42. Mylrea KC, Hameroff SR, Calkins JM, et al. Evaluation of peripheral nerve stimulators and relationship to possible errors in assessing neuromuscular blockade. Anesthesiology 1984;60:464–466.

43. Reference deleted.

44. Epstein RA, Wyte SR, Jackson SH, et al. The electromechanical response to stimulation by the block-aid monitor. Anesthesiology 1969;30:43–47.

45. Ali HH, Miller RD. Monitoring of neuromuscular function. In: Miller RD, ed. Anesthesia. 2nd ed. New York: Churchill Livingstone, 1986:871–887

46. Ali HH, Savarese JJ. Stimulus frequency and dose-response curve to d-tubocurarine in man. Anesthesiology 1980;52:36–39.

47. Heier T, Caldwell JE, Sessler KL, et al. The relationship between adductor pollicis twitch tension and core, skin and muscle temperature during nitrous oxide-isoflurane anesthesia in humans. Anesthesiology 1989;71:381–384.

48. Heier T, Caldwell JE, Sessler DI, et al. The effect of local surface and central cooling on adductor pollicis twitch tension using nitrous oxide/isoflurane and nitrous oxide/fentanyl anesthesia in humans. Anesthesiology 1990;72:807–811.

49. England AJ, Wu X, Feldman SA. Effect of temperature on the sensitivity of transducers used on human volunteers during neuromuscular stimulating experiments? Anaesthesia 1994;49:554.

50. Eriksson LI, Lennmarken C, Jensen E, et al. Twitch tension and train-of-four ratio during prolonged neuromuscular monitoring at different peripheral temperatures. Acta Anaesthesiol Scand 1991; 35: 247–252.

51. Donati F, Bevam JC, Bevan DR. Neuromuscular blocking drugs in anaesthesia. Can Anaesth Soc J 1984;31:324–335.

52. Ali HH, Utting JE, Gray C. Stimulus frequency in the detection of neuromuscular block in humans. Br J Anaesth 1970;42:967–978.

53. Lee CM. Quantitation of competitive neuromuscular block. Anesth Analg 1975;54:649–653.

54. Silverman DG, Connelly NR, O'Connor TZ, et al. Accelographic train-of-four at near-threshold currents. Anesthesiology 1992;76:34–38.

55. Ali HH, Savarese JJ, Lebowitz PW, et al. Twitch, tetanus and train-of-four as indices of recovery from nondepolarizing neuromuscular blockade. Anesthesiology 1981;54:294–297.

56. Brull SJ, Silverman DG. Visual assessment of train-of-four and double burst induced fade at submaximal stimulating currents. Anesth Analg 1991;73: 627–632.

57. Drenck NE, Ueda N, Olsen V, et al. Manual evaluation of residual curarization using double burst stimulation. A comparison with train-of-four. Anesthesiology 1989;70:578–581.

58. Gill SS, Donati F, Bevan DR. Clinical evaluation of double-burst stimulation. Its relationship to train-of-four stimulation. Anaesthesia 1990;45:543–548.

59. Saddler JM, Bevan JC, Donati F, et al. Comparison of double-burst and train-of-four stimulation to assess neuromuscular blockade in children. Anesthesiology 1990;73:401–403.

60. Tammisto I, Wirtavouri K, Linko K. Assessment of neuromuscular block: comparison of three clinical methods and evoked electromyography. Eur J Anaes 1988;5:1–8.

61. Viby–Mogensen J, Jensen NH, Engbaek J, et al. Tactile and visual evaluation of the response to train-of-four nerve stimulation. Anesthesiology 1985;63: 440–443.

62. Brull SJ, Silverman DC. Real time versus slow-motion train-of-four monitoring: a theory to explain the inaccuracy of visual assessment. Anesth Analg 1995; 80: 548–551.

63. Silverman DG, Sorin I, Brull J. Patterns on stimulation in neuromuscular block. In: Silverman DG, ed. Perioperative and intensive care. Philadelphia: JB Lippincott, 1994:37–50.

64. Ueda N, Viby-Mogensen J, Viby–Olsen N, et al. The best choice of double burst stimulation pattern for manual evaluation of neuromuscular transmission. J Anesth 1989;3:94–99.

65. Engbaek J, Ostergaard D, Viby–Mogensen J. Double burst stimulation (DBS). A new pattern of nerve stimulation to identify residual neuromuscular block. Br J Anaesth 1989;62:274–278.

66. Drenck NE, Ueda N, Olsen V, et al. Manual evaluation of residual curarization using double burst stimulation. A comparison with train of four. Anesthesiology 1989;71:578–581.

67. Saitoh Y, Nakazawa K, Tanaka H, et al. Double burst stimulation$_{2,3}$: a new stimulating pattern for residual neuromuscular block. Can J Anaesth 1996;43: 1001–1005.

68. Braude N, Vyvyan HAL, Jordan MJ. Intraoperative assessment of atracurium-induced neuromuscular block using double burst stimulation. Br J Anaesth 1991;67:574–578.

69. Reference deleted.

70. Kirkegaard-Nielsen H, Helbo-Hansen HS, Lindholm P, et al. Stabilization of the neuromuscular response when switching between different modes of nerve stimulation at surgical degrees of neuromuscular blockade. Journal of Clinical Monitoring 1995; 11:317–323.

71. Dupuis Y, Tessonnier JM. Clinical assessment of the muscular response to tetanic nerve stimulation. Can J Anaesth 1990;37:397–400.

72. Kopman AF, Epstein RH, Flashburg MH. Use of 100 Hz tetanus as an index of recovery from pancuronium-induced non-depolarizing neuromuscular blockade. Anesth Analg 1982;61:439–441.

73. Stanec A, Heyduk J, Stanec G, et al. Tetanic fade and post-tetanic tension in the absence of neuromuscular blocking agents in anesthetized man. Anesth Analg 1978;57:102–107.

74. Causton PR, Lennon RL, Jones KA. Assessment of residual blockade by 50 Hz and 100 Hz tetany. A comparison with train-of-four ratio. Anesth Analg 1992;74:S40.

75. Silverman DG, Brull SJ. The effect of a tetanic stimulus on the response to subsequent tetanic stimulation. Anesth Analg 1993;76:1284–1287.

76. Brull SJ, Connelly NR, O'Connor TZ, et al. Effect of tetanus on subsequent neuromuscular monitoring in patients receiving vecuronium. Anesthesiology 1991;74:64–70.

77. Saitoh Y, Masuda A, Toyooka H, et al. Effect of tetanic stimulation on subsequent train-of-four responses at various levels of vecuronium-induced neuromuscular block. Br J Anaesth 1994; 73:416–417.

78. Viby-Mogensen J, Howardy-Hansen P, Chraemmer-Jorgensen B, et al. Post-tetanic count (PTC). A new method of evaluating intense nondepolarizing neuromuscular blockade. Anesthesiology 1981;55: 458–461.

79. Viby-Mogensen J, Bonsu AK, Muchhal FK, et al. Monitoring of intense neuromuscular blockade caused by atracurium. Br J Anaesth 1986;58:68S.

80. Gwinnutt CL, Meakin G. Use of the post-tetanic count to monitor recovery from intense neuromuscular blockade in children. Br J Anaesth 1988;61: 547–550.

81. Eriksson LI, Lennmarken C, Staun P, et al. Use of post-tetanic count in assessment of a repetitive vecuronium-induced neuromuscular block. Br J Anaesth 1990;65:487–493.

82. Bonsu AK, Viby-Mogensen J, Fernando PUE, et al. Relationship of post-tetanic count and train-of-four response during intense neuromuscular blockade caused by atracurium. Br J Anaesth 1987;59: 1089–1092.

83. Fernandes LA, Stout RG, Silverman DG, et al. Comparative recovery of 50-Hz and 100-Hz post-tetanic twitch following profound neuromuscular block. J Clin Anesth 1997; 9:48–51.

84. Silverman DG, Sorin I, Brull J. Features of neurostimulation in neuromuscular block in perioperative and intensive care. Philadelphia: JB Lippincott, 1994: 23–26.

85. Lippmann M, Feilds WA. Burns of the skin caused by a peripheral-nerve stimulator. Anesthesiology 1974; 40:82–84.

86. Hunter JM, Kelly JM, Jones RS. Difficulties with neuromuscular monitoring. Anaesthesia 1985;40: 916.

87. Miller LR, Benumof JL, Alexander L, et al. Completely absent response to peripheral nerve stimulation in an acutely hypothermic patient. Anesthesiology 1989;71:779–781.

88. Booij LHDJ. Active reversal and monitoring of neuromuscular block. In: Booij LHDJ, ed. Neuromuscular transmission. London, England: BMJ Publishing Group, 1996:160–187.

89. Berger JJ, Gravenstein JS, Munson ES. Electrode polarity and peripheral nerve stimulation. Anesthesiology 1982;56:402–404.

90. Rosenberg H, Greenhow DE. Peripheral nerve stimulator performance. The influence of output polarity and electrode placement. Can Anaesth Soc J 1978; 25:424–426.

91. Brull SJ, Silverman DG. Neuromuscular block monitoring in Anesthesia Equipment, Principles and Applications. Ehrenwerth J, Eisenkraft JB, eds. St. Louis, MO: Mosby, 1993:297–318.

92. Brull SJ, Connelly NR, Sutherland D, et al. Visual assessment of fade with low intensity stimulating current. Anesthesiology 1990;73:A863.

93. Viby-Mogensen J. Clinical assessment of neuromuscular transmission. Br J Anaesth 1982;54:209–223.

94. Howardy-Hansen P, Viby-Mogensen J, Gottschau A, et al. Tactile evaluation of the post-tetanic count (PTC). Anesthesiology 1984;60:372–374.

95. Saitoh Y, Nakazawa K, Makita K, et al. Evaluation of residual neuromuscular block using train-of-four and double burst stimulation at the index finger. Anesth Analg 1997;84:1354–1358.

96. Donlon JV, Savarese JJ, Ali HH. Cumulative dose-response curves for gallamine: effect of altered resting thumb tension and mode of stimulation. Anesth Analg 1979;58:377–381.

97. Viby–Mogensen, Jensen E, Werner M, et al. Measurement of acceleration; a new method of monitoring neuromuscular function. Acta Anaesthesiol Scand 1988;32:45–48.

98. Ueda N, Muteki T, Poulsen A, et al. Clinical assessment of a new neuromuscular transmission monitoring system (Accelerograph). Jpn J Anesth 1989;3: 90–93.

99. Werner MU, Nielsen HK, May O, et al. Assessment of neuromuscular transmission by the evoked acceleration response. Acta Anaesthesiol Scand 1988;32: 395–400.

100. May O, Nielsen HK, Werner MU. The acceleration transducer—an assessment of its precision in comparison with a force displacement transducer. Acta Anaesthesiol Scand 1988;32:239–243.

101. Meretoja OA, Brown WA, Cass NM. Simultaneous monitoring of force, acceleration and electromyogram during computer-controlled infusion of atracurium in sheep. Anaesthesia and Intensive Care 1990; 18:486–489.

102. Itagaki T, Tai K, Katsumata N, et al. Comparison between a new acceleration transducer and a conventional force transducer in the evaluation of twitch responses. Acta Anaesthesiol Scand 1988;32:347–349.

103. Kern SE, Johnson JO, Westenskow DR, et al. An effective study of a new piezoelectric sensor for train-of-four measurement. Anesth Analg 1994;78: 978–982.

104. Loan PB, Paxton LD, Mirakhur RK, et al. The TOF-Guard neuromuscular transmission monitor. A comparison with the Myograph 2000. Anaesthesia 1995; 50:699–702.

105. Crofts SL, Hutchison GL. Clinical monitoring of neuromuscular function. Br J Hosp Med 1992;48: 633–638.

106. Itagaki T, Tai K, Katsumata N, et al. Comparison between a new acceleration transducer and a conventional force transducer in the evaluation of twitch responses. Acta Anaesthesiol Scand 1988; 32: 347–349.

107. McCluskey A, Meakin G, Hopkinson JM, et al. A comparison of acceleromyography and mechanomyography for determination of the dose-response curve of rocuronium in children. Anaesthesia 1997;52; 345–349.

108. Ansermino JM, Sanderson PM, Bevan DR. Acceleromyography improves detection of residual neuromuscular blockade in children. Can J Anaesth 1996;43: 589–594.

109. Calvey TN. Assessment of neuromuscular blockade by electromyography: a review. J Roy Soc Med 1984; 77:56–59.

110. Sakabe T, Nakashima K. The Datex relaxograph NMT-100. Anesthesiol Rev 1990;17:45–51.

111. Paloheimo M. Quantitative surface electromyography (qEMG): applications in anaesthesiology and critical care. Acta Anaesthesiol Scand 1990; (Suppl 93) 34:3–51.

112. Lekowski RW, Johnston JF. Clinical use of the relaxograph NMT-100. Anesth Review 1994;21:22–26.

113. Paloheimo M, Edmonds HL Jr. Minimizing movement-induced changes in twitch response during integrated electromyography. In reply. Anesthesiology 1988;69:143.

114. Pugh ND, Kay B, Healy TEJ. Electromyography in anaesthesia. A comparison between two methods. Anaesthesia 1984;39:574–577.

115. Pugh ND, Harper NJN, Healy TEJ, et al. Effects of atracurium and vecuronium on the latency and the duration of the negative deflection of the evoked compound action potential of the adductor pollicis. Br J Anaesth 1987;59:195–199.

116. Harper NJN, Pugh ND, Healy TEJ et al. Changes in the power spectrum of the evoked compound action

potential of the adductor pollicis with the onset of neuromuscular blockade. Br J Anaesth 1987;59: 200–205.

117. Smith DC, Booth JV. Influence of muscle temperature and forearm position on evoked electromyography in the hand. Br J Anaesth 1994;72:407–410.

118. Wood R, Ponthenkandath N, Steen SN, et al. Neuromuscular transmission monitoring: implications of changes in hand positions. Anesth Analg 1997;84: S281.

119. DeVries JW, Ros HH, Booij LHDJ. Infusion of vecuronium controlled by a closed-loop system. Br J Anaesth 1986;58:1100–1103.

120. Astley BA, Katz RL, Payne JP. Electrical and mechanical responses after neuromuscular blockade with vecuronium, and subsequent antagonism with neostigmine or edrophonium. Br J Anaesth 1987;59: 983–988.

121. Carter JA, Arnold R, Yate PM, et al. Assessment of the Datex relaxograph during anaesthesia and atracurium-induced neuromuscular blockade. Br J Anaesth 1986;58:1447–1452.

122. Donati F, Bevan DR. Muscle electromechanical correlations during succinylcholine infusion. Anesth Analg 1984;63:891–894.

123. Epstein RA, Epstein RM. The electromyogram and the mechanical response to indirectly stimulated muscle in anesthetized man following curarization. Anesthesiology 1973;38:212–223.

124. Engboek J, Ostergaard D, Viby–Mogensen J, et al. Clinical recovery and train-of-four ratio measured mechanically and electromyographically following atracurium. Anesthesiology 1989;71:391–395.

125. Katz RL. Electromyographic and mechanical effects of suxamethonium and tubocurarine on twitch, tetanic and post-tetanic responses. Br J Anaesth 1973; 45:849–859.

126. Kopman AF. The relationship of evoked electromyographic and mechanical responses following atracurium in humans. Anesthesiology 1985;63:208–211.

127. Kopman AF. The effect of resting muscle tension on the dose-effect relationship of *d*-tubocurarine; does preload influence the evoked EMG? Anesthesiology 1988;69:1003–1005.

128. Kopman AF. The relationship of evoked electromyographic and mechanical responses following atracurium in humans. Anesthesiology 1985;63:208–211.

129. Kopman AF. The dose-effect relationship of metocurine. The integrated electromyogram of the first dorsal interosseous muscle and the mechanomyogram of the adductor pollicis compared. Anesthesiology 1988;68:604–607.

130. Harper NJN, Bradshaw EG, Healy TEJ. Evoked electromyographic and mechanical responses of the adductor pollicis compared during the onset of neuromuscular blockade by atracurium or alcuronium, and during antagonism by neostigmine. Br J Anaesth 1986;58:1278–1284.

131. Shanks CA, Jarvis JE. Electromyographic and mechanical twitch responses following suxamethonium administration. Anaesthesia and Intensive Care 1980; 8:341–344.

132. Windsor JPW, Sebel PS, Flynn PJ. The neuromuscular transmission monitor. A clinical assessment and comparison with a force transducer. Anaesthesia 1985;40:146–151.

133. Weber S, Muravchick S. Electrical and mechanical train-of-four responses during depolarizing and nondepolarizing neuromuscular blockade. Anesth Analg 1986;65:771–776.

134. Weber S, Muravchick S. Monitoring technique affects measurement of recovery from succinylcholine. Journal of Clinical Monitoring 1987;3:1–5.

135. Engbaek J, Roed J. Differential effect of pancuronium at the adductor pollicis, the first dorsal interosseous and the hypothenar muscles. An electromyographic and mechanomyographic dose-response study. Acta Anaesthesiol Scand 1992;36:664–669.

136. Engbaek J, Roes J, Hangaard N, Viby–Mogensen J. The agreement between adductor pollicis mechanomyogram and first dorsal interosseous electromyogram. A pharmacodynamic study of rocuronium and vecuronium. Acta Anaesthesiol Scand 1994; 38: 869–878.

137. Engbaek J, Skovgaard LT, Fries B, et al. Monitoring of neuromuscular transmission by electromyography (II). Evoked compound EMG area, amplitude and duration compared to mechanical twitch recording during onset and recovery of pancuronium-induced blockade in the cat. Acta Anaesthesiol Scand 1993; 37:788–798.

138. Engbaek J, Skovgaard LT, Friis B, et al. Monitoring of the neuromuscular transmission by electromyograph (I). Stability and temperature dependence of evoked EMG response compared to mechanical twitch recordings in the cat. Acta Anaesthesiol Scand 1992; 36:495–504.

139. Mortier E, Moulaert P, de Somer A, et al. Comparison of evoked electromyography and mechanical activity during vecuronium-induced neuromuscular blockade. Eur J Anaesth 1988; 5:131–141.

140. Eisenkraft JB, Pirak L, Thys DM. Monitoring neuromuscular blockade. EMG versus twitch tension. Anesth Analg 1986;65:S47.

141. Johnson JO. Apiezo electric Neuromuscular monitor. In response. Anesth Analg 1994;79:1210–1211.

142. Roberts C, Dorsch JA. ParaGraph muscle stimulator: new approach to placement. Anesthesiology 1996; 85:1218–1219.

143. Kern SE, Westenskow DR, Orr JA, et al. Measurement of train-of-four ratio from a patient's hand tucked at their side. Anesthesiology 1992;77:A952.

144. Brandom BW, Lloyd ME, Woelfel SK, et al. Comparison of the Datex EMG and Paragraph monitors during recovery from pancuronium in anesthetized pediatric patients. Anesth Analg 1997;84:S228.

145. Hudes E, Lee KC. Clinical use of peripheral nerve stimulators in anaesthesia. Can J Anaesth 1987;34: 525–534.

146. Theroux MC, Brandom BW, Cook DR. Neuromuscular monitoring of the flexor hallucis brevis compared with the adductor pollicis in anesthetized children. Anesth Analg 1990;70:S408.

147. Graham DH. Monitoring neuromuscular block may be unreliable in patients with upper-motor-neuron lesions. Anesthesiology 1980;52:74–75.

148. Iwasaki H, Namiki A, Omote K. Response differences of paretic and healthy extremities to pancuronium and neostigmine in hemiplegic patients. Anesth Analg 1985;64:864–866.

149. Brull SJ, Gardia R, Halevy J, et al. Comparative EMG responses during ulnar nerve stimulation. Anesthesiology 1992;77:A566.

150. Gertel M, Shapira SC. Ulnar nerve palsy of unusual etiology. Anesth Analg 1987;66:1343.

151. Harper NJN. Comparison of the adductor pollicis and the first dorsal interosseous muscles during atracurium and vecuronium blockade: an electromyographic study. Br J Anaesth 1988;61:477–478.

152. Kalli I. Effect of surface electrode position on the compound action potential evoked by ulnar nerve stimulation during isoflurane anaesthesia. Br J Anaesth 1990;65:494–499.

153. Paloheimo MPJ, Wilson RCW, Edmonds HL, et al. Comparison of neuromuscular blockade in upper facial and hypothenar muscles. Journal of Clinical Monitoring 1988;4:256–260.

154. Meretoja OA, Werner MU, Wirtavuori K, et al. Comparison of thumb acceleration and thenar EMG responses in the pharmacodynamic evaluation of neuromuscular blockade. Anesthesiology 1988;69: A270.

155. Frank LP. But where will I put my twitch monitor? Anesth Analg 1986;65:419–425.

156. Sopher MJ, Sears DH, Walts LF. Neuromuscular function monitoring comparing the flexor hallucis brevis and adductor pollicis muscles. Anesthesiology 1988;69:129–131.

157. Kern SE, Johnson JO, Orr JA, et al. Clinical analysis of the flexor hallucis brevis as an alternative site for monitoring neuromuscular block from mivacurium. Journal of Clinical Anesthesia 1997;9:383–387.

158. Kitajima T, Ishii K, Ogata H. Assessment of neuromuscular block at the thumb and great toe using accelography in infants. Anaesthesia 1996;51: 341–343.

159. Kitajima T, Ishii K, Kobayashi T, et al. Differential effects of vecuronium on the thumb and great toe as measured by accelography and electromyography. Anaesthesia 1995;50:76–78.

160. Henthorn RW, Cajee RA. A neuromuscular block monitor using the toe flexors. Anesth Analg 1992; 74:774.

161. Jones K, Leslie K, Beemer GB. Supramaximal stimulation of the common peroneal nerve. Anaesthesia and Intensive Care 1997;25:191.

162. Kempen PM. Clinical use of peripheral nerve stimulators. Can J Anaesth 1988;35:542.

163. Caffrey RR, Warren ML, Becker KE. Neuromuscular blockade monitoring comparing the orbicularis oculi and adductor pollicis muscles. Anesthesiology 1986; 65:95–97.

164. Stiffel P, Hameroff SR, Blitt CD, et al. Variability in assessment of neuromuscular blockade. Anesthesiology 1980;52:436–437.

165. Gray JA. Nerve stimulators. Anesthesiology 1975;42: 231–232.

166. Ho LC, Crosby G, Sundaram P, et al. Ulnar train-of-four stimulation in predicting face movement during intracranial facial nerve stimulation. Anesth Analg 1989;69:242–244.

167. Rimaniol JM, Dhonneur GM, Sperry L, et al. A comparison of the neuromuscular blocking effects of atracurium, mivacurium, and vecuronium on the adductor pollicis and the orbicularis oculi muscle in humans. Anesth Analg 1996;83:808–813.

168. Pathak D, Sokoll MD, Barcellos W, et al. A comparison of the response of hand and facial muscles to non-depolarising relaxants. Anaesthesia 1988;43: 747–748.

169. Jones KA, Lennon RL, Black S. Methods of intraoperative monitoring of neuromuscular function and residual blockade in the recovery room. Anesthesiology 1989;71:A946.

170. Sharpe MD, Moote CA, Lam AM, et al. Comparison of integrated evoked EMG between the hypothenar and facial muscle groups following atracurium and vecuronium administration. Can J Anaesth 1991;38: 318–323.

171. Jones KA, Lennon RL, Hosking MP. Method of intraoperative monitoring of neuromuscular function

and residual blockade in the recovery room. Minnesota Med 1992;75:23–26.

172. Curran MJ, Ali HH, Savarese JJ, et al. Comparative evoked thumb and jaw force measurement using accelerometry. Anesthesiology 1988;69:A472.

173. Plumley MH, Bevan JC, Saddler JM, et al. Dose-related effects of succinylcholine on the adductor pollicis and masseter muscles in children. Can J Anaesth 1990;37:15–20.

174. Saddler JM, Bevan JC, Plumley MH, et al. Potency of atracurium on masseter and adductor policis muscles in children. Can J Anaesth 1990;37:26–30.

175. Smith CE, Donati F, Bevan DR. Differential effects of pancuronium on masseter and adductor pollicis muscles in humans. Anesthesiology 1989;71:57–61.

176. Meakin G. Stimulation of the spinal accessory nerve as a method of monitoring neuromuscular transmission. Anaesthesia 1993;48:85.

177. Hall IA. A complication of inappropriate use of peripheral nerve stimulation. Anaesthesia 1994;49:925.

178. Kopman AF. A safe surface electrode for peripheral nerve stimulation. Anesthesiology 1976;44:343–345.

179. Brull SJ, Connelly NR, Silverman DG. Succinylcholine-induced fasciculations: correlation to loss of twitch response at different stimulation frequencies. Anesthesiology 1990;73:A868.

180. Curran MJ, Donati F, Bevin DR. Onset and recovery of atracurium and suxamethonium-induced neuromuscular blockade with simultaneous train-of-four and single twitch stimulation. Br J Anaesth 1987;59:989–994.

181. Viby–Mogensen J. Monitoring of neuromuscular blockade: technology and clinical methods. In: Agoston S, Bowman WC, eds. Muscle relaxants. 2nd ed. New York: Elsevier, 1990:141–162.

182. Zorab JSM, Bettles ND, Lynn PA, et al. A computerized neuromuscular blockade monitor with visual-display unit. A preliminary report. Eur J Anaesth 1984;1:85–92.

183. Smith CE, Donati F, Bevan DR. Effects of succinylcholine at the masseter and adductor pollicis muscles in adults. Anesth Analg 1989;69:158–162.

184. Donati F, Meistelman C, Plaud B. Vecuronium neuromuscular blockade at the adductor muscles of the larynx and adductor pollicis. Anesthesiology 1991;74:833–837.

185. Fisher DM, Szerohradszky J, Wright PMC, et al. Pharmacodynamic modeling of vecuronium-induced twitch depression. Rapid plasma-effect site equilibration explains faster onset at resistant laryngeal muscles than at the adductor pollicis. Anesthesiology 1997;86:558–566.

186. Plaud B, Debaene B, Lequeau F, et al. Mivacurium neuromuscular block at the adductor muscles of the larynx and adductor pollicis in humans. Anesthesiology 1996;85:77–81.

187. Debaene B, Lieutaud T, Billard V, et al. ORG 9487 neuromuscular block at the adductor pollicis and the laryngeal adductor muscles in humans. Anesthesiology 1997;86:1300–1305.

188. Iwasaki H, Igarashi M, Namiki A, et al. Differential neuromuscular effects of vecuronium on the adductor and abductor laryngeal muscles and tibialis anterior muscle in dogs. Br J Anaesth 1994;72:321–323.

189. Smith CE, Donati F, Bevan DR. Differential effects of pancuronium on masseter and adductor pollicis muscles in humans. Can J Anaesth 1988;35:S214.

190. Donati F, Antzaka C, Bevan DR. Potency of pancuronium at the diaphragm and the adductor pollicis muscle in humans. Anesthesiology 1986;65:1–5.

191. Donati F, Meistelman C, Plaud B. Vecuronium neuromuscular blockade at the diaphragm, the orbicularis oculi, and adductor pollicis muscles. Anesthesiology 1990;73:870–875.

192. Meistelman C, Plaud B, Donati F. Rocuronium (ORG 9426) neuromuscular blockade at the adductor muscles of the larynx and adductor pollicis in humans. Can J Anaesth 1992;39:665–669.

193. Waund BE, Waund DR. The margin of safety of neuromuscular transmission in the muscle of the diaphragm. Anesthesiology 1972;37:417–422.

194. Ungureanu D, Meistelman C, Frossard J, Donati F. The orbicularis oculi and the adductor pollicis muscles as monitors of atracurium block of laryngeal muscles. Anesth Analg 1993; 77:775–779.

195. Plaud B, Laffon M, Ecoffey C, et al. Monitoring orbicularis oculi predicts good intubating conditions after vecuronium in children. Can J Anaesth 1997; 44:712–716.

196. Helbo-Hansen HS, Jensen B, Norreslet J, et al. Response to single twitch or single burst stimulation of the ulnar nerve as predictive guide for intubating conditions. Acta Anaesthesiol Scand 1995;39:498–502.

197. Sayson SC, Mongan PD. Onset of action of mivacurium chloride. A comparison of neuromuscular blockade monitoring at the adductor pollicis and the orbicularis oculi. Anesthesiology 1994;81:35–42.

198. Curran MJ, Donati F, Bevan DR. Onset and recovery of atracurium and suxamethonium-induced neuromuscular blockade with simultaneous train-of-four and single twitch stimulation. Br J Anaesth 1987;59:989–994.

199. McCoy EP, Mirakhur RK, Connolly FM, et al. The influence of the duration of control stimulation on the onset and recovery of neuromuscular block. Anesth Analg 1995;80:364–367.

200. Beale MD, Kellner CH, Lemert R, et al. Skeletal muscle relaxation in patients undergoing electroconvulsive therapy. Anesthesiology 1994;80:957.

201. Dorsch SE, Dorsch JA. Skeletal muscle relaxation in patients undergoing electroconvulsive therapy. Anesthesiology 1994;81:1309–1310.

202. Young ML, Hanson W III, Bloom MJ, et al. Localized hypothermia influences assessment of recovery from vecuronium neuromuscular blockade. Can J Anaesth 1994;41:1172–1177.

203. Helbo–Hansen HS, Bang U, Nielsen HK, et al. The accuracy of train-of-four monitoring at varying stimulating currents. Anesthesiology 1992;76:199–203.

204. Brull SJ, Silverman DG. Visual assessment of train-of-four and double burst-induced fade at submaximal stimulating currents. Anesth Analg 1991;73:627–632.

205. Silverman DG, Brull SJ. Assessment of double-burst monitoring at 10 mA above threshold current. Can J Anaesth 1993;40:502–556.

206. Brull SJ, Silverman DG. Stimulation with submaximal current for train-of-four monitoring. Anesthesiology 1990;72:629–632.

207. Thornberry EA, Mazumdar B. The effect of changes in arm temperature on neuromuscular monitoring in the presence of atracurium blockade. Anaesthesia 1988; 43:447–449.

208. Kern SE, Johnson JO, Westenkow DR, et al. A comparison of dynamic and isometric force sensors for train-of-four measurement using submaximal stimulation current. Journal of Clinical Monitoring 1995; 11:18–22.

209. Haraldsted VY, Nielsen JW, Joensen F, et al. Infusion of vecuronium assessed by tactile evaluation of evoked thumb twitch. Br J Anaesth 1988;61:479–481.

210. Rupp SM. Monitoring neuromuscular blockade. Twitch monitoring. Anes Clin N Amer 1993;11, 2:361–378.

211. Gibson FM, Mirakhur RK, Clarke RSJ, et al. Quantification of train-of-four responses during recovery of block from non-depolarizing muscle relaxants. Acta Anaesth Scand 1987;31:655–657.

212. Ali HH, Wilson RS, Savarese JJ, et al. The effect of tubocurarine on indirectly elicited train-of-four muscle response and respiratory measurements in humans. Br J Anaesth 1975;47:570–574.

213. Fernando PUE, Viby–Mogensen J, Bonsu AK, et al. Relationship between post-tetanic count and response to carinal stimulation during vecuronium-induced neuromuscular blockade. Acta Anaesthesiol Scand 1987;31:593–596.

214. Salathe M, Johr M. Use of post-tetanic train-of-four for evaluation of intense neuromuscular blockade with atracurium. Br J Anaesth 1988;61:123.

215. Tammisto T, Olkkola KT. Dependence of the adequacy of muscle relaxation on the degree of neuromuscular block and depth of enflurane anesthesia during abdominal surgery. Anesth Analg 1995; 80:543–547.

216. Saitoh Y, Kaneda K, Toyooka H, et al. Post-tetanic count and single twitch height at the onset of reflex movement after administration of vecuronium under different types of anaesthesia. Br J Anaesth 1994;72:688–690.

217. Bevan DR, Donati F, Kopman AF. Reversal of neuromuscular blockade. Anesthesiology 1992;77:785–805.

218. D'Honneur H, Guignard B, Slavov V, et al. Comparison of the neuromuscular blocking effects of atracurium and vecuronium on the adductor pollicis and the geniohyoid muscle in humans. Anesthesiology 1995; 82:649–654.

219. Iwasaki H, Igarashi M, Omote K, et al. Vecuronium neuromuscular blockade at the cricothyroid and posterior cricoarytenoid muscles of the larynx and at the adductor pollicis muscle in humans. J Clin Anesth 1994;6:14–17.

220. Saddler JM, Marks LF, Norman J. Comparison of atracurium-induced neuromuscular block in rectus abdominis and hand muscles of man. Br J Anaesth 1992;69:26–28.

221. Saitoh Y, Koitabashi Y, Makita K, et al. Train-of-four and double burst stimulation fade at the great toe and thumb. Can J Anaesth 1997;44:390–395.

222. Ali H, Kitz RJ. Evaluation of recovery from nondepolarizing neuromuscular block, using a digital neuromuscular transmission analyzer. Preliminary report. Anesth Analg 1973;52:740–745.

223. Ali HH, Savarese JJ. Monitoring of neuromuscular function. Anesthesiology 1976;45:216–245.

224. Brand JB, Cullen DJ, Wilson NE, et al. Spontaneous recovery from nondepolarizing neuromuscular blockade: correlation between clinical and evoked responses. Anesth Analg 1977;56:55–58.

225. Sharpe MD, Lam AM, Nicholas FJ, et al. Correlation between integrated evoked EMG and respiratory function following atracurium administration. Anesthesiology 1987;67:A608.

226. Isono S, Ide T, Mizuguchi T, et al. Effects of partial paralysis on the swallowing reflex in conscious humans. Anesthesiology 1991;75:980–984.

227. Kopman AF, Yee PS, Neuman GG. Relationship of the train-of-four ratio to clinical signs and symptoms of residual paralysis in awake volunteers. Anesthesiology 1997;86:765–771.

228. Eriksson LI, Milsson L, Witt H, et al. Videoradiographical computerized manometry in assessment of pharyngeal function in partially paralysed humans. Anesthesiology 1995; 83:A886.

229. Eriksson LI, Lennmarken C, Wyon N, et al. Attenuated ventilatory response to hypoxaemia at vecuronium-induced partial neuromuscular block. Acta Anaesthesiol Scand 1992;36:710–715.

230. Eriksson LI, Sato M, Severinghaus JW. Effect of a vecuronium-induced partial neuromuscular block on hypoxic ventilatory response. Anesthesiology 1993; 78:693–699.

231. Viby-Mogensen J. Clinical measurement of neuromuscular function: an update. Clin Anesthesiol 1985; 3(2):467–482.

232. Ali HH. Monitoring neuromuscular function. Semin Anesth 1989;8:158–168.

233. Brull SJ, Connelly NR, Silverman DG. Correlation of train-of-four and double burst stimulation ratios at varying amperages. Anesth Analg 1990;71:489–492.

234. Myyra R, Dalpra M, Globerson J. Electrical erythema? Anesthesiology 1988;69:440.

235. Pue AF. Disposable EKG pads for peripheral nerve stimulation. Anesthesiology 1976;45:107–108.

236. Sia RL, Straatman NJA. Thumb paresthesia after neuromuscular twitch monitoring. Anaesthesia 1985;40: 167–169.

237. Cheng ACK. Neuromuscular stimulator causes changes in electrocardiograph tracing. Anesth Analg 1993;76:919.

238. O'Flaherty D, Wardill M, Adams AP. Inadvertent suppression of a fixed rate ventricular pacemaker using a peripheral nerve stimulator. Anaesthesia 1993;48:687–689.

239. Lampotang S, Good ML, Heynen PMAM. Low-battery characteristic of the Professional Instruments NSCA nerve stimulator. Journal of Clinical Monitoring 1994;10:276.

QUESTIONS

1. The waveform for neuromuscular stimulation should be:
   A. Biphasic
   B. Rounded
   C. Monophasic
   D. Sloping
   E. Notched

2. The twitch frequency for the train-of-four stimulation is
   A. 1 Hz for 1 second
   B. 2 Hz for 2 seconds
   C. 2 Hz for 1 second
   D. 1 Hz for 2 seconds
   E. 3 HZ for 2 seconds

3. The duration of the waveform should be:
   A. Greater than 0.2 milliseconds
   B. Less than 0.6 milliseconds
   C. 0.04 milliseconds
   D. 0.2 milliseconds or less
   E. 0.4 milliseconds

4. The time interval between train-of-four stimulations should be at least
   A. 4 seconds
   B. 8 seconds
   C. 12 seconds
   D. 22 seconds
   E. 20 seconds

5. The frequency of single twitch stimulation should not exceed
   A. .01 Hz
   B. .1 Hz
   C. 1 Hz
   D. 1.5 Hz
   E. 10 Hz

Each question below contains four suggested answers of which one or more is correct.
Choose the answer:
A if 1, 2, and 3 are correct
B if 1 and 3 are correct
C if 2 and 4 are correct
D if 4 is correct
E if 1, 2, 3, and 4 are correct

6. Supramaximal stimulation refers to the
   1. Voltage used to stimulate the nerve
   2. Current used to stimulate a nerve
   3. Voltage above that necessary for maximal stimulation
   4. Current higher than that needed for maximal stimulation

7. Single twitch stimulation
   1. Cannot distinguish between depolarizing and nondepolarizing blocks
   2. Is useful for identifying satisfactory conditions for intubation
   3. Is not useful for assessing recovery from neuromuscular block
   4. Is not useful to determine supramaximal stimulus

8. Factors affecting the train-of-four (TOF) ratio include
   1. The nature of the neuromuscular block (depolarizing or nondepolarizing)
   2. Depth of the neuromuscular block
   3. Skin temperature
   4. The nerve being monitored

9. Advantages of train-of-four (TOF) stimulation include
   1. It is more sensitive than the single twitch
   2. It can detect phase II block
   3. It can distinguish between depolarizing and nondepolarizing blocks
   4. It is easy to detect fade with visual or tactile methods

10. Double burst stimulation (DBS)
    1. Consists of two short tetanic stimuli separated by 750 milliseconds
    2. Is primarily used to determine residual neuromuscular block
    3. Is more sensitive than train-of-four stimulation for determining fade
    4. Causes less discomfort than train-of-four (TOF) stimulation

11. With tetanic stimulation
    1. If no relaxants are present there will be a contraction followed by relaxation of the stimulated muscles
    2. If there is a depolarizing block, there will be a sustained contraction of lower magnitude

3. Profound block will show muscle movement after 10 seconds of stimulation
4. If a nondepolarizing block is present there will be a nonsustained contraction of the muscles

12. 50 Hz is most often used for tetanic stimulation because
   1. It is more physiologic
   2. If the frequency is greater than 50 Hz, the fade will be less pronounced
   3. If the frequency is less than 50 Hz the fade will be more pronounced
   4. It stresses the neuromuscular junction similar to a voluntary effort

13. Post-tetanic facilitation (PTF)
   1. Occurs with depolarizing blocks
   2. Is maximal in 5 seconds and lasts for up to 2 minutes
   3. Is more pronounced with lesser levels of neuromuscular block
   4. Is used to determine the depth of block in profoundly relaxed patients

14. Accelerography (ACG)
   1. Utilizes a piezoelectric sensor that produces an electronic signal proportional to the amount of movement
   2. Is useful in patients whose extremities are tucked
   3. Requires a preload
   4. Can be used with the facial nerve

15. The electromyograph (EMG)
   1. Is not useful in infants
   2. Measures a biphasic action is in each muscle stimulated
   3. Cannot be used with muscles which could not be used with the (MMG)
   4. Uses stimulating electrodes placed in a similar fashion as other monitoring technologies.

16. The facial nerve
   1. Is relatively resistant to muscle relaxants
   2. Can be used with accelerography (ACG)
   3. May show complete recovery when significant neuromuscular block (NMB) still exists
   4. Is useful in determining the relaxation of the jaw and diaphragm

17. During induction of anesthesia
   1. The stimulator should be applied prior to induction
   2. The facial nerve is most useful for determining the time for intubation
   3. Supramaximal stimulation should be determined after induction but before the administration of relaxant
   4. To determine optimal time of intubation, a nerve should be stimulated at 1 Hz

18. The post-tetanic count (PTC)
   1. Is the number of response after application of a tetanic stimulus of 50 Hz for 3 seconds
   2. Is directly proportional to the degree of neuromuscular block present
   3. Can only be used with a peripheral nerve
   4. Is useful for assessing deep neuromuscular block

19. Needle electrodes
   1. May be useful when the skin is cold
   2. Are useful with hyperthyroid patients
   3. Are used with currents of less than 10 mA
   4. Should be inserted perpendicular to the nerve to be stimulated

20. Clinical criteria useful to determine the adequacy of recovery from neuromuscular block include
   1. A inspiratory force of at least -20 cm H_2O pressure
   2. Sustained hand grip
   3. Sustained head life for 10 seconds
   4. Adequate tidal volume

ANSWERS

1.	C	11.	C
2.	B	12.	D
3.	D	13.	C
4.	C	14.	C
5.	C	15.	C
6.	B	16.	E
7.	A	17.	A
8.	A	18.	D
9.	A	19.	B
10.	A	20.	C

Temperature Monitoring

UNDER GENERAL ANESTHESIA, patients lose their normal mechanisms for regulating body temperature. Numerous studies have shown that significant temperature changes routinely occur in anesthetized patients. Normal core temperature is 36 to 37.5°C. This usually decreases by 0.5 to 1.5°C during the first 30 minutes of anesthesia (1).

INDICATIONS (2–4)

The monitoring guidelines of the American Society of Anesthesiologists state that there shall be a readily available means to measure continu-ously the patient's temperature (5). When changes in body temperature are intended, antici-pated, or suspected, the temperature shall be mea-sured. Temperature monitoring should be per-formed whenever large volumes of cold blood and/or intravenous fluids are administered, when the patient is deliberately cooled and/or warmed, for pediatric surgery of substantial duration, and in hypothermic or pyrexial patients or those with a suspected or known temperature regulatory problem such as malignant hyperthermia. Major surgical procedures, especially those involving body cavities, should be considered a strong indi-cation for temperature monitoring. There is a high incidence of perioperative hypothermia. Even mild hypothermia has adverse effects on pa-tient outcome, including an increased incidence of myocardial ischemia and cardiac morbidity, ar-rhythmias, interference with coagulation, in-creased blood loss, postoperative shivering, hyper-metabolism; mild hypothermia also has an increased risk of postoperative sepsis, surgical wound infections, prolonged postanesthetic re-covery (even when core temperature is not a dis-charge criterion), and prolonged hospitalization. Hyperthermia that may occur during sepsis, hy-perthyroidism, malignant hyperthermia, and drug or transfusion reactions needs to be recognized and treated promptly, as it can lead to life-threat-ening physiological disturbances.

TECHNOLOGY

A variety of technologies is available to measure temperature. None is not suitable for all situa-tions. Many devices simply display the tempera-ture. These are less than optimal, because a high or low temperature may go unnoticed for some

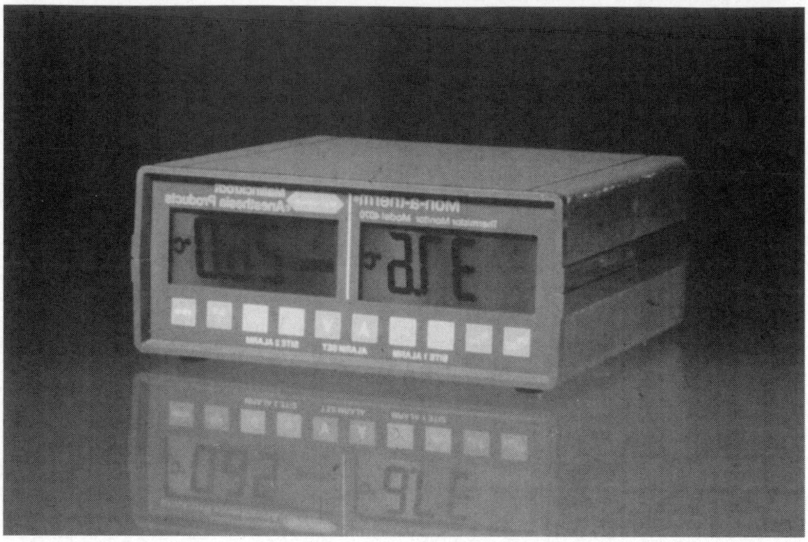

FIGURE 22.1. Monitor with capability for monitoring temperature at two sites and alarms. (Courtesy of Mallinkrodt, Inc.)

time. Most modern devices have alarms for high and low temperatures (Fig. 22.1). Those that are battery powered should have a means to indicate when battery power is low. Trend indicators are available on some instruments.

Thermistor

A thermistor is a substance whose electrical resistance varies with its temperature. There must be a source of current and a means to measure the current so that the resistance can be converted to a temperature (6). Advantages of thermistors include small sensors, rapid response, continuous readings, and sensitivity to small changes in temperature. They are fairly inexpensive. Probes can be made interchangeable and disposable. Most clinical thermistors have an accuracy of 0.1 to 0.3°C (7–9). There are disadvantages, however. The resistance gradually increases with age and will change if it is subjected to rapid or large changes of temperature (6). The resistance of a batch of thermistors tends to vary.

Thermocouple (10)

A thermocouple consists of an electrical circuit with two wires of different metals welded together at their ends. One junction is located in the tem-

perature probe and the other is kept at a standard reference temperature. A current flows in the circuit that is proportional to the temperature difference. Compared to thermistors, these devices have a less linear response to changes in temperature (6). Advantages of thermocouples include accuracy, small size, rapid response, continuous readings, stability, capability of remote reading, and interchangeability of probes. Most clinical thermocouples have an accuracy of approximately 0.1°C (7, 9). The materials are inexpensive so that sensor probes can be made disposable.

Platinum Wire

The electrical resistance of platinum wire varies almost linearly with temperature. By employing wire of extremely small diameter, rapid thermal equilibration is possible. The resistance is measured in a manner similar to a thermistor. These thermometers are accurate and give continuous readings. Probes can be made interchangeable. If a probe with a thermocouple, thermistor, or platinum wire is to be used inside the body, it must be ensheathed so it does not get wet. The end of the probe designed to be inserted into the patient is sealed, and the electrical connection made at the other end. The connection needs to be kept dry. If it becomes wet, erroneous readings can result (8, 11, 12).

Liquid Crystal (13–15)

Certain organic compounds in the thermal transformation from solid to liquid state pass through an intermediate phase that exhibits anisotropic (optically active) properties. The term *liquid crystal* is used to describe this state. When light shines on such a material, crystals at a certain temperature scatter some of the light, producing iridescent colors. The remaining portion of the incident light is transmitted by the crystals. By encapsulating the liquid crystals, the colors form letters and numbers. An absorptive black background prevents reflection of the transmitted light and enhances the resolution of the colors. Liquid crystal temperature monitors are shown in Figure 22.2. Each consists of a flexible adhesive-backed strip or disc with plastic-encased liquid crystals on a black background. To use, the covering over the adhesive is removed and the disc or strip placed on the skin. The liquid crystal thermometer (LCT) is available in two forms: one displays the skin temperature directly; the other has a built-in offset (see Fig. 22.1) so that the temperature displayed estimates core temperature (6, 15). Others have a second scale to indicate that temperature (16). LCT have a number of advantages. They are convenient, noninvasive, easy to apply and read, noninvasive, unbreakable, disposable, nonirritating,

and inexpensive. They give fast, continuous readings and involve no electronic circuitry. They can be applied before induction and are easily transferred with the patient. Disadvantages include the need for subjective observer interpretation and the inability to interface with a recording system. They are less accurate than other devices. Extremes of ambient temperature, humidity, and air movement can introduce inaccuracy (15). They are capable of measuring temperature only on the skin. If left in the sun for an extended period, an error indicating hyperthermia can be induced. Freezing can cause all the numbers to be visible at once (17). Infrared heating lamps may cause erroneously elevated readings (14). There is a report of failure of a liquid-crystal thermometer in which it gave a falsely high temperature (18).

Infrared (19–23)

The infrared thermometer is a noninvasive device that senses the infrared radiation emitted by a warm object such as the tympanic membrane or ear canal. The measurement is based on the difference between the thermometer's temperature and the temperature emanating from the target. The instrument has an otoscope-like probe (Fig. 22.3). Disposable plastic probe covers are used for hygiene and to prevent cerumen buildup. Temperatures between 15.5 and 43.3°C can be measured (24). One study showed this device had an accuracy of 0.1°C between 34.0 and 39.5°C

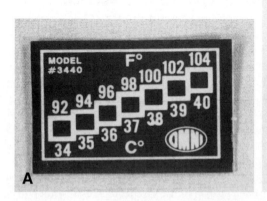

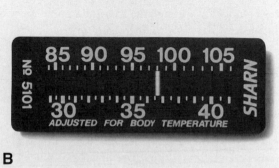

FIGURE 22.2.   The flexible adhesive-backed strips of these liquid-crystal temperature monitors have a black background. To use, the covering over the adhesive is removed, and the monitor is placed on the skin. (**B**, courtesy of Sharn Inc.)

FIGURE **22.3.** The infrared thermometer's probe is inserted into the external ear canal.

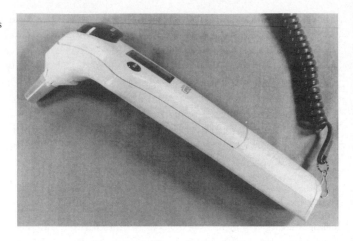

(25). Other studies have shown slightly less accuracy (26). These devices are well-tolerated by patients (20). They are stable over a wide range of patient and ambient temperatures (20). Because the device does not contact any surface, there should be no trauma associated with its use. Measurements are rapid (27). Disadvantages include the fact that measurement is intermittent. Poor penetration, improper aiming, and obstructions such as curvatures of the ear canal will result in significantly lower temperatures. Many have offsets to correct for these factors (19, 26).

SITES

Temperature can be monitored at a number of body sites. The temperature can vary considerably in different parts of the body at any time. Factors influencing temperature at any given site include the tissue's heat production, the temperature and rate of blood flow through the area, the amount of insulation from the environment, and any external influences on the site (28). During passive or active heating or cooling, one part of the body may be markedly warmer than another. It may then be helpful to monitor two sites. The difference between core and a second site can provide indirect information on blood flow (slow change = poor blood flow) and is helpful in guarding against an overshoot during warming or cooling. When significant changes in body heat are expected, core temperatures should be monitored. The core compartment is composed of well-perfused tissues with a uniform temperature. Core temperature reflects the amount of heat generated in the most central and vital body organs (heart, brain, liver, and kidney). Core tissues contribute 80 to 90% of the thermal input to the thermoregulatory system. Sites differ in how well they reflect core temperature and this may depend on the rate of temperature change. A site that reflects core temperature accurately when temperature change is slow may fail to reflect rapid changes, such as are seen with cardiac surgery. Some believe that the temperature of the hypothalamus should be regarded as the true core temperature because the control center for temperature regulation is located there (3).

Skin

Skin temperature can be measured using liquid crystal devices or flat metal discs containing thermocouples or thermistors (Fig. 22.4). Some skin probes have a special backing to insulate the sensor from ambient conditions and may have a coating to reflect radiant heat and light. Use of an opaque dressing and/or tape over the sensor may decrease the effect of environmental factors on the reading. Skin temperature is most commonly measured at the forehead, because this site has a fairly good blood flow and there is not much underlying fat. The back, chest, anterior abdominal wall, fingers, toes, and the inside of the elbow have also been used. The skin of the forehead gives a better correlation with core temperatures than neck skin (29). Skin temperature may be useful in evaluating the quality of a nerve block. A rise in temperature is

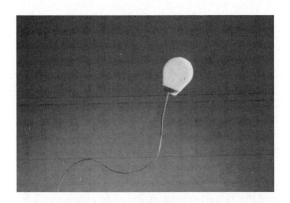

FIGURE 22.4. Disposable probe for measuring skin temperature. Note the backing that insulates the sensor from ambient conditions. (Courtesy of Mallinkrodt, Inc.)

an indication that the block is successful. Another use is in microsurgery. An increase in skin temperature may indicate that blood flow to that area has increased. The correlation of skin temperature with core temperature is controversial. In some studies it has been found to correlate well (13, 30–34). Other investigations have found that skin temperature does not accurately reflect core temperature and there may not be a relation between a change in skin temperature and a change in core temperature (7, 13, 35–47). Readings are affected by ambient temperature, use of skin-surface warming devices, intraoperative changes in cardiac output, and regional vasoconstriction (29, 48). Its usefulness as a screening device for malignant hyperthermia is limited, as cutaneous vasoconstriction may occur with this syndrome (38, 49). Monitoring skin temperature carries few risks, and the site is easily accessible. It may be useful in situations in which other means of obtaining a temperature cannot be used.

Axilla

To measure axillary temperature, the probe should be positioned over the axillary artery and the arm adducted (7). It should not be used on the same side as a blood pressure cuff on the upper arm. Equilibration may take 10 to 15 min (49). Axillary temperature monitoring is convenient, noninvasive, and carries little risk. It is most frequently used on infants and children. Readings

are influenced by contact with the probe, skin perfusion, and proximity of the probe to the axillary artery. Studies differ on how well temperatures measured at this site relate to core temperatures with some showing good (7, 39) and some poor (41, 47, 50–58) correlation.

Nasopharynx

The temperature of the nasopharynx is measured with the sensor in contact with the posterior nasopharyngeal wall. This should place it close to the hypothalamus. Readings taken with a probe in this position are normally not affected by the temperature of inspired gases, unless there is leakage around the tracheal tube (59, 60). Although some studies show a good correlation with core temperature (6, 37, 41, 47, 51), in others the correlation is less satisfactory (34, 60–63). An advantage of this site is that it is usually easily accessible during surgery. However, it cannot be used in nonintubated patients. Epistaxis may follow insertion of the probe (64).

Urinary Bladder

Urinary catheters with a temperature sensor near the patient end are available (Fig. 22.5). The temperature of the urinary bladder usually correlates well with those measured by tympanic membrane, pulmonary artery, and esophageal sensors (27, 55, 65–67), but may lag behind during rapid warming or cooling (26, 37, 39–41, 47, 68–72). The correlation will be increased with a high rate of urine flow (70). This method is useful in pa-

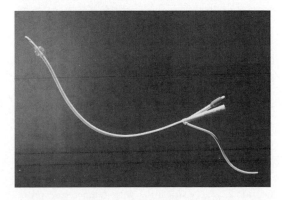

FIGURE 22.5. Urinary catheter with temperature sensor near the patient end. (Courtesy of Mallinkrodt, Inc.)

tients who need a urinary catheter during the postoperative period. It should not be used during genitourinary procedures (71).

Esophagus

Measurement of esophageal temperature can be accomplished using a simple probe, esophageal stethoscope with a temperature sensor (Fig. 22.6), or gastric tube with the temperature sensor some distance from the end of the tube (Fig. 22.7) (73). The temperature in the esophagus can vary up to 4°C (74, 75). It should be measured with the sensor located in the lower third or fourth of the esophagus (74, 76). At this depth, the esophagus lies between the heart and the descending aorta. Placement in this position will minimize

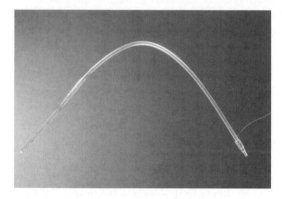

FIGURE 22.6. Esophageal stethoscope and temperature probe. (Courtesy of Mallinkrodt, Inc.)

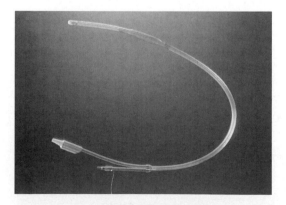

FIGURE 22.7. Gastric tube with temperature probe. This also functions as an esophageal stethoscope. (Courtesy of Mallinkrodt, Inc.)

(but not completely eliminate) the effect of the temperature of respired gases (7, 76). If the probe is placed higher in the esophagus, the reading will be lowered by inspired gases (60, 74, 75, 77–79). If the probe is placed in the stomach, it may record temperatures higher than core, reflecting liver metabolism. Also, the response time to changes in temperature is slow with the probe in this position. The probe is most accurately placed by using an electrocardiographic lead built into the probe (80). The positive lead is attached to the probe and the negative lead to the right shoulder. A biphasic P wave indicates that the probe tip is at the midatrial level. In adults, the ideal position is approximately 38 to 46 cm below the central incisors (75), 24 cm below the larynx (74, 77), and 45 cm from the nostril (81). Other formulas for determining the proper depth are as follows (82):

$$L \text{ (cm)} = 0.228 \times \text{(standing height)} - 0.194$$
$$\text{or } L \text{ (cm)} = 0.479 \times \text{(sitting height)} - 4.44$$

where L is the length from the opening to the nares. In children, the ideal distance in centimeters below the corniculate cartilages is approximated by the following formula (78):

$$10 + (2 \times \text{age in years})/3 \text{ cm.}$$

When the sensor is part of an esophageal stethoscope, one method of placement is to locate the point of maximum breath and heart sounds. The ideal depth of placement is 12 to 16 cm distal to the point of maximum heart sounds (6, 75, 83). Esophageal temperature follows quantitatively and quickly temperature changes in the pulmonary artery (84). Brain temperature may be adequately reflected by esophageal temperature during mild but not profound hypothermia (47, 62, 85). The esophagus is easily accessible during most general anesthesia. Probes are easily inserted without significant risk and are relatively inexpensive. Contraindications to use of an esophageal probe include procedures on the face, oral cavity, nose, airway, or esophagus. It is uncomfortable and poorly tolerated by awake patients. Correct placement may be difficult and probes may become displaced (86). Esophageal temperatures are unreliable during rapid transfusion of cold blood or fluids and during thoracic or upper abdominal surgery (67). Continuous gastric suctioning will cause a decrease in esophageal temperature (87). When an esophageal probe is used with the patient in the sitting or prone position, oral secretions can track down to the connection between the probe and monitor cable. This can lead to incorrect readings (8).

Tympanic Membrane

The anatomical position of the tympanic membrane deep within the skull and separated from the internal carotid artery by only the narrow air-filled cleft of the middle ear and a thin shell of bone makes it an attractive site for temperature measurements. Temperature can be measured by inserting a thermistor or thermocouple probe into the external auditory canal until it contacts the membrane (88). The anterior lower part of the membrane is recommended (42). Because of the danger of perforation of the membrane, clinicians tend not to place the probe far enough into the canal. If it does not touch the membrane, the readings will not be accurate (89). Tympanic membrane probes are shown in Figure 22.8. The sensor is enclosed in soft foam. It usually has a widened segment, piece of foam, or a feather or barb to hold it in place after insertion. After insertion the reading should stabilize quickly. If it does not, the probe should be slowly advanced until the reading stabilizes. Infrared temperature measurement is performed by inserting an otoscope-like probe into

the external ear canal (23). A tug on the ear to straighten the canal when taking a reading improves correlation with core temperatures (90). Numerous studies have shown a good correlation between tympanic membrane temperature and temperature measured in the esophagus or pulmonary artery (7, 26, 46, 55, 58, 81, 88, 91–94). However, with profound hypothermia, an accurate estimate of brain temperature may not be obtained (47). Ambient air temperature will influence the readings, but the effect is minimal if the probe is correctly placed (42, 95). Cerumen may render readings inaccurate using a probe, but not infrared technology because ear wax is essentially transparent to infrared energy (96–98). Acute otitis media will not influence the reading unless there is suppuration, in which case the reading will be increased slightly (97, 99–102). Advantages of tympanic membrane temperature monitoring include cleanliness and convenience. It is tolerated by conscious patients, making it useful for postoperative monitoring. The site is readily accessible during most surgical procedures. Complications have been reported. Oozing from the ear, trauma to the external auditory canal with subsequent otitis externa, and perforation of the membrane have been reported (81, 103–105), but these occurred before the advent of flexible cotton-tipped probes that appear to be much less traumatic (6). Recommended methods to avoid trauma include otoscopic inspection of the canal

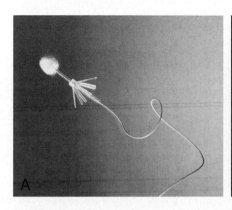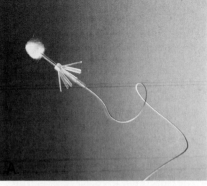

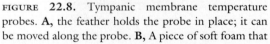

FIGURE 22.8. Tympanic membrane temperature probes. **A,** the feather holds the probe in place; it can be moved along the probe. **B,** A piece of soft foam that can be moved along the probe helps hold the probe in place. (**A,** courtesy of Mallinkrodt, Inc.)

and drum before insertion, stopping insertion as soon as resistance is felt, and placement in awake patients to assess discomfort. Care should be taken to make sure the probe is not pushed into the canal when the head is moved. Contraindications include any abnormality of the ear that would prevent correct placement, a skull fracture that passes through the osseous meatus, and perforation of the membrane (106).

Pulmonary Artery

Pulmonary artery temperature can be measured in patients who have a Swan-Ganz catheter in place. It generally correlates well with brain temperature even with rapid cooling and rewarming (51), although poor correlation with brain temperature has been found with profound hypothermic circulatory arrest (47). Pulmonary artery readings are not reliable during thoracotomy or cardiopulmonary bypass when there is no flow through the heart and lungs and may be directly affected by the cardioplegia used during cooling.

Oral Cavity

Oral temperature is measured by placing a probe in one of the pockets on either side of the frenulum of the tongue. Here the probe is in close proximity to branches of the lingual artery (28). Probe placement is critical; the temperature just a few centimeters away can vary significantly (19). The patient's mouth should be closed and enough time allowed for the reading to be accurate (6). Studies have found a close relationship with pulmonary artery and tympanic temperatures (39, 55, 107, 108). The temperature measured will be slightly higher with a tracheal tube in place (57). Respiratory rate, presence or absence of teeth, mouth position, and the temperature within the tracheal tube have no effect. An increase in oral temperature may be seen if the ambient environment is warm but cold does not appear to affect the reading (95).

Rectum

In the past, measurement of rectal temperature was commonly performed during anesthesia. Measurements are best made at a depth of 8 or more centimeters. In children, 3 cm is the sug-

gested depth (27). Rectal temperature is commonly higher than core temperature (25, 41, 51, 86, 109). Readings will be affected by blood returning from the lower limbs, peritoneal lavage and cystoscopy. Changes in temperature at this site tend to lag behind those at other sites because of the area's low blood flow and the presence of rectal contents that form a thermal reservoir so that it does not reflect core temperature (6, 34, 37, 47, 51, 54, 63, 70, 84, 86, 92, 104, 110, 111). This method is generally disliked by patients as uncomfortable, hospital personnel as cumbersome, and both as aesthetically objectionable. The probes are prone to extrusion during recovery. Other disadvantages are the relative inaccessibility during surgery and the risk of bacterial contamination. Contraindications include obstetric, gynecologic, and urologic procedures. Bowel perforation is a risk. A pararectal abscess has been reported associated with its use (112).

Trachea

Temperatures in the trachea can be measured with a tracheal tube with the sensor in the cuff (113). Temperatures measured at this site correlate well with temperatures measured at core sites (113–115).

USE

Reusable probes must be thoroughly cleaned and disinfected between uses. They are subject to wear and tear and must be checked before use. If the thermometer has a range that includes normal operating room temperature, a one-point calibration check can be performed. When unexpected and extreme temperature readings are seen, the accuracy should be verified by another means. It is important that the connection between the probe and the cable be kept dry to avoid incorrect readings (8,11). Use of waterproof tape is recommended.

HAZARDS OF THERMOMETRY
Damage to the Monitoring Site

Tympanic membrane and rectal perforation and trauma to the external auditory canal, rectum and esophagus have been reported (81, 103–105, 112, 116, 117). A wire may protrude from the tip of the probe (118). Epistaxis may occur with a nasopharyngeal probe.

Burns (119–121)

Burns can occur at the site of measurement if the probe acts as a ground for the electrosurgical apparatus. No insulation can completely block radiofrequency currents, and if there is no other satisfactory return path, the current can burn through insulation (122). Using a battery-operated device is no guarantee of electrical safety, because the chassis may be grounded through a metal support. Temperature probes should be examined before use to detect damage to the insulation. Esophageal burns may be avoided by inserting the probe via a small tracheal tube (123). The probe may be pulled back into the tube during periods of maximal electrical activity. A burn associated with temperature monitoring during magnetic resonance imaging has been reported (124). This occurred with a probe designed for use during magnetic resonance imaging.

Incorrect Information

A faulty probe can cause an incorrect temperature to be displayed (125–128). Secretions or fluids in the connection between the probe and reading instrument can result in falsely elevated readings (8, 11). It is important to use probes that are electronically compatible with the monitor used. Jacks that fit the receptacle but have internal electronics incompatible with the monitor can give false readings and may affect blood pressure and heart rate readings by the same instrument.

REFERENCES

1. Epstein BS. Generic quality screen guidelines and temperature monitoring. American Society of Anesthesiologists Newsletter 1992;56:30–1.
2. Holloway AM. Monitoring and controlling temperature. Anaesthesia and Intensive Care 1988;16:44–47.
3. Sessler DI. Temperature monitoring should be routine during general anesthesia. Anesthesiol Rev 1992;19:40–43.
4. Kaplan RF. Temperature monitoring need not be done routinely during general anesthesia. Anesthesiol Rev 1992;19:43–46.
5. Anonymous. Standards for basic intra-operative monitoring. Anesthesia Patient Safety Foundation Newsletter 1987;51,2:3.
6. Frank SM. Body temperature monitoring. Anesth Clin N Amer 1994;12:387–407.
7. Bissonnette B, Sessler KI, LaFlamme P. Intraoperative temperature monitoring sites in infants and children and the effect of inspired gas warming on esophageal temperature. Anesth Analg 1989;69:192–196.
8. Berman MF. The susceptibility of thermistor-based esophageal temperature probes to errors caused by electrically conductive fluids ("artificial saliva"). Journal of Clinical Monitoring 1992;8:107–110.
9. Imrie MM, Hall GM. Body temperature and anaesthesia. Br J Anaesth 1990;64:346–354.
10. Vrtis AM. Clinical temperature measurement. In: Marohn ML, Muldoon SM, eds. Problems in Anesthesia. 1994;8:11–22.
11. Berman MF. An unusual cause of misleading temperature readings. Anesthesiology 1990;72:208.
12. Wiegert PE. An unusual cause of misleading temperature readings. Anesthesiology 1990;72:208.
13. Burgess GE, Cooper JR, Marino RJ, et al. Continuous monitoring of skin temperature using a liquid-crystal thermometer during anesthesia. South Med J 1978;71:516–518.
14. Bjoraker DG. Liquid crystal temperature indicators. Anesthesiol Rev 1990;17:50–56.
15. MacKenzie R, Asbury AJ. Clinical evaluation of liquid crystal skin thermometers. Br J Anaesth 1994;72:246–249.
16. Shomaker TS, Bjoraker DG. Measurement offset with liquid crystal temperature indicators. Anesthesiology 1990;73:A425.
17. Enright CF. Colorful thermometers. ASTM Stand News. 1986;14(3):67.
18. Marsh ML, Sessler DI. Failure of intraoperative liquid-crystal temperature monitoring. Anesth Analg 1996;82:1102–1104.
19. Anonymous. Infrared thermometers. An earful of innovation. Technology for Anesthesia 1992;12(7):1–7.
20. Weiss ME, Pue AF, Smith J III. Laboratory and hospital testing of new infrared tympanic thermometers. J Clin Eng 1991;16:137–144.
21. Lopez M, Ozaki M, Sessler DI, et al. Clinical evaluation of the Oratemp 3000 and light touch infrared thermometers. Anesthesiology 1993;79:A524.
22. Matsukawa T, Ozaki M, Hanagata K, et al. A comparison of four infrared tympanic thermometers with tympanic membrane temperatures measured by thermocouples. Can J Anaesth 1996;43:1224–1228.
23. Edge G, Morgan M. The Genius infrared tympanic

thermometer. An evaluation for clinical use. Anesthesia 1993;48:604–607.

24. Ward L, Kaplan RM, Paris PM. A comparison of tympanic and rectal temperatures in the emergency department. Ann Emerg Med 1988;17:198.

25. Shinozaki T, Deane R, Perkins FW. Infrared tympanic thermometer. Evaluation of a new clinical thermometer. Crit Care Med 1988;16:148–150.

26. Nierman DM. Core temperature measurement in the intensive care unit. Crit Care Med 1991;19: 818–823.

27. Daneman HL. Fever thermometry. Medical Electronics 1991;68–73.

28. Blainey CG. Site selection in taking body temperature. Am J Nurs 1974;74:1859–1860.

29. Ikeda T, Sessler DI, Marder D, et al. Influence of thermoregulatory vasomotion and ambient temperature variation on the accuracy of core-temperature estimates by cutaneous liquid-crystal thermometers. Anesthesiology 1997;86:603–612.

30. Lees DE, Schuette W, Bull JM, et al. An evaluation of liquid-crystal thermometry as a screening device for intraoperative hyperthermia. Anesth Analg 1978; 57:669–674.

31. Allen GC, Horrow JC, Rosenberg H. Does forehead liquid crystal temperature accurately reflect "core" temperature? Can J Anaesth 1990;37:659–662.

32. Brull SJ, Cunningham AJ, Connelly NR, et al. Liquid crystal skin thermometry: an accurate reflection of core temperature? Can J Anaesth 1993;40:375–381.

33. Brull SJ, O'Connor TZ, Poglitsch E, et al. Comparison of crystalline skin temperature and esophageal temperature during anesthesia. Anesthesiology 1990; 73:A472.

34. Sakuragi T, Mukai M, Dan K. Deep body temperature during the warming phase of cardiopulmonary bypass. Br J Anaesth 1993;71:583–585.

35. Lacoumenta S, Hall GM. Liquid crystal thermometry during anaesthesia. Anaesthesia 1984;39:54–56.

36. Leon JE, Bissonnette B, Lerman J. Liquid crystalline temperature monitoring: does it estimate core temperature in anaesthetized paediatric patients? Can J Anaesth 1990;37:S98.

37. Moorthy SS, Winn BA, Jallard MS, et al. Monitoring urinary bladder temperature. Heart Lung 1985;14: 90–93.

38. Vaughan MS, Cork RC, Vaughan RW. Inaccuracy of liquid crystal thermometry to identify core temperature trends in postoperative adults. Anesth Analg 1982;61:284–287.

39. Ilsley AH, Rutten AJ, Runciman WB. An evaluation of body temperature measurement. Anaesthesia and Intensive Care 1983;11:31–39.

40. Earp JK, Finlayson DC. Urinary bladder/pulmonary artery temperature ratio of less than 1 and shivering in cardiac surgical patients. Am J Crit Care 1992;1: 43–52.

41. Cork RC, Vaughan RW, Humphrey LS. Precision and accuracy of intraoperative temperature monitoring. Anesth Analg 1983;62:211–214.

42. Brinnel H, Cabanac M. Tympanic temperature is a core temperature in humans. J Therm Biol 1989;14: 47–53.

43. Iaizzo PA, Zink RS, Kehler CH, et al. Skin and central temperatures during malignant hyperthermia in swine. Anesthesiology 1992;77:A569.

44. Mayfield SR, Bhatia J, Nakamura KT, et al. Temperature measurement in term and preterm neonates. J Pediatr 1984;104:271–275.

45. Patel N, Smith CE, Costello F, et al. Comparison of esophageal, tympanic and skin temperatures in adults. Anesthesiology 1994;81:A598.

46. Patel N, Smith CE, Pinchak AC, et al. Comparison of esophageal, tympanic, and forehead skin temperatures in adult patients. J Clin Anesth 1996;8: 462–468.

47. Stone JG, Young WL, Smith CR, et al. Do standard monitoring sites reflect true brain temperature when profound hypothermia is rapidly induced and reversed? Anesthesiology 1995;82:344–351.

48. Sessler DI, Moayeri A. Skin-surface warming: heat flux and central temperature. Anesthesiology 1990; 73:218–224.

49. Sladen RM. Temperature regulation and anesthesia (ASA Refresher Course #243). New Orleans: ASA, 1990.

50. Stewart SM, Luhan E, Ruff CL. Incidence of adult hypothermia in the post anesthesia care unit. Perioper Nurs Q 1987;3:57–62.

51. Stone JG, Young WL, Smith CR, et al. Do temperatures recorded at standard monitoring sites reflect actual brain temperature during deep hypothermia. Anesthesiology 1991;75:A483.

52. Kamal GD, Hasell RH, Pyle SM, et al. Inconsistent relationship between axillary and tympanic temperature following general anesthesia. Anesth Analg 1992;74:S155.

53. Casey WF, Broadman LM, Rice LJ, et al. Comparison of liquid crystal skin temperature probe and axillary thermistor probe in measuring core temperature trends during anaesthesia in paediatric patients. Can J Anaesth 1989;36:S62–S63.

54. Allen GC, Horrow JC, Rosenberg H. Does forehead liquid crystal temperature accurately reflect "core" temperature? Can J Anaesth 1990;37:659–662.

55. Erickson RS, Kirklin SK. Comparison of ear-based, bladder, oral and axillary methods for core temperature measurement. Crit Care Med 1993;21: 1528–1534.

56. Kamal GD, Hasell RH, Pyle SM, et al. Inconsistent relationship between axillary and tympanic temperature following general anesthesia. Anesth Analg 1992; 74:S155.

57. Konopad E, Kerr JR, Noseworthy T, et al. A comparison of oral, axillary, rectal and tympanic-membrane temperatures of intensive care patients with and without oral endotracheal tube. J Adv Nurs 1994;20: 77–84.

58. Summers S. Axillary, tympanic, and esophageal temperature measurement: descriptive comparisons in postanesthesia patients. J Post Anesth Nurs 1991;6: 420–425.

59. Siegal MN, Gravenstein N. Use of a heat and moisture exchanger partially improves the correlation between esophageal and core temperature. Anesthesiology 1988;69:A284.

60. Whitby JD, Dunkin LJ. Cerebral esophageal and nasopharyngeal temperatures. Br J Anaesth 1971;43: 673–676.

61. Grocott HP, Croughwell ND, Lowery E, et al. Comparison between jugular venous bulb and nasopharyngeal temperatures during cardiac surgery. Anesth Analg 1996; 82:SCA85.

62. Hindman BJ, Dexter F. Estimating brain temperature during hypothermia. Anesthesiology 1995;82: 329–330.

63. Kern FH, Greeley WJ. Con: Monitoring of nasopharyngeal and rectal temperatures is not an adequate guide of brain cooling before deep hypothermic circulatory arrest. J Cardiothor Vasc Anesth 1994;8: 363–365.

64. Singleton RJ, Ludbrook GL, Webb RK, et al. Physical injuries and environmental safety in anaesthesia: an analysis of 2000 incident reports. Anaesthesia and Intensive Care 1993;21:659–663.

65. Earp JK, Finlayson DC. Relationship between urinary bladder and pulmonary artery temperatures: A preliminary study. Heart and Lung 1991;20:265–270.

66. Imaizumi H, Tsunoda K, Ichimiya N, et al. Urinary bladder temperature monitoring in extensively burned patients. Journal of Clinical Monitoring 1993;9:99–100.

67. Russell SH, Freeman JW. Comparison of bladder, esophageal and pulmonary artery temperatures in major abdominal surgery. Anaesthesia 1996;51: 338–340.

68. Mravinac CM, Dracup K, Clochesy JM. Urinary bladder and rectal temperature monitoring during clinical hypothermia. Nurs Res 1989;38:73–76.

69. Lilly JK, Boland JP, Zekan S. Urinary bladder temperature monitoring. A new index of body core temperature. Crit Care Med 1980;8:742–744.

70. Horrow JC, Rosenberg H. Does urinary catheter temperature reflect core temperature during cardiac surgery? Anesthesiology 1988;69:986–989.

71. Glosten B, Sessler DI, Faure E, et al. Bladder versus tympanic core temperature measurement during cesarean section. Anesthesiology 1990;73:A960.

72. Bone ME, Feneck RO. Bladder temperature as an estimate of body temperature during cardiopulmonary bypass. Anaesthesia 1988;43:181–185.

73. Koyama K, Takahashi J, Ochiai R, et al. Evaluation of esophageal temperature measured by gastric tube with thermistor. Can J Anaesth 1990;37:S111.

74. Whitby JD, Dunkin LJ. Temperature differences in the oesophagus. Br J Anaesth 1968;40:991–995.

75. Kaufman RD. Relationship between esophageal temperature gradient and heart and lung sounds heard by esophageal stethoscope. Anesth Analg 1987;66: 1046–1048.

76. Bloch EC, Ginsberg B, Binner RA. The esophageal temperature gradient in anesthetized children. Journal of Clinical Monitoring 1993;9:73–77.

77. Whitby JD, Dunkin LJ. Temperature differences in the oesophagus. Br J Anaesth 1969;41:615–618.

78. Whitby JD, Dunkin LJ. Esophageal temperature differences in children. Br J Anaesth 1970;42: 1013–1015.

79. Siegel MN, Gravenstein N. Passive warming of airway gases (artificial nose) improves accuracy of esophageal temperature monitoring. Journal of Clinical Monitoring 1990;6:89–92.

80. Brengelmann GL, Johnson JM, Hong PA. Electrocardiographic verification of esophageal temperature probe position. J Appl Physiol 1979;47:638–642.

81. Webb GE. Comparison of esophageal and tympanic temperature monitoring during cardiopulmonary bypass. Anesth Analg 1973;52:729–733.

82. Mekjavic IB, Rempel ME. Determination of esophageal probe insertion length based on standing and sitting height. J Appl Physiol 1990;69:376–379.

83. Freund PR, Brengelmann GL. Placement of esophageal stethoscope by acoustic criteria does not consistently yield an optimal location for the monitoring of core temperature. Journal of Clinical Monitoring 1990;6:266–270.

84. Shiraki K, Konda N, Sagawa S. Esophageal and tympanic temperature responses to core blood temperature changes during hyperthermia. J Appl Physiol 1986;61:98–102.

85. Baker KZ, Stone JG, Osipov AE, et al. Core body temperature correlates with brain parenchymal temperature during mild hypothermia for neurosurgery. J Neurosurg Anesth 1996;8:345.

86. Benzinger M. Tympanic thermometry in surgery and anesthesia. JAMA 1969;209:1207–1211.

87. Nelson EJ, Grissom TE. Continuous gastric suctioning decreases measured esophageal temperature during general anesthesia. Journal of Clinical Monitoring 1996;12:429–432.

88. Walpoth BH, Galdikas J, Leupi F, et al. Assessment of hypothermia with a new "tympanic" thermometer. Journal of Clinical Monitoring 1994;10:91–96.

89. Sharkey A, Elliott P, Giesecke AH, et al. Relations between temperature of the external auditory meatus and the esophagus during anesthesia. Anesthesiology 1986;65:A530.

90. Pransky SM. The impact of technique and conditions of the tympanic membrane upon infrared tympanic thermometry. Clin Pediatr 1991;30(Suppl 4):50–52.

91. Ferrara–Love R. A comparison of tympanic and pulmonary artery measures of core temperatures. J Post Anesth Nurs 1991;6:161–164.

92. Milewski A, Ferguson KL, Terndrup TE. Comparison of pulmonary artery, rectal, and tympanic membrane temperatures in adult intensive care unit patients. Clin Pediatr 1991;30 (Suppl 4):13–16.

93. Romano MJ, Fortenberry JD, Autreu E, et al. Infrared tympanic thermometry in the pediatric intensive care unit. Crit Care Med 1993;21:1181–1185.

94. Rotello LC, Crawford L, Terndrup TE. Comparison of infrared ear thermometer derived and equilibrated rectal temperatures in estimating pulmonary artery temperatures. Crit Care Med 1996;24:1501–1506.

95. Zehner WJ, Terndrup TE. The impact of moderate ambient temperature variance on the relationship between oral rectal and tympanic membrane temperatures. Clin Pediatr 1991;30(Suppl 4):61–64.

96. Morley-Forster PK. Unintentional hypothermia in the operating room. Can Anaesth Soc J 1986;33:516–527.

97. Kenney RD, Fortenberry JD, Surratt SS, et al. Evaluation of an infrared tympanic membrane thermometer in pediatric patients. Pediatrics 1990;85:854–858.

98. Beach PS, McCormick DP. Editorial comment. Clinical applications of ear thermometry. Clin Pediatr 1991;30(Suppl 4):3–4.

99. Terndup TE, Wong A. Influence of otitis media on the correlation between rectal and auditory canal temperatures. Am J Dis Child 1991;145:75–78.

100. Treloar D, Muma B. Comparison of axillary, tympanic membrane, and rectal temperatures in young children. Ann Emerg Med 1988;17:198.

101. Muma BK, Treloar DJ, Wurmlinger K, et al. Comparison of rectal, axillary, and tympanic membrane temperatures in infants and young children. Ann Emerg Med 1991;20:41–44.

102. Kelly B, Alexander D. Effect of otitis media on infrared tympanic thermometry. Clin Pediatr 1991;30(Suppl 4):46–48.

103. Tabor MW, Blaho DM, Schriver WR. Tympanic membrane perforation. Complication of tympanic thermometry during general anesthesia. Oral Surg 1981;51:581–583.

104. Dickey WT, Ahlgren EW, Stephen CR. Body temperature monitoring via the tympanic membrane. Surgery 1970;67:981–984.

105. Wallace CT, Marks WE, Adkins WY, et al. Perforation of the tympanic membrane. A complication of tympanic thermometry during anesthesia. Anesthesiology 1974;41:290–291.

106. Anonymous. Tympanic thermometry during anesthesia. Arch Otolaryngol 1969;90:28.

107. Audiss D, Brengelmann G, Bond E. Variations in the temperature differences between pulmonary artery and sublingual temperatures. Heart Lung 1989;18:294–295.

108. Erickson RS. Comparison of tympanic and oral temperatures in surgical patients. Nurs Res 1991;40:90–93.

109. Nilsson K. Maintenance and monitoring of body temperature in infants and children. Pediatr Anaesth 1991;1:13–20.

110. Benzinger TH. Clinical temperature. JAMA 1969;209:1200–1206.

111. Estebe J-P. Use of a pneumatic tourniquet induces changes in central temperature. Br J Anaesth 1996;77:786–788.

112. Di Paola I, Macneil P. Rectal thermometer complication. Anaesthesia and Intensive Care 1985;13:441.

113. Hayes JK, Collette DJ, Peters JL, et al. Monitoring body-core temperature from the trachea: comparison between pulmonary artery, tympanic, esophageal and rectal temperatures. Journal of Clinical Monitoring 1996;12:261–269.

114. Yamakage M, Kawana S, Wantanabe H, et al. The utility of tracheal temperature monitoring. Anesth Analg 1993;76:795–799.

115. Kawano Y, Imai M, Komura Y, et al. Tracheal cuff as a new core temperature site. Anesthesiology 1992;77:A563.

116. Greenbaum EI, Carson M, Kincannon WN, et al. Rectal thermometer-induced pneumoperitoneum in the newborn. Pediatrics 1989;44:539–542.

117. Merenstein GB. Rectal perforation by thermometer. Lancet 1970;1:1007.

118. Anonymous. "Tissue agitation" cited in temperature probe recall. Biomedical Safety & Standards 1989; 19:67–68.

119. Parker EO. Electrosurgical burn at the site of an esophageal temperature probe. Anesthesiology 1984; 61:93–95.

120. Schneider AJL, Apple HP, Braun RT. Electrosurgical burns at skin temperature probes. Anesthesiology 1977;47:72–74.

121. Wald AS, Mazzia VDB, Spencer FC. Accidental burns. JAMA 1971;217:916–921.

122. Anderson GD. Electrosurgery units, not temperature probes, must be corrected to prevent burns. Anesthesiology 1985;62:834.

123. Weis FR, Kaiser RE. Technique of avoiding esophageal burns. Anesthesiology 1985; 62:370.

124. Hall SC, Stevenson GW, Suresh S. Burn associated with temperature monitoring during magnetic resonance imaging. Anesthesiology 1992;76:152.

125. Chapin JW, Moravec M. Faulty temperature probe. Anesthesiology 1980;52:187.

126. Davies AO. Malignant temperature probe. Can Anaesth Soc J 1980;27:179–180.

127. Anonymous. Inaccurate temperature displays with Sheridan Sonatemp temperature monitors and defective YSI 400/700 probes. Health Devices 1994;23: 145–146.

128. Cohen JA, Winston RS. Assessment of masseter spasm complicated by a faulty temperature probe. J Clin Anesth 1994;6:521–524.

QUESTIONS

Each question below contains four suggested answers of which one or more is correct. Choose the answer:

A. if 1, 2, and 3 are correct
B. if 1 and 3 are correct
C. if 2 and 4 are correct
D. if 4 is correct
E. if 1, 2, 3, and 4 are correct.

1. Consequences of hypothermia include
   1. Cardiac arrhythmias
   2. Hypermetabolism
   3. Increased risk of postoperative sepsis
   4. Decreased incidence of myocardial ischemia

2. Hyperthermia may be caused by
   1. Sepsis
   2. Drug reactions
   3. Malignant hyperthermia
   4. Hypothyroidism

3. Advantages of thermistors include
   1. Stable resistance with rapid and too large changes in temperature
   2. Interchangeable and disposable probes
   3. Stable resistance over a long time span
   4. Rapid response

4. With the platinum wire thermometer
   1. Current flows in proportion to the temperature difference
   2. Rapid thermal equilibration is possible because of the diameter of the wire
   3. Two wires of different metals are welded together at their ends
   4. Resistance of the wire varies with temperature

5. Advantages of the liquid crystal thermometers include
   1. Fast, continuous readings
   2. Infrared lamps do not interfere with their readings
   3. They can be applied prior to induction
   4. Accuracy even at the extremes of ambient temperature.

6. Advantages of the infrared temperature monitors include
   1. They do not contact the eardrum directly
   2. Stability over a wide range of ambient temperatures
   3. Rapid measurement
   4. Continuous measurement.

7. Concerning core temperature
   1. The core compartments are composed of the well-perfused tissues of uniform temperature
   2. Core tissues contribute 60 to 75% of the thermal input to the thermo-regulatory system
   3. Core temperature reflects the amount of heat generated in the heart, brain, liver, and kidney
   4. The hypothalamus contains the center for core temperature regulation

8. The accuracy of axillary temperature determinations is influenced by
   1. Proximity to the axillary artery
   2. Perfusion of the skin
   3. Skin contact with the probe
   4. Patient age

9. Factors influencing the temperature reading in the nasopharynx include
   1. Temperature of the inspired gases
   2. Leak in the tracheal tube cuff
   3. Epistaxis
   4. Temperature in the hypothalamus

10. For correct use of the esophageal temperature monitor
   1. The sensor should be located in the lower third to quarter of the esophagus
   2. Stomach placement of the probe will provide temperatures lower than core
   3. The probe should be placed 12 to 16 cm distal to the point of maximum heart sounds
   4. Temperature of the respired gases is not a factor in the lower third of the esophagus

11. Factors that can cause esophageal temperatures to be unreliable include
    1. Rapid transfusion of cold blood
    2. Upper abdominal surgery
    3. Continuous gastric suction
    4. Patient in the sitting position

12. When using the tympanic membrane to measure temperature
    1. The probe need not actually contact the membrane
    2. Perforation of the membrane can occur
    3. Readings will be stable if the probe is in close proximity to the membrane
    4. The probe should have a means to hold it in place

13. Factors which will cause incorrect readings from the tympanic membrane include
    1. Cerumen

    2. Ambient air temperature
    3. Otitis media with suppuration
    4. Otitis media without suppuration

14. Factors affecting the temperature measured in the rectum include
    1. Cystoscopy
    2. Peritoneal lavage
    3. Rectal contents
    4. Colon pathology

ANSWERS

1.	A	8.	A
2.	A	9.	C
3.	C	10.	B
4.	C	11.	E
5.	B	12.	C
6.	A	13.	A
7.	A	14.	A

Alarm Devices

ALARMS ARE WARNING signals generated by equipment to indicate abnormal or unusual conditions. The purposes of an alarm are to get attention, transfer information, enhance vigilance, and warn of an existing or developing adverse condition (1–4). Another may be to transfer legal responsibility from the manufacturer to the user (5). It is essential that there be means of alerting personnel to a change in the anesthesia machine, breathing system, or patient for there will always be occasions when his or her vigilance will be lowered or attention reduced by the need to perform other tasks (6). The number of alarms in the anesthetizing areas has increased greatly. To add further confusion, alarm-like sounds may come from sources other than from anesthesia apparatus including electrosurgical apparatus, lasers, warming devices, hearing aids, beepers, blankets, and infusion pumps (7, 8).

STANDARDS

In 1993, an American standard for electronically generated alarm signals for use in anesthesia and respiratory care was published (9). Some of its specifications are shown in Table 23.1. Two international standards are also available and a third one is in preparation (10–12).

AUDIBLE SIGNAL

An audible signal attracts attention faster and more reliably than a visual one (13–15). Ideally, it should do this without startling anybody. Unfortunately, the qualities that cause sounds to attract attention also tend to make them annoying. Some are so unpleasant that the principal response may be to want to make the offensive noise go away rather than address the condition that generated the alarm. Manufacturers may deliberately make alarm sounds intrusive to ensure that their equipment will not be faulted for failing to alert the clinician to a deteriorating situation.

There are a number of options available in alarm sound technology, including variations in pattern, pitch, tone, frequency, and loudness (4). Fundamental frequency, harmonic series, amplitude envelope shape, and delayed harmonics as well as speed, rhythm, pitch range, and melodic structure all have clear and consistent effects on perceived urgency (16, 17). The American Society for Testing and Materials (ASTM) standard requires audible sounds to have a fundamental frequency between 150 and 1000 Hz based on standard musical pitches. There must be at least four frequency components ranging from 300 to 4000 hertz (Hz) and these must be related so that they form a distinct sound. To avoid startling, a low

TABLE 23.1. **Alarm Signals**

Alarm Category	Operator Response	Audible Indicators	Indicator Color	Flashing Frequency
High priority	Immediate	Not medium or low priority	Red	1.4 to 2.8 Hz
Medium priority	Prompt	Not high or low priority	Yellow	0.4 to 0.8 Hz
Low priority	Awareness	Not high or medium priority	Yellow	Constant

From American Society for Testing and Materials. Specification for alarm signals in medical equipment used in anesthesia and respiratory care, (F1463-93) Philadelphia: ASTM, 1993.

onset and offset is required. Adjustable alarms must have a volume between 45 and 85 decibels. Those with fixed intensity must be between 70 and 85 decibels. One of the problems associated with alarm sounds is that clinicians may not hear them. Background noise and other alarms can interfere with alarm detection (18–20). If an audible signal is allowed to sound continuously, other audible alarms may not be noticed (21, 22). An anesthesia provider with a hearing deficit may have difficulty determining the source of sounds. One study showed that 67% of anesthesiologists had an abnormal audiogram with 18% having one or more alarm intensities under their detectability threshold (20). An approach favored in Europe is the Patterson sounds. These tones, originally developed for aviation, were modified for medical equipment. There are three general sounds for advisory, caution, and warning and six categories for ventilation, oxygenation, cardiovascular, artificial perfusion, drug administration, and temperature. Concerns about these sounds have been raised, stemming from questions about their applicability to the operating room setting in view of advances that have been made in monitoring devices and technology, and concern that their use will worsen noise pollution in the operating room (4, 23). Another approach is to have alarm tones play themes from popular songs (24).

AUDIBLE SIGNAL IDENTIFICATION

Once an audible signal is activated, the next step is to identify its origin. This is important because many monitors are not in the clinician's immediate field of view and he or she cannot always turn around. Many anesthesia providers have trouble identifying audible alarms (16, 19, 25–28). The high noise levels in the operating

room may cause some alarm tones to be misidentified. Inability to identify an alarm may delay or prevent the appropriate remedial action (2, 6, 22). The time from onset of an alarm to recognition varies (29). One study determined that the average time to recognition was 61 seconds. Sixteen percent of alarms were unrecognized after 5 minutes. Response times were shorter with healthy patients as opposed to sick ones.

VISUAL SIGNAL

While sounds draw attention to a problem, visual signals give more specific information. Their principal drawback is that they can go unrecognized for a much longer time than audible signals (14, 30). In a situation where the individual responsible for reacting to an alarm is required to use his or her vision for other tasks, a visual message may go unnoticed (25). It may not be possible for the individual to turn and look at the alarm (e.g., during laryngoscopy).

Alarm lights can be coded by color, brightness, size, location, and flashing frequency (4) (Fig. 23.1). Flashing lights are more noticeable and have traditionally been used for more crucial information The standard requirements for visual signals are shown in Table 23.1. Alphanumeric or computer-generated graphic displays of alarm messages, including centralized alarm displays, are exempt from the color and flashing frequency requirements shown in the table. Visual signals must be legible at a distance of 1 m and an angle of 30° from either side of the center of the display or control panel. High- and medium-priority signals must be distinguishable at 4 m.

ALARM PRIORITIZATION

All alarms are not equally important. The information that an alarm conveys may represent an

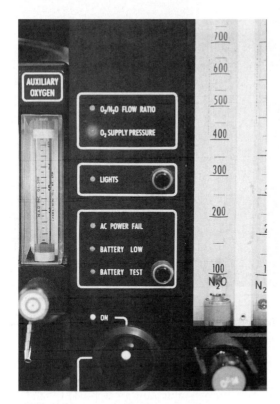

FIGURE **23.1.** A light identifies the source of an audible signal. A flashing light draws more attention than a continuous one.

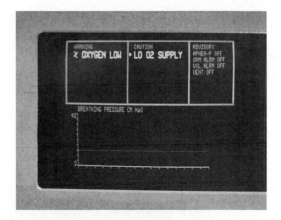

FIGURE **23.2.** One type of alarm organization. The three alarm categories are shown. The single integrated display connects to various monitors. Alarm conditions can be identified in this area.

emergency, the potential for an emergency, or just an unusual condition. Frequently, there is no correlation between an alarm sound and the urgency of the condition it annunciates. Prioritized alarms help to differentiate life-threatening situations from less urgent warnings. The alarm standard divides alarms into three priorities: high, medium, and low (Fig. 23.2). A high-priority alarm indicates a condition that requires immediate action. Medium priority implies a potentially dangerous situation that requires a prompt response. A low-priority alarm indicates that only operator awareness is required. It may or may not have an audible signal. It may be possible to alter alarm priorities, but the priority may only be increased. The object of prioritization is to minimize distraction from less important alarms during an emergency. It has been suggested that only the alarm sound corresponding to the most urgent of the prevailing alarm conditions should be annunciated; all other

sounds should be temporarily suppressed (2). Once the most urgent alarm condition is resolved, the sound corresponding to the next highest priority condition would then be initiated. This priority interlock should be limited to audible annunciation; lower-priority alarm visual indications need not be suppressed because they are unobtrusive.

ORGANIZATION OF ALARMS

Frequently in a monitoring environment, alarm messages arrive in an unorganized pattern. The single integrated display (Fig. 23.2 and Fig. 23.3) is designed to aid alarm identification (2). It is connected to various monitors. Alarm conditions can be identified in this area. Thus anesthesia personnel need look in only one place to identify problems. This area should be repeatedly observed during an alarm situation (21). A disadvantage of this is that a crowded display may be difficult to read during a crisis. Also, it may not be possible to integrate all monitors into a single display.

ALARM SET POINTS

The criteria that determine when an alarm is activated are called the set points (threshold values, limits, thresholds, settings). They should be displayed continuously or be capable of being displayed at the user's discretion so that it can be

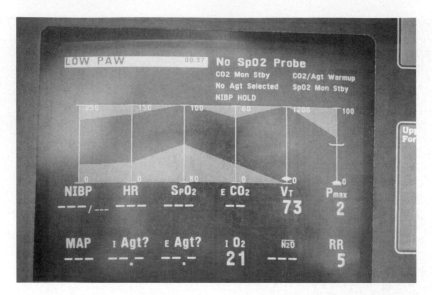

FIGURE 23.3. Another type of alarm organization. Warnings, advisories, and cautions are displayed on the top of the screen. Data from various monitors are displayed both numerically and graphically. Numerical data are at the bottom. Above, measured data are displayed relative to the alarm limits.

determined if the set values are appropriate for the patient and procedure (Figs. 23.4 and 23.5). Limits can be set by either the manufacturer or the user. Those set by the manufacturer may be default values (those that the monitor automatically assumes when it is turned on) or the monitor may analyze data collected for a certain period of time after monitoring has commenced and set the limits based on measured values (6). This is known as a baseline alarm system. Default limits should be set at values likely to provide reasonable protection to most patients. Most monitors allow the user to alter the default settings. Ensuring that an alarm sounds before a dangerous condition has occurred without creating frequent spurious signals requires intelligence on the part of both the alarm system and the user (4, 31). Some operators set limits to wide extremes unlikely to be encountered clinically. Others simply use the limits set by the last person who used the device. Others keep the thresholds close to the safe limits, changing the thresholds often to prevent the occurrence of false alarms. Unfortunately, this may lead the user to disable the alarm (4, 32). Using unrealistic set points can result in an increase in false-positive or false-negative alarms (6). The farther thresholds

are from normal values, the greater the probability that a dangerous condition will occur without activating the alarm. On the other hand, the closer the thresholds are to normal values, the more likely it is that false alarms will be produced. It is good practice to record alarm set points on the anesthesia record. This provides evidence that the alarms were activated. It may also increase the operator's awareness of the alarms and/or make it more likely that appropriate limits will be set.

FALSE ALARMS (33)

If an alarm fails to generate a signal when it should (false negative), the patient's well-being will be threatened. If it is activated without proper cause (false positive), it is annoying and this may lead to its being ignored, silenced, or turned off.

False-Positive Alarms

Many alarms are spurious and only a small number indicate actual risk (34–41). A false alarm requires time and effort to check the actual conditions. This will result in less attention to other tasks and may lead to an inappropriate action which will take additional time and potentially pose a risk to patient safety (4). False alarms are

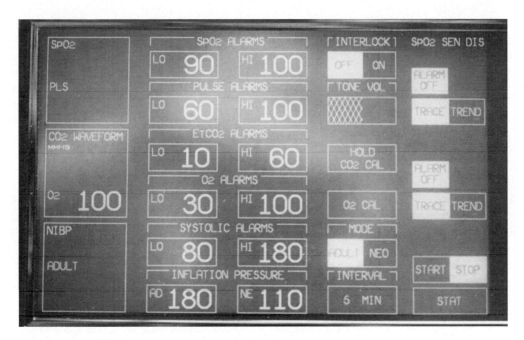

FIGURE 23.4. Alarm set points that can be displayed allow the user to determine if they are appropriate. These can be altered on the screen.

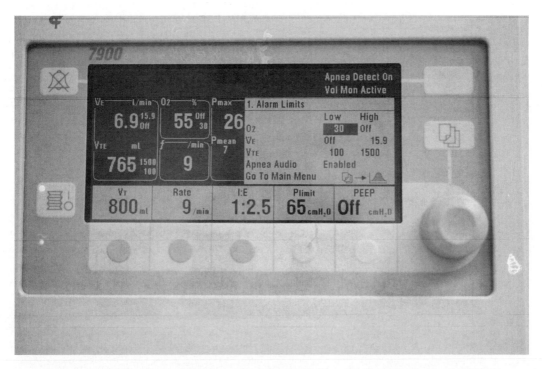

FIGURE 23.5. This alarm set points menu allows the limits to be viewed and altered. Note the temporary silencing touch key at the upper left.

a source of irritation and a threat to patient care, because the anesthesia practitioner becomes increasingly likely to ignore the signals, disable the entire alarm system, silence the alarm without looking for the cause, or set the alarm limits at extreme values (42–44).

There are a number of reasons for false alarms (13). These include alarm malfunction, alarm activation by an inappropriate device, artifacts, extraneous sounds being mistaken for alarm signals, and inappropriate set points. The manufacturer may incorporate narrow default limits to protect itself. The user can reduce the number of false alarms by carefully preparing the patient interface, securely attaching probes and selecting warning devices with artifact rejection capabilities. Setting wide set points and delaying the time between detection of a condition and alarm signal activation will help (32, 45–47). They can be reduced further by changing alarm set points at certain times, since clinical ranges vary during different phases of anesthesia (48). For example, the heart rate limits should be wider during intubation than

maintenance. Another way is to smooth data by repeatedly calculating the median of a number of values in a variable (47). On some pulse oximeters, the time over which signals are averaged can be varied. Increasing the averaging time will decrease the number of false alarms. Comparing data from more than one monitor can reduce the incidence of false alarms (49, 50). False alarms can be reduced by integration of monitors. An example is synchronizing the pulse oximeter and noninvasive blood pressure monitors. If the oximeter probe is on the same arm as the blood pressure cuff, no alarm will sound if no pulse is detected when the cuff is inflated. Another example is the pulse oximeter and electrocardiogram. SpO_2 values are rejected unless the pulse rate measured on the oximeter matches that on the EKG.

False-Negative Alarms

False-negative alarms may be caused by setting the limits too widely, silencing the alarm indefinitely, turning the alarm off, or turning the audible volume so low that it cannot be heard.

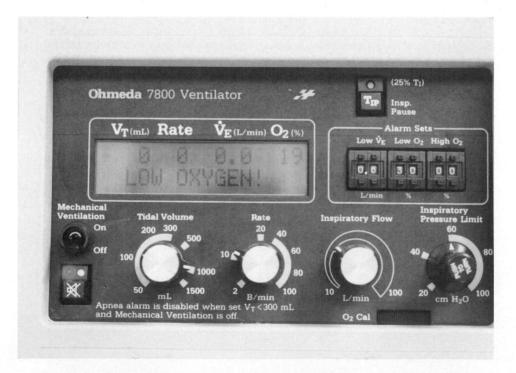

FIGURE **23.6.** The temporary silencing button is at the lower left. The light above it flashes to indicate that silencing is in effect.

ALARM SILENCING
Temporary

After an audible alarm signal has succeeded in capturing the user's attention, silencing (muting, resetting, pausing) it will provide time to correct the situation. The visual component of the alarm indicator and associated functions should still be activated until the condition that triggered the alarm is corrected. If another alarm condition occurs while an alarm is silenced, the additional alarm should have an audible and visual indicator. Most manufacturers provide a means to temporarily silence the auditory signal (Figures 23.6 and 23.7). The silencing time varies with the instrument and can sometimes be varied. Some monitors indicate the elapsed time. The alarm standard requires that there be a visual indication that a high- or medium-priority alarm signal has been silenced.

Indefinite

Some alarms can be turned off (defeated, disabled) for an unlimited time (Figure 23.7). On some the volume control can be decreased to a point where it cannot be heard. The visible signal is still present (51). Some users silence alarms to avoid a startle reaction in the surgeon.

ALARM ENABLING

A feature present on many monitors is automatic enabling. Once the parameter to be monitored is sensed, the alarm is enabled. This eliminates the problem of the user forgetting to turn an alarm back on or not being aware that an alarm has been turned off by someone else.

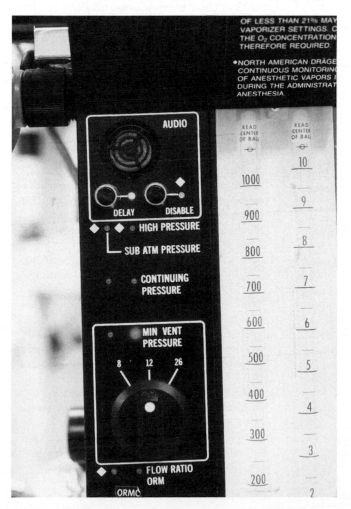

FIGURE 23.7. Pushing the button marked "delay" will result in temporary silencing of audible signals. Pushing the button marked "disable" will cause indefinite silencing of certain alarms.

SMART ALARMS (33, 41, 48, 52–59)

With a smart (expert, intelligent) alarm system, when an alarm condition is sensed, the smart alarm, a neural network, or rule-based system identifies the source, analyzes the data using algorithms, provides the operator with a list of conditions that could have triggered the alarm(s), and presents information helpful in dealing with the condition that triggered the alarm. When several alarm conditions occur simultaneously, a smart alarm system can distinguish between them and decide whether one alarm is more important than another. Smart alarms can reduce the number of false alarms by discriminating between artifacts and truly threatening conditions. Human response times are longer and have greater variability with conventional alarms than intelligent alarms (60, 61). They may help free up the anesthesia provider to focus efforts on the patient while the alarm system finds or identifies technical problems (62). A problem with developing and using smart alarms is integrating stand-alone monitors. One solution is to purchase all monitors from a single vendor. Another is to incorporate the smart alarm into a data management system.

REFERENCES

1. Beneken JEW, van der Aa JJ. Alarms and their limits in monitoring. Journal of Clinical Monitoring 1989; 5:205–210.
2. Schreiber PJ, Schreiber J. Structured alarm systems for the operating room. Journal of Clinical Monitoring 1989;5:201–204.
3. Quinn ML. Semipractical alarms. A parable. Journal of Clinical Monitoring 1989;5:196–200.
4. Weinger MB, Smith NT. Vigilance, alarms, and integrated monitoring systems. In: Ehrenwerth J, Eisenkraft JB, Eds. Anesthesia equipment, principles and applications. St. Louis: CV Mosby, 1993:350–384.
5. Hayman WA, Drinker PA. Design of medical device alarm systems. Med Instrum 1983;17:103–106.
6. Sykes MK. Panel on practical alarms. Journal of Clinical Monitoring 1989;5:192–193.
7. Elliott B, Chestnut J. Dangers of alarms. Anaesthesia 1996;51:799–800.
8. Zmyslowski WP, Ravi VS, Chua M, et al. Spurious anesthesia alarm in an anesthetized patient. Anesthesiology 1993;79:1150–1151.
9. American Society for Testing and Materials. Specification for alarm signals in medical equipment used in anesthesia and respiratory care (F1463–93). Philadelphia, PA: ASTM; 1993.
10. International Standards Organization. Anaesthetic and respiratory care alarm signals—Part I: Visual alarm signals. (ISO 9703–1:1992). Geneva: ISO, 1992.
11. International Standards Organization. Anaesthetic and respiratory care alarm signals—Part II: Auditory alarm signals. (ISO 9703–2:1994). Geneva: ISO, 1994.
12. Welyczko GL, Graber MD. International standards for visual and auditory alarm signals for medical devices. Biomed Instrum Technol 1994;24:228–231.
13. Morgan CT, Cook JS III, Chapanis A, et al. Eds. Human engineering guide to equipment design. New York: McGraw-Hill, 1963.
14. Morris R, Montano S. Monitoring the monitors: how quickly do anaesthetists react to an alarm. Anaesthesia and Intensive Care 1993;21:241–242.
15. Morris RW, Montang SR. Response times to visual and auditory alarms during anaesthesia. Anaesthesia and Intensive Care 1996;24:682–684.
16. Finley GA, Cohen AJ. Perceived urgency and the anaesthetist: responses to common operating room monitor alarms. Can J Anaesth 1991;38:958–964.
17. Edworthy J, Loxley S, Dennis I. Improving auditory warning design: relationship between warning sound parameters and perceived urgency. Human Factors 1991;33:205–231.
18. Stanford LM, McIntyre JWR, Hogan JT. Audible alarm signals for anaesthesia monitoring equipment. Journal of Clinical Monitoring 1985;1:251–256.
19. Momtahan K, Hetu R, Tansley B. Audibility and identification of auditory alarms in the operating room and intensive care unit. Ergonomics 1993;36:1159–1176.
20. Wallace MS. Ashman MN, Matjasko MJ. Hearing acuity of anesthesiologists and alarm detection. Anesthesiology 1994;81:13–28.
21. Chui PT, Gin T. False alarms and integrated alarm system: report of a potential hazard. Anesth Analg 1994;79:192–193.
22. Jones D, Lawson A, Holland R. Case reports. Integrated alarms and 'alarm overload.' Anaesthsia and Intensive Care 1991;19:101–102.
23. Weinger MB. Proposed new alarm standards may make a bad situation worse. Anesthesiology 1991;74:791–792.
24. Block FE. Evaluation of users' abilities to recognize musical alarm tones. Journal of Clinical Monitoring 1992;8:285–290.
25. Griffith RL, Raciot BM. A survey of practicing anesthesiologists on auditory alarms in the operating room. In: Hedley-Whyte, J, Ed. Operating room and intensive care alarms and information transfer (STP 1152). Philadelphia, PA: ASTM, 1992:10–18.

26. Loeb RG, Jones BR, Leonard RA, et al. Recognition accuracy of current operating room alarms. Anesth Analg 1992;75:499–505.

27. Samuels SI. An alarming problem. Anesthesiology 1986;64:128–129.

28. Schmidt SI, Baysinger CL. Alarms: help or hindrance? Anesthesiology 1986;64:654–655.

29. Loeb RG. A measure of intraoperative attention to monitor displays. Anesth Analg 1993;76:337–341.

30. Morris RW, Montano SR. Response times to visual and auditory alarms during anaesthesia. Anaesthsia and Intensive Care 1996;24:682–684.

31. Kerr JH. Alarms and excursions [Editorial]. Anaesthesia 1986;41:807–808.

32. Anonymous. Delay circuit may reduce pulse oximetry false alarms. Biomedical Safety & Standards 1992;22:162–163.

33. Kerr JH. Warning devices. Br J Anaesth 1985;57:696–708.

34. Koski EMJ, Makivirta A, Sukuvaara T, et al. Frequency and reliability of alarms in the monitoring of cardiac postoperative patients. Int J Clin Monit Comput 1990;7:129–133.

35. Wiklund L, Hok B, Jordeby-Jonsson A, et al. Postanesthesia monitoring. More than 75% of pulse oximeter alarms are trivial. Anesthesiology 1992;77:A582.

36. Watt RC, Miller KE, Navabi MJ, et al. An approach to "smart alarms" in anesthesia monitoring. Anesthesiology 1988;69:A241.

37. Schaaf C, Block FE. Evaluation of alarm sounds in the operating room. Journal of Clinical Monitoring 1989;5:300–301.

38. O'Carroll TM. Survey of alarms in an intensive therapy unit. Anaesthesia 1986;41:742–744.

39. Kestin IG, Miller BR, Lockhart CH. Auditory alarms during anesthesia monitoring. Anesthesiology 1988;69:106–109.

40. Lawless ST. Crying wolf: False alarms in a pediatric intensive care unit. Crit Care Med 1994;22:981–985.

41. Tsien CL, Fackler JC. Poor prognosis for existing monitors in the intensive care unit. Crit Care Med 1997;25:614–619.

42. McIntyre JWR. Ergonomics. Anaesthetists' use of auditory alarms in the operating room. Int J Clin Monit Comput 1985;2:47–55.

43. Anonymous. Critical alarms: patients at risk. Technology Anesthesia 1987;7(10):1–6.

44. Sury MRJ, Hinds CJ, Boustred M. Accidental disconnection following inactivation of Servo ventilator alarm. Anaesthesia 1986;41:91.

45. Pan PH, James CF. Effects of default alarm limit settings on alarm distribution in telemetric pulse oximetry network in ward setting. Anesthesiology 1991;75:A405.

46. Anonymous. Noise pollution in the operating room from monitor alarms. Technology for Anesthesia 1993;13(10):3.

47. Makivirta A, Koski EMJ. Alarm-inducing variability in cardiac postoperative data and the effects of pre-alarm delay. Journal of Clinical Monitoring 1994;10:153–154.

48. Mylrea KC, Orr JA, Westenskow DR. Integration of monitoring for intelligent alarms in anesthesia: neural networks—can they help? Journal of Clinical Monitoring 1993;9:31–37.

49. Raison JCA, Beaumont JO, Russell JAG, et al. Alarms in an intensive care unit: an interim compromise. Comput Biomed Res 1968;1:556–564.

50. Navabi MJ, Watt RC, Hameroff SR, et al. Integrated monitoring can detect critical events and improve alarm accuracy. Clin J Eng 1991;16:295–306.

51. Anonymous. Critical alarms: patients as risk. Tech for Anesth 1996;16(10):1–6.

52. Anonymous. Alarms in the operating room. Can J Anaesth 1991;38:951.

53. Egbert TP, Westenskow DR. Detection of artifact in pulse oximetry signals using a neural network. Anesthesiology 1992;77:A521.

54. Fukui Y, Masuzawa T. Knowledge-based approach to intelligent alarms. Journal of Clinical Monitoring 1989;5:211–216.

55. Orr JA, Westenskow DR. Evaluation of a breathing circuit alarm system based on neural networks. Anesthesiology 1990;73:A445.

56. Pan PH. False alarms distribution in intraoperative pulse oximetry. Anesthesiology 1992;77:A494.

57. Farrell RM, Orr JA, Kuck K, et al. Differential features for a neutral network based anesthesia alarm system. Biomed Sciences 1992;28:99–104.

58. Orr JA, Westenskow DR. A breathing circuit alarm system based on neural networks. Journal of Clinical Monitoring 1994;10:101–109.

59. Watt RC, Maslana ES, Mylrea KC. Alarms and anesthesia. Challenges in the design of intelligent systems for patient monitoring. IEEE Engineering in Med and Biol 1993;(Dec):34–41.

60. Westenskow DR, Orr JA, Simon FH, et al. Intelligent alarms reduce anesthesiologist's response time to critical faults. Anesthesiology 1992;77:1074–1079.

61. Orr JA, Simon FH, Bender H-J, et al. Response time with smart alarms. Anesthesiology 1990;73:A447.

62. Dueck R. Respiratory monitoring. Cur Opin Anaesthesiology 1993;6:946–51.

QUESTIONS

Each question below contains four suggested answers of which one or more is correct. Choose the answer:

A. if 1, 2, and 3 are correct
B. if 1 and 3 are correct
C. if 2 and 4 are correct
D. if 4 is correct
E. if 1, 2, 3, and 4 are correct.

1. Purposes of an alarm include
    1. Warning of an existing or developing adverse condition
    2. Getting attention
    3. Transferring information
    4. Transferring legal responsibility from the manufacturer to the user

2. Problems associated with determining the source of an alarm include
    1. The hearing of the anesthesia provider
    2. Difficulty in recognizing tone patterns
    3. Noise levels in the operating room
    4. Sounds that do not sound continuously

3. Visual signals
    1. Give less specific information than audible signals
    2. May go unrecognized for a longer period of time than audible signals
    3. Use continuous lights for more crucial information
    4. Require the anesthesia provider to be looking at the monitor instead of the patient

4. Causes of false positive alarms include
    1. Activation by an inappropriate device
    2. Extraneous sounds which sound like an alarm signal
    3. Alarm malfunction
    4. Widely set limits

5. Means to reduce the incidence of the false positive alarms include
    1. Altering set points during the procedure
    2. Synchronizing monitors
    3. Delaying the time between detection of an alarm condition and alarm activation
    4. Decreasing the averaging time

6. Concerning alarm prioritization
    1. A low-priority alarm may not have an audible signal
    2. A high-priority alarm requires a prompt response
    3. The alarm standard requires high- and medium-priority visual signals be legible at 4 m
    4. Priorities can be increased or decreased by the user

7. Advantages of smart alarms include
    1. Enhanced ability to recognize artifacts
    2. They may be incorporated into a data management system
    3. They may give the anesthesia provider a list of conditions which could have triggered the alarm
    4. They may be used for stand-alone monitors

ANSWERS

1. E
2. B
3. C
4. A

5. A
6. B
7. A

Automatic Noninvasive Blood Pressure Monitors

INTRODUCTION

Frequent determination of blood pressure (BP) is routine during anesthesia. It serves to aid in drug titration and fluid management and to provide warning of conditions that could affect patient safety. Devices that automatically measure BP noninvasively (indirectly) are widely used. The original devices were stand-alone monitors. All modern physiological monitors and anesthesia workstations incorporate an automatic noninvasive BP (ANIBP, NIBP) monitor.

INTERMITTENT TECHNIQUES

Intermittent noninvasive measurement of BP requires a distensible cuff or a distensible bladder enclosed in an unyielding cuff. The cuff is inflated and blood flow through the underlying artery obstructed. The cuff is then deflated in a controlled manner, causing the pressure applied to the artery to decrease. Pulsations are detected and the results displayed or recorded as BP. In addition, most devices display pulse rate.

An American standard on automated sphygmomanometers was published in 1992 (1). Among its provisions are the following:

1. BP measurements by the device must be evaluated against either those obtained by a trained observer using the cuff/stethoscope auscultation method, those obtained by intraarterial measurement or both.
2. For systolic and diastolic pressures, the mean difference between pressures obtained with the monitor and the comparison device shall be 5 mm Hg or less with a standard deviation of 8 mm Hg or less.
3. The cuff pressure shall not exceed 330 mm Hg or 30 mm Hg above the upper limit of the manufacturer's stated operating range, whichever is higher.
4. The device must incorporate a means to ensure that cuff pressure will not be maintained above 10 mm Hg for longer than 5 min.

The British Hypertension Society has developed a protocol to validate automated BP devices using a cuff/stethoscope auscultatory method (2–4). There are a number of differences in the American and British protocols (4).

The majority of automated noninvasive monitors employs some variant of oscillometry although some have a microphone or ultrasound transducer in the cuff (5). The artery is held in partial occlusion by an air-filled cuff, pressure pulsations (oscillations) caused by movement of the arterial wall are transmitted to the cuff. The cuff is wrapped around an extremity. BP is determined by a sequence that is initiated either manually or automatically when the user-set time between determinations lapses.

The cuff is first inflated to a predetermined pressure that is held constant while oscillations in it are sampled. If significant pulsations are still present, the cuff is inflated further until no significant pulsations are sensed. If the steps are small, the resolution is greater. When first turned on, most automatic BP monitors stop inflation at 160

torr or less (5). On pediatric units, a lower pressure is used. If the initial cuff pressure is greater than necessary to determine systolic pressure, the monitor may decrease this pressure during the next cycle. If the initial pressure was too low, the monitor will increase it during the next cycle.

When no oscillations are detected, the pressure in the cuff is decreased in a stepwise or linear manner (Fig. 24.1). This varies among the various monitors. The resolution depends on the size of the step.

As cuff pressure decreases, blood starts to flow in the previously occluded artery and pressure oscillations are superimposed on the cuff pressure. The magnitude of these oscillations increases to a maximum, then decreases. The monitor measures these oscillations. After the determination is completed, the remaining air in the cuff is rapidly exhausted.

These monitors rely on measurement, extrapolations, and clinically tested algorithms to arrive at values for mean, systolic, and diastolic pressures (5–7). The point of maximum amplitude is often considered to be the mean pressure (8). On some instruments it is calculated using an algorithm based on the systolic and diastolic pressures. Systolic and diastolic pressures can be estimated by identifying the region where the amplitudes of oscillations increase or decrease rapidly (5). On some monitors the point of oscillation detection is considered to be the systolic pressure. Diastolic pressure may be derived mathematically from the systolic and mean pressures or from the characteristics of the oscillations at low pressures (9). Because the ways of arriving at these values differ among monitors, measurements by different devices do not yield the same pressures (10). Most machines have an algorithm that can reject most artifacts caused by patient movement or external interference.

With oscillometry, accurate placement over an artery is not necessary and risk of dislodgment is minimal. These monitors do not require a low-noise environment. They are not sensitive to electrosurgical interference. They work well when there is peripheral vasoconstriction. There is little effect on their accuracy if venous engorgement is not allowed to subside (5).

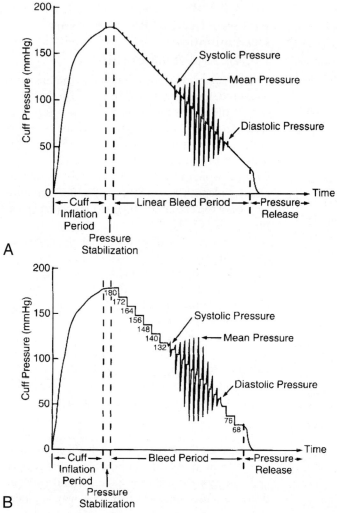

FIGURE 24.1. A and B: Sequence of oscillometric blood pressure determination. Cuff deflation may be linear (**A**) or in steps (**B**). Pressure oscillations increase in magnitude then decrease. The oscillations are analyzed to determine systolic, mean, and diastolic pressures. (Reprinted with permission from Nellcor Puritan Bennett, Pleasanton, California.)

EQUIPMENT

These monitors use electricity, either line voltage or battery, as the power source. Many manufacturers offer different models for different sized patients.

Inflatable Cuff

Cuffs come in different sizes. Disposable cuffs are available (11).

Pressure Tubing(s)

One or two tubings serve as a means to inflate the cuff and sense the pressure within the cuff.

Use of a Y-piece near the cuff to mix single- and two-hose systems was found to have no adverse effect on the performance of the monitor (12).

Cuff Inflation Mechanism

The cuff inflation mechanism consists of a pump plus a reservoir that holds a quantity of air that can be quickly released into the cuff.

Deflation Valve

A bleed valve deflates the cuff. The speed and manner of deflation vary from manufacturer to manufacturer. Some adjust the rate as a function of pressure.

Pressure Sensing Mechanism

A pressure transducer detects the pressure in the cuff and transforms the input into electrical currents that can be measured. In some monitors, the pressure sensing mechanism is built into the cuff.

An autozero valve periodically opens the transducer to atmosphere, automatically establishing zero pressure (5).

Timing Circuitry

The timing circuitry regulates the frequency of the determinations. Most have a provision for manual as well as automatic initiation of a cycle. Most offer a STAT mode which allows a number of determinations in quick succession.

Control Circuitry

The control circuitry determines such parameters as the maximum inflation pressure in the cuff, artifact rejection, electrosurgical suppression, deflation rate, and automatic cutoff. The overpressure switch may be set differently for adult and pediatric models. Some machines have automatic cuff deflation when the cycle time exceeds a predetermined limit.

Alarms

Monitors vary, according to which parameter(s) will trigger an alarm. Alarms may be set around the systolic, diastolic or mean BP(s) and heart rate. Some monitors automatically set alarms around the initial values. Some have default alarms which can be changed by the operator. In addition, some alarm when they are unable to determine the BP. Most alarms are both visual and audible. The alarm volume needs to be high enough that the anesthesia provider can hear it. The ability to make the alarm volume inaudible is dangerous (8).

Printer

Many units are equipped with connections for printers. Some printers can display trends graphically.

ACCURACY

Factors Affecting Blood Pressure Determinations

Cuff/Arm Relationship

Cuff (or bladder) size influences the pressures measured. Cuff size should be based on the thickness of the extremity where the BP is being measured; the length of the extremity is not as important (13). A cuff that is 125 to 150% of the diameter (40 to 50% of the circumference) of the limb on which it is used at the limb's midpoint and has a length that is 80 to 100% of the circumference of the extremity will provide accurate measurements (13–15).

An undersized cuff will cause falsely high readings and an oversized cuff falsely low ones (16–20). Too small a bladder will cause falsely elevated readings even if the cuff size is correct (21). The error caused by a cuff which is too large is less than if a cuff that is too small is used. Since this error is smaller and since most adults have large arms, it has been recommended that large cuffs be used routinely (16, 17, 19, 22). If a sufficiently large cuff is not available, it may be possible to place a cuff more distally on the limb.

Site

The site of cuff placement will affect the pressure measured. As the site becomes more peripheral, the systolic pressure increases and diastolic decreases. Increased vascular tone may augment this increase in pulse pressure. Vascular disease and peripheral vasoconstriction may cause reduced pressures at distal locations.

Hydrostatic Factors

If the cuff and the patient's heart are not at the same level, hydrostatic pressure will affect the reading and a correction must be made (23). For each 10 cm of vertical height above or below the heart level, 7.5 mm Hg must be added to or subtracted from the pressures observed (8).

Correlation with Other Methods of Blood Pressure Determination

Direct Methods

Many feel that the standard of comparison should be the pressure measured directly in an artery, most commonly the radial. However, indirect pressure readings will never correlate exactly with invasive pressures. One problem is that simultaneous measurements often cannot be taken. Despite these problems many studies have compared pressures obtained with NIBP monitors with those obtained directly in adults (24–39). Unfortunately, differences in study populations, models and ages of instruments, sites for taking measurements, methods of disclosing findings, statistical procedures, and protocols make comparison of these studies difficult (40). Another problem is that modifications to software are often made without a new model being issued.

In general these instruments are most accurate in normal healthy patients and least accurate at the extremes of BP. Although errors can occur in either direction, oscillometric devices tend to overestimate low pressures and underestimate high pressures.

The STAT mode was found not to denigrate the BP values and to be subject to the same variations as measurements taken under normal circumstances (41).

In hypertensive patients, the systolic pressure measured noninvasively is significantly lower than that measured directly (42). However, in a study in patients with severe pre-eclampsia, the oscillometer showed good accuracy compared with auscultatory methods (43).

In obese patients, studies have found that diastolic pressure was underestimated but dynamic changes were reflected accurately (44). Cuff size is important in these patients. If the cuff is too small, the measured pressures will be falsely elevated. (45)

The correlation between invasive and noninvasive BP has been studied in the pediatric population. (17, 37, 46–53). In general, good correlation was found between direct and indirect measurements.

In critically ill patients, studies have concluded that while there is generally good correlation between direct and oscillometrically measured pressures, a NIBP monitor is not good enough to use if vasoactive drugs are being administered (54). Accuracy and reproducibility are diminished during periods immediately surrounding cardiopulmonary bypass (39, 55).

The correlation between direct and oscillometric BP during hypotension has been studied in adults (25, 29) and infants (50, 56). The investigators concluded that oscillometric BP were useful for trending purposes but if absolute numbers were required, direct measurements were preferable. Another problem is that with moderate to severe hypotension, the automated machine often cycles repeatedly before indicating a failure to measure (57).

Manual Auscultatory Methods

Auscultatory measurements are considered by many to be the standard to which automated devices should be compared. A number of factors affect the determination of BP by this method, including variable hearing acuity, rates of cuff deflation and inflation, differing concepts of diastolic end points, and placement of the stethoscope.

Many studies have compared auscultatory and oscillometric techniques (35, 37, 52, 58–65). Results were similar to those comparing oscillometric and direct pressures.

PROPER USE (5)

If possible, the cuff should not be applied to the limb in which the intravenous infusion is placed as infusion of fluids and drugs will be slowed or blocked and the increased pressure may cause blood to flow retrograde into the infusion set tubing or cause extravasation. A simple method to reduce these problems is to route the infusion set tubing through the BP cuff (66, 67). In some cases it may be possible to place the cuff distal to the site of the infusion. Some intravenous infusion sets have one-way valves to prevent retrograde flow.

If used on the arm, the cuff should be placed as high as possible and the inflation tubes should exit proximally (68–70). If the upper arm is very large or conically shaped, measurements can be made at locations such as the ankle, thigh, or forearm (71, 72). The superficial temporal and supraorbital arteries have also been used (73–75). The cuff should not be applied over a superficial nerve, bony prominence, or joint.

If a site other than the proximal arm is to be used, it may be desirable to check the pressures in both the arm and the alternative site to see how well they correlate. Studies have shown that the arm and forearm are interchangeable in obese patients. (76, 77)

Neonatal BP cuffs have been used on digits of larger patients (78). In children and young adults, this provides a reliable estimate of systolic, but not of mean or diastolic pressures (79). In adults, studies show varying results, with the best correlation reported with mean BP in normotensive patients (78, 80, 81).

Prior to application of the cuff all residual air should be expelled. The portion of the limb over which the cuff is to be placed should be covered with padding (82, 83). The cuff should be applied snugly enough to allow only one finger to be slipped under it (5). Too tight a cuff may cause discomfort and venous distention. Too loose a cuff may cause falsely elevated readings and may result in failure of the monitor to determine BP. However, one study demonstrated that loosely wrapped cuffs still generated clinically acceptable data, provided the cuff was not too small (84).

The cuff should be placed and several inflations allowed to occur while the patient is awake to elicit complaints.

BP measurements should be made no more frequently than clinically necessary. The cuff site and extremity should be inspected periodically during prolonged applications. A good practice is to remove the cuff occasionally and switch it to another site if possible.

COMPLICATIONS
Petechiae, Edema, Thrombophlebitis, Skin Avulsion

Several of these cases have been reported (85–90). Predisposing factors to the development of petechial hemorrhages include patients taking nonsteroidal anti-inflammatory drugs, steroids, and anticoagulants and patients with large arms or redundant skin (82, 83).

Nerve Palsies

Neuropathies of the median, ulnar, and radial nerves following use of an ANIBP monitor have been reported (68, 69). All resolved spontaneously.

If there is excessive movement which would make it difficult for the device to determine pres-

sures, the device will cycle more often, possibly to higher pressures. This can contribute to nerve injuries (68).

Compartment Syndrome

Three cases of compartment syndrome requiring fasciotomies associated with prolonged use of ANIBP monitors have been reported. In one case the patient had hyperactivity and tremor. This caused the instrument to take repeated measurements at increased pressures (91). In another case the BP was labile, causing the monitor to cycle longer and with higher pressures than usual (92). In the third case the cuff was applied across the antecubital fossa with arm flexion (93).

Mechanical Problems

Failure of an NIABP monitor is not uncommon and may be associated with serious morbidity or mortality (94). A common problem is a cuff, hose, or connector that leaks (5). Other reported problems include a partially obstructed cuff vent that caused an erroneous zero setting for the pressure transducer, and resulted in lower-than-actual readings and failure of the cuff to deflate (6). In one reported case the module locked up, failed to make any more BP determinations, displayed the last value, and did not give an indication that there was a malfunction. (95)

Artifacts

Oscillometric devices are sensitive to pulsatile signals caused by both intrinsic or extrinsic motions. Most models reliably reject extraneous signals, but they can be fooled. Before any intervention is made in response to a measurement, it should be confirmed by repeating it.

Intrinsic motion artifacts are caused by movement of the patient such as shivering, tremors, convulsions, restlessness or vigorous skin preparation (96). A patient tapping her finger to music was found to have artifactual hypertension (97). Massaging of the arm where the BP cuff is located may result in underestimation of the BP (98). Extrinsic motion artifacts are caused by actions that compress the cuff such as bumping by personnel or an ambulance ride (5).

BP readings were reported in a patient where the cuff was under the patient's head (99). It is surmised that movements of the head provided enough motion in the cuff to produce the artifactual readings. In another case a cuff became unfastened but the bladder remained between the arm and the thorax (100). It was still able to detect oscillations and displayed a fictitiously low pressure.

ADVANTAGES
Automaticity

The chief advantage of these devices is that they can determine pressures regularly and frequently on an automatic basis. During busy times, it is very helpful to have the current pressure displayed.

Objectivity

Automatic devices eliminate most of the factors that cause errors when BP are determined manually, such as variable concentration, reaction times, hearing acuity, ambient noise, confusion of auditory and visual cues, variable deflation rates, background noise, variable interpretation of sounds, preference for certain digits, and bias due to knowledge of previous readings. They may eliminate some of the mistrust some individuals have when other people measure the BP manually.

Simplicity of Use

ANIBP monitors are simple to use. They do not require extensive training to set up or maintain.

Noninvasiveness

In comparison with direct measurements, they are less expensive, cause less discomfort, and avoid the risks (ischemic damage, emboli) associated with direct techniques.

Reliability

These are generally reliable devices that do not require a lot of maintenance or experience a lot of down-time.

Usefulness in Difficult Situations

Some will work in certain patients (such as those with obesity, medial calcified sclerosis and infants), in whom an accurate pressure cannot be obtained using the Korotkoff sounds (101). They

will read accurately through bulky dressings (102).

Patient and Personnel Acceptance

Acceptance of ANIBP monitors by users and patients has been very positive (103).

Many Sites Suitable for Measurement

Oscillometric BP measurements can be taken anywhere there is an artery over which a cuff can be wrapped.

DISADVANTAGES
Unsuitability for Rapid Changes in Blood Pressure

While an ANIBP monitor is helpful in establishing trends, it is unsuitable for detecting rapid changes or critical events. If rapid changes are anticipated, a continuous method of measurement should be used.

Patient Discomfort

Some patients note discomfort, often associated with a prolonged cycle time. Cycle time will be prolonged with large cuffs, hypertensive patients, poor peripheral circulation, a leak in the monitor, low BP, dysrhythmias, or motion artifacts.

Clinical Limitations

Automated BP devices may not work well with extreme heart rates and pressures and various dysrhythmias (25, 104). Shock and low pulse pressure can reduce the cuff oscillations to the point where only mean pressure is measurable (5). In the extreme, even mean pressure may not be measurable.

Loss of Hands-On Diagnostic Information

An advantage of manual techniques is the ability to detect physical signs such as cold, hot, clammy, or dry skin. Automatic methods distance the anesthesia provider from the patient.

Decreased Vigilance

While one study concluded that use of ANIBP monitors was associated with a decrease in vigilance (105), another found that detection of hypotension improved after the ANIBP devices were introduced (106).

Limited Usefulness during Patient Transport

Studies involving ambulance and helicopter transport have shown that in critically ill patients, these monitors are not as reliable as direct measurements (107–109).

REFERENCES

1. ANSI/AAMI SP10-1992, Electronic or automated sphygmomanometers. Arlington, VA: Association for the Advancement of Medical Instrumentation, 1992.
2. O'Brien E, Mee F, Atkins N, et al. Short report: Accuracy of the Dinamap portable monitor, model 8100 determined by the British Hypertension Society protocol. J Hypertens 1993;11:761–763.
3. O'Brien E, Petrie J, Littler W, et al. Short report: An outline of the revised British Hypertension Society protocol for the evaluation of blood pressure measuring devices. J Hypertens 1993;11:677–679.
4. O'Brien E, Petrie J, Littler W, et al. The British Hypertension Society protocol for the evaluation of automated and semi-automated blood pressure measuring devices with special reference to ambulatory systems. J Hypertens 1990;8:607–619.
5. Vig Ramsey M III. Blood pressure monitoring: automated oscillometric devices. Journal of Clinical Monitoring 1991;7:56–67.
6. Anonymous. Automatic sphygmomanometers. Technol for Anesth 1986;7,3:1–4.
7. Amoore JN. Assessment of oscillometric non-invasive blood pressure monitors using the Dynatech Nevada CuffLink analyser. J Med Eng Technol 1993;17:25–31.
8. Anonymous: Automated sphygmomanometers. Health Devices 1986;15:187–208.
9. Quill TJ. Blood pressure monitoring in anesthesia equipment. principles and applications. J Ehrenwerth, JB Eisenkraft, eds. St. Louis: Mosby, 274–283.
10. Kaufmann MA, Pargger H, Drop LJ. Oscillometric blood pressure measurements by different devices are not interchangeable. Anesth Analg 1996;82:377–381.
11. Alpert BS, Cohen ML. The PAPERCUFF, a new disposable blood pressure cuff. Am J Cardiol 1996;77:531–532.
12. Amoore JN, Scott DHT. Noninvasive blood pressure measurements with single and twin-hose systems—do mixtures matter? Anaesthesia 1993;48:799–802.
13. Park MK, Guntheroth WG. Accurate blood pressure measurement in children. Am J Noninvas Cardiol 1989;3:297–309.
14. Report of the second task force on blood pressure control in children, 1987. Pediatrics 1987;79:1–25.
15. Frohlich ED, Grim C, Labarthe DR, et al. Recommendations for human blood pressure determination by sphygmomanometers. Report of a special task force appointed by the Steering Committee, American Heart Association. Circulation 1988;77:501A–514A.
16. Iyriboz Y, Hearon CM, Edwards K. Agreement between large and small cuffs in sphygmomanometry: a quantitative assessment. Journal of Clinical Monitoring 1994;10:127–133.
17. Kimble KJ, Darnall RA, Yelderman M, et al. An automated oscillometric technique for estimating mean arterial pressure in critically ill newborns. Anesthesiology 1981;54:423–425.
18. Manning DM, Kuchirka C, Kaminski J. Miscuffing. Inappropriate blood pressure cuff application. Circulation 1983;68:763–766.
19. van Montfrans GA, van derf Hoeven GMA, Karemaker JM, et al. Accuracy of auscultatory blood pressure measurement with a long cuff. BMJ 1987;295:354–355.
20. Whincup PH, Cook DG, Shaper AG. Blood pressure measurement in children: the importance of cuff bladder size. J Hypertens 1989;7:845–850.
21. Schulman SR. Blood pressure monitoring in infants. Journal of Clinical Monitoring 1991;7:280.
22. Russell AE, Wing LMH, Smith SA, et al. Optimal size of cuff bladder for indirect measurement of arterial pressure in adults. J Hypertens 1989;7:607–613.
23. Webster J, Newnham D, Petrie JC, et al. Influence of arm position on measurement of blood pressure. BMJ 1984;288:1574–1575.
24. Borow KM, Newburger JW. Noninvasive estimation of central aortic pressure using the oscillometric method for analyzing systemic artery pulsatile blood flow: Comparative study of indirect systolic, diastolic, and mean brachial artery pressure with simultaneous direct ascending aortic pressure measurements. Am Heart J 1982;103:879–886.
25. Hutton P, Dye J, Prys-Roberts C. An assessment of the Dinamap 845. Anaesthesia 1984;39:261–267.
26. Davis RF. Clinical comparison of automated ausculatory and oscillometric and catheter-transducer measurements of arterial pressure. Journal of Clinical Monitoring 1985;1:114–119.
27. Loubser PG. Comparing direct and indirect arterial blood pressures. Anesthesiology 1985;63:566–567.

28. Nystrom E, Reid KH, Bennett R, et al. A comparison of two automated indirect arterial blood pressure meters: with recordings from a radial arterial catheter in anesthetized surgical patients. Anesthesiology 1985; 62:526–530.

29. Gourdeau M, Martin R, Lamarche Y, Tetreault L. Oscillometry and direct blood pressure: a comparative clinical study during deliberate hypotension. Can Anaesth Soc J 1986;33:300–307.

30. Gorback MS, Quill TJ, Lavine ML. The relative accuracies of two automated noninvasive arterial pressure measurement devices. Journal of Clinical Monitoring 1991;7:13–22.

31. Johnson CJH, Kerr JH. Automatic blood pressure monitors. A clinical evaluation of five models in adults. Anaesthesia 1985;40:471–478.

32. Van Egmond J, Hasenbos M, Crul JF. Invasive versus Non-invasive measurement of arterial pressure. Comparison of two automatic methods and simultaneously measured direct intr-arterial pressure. Br J Anaesth 1985;57:434–444.

33. Ramsey M III. Noninvasive automatic determination of mean arterial pressure. Med Biol Eng Comput 1979;17:11–18.

34. Rutten AJ, Ilsley Ahm Skowronski A, Runciman WB. A comparative study of the measurement of mean arterial blood pressure using automatic oscillometers, arterial cannulation and auscultation. Anaesthesia and Intensive Care 1986;14:58–65.

35. Manolio TA, Fishel SC, Beattie C, et al. Evaluation of the Dinamap continuous blood pressure monitor. Am J Hypertens 1988;1:161S–167S.

36. Pace ML, East TD. Simultaneous comparison of intraarterial, oxcilometric and Finapres monitoring during anesthesia. Anesth Analg 1991;73:210–220.

37. Sun M, Tien J, Jones R, Ward R. A new approach to reproducibility assessment: clinical evaluation of SpaceLabs medical oscillometric blood pressure monitor. Biomed Instrum Technol 1996;30:439–448.

38. Yelderman M, Ream AK. Indirect measurement of mean blood pressure in the anesthetized patient. Anesthesiology 1979;50:253–256.

39. Whalen P, Ream AK. A quantitative evaluation of the Hewlett-Packard 7835A noninvasive blood pressure meter. Journal of Clinical Monitoring 1988;4: 21–30.

40. Iyriboz Y, Hearon CM. A proposal for scientific validation of instruments for indirect blood pressure measurement at rest, during exercise, and in critical care. Journal of Clinical Monitoring 1994;10: 163–177.

41. Gorback MS, Quill TJ, Graubert DA. The accuracy of rapid oscillometric blood pressure determination. Biomed Instrum Technol 1990;24:371–4.

42. Loubser PG. Comparison of intra-arterial and automated oscillometric blood pressure measurement methods in postoperative hypertensive patients. Med Instrum 1986;20:255–259.

43. Shennan A, Halligan A, Gupta M, et al. Oscillometric blood pressure measurements in severe pre-eclampsia: validation of the Space Labs 90207. Br J Obstet Gyn 1996;103:171–173.

44. Dorman BH, Spinale FG, Haynes GR, et al. Is noninvasive blood pressure monitoring accurate in obese and morbidly obese patients? Anesthesiology 1994; 81:A506.

45. Maxwell MH, Waks AU, Schroth PC, et al. Error in blood-pressure measurement due to incorrect cuff size in obese patients. Lancet 1982;2:33–35.

46. Baker MD, Maisels J, Marks KH. Indirect BP monitoring in the newborn. Evaluation of a new oscillometer and comparison of upper- and lower-limb measurements. AJDC 1984;138:775–778.

47. Baker LK. DINAMAP monitor versus direct blood pressure measurements. Dimens Crit Care Nurs 1986;5:228–235.

48. Colan SD, Fujii A, Borow KM, et al. Noninvasive determination of systolic, diastolic and end-systolic blood pressure in neonates, infants and young children: comparison with central aortic pressure measurements. Am J Cardiol 1983;52:867–870.

49. Cullen PM, Dye J, Hughes DG. Clinical assessment of the neonatal Dinamap 847 during anesthesia in neonates and infants. Journal of Clinical Monitoring 1987;3:229–34.

50. Chia F, Ang AT, Wong T-W, et al. Reliability of the Dinamap non-invasive monitor in the measurement of blood pressure of ill Asian newborns. Clin Ped 1990;29:262–267.

51. Dellagrammaticas HD, Wilson AJ. Clinical evaluation of the Dinamap non-invasive blood pressure monitor in pre-term neonates. Clin Phys Physiol Meas 1981;2:271–6.

52. Park MK, Menard SM. Accuracy of blood pressure measurement by the Dinamap monitor in infants and children. Pediatrics 1987;79:907–914.

53. Reder RF, Dimich I, Cohen ML, et al. Evaluating indirect blood pressure measurement techniques: a comparison of three systems in infants and children. Pediatrics 1978;62:326–330.

54. Venus B, Mathru M, Smith RA, et al. Direct versus indirect blood pressure measurements in critically ill patients. Heart & Lung 1985;14:228–231.

55. Gravlee GP, Brockeschmidt JK. Accuracy of four indirect methods of blood pressure measurement, with hemodynamic correlations. Journal of Clinical Monitoring 1990;6:284–298.

56. Diprose GJ, Evans DH, Archer LNJ, et al. Dinamap fails to detect hypotension in very low birthweight infants. Arch Dis Child 1986;61:771–773.

57. Cockings JGL, Webb RK, Klepper ID, et al. Blood pressure monitoring-applications and limitations: an analysis of 2000 incident reports. Anaesthesia and Intensive Care 1993;21:565–569.

58. Bassein L, Borghi C, Costa FV, et al. Comparison of three devices for measuring blood pressure. Statistics in Medicine 1985;4:361–368.

59. Bassein L, Borghi C, Costa FV, et al. Comparison of two automatic devices and the standard mercury sphygmomanometer in hypertensive patients. Clin Exper Theory Pract 1985;A7(2 & 3):387–390.

60. Harrison DW, Crews WD. The Takeda Model Ua-751 blood pressure and pulse rate monitor. Biomed Instrum Technol 1992;26:325–327.

61. Kawahara M. Evaluation of the accuracy of non-invasive automatic blood pressure monitors. Anesth Prog 1990;37:244–247.

62. Ornstein S, Markert H, Litchfield L, et al. Evaluation of the DINAMAP blood pressure monitor in an ambulatory primary care setting. J Family Practice 1988;26:517–521.

63. Pessenhofer H. Single cuff comparison of two methods for indirect measurement of arterial blood pressure: standard auscultatory method versus automatic oscillometric method. Basic Res Cardiol 1986;81:101–109.

64. Weaver MG, Park MK, Lee D-H. Differences in blood pressure levels obtained by auscultatory and oscillometric methods. Am J Dis Child 1990;144:911–914.

65. Wattigney WA, Webber LS, Lawrence MD, et al. Utility of an automatic instrument for blood pressure measurement in children. The Bogalusa heart study. Am J Hypertens 1996;9:256–262.

66. Brin EB, Lewis TC, Brin A J. A simple method for reducing backup of blood into intravenous lines caused by inflation of a blood pressure cuff. Anesth Analg 1990;71:569.

67. Wait CM. Blood pressure measurements and intravenous infusions. Anaesthesia 1992;47:1012.

68. Bickler PE, Schapera A, Bainton CR. Acute radial nerve injury from use of an automatic blood pressure monitor. Anesthesiology 1990;73:186–188.

69. Sy WP. Ulnar nerve palsy possibly related to use of automatically cycled blood pressure cuff. Anesth Analg 1981;60:687–688.

70. Ward CF. An update on pediatric monitoring. Journal of Clinical Monitoring 1985;1:172–179.

71. Schulte GT, Block FE Jr. Comparison of non-invasive blood pressure measurements on the arm and ankle. Anesthesiology 1989;71:A408.

72. Zornow MH, Schubert A, Todd MM. Intraoperative oscillometric arterial blood pressure monitoring using non-standard cuff locations. Anesthesiology 1986;65:A135.

73. Lee T-K, Egbert TP, Westenskow DR. Supraorbital artery as an alternative for oscillometric blood pressure measurement. Journal of Clinical Monitoring 1996;12:293–297.

74. Narus S, Egbert Y, Lee T-K, et al. Noninvasive blood pressure monitoring from the supraorbital artery using an artificial neural network oscillometric algorithm. Journal of Clinical Monitoring 1995;11:289–297.

75. Lee T-K, Silva FH, Egbert TP, et al. Optimal sites for forehead oscillometric blood pressure monitoring. Journal of Clinical Monitoring 1995;11:298–304.

76. Bowen M, Cho D, Stevens W. Arterial pressure in obese patients: comparison of measurements at the arm, forearm and with a radial artery catheter. Anesthesiology 1995;83:A482.

77. Latman NS, Coker N, Teague C. Evaluation of an instrument for noninvasive blood pressure monitoring in the forearm. Biomed Instrum Technol 1996;30:160–163.

78. Green DW. Use of a neonatal noninvasive blood pressure module on adult patients. Anaesthesia 1996;51:1129–1132.

79. Lyew MA, Jamieson JW. Blood pressure measurement using oscillometric finger cuffs in children and young adults. A comparison with arm cuffs during general anaesthesia. Anaesthesia 1994;49:895–899.

80. Jahr JS, Hester ZR, Davis JJ, et al. Comparison of two sites for noninvasive arterial blood pressure monitoring. Am J Anesth 1995;22:32–36.

81. Gorback MS, Quill TJ, Bloch EC, et al. Oscillometric blood pressure determination from the adult thumb using an infant cuff. Anesth Analg 1989;69:668–670.

82. Schinelli A, Shultes PD, Gravenstein JS. Reducing the incidence of petechial hemorrhages under noninvasive blood pressure cuffs. Anesthesiology 1992;77:A546.

83. Ramsey M III. Automatic oscillometric NIBP versus manual auscultatory blood pressure in the PACU. Journal of Clinical Monitoring 1994;10:136–139.

84. Banner TE, Gravenstein JS. How tightly to wrap a blood pressure cuff. Anesthesiology 1989;71:A352.

85. Bause GS, Weintraub AC, Tanner GE. Skin avulsion during oscillometry. Journal of Clinical Monitoring 1986;2:262–263.

86. Creevy PC, Burris JF, Mroczek WJ. Phlebitis associated with noninvasive 24-hour ambulatory blood pressure monitor. JAMA 1985;254:2411.

87. White WB. The Rumpel-Leede sign associated with a noninvasive ambulatory blood pressure monitor. JAMA 1985;253:1724.

88. de Silva PHDP, Mostafa SM. Assessment of the Dinamap 845. Anaesthesia 1985;40:817.

89. Nicholls BJ, Ryan DW. Petechial rashes and automatic blood pressure measurements. Anaesthesia 1986;41:88.

90. Showman A, Betts EK. Hazard of automatic noninvasive blood pressure monitoring. Anesthesiology 1981;55:717–718.

91. Celoria G, Dawson JA, Teres D. Compartment syndrome in a patient monitored with an automated blood pressure cuff. Journal of Clinical Monitoring 1987;3:139–141.

92. Vidal P, Sykes PJ, O'Shaughnessy M, et al. Compartment syndrome after use of an automatic arterial pressure monitoring device. Br J Anaesth 1993;71: 902–904.

93. Sutin KM, Longaker MT, Wahlander S, et al. Acute biceps compartment syndrome associated with the use of a noninvasive blood pressure monitor. Anesth Analg 1996;83:1345–1346.

94. Webb RK, Russell WJ, Klepper I, et al. Equipment failure: an analysis of 2000 incident reports. Anaesthesia and Intensive Care 1993;21:673–677.

95. Anonymous. Defective NIBP modules can affect anesthesia systems displays. Biomed Safe Stand 1993; 23:100–101.

96. de Courcy JG. Artefactual 'hypotension' from shivering. Anaesthesia 1989;44:787–788.

97. Das PA. Artefactual hypertension from rhythmic finger tapping. Anaesthesia 1994;49:262–263.

98. Healzer JM, Pearl RG. Husband-induced hypotension. Anesthesiology 1995;82:323.

99. Ehlers KC, Grabenbauer SA. Erroneous blood pressure measurements with a noninvasive blood pressure monitor. Anesthesiology 1991;74:967.

100. Blue D, Hannallah M. An unusual cause of an erroneous noninvasive blood pressure reading. Anesthesiology 1993;78:1196–1197.

101. Paulus DA. Noninvasive blood pressure measurement. Med Instrum 1981;15:91–94.

102. Bainbridge LC, Simmons HM, Elliot D. The use of automatic blood pressure monitors in the burned patient. Br J Plast Surg 1990;43:322–324.

103. Campbell-Heider N, Knapp TR. Nurses' attitudes toward conventional and automated vital signs measurement methods. Med Instrum 1988;22:257–262.

104. Weinger MB, Scanlon TS, Miller L. A widely unappreciated cause of failure of an automatic noninvasive blood pressure monitor. Journal of Clinical Monitoring 1992;8:291–294.

105. Kay J, Neal M. Effect of automatic blood pressure devices on vigilance of anesthesia residents. Journal of Clinical Monitoring 1986;2:148–1450.

106. Kross R, Shah N, Shah S, et al. Improved detection of hypotension by automated, non-invasive BP monitoring. Anesthesiology 1989;71:A943.

107. Low RB. Accuracy of blood pressure measurements made aboard helicopters. Ann Emerg Med 1988;17: 604–612.

108. Runcie CJ. Reeve WG, Reidy J, et al. Blood pressure measurement during transport. A comparison of direct and oscillotonometric readings in critically ill patients. Anaesthesia 1990;45:659–665.

109. Morley AP. Prehospital monitoring of trauma patients: experience of a helicopter emergency medical service. Br J Anaesth 1996;76:726–730.

QUESTIONS

Each question below contains four suggested answers of which one or more is correct. Choose the answer:

A. if 1, 2, and 3 are correct
B. if 1 and 3 are correct
C. if 2 and 4 are correct
D. if 4 is correct
E. if 1, 2, 3, and 4 are correct.

1. Automated blood pressure machines are evaluated by
   1. Using a trained observer with a cuff and stethoscope
   2. Auscultation
   3. Intraarterial measurement
   4. Oscillometric measurement

2. What points during the measurement cycle are used to determine the blood pressure?
   1. The point of maximum amplitude is considered the systolic pressure
   2. Systolic and diastolic pressures may be estimated by identifying the region where amplitudes of oscillations increase and decrease rapidly
   3. The diastolic pressure is the point where oscillations cease
   4. Mean pressure may be calculated using an algorithm based on the systolic and diastolic pressures

3. Which statements regarding accuracy of noninvasive blood pressure monitors are correct?
   1. Since most use oscillometric technology, there is close agreement between different instruments
   2. Placement of the cuff over the artery is important
   3. Patient movement causes a great deal of artifact to an oscillometric technique
   4. The risk of dislodgment from the proper placement is minimal

4. Accuracy of the automatic blood pressure monitor may be affected by
   1. Electrosurgical interference
   2. Venous engorgement
   3. Peripheral vasoconstriction
   4. A noisy environment

5. Which factors characterize the relationship between the size of the cuff and the size of the arm.
   1. Undersized cuffs give falsely low readings
   2. The cuff width should be 125 to 150% of the diameter of the limb on which it is used
   3. Oversized cuffs give falsely high readings
   4. The cuff length should be 80 to 100% of the circumference of the limb

6. In which patients will there be good correlation between blood pressure measured directly and indirectly?
   1. Critically ill patients on vasoactive drugs
   2. Pediatric patients
   3. Obese patients
   4. Pre-eclamptic patients

7. Factors that can affect the determination of blood pressure by the auscultatory method include
   1. Rate of cuff deflation
   2. Rate of cuff inflation
   3. Hearing acuity
   4. Standardized concept of systolic and diastolic end point

8. Which techniques constitute proper cuff placement?
   1. The cuff should be placed tightly on the limb
   2. A loosely applied cuff will usually cause false readings
   3. The cuff should be kept on the same arm even during long procedures
   4. The limb should be wrapped with padding where the cuff is to be placed

9. Patients are at risk for developing petechiae include
   1. Those on anticoagulants
   2. Those taking steroids
   3. Those taking nonsteroidal anti-inflammatory drugs
   4. Those with redundant skin

10. Contributing causes of a compartment
syndrome include
1. Tremor involving the limb on which
the cuff is placed
2. Hyperactive patient
3. Low placement of the cuff
4. Stable blood pressures

ANSWERS

1. A	**6.** C
2. C	**7.** A
3. D	**8.** C
4. B	**9.** E
5. C	**10.** A

Electronic Recordkeeping and Perioperative Information Management Systems

INTRODUCTION

At present, most anesthesia departments add information to the anesthesia record manually. This is slow, labor intensive, and diverts attention from more important tasks. Manual records are often inaccurate, incomplete and illegible and require huge amounts of storage space. Much data entry can be automated using existing technology.

DEFINITIONS (1)

Anesthesia information system (AIS or AIMS): A system that manages information throughout the perioperative period.

Applications: Computer programs, usually of a similar type.

Analog Data: Continuous data which can, within limits, assume any value. An analog computer cannot handle alphanumeric data (letters and numbers) but can process waveforms. Analog is the opposite of digital.

Artifact: Data that are not a true representation of a condition.

Automated anesthesia record keeper (AARK): A device that keeps an electronic record during anesthesia.

Back-up: An electronic copy of a file.

CD-ROM: (Compact Disk Read-Only Memory): A metal platter on which data are recorded by creating tiny pits along a circumferential track.

Central Processing Unit (CPU): A microprocessor that controls everything in the computer.

Closed architecture or system: Equipment designed to work only with accessories made by one company.

Database: A collection of data, often in storage for later access.

Digital: A way of storing information using numbers. Digital is the opposite of analog.

Disk: A storage device for computer information. Disks are of two types: hard and floppy.

Editing: Changing a recorded value, comment, annotation, or event after it has been made part of the record.

File: A collection of information in a format designed for computer use.

Fileserver (server): The master computer into which all the other computers on a network hook. The fileserver stores programs, processes and stores data in a database, and runs the network operating system.

Hard Copy: A paper record created by a computer output device.

Hard Disk: A long-term storage device for a computer. Hard disks are faster and store more information than floppy disks.

Hardware: The physical parts of a computer, e.g., printer, screen, keyboard, electronic components.

Input Device: A device used to manually enter data or control a computer. Examples include a keyboard, mouse, trackball, light pen, bar code scanner, touch screen, voice recognition device, and pen pad.

Interface: The common boundary between computers, between computers and their peripheral devices or between two peripheral devices.

Local area network (LAN): A network that is limited to a local area such as a department. A LAN can be integrated into a larger network.

Macro: A tool used to automate tasks or procedures within a program. An example would be pretyped notes for easy entry into the record.

Medical Information Bus (MEDIBUS, MIB) (2): A family of hardware, software, and transmission protocols for medical electronic equipment developed by the Association for the Advancement of Medical Information and the Institute of Electrical and Electronics Engineers. The purpose of the MIB is to allow a wide variety of medical devices to interface with minimal effort and to standardize information exchange between these devices.

Microprocessor (processor, CPU): The computer's main processing chip, where all calculations take place and the control center for the entire computer.

Network: A group of computers connected together.

Non-volatile: Stored electronically in such a way that the loss of electric power will not alter the data. Examples include hard disks, magnetic tape, magneto-optical drives, and CD-ROMs.

Open Architecture: The practice of making the design and engineering of computers or programs public knowledge.

Operating System: Software that controls how a computer performs its functions.

Output Device: A device that presents data from a computer system to a user for viewing or storage. Examples include printers and screens.

Parallel Port: A port over which data are sent eight or more bits abreast. Parallel ports are good for high-speed data transfer, but they don't work well over long distances.

Peripheral: A general term for any of the devices by which a computer gathers its input and disseminates its output.

Port: A connector on a computer to which external items can be attached. Ports are usually either serial or parallel.

Protocol: A set of standards that enables communication or file transfer between two computers.

Serial Port: A port that transmits data one bit after another through a single cable. The advantage of serial ports is that information can be sent over longer distances.

Software: Programs that control the hardware and determine the functions performed by a computer.

ELEMENTS OF AN INFORMATION MANAGEMENT SYSTEM (1,2)

A typical AIS is shown in Figure 25.1. It consists of a central fileserver and a network connecting the components. Each computer handles certain tasks. In a properly designed system, failure of an individual computer will not disable the entire system, but affect only those functions it was performing.

An information system may be closed or open (3). With a closed system, all software and hardware are supplied by a single manufacturer. This helps to ensure that all components work together and allows the institution to deal with only a single vendor. However, a closed system may not work well with components from other manufacturers.

In an open system, components from various vendors are used. This enables each department to choose the best components for its needs, while still allowing the information to be accessed by other systems in the facility. Institutions selecting an open system must make sure that new components will interface with their network.

Fileserver

The fileserver processes and stores data in a database, stores application programs, and runs the network operating system.

Input Sources
Automated Anesthesia Record Keepers

The AARK collects information from various sources, processes the data, presents selected values and trends on a screen, and transports data to other parts of the system. It may perform additional functions such as integration of information and alarms. A choice of displays on the screen is usually available.

The AARK may be mounted on the machine, a cart, the floor, or the ceiling system. Some are an integral part of the anesthesia workstation.

The AARK must provide a means for entry of data that cannot be transferred automatically and to navigate between screens. A variety of devices has been used, including keypads, bar-code readers, touch screens, light pens, mouse, trackballs, voice activation, and electronic handwriting tablets (4–8). Manual entry should be as easy as possible. If it is difficult or takes time away from patient care, it will often be incomplete or incorrect. Pretyped notes for frequently used entries and macros that incorporate many items of information can be used to facilitate manual entry.

Because it is not always possible to enter all information at the time it occurred, there needs to be a means to add it after the fact and to indicate when it took place. Available systems handle back dating differently. A common method is to allow the timing of an entry in the past with an indication of when the entry was made.

Other Inputs

Connecting the network to other departments will enable personnel in the operating room to acquire records (laboratory, X-ray, etc.), consults and sources of information such as electronic textbooks and local information (protocols, drug pricing, telephone and beeper lists, call/staffing schedules, etc.).

Printer

If a printed (hard) copy of the anesthesia record or other information (such as the total quantities and costs of drugs used) is desired, a device capable of printing both graphics and text will be needed. Frequently the printing is performed at a location such as the postanesthesia care unit (PACU) or an office.

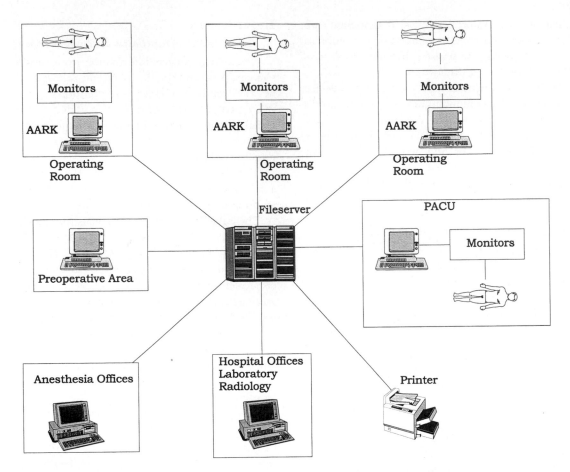

FIGURE 25.1.   Typical Anesthesia Information System (AIS). Workstations and peripheral devices are physically connected to each other and to the fileserver by wires or cables to form a local area network (LAN). Part of the network operating system resides in the fileserver and part at each user workstation. Applications software which runs the automated anesthesia record keepers (AARK) may reside in the fileserver but are executed in the AARKs. An AARK can be located in other places beside the operating room. PACU, postanesthesia care unit.

An important consideration is whether the printed record generated as data becomes available immediately or at the completion of the case, or both. If the record can only be printed at the end of the case, data can be lost should the AARK malfunction. Frequent back up will limit the loss. With a real-time copy the record can be removed from the printer and completed by hand should the automated system fail (8). Other benefits are that additional data and messages and correction of erroneous data can be done by hand.

RECORDS (9–11)

It may be advisable to have separate preoperative, intraoperative, and postoperative records. Each should have patient identification.

Pre-Anesthesia

Before anesthesia is begun, the patient needs to be assessed and a plan formulated. Needed information includes vital signs, history (including previous anesthetics), family history as far as it is of interest to the anesthesia provider (malignant hyperthermia, atypical pseudocholinesterase, etc.), medications, demographics and consent. Laboratory data, various reports (radiology, echocardiography, electrocardiography, treadmill, bronchoscopy, etc.) and consultations are also needed.

Manual recording of this information is time consuming and adds little to patient care. It can be automated by installing computers in the pre-anesthetic evaluation clinic (12). Programs to guide pre-anesthetic procedures are available with many data management systems.

Intraoperative

Intraoperative data are typically displayed in a form that emulates the traditional anesthesia record. Data can be presented in three ways: text, lists, and graphics. Text includes information in sentences, words, or phrases. Lists include tables, symbols for events, or numbers showing changes over time. Graphics are plots of data on a grid with the value of the variable plotted against time. Graphic displays may exhibit a trend which may not be evident from a list. Advances in hardware and software may permit video displays in future systems (13).

Patient Variables

The bulk of entries are objective patient variables (blood pressure, heart rate, oxygen saturation [SpO_2], carbon dioxide concentrations, end-tidal oxygen and anesthetic agent concentrations, central venous and arterial pressures, directly-measured blood gases, mixed venous SpO_2, intracranial pressure, cardiac output, tidal and minute volumes with spontaneous respiration, compliance, resistance, temperature, electrocardiogram, electroencephalogram). Most of this information can be transferred automatically.

Different systems handle editing of automatically captured patient variables in various ways. Some will not permit editing and require a note to explain an artifact. Others require the operator to approve variables before they are recorded, offer a window of time for editing or make the variables editable at any time.

Workstation Variables

Many of the variables measured by components of the anesthesia workstation and vigilance aids (composition of respiratory gases, breathing system pressure, tidal and minute volumes, respiratory rate, I:E ratio, breathing system pressures and flows, whether alarms are armed or disarmed and their settings, drugs administered by infusion pumps) can be transferred automatically to an electronic record. This can be automated totally or in part.

For some variables, such as gas flows and vaporizer settings, suitable transducers and interfaces are not yet available, so this information must be entered manually. New developments such as electronic flowmeters should make more automatic transfer of more information possible. From an anesthetic standpoint the end-tidal concentrations are more important than the settings. If the anesthetic agent monitor does not have automatic agent identification, this will need to be hand entered. It may be useful to include a prompt to remind the provider to enter this information.

Information from Anesthesia Care Provider

Some information, including observations and interventions, is available only from the anesthesia care provider. These should always be time stamped by the system. Entry of much of this information can be facilitated by macros. Important information includes pre- and postoperative diagnoses; premedication-type, amount, time given and effects; operation(s) performed; position of tracheal tube; difficulties encountered with intubation; heart and lung sounds; echocardiography information; patient appearance (e.g., pale, flushed, sweaty, wrinkled); estimated blood loss; urine output; the type of breathing system; special safety precautions; and checks of equipment.

Routine procedures, including positioning, padding of pressure points and eye care need to be included. Special procedures such as introduction of a central or arterial line or performance of a block with information on how it was performed and any problems that occurred should be recorded. Events that need to be entered (along with the time) include surgery start and stop times, tourniquet inflation and release, clamping and declamping of major vessels and cardiopulmonary bypass beginning and end. Many of these can be chosen from a preformed list.

The site, size, and type of intravenous catheter(s) and the type, amount and time of fluid administration need to be noted. If an infusion pump is being used, this can often be interfaced to the AARK. When a pump is not being used it is necessary to enter this data manually.

Laboratory Information

Laboratory information such as hemoglobin, blood gases, clotting values, and electrolytes are often needed during the course of an anesthetic. If the AIMS is connected to the laboratory computer, this information should be quickly available. Test results should be entered on the record at the time of sampling. For legal reasons, the time of arrival of results should be recorded as well.

If the information on a blood container could be scanned into a computer, this could be recorded on the record. If the electronic record is interfaced to the blood bank, the information on the container could be checked to determine if the blood was being administered to the correct patient (5).

Miscellaneous Measurements

Some information may be automatically transferred or may need to be entered manually totally or in part, depending on the institution.

Status of Neuromuscular Relaxation

Most neuromuscular stimulators depend on the anesthesia provider to assess the response so manual entry will be required. However, some instruments both stimulate and assess the response. These can be interfaced to the electronic record for automatic transfer of data.

Administration of Drugs

The record should contain the dosages and times of all medications administered. The complete record can then measure and display the total quantity of each drug given. Various methods have been used to at least partially automate these entries.

For convenience, most anesthesia drugs can be divided into categories by their actions (14). The specific medication can then be selected from a menu and its dosage entered.

Labels carrying the drug names and bar code

numbers can be attached to syringes. When the anesthesia provider picks up the syringe marked with a precoded label, he presents the label to the automatic reader (14).

Postanesthesia

Preoperative patient information and the record made during the intraoperative period should be immediately available to the PACU. It can then be continued in a different format during the patient's stay in that area.

USES OF DATA MANAGEMENT SYSTEMS

Log of Perioperative Events

An AIS can provide a timely and accurate record of patient care through the entire perioperative period.

Performance Assessment (15)

The electronic record can assist in studying outcomes. When a problem with a patient occurs, manual charting is often incomplete or inaccurate. AARK systems typically record information more frequently and accurately so that the relationship between events or interventions and the onset or continuation of a problem can be examined.

Research (15, 16)

Large retrospective studies are difficult to handle manually and may reflect the bias of the reviewer. If the record is electronic, it will be easier to look for the variables being studied. The database can be searched by procedure, patient characteristics, drugs, or other parameters. After the database has been established, the effects of a change in some aspect of care can be studied.

Education (15, 17, 18)

As departments institute various practice guidelines (e.g., preoperative testing, intraoperative medications and procedures, and postoperative care) the availability of these online may improve and simplify their implementation.

In a training program, an automated record can be used to review and refine the trainee's skills. An AIMS can provide a record of procedures performed by each trainee.

Billing (15, 19, 20)

Information necessary for billing includes patient demographics, insurance information, case-specific facts, and concurrency (the number of anesthetics supervised at one time). A data management system can be programmed to recognize these and to assign the proper billing codes.

Administrative Functions (20, 21)

The electronic record can provide information on utilization of facilities, personnel, equipment, and supplies. It may be used to facilitate case scheduling. It can also be used to obtain summaries of an anesthesia provider's or a group's practice patterns, e.g., the number of cases of a particular type done in a given period of time. In a group practice, questions often arise as to how the work is divided, time off, call, and number of nights and hours worked. The AIMS can be used to track these variables.

Quality Assurance (15, 22–26)

Data management systems can facilitate and improve quality assurance programs by scanning records electronically. Voluntary reporting of indicators has been shown to be unreliable (26, 27).

When an incident occurs, the relationships to drugs or procedures can be determined more accurately from an electronic record. In one reported case, it would have not been possible to determine the cause of a critical incident from the manual record. Fortunately there was also an electronic record that indicated the problem (28).

ADVANTAGES (7, 15, 29–31)
Accuracy (15, 32, 33)

The accuracy of handwritten records leaves much to be desired. (34, 35). There is a bias towards recording more normal values (36, 37). Electronic transfer reduces errors (38–41).

Studies show a high number of errors are made during telephone reporting of blood gas analysis in the operating room (42). Electronic transfer of this information should be more accurate.

Timeliness (15, 32)

Clinicians are not always able to make timely notations in the written record while responding to emergencies, and their memories are not completely reliable when recording after an incident. The result is that there is often an incomplete record during the periods of significant and rapid physiological changes and during which increased physical and pharmacological manipulations occur. With an electronic recordkeeper, recording will continue during these times.

Completeness (15, 33, 39, 43)

The automated record is more complete than the hand-written one (5, 39, 44). It is unusual to have vital signs recorded on a written record more often than every 5 minutes. Computerized records capture much more data.

Legibility (15, 32, 33)

Legibility is often a problem with manual records (5, 43). It can also be a problem with electronic records. The record needs to be configured in a format that is easily readable.

Standardization of Records

If the specialty of anesthesia is to conduct studies involving large numbers of patients, a standardized method of recording information will be needed. This will be easier to accomplish with electronic records. Standardization will allow subsequent care givers to determine all the facts of an anesthetic with minimal time and effort.

Decreased Paper Use (15)

Decreased paper use is a goal of electronic records. It is possible that in the future a paper printout will be unnecessary since it will be possible to call up all records on a computer.

Accessibility (15, 19)

Anesthesia providers need access to the record of previous anesthetics, especially if there has been an adverse drug reaction, difficult intubation, or nausea or vomiting. In the past, this necessitated having someone locate the old chart. This can be time consuming and may not be possible during off hours. If the record is stored electronically, it should be readily available at any time at all locations where access to patient data is required. In the future it may even be possible to transfer records between institutions.

Integration of Monitored Variables and Alarms

The operating room is an information-intensive situation with data frequently provided by a heterogeneous mix of independent devices. As a result, it may be difficult to compare variables and to determine the relationship between them. Trends that require the initiation of therapeutic measures may be overlooked. The electronic record may make it easier to present the data in a format that allows rapid and accurate identification of developing patterns and allows examination of the relationship between various interventions and responses.

Another problem in the operating room is that several different alarms are often enunciated at once. This may result in confusion as to the source and importance of the alarms. An integrated system can generate more specific and descriptive alarm messages. Ideally, all alarms would be displayed on one central panel designed for maximal visibility and readability, and the alarms on the primary monitors could be turned off. This would speed the process of determining what condition(s) required attention. The AARK could then analyze the data and suggest diagnoses and even treatments.

Legal Protection for the Provider (15, 32, 43, 45–49)

Every anesthetic record has the potential to become a legal document. No case will come to trial or settlement without a detailed analysis of it. A full and accurate record can make a difference in a claim for damages. Incomplete or illegible medical records create the impression that care was careless, superficial, or substandard—even if, in truth, it was reasonable. Clear, complete, and timely anesthesia records will almost always help to defend a case that was properly managed, although they will not help with one that was handled poorly. They may also help defend providers who make errors by helping to determine what occurred (9). An automated record can facilitate documentation of protective activities by presenting the clinician with a checklist of relevant safety items. The electronic record has more data than the written record and those data are more objective since they were not entered with the bias which an anesthesia provider might have.

These arguments are largely blunted if there is much artifact in the record or there is a way that the operator can alter the record. The medicolegal significance of the electronic record has yet to be determined since there have not been a large number of legal proceedings in which they were involved. While it is possible that the automated record will be a positive development in the defense of claims against anesthesia personnel, evidence that it reduces liability is not good (50). It is likely that each side is going to lose some cases it might have won with poorly decipherable records but on balance, the use of electronic records should promote justice and lead to more reasonable settlements.

Beneficial Effects on Anesthesia Provider's Time

Automation of data collection may make more time available for direct patient care. The time savings may be offset, however, if manual entry is difficult. Evidence that the electronic record has a beneficial impact on the provider's time is contradictory. Some studies have determined that charting time was not statistically different (51). Other studies have shown that charting time was modestly less with the electronic record (44, 52, 53).

Discovery of Discrepancies

It may be possible to pick up discrepancies between settings and readings using a computerized data system (54).

PROBLEMS (55)
Artifacts (5, 15, 32, 56–58)

A common source of concern with electronic records is fear that artifacts will be held against the practitioner if there is an untoward occurrence. Reducing artifacts is important not only because it avoids false data, but also will reduce the number of false-positive alarms and the possibility that incorrect information will be used to alter patient management. Artifacts may be caused by mechanical or electrical disturbances (e.g., external pressure on the blood pressure cuff; electrocautery interference on the electrocardiograph, oxygen monitor or pulse oximeter; malposition, ambient light, or motion on the pulse oximeter probe; line flushing or sampling on invasive pressures; and plugging of a sampling gas line). Another source of artifacts is logging errors by the anesthesia provider (59).

Artifacts can be reduced by using newer monitors with more resistance to interference and artifact rejection capability. Another method is to utilize the data comparison capabilities of the AARK. For example, heart rate is measured by several different monitors. The computer could compare these measurements and reject one that does not match the others.

When an erroneous value is not filtered out, manual entry of notes can be used to explain the questionable reading. Many artifacts can be addressed with prewritten notes from a prepared list of common causes of artifacts (e.g., SpO_2 affected by electrocautery). The practitioner may want to add an explanation as to why he feels that these data are artifactual.

Physical Layout

Contemporary operating rooms are often crowded, so the bulk of the AARK may pose problems. Careful consideration should be given to where the equipment and cables are placed. They should be in a location that is ergonomically practical and does not interfere with the function of other equipment.

Interfacing (2, 15, 59)

Interfacing some equipment to the electronic record can be difficult. Some devices must be modified and unless this is done correctly they may be rendered unsafe. Also the warranty may become void (60). A customized interface may make it difficult to exchange monitors.

One proposed solution to interfacing problems is the MIB (2, 59, 61, 62). The MIB provides a connection-oriented communication service between medical devices or between medical devices and computers. This will allow pieces of equipment that adhere to the standard to communicate with each other more easily and at a more rapid rate. Clinicians can make a vendor-independent selection of monitors and other devices. Retrofit-

ting current systems will require a "black box" converter between the port of each device and the computer.

Adverse Effects on Operator Vigilance (15)

A proposed argument against the AARK is that the clinician will not look at the monitors since there is no need to record the values shown on them (63). The thinking is the process of entering data on the record causes the anesthesia provider to mentally absorb that information (18). However, it has also been hypothesized that vigilance may be enhanced by the electronic record by presenting data in an integrated trending format and by eliminating much of the time devoted to record keeping (31, 33).

One study showed that anesthesia providers using an AARK demonstrated a significantly greater number of vigilance errors than those charting manually (64) Other studies have found that vigilance is not adversely affected by use of an electronic record (51, 52, 65).

User Attitude (15)

An anesthesia provider who finds computers intimidating or who has the perception that automated records invite lawsuits may be reluctant to invest the time and energy necessary to learn to use an information system. Since the electronic record is in development, there will be frequent upgrades, which can be a source of irritation. For a system to be successful, equipment needs to be dependable and there needs to be resources available at all times to straighten out glitches. Involving the users in choosing and configuring the system will help win support. A team to carry out implementation of an information system should be put together prior to its introduction (66). Detailed education in both the reasons for the conversion and the mechanical operation of the system will be necessary.

The method of introduction will affect acceptance (67). A common mistake is to introduce a system gradually and operate with two systems, paper and electronic, during the transition. Experience suggests that in most cases it is best is to make a quick, clean break with the old system and require all providers to use the new one (67).

Security (1, 47)

There needs to be a means to prevent intentional or accidental alteration of the record as well as a way of determining when and by whom alterations in the record have been made.

Confidentiality (1, 7, 47, 68)

The system must provide tools to safeguard the secrecy of the collected data yet make it easily retrievable to select users. The anesthesia record will be used by other health care providers and administrators, including nurses, physicians, technicians, billing personnel, pharmacy, peer review, and other anesthesia providers. All these individuals need certain information but not necessarily all that is on the record. It may be advantageous to make the record available in different formats that include only the information needed for their purposes (10).

Training (18, 24, 30, 66, 69)

Implementing an automated recordkeeping system requires an initial investment of time for user education. An inadequately prepared provider can cause records to be inaccurate or unusable. Training cannot be hit or miss. All providers must receive instruction before being allowed to use the electronic record. This can be difficult, especially if there are providers who work at different facilities.

Mechanical Problems

The operating room can be a hostile environment for computers. Damage may be caused by other equipment or user abuse. Cleanliness can be a problem. Bloody gloves may be used to make entries. Liquids may find their way into the mouse or keyboard. There is a great deal of other electrical equipment that could cause interference. Computer components are very sensitive to variations in temperature, humidity, and line voltage.

Electrical fluctuations can damage computer components, impair performance, and destroy data. The system should not be affected by power fluctuations, brownouts, or blackouts (66). Preventive measures include an uninterruptible power supply, and a line conditioner to prevent fluctuations in voltage. While special programs may help the user solve the most common problems, there must be support staff who can deal with other difficulties.

The information on the electronic record needs to be backed up at frequent intervals and stored in a manner which will ensure that it will not be lost. There needs to be a means to record data even if the computer fails during an anesthetic.

Inability to Deal with Certain Information

No devices are available for quantifying or measuring parameters such as pupillary size and reactivity, sweating, or blood loss.

Difficulty in Adapting to Special Situations (15)

In the operating room, the equipment is located in one or two locations. This means that connections between monitors and the electronic record and between the electronic record and the network do not need to be altered frequently. When anesthesia is administered in the radiology department, catheterization laboratory, or other remote area, the monitors in that location will probably not interface with the electronic record. This will necessitate taking the entire anesthesia machine with its monitors and electronic record to the location. This is inconvenient and can result in damage to the equipment. The information will need to be stored in the AARK until it can be connected to the network and the information downloaded for storage and printing.

Electroconvulsive therapy poses other problems. This is usually performed in a psychiatry suite or PACU. In this situation, several patients can be lined up and the anesthesia administered. The total time per patient is only several minutes and an anesthesia machine is usually not used. To use an electronic record in these cases, monitors would need to be connected and disconnected every few minutes and the record restarted for the next patient and demographic information added for each patient. A large anesthesia machine would need to be used. Many anesthetics would need to be stored on the electronic record until such time as downloading was possible. All this would greatly extend the time required. It is not likely that the electronic record will save time and make performing anesthesia for electroconvulsive therapy more efficient (70).

FINANCIAL CONSIDERATIONS (3, 30, 66)

If an institution is to survive, expenditures have to be controlled. All costs incurred and savings generated must be carefully taken into account.

Costs

The initial cost of a data management system will range between $12,000 and $35,000 per location, depending on the number of operating rooms and what equipment and infrastructure is already in place (71). The more sophisticated the system, the higher the cost. The cost will also depend on the wiring requirements and ability of existing monitors and other equipment to interface with the system. There are costs involved in training users and support personnel. Both the cost of the training and that of lost work must be considered. These will be incurred each time there is a revision in the program.

After purchase and installation, ongoing costs include hardware and software maintenance and support personnel. Software maintenance, including upgrades, can range from 5 to 20% of the initial purchase price of the system each year (66). Other costs to be considered include paper and cartridges for the printer and the cost of adding bar codes. If the system is difficult to operate, mistakes may result in lost billings.

Savings

The electronic record makes it easier to look at costs (72, 73). By combining the costs of drugs and disposable items with those of monitoring and other equipment used, the actual cost of an anesthetic can be determined. After each case the caregiver can be presented with the costs of drugs and other items used. Items can then be examined to determine if they were truly necessary and if other less costly ones could be used. The costs of different techniques can also be compared.

Savings may be achieved by using the record to assist in the implementation of pharmaceutical practice guidelines (72). The system can alert the user to the cost of different drugs and determine the most cost-effective. Further savings can be achieved by reducing last minute delays or cancellations of surgery, and improving operating room staffing and utilization.

Automated records should reduce losses due to uncaptured drug and supply charges and inaccurate coding or time billing. Other possible savings include reductions in administrative and overhead costs in billing and medical records. Savings can be achieved on quality assurance and compliance with Joint Commission on Accreditation of Healthcare Organizations (JCAHO) and other regulatory requirements by reducing secretarial time (19). Improved inventory control for disposable items and medications may save money.

Savings can be achieved if automated records aid physicians and institutions in professional liability litigation. One insurance company has offered a discount for use of automated records (49). Some problems that result in lawsuits, such as injecting the wrong, drug may be avoided.

If central trending and alarm functions are assumed by the automated record system, barebones monitors without trending and alarms are all that are necessary and these cost less than the top-of-the-line models with every possible feature (43).

Whether data management systems will be cost effective remains to be demonstrated (71). While some centers have reported savings (30), cost reductions sufficient to justify the high cost of AARKs have been difficult to document.

In summary, the electronic record offers many advantages as well as a number of disadvantages. Some institutions have used them for a time and then stopped, because the work of supporting them was too demanding (9). Systems presently available are still somewhat rudimentary in relation to their potential, but they are becoming more powerful, easier to use and less expensive. Despite the fact that there are little hard data to support the superiority of automated records, it seems likely that in the future all medical records will be computerized and integrated.

REFERENCES

1. Anonymous. An overview of anesthesia information management systems. Technology for Anesthesia 1995;16(4):1–5.

2. Anonymous. The medical information bus: Is the clinician-friendly device interface standard commercially viable? Journal of Clinical Monitoring 1995;11:260.

3. Anonymous. Understanding and implementing hospital information systems, Part 1. Technology for Anesthesia 1995;15(10):1–8.

4. Block FE Jr. Entry of drug administration data. In: Gravenstein JS, Newbower TS, Ream AK, et al., eds. The automated anesthesia records and alarm systems. Boston, MA: Butterworth, 1987;93–98.

5. Abenstein JP, DeVos CB, Tarhan A, et al. Eight years' experience with automated anesthesia record keeping: Lessons learned—new directions taken. Int J Clin Monit Comput 1992;9:117–129.

6. Smith NT, Brien RA, Pettus DC, et al. Recognition accuracy with a voice-recognition system designed for anesthesia record keeping. Journal of Clinical Monitoring 1990;6:299–306.

7. Weiss YG, Cotev S, Drenger B, et al. Patient data management systems in anaesthesia: an emerging technology. Can J Anaesth 1995;42:914–921.

8. Feldman JM. Computerized anesthesia recording systems. Adv Anes 1989;6:325–354.

9. Ream AK. Automating the recording and improving the presentation of the anesthesia record. Journal of Clinical Monitoring 1989;5:270–283.

10. Gravenstein JS. The uses of the anesthesia record. Journal of Clinical Monitoring 1989;5:256–263.

11. Ream AK. Computerization of anesthesia information management. Information management: What is it? How is it done? Journal of Clinical Monitoring 1991;7:75–77.

12. Gibby GL, Lemeer G, Jackson K. Use of data from a hospital online medical records system by physicians during preanesthetic evaluation. Journal of Clinical Monitoring 1996;12:405–408.

13. Perrino AC, Luther MA, Phillips DB, et al. A multimedia perioperative record keeper for clinical research. Journal of Clinical Monitoring 1996;12:251–259.

14. Apple HP, Schneider AJL, Fadel J. Design and evaluation of a semiautomatic anesthesia record system. Med Instrum 1982;16:69–71.

15. Anonymous. Automated record keeping in anesthesia. Health Devices 1988;17:30–31.

16. Stanley TE III. Clinical research applications of automated anesthesia information management systems. Journal of Clinical Monitoring 1991;7:357–358.

17. Booij LDHJ. Use of the anesthesia database for supervision and training. Journal of Clinical Monitoring 1991;7:356–357.

18. Heinrichs W. Automated anaesthesia record systems, observations on future trends of development. Int J Clin Monit Comput 1995;12:17–20.

19. Eichhorn JH, Edsall SW. Computerization of anesthesia information management. Journal of Clinical Monitoring 1991;7:71–82.

20. Phillips CA III. Using the database for billing and administrative purposes. Journal of Clinical Monitoring 1991;7:355–356.

21. Krucylak PE, Foroughi V, Eaton F, et al. Anesthesia data management systems as a tool for total quality management of operating rooms. Anesth Analg 1997; 84:S41.

22. Eichorn JH. Computerization of anesthesia information management. Quality assurance: no longer a separate process. Journal of Clinical Monitoring 1991;7: 79–81.

23. Edsall DW. Using the database for quality assurance and risk management. Journal of Clinical Monitoring 1991;7:351–358.

24. Edsall DW. Quality assessment with a computerized anesthesia information management system (AIMS). QRB 1991;17:182–93.

25. Feldman JM. Anesthesia recordkeepers into the next century. American Society of Anesthesiologists Newsletter 1993;57:24–27.

26. Sanborn KV, Castro J, Kuroda M, et al. Detection of intraoperative incidents by electronic scanning of computerized anesthesia records. Anesthesiology 1996;85: 977–987.

27. Sanborn KV, Castro J, Kuroda M, et al. Computerized detection of quality assurance incidents using an automated anesthesia record-keeping system. Journal of Clinical Monitoring 1995;11:276–277.

28. Thrush DN. Automated anesthesia records and anesthetic incidents. Journal of Clinical Monitoring 1992; 8:59–61.

29. Queram BJ. Development of automated anesthesia recordkeeper: past, present, future. Journal of Clinical Monitoring 1987;3:307–308.

30. Tuohy GF. Advantages and disadvantages of automated anesthesia records. American Society of Anesthesiologists Newsletter 1995;59:17–20.

31. Whitcher C. Advantages of automated record keeping in safety and cost containment in anesthesia. In: Gravenstein JS, Holzer JF, eds. Safety and cost containment in anesthesia. Boston: Butterworth, 1988;207–221.

32. Kroll M. Computerization of anesthesia information management. The automated record: legal helper or Pandora's box. Journal of Clinical Monitoring 1991; 7:77–78.

33. Hamilton WK. The automated anesthesia record is in-

evitable and valuable. Journal of Clinical Monitoring 1990;6:333–334.

34. Rowe L, Galletly DC, Henderson RS. Accuracy of text entries within a manually compiled anaesthetic record. Br J Anaesth 1992;68:381–387.

35. Thrush DN, Are automated anesthesia records better? J Clin Anesth 1992; 4:386–389.

36. Cook R, McDonald JS, Nunciata E. Differences between handwritten and automatic blood pressure records. Anesthesiology 1989;71:385–390.

37. Devitt JH, Kurrek MM, Cohen MM, et al. Peaks and valleys of anaesthetic charting. Can Anaesth Soc J 1997;44:A49.

38. Dirksen R, Lerou JGC, van Daele M, et al. The clinical use of the Ohmeda automated anesthesia record keeper integrated in the Modulus II anesthesia system. Int J Clin Monit Comput 1987;4:135–139.

39. Lerou JGC, Dirksen R, van Daele M, et al. Automated charting of physiological variables in anesthesia: a quantitative comparison of automated versus hand-written anesthesia records. Journal of Clinical Monitoring 1988;4:37–47.

40. Paulus DA, van der Aa JJ, McLaughlin GM, et al. A semiautomated anesthesia record keeper—clinical evaluation. Journal of Clinical Monitoring 1985;1: 286–287.

41. Gravenstein JS, Paulus DA, Eames S, et al. The electronic clipboard: a semiautomatic anesthesia record. Int J Clin Monit Comput 1987;4:153–159.

42. Gaiser R, Hayes T, Castro A. Telephone reporting of blood analysis into the operating room. Anesth Analg 1996;82:1284–1286.

43. Eichhorn JH. Anesthesia record keeping. Int J Clin Monit Comput 1993;10:109–1015.

44. Edsall DW, Deshane P, Giles C, et al. Computerized patient anesthesia records: less time and better quality than manually produced anesthesia records. J Clin Anesth 1993;5:275–283.

45. Ferrari HA. Defending anesthesia malpractice claims: role of computerized records. American Society of Anesthesiologists Newsletter 1995;59:14–16.

46. Gibbs RF. The present and future medicolegal importance of record keeping in anesthesia and intensive care: the case for automation. J Clin Monit 1989;5: 251–255.

47. Kroll DA. The legal implications of computerized anesthesia records: an admittedly biased review. Seminars in Anesthesia 1991;10:30–35.

48. Meijen AP, Beneken JEW. Data acquisition and display. A system with centralized display, automated record keeping and intelligence alarms. In: Gravenstein JS, Newbower RS, Ream AK, et al., eds. The auto-

mated record and alarm systems. Boston: Butterworths, 1987;229–245.

49. Schoenstadt DA. Computerized anesthesia records: an insurance company's perspective. Seminars in Anesthesia 1991;10:41–47.

50. Zeitlin GL. Automated records do not reduce anesthesia liability. American Society of Anesthesiologists Newsletter 1995;59:21–23.

51. Allard J, Dzwonczyk R, Yablok D, et al. Effect of automatic record keeping on vigilance and record keeping time. Br J Anaesth 1995;74:619–626.

52. Herndon OW, Weinger MB, Zornow MH, et al. The use of automated record keeping saves time in complicated anesthetic procedures. Anesth Analg 1993; 76: S140.

53. Weinger MB, Herndon OW, Gaba DM. The effect of electronic record keeping and transesophageal echocardiography on task distribution, workload, and vigilance during cardiac anesthesia. Anesthesiology 1997; 87:144–155.

54. Gilmour IJ, Gove K. Safety and efficacy of a ventilator database interface. Journal of Clinical Monitoring 1995;11:183–185.

55. Eichhorn JH. Disadvantages of automated anesthesia records. In: Gravenstein JS, Holzer JF, eds. Safety and cost containment in anesthesia. Boston: Butterworth, 1988;223–232.

56. Westenskow DW. Computerization of anesthesia information management. Artifacts and alarms: problems and benefits. Journal of Clinical Monitoring 1991;7:76–77.

57. Jones BR, Smith NT. Type and frequency of artifacts recorded on automated anesthesia records. Anesth Analg 1990;70:S180.

58. Saunders RJ. The automated anesthetic record will not automatically solve problems in record keeping. Journal of Clinical Monitoring 1990;6:334–337.

59. Gardner RM, Prakash O. Challenges and opportunities for computerizing the anesthesia record. J Clin Anesth 1994;6:333–341.

60. Roessler P, Brenton MW, Lambert TF. Problems with automating anaesthetic records. Anaesthesia and Intensive Care 1986;14:443–447.

61. Fiegler A, Stead S. The medical information bus. Biomed Instrum Technol 1990; 24:101–111.

62. Weinger MB, Smith NT. Vigilance, alarms, and integrated monitoring systems. In: Ehrenwerth J, Eisenkraft JB, eds. Anesthesia equipment, principles and applications. St. Louis: Mosby, 1993;350–384.

63. Noel TA. Computerized anesthesia records may be dangerous. Anesthesiology 1986; 64:300.

64. Yablok DO. Comparison of vigilance using automated

versus hand written records. Anesthesiology 1990;73: A416.

65. Loeb RG. Manual record keeping is not necessary for anesthesia vigilance. Journal of Clinical Monitoring 1995;11:9–13.

66. Anonymous. Understanding and implementing hospital information systems, Part II. Technology for Anesthesia 1995;15(11):1–7.

67. McDonald JS, Block FE Jr, Minic K. Will automated anesthesia recordkeeping work in a large university hospital setting? Anesth Analg 1990;70:S263.

68. Woodward B. The computer-based patient record and confidentiality. N Engl J Med 1995;333:1419–1422.

69. Stanley TE. Automated anesthesia records—worth the effort? IARS Review Course Lecture, Orlando, FL, March 1994.

70. Gage JS, Litman SJ, Bicker A, et al. Automated record keeping for electroconvulsive therapy. Br J Anaesth 1995;74:24.

71. Anonymous. Anesthesia information systems used to track costs, outcomes. Technology for Anesthesia 1994;14(12):1–3.

72. Lubarsky DA, Sanderson IC, Gibert WC, et al. Using an anesthesia information management system as a cost containment tool. Description and validation. Anesthesiology 1997;86:1161–1169.

73. Sanderson IC, Coleman RL, Lubarsky DA, et al. In defense of the ARKIVE. Br J Anaesth 1995;75: 502–503.

QUESTIONS

1. Which of the following definitions is incorrect?
   A. Analog data are continuous data that can, within limits, assume any value
   B. Closed architecture refers to equipment designed to work only with accessories made by one manufacturer
   C. Analog is a way of storing information using numbers
   D. A serial port transmits data one bit after another through a single cable
   E. A macro is a tool used to automate tasks within a program

Each question below contains four suggested answers of which one or more is correct.
Choose the answer:
A if 1, 2, and 3 are correct
B if 1 and 3 are correct
C if 2 and 4 are correct
D if 4 is correct
E if 1, 2, 3, and 4 are correct

2. Uses of a data management system in anesthesia include
   1. Education
   2. Quality assurance
   3. Research
   4. Billing

3. Proven benefits of automated records include
   1. Legal protection for the anesthesia provider
   2. Financial savings
   3. Beneficial effect on anesthesia provider's time
   4. Accuracy

4. Functions of the automated record keeper include
   1. Collecting information from various monitors
   2. Presenting trends on a screen
   3. Integrating alarms
   4. Storing data in a database

5. Data can be entered into the automated record keeper
   1. Using bar codes
   2. Electronically from a clinical laboratory
   3. Using voice activation
   4. Manually from a keyboard

6. Problems associated with data management systems include
   1. Artifactual data
   2. Integration of monitored variables and alarms
   3. Increased paper use
   4. Interfacing monitors

7. Principles in successful introduction of a data management system include
   1. Technical support
   2. Gradual introduction of the system
   3. User friendliness
   4. During introduction of the electronic system, the paper record should also be used

8. Factors that will ensure a minimum of mechanical problems include
   1. Cleanliness when working with components
   2. Uninterruptible power supply
   3. Frequent backup of data
   4. Constant temperature

9. Factors that must be considered in the cost of a data management system include
   1. Billing errors
   2. Initial cost of $35,000 to $45,000 per anesthetizing location
   3. Continuing technical support
   4. Software maintenance of up to 5% of the initial cost

10. Financial benefits of the data management system include
    1. Determining actual costs of the materials and medications used for an anesthetic
    2. Decreased liability insurance premiums
    3. Implementation of pharmaceutical practice guidelines
    4. Better staffing utilization

ANSWERS

1. C
2. E
3. D
4. E
5. E
6. E
7. B
8. E
9. B
10. E

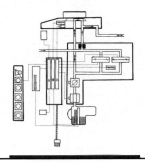

EQUIPMENT CARE AND PLANNING

CHAPTER 26

Equipment Checking and Maintenance

INTRODUCTION

The purpose of a checkout procedure analogous to the preflight check for airline pilots is to determine whether the equipment is functioning properly and ready for use (1–3). Failure to check equipment properly may be a factor in up to 33% of critical incidents (4–10). Defects may be found even just after preventive maintenance is performed (11).

Checking equipment properly can help to prevent equipment-related morbidity and mortality, improve preventive maintenance and educate the anesthesia provider about equipment (1, 4, 12–14).

Unfortunately, failure to perform a proper check before use is common (8, 15–21), and many anesthesia personnel are unable to identify intentionally created faults (22–26). With intensive training, performance is improved but high rates of completion are not achieved (27). It is recognized that it may not be possible to carry out a full check in an emergency situation, but it would seem reasonable to document the circumstances when time permits (1).

The 1988 anesthesia machine standard that was reapproved in 1994 (28) requires that an outline of operational checks to be carried out before use be provided by the manufacturer and be located on the machine. User manuals provided by manufacturers for newer machines have fairly complete and detailed directions for checking. These should be read carefully, and the suggested procedures followed.

The Food and Drug Administration (FDA), working with representatives of the anesthesia community and industry, developed a general pre-use checkout and inspection procedure, which was published in 1986 (29). Unfortunately, this list was too complicated for most users. Also, a study showed that the introduction of this checklist did not improve the ability to detect faults (23). A simplified, more user-friendly version was published in 1993 (30). This is shown in Table 26.1. An attempt was made to retain or add checks of components that fail more frequently than others and that quickly injure the patient when they do fail (31). Components that fail infrequently and that do not immediately jeopardize the patient when they do fail are not included in the 1993 version, but must still be checked during routine preventive maintenance of the anesthesia machine. The steps follow a logical sequence as they parallel the flow of gas through the anesthesia machine.

This list is designed for workstations with a circle system, ventilator with a standing bellows and a capnograph, pulse oximeter, oxygen analyzer, respiratory volume meter, and airway pressure monitor with high and low pressure alarms. Clinicians using equipment that does not conform to this configuration will need to modify the procedure. For example, if a Mapleson system is to be used, the checking procedure should include this fact. The manufacturer's user's manual should be consulted for special procedures. Local modifications should have appropriate peer review.

A copy of the checkout procedure should be kept in the drawer of the anesthesia machine or cart or attached to one of these. A record that the checklist was used should be made and kept for several years. A general rule says, "If it isn't written down, it wasn't done" (32).

This chapter is constructed along the outline of the FDA checkout procedure. These recommendations should be regarded as the minimum that should be performed. Other suggested tests are given here to give the reader a choice. When an alternate test is given, an attempt will be made to point out the advantages and deficiencies of the various tests. The user should read the manufacturer's suggested checking procedures and incorporate specific points into the generic checkout.

A printed checklist presents a more organized and systematic approach than if the anesthesia

---

TABLE 26.1. **Anesthesia Apparatus Checkout Recommendations, 1995**

This checkout, or a reasonable equivalent, should be conducted before administration of anesthesia. These recommendations are only valid for an anesthesia system that conforms to current and relevant standards and includes an ascending bellows ventilator and at least the following monitors: capnograph, pulse oximeter, oxygen analyzer, respiratory volume and monitor (spirometer), and breathing system pressure monitor with high and low pressure alarms.

Emergency Ventilation Equipment
*1. Verify backup ventilation equipment is available and functioning.

High Pressure System
*2. Check oxygen cylinder supply.
    a. Open O_2 cylinder and verify at least half full (about 1000 psi).
    b. Close cylinder.
*3. Check central pipeline supplies.
    Check that the hoses are connected and pipeline gauges read about 50 psi.

Low Pressure System
*4. Check initial status of low pressure system.
    a. Close flow control valves and turn vaporizers off.
    b. Check fill level and tighten vaporizers' filler caps.
*5. Perform leak check of machine low pressure system.
    a. Verify that the machine master switch and flow control valves are OFF.
    b. Attach "suction bulb" to common (fresh) gas outlet.
    c. Squeeze bulb repeatedly until fully collapsed.
    d. Verify bulb stays *fully* collapsed for at least 10 seconds.
    e. Open one vaporizer at a time and repeat 'c' and 'd' as above.
    f. Remove suction bulb, and reconnect fresh gas hose.
*6. Turn on machine master switch and all other necessary electrical equipment.
*7. Test flowmeters.
    a. Adjust flow of all gases through their full range, checking for smooth operation of floats and undamaged flowtubes.
    b. Attempt to create an hypoxic O_2/N_2O mixture and verify correct changes in flow and/or alarm.

Scavenging System
*8. Adjust and check scavenging system.
    a. Ensure proper connections between the scavenging system and both adjustable pressure-limiting (APL) (pop-off) valve and ventilator relief valve.
    b. Adjust waste gas vacuum (if possible).
    c. Fully open APL valve and occlude Y-piece.
    d. With minimum O_2 flow, allow scavenger reservoir bag to collapse completely and verify that absorber pressure gauge reads about zero.
    e. With the O_2 flush activated, allow the scavenger reservoir bag to distend fully, and then verify that absorber pressure gauge reads <10 cm H_2O.

Breathing System
*9. Calibrate O_2 monitor.
    a. Ensure monitor reads 21% in room air.
    b. Verify low O_2 alarm is enabled and functioning.
    c. Reinstall sensor in circuit and flush breathing system with O_2.
    d. Verify that monitor now reads greater than 90%.

(continued)

TABLE **26.1. (continued)**

10. Check initial status of breathing system.
  a. Set selector switch to "Bag" mode.
  b. Check that breathing circuit is complete, undamaged, and unobstructed.
  c. Verify that CO_2 absorbent is adequate.
  d. Install breathing circuit accessory equipment (e.g., humidifier, positive end–expiratory pressure (PEEP) valve) to be used during the case.
11. Perform leak check of the breathing system.
  a. Set all gas flows to zero (or minimum).
  b. Close APL (pop-off) valve and occlude Y-piece.
  c. Pressurize breathing system to about 30 cm H_2O with O_2 flush.
  d. Ensure that pressure remains fixed at least 10 seconds.
  e. Open APL (pop-off) valve and ensure that pressure decreases.

Manual and Automatic Ventilation Systems
12. Test ventilator systems and unidirectional valves.
  a. Place a second breathing bag on Y-piece.
  b. Set appropriate ventilator parameters for next patient.
  c. Switch to automatic ventilation (Ventilator) mode.
  d. Turn ventilator ON and fill bellows and breathing bag with O_2 flush.
  e. Set O_2 flow to minimum, other gas flows to zero.
  f. Verify that during inspiration, bellows delivers appropriate tidal volume and that during expiration bellows fills completely.
  g. Set fresh gas flow to about 5 l/min.
  h. Verify that the ventilator bellows and simulated lungs fill and empty appropriately without sustained pressure at end expiration.
  i. Check for proper action of unidirectional valves.
  j. Exercise breathing circuit accessories to ensure proper function.
  k. Turn ventilator OFF and switch to manual ventilation (Bag/APL) mode.
  l. Ventilate manually and ensure inflation and deflation of artificial lungs and appropriate feel of system resistance and compliance.
  m. Remove second breathing bag from Y-piece.

Monitors
13. Check, calibrate and/or set alarm limits of all monitors.
  Capnometer   Pulse oximeter
  Oxygen analyzer   Respiratory volume monitor
  (spirometer)
  Pressure monitor with high and low airway alarms

Final Position
14. Check final status of machine.
  a. Vaporizers off.
  b. APL valve open.
  c. Selector switch to "Bag"
  d. All flowmeters to zero.
  e. Patient suction level adequate.
  f. Breathing system ready to use.

---

* If an anesthesia provider uses the same machine in successive cases, these steps need not be repeated or may be abbreviated after the initial checkout.
APL = adjustable pressure limiting.

provider uses a mental list and may result in improved detection of faults (26). A pictorial checkout may be easier to read and follow than a typewritten list (9).

Electronic checklists have been developed (4, 33). They may provide more extensive checking and support information than a paper checklist (4). They may also include other protocols and problem-solving information.

As anesthesia machines become more electronic, more checking will be performed automatically and will include such things as system compliance and leakage. Electronic checklists designed for particular pieces of equipment will be developed and displayed during startup. Minimal user interaction will be necessary during the checking procedure. It will be necessary to perform specific checkout procedures before the equipment can be used. Whether a full check was carried out or some parts were omitted will be automatically recorded.

DAILY CHECKS BEFORE BEGINNING ANESTHESIA
Emergency Ventilation Equipment (31)
Manual Resuscitator

A backup ventilation system must be readily available and functioning and should not require oxygen from the anesthesia machine. Though rare, certain malfunctions can render the anesthesia machine inoperative (31). Sometimes a problem occurs that cannot be diagnosed quickly. In these cases, a manual resuscitator will allow the user to generate a positive pressure and ventilate the patient while the problem is corrected or the machine replaced.

These requirements can be fulfilled by a self-inflating resuscitation bag (see Chapter 9, "Manual Resuscitators"). An oxygen flowmeter that can be attached to the pipeline outlet (Fig. 26.1) will provide a source of oxygen if the anesthesia machine cannot be used. The resuscitation bag should be inspected for signs of wear such as cracks or tears. Next, the patient port should be occluded and the bag squeezed (Fig. 26.2). Pressure should build up rapidly to a point at which the bag can no longer be compressed. If there is a pressure-limiting device, it can be checked by connecting a pressure manometer between the patient port and the bag, using a T fitting. If there is an override mechanism on the pressure-limiting device, this should be checked.

To check the bag refill valve, the bag should be squeezed, then the patient port occluded, then

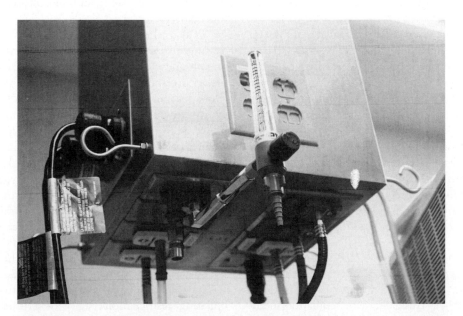

FIGURE 26.1. A flowmeter separate from the anesthesia machine can provide a source of oxygen in an emergency.

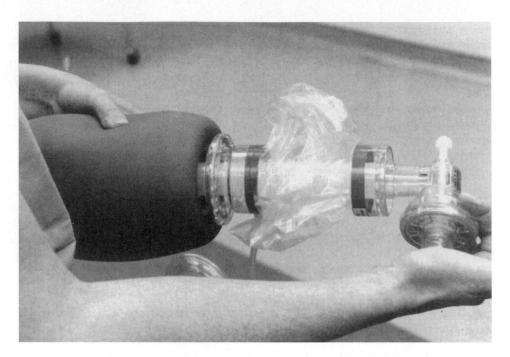

FIGURE 26.2. Squeezing the resuscitation bag with the patient port occluded.

the bag released. The bag should reexpand rapidly.

If the resuscitator has a reservoir, its function can be checked by performing several compression-release cycles with no oxygen flow into the reservoir. The reservoir should deflate, but the resuscitation bag should continue to expand.

A reservoir bag should be placed over the patient port (Fig. 26.3). Squeezing the resuscitation bag should cause the reservoir bag to inflate. After the resuscitation bag is released, patency of the exhalation path should be confirmed by squeezing the reservoir bag. It should deflate easily.

A Mapleson D system (see Chapter 7, "Breathing Systems II: Mapleson Systems") with a separate oxygen source may also be used for emergency ventilation. This system must also be checked for obstructions and leaks.

Equipment for the Difficult Airway

There should be immediately available a means to deal with the cannot ventilate/cannot intubate situation (34). Three alternate ventilation methods that can be instituted blindly and quickly and that appear to have a low risk:benefit ratio have

been described: the Combitube (discussed in Chapter 17, "Tracheal Tubes"); the laryngeal mask airway (discussed in Chapter 15, "The Laryngeal Mask Airway"); and transtracheal ventilation devices.

Transtracheal ventilation is performed by inserting a large catheter through the cricothyroid membrane and connecting it to a source of oxygen under pressure (35). There are three systems that work reliably and can be easily and inexpensively assembled. The first is a jet injector (blow gun) powered by regulated or unregulated pipeline oxygen pressure (Fig. 26.4). The second is a jet injector powered by an oxygen cylinder regulator. The third uses the anesthesia machine oxygen flush valve. The fresh gas outlet of the anesthesia machine is connected to noncompliant tubing by a standard 15 mm tracheal tube connector. The other end of the tubing is connected to the transtracheal catheter. This can be accomplished in several ways. One is shown in Figure 26.5. **NOTE:** Using the anesthesia breathing system or a self-inflating resuscitation bag with a transtracheal catheter *will not* produce effective ventilation (35).

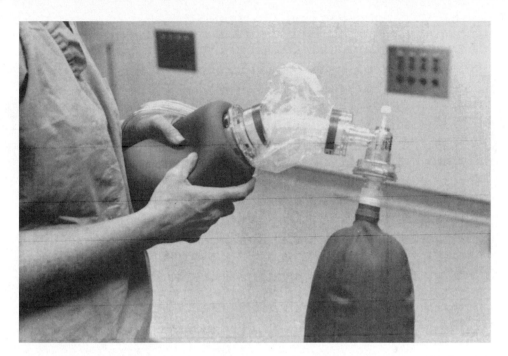

FIGURE 26.3. The resuscitation bag is further checked by placing a reservoir bag over the patient port. Squeezing the resuscitation bag should cause the reservoir bag to inflate. The reservoir bag should then deflate easily when it is squeezed.

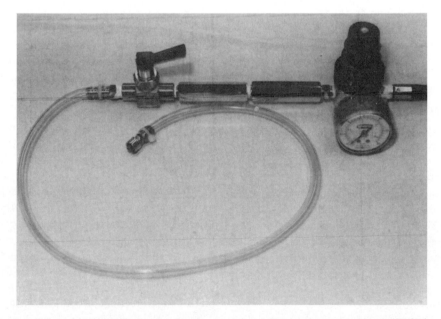

FIGURE 26.4. This system is designed to deliver oxygen at high flow through a small tubing. The regulator at the right is attached to a 50-psig oxygen source such as the pipeline system. The pressure delivered can be adjusted by turning the knob. The flow is controlled by the toggle switch downstream of the regulator. The tubing is attached to a large-bore needle or other device placed percutaneously through the cricothyroid membrane.

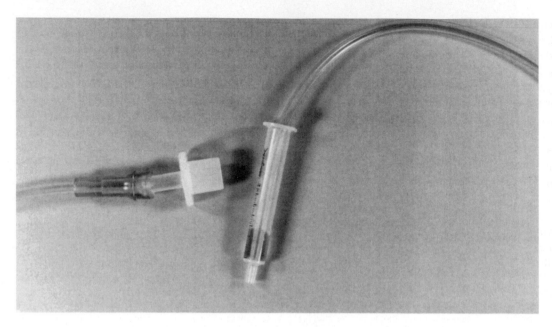

FIGURE 26.5. One end of the tubing has a 15-mm adaptor for attachment to the machine fresh gas outlet. The other end is firmly glued into the barrel of a 3-ml syringe. This end attaches to a large-bore intravenous catheter inserted percutaneously through the cricothyroid membrane.

Some authors recommend before any checking of the anesthesia machine is done that the user smell the gas from the fresh gas outlet to see if vapor has been leaking from a vaporizer.

High Pressure System
Cylinder Gas Supply

Oxygen cylinders must be checked for correct mounting and adequate content. Leaks from inadequately tightened yoke screws are frequently detected at this time.

Before gas supplies are checked, all flow control valves should be closed by turning them completely clockwise. Excessive torque should be avoided. Opening a cylinder or connecting a pipeline hose when a flow control valve is open may cause the flowmeter indicator to shoot up to the top of the tube and perhaps be damaged, stuck at the top, or not noticed (36–38).

Cylinder gauges should be checked to make certain that they read zero. Yokes should be scanned to make certain any not containing a cylinder are fitted with a yoke plug. All tags should indicate *full* or *in use*.

The pressure in an oxygen cylinder is checked by turning the valve slowly counterclockwise while observing the related pressure gauge. If a hissing sound occurs, the cylinder should be tightened in the yoke. If the machine is equipped with a double yoke, the pressure in the second cylinder should be checked. The valve on the first cylinder should be closed and the oxygen flush used to release the pressure from the first cylinder. The second cylinder is then opened and its pressure checked.

The cylinder(s) should contain sufficient gas so that in the event of a problem with the pipeline supply, life support can be maintained until the pipeline problem can be corrected or more cylinders obtained. Whether a less-than-full cylinder is acceptable will depend on the particular circumstances. A full E cylinder will contain about 625 liters. Therefore, one full cylinder will last less than 4 hr at a flow of 3 l/min. How low a pressure is acceptable will depend on whether additional cylinders are readily available and how low a fresh gas flow the user is willing to use. Hand ventilation as opposed to automatic ventilation will conserve gas. The FDA checklist recommends that the cylinder be at least half full (about 1000 psig [6800 kPa]). If there are two cylinders and one is completely full, a lower pressure in the second cylinder may be acceptable. Even if there is only one cylinder and it is 25% full, it will deliver oxygen at 1 l/min for over 2 hours if a ventilator is not in use. The authors feel that having 500 psig (3400 kPa) in a cylinder is adequate provided the anesthesia provider is aware of the steps needed to conserve oxygen until a full cylinder can be procured.

If pipeline oxygen pressure is lost, a half-full E cylinder of oxygen will run the anesthesia machine and mechanical ventilator for approximately 10 to 30 minutes, depending on the type of ventilator.

It has been suggested that merely checking a cylinder for adequate pressure is not enough. The check valve that prevents cylinder gas from being used when the pipeline is connected may stick, preventing flow from the cylinder if the pipeline is not in use. To check this valve, the pipeline should be disconnected and flow demonstrated after the cylinder is turned ON (39).

Empty or near-empty cylinders should be labeled as empty and replaced with full ones.

The 1993 FDA recommendations do not mention checking cylinders containing gases other than oxygen, because these are not essential for life support. If it is planned to use one of these gases, it is reassuring to know that reserve supplies are available on the machine. As discussed in Chapter 1, "Compressed Gas Containers," the contents of a nitrous oxide cylinder may not be reflected by the pressure. The pressure gauge will continue to read 745 psig (5066 kPa) until all of the liquid has been consumed. If the pressure is less than 600 psig (4080 kPa), the nitrous oxide cylinder is nearly empty and should probably be replaced. Air cylinders should be replaced around 1000 psig (6800 kPa), carbon dioxide around 600 psig (4080 kPa), and oxygen-helium around 1000 psig (6800kPa) (40).

After the pressures are checked, all cylinder valves should be closed. If this is not done, leaks may cause loss of the entire supply. During use, there will be pressure fluctuations in the machine and the pipeline hoses. This is especially true of oxygen when a ventilator is in use. As the ventila-tor cycles, there will be a transient lowering of pressure in the machine. If the pressure falls below that at the regulator outlet while the cylinder valve is open, gas will be drawn from the cylinder until the pressure increases. Eventually, the cylinder will empty and there may be no emergency supply available.

When piped gases are not going to be used, there should be one full cylinder of each gas to be used and the valve on any cylinder not to be used should be closed after the pressure has been checked. The cylinders of gases which are to be used should be checked to make certain they have adequate contents for the intended procedure and the valves on these cylinders left fully open.

Pipeline Gas Supply

Many institutions disconnect the pipeline hoses from the machine at night to prevent leakage from the hoses and to allow the machine to be moved for cleaning. If this is the case, the hoses need to be reconnected to the pipeline system. Fittings should hold firmly, no leaks should be audible and the hoses should be arranged to prevent occlusion. The pipeline pressure indicators (gauges) should read 345 to 380 kPa (50 to 55 psig).

As discussed in Chapter 4, "Anesthesia Machines," a pipeline pressure gauge will register only pipeline pressure if it is positioned upstream of the check valve at the pipeline inlet, as required by the 1988 American Society for Testing and Materials (ASTM) machine standard (28). If it is located downstream of the check valve, as it is on some older machines, the pressure registered will reflect the pressure in the machine (41).

Low Pressure System (31)
Initial Status

The check of the low-pressure system is begun by making sure that all vaporizers and flow control valves are turned off. The liquid level in each vaporizer should be checked, adding more if needed. Filler caps and drain valves should be checked for tightness.

Leak Checks of Machine Low-Pressure System (42–44)

Leaks in the low-pressure system of the anesthesia machine can cause hypoxia or patient awareness. Profound hypercarbia can occur if a Mapleson system is in use (45).

Selecting an appropriate leak check can be confusing because some anesthesia machines have a check valve at the common gas outlet while others do not. This check valve prevents gas under positive pressure from moving retrograde into the low pressure system of the machine and out through a leak, if present.

As a result, leaks in the machine may go undetected. Application of a positive-pressure test to a machine equipped with a check valve can lead to a false sense of security despite the presence of a leak in components upstream of the check valve.

Negative Pressure Test (43, 46)

The FDA checkout recommends using a suction bulb to create a negative pressure in the machine. The bulb is attached to a hose with a 15-mm adapter, which will fit the anesthesia machine common gas outlet (Fig. 26.6). This device can be constructed by taking a sphygmomanometer

bulb and reversing the valve in the end. One end of a tubing is connected to the bulb and the other to a tracheal tube adaptor. When reversed, the valve will pull air from the machine side of the bulb. Another device constructed from the bulb pump of a disposable intravenous blood administration set has been described (47).

To perform the test, all flowmeters are turned off. A machine with a minimum mandatory flow must be turned off at the master switch. Squeezing the bulb until it is collapsed creates a negative pressure in the machine. If the bulb remains fully collapsed for 10 seconds, there is no significant leak present. If there is a leak, the bulb will inflate. This test is repeated with each vaporizer individually turned on because internal vaporizer leaks can be detected only with the vaporizer turned ON. The suction bulb should then be removed and the fresh gas hose reconnected.

This negative pressure leak test will work for all makes and models of machines, whether there

FIGURE 26.6. The suction bulb is attached to the common gas outlet and squeezed until it is collapsed. It should remain collapsed for at least 10 seconds. Following this each vaporizer in turn should be opened and the maneuver repeated.

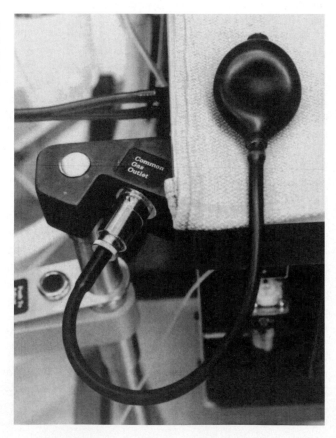

is a check valve or not, and can be performed on machines that have a minimum mandatory flow (43). For this reason it is sometimes called the universal leak test. It is sensitive enough to detect leaks as small as 30 cc/min. Comparisons of this test with the positive pressure tests have shown that this test was more sensitive (43, 44). Another advantage of this test is that it differentiates between breathing system leaks and leaks in the machine.

It is possible that the negative pressure could close some leaks and give a false-negative result. Also an unintentional continuous flow of gas will result in a false-positive test (44).

Positive Pressure Tests

There are methods of testing for leaks in the machine using a positive pressure. When performing a positive pressure test, care must be taken that the pressures do not increase beyond the prescribed limits. There is little room for compression in the machine tubing and no bag to buffer pressure increases. It is possible that the pressure could increase to a point at which a flowmeter or other part of the machine could be damaged.

Pressure gauge test (44, 48). A pressure gauge (the gauge from a standard sphygmomanometer will do) is attached to the common gas outlet (Fig. 26.7), and a flow control valve is slowly opened until the pressure on the gauge reaches 30 cm H_2O (22 mm Hg). The flow is then lowered until a steady pressure reading is achieved. The flow rate on the flowmeter is then equal to the leak rate in the machine. It should be less than 50 ml/min. This check should be repeated with each vaporizer turned on.

Fresh gas line occlusion test. With this test a flow of 50 ml/min or the minimum mandatory flow is set on the oxygen flowmeter and the fresh gas line kinked. The indicator in the flowmeter should move downward. An advantage of this test is that it can be performed during a case (43).

Elapsed time pressure test. If the machine does not have a flowmeter that reads as low as 50 ml/min, the following test may be used. A pressure gauge is attached to the machine outlet. The oxygen flowmeter is slowly turned on until a pressure of 30 cm H_2O is registered on the gauge. The flow is then turned off and the time it takes for the pressure to drop to 20 cm H_2O is measured. The time should be at least 10 seconds. A shorter time implies an unacceptably high leak rate. This

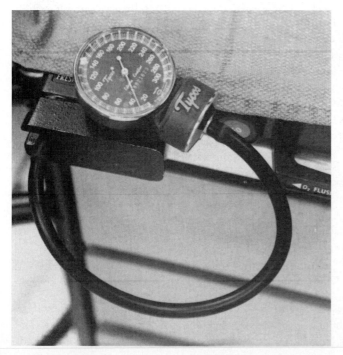

FIGURE 26.7. A pressure gauge from a blood pressure cuff is attached to the delivery hose from the machine. Sufficient flow is established on a flowmeter to maintain a pressure of 22 mm Hg on the pressure gauge. The flow required to maintain that pressure should be less than 50 ml/min.

test should also be repeated with each vaporizer turned on.

Combination breathing system and machine leak tests. The following tests can be used to check for leaks in the breathing system and parts of the machine downstream of the check valve.

RETROGRADE FILL TEST. The adjustable pressure limiting (APL) valve is closed and the patient port occluded. A vaporizer is turned on. The oxygen flush or a high flow on the flowmeter is used to fill the reservoir bag. As the bag begins to distend, the pressure on the manometer begins to rise. As the pressure starts to rise, the flowmeter flow is decreased until the pressure remains at 30 cm H_2O. If this pressure is overshot, the APL valve should be opened briefly. The flow necessary to maintain a steady pressure in the breathing system should be no greater than 350 ml/min.

The advantages of this test are that it can be performed quickly without accessory equipment and that it checks the breathing system as well as the low-pressure parts of the machine in those models that do not have a check valve (49). It also allows checking of the continuous positive pressure airway alarm. A disadvantage is that it is relatively insensitive to small leaks. It also does not localize the source of the leak.

SQUEEZE BULB TEST. With the machine master switch, flow control valves, and vaporizers off, the ports of the inspiratory and expiratory valves are connected with a hose. The manual/automatic selector is set to "bag," and the APL valve closed. A suction bulb is connected to the breathing bag mount, and squeezed repeatedly until the breathing system pressure gauge reads 50 cm H_2O. The pressure gauge is observed. If a drop in pressure from 50 to 30 cm H_2O takes 30 seconds or longer the leak rate is acceptable. After the test is performed, the hose, squeeze bulb, and test terminal are removed. This test may miss leaks in the machine upstream of the check valve.

IN-USE TEST. During use, a leak in the machine or breathing system can be tested for by lowering the fresh gas flow (50). If the ventilator bellows or reservoir bag should continue to fill, the leak rate is less than the fresh gas flow.

When the leak test of the machine is complete, residual vapors should be flushed out of the machine by turning on oxygen at 1 l/min for 1 min

with all vaporizers off (49). Using the oxygen flush will not drive vapors out of the machine, because its flow enters the fresh gas flow downstream of the vaporizers. There should be no noticeable odor in the gas coming from the common gas outlet.

Turn on the Machine's Master Switch

To continue the machine checkout, the on-off switch on the machine needs to be turned ON to enable the pneumatics and electronics. It is a good idea to turn ON all the monitors and electrical equipment to allow them to warm up prior to further checks.

Tests of Flowmeters

Flowmeters should be examined with no flow to make certain that the indicator is at the zero position (or at minimum mandatory flow if so equipped). Each flow control valve should be slowly opened and closed while observing the indicator as it rises and falls within the tube. It should move smoothly and respond to small adjustments of the flow control valve. If the indicator is a rotameter or ball it should rotate freely. An indicator with erratic movement or that fails to return to zero may be displaying erroneous flow rates and the machine should be taken out of service until the problem is corrected.

To test the proportioning system, an attempt should be made to create a hypoxic mixture by adjusting the nitrous oxide flow up or the oxygen flow down while nitrous oxide is flowing. Turning the nitrous oxide flow up should cause the oxygen flow to increase so that a concentration of at least 25% oxygen is maintained. Similar results should occur if the oxygen flow is adjusted downward. If the machine has a ratio alarm, it should be activated.

Scavenging System and APL Valve (31)

The scavenging system should be checked to make certain the APL valve and ventilator are connected to the interface. If an active disposal system is being used, the flow should be adjusted. The manufacturer's instructions should be consulted.

APL Valve

Functioning of the scavenging system and APL valve are checked by closing the APL valve, occluding the patient port, and filling the system using the oxygen flush so that the breathing system pressure gauge reads 50 cm H_2O. The APL valve is then opened. There should be a gradual loss of pressure from the system. This establishes proper functioning of the APL valve and patency of the transfer tubing. If the scavenging system interface has a reservoir bag, it should inflate when the APL valve is opened then deflate (51).

If the pressure is released by removing the occlusion at the patient port, the APL valve and scavenging system patency will not be checked. In addition, this may cause a cloud of absorbent dust to enter the breathing system (52, 53).

Closed Scavenging System

Check of the Air Intake Valve

With minimal flow from the anesthesia machine, the APL valve should be fully open and the Y-piece occluded. Suction should be applied to the scavenging system. The negative pressure in the interface should cause the bag to collapse. The breathing bag in the breathing system may also collapse. At this point the breathing system pressure indicator should show not more than a few centimeters of water negative pressure.

Check of Positive Pressure Relief

To test the positive pressure relief valve on the scavenging interface the APL valve is opened fully and the Y-piece of the breathing system occluded. The oxygen flush is activated. The breathing system pressure indicator should read less than 10 cm H_2O.

Open Scavenging System

An open scavenging system should be checked to verify that all connections are in place. To check for negative pressure relief, the absorber inlet and outlet are connected with a 22-mm hose, the APL valve fully opened, and suction applied to the scavenging system. All flow control valves should be turned OFF. Occluding the bag mount on the breathing system should result in a pressure of 0 ± 2 cm H_2O on the breathing system pressure indicator (40).

Breathing System (31)

Calibration of the Oxygen Monitor

The oxygen monitor sensor must be removed from the system and enough time allowed for it to adjust to room air. It should be calibrated to 21%, and the low oxygen alarm checked by setting it above 21%. The sensor should then be placed securely in its mount in the breathing system. Repeated flushing with oxygen should result in a reading over 90%. The oxygen monitor should not be recalibrated at a high oxygen concentration, because greater accuracy is needed at low concentrations (31). Some checklists recommend that gas flows be set for 50% oxygen and the reading checked. This also checks the flowmeters.

Many clinicians use oxygen monitors which are part of the physiologic monitor. Often these do not have daily calibration procedures. The instruction manual needs to be consulted to determine what calibration is necessary and how often it should be carried out.

Initial Status Check of the Breathing System

The breathing system should be inspected to determine that no parts are damaged or missing. If a diverting gas monitor is to be used, the sampling line should be checked for kinks or occlusion and connected to the breathing system, but the gas monitor not turned on. Transparent breathing tubes should be checked for the presence of foreign bodies (54). The bag-ventilator selector switch should be in the bag position. The pressure gauge should be observed to determine that it reads zero. If there is an absorber bypass, it should be in the position that does not allow gas to bypass the absorber chamber.

The absorbent color should be noted. If color change extends into the second chamber, the upstream canister should be replaced by the partially charged canister and the exhausted absorbent should be discarded and replaced with fresh absorbent. Accumulated absorbent dust and water should be removed from the absorber dust cup, taking care not to spill either.

At this point, accessory equipment such as a humidifier, heat and moisture exchanger, filter, or positive end–expiratory pressure (PEEP) valve should be added to the breathing system. If these are added just before or after the start of the case they will not be included in the checkout procedure and faults or improper installation will not be discovered until a problem has surfaced.

Breathing System Leak Check

To initiate the breathing system leak test, all gas flows should be zero. The APL valve should be closed and the patient port occluded. The breathing system should be pressurized to 30 cm H_2O using the oxygen flush (Fig. 26.8). The pressure should remain at this level for at least 10 seconds. The APL valve is then opened. The pressure should decrease.

Another test is to connect the ports on the absorber with a 22-mm hose. The APL valve should be closed. The pressure in the system is increased to 50 cm H_2O using a squeeze bulb attached to the reservoir bag mount. The pressure should not drop more than 20 cm H_2O in 30 seconds (40). This method does not check for leaks in the breathing tubes or other accessories which may be present in the breathing system.

The leak can be quantified by adjusting the oxygen flowmeter to maintain a certain pressure. The breathing system standard requires that this not exceed 300 ml/min at a pressure of 3.0 kPa (30 cm H_2O) (55).

Mapleson Breathing Systems

A Mapleson breathing system should be connected to the fresh gas source and the APL valve closed. With the patient port occluded, the system should be pressurized to 30 cm H_2O using the oxygen flush. If there is no leak, the pressure will remain at this level for at least 10 seconds. The pressure should be released by opening the APL valve. The leak rate can be quantified by attaching a manometer to the patient port and determining the flow needed to sustain a certain pressure (56).

Test of Inner Tube of the Bain System

The integrity of the inner tube of the Bain breathing system is essential in avoiding excessive

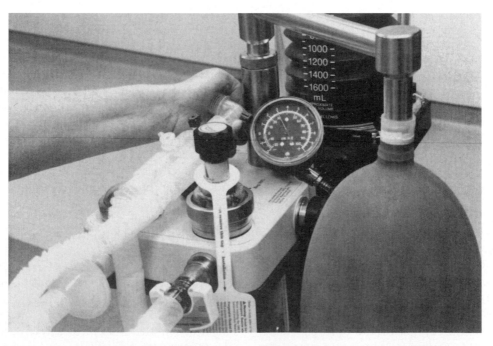

FIGURE 26.8. Test for leaks in the breathing system. With all gas flows set to zero or minimum, the APL valve is closed and the patient port occluded. The reservoir bag is filled using the oxygen flush until a pressure of 30 cm H_2O is shown on the gauge. With no additional gas flow, the pressure should remain at this level for at least 10 seconds.

dead space. Profound hypercarbia can occur if the inner tube has a hole, is detached at its proximal end, or does not extend to the patient end of the outer tubing.

Inner Tube Occlusion Test (57–59)

1. A 2 L/min flow is set on one of the flowmeters.
2. The plunger from a small syringe or a finger is inserted into the distal (patient) end of the outer tube, occluding the inner tube (Fig. 26.9). The flowmeter indicator should fall. The machine relief valve, if present, should open. This test can detect holes in the inner tubing as small as 1 mm (60). A variation of this is to attach a manometer to the end of the inner tube and determine the flow needed to cause a sustained pressure (56). **NOTE:** If the system has side holes or slots at the patient end of the inner tubing, this test *will not* work (61–63)

Oxygen Flush Test (64)

1. The reservoir bag is filled.
2. The patient port is left open to atmosphere.

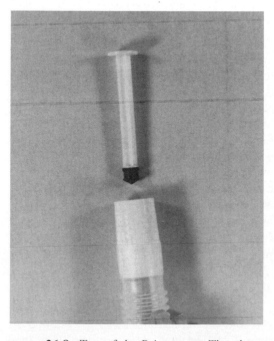

FIGURE 26.9. Test of the Bain system. The plunger from a small syringe is inserted into the patient end of the system over the end of the inner fresh gas delivery tubing. The flowmeter indicator should drop.

3. The oxygen flush valve on the machine is activated. The high flow of gas through the inner tube will produce a Venturi effect, which lowers the pressure in the outer tube. If there are no problems with the inner tube, the bag should deflate slightly. If the bag does not deflate or inflates slightly, the inner tube should be checked. This test may fail to detect major faults that can be detected by the inner tube occlusion test (60, 65–67).

Test of the Inner Tube of the Lack System (68, 69)

To test the integrity of the inner limb of the Lack system, a tracheal tube can be inserted to fit over the inner tubing at the patient end (68). Blowing down the tracheal tube with the APL valve closed will produce movement of the bag if there is leakage between the inner and outer limbs.

An alternative method is to occlude both the inner and outer limbs with the APL valve fully open (69). There should be no gas escape on applying pressure to the reservoir bag. If the inner limb is defective, gas will escape through the APL valve and the bag will collapse.

A third test is to insert a 7.5 tracheal tube into the patient end until the cuff abuts the opening of the inner tube and slight resistance is felt (70). The cuff is inflated firmly to obstruct the opening between the outer and inner tubes. With the APL valve fully open, the reservoir bag should be filled using the oxygen flush through a small flow set on the oxygen flowmeter. Squeezing the bag should cause the flowmeter indicator to drop, but no gas should be released through the APL valve.

Still another test uses a pressure manometer, and inflating bulb (48). A 7-mm nasal airway is inserted into the inner tube of the breathing system. The inflating bulb is used to pressurize the inner tube to 50 cm H_2O. There should be minimal decline in pressure over 30 seconds.

Manual and Automatic Ventilation Systems (31)

Functional Test of the Ventilator

The first step is to detect leaks in the ventilator or ventilator hose. A second reservoir bag should

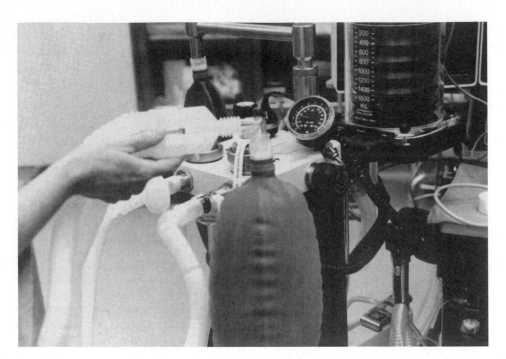

FIGURE 26.10. Test of ventilator. A reservoir bag is placed on the patient port. The oxygen flowmeter is set for a flow of 300 ml/min. Ventilator parameters appropriate for the next patient are set. The bag-ventilator selector switch should be in the ventilator position. The bellows and reservoir bag are filled, and the ventilator is turned on. The bellows should move freely and fill completely as the ventilator cycles. The unidirectional valves should be observed to make certain the discs move properly.

be placed on the patient port (Fig. 26.10). Ventilator parameters appropriate for the next patient are set. The oxygen flowmeter should be set at the minimum flow. The bag-ventilator selector switch should be set in the ventilator mode. The bellows and reservoir bag are filled using the oxygen flush, and the ventilator is turned on. The appropriate tidal volume should be delivered and the bellows should fill completely during expiration. If the bellows does not fill, a leak in the ventilator or hose should be suspected.

Leak Test for the Bellows and Transfer Tubing

Another check for a leak in the bellows or transfer tubing is to fill the bellows then occlude the patient port and turn off the flowmeters. Alternately, the bag-ventilator selector switch can be set to bag. The bellows should stay inflated. If it falls, there is a leak.

To check for a leak in a ventilator with a hanging bellows (Fig. 26.11), all flowmeters should be turned off or to the minimum flow. The APL valve is closed and the ventilator turned on. When the bellows is fully contracted against the head of the bellows assembly, the patient port is occluded (or the bag-ventilator selector switch is put in the bag position) and the ventilator switched off. The bellows should remain at the top of the housing. If it expands downward, a leak is present. Another way of performing this test is to occlude the patient port (or put the bag-ventilator selector switch in the bag position) with the ventilator turned off and lower the bellows stop. The bellows should not expand downward.

Alarm Check

The bag should be removed from the patient port and the ventilator allowed to continue cycling (71). The low airway pressure alarm (and volume monitor alarm, if present) should sound after an appropriate delay.

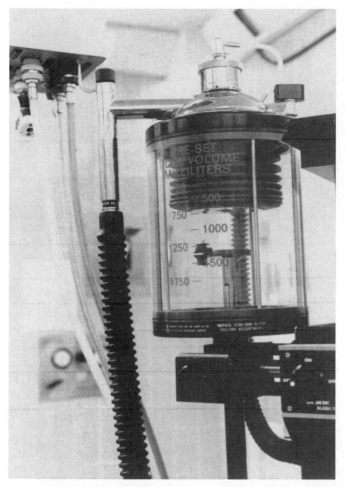

FIGURE **26.11.** Test for leak in ventilator with hanging bellows. The flowmeters should be turned off or at minimum flow. The adjustable pressure limiting (APL) valve is closed and the ventilator turned on. When the bellows is fully contracted against the head of the bellows assembly, the patient port is occluded (or the bag-ventilator selector switch is put in the bag position) and the ventilator is turned off. The bellows should remain at the top of the housing for at least 10 seconds.

Check of Ventilator Safety-Relief Valve

With the patient port occluded, the ventilator should be turned on. The breathing system pressure should rise no higher than the safety-relief pressure of the ventilator, usually 65 to 80 cm H_2O.

Tests of the Unidirectional Valves

The FDA checklist does not specify how the unidirectional valves are to be checked for proper function. Many practitioners feel that watching the inhalation valve disc rise during inhalation and the exhalation valve rise during exhalation while the ventilator is cycling is adequate. This verifies that they open, but not that they close completely.

During use incompetent unidirectional valves can be detected by an inspired carbon dioxide greater than zero when using a capnograph (see Chapter 18, "Anesthesia Gas Monitoring"). Some respirometers can detect reverse flow. Preoperatively, unidirectional valves may be checked by several tests.

Breathing Method

With the APL valve closed, the inspiratory limb of the breathing system is detached from the absorber and occluded. Wearing a mask, the tester tries to breath through the Y-piece (Fig. 26.12 Top). It should be possible to exhale freely but not inhale. Next the exhalation tube is detached and occluded. The tester should be able to inhale but not exhale (Fig. 26.12 Bottom).

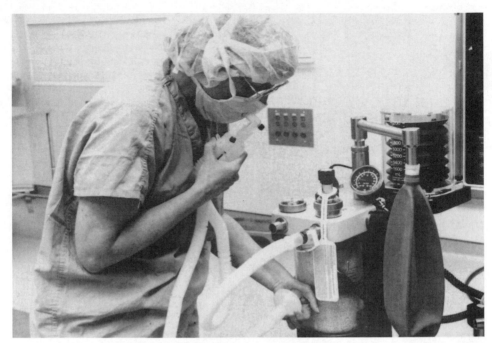

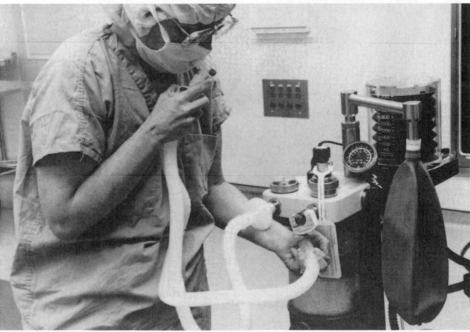

FIGURE **26.12.** Checks for incompetent unidirectional valves. **Top,** The inspiratory limb is detached and occluded. The tester tries to breathe through the Y piece. It should be possible to exhale freely but not inhale. **Bottom,** The exhalation tubing is detached and occluded. The tester should be able to inhale from the Y piece but not exhale.

Pressure Method

The inspiratory valve is checked by connecting a reservoir bag at the bag mount site and a corrugated tube to the inhalation outlet. While the exhalation inlet is covered, positive pressure is applied to the corrugated tube. No gas should flow into the tube and the reservoir bag should not fill.

To check the exhalation valve, a reservoir bag is connected to the expiratory limb connection and a corrugated tube to the reservoir bag connection. While the inhalation outlet is covered, positive pressure is applied to the corrugated tube. No gas should flow into the tube and the reservoir bag should not fill.

Valve Tester (72, 73)

This method utilizes a device consisting of a bulb with a 22-mm female fitting which can attach to the inspiratory and exhalation ports. To check the expiratory valve, the tester is attached with the bulb in the relaxed state. If the valve works properly, the bulb should compress easily then remain collapsed. To test the inspiratory valve, the compressed bulb is attached to the inspiratory port. It should immediately reinflate. When the bulb is compressed, firm resistance should be felt.

Pressure Decline Method (74)

In this method the outlet of the inhalation unidirectional valve is occluded and the breathing system pressurized to 30 cm H_2O using the oxygen flush. This pressure should be maintained. A rapid decline in pressure indicates a leak in the expiratory unidirectional valve.

To check the inhalation check valve, a reservoir bag is connected to the inhalation port and filled using the oxygen flush The pressure in the bag should be maintained.

At this point breathing system accessories (e.g., PEEP valve, heated humidifier) should be turned on and their proper function verified. The ventilator should be turned off and the selector switch placed in the manual (bag) mode.

The bag-ventilator selector switch should be put in the bag position. As the reservoir bag in the breathing system is squeezed, inflation and deflation of a bag on the patient port (artificial lungs) should occur (Fig. 26.13). System resistance and

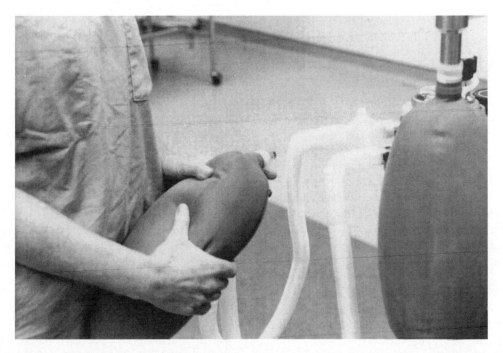

FIGURE **26.13.** Test for manual ventilation system. A reservoir bag is placed on the patient port. The bag-ventilator switch is turned to the bag position. As the reservoir bag in the breathing system is squeezed, the bag on the port should inflate. Squeezing the bag on the patient port should cause the reservoir bag in the breathing system to inflate.

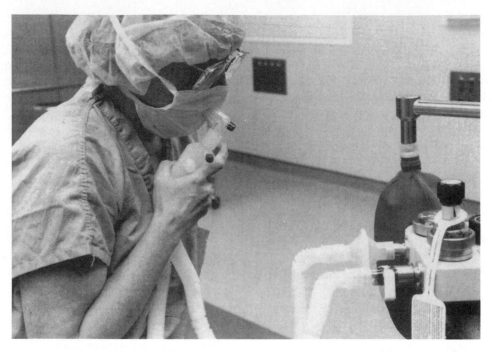

FIGURE 26.14. Breathing system patency can be confirmed by inhaling and exhaling through the patient port.

compliance should be evaluated. This is useful to detect inadvertent PEEP or an obstruction in the system (75).

These problems can also be detected by having the patient breathe 100% oxygen using a mask before induction of anesthesia, provided a tight mask fit is achieved (76). This can also be done by anesthesia personnel (wearing a mask of course) (Fig. 26.14). Negative pressure will reveal an obstruction in the inspiratory limb; positive pressure will reveal an obstruction in the expiratory limb (77). While this is being done, the capnograph should be checked to make certain a waveform appears, the reservoir bag should inflate and deflate and the breathing system pressure indicator show no PEEP.

Monitors (31)

All monitors should be turned on and calibrated if required; alarms should be tested and appropriate alarm limits set.

Final Machine Status (31)

The final status of all controls should be checked before the machine is put in use. This includes having all flow control valves closed, all flowmeters indicating zero flow, all vaporizers in the off position, the bag-ventilator selector switch set to bag, the PEEP valve closed and the APL valve open.

A rigid suction catheter should be present. The adequacy of suction can be checked by placing the end of the suction tubing on the underside of the finger (Fig. 26.15). The tubing should stay without support.

SUBSEQUENT CHECKS ON THE SAME MACHINE ON THE SAME DAY

If a thorough check is performed before the first case of the day, a less complete procedure can be followed before subsequent cases. Those steps are indicated in Table 26.1.

PROCEDURES AT THE END OF THE CASE

At the conclusion of a case, flowmeters, vaporizers, and suction should be turned off. Monitors that would need recalibration if turned off should be left on or put in a standby mode. The absorbent should be checked for signs of exhaustion and

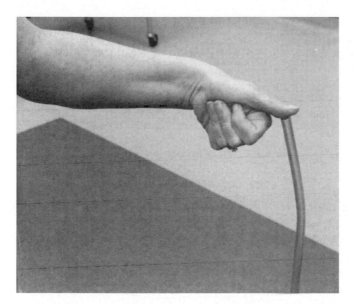

FIGURE **26.15.** Suction check. The strength of the vacuum is tested by determining that the weight of the suction tubing can be supported at waist height by the seal between the tubing and the underside of a finger. If the vacuum is unsatisfactory, the tubing will not remain in contact with the finger.

changed if indicated (see Chapter 8, "Breathing Systems III: Circle System").

OTHER MACHINE AND BREATHING SYSTEM CHECKS

While the FDA checkout recommendations are adequate for daily use, other parts may need to be checked either daily or as the need arises. This is especially true after the machine has been altered or serviced.

Oxygen Pressure Failure Alarm

Most machines are now equipped with an oxygen pressure failure alarm, which is activated if there is no or low oxygen pressure in the machine while the master on-off switch is turned on. To test this alarm, the oxygen pipeline hose is disconnected and all cylinders closed. Any pressure remaining in the machine should be bled off using the oxygen flush. The alarm should sound. This step was not included in the 1992 FDA checkout recommendations because isolated failure of this component will not injure a patient (31).

Leakage at the Yoke

If a cylinder is not properly tightened in a yoke there will be leakage of gas when the cylinder valve is opened. If there is a large leak, it will be quite apparent. If the leak is small, it will not be heard but could cause significant loss of gas. To check for leakage at the yoke, after the cylinder pressures have been checked and the valves closed, the cylinder pressure indicators should be observed for 2 to 5 minutes, with no flow on the flowmeters. A drop of more than 50 psig (340 KPa) indicates significant leakage.

Oxygen Failure Safety Valve

The oxygen failure safety valve was included as a routine test in the first edition of the FDA checkout but was not made part of the newest version because failures of it are rare and there are many other methods of detecting the problem (31). This test can be performed using either the pipelines or cylinders as the gas source. A cylinder of each gas on the machine is turned on, leaving the pipeline hoses disconnected. Flows of 2 l/min are established on the flowmeters for each gas. The oxygen cylinder is then turned off. As the pressure of the oxygen falls, the flows of all other gases, except possibly air, should decrease in proportion to the decrease in oxygen flow and eventually shut off. Restoring the oxygen pressure should cause the indicators to return to their previous positions.

To perform the test using pipeline gases, all cylinder valves should be closed and the flow control valves opened until the cylinder pressure indicators register zero. The pipeline hoses are then connected and flows established on all flow-meters. The oxygen hose is then disconnected. The indicators of the anesthetic gas flowmeters should fall with the oxygen indicator.

Spare Components

Extra components of the breathing system should be immediately available. These include an additional disposable system or individual components of reusable systems (Y piece, tubings, bag).

Electrical System

The electrical system of the anesthesia machine is described in detail in Chapter 4, "Anesthesia Machines." Specific tests for the electrical system vary with different machines. Most have a means to test the reserve battery. In addition there is usually an indication that the machine is working on the battery power. To check this, the machine is disconnected from the mains power. The battery power indicator should be activated.

Vaporizer Exclusion System

Modern anesthesia machines have a mechanism to allow only one vaporizer to be turned ON at a time. This is discussed in more detail in Chapter 5, "Vaporizers." To test the vaporizer exclusion system, one vaporizer should be turned ON and an attempt made to turn ON each of the other vaporizers, one at a time. If this can be accomplished, the exclusion system is not functioning properly.

CHECKING OTHER EQUIPMENT
Tracheal Tubes

A tracheal tube of the size appropriate for the patient should be ready for use. Patency of the lumen should be checked. With clear tubes, simple observation will suffice. With other tubes, it is necessary to look in both ends or insert a stylet. The cuff should be held inflated for at least 1 minute to verify that there are no leaks. It should inflate evenly and not stick to the wall of the tube or decrease the size of the lumen. One larger and one smaller tracheal tube should be readily available.

Laryngoscopes

Laryngoscope malfunction is a frequent problem. At least two handles should be present, each fitted with the type of blade the user anticipates will be best for the patient. The lights should be checked for adequate intensity. Blades of other sizes and shapes should be immediately available and checked for proper function.

Accessory Intubation Equipment

A stylet should be immediately available. If a rapid sequence intubation is planned, it should be fitted to the tracheal tube. An intubating forceps should be immediately available. If a difficult intubation is anticipated, specialized equipment for difficult intubation described in Chapters 16, "Laryngoscopes," Chapter 17, "Tracheal Tubes," and Chapter 28, "Operating Room Design and Equipment Selection" should be assembled.

Masks and Airways

An assortment of masks and airways in a variety of sizes should be readily available.

Other Equipment

Special equipment required for particular cases such as extension pipeline hoses, a hot air warming system, etc., should be present and checked before use.

CARE AT THE END OF THE DAY

Following the last case, the pipeline hoses should be disconnected at the wall or ceiling (not at the back of the machine) and coiled over the machine. If the hoses are disconnected at the back of the machine, they will continue to be pressurized and gas may be lost into the room through leaks. Cylinder valves should be closed. Each flow control valve should be opened until the cylinder and pipeline pressure gauges read zero, then closed. Closing the flow control valves will not conserve gas, but if they are left open, restoration of the gas supply may forcibly raise the indicator to the top of the tube, causing damage.

Vaporizers should be filled at the conclusion of the day after most operating room personnel have left the room. This will decrease exposure to trace amounts of anesthetic agents.

Liquid should be drained from the base of the absorber. Care must be exercised as the liquid is caustic and should not come in contact with skin.

CHECKING NEW OR MODIFIED EQUIPMENT

Each new anesthesia machine, ventilator, or other complex piece of equipment should be checked for proper functioning before being put to use. Often this is best performed by a manufacturer's representative. Often this person will give in-service instructions. A document certifying that the equipment has been checked for proper assembly and function should be obtained and kept.

A manual that contains assembly and installation instructions, maintenance requirements, checking procedures, and instructions for use should be supplied with each piece of equipment. This should be read carefully and reviewed periodically. A copy should be kept in the central equipment files and with the equipment itself.

PREVENTIVE MAINTENANCE

Many items in an anesthesia machine and ventilator deteriorate with time and use. Preventive maintenance is designed to anticipate predictable failures and replace weakened components before they fail. In some cases an improved part has become available and can be substituted for one likely to fail. It has been shown to be effective in preventing equipment failure (78). Lack of a preventive maintenance program may lead to an unacceptably high rate of breakdowns, premature replacement of major equipment, and unnecessary accidents and hazards (79).

Equipment Manufacturer Under Service Contract

With a service contract, the manufacturer's agent comes to the healthcare facility. Often different levels of service are available. The cost will depend on the number of parts covered, the frequency of the visits and the response time.

Independent Service Company

Independent companies not associated with a particular manufacturer may perform service on certain equipment on a contractual basis. It may be difficult for the anesthesia provider to determine the qualifications of an independent service provider. Some manufacturers certify independent providers to service their particular equip-

ment. To become certified, they must satisfactorily complete the same courses as the company's own service technicians. It may not always be possible for an independent company to procure manufacturer-approved parts unless the service technician has been certified by the manufacturer.

The contract with an independent service organization must be reviewed by the lawyer for the healthcare facility. There should be no hold-harmless provisions in favor of the contractor. Proof of liability insurance or a performance bond should be provided.

Laws recently enacted in at least one state (New Jersey) require that the credentials of each servicing person be approved by the machine manufacturer or determined by the physician director of the anesthesia department to be equivalent to the credentials of the manufacturer's service person.

In-House Biomedical Services

In-house biomedical services may be a satisfactory option for much equipment. Biomedical technicians can attend courses and become certified to service specific equipment.

Advantages of in-house biomedical maintenance include minimal response time to trouble calls and observation of problems while the equipment is in use. The intensity of service from outside sources and down time for equipment can be reduced. The biomedical technicians can assist with clinical education, provide a single liaison between users and manufacturers, help with equipment selection, and keep abreast of modifications and service bulletins issued by manufacturers.

The question of liability exposure must be addressed when considering in-house service (80). If a problem occurs as a result of the actions of a biomedical technician, the facility will have to accept the liability.

RECORD KEEPING

Record keeping on equipment has frequently been neglected in the past. Often it is assumed that the manufacturer's service representative who does periodic preventive maintenance will take care of this task. Common experience does not support this. Record keeping is important for several reasons.

1. It provides proof that an effort has been made to keep the equipment in proper working order. This could have medicolegal significance.
2. It provides a means of communication with the service representative. Representatives frequently come in the late afternoon or evening when anesthesia personnel have left. If there is no written record of problems that have occurred with the equipment, the service representative may not perform the indicated repair(s).
3. It provides a complete, up-to-date record for each piece of equipment. If one piece of equipment malfunctions more frequently than others, consideration should be given to replacing it.
4. It provides a written record that maintenance by a service representative was performed and shows what was done. Service representatives may present only a bill for service and parts and no record of what was actually done.
5. It provides a check on the service rendered by the representative. After equipment is serviced, it should perform well. If a machine develops a problem soon after servicing or if there is an increased frequency of repairs that can be traced to a change in service representatives, one may wish to question that representative's effectiveness.
6. With pieces of equipment such as vaporizers that need to be sent to the manufacturer periodically for servicing, or oxygen analyzers that need to have certain components replaced at intervals, it serves to remind the user when the equipment needs to be serviced or a component replaced. After a vaporizer is serviced, it may be held in reserve before being put into use. This would extend the time before servicing would be due. This can be noted on the form by recording the time when a vaporizer is received from the manufacturer and when it is actually put into service on a machine.

A record should be kept for each piece of complex equipment such as an anesthesia machine, ventilator, vaporizer, or monitor. This should include identification information; date of purchase; instructions for servicing; and the name, address, and telephone number of the service representative. If a problem with the equipment arises, the date, problem, and corrective action should be recorded. When routine servicing is performed, this should be noted, along with any problems or parts replaced. Each entry should be signed by the person making it. Laws recently enacted in at least one state stipulate that records must be kept of each machine, including the name of the service person, work performed, and date the work was performed.

ACCIDENT INVESTIGATION (81–85)

Any time a patient has an unexplained problem, equipment malfunction or misuse should be suspected and the apparatus not used again until this has been disproved.

When there has been an injury to a patient, the hospital safety officer (risk manager) should be contacted at once to supervise investigation of the incident. An established protocol should be followed so that all important areas are covered systematically. All individuals involved in the incident should document their observations soon after the event, while details are still fresh in their minds. This should be a simple statement of facts, without judgments about causality or responsibility.

The following questions need to be asked:

1. What was the date and time of the problem?
2. In what area did the problem occur?
3. What monitors were being used?
4. What were the set alarm limits?
5. What was the first indication that there was a problem?
6. At what time did this occur?
7. Who first noted the problem?
8. What changes attracted attention? Were any alarms activated?
9. What signs or symptoms did the patient exhibit?
10. Had there been any recent modifications to the electrical system or gas pipelines in that area?
11. Was anything altered shortly before the incident?
12. Was this the first case performed in that area that day?

13. Were there any problems during previous cases performed in that area that day or the previous day?
14. Were there any unusual occurrences in other areas that day or the previous day?
15. Had any equipment been moved into that area recently? Were there any problems noted in the room where it was previously used?
16. What preuse checks were made of the anesthesia equipment?
17. Who last filled the vaporizers on the anesthesia machine?
18. If a vaporizer was recently attached to the machine, were precautions taken to prevent liquid from being spilled into the outflow tract?
19. After the initial indication of a problem, what was the sequence of events that occurred?

An important step involves construction of a time line, on which all events are listed in chronological order (81). This will help to sort out events and may lead to identification of missing data.

Numerous photographs should be taken of the area from various angles, with all equipment situated where it was at the time of the incident. Each piece of equipment should be photographed separately.

After pictures have been taken, all supplies and equipment associated with the case should be saved and sequestered in a secure location and labeled "DO NOT DISTURB" (86). Settings should not be changed. Relevant identifying information such as the manufacturer and lot and/or serial numbers should be recorded.

If, after all this has been done, it appears possible that the equipment may be implicated in causing the problem, a thorough inspection of the equipment in the presence of the primary anesthesia personnel, insurance carrier, hospital safety officer, patient representative, and equipment manufacturers should be conducted. The investigation should consist of an in-depth examination of the equipment similar to the checking procedures described earlier in this chapter. Vaporizers should be calibrated and checked to determine if vapor is delivered in the OFF position. An analysis should be made of the vaporizers' contents. Following the investigation, a report should be made, detailing all facts, analyses, and conclusions.

If a problem with the equipment is found, an attempt should be made to reconstruct the accident if this can be done without danger to anyone, and the equipment should again be locked up until any litigation is settled. If the investigation reveals no problems, the equipment can be returned to service with the consent of all parties.

The Safe Medical Devices Act of 1990 requires medical device user facilities to report incidents that reasonably suggest there is a probability that a medical device has caused or contributed to the death, serious injury, or serious illness of a patient (87). The report is due as soon as possible but no later than 10 working days after the user facility becomes aware of the incident.

ACCIDENT PREVENTION
Selection of Equipment

Prevention of accidents associated with anesthesia equipment should start with proper selection. Reliability, safety, and cost should all be considered. Standardization of equipment, both within the anesthesia department and with other hospital areas, may help decrease mishaps.

Replacement of Obsolete Equipment (88–90)

Replacement of outdated equipment is a necessary ongoing process. Apparatus that was the best available at one time may become unacceptable as improved models become available. Age alone is not a determinant of obsolescence. Answers to the following questions may be helpful in determining when a piece of equipment needs to be replaced. If they cannot be answered in the affirmative, replacement should be considered.

1. Can the equipment perform its functions within the manufacturer's specified tolerances?
2. Are the manufacturer's tolerances satisfactory for current practice? Practice techniques change and may result in new demands being placed on the equipment. An example is the trend toward use of lower fresh gas flows. Vaporizers that are accurate at high but not low flows may be within the manufacturer's specifications but not suitable for this application.

3. Is the potential for human error unacceptable? Most newer machines incorporate features designed to limit errors. Use of such equipment may prevent accidents. Examples include features to prevent dialing a hypoxic mixture on an anesthesia machine and a bag-ventilator selector valve that isolates the APL valve.

Anesthesia providers may make mistakes when switching from one type of anesthesia machine to another. It may be safer to have a similar model of anesthesia machine in all anesthetizing locations.

4. Can the equipment be upgraded to meet current needs and safety standards? Although it may not be possible to upgrade equipment to meet new standards, there may be things that can be done to make it safer (91).

5. Can the equipment be serviced by qualified personnel with proper components? In most cases this means the manufacturer's representative. If the manufacturer is no longer in existence or will no longer service the equipment, it will be necessary to replace it.

6. Will recent anesthesia trainees be able to use the equipment safely? Some may not be acquainted with older equipment. This could lead to mistakes.

7. Can the addition of monitoring equipment make the machine safer? Monitors such as oxygen analyzers, carbon dioxide monitors, agent monitors, pressure alarms, and respirometers may allow the anesthesia provider to detect problems which, although they might be avoided with more modern equipment, would be caught before any harm would have occurred.

8. Does the equipment meet current standards? Equipment standards are made to guide the production of new equipment and are not meant to be retroactive to equipment produced before their adoption.

9. Does the equipment have a reasonable maintenance history? Records must be kept on maintenance for each piece of equipment. If a particular piece has an high failure rate and requires frequent repair, it may be a candidate for replacement.)

Use of Vigilance Aids

Use of vigilance aids (described in Chapters 18 through 24) can provide warning of problems before the patient suffers harm.

Education and Communication

It is essential that all members of the department receive proper instruction in how to use equipment properly. Manuals that come with equipment should be reviewed thoroughly.

Proper communication among members of the department is important. Information about equipment modifications or problems should be conveyed to each member. Accidents and near accidents should be discussed at department meetings, so that steps can be taken to prevent such occurrences in the future.

REFERENCES

1. Charlton JE. Checklists and patient safety [Editorial]. Anaesthesia 1990;45:425–426.
2. Cundy J, Baldock GJ. Safety check procedures to eliminate faults in anaesthetic machines. Anaesthesia 1982; 37:161–169.
3. Chopra V, Bovill JG, Spierdijk J. Checklists: Aviation shows the way to safer anesthesia. Anesthesia Patient Safety Foundation Newsletter 1991;6:26–29.
4. Cooper JB, Newbower RS, Kitz RJ. An analysis of major errors and equipment failures in anesthesia management: considerations for prevention and detection. Anesthesiology 1984;60:34–42.
5. Craig J, Wilson ME. A survey of anaesthetic misadventures. Anaesthesia 1981;36:933–936.
6. Cobcroft MD. More misconnected Boyle circuit tubings. Anaesthesia and Intensive Care 1978;6: 170–171.
7. Chopra V, Bovill JG, Spierdijk J, et al. Reported significant observations during anaesthesia: a prospective analysis over an 18 month period. Br J Anaesth 1992; 68:13–17.
8. Witham–Wilson MJ. FDA preuse equipment checklist spurred by accidents, studies. Anesthesia Patient Safety Foundation Newsletter 1991;6:27.
9. Adams AP, Morgan M. Checking anaesthetic machines—checklists or visual aids? Anaesthesia 1993;48: 183–46.
10. Short TG, O'Regan A, Lew J, et al. Critical incident reporting in an anaesthetic department assurance programme. Anaesthesia 1992;47:3–7.

11. Drews JH. Hazardous anesthesia machine malfunction occurring after routine preventive maintenance inspection. Anesth Analg 1983;62:701.

12. Kumar V, Barcellos WA, Mehta MP, et al. Analysis of critical incidents in a teaching department for quality assurance. A survey of mishaps during anaesthesia. Anaesthesia 1988;43:879–883.

13. Barthram C, McClymont W. The use of a checklist for anaesthetic machines. Anaesthesia 1992;47:1066–1069.

14. Hunziker P, Koch JP, Devitt JH. Formalization and implementation of an institutional preanesthetic checklist. Can J Anaesth 1990;37:S9.

15. Mayor AH, Eaton JM. Anaesthetic machine checking practices. Anaesthesia 1992;47:866–868.

16. Anonymous. FDA re-examines anesthesia safety & equipment check procedures. Biomedical Safety & Standards 1991;21:17–19.

17. Ewell MG, Pennant JH, Shearer VE. Spot assessment of the daily anesthesia check—human factors analysis. Journal of Clinical Monitoring 1992;8:188–189.

18. Higham H, Beck GN. Checking anaesthetic machines. Anaesthesia 1993; 48:536.

19. Reference deleted.

20. Klopfenstein CE, Bernstein M, Van Gessel E, et al. Preoperative checking of the anaesthetic machine. A survey in a university department of anaesthesia. Br J Anaesth 1994; 72(Suppl 11):A20.

21. Mayor AH, Zuckerberg AL. Pre-operative checking of anesthesia equipment: A survey of practice. Anesthesiology 1993; 79:A447.

22. Buffington CW, Ramanathan S, Turndorf H. Detection of anesthesia machine faults. Anesth Analg 1984; 63:79–82.

23. March MG, Crowley JJ. An evaluation of anesthesiologists' present checkout methods and the validity of the FDA checklist. Anesthesiology 1991;75:724–729.

24. Jackson IJB, Wilson RJT. Association of Anaesthetist's checklist for anaesthetic machines: problems with detection of significant leaks. Anaesthesia 1993; 48:152–153.

25. Berge JA, Gramstad L, Grimes S. An evaluation of a time-saving anaesthetic machine checkout procedure. Eur J Anaesthesiol 1994;11:394–398.

26. Groves J, Edwards N, Carr B. The use of a visual aid o check anaesthetic machines. Is performance improved? Anaesthesia 1994;49:122–125.

27. Olympio MA, Goldstein MM, Mathes DD. Instructional review improves performance of anesthesia apparatus checkout procedures. Anesth Analg 1996;83:618–622.

28. American Society for Testing and Materials. Standard specification for minimum performance and safety requirements for components and systems of anesthesia gas machines (F1161–1188 reapproved 1994). Philadelphia: ASTM, 1994.

29. Carstensen P. FDA issues pre-use checkout. Anesthesia Patient Safety Foundation Newsletter 1986;1:13–20.

30. Morrison JL. FDA anesthesia apparatus checkout recommendations, 1993. American Society of Anesthesiologists Newsletter 1994;58(6):25–26.

31. Anonymous: FDA publishes final version of revised apparatus checkout. Anesthesia Patient Safety Foundation Newsletter 1994;9:35.

32. American Society of Anesthesiologists. Professional liability and the anesthesiologist. Park Ridge, IL: ASA, 1987.

33. Blike G, Witherell P, Biddle C. Anesthesia equipment fault detection by anesthesia providers: A comparison of an electronic equipment checklist against a standard checklist recommended by the FDA. Journal of Clinical Monitoring 1996;12:467–468.

34. Benumof JL. Management of the difficult adult airway. Anesthesiology 1991;75:1089–1110.

35. Benumof JL, Scheller MS. The importance of transtracheal jet ventilation in the management of the difficult airway. Anesthesiology 1989;71:769–778.

36. Dinnick OP. Accidental severe hypercapnia during anaesthesia. Br J Anaesth 1968;40:36–45.

37. Lomanto C, Leeming M. A safety signal for detection of excessive anesthetic gas flows. Anesthesiology 1970; 33:663–664.

38. Prys–Roberts C, Smith WDA, Nunn JF. Accidental severe hypercapnia during anaesthesia. Br J Anaesth 1967;39:257–267.

39. Reimer DH. Oxygen tank check. Can J Anaesth 1995; 42:657–658.

40. North American Drager Educational Services, Daily checkout Procedure Narkomed 2C Operators Manual Sec. 3, 1994

41. Wilson AM. The pressure gauges on the Boyle international anaesthetic machine. Anaesthesia 1982;37:218–219.

42. Andrews JJ. Understanding your anesthesia machine. American Society of Anesthesiologists 1996 Annual Refresher Courses, Atlanta.

43. Myers JA, Good ML, Andrews JJ. Comparison of tests for detecting leaks in the low-pressure system of anesthesia gas machines. Anesth Analg 1997;84:179–184.

44. Somprakit P, Soontranan P. Low pressure leakage in anaesthetic machines. Evaluation by positive and negative pressure tests. Anaesthesia 1996;51:461–464.

45. Berner MS. Profound hypercapnia due to disconnec-

tion within an anaesthetic machine. Can J Anaesth 1987;34:622–626.

46. Myint Y. Detection of leaks in anaesthetic machines. Anaesthesia 1993; 48:729–730.

47. Targ AG, Andrews BW. A new device to check the anesthesia machine low-pressure system. Anesthesiology 1993;79:629–630.

48. Strong TS, Barrowcliffe MP. Pressure testing the anaesthetic machine and breathing system. Anaesthesia 1996;51:88–89.

49. Eisenkraft JB. The anesthesia delivery system. Part II: Progress in Anesthesiology 1989;3:1–12.

50. Ghani GA. Test for a leak in the anesthesia circle. Anesth Analg 1983;62:855–856.

51. Eisenkraft JB, Sommer RM. Flapper valve malfunction. Anesth Analg 1988;67:1132.

52. Debban DG, Bedford RF. Overdistention of the rebreathing bag, a hazardous test for circle-system integrity. Anesthesiology 1975;42:365–366.

53. Ribak B. Reducing the soda-lime hazard. Anesthesiology 1975;43:277.

54. Babarczy A. Checking the anaesthetic machine. Anaesthesia and Intensive Care 1994;22:497.

55. American Society for Testing and Materials. Standard specification for minimum performance and safety requirements for anesthesia breathing systems (F1208–1989). Philadelphia: ASTM, 1989.

56. Berge JA, Gramstad L, Bodd E. Safety testing the Bain circuit: A new test adaptor. Eur J Anaesthesiol 1991; 8:309–310.

57. Foex P, Crampton Smith A. A test for co-axial circuits. Anaesthesia 1977;32:294.

58. Ghani GA. Safety check for the Bain circuit. Can Anaesth Soc J 1984;31:487–488.

59. Jackson IJB. Tests for co-axial systems. Anaesthesia 1988;43:1060–1061.

60. Podraza AG, Prekezes C, Salem MR. Testing the integrity of the Bain breathing circuit. Anesthesiology 1995;83:A471.

61. Robinson S, Fisher DM. Safety check for the CPRAM circuit. Anesthesiology 1983;59:488–489.

62. Jones GN. Mapleson D coaxial breathing system integrity testing. Anaesthesia 1993;48:917–918.

63. Theaker NJ, van Hasselt G. Equipment safety checks. Anaesthesia 1993; 48:837–838.

64. Pethick SL. Correspondence. Can Anaesth Soc J 1975; 22:115.

65. Heath PJ, Marks LF. Modified occlusion tests for the Bain breathing system. Anaesthesia 1991;46: 213–216.

66. Petersen WC. Bain circuit. Can Anaesth Soc J 1978; 25:532.

67. Beauprie IG, Clark AG, Keith IC, et al. Pre-use testing of coaxial circuits: the perils of Pethick. Can J Anaesth 1990;37:S103.

68. Furst B, Laffey DA. An alternate test for the Lack system. Anaesthesia 1984;39:834.

69. Martin LVH, McKeown DW. An alternative test for the Lack system. Anaesthesia 1985;40:80–92.

70. Normandale JP, Found P. Checking the Lack breathing system. Anaesthesia 1994; 49:735.

71. Campbell RM, Sheikh A, Crosse MM. A study of the incorrect use of ventilator disconnection alarms. Anaesthesia 1996;51:369–370.

72. Eappen S, Corn SB. The anesthesia machine valve tester: A new device and method for evaluating the competence of unidirectional anesthetic valves. J Clin Anesth 1996;12:305–309.

73. Corn SB. A method and apparatus for testing the anesthesia machine circuit unidirectional valves. Journal of Clinical Monitoring 1996;8:261–262.

74. Kitagawa H, Sai Y, Nosaka S, et al. A new leak test for specifying malfunctions in the exhalation and inhalation check valve. Anesth Analg 1994; 78:611.

75. James RH. Checking the expiratory limb of anaesthetic breathing systems. Anaesthesia 1994;49:646–647.

76. Olympio MA, Stoner J. Tight mask fit could have prevented "airway" obstruction. Anesthesiology 1992; 77:822–825.

77. Grundy EM, Bennett EJ, Brennan T. Obstructed anesthetic circuits. Anesthesiol Rev 1976;3:35–36.

78. Holley HS, Carroll JS. Anesthesia equipment malfunction. Anaesthesia 1985;40:62–65.

79. Tamse JG. Preventive maintenance of medical and dental equipment. Paper presented at the AAMI 13th annual meeting, Washington, DC, March 28–April 1, 1978.

80. Welch JP. Clinical engineering in anesthesia. Med Instrum 1985;3:109–112.

81. Armstrong JN, Davies JM. A systematic method for the investigation of anaesthetic incidents. Can J Anaesth 1991;38:1033–1035.

82. Eagle CJ, Davies JM, Reason J. Accident analysis of large-scale technological disasters applied to an anaesthetic complication. Can J Anaesth 1992;39:118–122.

83. Cooper JB, Cullen DJ, Eichhorn JH, et al. Administrative guidelines for response to an adverse anesthesia event. J Clin Anesth 1993;5:79–84.

84. Forsell RD. The clinical engineer's role in incident investigation. Biomed Instrum Technol 1993;27: 378–383.

85. Lee RB. Reply to guidelines and techniques for the investigation of anesthetic accidents. J Clin Anesth 1994;6:171–172.

86. Anonymous. Impounding incident-related devices. Technology for Anesthesia 1984;4(10):1.

87. Anonymous. FDA proposed rule on user facility and manufacturer reporting under the Safe Medical Devices Act of 1990. Biomedical Safety & Standards 1991;14(Suppl):1–16.

88. Petty WC. Letter to the Editor: Questions help decide when to replace machines. Anesthesia Patient Safety Foundation Newsletter 1996;11:14–15.

89. Schreiber P: Anesthesia machine maker responds to question of obsolescence. Anesthesia Patient Safety Foundation Newsletter 1996;11:15–17.

90. Schreiber PJ. Con: There is nothing wrong with old anesthesia machines and equipment. Journal of Clinical Monitoring 1996;12:39–41.

91. Schneider AJL. Older anesthesia machines targeted for component replacement. Anesthesia Patient Safety Foundation Newsletter 1989;4:25–27.

QUESTIONS

Each question below contains four suggested answers of which one or more is correct.
Choose the answer:
A if 1, 2, and 3 are correct
B if 1 and 3 are correct
C if 2 and 4 are correct
D if 4 is correct
E if 1, 2, 3, and 4 are correct

1. Which equipment can provide an alternate ventilation method for the patient with a difficult airway?
   1. Laryngeal mask
   2. Combitube
   3. Transtracheal ventilation device
   4. Assortment of laryngoscope blades

2. Which of the following can provide satisfactory transtracheal ventilation?
   1. Jet injector attached to pipeline oxygen outlet
   2. A self-refilling resuscitation bag with a transtracheal catheter
   3. Jet injector attached to an oxygen tank regulator
   4. A noncompliant tubing attached to the Y-piece of the breathing system and activated with the oxygen flush

3. If there is a loss of pipeline oxygen, which steps should be taken to conserve oxygen from the cylinder?
   1. Discontinue using nitrous oxide
   2. Discontinue using the ventilator
   3. Use air and intravenous agents
   4. Use a low oxygen flow

4. When checking gas cylinders
   1. 500 psig should be the minimum pressure in the oxygen cylinder
   2. The cylinder valve should be left open to supply gas if the pipeline fails
   3. The check valve in the yoke should also be checked
   4. The pressure in the nitrous oxide cylinder reflects contents in the cylinder

5. The following test(s) will check the low pressure system in all anesthesia machines for leaks:
   1. Negative pressure test
   2. Elapsed time pressure test
   3. Fresh gas line occlusion test
   4. Retrograde fill test

6. What tests can be used to check a closed scavenging interface?
   1. The APL valve is closed and suction is turned on, the interface bag should collapse
   2. The APL valve is opened and the bag on the scavenging interface and the bag in the breathing system should be fully inflated
   3. When the suction is turned on, no negative pressure is applied to the breathing system
   4. With the oxygen flush activated there should be less than 10 cm H_2O in the breathing system with the APL valve fully open

7. When an open scavenging system is checked
   1. The bag mount should be occluded
   2. A minimum flow of 5 l/min should be registered on the flowmeters
   3. The absorber inlet and outlet are connected with a hose
   4. The pressure on the breathing system pressure gauge should be 0 ± 5 cm H_2O

8. When the oxygen analyzer is calibrated
   1. The low setting should be calibrated using room air
   2. The low oxygen alarm should be checked
   3. Repeated oxygen flushing should cause the analzyer to read over 90%
   4. The high setting should be calibrated at 100% oxygen

9. Tests used to test the integrity of inner tube on the Bain System?
   1. Occluding the inner tube with a plunger

2. Pressure variation test for systems with holes near the patient end of the inner tube

3. Activating the oxygen flush is activated while the bag is open to atmosphere

4. Pressurizing the inner tube to 30 cm H_2O

10. Leaks in the ventilator bellows and transfer tubing can be detected by which of the following tests?
   1. Isolating these parts with the bag/ventilator selector switch
   2. Varying the fresh gas flow and observing the delivered volume
   3. Using a minimum flow from the oxygen flowmeter and observing the bellows return to the fully inflated position
   4. Observing the excursion of the bellows during inspiration

11. Competency of the unidirectional valves can be checked by the following methods
   1. Observing the motion of the leaflet as the ventilator cycles
   2. Occluding the inspiratory tubing and not being able to inhale through the expiratory tube
   3. Removing the valve leaflet to inspect for damage to leaflet or its seat
   4. Occluding the expiratory tubing and not being able to exhale through the inspiratory tube

12. Actions which should be taken if a piece of equipment is suspected to have caused harm to a patient include
   1. Documenting the circumstances surrounding the time the problem first occurred
   2. Determining if similar problems had occurred in other operating rooms at the same time
   3. Isolating the equipment until the problem can be investigated
   4. Having the company service representative service the equipment

13. The following are required by the Safe Medical Devices Act
   1. Problems which must be reported include death of a patient
   2. Reporting is done by the clinician who experienced the problem
   3. Serious injury resulting from equipment must be reported
   4. Incidents must be reported within 20 working days

14. Criteria that would make an equipment obsolete include
   1. Replacement parts not available
   2. Inability to meet requirements for current practice
   3. Recent trainees have not trained to use the equipment properly
   4. Age

ANSWERS

1.	A	8.	A
2.	B	9.	B
3.	C	10.	B
4.	B	11.	C
5.	A	12.	A
6.	D	13.	B
7.	B	14.	A

CHAPTER
27

Cleaning and Sterilization

ALL ANESTHESIA PRACTITIONERS need to be interested in the cleanliness of their equipment. This is important both to prevent spread of infection between patients but also to ensure that the anesthesia provider does not contract infection from the equipment. There is no one way to care for every piece of equipment and to that end this chapter will discuss the various methods which are suitable to care for the different equipment used.

DEFINITIONS

Antiseptic: A substance that has antimicrobial activity and that can be safely applied to living tissue.

Bacteria: Minute unicellular organisms. This term is usually applied to the vegetative (growing) forms.

Bacteriostat: An agent that will prevent bacterial growth but does not necessarily kill the bacteria. Bacteriostatic action is reversible; when the agent is removed the bacteria will resume normal growth.

Bioburden (Bioload, Microbial Load): The number and types of viable organisms with which an object is contaminated.

Biologic Indicator: A sterilization-process monitoring device consisting of a standardized, viable population of microorganisms (usually bacterial spores) of high resistance to the mode of sterilization being monitored. Subsequent growth or failure of the microorganisms to grow under suitable conditions indicates whether or not conditions were adequate to achieve sterilization.

Chemical Indicator (Chemical Monitor, Sterilizer Control, Chemical Control Device): A sterilization process monitoring device designed to respond with a characteristic chemical change to one or more process parameters of a sterilization cycle.

Chemosterilizer (Chemical Sterilant): A chemical used for the purpose of destroying all forms of microbiologic life, including bacterial spores.

Cleaning: Removal of visible extraneous material from objects.

Contamination: The state of actually or potentially having been in contact with microorganisms.

Decontamination: This term has a number of definitions.

1. The process by which contaminated items are rendered safe for personnel who are not wearing protective attire to handle, that is, reasonably free of the probability of transmitting infection (1–5). In some cases, the decontamination process is also sufficient to render the items safe for reuse in patient care.
2. The reduction of microbial contamination to an acceptable level (6, 7).
3. Any process that eliminates harmful substances (8).

A decontamination procedure can range from sterilization to simple cleaning.

Disinfectant: A chemical germicide that is formulated to be used solely on inanimate objects. The Environmental Protection Agency (EPA) has divided disinfectants into those with labels that claim tuberculocidal activity and those with no claim for tuberculocidal activity.

Disinfection: The destruction of many, but not all, microorganisms on inanimate objects. The Centers for Disease Control and Prevention (CDC) have adopted a classification that includes three levels of disinfection (1) as shown in Table 27.1.

1. *High-Level Disinfection.* A procedure that kills all organisms with the exception of bacterial spores and certain viruses, such as the Creutzfeldt-Jakob virus (2). High-level disinfectants are registered with the EPA as sterilant/disinfectants, sporicidal hospital disinfectants, or sterilants (3). Most high-level disinfectants can produce sterilization with sufficient contact time.

TABLE **27.1. Levels of Disinfection**[a,b]

Levels	Bacteria				Lipid and Medium Size	Nonlipid and Small Size
	Vegetative	Tubercle	Spores	Fungi		
High	+	+	+[c]	+	+	+
Intermediate	+	+	±[d]	+	+	±[e]
Low	+	−	−	±[f]	+	−

[a] From American National Standards Institute. Good hospital practice: handling and biological decontamination of reusable medical devices (ST35-1991). Arlington, VA: Association for the Advancement of Medical Instrumentation, 1991.
[b] +, a killing effect can be expected when the normal-use concentrations of chemical disinfectants or pasteurization are properly employed; −, little or no killing effect.
[c] Only with extended exposure times are high-level disinfectant chemicals capable of actual sterilization.
[d] Certain intermediate-level disinfectants can be expected to exhibit some sporicidal action.
[e] Some intermediate-level disinfectants may have limited virucidal activity.
[f] Some low-level disinfectants may have limited fungicidal activity.

2. *Intermediate-Level Disinfection.* A procedure that kills bacteria, including *Mycobacterium tuberculosis,* some fungi, and most viruses but not bacterial spores. Chemical germicides that cause intermediate-level disinfection correspond to EPA-approved "hospital disinfectants" that are also "tuberculocidal."

3. *Low-Level Disinfection.* A procedure that kills most bacteria but not mycobacteria, some fungi, some viruses, or spores.

Disposable: A device intended for single use or single-patient use.

Fungicide: An agent that kills fungi.

Germicide: An agent that destroys microorganisms.

Mechanical Control (Physical) Monitors: Sterilizer components that gauge and record time, temperature, humidity, or pressure during a sterilization cycle.

Microbicidal Process: A process designed to provide an appropriate level of microbial lethality (kill). Depending on the level of decontamination, this process may be sanitization, disinfection, or sterilization (1).

Microbiocide: An agent that kills all organisms.

Nosocomial: Pertaining to a healthcare facility.

Sanitization: The process of reducing the number of microbial contaminants to a safe or relatively safe level. The term is generally used in connection with cleaning.

Sanitizer: A low-level disinfectant with no claim for tuberculocidal activity (9)

Spore: The normal resting stage in the life cycle of certain bacteria.

Sporicide: An agent that kills spores.

Sterilant/disinfectant: Term applied by EPA to a germicide that is capable of sterilization or high-level disinfection

Sterile/sterility: The state of being free from all living microorganisms. Sterility is usually described in terms of the probability that a microorganisms will survive treatment (10, 11).

Sterility Assurance Level (SAL): The probability of survival of microorganisms after a terminal sterilization process and a predictor of the efficacy of the process. A SAL of 10^{-6} means that the possibility of a nonsterile items exists, but is no greater than 1×10^{-6} or 1 in 1,000,000.

Sterilization: Destruction of all viable forms of microorganisms.

Terminal Sterilization: A sterilization process that is carried out after an item has been placed in its final packaging (1).

Viricide: An agent that kills viruses. The label on a product should indicate which viruses an agent will inactivate.

Viruses: Submicroscopic, noncellular parasitic particles composed of a protein shell and a nucleic acid core.

ROLE OF THE FEDERAL GOVERNMENT IN DISINFECTION AND STERILIZATION (5, 9)

The primary U.S. federal government agency involved with disinfection and sterilization devices and procedures is the EPA, which requires that chemical germicides be registered and regulated. The EPA requires manufacturers to test formulations of chemical germicides for microbicidal activity, stability, and toxicity to humans. It also approves sterilization devices.

If a chemical germicide is advertised and marketed for use on a specific medical device, then it falls under the additional regulatory control of the Food and Drug Administration (FDA). The FDA also requires that the manufacturer of a device that is marketed as reusable provides the user with adequate instructions for cleaning and disinfecting or sterilizing the item.

Occupational exposure to chemical disinfectants and sterilizers is regulated by the Occupational Safety and Health Administration (OSHA).

The CDC does not approve, regulate, or test germicides or sterilizers. Rather, it recommends broad strategies to prevent transmission of infections in the healthcare environment (12).

RESISTANCE OF MICROORGANISMS TO DISINFECTION AND STERILIZATION

Microorganisms can be categorized into several general groups according to their innate resistance to a spectrum of physical processes or chemical germicidal agents. These groups are listed in broad descending order in Table 27.2.

TABLE 27.2. **Descending Order of Resistance to Germicidal Chemicals**

Bacterial Spores
Mycobacteria (including Mycobacterium tuberculosis)
Nonlipid or small viruses
Fungi
Vegetative bacteria (including Pseudomonas aeruginosa and Staphylococcus aureus)
Lipid or medium-sized viruses (including hepatitis B and human immunodeficiency viruses)

The most resistant types are bacterial spores, some of which are quite resistant to both chemical and physical stresses. In descending order of relative resistance, considerably below bacterial spores, are the mycobacteria, small or nonlipid viruses, fungi, vegetative bacteria, and medium-sized or lipid-containing viruses.

Resistance to disinfection and sterilization is not equivalent to resistance to antibiotics. Antibiotic-resistant strains of staphylococci do not appear to be more resistant to chemical germicides than ordinary bacteria (9).

CLEANING OF EQUIPMENT

The first and most important step in decontamination is thorough cleaning and rinsing. If an article is not clean, retained soil could inactivate chemical germicides or protect microorganisms from destruction during the disinfection or sterilization processes. Even if the item is rendered sterile, a patient may have a reaction to the residue.

The manufacturer's instructions should be consulted to determine the appropriate cleaning methods and agents. Immersible devices should be cleaned under water to prevent aerosolization of microorganisms. Items that do not lend themselves to cleaning by immersion often may be cleaned by a cloth soaked in detergent and water.

Cleaning should be performed in a designated location that is divided into dirty and clean areas (6). Personnel should wear protective attire (masks, protective eye wear, waterproof aprons, and gloves) and be careful not to injure themselves with contaminated instruments. Brushes and other cleaning implements should be disinfected or sterilized daily.

To facilitate cleaning, devices composed of more than one part must be disassembled and jointed instruments must be opened. Tape should be removed. Adhesive residue should be dissolved using a special solvent.

An initial water rinse or soaking with a specialized product (e.g., a protein-dissolving solution) is sometimes recommended to prevent coagulation of blood and remove gross debris.

After the equipment has soaked long enough to loosen organic matter, it should be scrubbed thoroughly inside and out. Particular attention should be paid to corners and grooves in which debris may be hidden. Cleaning may be accomplished manually, mechanically, or by a combination of the two methods. Using mechanical equipment may increase productivity, improve cleaning effectiveness, and/or promote employee safety.

Cleaning must remove residual organic soil without damaging the device. The appropriate cleaning agent (i.e., one that is compatible with the materials of which the device is composed and with the cleaning method selected) should be used in accordance with the instructions of the manufacturer of the cleaning agent. Commercial products (e.g., blends of quaternary ammonium compounds with other additives) that provide the double action of cleaning and preliminary disinfection, thereby reducing employee hazards during decontamination, are available.

A variety of machines for washing equipment is available (13–17). They include ultrasonic cleaners, washer/sanitizers, pasteurization equipment, washer/disinfectors, and washer/sterilizers. Use of these may result in greater productivity and better economics for some institutions.

Equipment that has joints, crevices, lumens, and other areas that are difficult to clean by other methods can be treated in an ultrasonic cleaning system after gross soil has been removed. In an ultrasonic cleaner, high-frequency electrical energy is converted into mechanical energy in the form of sound waves. The waves, passing through a solvent, produce submicroscopic bubbles. These bubbles collapse on themselves, generating tiny shock waves that knock debris off surfaces. A detergent is often added to the ultrasonic liquid. Ultrasonic cleaning tanks are available in a variety of sizes and configurations (18). The equipment to be cleaned is placed in a basket or tray and into the ultrasonic tank for a preset period of time—usually 3 to 6 minutes. Ultrasonic cleaning is sometimes superior to scrubbing by hand, because it can remove soil in hard-to-reach areas. It may be the most economical way of cleaning some articles. Some manufacturers of delicate instruments recommend that they not be subjected to sonic cleaning because the process may loosen fine screws and adversely affect alignment (19).

After cleaning has been performed, rinsing is important to remove soil and residual detergent and keep them from resettling on the equipment. After rinsing, each item should be inspected for the absence of foreign matter.

Unless steam sterilization, pasteurization, or the Steris system is to be used, the cleaned item should be thoroughly dried. Even if an item is to undergo no further disinfection, drying is important because a humid environment may encourage the growth of Gram-negative organisms (6). If a liquid chemical agent is to be used, water on the equipment will dilute the agent and make it less effective. If water droplets are left on equipment that is to be gas sterilized, ethylene oxide (EtO, EO) will dissolve in the water and form ethylene glycol, which is both toxic and difficult to remove. Most items may be towel or air dried. Air-drying cabinets and hot-air ovens are available (see Fig. 27.1). If an item is to undergo EO sterilization, unheated air should be used.

METHODS OF DISINFECTION AND STERILIZATION
Pasteurization

With pasteurization, the equipment is immersed in water at an elevated temperature (but below 100°C) for a given time period. The time and temperature recommended vary. Contact time is inversely related to temperature, i.e., for equivalent microbial kill, a longer exposure time may be required when the temperature is reduced.

Pasteurizing machines come in different sizes and capacities (Fig. 27.2). They are simple to load and operate. Special dryers equipped with filters are available.

This is a disinfecting process but cannot be depended on for sterilization. CDC guidelines refer to pasteurization as a high-level disinfection process, although this is inconsistent with its classification system because of the inability of the procedure to reliably kill spores and viruses (6).

Pasteurization has been used for breathing tubes, reservoir bags, tracheal tubes, face masks, airways, laryngoscope blades, and ventilator bellows (4). It may produce tubings as clean as those of a disposable breathing system (4).

The biggest advantage of this method is that the lower temperature is less damaging to equipment than the higher temperatures employed in autoclaving. There are no toxic fumes or residues. It is simple, inexpensive, and reliable. Its use may result in considerable cost savings compared to throwing equipment away. The main disadvantage is that the treated equipment is wet and must still be dried and packaged, during which it may again become contaminated. Some materials may be damaged by the heat.

Steam Sterilization (17)

Steam sterilization (autoclaving), which uses saturated steam under pressure, is commonly used for sterilization in healthcare facilities.

Equipment to be sterilized is first cleaned and then packaged in muslin, linen, or paper. The steam easily penetrates these materials. After sterilization, the packaging material prevents recontamination during subsequent handling and storage.

The chamber is the portion of the sterilizer in which materials are placed and through which steam is circulated (20). The jacket is the portion surrounding the chamber that functions to maintain the temperature in the chamber.

The items are placed on a shelf in the chamber, and the door closed and secured. Autoclaves have automatic controls that ensure that the correct sequence is followed. Before the sterilization cycle begins, air is evacuated from the chamber. If this is not done, the quantity of steam entering the autoclave is reduced and, with this, the temperature achieved. As steam enters the chamber, it enters the load to be sterilized and gives up its latent heat. Once the intended temperature is reached, the duration of sterilization is set. At the end of this period the steam is exhausted from the autoclave to avoid condensation of water on the load when cool air is admitted.

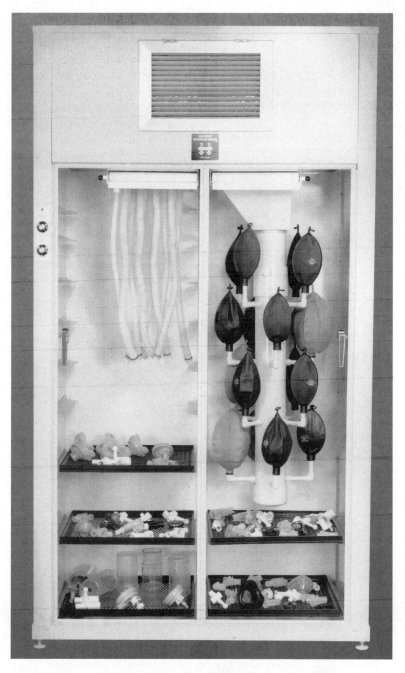

FIGURE **27.1.** Forced-air drying cabin for equipment. (Courtesy of Olympic Medical.)

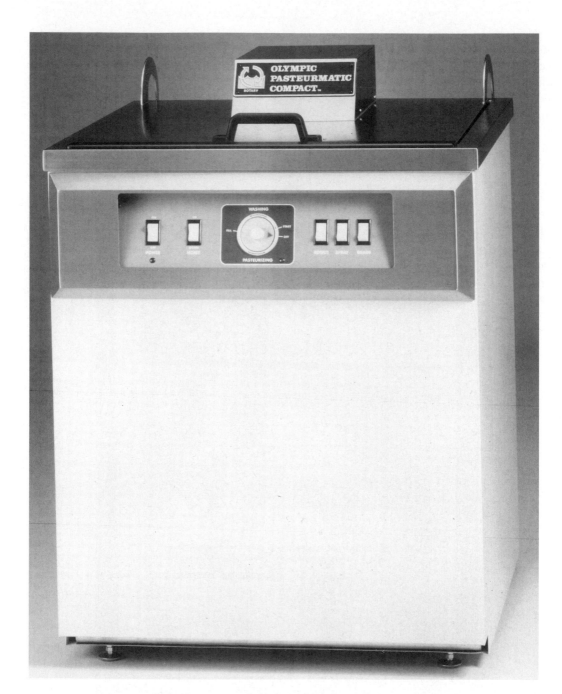

FIGURE 27.2. Pasteurization machine. (Courtesy of Olympic Medical.)

Variables in Steam Sterilization

Autoclaving is extremely effective because the saturated steam rapidly transfers heat to materials. Microbial destruction will be most effective at locations where saturated steam can contact the microorganisms. At locations inaccessible to steam penetration (as might occur with complex medical devices, improperly packaged items or incorrect load configurations), some microbial destruction may occur as a result of dry heat, but dry heat is not as efficient at sterilizing as saturated steam.

Temperature

At sea level, water boils at 100°C. When it is boiled within a closed vessel at increased pressure, the temperature at which it boils and that of the steam it forms will exceed 100°C. The increase in temperature depends on the pressure within the chamber. This is the basic principle of the autoclave. Pressure per se has little or no sterilizing effect. It is the moist heat at a suitable temperature, as regulated by the pressure in the chamber, that brings about sterilization.

Time

The higher the temperature, the more rapidly sterilization can be accomplished. The minimum time for steam sterilization at 121°C is 15 minutes (21). If the temperature is 126°C, the time is reduced to 10 minutes. It is 3.5 minutes at 134°C and only a few seconds at 150°C (22).

Flash sterilization refers to steam sterilization of items for immediate use (23). The items to be processed are usually unwrapped, although a single wrap may be used in certain circumstances. The cycle time and temperature settings will depend on the sterilizer and the configuration of the load (23). The processed items can be assumed to be wet and must be transferred immediately from the sterilizer to the actual point of use, usually the sterile field in an ongoing surgical procedure.

Characteristics of the Steam (11)

Less-than-optimum steam characteristics reduce the efficiency of heat transfer and jeopardize the sterility. Steam should contain no air, liquid water, or solid particles. A filter that removes liquids and solid particles should be installed in the steam line just upstream of the autoclave.

Problems with Steam Sterilization (11)

Steam Quality

Steam quality or saturation refers to the level of moisture in steam. Liquid water may be present in the form of "fog" or water droplets. "Wet" steam may condense onto cool surfaces and impede the transfer of heat to items being sterilized. Current standards call for a steam quality greater than 97% (less than 3% liquid water). Low-quality ("wet") steam is one cause of wet packs. It may result from problems in the steam supply itself, or may occur locally within the chamber when steam contacts a cold load.

Steam Saturation

Steam is said to be saturated when it has the proper balance of pressure and temperature. If the pressure is too great, the steam will change to rain, causing packs to become wet; if the pressure is too low, the steam will be superheated. Superheated steam is less able than saturated steam to transfer its heat energy to the cooler items being sterilized and will make it difficult to attain a uniform temperature in the chamber. Superheating may be caused by the materials being processed. Packs that are overly dry, because they have been accidentally processed twice, or that are reprocessed without laundering or other means of humidification may cause superheating by removing moisture from the steam.

Steam Supply

Variations in steam pressure may affect the time to attain the proper temperature and temperature uniformity within the chamber. Pressure variations may be caused by clogged filters, poorly engineered piping or excessive demands on the steam supply. It is not unusual for problems to occur at the start of winter in cold climates; these problems can often be traced to a marginal steam supply that is overloaded when it is used to heat the building.

Air in the Autoclave Chamber (11)

The presence of air in the chamber will impair sterilization. Air is a poor conductor of heat and retards the penetration of steam (24). The autoclave evacuates much of the air by gravity displacement by the steam, one or more vacuum excursions at the beginning of the cycle or a repeated sequence of steam flushes and pressure pulses (17).

Equipment Malfunction (11)

Examples of equipment malfunction include out-of-calibration temperature or pressure gauges and controllers, incorrect steam supply pressure, faulty or maladjusted control valves, leaks, clogged vent lines or drain screens, faulty vacuum pumps, defective steam traps, and malfunctioning cycle sequence controllers.

Personnel Errors

Personnel errors include inadequate cleaning of equipment, incorrect pack preparation and packaging methods, and poor loading techniques. There is also the possibility that an entire load could inadvertently not be processed.

Steam Sterilization Process Monitoring

There is no monitor or indicator that can give assurance that each item in a load is sterile, but there are devices that will give a high level of assurance.

Mechanical, biological, and chemical indicators are all used to determine whether the conditions were adequate to achieve sterilization (17, 23). Using these in concert will give the greatest possible confidence that individual items are sterile.

Mechanical Monitors

Mechanical monitors are devices or gauges that indicate the time, temperature, and pressure. They will detect major equipment malfunctions while the cycle is in progress. Most autoclaves provide a permanent record in the form of chart recordings or computer-driven printouts.

Biological Indicators (11, 25, 26)

Biological indicators are standardized preparations of microorganisms resistant to a particular sterilization process. For steam sterilization, paper strips impregnated with spores or ampules of spores are most often used. The strips or ampules are placed in the chamber, within a special test pack or within packaged items. They are then exposed to the sterilization cycle, retrieved, incubated, and examined for microbial growth.

The CDC recommends use of biological monitors at least once a week (12). The main problem with biological indicators is that time is needed for incubation.

Chemical Indicators (11)

A chemical indicator is a sterilization-process monitoring device designed to respond to one or more of the physical conditions (temperature, time, or pressure) within the sterilization chamber. They are a more practical means of detecting local conditions within the load than biological indicators. They can reveal potential problems immediately (or at least before an item is used), whereas biological indicator results are usually not available for several days.

The CDC and all major U.S. organizations that issue sterilization-related standards or guidelines advocate that a chemical indicator be attached to every package that goes through a sterilization cycle (12).

Advantages and Disadvantages

Autoclaving can kill all bacteria, spores, and viruses. Advantages include speed, good penetration, economy, ease of use, absence of toxic products or residues, and reliability. The material can be prepackaged and kept sterile until used. It allows the interior of a wrapped package to be sterilized. A major advantage is that at least one autoclave is available in every modern operating theater.

The principal disadvantage of autoclaving is that many pieces of equipment made from heat-sensitive materials are damaged if subjected to steam. Autoclaving can cause blunting of cutting edges, corrosion of metal surfaces, and shortened life of electronic components.

Chemical Disinfection and Sterilization

Chemical (cold) disinfection and sterilization utilize liquid chemical agents and is especially useful for heat-sensitive equipment. Cold disinfection/sterilization is often performed by soaking an item in a solution. It can also be accomplished by automated equipment called washer/disinfectors or washer/sterilizers, which typically provide a cycle of cleaning, rinsing, disinfection, rinsing, and sometimes drying.

Regulation of Chemical Germicides (5)

The EPA regulates formulations and labeling of chemical germicides. The labeling must provide information relating to safe and effective use, including required contact time, use temperature, reuse pattern, and shelf life.

The EPA requires the label of a hospital disinfectant to show the ability of the chemical agent to destroy *M. tuberculosis* and the time and temperature required. If the product is effective against this organism, the label will say "tuberculocidal." Similarly, if a disinfectant product is capable of destroying *Pseudomonas aeruginosa*, the label will state that it is pseudomonacidal. If the product is effective against the human immunodeficiency virus (HIV), the label must state this.

Safety Considerations in Chemical Disinfection

OSHA has established limits on occupational exposure to glutaraldehyde, formaldehyde, and other chemical disinfectants and sterilants (see Table 27.3). The user should consult the information supplied by the disinfectant manufacturer and observe recommended safety precautions. The following general measures should be implemented:

1. Centralizing chemical germicide use in a few key areas.

TABLE 27.3. **Occupational Exposure Limits for Some Chemical Sterilants and Disinfectants**[a,b]

Chemical Agent	OSHA Requirements[c]
Alcohols	Varying PEL
Chlorine dioxide	0.1 ppm 8-hr TWA/0.3 ppm STEL
Ethylene oxide	1.0 ppm 8-hr/TWA 5 ppm STEL
Formaldehyde	0.75 ppm 8-hr TWA/2 ppm STEL
Glutaraldehyde	0.2 ppm 8-hr TWA
Hydrogen peroxide	1.0 ppm 8-hr TWA
Peracetic acid	No limits established
Phenol	5.0 ppm 8-hr TWA

[a] From American National Standards Institute. Good hospital practice: handling and biological decontamination of reusable medical devices (ST35-1991). Arlington, VA: Association for the Advancement of Medical Instrumentation, 1991.
[b] Standard ST35-1991 has been in effect since 1989, but until the end of 1993, compliance methods such as work practices and protective personal equipment suffice. After this, administrative and engineering controls must have been implemented whenever feasible. A ceiling limit is the highest concentration an employee may be exposed to during any part of the workday.
[c] PEL, permissible exposure limit; TWA, time-weighted average; STEL, short-term excursion limit (TWA for 15 minutes).

2. Adequate ventilation and, if possible, a fume hood in the disinfection area.
3. Use of containers with lids for the disinfectant solution.
4. Protective clothing and devices such as gowns, gloves, eye protection, and masks for personnel.
5. Neutralization of solutions in the hood before removal for disposal.
6. Use of special devices to avoid exposure when the germicide is discarded.
7. Use of monitoring badges and alarms to detect high levels.
8. Establishment of a plan of action for a germicide spill.

Factors Influencing Chemical Disinfection
Concentration of the Chemical

Generally, the rate of kill of bacteria varies directly with the concentration of the disinfectant (27). An exception is the alcohols. Concentration will also influence the ability of a chemical agent to kill or inactivate certain microorganisms. A chemical in low concentrations may kill certain organisms, whereas a higher concentration is required to inactivate others. A strong solution may be more irritating and/or injurious to the item being disinfected.

Water left on equipment will dilute the liquid agent and render it less effective. For this reason, most equipment should be dried after it is cleaned. Dilution can become significant with frequent reuse and can reduce the concentration to a level too low to be effective.

Several products registered with the EPA as sterilant/disinfectants can be used for sterilization with a concentrated or slightly diluted product, and for disinfection with higher dilutions that exceed the product's ability to inactivate spores (9).

Temperature

Although these agents are designed to be used at room temperature, increasing the temperature usually increases their effectiveness (28). Special devices are available for heating some chemical solutions. The product label will usually tell what temperature should be used. The temperature should not be high enough that the active ingredients evaporate appreciably, or that the germicide itself is degraded

Evaporation and Light Deactivation

If the solution is in an uncovered container, evaporation can occur. Generally, evaporation is not as critical as dilution. However, if the chemical agent is more volatile than the diluent, then loss of the agent by evaporation can be very important. Chlorine products are especially susceptible to evaporation. Exposure to light may adversely affect chlorine disinfectants.

pH

Some disinfectants may be formulated over a range of pHs. Some are more effective in killing microorganisms under alkaline conditions while others work best with acidic conditions. The presence of detergents in the disinfectant solution, which may occur if the device is inadequately rinsed after cleaning, can alter the pH of the solution and reduce its effectiveness.

Bioburden

The effectiveness of the disinfectant depends on the nature and number of contaminating microorganisms. In general, the higher the level of microbial contamination, the longer the exposure to the chemical germicide necessary before the entire microbial population is killed. Liquid agents vary widely in their effectiveness against various types of microorganisms. Table 27.4 shows the capabilities of some commonly used disinfectant agents.

Characteristics of the Item to Be Disinfected

A disinfectant solution will be effective only if it can contact all surfaces of the item to be disin-fected. Uneven or porous surfaces resist chemical disinfection (27). Air entrapment prevents contact between the liquid and bubble-covered regions.

Use Pattern and Use Life

The product label should be examined for information on the use pattern, use life, and storage life of the product. It is important to distinguish between the use life and use pattern. The use life commonly applies, but is not limited, to disinfectant products that require the mixing of two ingredients for activation. Once a disinfectant solution is mixed, there may be a limited period of time during which the activated solution may be used. That time is its use life. The use pattern refers to how many times the solution can be used. The storage life is the time period after which the unused and/or unactivated product is no longer deemed effective.

Time

The time required for different chemical agents to function effectively varies from seconds to hours and will depend on the factors just mentioned. Some microorganisms are killed faster than others. Contact time may make the difference between sterilization and high-level disinfection with a specific chemical germicide.

Sterilization Monitors

Test methods are available to determine the efficacy of sterilizing chemical agents. These tests employ standardized carriers onto which the test organism is deposited. The inoculated carrier is then exposed to the sterilizing agent under the

---

TABLE 27.4. **Capabilities of Disinfecting Agents**[a,b]

Disinfectant	Gram-Positive Bacteria	Gram-Negative Bacteria	Tubercle Bacillus	Spores	Viruses	Fungi
Quats	+	±	0	0	±	±
Alcohols	+	+	+	0	±	±
Glutaraldehydes	+	+	+	±	+	+
Hydrogen peroxide–based compounds	+	+	+	±	+	+
Formaldehyde and other agents	+	+	+	−	+	+
Phenolic compounds	+	+	±	0	±	±
Chlorine	+	+	+	−	+	+

[a] From Chatbum RL. Decontamination of respiratory care equipment: what can be done, what should be done. Respir Care 1989;34:98; and Berry AJ. Infection control in anesthesia. Anesth Clin North Am 1989;7:967–981.

[b] +, good; ±, fair; 0, little or none.

conditions recommended for its routine use (exposure time, concentration, temperature, etc.).

Following exposure, the carrier is placed in a growth media and incubated. Growth in the media indicates that the sterilization process failed to destroy the test organisms. No growth indicates that the sterilization process was effective.

Agents (2)

No single chemical germicide is adequate for all purposes and a number of factors that should be considered in selecting among those available, including the degree of microbial killing required; the nature and composition of the item being treated; whether the item is critical, semicritical, or noncritical; and the cost, safety, and ease of use (9).

Formaldehyde

Formaldehyde is used principally in a water-based solution called formalin. It is noncorrosive and is not inactivated by organic matter (29). Although formaldehyde-alcohol is a chemosterilizer and formalin is a high-level disinfectant, its uses are limited by its pungent odor and fumes, which irritate the skin, eyes, and respiratory tract at very low levels (30). The National Institute for Occupational Safety and Health (NIOSH) has indicated that formaldehyde should be handled as a potent sensitizer and probable carcinogen and has set exposure limits (see Table 27.3). Sterilization with low temperature steam and formaldehyde is used in some countries (16).

Quaternary Ammonium Compounds (2, 6)

Quaternary ammonium compounds (quats) are low-level disinfectants (29). They are bactericidal, fungical, and viricidal at room temperature within 10 minutes, but have not demonstrated sporicidal effects. If a spore is coated with a quaternary ammonium compound, it will not develop into a vegetative cell as long as the coating of the germicide remains, but if the coating is removed, the cell can germinate (31, 32). These compounds are more effective against Gram-positive than Gram-negative bacteria and are only marginally effective against *P. aeruginosa*. Quats inactivate HIV but some do not inactivate the hepatitis virus (2). Recently hepacide quat–based disinfectants have become available.

Early generation quats were affected by factors such as hard water, soap, and anionic residues and were inactivated by organic materials (e.g., cork, cotton, and gauze pads). Some, either used in insufficient concentrations or in solutions that have deteriorated from age or the presence of organic soil, not only failed to kill some microbes, but actually supported their growth (9). Newer ones are mixed with various substances to produce synergistic antimicrobial and detergent activities greater than that of the individual components while maintaining the hard water, protein, and anionic tolerance necessary in environmental disinfectants (2, 6). They are quick acting, relatively nontoxic and noncaustic, and do not produce noxious fumes. They are useful for cleaning as well as disinfection (6).

Reported problems include an allergic reaction of the tracheal mucosa after use of a quaternary ammonium compound to clean a tracheostomy tube (33) and contact dermatitis (34).

Phenolic Compounds (2, 6)

Phenolic compounds (phenolics) are derived from carbolic acid (phenol), one of the oldest germicides. They are good bactericides and are active against fungi. They are sometimes virucidal but are not sporicidal except at or above 100°C. They are active in the presence of organic matter and soap (35). They are sometimes combined with detergents to form detergent germicides. Phenols are very stable and remain active after mild heating and prolonged drying. Application of moisture to a surface previously treated with a phenolic compound can redissolve the chemical so that it again becomes bactericidal. Phenolics remain active in contact with organic soil and for this reason are often one of the disinfectants of choice when dealing with gross organic contamination in general housekeeping or for environmental disinfection in laboratory areas.

Most phenolic compounds have a bad odor and are irritating to skin (31, 36). They are absorbed by rubber and may damage skin or mucous membranes they contact. Phenols are generally difficult to rinse from most materials and residual disinfectant may cause tissue irritation (2, 9).

Phenols are considered intermediate- to low-level disinfectants (31). They are not recommended for semi-critical items because of the lack of published efficacy data for many of the available formulations and because residual disinfectant may cause tissue irritation even after thorough rinsing (2). They are used mainly on environmental surfaces and for noncritical devices. They have been used for reservoir bags but are absorbed by rubber and may irritate the anesthesia provider's hand. Facial burns may result from their use on masks (37). Skin depigmentation has been reported (38).

Alcohols

Ethyl alcohol is bactericidal in 60 to 90% concentrations (70% is best) and isopropyl alcohol in 60% or greater concentration (90% is best). Both kill most bacteria, including mycobacteria during an exposure of 1 to 5 minutes (35, 39). They do not kill spores. Their action against viruses is variable, with ethyl alcohol superior to isopropyl alcohol (30). The CDC recommends exposure to 70% ethanol for 15 minutes to inactivate the hepatitis virus, but 1 minute should be adequate for HIV (40). Neither will inactivate the Creutzfeldt-Jakob virus (41).

Ethyl and isopropyl alcohol are relatively inexpensive intermediate-level disinfectants. Their effectiveness is limited because of their rapid evaporation that results in short contact times unless the items are immersed and because they lack the ability to penetrate residual organic material. Items to be disinfected with alcohols should be carefully precleaned and then totally submerged for an appropriate exposure time.

They are sometimes combined with other agents to form a tincture.

Alcohols have a cleansing action. They are inactivated by protein, but not by soap (2, 29). It is not necessary to rinse items soaked in alcohol because it evaporates rapidly. For this reason an alcohol flush cycle is used in some automatic processing machines. They are sometimes used to disinfect external surfaces of equipment (e.g., stethoscopes and ventilators) (2). They have been used to clean fiberoptic cables (42).

Alcohols can damage the mounting of lensed instruments and tend to swell and harden rubber and certain plastics after prolonged and repeated use (30, 43).

Alcohols are flammable so care must be taken not to use them in the presence of a heat source that could ignite the vapor.

Alcohol and agents containing alcohol must not be allowed to seep into sampling lines as this can lead to incorrect results when measuring anesthetic agents.

Iodophors

An iodophor is a combination of iodine and a solubilizing agent or carrier with the resulting complex providing a sustained-release reservoir of iodine and releasing a small amount of free iodine in aqueous solution. They are bactericidal, viricidal, and tuberculocidal but may require prolonged contact time to kill certain fungi and bacterial spores.

Iodophors are used principally as antiseptics but are capable of intermediate-level and low-level disinfection (30). Iodophors formulated as antiseptics are not suitable for disinfecting medical instruments or environmental surfaces (9). Some iodophors are unstable in the presence of very hard water, heat, and organic soil, but are reliable general-purpose disinfectants if used in concentrations recommended by the manufacturer (9). Some metallic instruments can be corroded if they are routinely disinfected with iodophors for long periods; nonmetallic items are seldom damaged but may become stained or discolored.

Peracetic (Peroxyacetic) Acid

Peracetic acid is acetic acid with an extra oxygen atom. It is bactericidal, sporicidal, fungicidal, and viricidal at low temperatures (44). It remains effective in the presence of organic material. One problem is that it is corrosive and irritating to skin in a concentrated solution.

Peracetic acid is the active ingredient in the Steris sterilant. This is a single-use concentrate of 35% peracetic acid plus corrosion and degradation inhibitors, which are contained in a sealed single-use container. The concentrate is automatically diluted with sterile water before exposure to the instruments to be processed. The concentrate should be used only in the Steris processing system. It is not intended for manual open-pan techniques.

The Steris system is shown in Figure 27.3. Equipment to be sterilized, which must be clean but need not be dry, is placed in a special tray, which is then placed in the tabletop processor.

Each tray has holes in the bottom for fluid entry and drainage. Different types of trays are available for different equipment. The trays are designed so that there is a continuous flow of steri-

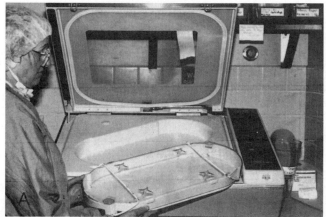

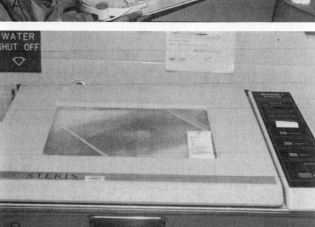

FIGURE 27.3. The Steris system. **A,** Items to be sterilized are cleaned, then placed in a tray. The tray is then placed in the sterilizer. **B,** After the lid is closed and the processing cycle started, the processor automatically opens the sterilant concentrate and mixes it with filtered water. The use dilution of the sterilant enters the tray, covering the instruments, and is circulated for 12 minutes. It is then drained from the chamber, and the chamber and tray are rinsed four times with sterile water. Next, sterile air is pumped into the chamber to displace the rinse water. A printout confirming that the sterilization parameters were met is provided.

lant on exposed surfaces and internal channels of instruments. Trays can be transported to the sterile field following processing.

After the tray is positioned in the sterilizer, a package of sterilant concentrate is placed in the sterilizer. The lid is closed, and the processing cycle started. During the cycle, the lid is sealed so that there is no exposure of personnel to the sterilant. The processor automatically opens the sterilant concentrate and mixes it with a controlled volume of filtered sterile water heated to 50 to 55°C (122 to 132°F). The diluted sterilant enters the tray, covers the instruments, and is circulated for 12 min. It is then drained from the chamber and the chamber and tray are filled with sterile water. The instruments and chamber are rinsed four times with sterile water, then sterile air is pumped into the chamber to displace the rinse water. The cycle takes from 20 to 30 minutes,

depending on the initial temperature of the water and how extensively the local water supply must be filtered. After the cycle is complete, the unit flushes the diluted sterilant and rinse water directly into a drain.

The processor is an automatic microcomputer-controlled device that monitors and maintains the parameters necessary to ensure sterile processing. It will stop the cycle if a process error is detected. At the end of each cycle, a printout confirming that the sterilization parameters were met is provided for quality assurance records.

This system provides a quick method of sterilizing a wide variety of heat-sensitive totally immersible instruments, including some fiberscopes. It is less damaging to delicate instruments than steam sterilization and is compatible with a wide variety of materials, including plastics, rubber, and most heat-sensitive items.

The Steris system is especially useful for items requiring a quick turnaround time. It is faster than sterilization with EO or glutaraldehyde and can be used on wet or dry items. No dilution of the sterilant by personnel is necessary, and the rinse is automatic so personnel are not exposed to any toxic chemicals. Consequently it can be situated in the operating room suite.

The Steris system does have some disadvantages. Only items that can be totally immersed can be sterilized. Only one scope or a small number of instruments can be processed in a cycle. The use of instruments sterilized in this system should be consistent with "just-in-time" processing and delivery. The processor and trays cannot be used as extended storage devices.

Chlorine and Chlorine Products

Hypochlorites are the most widely used of the chloride disinfectants. They are available in both liquid (e.g., sodium hypochlorite) and solid (e.g., calcium hypochlorite) forms. They are inexpensive and fast acting. Other compounds that release chlorine and are used in the healthcare setting include demand-release chlorine dioxide and chloramine-T (2). These retain chlorine longer and so exert a more prolonged bactericidal effect than the hypochlorites.

Most chlorine compounds are intermediate level disinfectants. They are active against all bacteria and viruses but not bacterial spores. Their disinfecting efficacy decreases with an increase in pH.

Household bleach is an inexpensive and excellent source of sodium hypochlorite. A 1:100 to 1:1000 dilution is effective against the human immunodeficiency virus (45, 46). A 1:5 to 1:10 dilution will destroy the hepatitis virus (4) and will inactivate the virus of Creutzfeldt-Jakob disease with an exposure time of 1 hour (41, 47, 48). High concentrations are corrosive as well as irritating to personnel and their use should be limited to situations in which organic material is difficult to clean or contains unusually high concentrations of microorganisms (9).

Inorganic chlorine solutions are useful for spot disinfection of countertops and floors. A 1:10 dilution of 5.25% sodium hypochlorite has been recommended by the CDC for cleaning blood spills (9). Their use is limited by their corrosiveness,

inactivation by organic matter and relative instability (2, 29). They may leave a residue and are irritating to skin, eyes, and the respiratory tract. A potential hazard is the production of the carcinogen *bis*-chloromethyl ether when hypochlorite solutions come into contact with formaldehyde. A mixture of sodium hypochlorite with acid will cause rapid evolution of toxic chlorine gas (9).

Hydrogen Peroxide (2, 6)

Hydrogen peroxide is an effective bactericide, fungicide, viricide, and sporicide (49–52). Synergistic sporicidal effects have been observed with a combination of hydrogen peroxide and peracetic acid (53). It is commercially available in a 3% solution but can be used in up to a 25% concentration (2, 29). It is noncorrosive and is not inactivated by organic matter but is an irritant to the skin and eyes (29). It is said to be safe for use with rubber, plastic, and stainless steel. It is used with plasma sterilization. The residuals after such treatment are water and oxygen.

Glutaraldehyde (Pentanedial) (2, 6, 9, 13, 14, 35, 40, 54–67)

Glutaraldehyde is a saturated dialdehyde that is available in a number of formulations. Glutaraldehyde-based solutions have been widely used because of their excellent biocidal properties, activity in the presence of organic matter, non-corrosiveness with most equipment, and non-coagulation of proteinaceous material.

Dilution of glutaraldehyde commonly occurs during use, and it is important to ensure that semicritical equipment is disinfected with an acceptable concentration: 1.0% glutaraldehyde is the minimum effective concentration when used as a high-level disinfectant (68, 69). Means to check the concentration are available. The time recommended for disinfection will vary, depending on the formulation, the temperature, and additives. Thorough rinsing of all exposed materials is mandatory, because residual glutaraldehyde is irritating to tissues.

Glutaraldehyde-based germicides are noxious and irritating and may result in a variety of toxic reactions in healthcare workers if proper ventilation and personal barriers (e.g., gloves, face protection) are not consistently used. Glutaraldehyde user stations in which the containers are enclosed in a device with transparent front door and sides are available (70). Fumes are drawn away from the operator into a filter where they are neutralized.

Disinfection can be carried out in a special automatic machine that performs both cleansing with a detergent and cold disinfection with glutaraldehyde (13, 14, 71). The glutaraldehyde is held in a side tank and is automatically pumped into the tub. Upon completion of the disinfection cycle, the solution is returned to the side tank for reuse.

Pseudomembranous laryngitis has been linked to disinfection of tracheal tubes with glutaraldehyde (72). Contact dermatitis has also been reported (67). Sticking of adjustable pressure limiting (APL) valves may occur (73).

Advantages and Disadvantages

Advantages of liquid chemical disinfection include economy, speed, and simplicity. The chief hazard is that the chemicals employed can be absorbed onto the items, causing harm to the patient. It cannot be used for all types of equipment. Many devices cannot be soaked. Prepackaging is not possible and the equipment will be wet. There is an opportunity for recontamination during subsequent rinsing, drying, or wrapping. With most agents, sterility cannot be guaranteed because some resistant organisms and spores may not be killed.

Some solutions are irritating to tissues and have unpleasant odors. Personnel handling them must take precautions to avoid prolonged skin contact or inhalation of the vapor.

Gas Sterilization

EO is a colorless, poisonous gas with a sweet odor. It is a liquid below 11°C (51°F). It is available in high-pressure tanks and unit-dose ampules and cartridges. Both the liquid and the gas are flammable in concentrations of 3% or greater. Manufacturers have dealt with this hazard in two ways. EO may be mixed with carbon dioxide or hydrochlorofluorocarbons (74). Mixtures containing up to 12% EO in these inert diluents are nonflammable, but retain their sterilizing capacity. Other manufacturers use 100% EO, but design equipment specially for gas containment and to minimize the risk of explosion.

EO kills bacteria, spores, fungi, and viruses. As a gas, it penetrates into crevices and through permeable bags. Items can be packaged before sterilization and stored sterile for extended periods of time. Because EO sterilization is a more complex and expensive process than steam sterilization, it is usually restricted to objects that might be damaged by heat or excessive moisture.

A number of standards have been approved for the use of EO sterilization in healthcare facilities (75–80).

Preparation for Ethylene Oxide Sterilization

It is important to verify that the product is suitable for sterilization by EO. The manufacturer's instructions for each device should be consulted. Some devices need to be sterilized at a lower temperature.

Before packaging, items must be disassembled, cleaned, and dried. Disassembly is important because all barriers to the gas's free movement must be removed to allow it to penetrate throughout the whole product. Caps, plugs, valves, and/or stylets must be removed. Hollow-bore products such as needles and tubes must be open at both ends and inspected to ensure an unobstructed lumen.

Items for gas sterilization must be free of water droplets. They should be towel dried or allowed to dry in ambient air. The use of heated air should be avoided, because EO sterilization depends on the presence of adequate (but not excessive) moisture. A relative humidity of 35% to 70% and a temperature of 18 to 22°C (64 to 72°F) throughout the processing and storage facility (75, 78) are recommended.

Items to be sterilized are placed in wire baskets, metal sterilizer carts, or other carriers that do not absorb EO. The sterilizer manufacturer's instructions for loading should be carefully followed. Items should be loaded loosely to allow penetration of gas throughout the load. Items should be loaded in such a fashion that packages will not contact the operator's hands when the baskets are transferred from the sterilizer to the aerator.

Sterilization

Factors Affecting Ethylene Oxide Sterilization
Gas concentration (81). The solubility of EO in the product and the gas diffusion rate through the

product will influence the sterilant concentration. The operating pressure of the EO cycle will greatly influence the gas diffusion rate. Packaging can also be critical.

Temperature. Exposure time can be decreased by increasing the temperature. Operating temperatures in automatic sterilizers are usually preset by the manufacturer. Some sterilizers provide a selection of temperatures, generally 120 to 145°F (49 to 63°C) for a warm cycle and 85 to 100°F (29 to 38°C) for a cold cycle. Some conduct sterilization at room temperature. This is equally efficacious if other factors (exposure time and concentration) are adjusted.

Humidity. Moisture hydrates microbes, making them more susceptible to destruction by EO. In most automatic sterilizers, humidity is injected into the sterilizer before the EO is admitted.

Protective barriers. Blood and other proteinaceous materials can act as barriers to EO. Therefore, equipment must be thoroughly cleaned and rinsed before sterilization.

Packaging. The wrapping must be permeable to EO gas and water vapor and allow for proper aeration. In sterilizers that have a vacuum cycle, the material must allow the air inside the packages to escape.

Exposure time. The time needed for sterilization will depend on the factors mentioned above. In automatic sterilizers, the time generally ranges from 1.5 to 6 hours. Up to 12 hours may be required.

Sterilizers (75)

EO sterilizers are of two types (77): general purpose and special purpose. A general-purpose sterilizer is a chamber-type system that injects water vapor for humidity adjustment during the cycle and generally uses excursions in pressure from atmospheric levels. A special-purpose sterilizer requires prehumidification of items to be sterilized, does not inject water vapor during the cycle, generally operates at atmospheric pressure, and may or may not have limitations placed by the manufacturers on the items that can be processed.

General-purpose EO sterilizers are sophisticated units with a number of automatic cycles. A source of EO gas is provided (by attachment of a cylinder of an EO mixture or insertion of a unit dose cartridge of 100% EO) and then a steriliza-

tion cycle is selected and begun. After the sterilizer chamber is tightly sealed and the controls set, a typical cycle includes the following: (*a*) warming the chamber; (*b*) evacuating air; (*c*) introducing moisture and maintenance for a "dwell" period; (*d*) introducing the EO; (*e*) raising the chamber pressure (in some sterilizers); (*f*) raising the temperature (if required); (*g*) exposing for the time required; (*h*) releasing the pressure in the chamber; and (*i*) removing the EO mixture under vacuum. This is called a purge cycle or phase; some sterilizers are provided with several successive purge phases. Sterilizers without purge cycles can release a cloud of EO gas when the sterilizer door is opened. This necessitates an extraction hood above the door with a dedicated exhaust system and potentially exposes the operator to EO gas (4). The last phase is (*j*) reestablishing atmospheric pressure by introduction of filtered air into the chamber.

Units that carry out sterilization at room temperature and ambient humidity are available (82). Special ventilation cabinets are available for exhausting the EO from these units to atmosphere (83).

Indicators (84)

Because of the many variables that affect EO sterilization, it advisable to have evidence that sterilization is being achieved. Three types of indicators (monitors) are available. For maximum value, they should be used in combination.

Physical Monitors

Physical (mechanical control) monitors include all sterilizer components that measure exposure time, temperature, humidity, and/or pressure during each cycle. They should be examined for proper function at the beginning, middle, and end of each cycle.

Chemical Indicators (12)

Chemical indicators change color when certain conditions necessary for sterilization have been met. Color change varies with the product. They are available as tapes, strips, cards, and sheets. They may be implanted or attached to packaging material or enclosed in packages.

Chemical indicators are not sterility indicators and should not replace biological monitors. They only indicate that the package has been subjected to some parameters of the sterilization cycle and may change color under conditions inadequate for sterilization.

It is recommended that a chemical indicator be used with each package that undergoes EO sterilization. The user of an EO sterilized item should always check the indicator for color change before use.

Biological Indicators (77)

A biological indicator is a calibration of microorganisms on or in a carrier, placed in a package that maintains the integrity of the inoculated carrier and serves to demonstrate whether sterilization conditions were met (77).

The CDC recommends their use at least once a week (12). They should always be used after installation of a sterilizer, after any repairs or modifications to the sterilizer, and any time there are changes in packaging procedures or materials or the composition of the load (77). They should be placed in the most inaccessible location in the sterilized load (77). It should be noted that if the articles to be sterilized have not been properly cleaned before packaging, a biological indicator will not be a valid tool for determining sterility.

Aeration

EO not only comes in contact with all surfaces of articles being sterilized but also penetrates some items, which then retain varying amounts. These items need special treatment called aeration (degassing, desorption) to remove EO to a level safe for both personnel and patient use. Aeration may be done passively in air (ambient aeration) or actively in a mechanical aerator.

Ambient Aeration

Ambient aeration is highly variable because of the lack of control of temperature and air flow. The temperature in the aeration area should be at least 18°C (78). It results in a slower reduction of residual EO than mechanical aeration. Items that require 8 to 12 hours of mechanical aeration may require 7 days of ambient aeration (85, 86). Some items take 5 to 6 weeks. It is possible that some of the toxicity problems encountered in the early use of EO resulted from failure to recognize

this. The facility must maintain a large and often costly inventory of items.

Ambient aeration may result in hazardous exposure of workers to EO. If ambient aeration is unavoidable (for heat-sensitive items that cannot withstand the elevated temperatures of conventional aerator cabinets or when a closed vented cabinet especially designed for that purpose is not available), measures to minimize traffic in the aeration area and to ensure that personnel who must enter the area are not exposed to EO at hazardous concentrations should be taken.

Mechanical Aeration

In mechanical aerators, a stream of filtered air is directed over the sterilized items. This reduces the necessary aeration time. An EO sterilizer may be combined with an aerator so one chamber is used for both processes.

Factors Affecting Aeration

Composition, thickness, configuration, and weight of the device and its wrapping material. The amount of residual EO and the length of time needed for it to dissipate depend on the type of material being sterilized. Thicker objects require longer aeration times than thin ones. Unwrapped nonporous metal and glass items do not absorb EO and require little or no aeration. Plastics, rubber, cloth, paper, and muslin may absorb significant quantities. Items that consist of a combination of absorbent and nonabsorbent materials (e.g., a metal item with rubber parts) must be treated as though they were made entirely of absorbent material. Metal and glass items that are wrapped in EO-absorbent material must be aerated.

The most common material retaining large amounts of EO is polyvinyl chloride (PVC). The type and amount of plasticizer in the PVC will strongly influence the amount absorbed. Rubber absorbs less, and polyethylene and nylon still less. Teflon absorbs very little EO. When the composition of a device is in doubt, it should be treated as if it were PVC.

Size and arrangement of packages in the aerator (87). Arranging items loosely in the aerator will allow easier diffusion.

Diluent. Gas mixtures with a fluorocarbon require a longer aeration time than those diluted with carbon dioxide.

Wrappings. The packaging material should allow the easy transfer of gas. Most wrappings allow free transfer of EO and do not present any problem with gas retention.

Temperature at which aeration occurs. Increasing the temperature accelerates the removal of EO from items. The usual aeration temperature is 50 or 60°C. If these temperatures would be damaging to a device, aeration can be carried out at room temperature in a closed ventilated cabinet especially designed for that purpose or ambient aeration can be used.

Air flow. Aeration is affected by the rate of air exchange and the air flow pattern.

Characteristics of EO sterilizer used. Use of sterilizers that subject materials to hot gases under elevated pressure can result in higher levels of EO in the items sterilized (88).

Intended use of the device. Whether the item is to be external to the body, within a body cavity, intravascular, or implanted will affect the acceptable level of residual EO.

Time. Because of the many aeration process variables, the recommend minimum aeration time varies. Most device manufacturers provide recommendations for their devices.

The minimum recommended times for devices that are difficult to aerate are 8 hours at 60°C (140°F), 12 hours at 50°C (120°F), and 7 days at room temperature (21°C) (70°F) (80). When in doubt about a particular device, these recommendations should be followed. It should be noted, however, that some items may require even longer periods.

Complications of Ethylene Oxide Sterilization

Patient Complications

Complications of EO sterilization stemming from residuals on sterilized items include skin reactions and laryngotracheal inflammation (89–92). When blood is exposed to EO treated materials, destruction of the red blood cells can occur (93–95). Sensitization and anaphylaxis from exposure to products sterilized with EO have been reported (96). The risk of patients developing cancer or suffering other adverse health effects from exposure to residual EO is negligible (97).

These problems are caused by excessive levels of EO or its byproducts, ethylene glycol, and ethylene chlorhydrin. Ethylene glycol is formed by the reaction of EO and water. Because even dry materials contain some moisture, some glycol formation is unavoidable. Traces of glycol are generally regarded as relatively harmless (98). Removing all visible water droplets from equipment before sterilization should prevent formation of excessive glycol.

Ethylene chlorhydrin is formed when EO comes into contact with chloride ions that may be present in previously γ-irradiated PVC items. The American National Standards Institute at one time recommended that PVC items that have been γ-irradiated never be resterilized with EO (86). Doubt has been cast on this, however, by some workers who have found very low levels of byproducts in γ-irradiated products treated with EO (99–101). Resterilization of γ-irradiated PVC tubes may be acceptable if strict attention is paid to aeration.

Alterations in Equipment

Repeated exposure of some plastics to EO and heat may leach out plasticizers and weaken the structural integrity (102). Rubber and some plastic tracheal tubes may soften and kink more easily (103) or become sticky. Blisters between layers in the walls of latex tracheal tubes with embedded spiral wires can occur, resulting in narrowing of the lumen (103). It is recommended that these tubes not be sterilized by this method (104). Detachment of the balloon on a disposable esophageal stethoscope sterilized with EO has been reported (102).

Personnel Complications

Possible hazards of exposure to EO (78). The presence of gaseous EO in very high concentrations is easily detected, because it is irritating to the eyes and mucous membranes, but this should not be depended upon. Odor is also not a reliable indicator of EO's presence and does not provide adequate warning of hazardous concentrations. It is possible to be in a room with dangerously high EO concentrations without being aware of it (105).

Exposure to liquid EO can cause burns or severe irritation of the skin (106, 107). The gas is heavier than air and can cause asphyxiation in enclosed, poorly ventilated, or low-lying areas. Another possible hazard is the danger of fires and explosions.

Acute exposure to significant levels of EO gas commonly provokes an irritant response (108, 109). Upper respiratory complaints, eye irritation, headache, blunting of taste or smell, a metallic taste, and coughing are common. With higher concentrations, nausea, vomiting, diarrhea, increased fatigability, memory loss, drowsiness, weakness, dizziness, incoordination, chest discomfort, shortness of breath, difficulty swallowing, cramps, and convulsions have been reported (110, 111). Respiratory paralysis and peripheral nerve damage have been reported after massive exposure. The onset of neurological signs and symptoms may be delayed for 6 hours or more after exposure.

Chronic exposure can affect the eyes (corneal burns, cataracts, epithelial keratitis), nervous system (sensorimotor polyneuropathy), and skin (irritant and allergic reactions) (108, 111–113). Respiratory infections, anemia, and impaired cognitive function may occur (98). In addition there are concerns that EO may be mutagenic or carcinogenic and that it may adversely affect the reproductive system. (114–117).

In some persons, EO exposure may result in allergic sensitization and further exposure may cause hives or a life-threatening allergic reaction.

OSHA regulations limit worker exposure to an 8-hour time-weighted average (TWA) of 1 ppm (118) with a short-term excursion limit (STEL) of 5 ppm averaged over 15 minutes. In facilities where worker exposure may exceed these levels, employers must institute numerous measures to meet OSHA regulations. However, a facility is excused from these requirements if it can document that the EO sterilization system employed will not expose workers to TWA levels above 0.5 ppm during 8 hours (the action level) and 5 ppm during 15 minutes (the short term exposure limit).

OSHA requires employers to provide respiratory protection and personal protective equipment in work operations such as maintenance, repair, or other activities, where engineering and work practice controls are not feasible.

The OSHA standard requires performance of initial (baseline) monitoring (119). If the 8-hour time-weighted airborne concentration of EO is at or exceeds the action level, employers must begin periodic exposure monitoring and medical surveillance. Below 0.5 ppm no action is required except when there has been a change in equipment, personnel or work practices. If the TWA exceeds 1 ppm, quarterly monitoring must be instituted in conjunction with exposure reduction measures. If the TWA is between 0.5 and 1 ppm, semiannual monitoring is required.

In addition, federal law requires exposure monitoring whenever there has been a change in the equipment, personnel, or work practices that may result in new or additional exposure to EO or there is reason to suspect that a change may result in new or additional exposure.

Sources of EO exposure. There are eight principal sources of EO exposure: the area in front of the sterilizer when the door is opened upon completion of the sterilization cycle, the freshly sterilized goods themselves, the aeration cabinet, the sterilizer, the floor drain, the procedure for changing the tank and/or cartridge, the safety valve, and the supply tanks and cartridges.

Recommendations to reduce exposure (66, 78, 82, 120–122). The EPA has made specific recommendations for workplace design and practice modifications in healthcare facilities where EO is used. Specific procedures have been developed for spills, leaks and disposal.

1. Unnecessary use of EO should be avoided. It should be reserved for products that must be sterilized and cannot withstand other methods of sterilization.
2. There should be strict adherence to the manufacturer's installation and operating instructions for sterilizers and aerators. Each sterilizer and aerator should have regular preventive maintenance to ensure that malfunctions, especially leaks, are minimized and that any malfunctions that occur are detected and corrected. Records should be kept on all malfunctions and repairs.
3. Cylinders of EO should be stored in a designated area that meets building codes and OSHA regulations, conforms to the temperature specifications of the gas supplier/manufacturer and is out of the way of traffic. Tanks

should not stand free but be chained upright to a solid structure and the protection cap should be in place when the tank is not in use. The storage area should be ventilated to prevent the buildup of a significant EO concentration in the event that a container has a leak.

4. Caution should be exercised to avoid exposure to personnel when changing tanks and filters. Protective attire (e.g., goggles or a face shield, heavy-duty gloves, full-body suits) should be worn. There should be check or shutoff valves in the lines close to the connection point to limit the release of EO into the atmosphere during cylinder changes.

5. A local exhaust hood should be installed near the EO cylinder connection area to capture EO released to the air during changeover and leakage around line connections. It should exhaust the EO to the outside atmosphere or to an emission control system.

6. Sterilizers and aerators should be located in well-ventilated areas with limited access, away from work stations and storage areas. Personnel traffic patterns should be routed away from the areas.

   The room(s) in which the sterilizer and aerator are located should be large enough to ensure adequate EO dilution and to accommodate the loading, unloading, and maintenance of the equipment. The ventilation system should allow at least 10 air changes per hour and be designed to allow air to flow over the sterilizer door opening and ultimately to an exhaust fan or blower system that carries the room air and any EO to the outside or an emission control system. Ventilation rates should be monitored and documented at least every 3 months.

7. Entrances to areas where EO is used should be posted with signs warning that high levels of EO are possible. No supplies or unnecessary equipment should be stored in the vicinity of sterilization/aeration equipment, and a minimum number of personnel should be permitted in those areas.

8. All EO sterilizers and sterilizer relief valves must be vented out of the workplace to the outside atmosphere, an emission control sys-

tem, or a sanitary floor drain. Running vent lines in ways that would either release EO within the building or allow the reentry of EO-contaminated air into the building and releasing EO near pedestrian traffic must be prohibited. The aerator must also be vented to provide proper exhaust ventilation.

9. EO sterilizers should meet the following requirements (81). (*a*) The sterilizer should be constructed so that the cycle cannot be initiated or allowed to continue unless all doors are closed and secured. It should not be possible to open the door when the chamber is under pressure or before the postevacuation cycle is completed. (*b*) The sterilizer should have purge (air flush) cycles to reduce the amount of residual EO on goods that will be removed from the sterilizer. (*c*). The sterilizer should be equipped with a means of detecting leaks.

10. Local exhaust ventilation systems should be installed to capture EO before it can escape into the general work environment. EO can be collected as close to the source as possible and exhausted to the outside atmosphere. The following are the most common areas where high EO concentrations occur and where local exhaust systems are recommended: (*a*) close to the sterilizer, preferably 1 to 2 inches from the top of the door; (*b*) the sterilizer pressure relief valve; (*c*) for sterilizers that discharge to a sanitary system, the area immediately above the line that drains into the sanitary sewer; and (*d*) the EO cylinder connection points.

11. Employees operating sterilizers or aerators should be properly instructed in the hazards of EO oxide and appropriate safety procedures. A continuing education program should be established, and all personnel working around EO should be required to participate in the program.

12. When feasible, workers should be isolated from direct contact with the work environment by the use of automated equipment operated by personnel observing from a closed control booth or room.

13. A combination sterilizer/aerator will reduce

EO exposure associated with opening the sterilizer door and removal of items from the sterilizer.

14. Occupational exposure to EO can be avoided by using a loading cart and/or wire baskets (82). These can be moved into and from the sterilizer, then directly into and from the aerator. Items should be loaded in such a manner that they will not touch the operator's hands when the cart or basket is transferred from the sterilizer to the aerator.

15. The single greatest source of EO exposure occurs when the sterilizer door is opened after completion of a sterilization cycle (123–125). Materials should not be left in a closed sterilizer after the cycle is complete, as this will allow high concentrations of EO to build up in the sterilizer and be released into the room when the door is first opened. The chamber door should be opened 6 inches immediately following a cycle (125). A door-opening device on some large sterilizers allows the operator to push a button, then walk away, while the sterilizer door slowly opens (98). The operator should leave the immediate sterilizer area for a minimum of 15 min after opening the door (78, 126).

    The purge characteristics of some newer sterilizers will prevent the buildup of EO inside the chamber (78). These should be unloaded immediately upon opening the door, because it is at this time that the EO concentration within the chamber is lowest. When in doubt, the manufacturer's instructions should be consulted.

16. Sterilized items should be transferred rapidly to the aerator. Goods should never be handled directly. Transfer carts should be used to remove items from large sterilizers and gloves and forceps for items in small sterilizers. Carts should be pulled, rather than pushed, to the aerator so that personnel are not upwind of the degassing goods. Items should be placed in the aerator without delay. Unaerated items should never be left outside the aerator where they might contaminate the environment or be used inadvertently.

17. Special-purpose sterilizers should be used only in a well-ventilated room. If a sterilizer does not have a venting mechanism other than the door or lid the healthcare facility must determine that the system effectively minimizes employee exposure to EO gas. Possible options include using local exhaust ventilation (such as a laboratory hood) and adding a chemical neutralization system or EO sorbent to the sterilizer. Ventilation cabinets designed for special-purpose EO sterilizers are available (127).

18. All EO-sterilized items should be aerated before handling. A mechanical aerator is best. If ambient aeration is unavoidable, the aeration area should be segregated from general work areas and have limited access. It should have good ventilation and be at a negative pressure with respect to adjoining areas. Storage of supplies in the area must be prohibited.

19. Personnel and environmental monitoring similar to that discussed in Chapter 12, "Controlling Trace Gas Levels," must be practiced to ensure that recommended levels are not exceeded (78, 128–140). Leak checks must be performed regularly. The frequency of monitoring required by OSHA depends on the levels found in the work environment (78). Badges that can be worn by employees are available, as are instruments to aid in instantaneous leak detection.

20. A system to detect ventilation system failures and to alert personnel with audible and/or visual alarms should be installed.

21. The seals on sterilizer and aerator doors should be inspected for cracks, tears, and foreign substances before each load. Sterilizer and aerator valves and fittings should be inspected at least every 2 weeks and replaced as necessary. Intake air filters for the restricted access area should be inspected and cleaned regularly.

22. Sterilizers, aerators, and the EO gas line entrance port to the sterilizer should be tested for leaks at least every 2 weeks.

23. Only 1 day's supply of EO cartridges should be stored in the immediate area of the sterilizer (78).

24. Each facility in which EO is used should have a written emergency plan for dealing with EO

leaks and spills (78, 141, 142). The facility should form an action team responsible for the development and exercise of the written procedures to handle EO leaks and spills (78).

Environmental Problems

Once EO is emitted, it remains in the air without breaking down for long periods of time. People who live near facilities with sterilizers or aerators may, therefore, be exposed to airborne EO. Some state and local agencies limit the amount of EO that can be emitted into the air (74). Catalytic convertors that break EO down into carbon dioxide and water are available. Other systems are available that absorb the EO and react it with water, producing ethylene glycol (143).

Advantages and Disadvantages

EO sterilization has many advantages. It is effective against all organisms. It is very reliable, because the gas penetrates into crevices and regions blocked to liquids. It can be used on a wide variety of items, including those that would be damaged by heat or high concentrations of moisture. Damage to most equipment is minimal. Items can be prepackaged and the package sealed. This eliminates the danger of recontamination that can occur during rinsing and packaging following cold sterilization and allows the items to remain sterile during long-term storage.

EO has a number of disadvantages. Fires and explosions involving sterilizers have been reported (144, 145). Even with diluted EO mixtures, care must be exercised, because there is a possibility that the gas mixture may become stratified and create a fire or explosion hazard (103).

A major disadvantage is that it may require at least 24 hours for turnaround time. This may make it necessary to have a larger stock of equipment.

It is more costly than most other types of disinfection. Installation of the necessary equipment is expensive and if large items are to be sterilized the equipment will take a great deal of space. Personnel need to be highly trained and supervised to ensure proper sterilization and prevent complications. Frequent biological monitoring is required.

Equipment to be sterilized needs to be dry, which can be difficult to achieve with items such as corrugated tubings. Some materials deteriorate after repeated sterilization, especially at elevated temperatures. It cannot be used to sterilize devices that have petroleum-based lubricants in or on them, because EO cannot permeate these substances (146).

Radiation Sterilization (147)

Radiation sterilization is the dominant process for sterilizing disposable products from manufacturers. Gamma-radiation (γ-rays) is an electromagnetic wave produced during the disintegration of certain radioactive elements. If the dosage applied to a product is large enough, all microorganisms, including bacterial spores and viruses, will be killed (6).

There are many advantages to γ-radiation (8). The product can be prepackaged in a wide variety of impermeable containers before treatment. The package will not interfere with the sterilization process. The treated items remain sterile indefinitely until the packaging seal is broken. As there is virtually no temperature rise during treatment, thermolabile materials can be sterilized and thermolabile packaging can be used. Equipment may be used immediately after γ-radiation treatment with no risk from retained radioactivity.

γ-Radiation is not practical for everyday use in healthcare facilities. It requires expensive equipment and is used only by large manufacturers to sterilize disposable equipment (148). Many healthcare facilities send their own packs for treatment. The importance of γ-radiation is that it does cause changes in some plastics, especially PVC. When PVC is sterilized by γ-radiation, chloride ions are liberated. It was once thought that a γ-radiated tracheal or tracheostomy tube should not be resterilized with EO (149). Evidence now confirms that previously γ-radiated tubes can be resterilized with EO (100, 101). As always, aeration times must be strictly enforced.

Gas Plasma Sterilization

Gas plasma sterilization uses a gaseous chemical germicide (peracetic acid, hydrogen peroxide) and gaseous plasma. Gaseous plasma is sometimes described as the fourth state of matter consisting of a cloud of reactive ions, electrons, and neutral atomic and molecular species. This can be produced through the action of an electric or magnetic field on a gas under a deep vacuum. The reactive species in the plasma cloud interact with molecules essential for the normal metabolism and reproduction of living cells.

Gas plasma can be an effective sterilant for a variety of medical device applications, including most packaging materials, plastics, and stainless-steel instruments. It has the potential to displace EO and steam from many uses in healthcare facilities since it offers rapid low-temperature sterilization and does not have the environmental problems associated with EO. No personnel or exhaust monitoring or protective equipment for changing tanks are needed.

This technology does require supplies (e.g., indicators, trays, wraps) that are compatible with the system. It may also require modification of some packaging techniques.

Sterrad System

In the Sterrad system, hydrogen peroxide is the precursor of the active species of the plasma. After the activated components have reacted with organisms or each other, they lose their high energy and recombine to form oxygen, water and other nontoxic byproducts.

Preparation of instruments for sterilization is similar to that for other methodologies: cleaning, reassembly, and wrapping in porous material. The system requires the use of non-woven polypropylene wraps and a special tray and container system.

The hydrogen peroxide solution is supplied in premeasured ampules in a sealed cassette. After the cassette has been placed in the sterilizer the ampules are automatically opened.

The items to be sterilized are placed in the sterilization chamber, the chamber closed, and a vacuum drawn. Vaporized hydrogen peroxide is injected and allowed to diffuse throughout the chamber, and thereby come into close proximity with the items to be sterilized. After reduction of the pressure in the chamber, gas plasma is generated by applying radiofrequency energy to create an electrical field. The plasma is maintained for a sufficient time to ensure sterilization. At the completion of the process, the radiofrequency energy

is turned off, the vacuum is released and the chamber is returned to atmospheric pressure by the introduction of filtered air. Total processing time is a little over 1 hour. There is a printout of the cycle for quality assurance (QA) documentation.

During the evacuation prior to plasma treatment and after a cycle has been completed, all vapor removed from the chamber passes through a filter specially designed to decompose the hydrogen peroxide.

This technology can be used for most items sterilizable by EO or steam, with the exception of cellulosic materials (e.g., cotton, linens, paper), powders, liquids, implants, and devices containing long, narrow, dead-end lumens. Devices to be sterilized must be able to withstand a vacuum. Items whose design permits the surfaces to collapse onto each other (e.g., bags) should not be processed in the sterilizer, unless some method is used to keep the surfaces separated. It is not recommended for flexible endoscopes.

It is well suited to heat- and moisture-sensitive instruments since the temperature does not exceed 50°C and sterilization occurs in a low moisture environment. It produces less effect on metal items than steam sterilization. It can be used with a variety of hinged and nonhinged instruments, plastic devices such as airways, devices with lumens (not dead-end), electric and fiberoptic cables, batteries, and rigid endoscopes.

Although these are small-capacity systems, the volume of products processed per unit of time may be equivalent to that of large capacity EO sterilizers. No venting or special installation is required. It is simply plugged into an electrical outlet.

The process requires no aeration, and there are no toxic residues or emissions. The color of anodized aluminum may fade after repeated cycles.

Plasmalyte System

With this technology, the gas plasma is produced in a separate plasma chamber where the gas mixture of hydrogen, oxygen, and argon is exposed to a microwave electromagnetic field. This plasma then flows through a gas distribution manifold into the sterilization chamber.

Preparation of instruments is similar to other technologies: cleaning, reassembly, and wrapping.

It is effective with all types of current wraps and sterilization containers.

Peracetic acid with a small amount of water and hydrogen peroxide is supplied in a sealed bottle that is placed in the sterilizer. After devices are loaded into the sterilization chamber, a vacuum is drawn. Peracetic acid vapor is then introduced into the chamber and allowed to diffuse through for 20 minutes. The chamber is then evacuated. Next, with the vacuum pump still withdrawing gas from the chamber, the plasma feed gas valve is opened. The gas flows from the plasma generator, through the gas distribution manifold, through the sterilization chamber where it diffuses through packaging, exposing items to the sterilization process and out through the pump. New plasma is continuously created throughout the cycle. After approximately 10 minutes, the electromagnetic field is turned off, the plasma feed valve is turned off, and the vacuum pump removes the remaining gas. The reactive components of the gas evacuated from the chamber recombine with one another to form oxygen, hydrogen, and water vapor, which can be released to the atmosphere without further treatment. This is followed by an additional peracetic acid vapor treatment, then another plasma treatment and so on. There are six sequential repetitions of the evacuation, vapor, and plasma phases. Upon completion of the six repetitions filtered air flows through the chamber for 10 minutes.

Sterilization is carried out at or below 55°C. The duration of the entire cycle varies from $3\frac{1}{2}$ to 4 hours. The time is determined in part by the items contained. Items that will absorb peracetic acid (such as cellusic materials) will cause the time to be prolonged.

This technology can be used for any items that can be sterilized by EO. It is not recommended for liquids, powders, non-vented containers or flexible endoscopes. Instruments containing brass must be dried before going into the sterilizer, or a light, turquoise film may form on the brass (150).

The sterilization chamber is larger than the one in the Sterrad system, so more items can be processed at one time. A special venting system must be installed from the sterilizer to the general exhaust.

A PROGRAM FOR ANESTHESIA EQUIPMENT
The Sterilization Dilemma (91, 151–153)

Those concerned with anesthesia equipment find themselves faced with a dilemma as to how much time, effort, and money should be expended to try to prevent transmission of infection to patients. Those who argue that vigorous approaches are not needed and feel that many of the measures being advocated are unreasonable advance the following arguments.

1. Documented cases of cross-infection by contaminated anesthesia equipment are rare. Studies have cast doubt on the likelihood that the breathing system causes postoperative respiratory infections (154, 155).
2. Decontamination is difficult, costly, and entails certain dangers to patients and personnel. It entails a heavy capital outlay for equipment, increased work for personnel, and increased space. Considerable training of staff is necessary.
3. The nature of many maneuvers required in anesthesia makes sterility impractical.
4. Many forms of sterilization can damage equipment. Liquid and gas chemical sterilization may leave residues that can subsequently harm a patient. Mistakes may be made during reassembly.

Proponents for more vigorous attempts at sterilization argue as follows:

1. Cases of cross-contamination caused by anesthesia equipment have been reported (156, 157).
2. The risk of cross-contamination may be greater than is commonly believed. The lack of documentation of nosocomial infection secondary to anesthetic practice may reflect a long incubation period or lack of follow-up (158). Patients undergoing anesthesia and surgery are more likely to develop respiratory infections than the normal population. Anesthesia interferes with ciliary and mucus activity and surgery can impair the patient's ability to cough and breathe deeply. Anesthesia care providers are caring for immunocompromised patients

more often and this group may be unable to protect itself against what formerly were thought to be harmless environmental organisms or insignificant innoculums (7).

3. Although there is general agreement that sterilization of equipment is essential after use in a patient with a respiratory infection or a particularly virulent organism, it is frequently impossible to identify these patients. Any organism is a potential cause of infection. Therefore, all equipment is suspect.

4. Even if the incidence of postoperative respiratory infections resulting from anesthesia apparatus is low, the cost of a single such infection in terms of mortality, morbidity, and economics is high (159).

CDC Rationale for Cleaning, Disinfection, and Sterilization

The CDC has published guidelines on how to prevent or control specific nosocomial infection problems. As shown in Table 27.5, they have divided items into three categories, based on the potential risk of infection involved in their use.

Critical Items

Critical items are those that penetrate the skin or mucous membranes or are in contact with normally sterile areas of the body. This includes vascular needles and catheters and regional block needles and catheters. These items must be sterile at the time of use. If an item's sterility is in doubt, it should not be used.

Semicritical Items

These are devices that come in contact with intact mucous membranes, but do not ordinarily penetrate body surfaces. Equipment that falls into this category includes endoscopes; laryngoscope blades; reusable rectal, nasopharyngeal and esophageal temperature probes; face masks; oral and nasal airways; resuscitation bags; breathing tubes and connectors; oxygen masks; esophageal stethoscopes; and tracheal and double-lumen tubes (3). Sterilization is desirable for these items, but if not easily possible, a high level of decontamination is acceptable (2, 9, 12). In most cases, meticulous cleaning followed by high-level disinfection gives a reasonable degree of assurance. Evidence that sterilization reduces the risk of infection is lacking (2).

Noncritical Items

Noncritical items are those that do not ordinarily touch the patient or only touch intact skin. Items in this category include stethoscopes (not esophageal); blood pressure cuffs and tubing; intravenous arm boards; pulse oximeter sensors and cables; electrocardiogram (ECG) cables; reusable skin temperature probes, temperature monitor cables; head straps; blood warmers; carbon dioxide absorber assemblies; T-adapters for oxygen sensors; and the exteriors of the anesthesia machine, ventilator, humidifiers, scavenging system, resuscitation bags, monitors, and equipment carts. Since intact skin normally acts as an effective barrier to most microorganisms these items need only intermediate-> or low-level disinfection. It has been suggested that these be disinfected at the end of the day or whenever visibly contaminated (3). Others have suggested that these devices should have high-level disinfection (160).

Some experts add another category, that of en-

TABLE **27.5. Classification of Devices, Processes, and Germicidal Products**

Critical	Sterilization: sporicidal chemical, prolonged contact	Sterilant/disinfectant
Semicritical	High-level disinfection: sporicidal chemical, short contact	Sterilant/disinfectant
Noncritical	Intermediate-level disinfection	Hospital disinfectant with tuberculocidal activity
	Low-level disinfection	Hospital disinfectant without tuberculocidal activity

vironmental surfaces (9). This consists of a wide variety of surfaces that do not ordinarily come into direct contact with the patient, but if they do, it is only with intact skin. These surfaces may potentially contribute to secondary cross-contamination by healthcare workers or by contact with medical instruments that will subsequently come into contact with patients. These surfaces can be further divided into *medical equipment surfaces* such as frequently touched adjustment knobs or handles and *housekeeping surfaces* such as floors, walls, and window sills.

Blood contamination of surfaces of anesthesia equipment is common (160). Visual inspection is not a reliable means for detecting blood.

Adequate levels of safety for surfaces of medical equipment may be achieved by thorough cleaning with detergent and water, followed by application of an intermediate- to low-level germicide (9). Adequate safety levels for housekeeping surfaces can be achieved by maintaining them in a state of cleanliness by using water and a detergent or a hospital grade disinfectant/detergent designed for general housekeeping purposes. Only when there has been a significant spill of blood or other potentially infectious body fluid should the added use of an intermediate-level chemical disinfectant be necessary (9).

Organization (1)

Each anesthesia department should have an infection control plan that documents procedures and policies to prevent transmission of infectious agents to patients and to minimize exposure of anesthesia personnel to occupational infectious hazards (29).

Considerations before Anesthesia
Use of Filters

Filters can be used to protect patients or equipment from contamination. A variety is available (see Chapter 6, "Breathing Systems I: General Considerations," and Chapter 10, "Humidification Equipment,"). While some early studies indicated that routine use of filters did not prevent postoperative pulmonary infections (155, 161–163), these involved filters of limited efficiency placed in the expiratory or inspiratory limbs. More recent studies show that use of an

effective filter at the patient port will protect the breathing system and environment from contamination (164, 165). The Association of Anaesthetists of Great Britain and Ireland and the Australian and New Zealand College of Anaesthetists have recommend that a filter be placed in this position (166, 167). When a patient with a known respiratory infection is anesthetized, one of these should be placed between the patient port of the breathing system and the patient. It has been suggested that such a filter be used with each patient and, as a cost-saving measure, the anesthesia circuit be used multiple times without changing. If a filter is used, it must be discarded or sterilized after each patient and the part of the breathing system between the patient and the filter should be discarded or cleaned and sterilized.

Choice of Equipment
Reusable versus disposable equipment (168–170). Most departments have struck a balance between disposable and reusable items. The balance, however, needs to be continually reassessed in light of changing technologies, costs, universal precautions, and waste management problems. Most departments keep at least some disposable items available for use with known infected cases.

Disposables ensure that the patient will always receive a sterile or clean item, and there is no need for decontamination after use. If labor costs are high, this may be an important consideration. Among the disadvantages of disposables are the costs of keeping sufficient inventory. Storage space can be a problem. The ecological problems of getting rid of disposable items after use and uncertain availability of petroleum products must be considered (8).

Reusable products cut down on the waste generated by a facility. However, a reusable device often requires disassembly, cleaning, drying, reassembly, repackaging, and disinfection, or sterilization before reuse (169). While equipment is being cleaned it cannot be used. This necessitates a larger inventory. The increased handling increases the risk of injury to the handler. It must be remembered that there is a limited life span for reusable equipment.

Reuse of disposable equipment. In an effort to reduce costs, up to 65% of healthcare facilities regularly reuse disposable devices (169, 171). This shifts the liability for the safety and effectiveness of the product from the manufacturer to the institution (29).

The healthcare facility must formulate a policy to assure the cleanliness and physical integrity of the device after reprocessing. It is recommended that an interdisciplinary committee within each institution be developed to assess all requests to resterilize and reuse any device labeled single-use or disposable by the manufacturer. Both the safety and efficacy of the reprocessing procedure and the likelihood that the device will function as intended after reprocessing must be considered.

The CDC does not recommend against all types of reuse (12). The American Society of Anesthesiologists Task Force on Infection Control does not recommend the reuse of disposable equipment (172).

Intraoperative Considerations
Care of Equipment
Anesthesia personnel should always work from a clean surface. At the start of a case only those articles that are reasonably likely to be used on that patient should be placed there. It is important to establish a routine whereby an article not used is kept separate from those that have been. Disposable items should be discarded in suitable containers. Contaminated reusable articles should be placed in a special receptacle. It may contain water with detergent to prevent drying of secretions. Additional isolation of dirty equipment such as laryngoscope blades can be achieved by wrapping them in a glove or packaging from a tracheal tube (173). At the end of the case, the receptacle for dirty equipment should be taken as soon as possible to the decontamination area, with care taken to confine the contaminated items during transport.

Decontaminating Spills of Blood and Body Fluids
Spills of blood or body fluids on equipment or environmental surfaces should be cleaned and decontaminated as soon as practical. Visible material should be removed with water and detergent followed by decontamination using a EPA-approved hospital disinfectant that is classified as tuberculocidal (29). A 1:10 to 1:100 dilution of 5.25% sodium hypochlorite has been recom-

mended by the CDC for cleaning blood spills (174, 175).

Decontamination of Reusable Equipment
A program that meets the needs of a given facility usually results from tailoring several techniques to that facility's needs. Factors to be considered include cost, types of equipment employed, and available facilities. Whatever plan is devised, it is important that alternate methods be available in the event the primary system fails.

Physical Arrangements (2)
The decontamination area should be physically separate from other areas of the department. However, spatial separation may be adequate if splashing and contamination of clean items and work surfaces can be avoided. Sinks should be large enough to contain large instruments and there should be enough sinks to accommodate concurrent soaking, washing, and rinsing. Sinks should have attached counters or adjacent work surfaces on which to place soiled and clean items separately. Signs showing where dirty equipment should be placed should be prominently displayed.

Airborne microbial and particulate contamination is likely to be high in the decontamination area. Therefore it is recommended that the ventilation system for the area be designed to maintain negative air pressure relative to surrounding spaces and to remove toxic vapors. Air from this area should be exhausted to the outside without recirculation or to a filtered partial recirculating system.

Good traffic control in the decontamination area will protect personnel and visitors. The area should be restricted as much as possible to authorized personnel. Hand washing facilities should be conveniently located in or near the decontamination area. They should be separate from sinks used in cleaning or rinsing items to be decontaminated.

There should be at least daily cleaning and disinfection of horizontal work surfaces. Floors should be cleaned daily and, when necessary, disinfected. Other surfaces, such as walls and storage shelves, should be cleaned on a regular basis.

Personnel (1)
The responsibility for decontamination of anesthesia equipment should be vested in one indi-

vidual who devises and administers a comprehensive program. This person should be a member of the infection control committee.

It is imperative that cleaning and disinfection or sterilizing of anesthesia equipment be delegated to conscientious, well-trained individuals who understand the principles of containment of contamination and the disinfecting or sterilizing processes (1, 176).

Most nurses are well-indoctrinated in the principles of aseptic technique. But frequently technicians caring for equipment are without a clinical background. Such people need considerable indoctrination before they can be relied on in practice.

Appropriate attire will minimize the transfer of microorganisms from contaminated items to personnel. Heavy-duty fluid-resistant protective gloves, a long-sleeved fluid-resistant covering, a face mask, and eye protection (goggles or safety glasses) should be worn. Gloves do not offer absolute protection because they may develop leaks. Therefore, it is important that hand washing be performed immediately after cleaning to prevent any further contamination of the worker or environment.

Surveillance

The third factor necessary for a successful decontamination program is surveillance to check the efficiency of decontaminating techniques. CDC guidelines do not recommend monitoring by routine cultures (12). Cultures need only be taken if a problem becomes evident. This should result in considerable cost savings (177).

Consideration of Individual Items

The level of decontamination required for a particular device depends on the potential hazard arising from its most recent and its intended subsequent use.

Anesthesia Carts

Anesthesia carts are used as a repository for equipment and drugs. Attention should be paid to the placement of equipment in the drawers. For instance, a blood pressure cuff that is used on several patients with no attempt to decontaminate it between cases should not be placed in the same drawer as airways or masks that are not kept in

sterile containers, but it may be placed in a drawer containing items such as suction catheters and syringes that are kept in disposable wrappers. Equipment such as airways and masks that are not kept in sterile containers should be placed in drawers that are less frequently opened, i.e., not in the same drawer as frequently used drugs. Containers used to hold drugs, syringes, and needles should be made of metal or plastic rather than cardboard to facilitate cleaning.

Horizontal surfaces should be cleaned of visible material between cases and at the conclusion of the workday. It may also be prudent to disinfect with an intermediate-level germicide (9). A clean covering should be placed on the top at the start of each case. Vertical surfaces should be cleaned at the end of the workday or if there is obvious contamination.

At least once a month, the entire cart should be cleaned. All equipment should be removed and the drawers and containers washed with detergent and water, then wiped or sprayed with a germicide.

Gas Cylinders

Gas cylinders are transported to the facility in open trucks and are frequently stored outside. They should be considered dirty when received in the operating room area. Some are provided with plastic or paper wrappers. Before taking a cylinder into an operating room, the wrapper, if present, should be removed. The cylinder should be washed with water and detergent and wiped with a cloth soaked in germicide or sprayed with a germicidal spray. After placing the cylinder on the anesthesia machine, it should be considered part of the machine and treated accordingly.

Anesthesia Machines

Anesthesia machines are often used to store drugs and equipment and may provide the "clean" and/or "dirty" areas for equipment. The same principles apply to machines as to carts. The work space should be supplied with a fresh, clean cover for each patient and should be wiped between cases and at the end of the workday. Spraying or wiping with an intermediate-level germicide may be prudent. Care should be taken not to get liquid in the vaporizer filling funnels. At least once a month equipment should be removed from the drawers and the drawers cleaned and disinfected by spraying or wiping.

Anesthesia Ventilators

The outside of ventilators should be treated similarly to the outside of anesthesia machines. The inside can be protected from contamination by use of a filter in the ventilator hose. This will also protect the patient from a contaminated ventilator.

The ventilator tubing and bellows should be cleaned and disinfected at regular intervals (3). Parts of the ventilator may be autoclavable. An important feature of the next generation of anesthesia ventilators is that all the parts which come in contact with respiratory gases can be easily removed and steam autoclaved (Fig. 27.4). This could be accomplished for each patient. Most rubber bellows and tubings can be sterilized using EO.

Absorber, Unidirectional Valves, and APL Valve

The outside of absorbers, APL valves and unidirectional valves should be cleaned of visible material. Use of an intermediate-level germicide may be prudent.

Carbon dioxide absorbent has a potent cidal effect on microorganisms and only a low number of resistant spores pass through the absorber (178, 179). Studies strongly suggest that patients rarely contaminate these parts with significant levels of bacteria (154, 180). Disposable absorbers are available, but offer no more protection against contamination of breathing systems than reusable ones (181).

The manufacturer's instructions should be consulted with respect to disassembling, cleaning, and disinfection. Canisters should be cleaned when the absorbent is changed. The screens should receive particular attention as they are susceptible to obstruction. Some canisters can be autoclaved and some can be sterilized using EO. Unidirectional valves are usually easily disassembled and cleaned by wiping the disc, the inside of the plastic dome, and the valve seat with alcohol or a detergent. APL valves can be cleaned by wiping with a detergent.

Some canisters can be disinfected by immersion in a liquid such as glutaraldehyde, as can most APL valves. However, use of glutaraldehyde on APL valves has been reported to cause stickiness and increase the opening pressure (73). Some APL valves may be autoclaved and some can be pasteurized (182, 183).

The next generation of breathing systems will have fully autoclavable canisters. They will be able to be easily disassembled and steam autoclaved (Fig. 27.5).

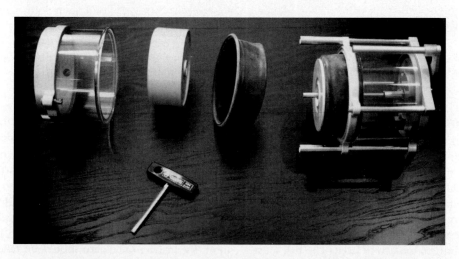

FIGURE 27.4. Drager-Divan ventilator disassembled for steam autoclaving.

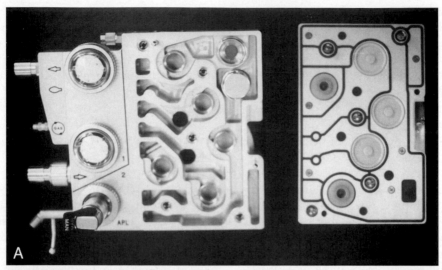

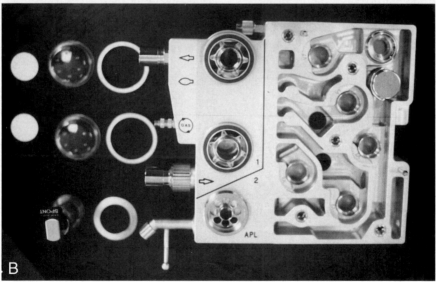

FIGURE 27.5. A, Absorber assembly partly disassembled. **B,** Adjustable pressure-limiting (APL) and unidirectional valves are also disassembled. The entire assembly can now be steam autoclaved.

The Reservoir Bag

Bags can be cleaned manually or in an automatic washing machine. EO is probably the most satisfactory means of sterilizing the bag. Aeration times should be carefully observed and the bag filled and emptied a few times before use on a patient. Some bags may be pasteurized although this will result in gradual deterioration (183). Chemical disinfection can be used. The bag must be filled with liquid to remove pockets of air (184). Of the various agents used, glutaraldehyde is probably the most satisfactory, provided adequate rinsing is performed.

Breathing Tubings

Corrugated tubing presents a difficult problem. Studies have shown that this tubing is contaminated after use (178). The closer to the patient, the heavier the contamination (185). Water commonly condenses in the expiratory tubing. If the tubings are lifted up, this water may run down into the patient.

Disposable tubings are usually used today. This may present a storage problem if frequent changes are made. One study showed that use of sterile tubings did not prevent postoperative pulmonary infections (155).

Because of their bulk and construction, tubings are difficult to clean and disinfect. Reusable tubings should be rinsed soon after use to prevent drying. They may then be soaked in a large container containing water and detergent.

The long length and ridges preclude a brush's being effective in cleaning. Ultrasonic cleaning has been used to remove debris (186). A washing machine may be used (187). After washing, the tubings should be thoroughly dried unless they are to undergo pasteurization. Special tube dryers are available.

Pasteurization has been used for corrugated tubings (185, 188). The Y piece should be removed beforehand. Otherwise, a loose fit may result.

Chemical disinfection can be carried out using an automatic washing machine or by immersion in a liquid agent (188). It is important that the tube be inserted vertically, making sure it is filled on the inside and there are no air pockets. One study found that machine-assisted chemical disinfection with glutaraldehyde was superior to pasteurization for tubings (187).

Y Piece

Y pieces are contaminated in a high percentage of cases. Fortunately, they are relatively easy to clean and sterilize. Disposable Y pieces attached to disposable tubings are commonly used.

After use, the Y piece should be removed from the corrugated tubings and rinsed under running water. They should then be placed in a solution of water and detergent to soak. They can be scrubbed manually or placed in a washing machine. If chemical or EO sterilization is to be used, the Y piece should be thoroughly dried. Y pieces may be pasteurized, immersed in liquid agents, or sterilized with EO.

Mapleson Systems

The Bain and Lack coaxial circuits present problems with cleaning because of the central tub-

ing. After use, these systems should be disassembled and the components cleaned. The components may be disinfected or sterilized by one of the methods discussed. Metal components can undergo autoclaving. Rubber and plastic parts can undergo gas sterilization or a liquid chemical agent may be used to disinfect or sterilize.

Adapters

Adapters used near the patient are contaminated in a high percentage of cases. Fortunately, they are usually not difficult to clean or sterilize. After use, adapters should be rinsed under a running tap, then placed in a solution of detergent and water and soaked. They may be washed manually or in a washing machine. Rubber and plastic adapters may be sterilized with EO or in a liquid such as glutaraldehyde. Metal adapters may be autoclaved or pasteurized.

Scavenging Equipment

A satisfactory method of treating scavenging equipment is to wash the device in a detergent solution monthly and to change the plastic hoses that connect the device to the breathing system and ventilator at the same time (182).

Face Masks

Face masks are among the most heavily contaminated pieces of equipment. Because of their proximity to the patient, transmittal of infection is a definite possibility. For obviously contaminated cases, disposable masks should be used.

Asepsis should be practiced in the use of face masks. They should not be allowed to drop onto the floor or be exposed to obvious contamination. After use, the mask should be kept near the patient's head or with the dirty equipment.

Immediately after use, the connector should be removed and the mask rinsed in cool tap water, then soaked and scrubbed. It may be cleaned automatically in a washing machine. Masks should always be thoroughly rinsed and carefully dried, especially if EO is to be used for sterilization.

With gas sterilization the mask can be maintained sterile for long periods of time. Aeration must be adequate or facial burns may result (89). Most automatic EO sterilizers employ a vacuum at least once during the sterilization cycle. This vacuum may cause the pneumatic cushion of the mask to be damaged (91). This can be prevented by removing the plug that seals the cushion or by using a sterilizer that does not have a vacuum phase.

Autoclaving is sometimes used for face masks. This will shorten their life. Neoprene face masks that will withstand steam sterilization are available (188). Autoclaving involves a vacuum phase that will damage the inflated cushion, so before autoclaving, the plug should be removed. Pasteurization also has been used for face masks (191, 192).

Liquid chemical agents are widely used for face masks. Thorough rinsing is important to remove residual detergent. Facial injury can be caused by a mask improperly sterilized with liquid agents. Phenolic compounds should not be used because they are absorbed by the rubber. Any cracks in the cushion of the mask can allow liquid agent to enter the airspace. When placed on a patient's face, the liquid can be squeezed out, possibly into the eyes.

Head Straps

Head straps should be subjected to cleaning with a detergent, then soaked in a disinfectant solution or sterilized with EO after use.

Airways

Before use, airways should be treated as clean objects and not allowed to drop on the floor. As soon as possible after use, they should be rinsed with cold water, then placed in a solution of water and detergent. They should be washed manually or in a machine (13, 14, 193). They should be thoroughly rinsed to remove residual detergent.

Pasteurization, liquid chemical disinfection, and EO sterilization have been used for airways. Rubber airways may be autoclaved, but this will shorten their useful life.

Rigid Laryngoscopes, Stylets, and Intubating Forceps (183)

Laryngoscope blades, stylets, and forceps should be stored under clean conditions. Many believe stylets should be kept sterile, because they are placed inside a tracheal tube.

Disposable laryngoscope blades and covers that fit over the handle and/or blade are available (194, 195) (Fig. 27.6). Their use may be worthwhile since contamination of both blades and handles is common (196–200).

The outside of the laryngoscope handle can be wiped with isopropyl alcohol. It can be sterilized by removing the batteries, then using autoclaving or gas sterilization. No aeration is required after gas sterilization.

All these items will be contaminated after use and should be treated as dirty and not placed on the clean surfaces of the anesthesia machine or anesthesia cart. The glove the operator is wearing may be inverted over the blade after use to prevent spreading of contamination (201).

As soon as possible after use, the laryngoscope blade, stylet, or forceps should be rinsed under a running tap then immersed in water and detergent. They should be washed mechanically with particular attention given to the area around the light bulb.

Blades, stylets, and forceps may be autoclaved at temperatures up to 134°C, gas sterilized, or treated with liquid chemicals. Of the liquid chemical agents, alcohol and glutaraldehyde are used most frequently. If EO is used for sterilization, no aeration time is required. Many fiberoptic blades can be steam sterilized.

Fiberoptic Scopes

Because they touch mucous membranes or are placed into normally sterile areas of the body, fiberscopes are considered to be semi-critical-to-critical instruments. The majority of all flexible endoscopic procedures is done with disinfected rather than sterilized instruments (9, 202).

There have been several reports of contaminated fiberscopes causing infections as a result of inadequate cleaning, improper selection of a disinfecting agent, insufficient exposure time, or failure to expose a portion of the equipment to the disinfectant (4, 203–207). Pseudoepidemics also have been reported (204, 207, 208). This can lead to unnecessary diagnostic and therapeutic interventions.

Automated machines that will handle one or two endoscopes are available. Some will use a variety of disinfectant/sterilants.

The manufacturer's instructions must be con-

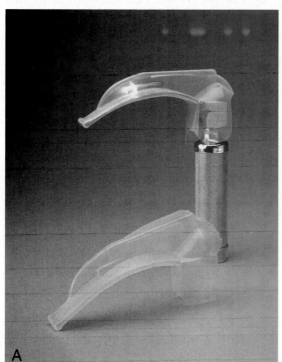
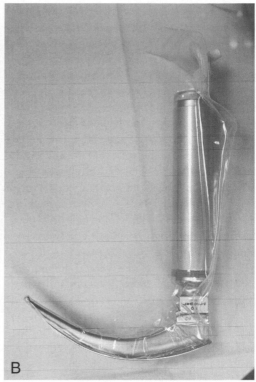

FIGURE 27.6.   Disposable laryngoscope covers. **A,** Coverings for blade only. (Courtesy of Blue Ridge Medical, Inc.) **B,** Covering for both blade and handle.

sulted as to cleaning procedures. In most cases, immediately after a scope is removed from the patient the air-water channel should be flushed with water and the scope's surfaces wiped with 70% alcohol or dry gauze. The scope's channels should be flushed with a detergent solution, then the scope soaked in detergent to break down organic soil. Special cleaning brushes can be inserted into the channels to remove debris loosened by the detergent. The fiberscope and all of its channels should be thoroughly rinsed with water to remove detergent residue. Excess water should then be removed from the channels. The exterior of the scope should be dried with a soft cloth.

Following cleaning, fiberoptic scopes should be sterilized or receive high-level disinfection (2). Endoscopic instruments are particularly difficult to disinfect and easy to damage because of their intricate design and delicate materials. The manufacturer's recommendations should be followed.

Chemical disinfectants used have included alcohol, iodophors, glutaraldehydes, a hydrogen peroxide-based formulation, and a quaternary ammonium compound followed by alcohol (8, 209–211). The Steris system uses peracetic acid. All lumens and/or channels must be filled with—and the device then immersed in—the disinfectant. After disinfection, the device must be thoroughly rinsed with sterile water or rinsed with tap water, then with 70% alcohol.

Gas sterilization at low temperatures may be used on some instruments (29). It is effective but will keep the instrument out of service for the period necessary for processing and aeration.

Tracheal and Double-Lumen Tubes and Connectors

The tracheal tube is placed into an area of the body that is normally sterile. The Subcommittee on Infection Control Policy of the American Society of Anesthesiologists has recommended that tracheal and bronchial tubes be kept sterile until the time of use (3). Disposable sterile tubes are available at relatively low cost. These are used routinely in most institutions. The tube should be kept in its package until just before use and the patient end should not be touched. Studies indicate that tracheal tubes can be kept up to 5 days after being opened (212). Sterile lubricant should be used. If possible, the tube should not touch any part of the mouth or pharynx during insertion.

After use, the tube should be treated as a dirty piece of equipment. If the tube is to be disinfected, it is important that secretions be prevented from drying by rinsing in cold running water and soaking in a detergent and water solution. Before immersion, the inflating tube should be plugged to prevent water from entering the inflating tube and cuff. The connector should be removed and tape, etc., taken off. The tube should then be washed inside and out, with care not to catch the cuff on any sharp object. Tracheal tubes may also be cleaned in a washing machine.

The tube should be rinsed thoroughly, making sure to flush the lumen. Thorough drying is important before chemical disinfection or gas sterilization. Unless the tube is to be autoclaved or pasteurized, the connector should be reinserted after cleaning.

Use of EO is a popular method for sterilizing tracheal tubes. The tube and connector must be free of water droplets. The end of the inflating tube should be open. With repeated gas sterilization, rubber and some plastic tracheal tubes become softened and kink more easily (103, 213). Spiral latex tracheal tubes should not be gas sterilized or steam sterilized with a vacuum applied in the sterilizing cycle, as the latex layers can separate. During anesthesia, anesthetic gases, especially nitrous oxide, may penetrate into the layers, resulting in partial or total occlusion of the lumen of the tube (104).

Steam sterilization has been used in the past for tracheal tubes. However, repeated autoclaving makes them more likely to kink and causes a decrease in the elasticity of the rubber composing the cuffs. Spiral embedded tubes are especially susceptible to damage from autoclaving. Most of the newer tracheal tubes made of plastic will not withstand the high temperatures involved in autoclav-ing. Pasteurization also has been used for tracheal tubes (185).

Liquid chemical disinfection of tracheal tubes has been used. The inflating tube should be closed during immersion to prevent the solution from entering the cuff. The tube will frequently float and needs to be held down with an object that does not distort it or prevent the solution from reaching all surfaces. Thorough rinsing is necessary after all agents except alcohol. Otherwise, tracheitis may result (214, 215).

Suction Catheters

Flexible suction catheters should be discarded immediately after use. A contaminated Yankauer suction that is still needed should be returned to its packaging after use, not placed under the mattress of the operating room table or draped over the carbon dioxide absorber.

Spray Applicators

Multidose spray applicators are frequently contaminated (216). Consideration should be given to using disposable dispensers. If a multidose applicator is used the nozzle should be cleaned and sterilized after use.

Resuscitation Bags

Resuscitation bags have been implicated as the source of epidemics (217–219). Disposable resuscitation bags are available. The primary source of contamination is the valve. This should be disassembled and cleaned, and if possible, disinfected or sterilized after each use or on a regular basis if dedicated to a single patient. The manufacturer's instructions should be followed.

Blood Pressure Cuffs and Stethoscopes

Blood pressure cuffs can be a reservoir of bacteria and frequently are contaminated with blood (160, 220, 221). Protective covers for cuffs are available (222). Reusable cuffs should be cleaned with a detergent at the end of the day and when visibly contaminated (3). More vigorous treatment has been recommended (160).

Periodic disinfection or sterilization is advisable. Most cuffs can be soaked in disinfectant solution. After rinsing, the bladder can be reinserted, air pumped into it, and the cuff dried. After drying, the cuff may be subjected to gas sterilization. Nonfabric cuffs can be sterilized using gas plasma sterilization.

Stethoscopes can be washed with soap and water and wiped with alcohol. Ear plugs can be cleaned with an alcohol-saturated applicator.

Pulse Oximeter Probes and Cables

These are frequently contaminated with blood and organisms (160, 223). They should be cleaned at the end of the day or when visibly contaminated (3). Simply wiping with an isopropyl alcohol solution may not be sufficient (224). Cables can be sterilized using gas plasma sterilization.

AIDS, HEPATITIS, TUBERCULOSIS AND CREUTZFELDT-JAKOB DISEASE

The CDC has determined that standard disinfection and sterilization procedures are adequate for devices contaminated by patients infected with HIV, hepatitis B virus (HBV) or tuberculosis. It should be noted that 50% of surfaces from which HBV antigen can be recovered do not have visible blood contamination.

Table 27.6 shows inactivation of HIV and HBV by chemical agents. A variety of intermediate to high-level disinfectant chemicals effectively inactivate HBV in relatively short exposure times and at low temperatures (9). HIV is relatively unstable in the environment and is rapidly inactivated by a wide range of chemical germicides, even

those that are classified as low level. Disinfectants classified as tuberculocidal are adequate for inactivation of HBV and HIV (29).

The CDC has published specific recommendations for handling patients with tuberculosis in the operating room environment (225, 226).

An infectious agent that requires unique decontamination procedures is the virus of Creutzfeldt-Jakob disease or other related infectious agents responsible for certain fatal degenerative diseases of the central nervous system (30, 41). These viruses are extremely resistant to most methods of disinfection and sterilization. After cleaning, steam sterilization for 1 hour at a temperature of 132°C is recommended for contaminated equipment. When steam sterilization cannot be used, items should be immersed in 1 N sodium hydroxide for 1 hour at room temperature. Noncritical patient care items or surfaces may be disinfected with either bleach (up to 1:10 dilution) or 4% sodium hydroxide at room temperature for 15 minutes (30).

PREVENTION OF OCCUPATIONAL TRANSMISSION OF INFECTION TO ANESTHESIA PERSONNEL (3)

Use of Barriers

Appropriate barrier precautions such as gloves, fluid-resistant masks, eye protection, and gowns

---

TABLE 27.6. Inactivation of Hepatitis B Virus and Human Immunodeficiency Virus by Disinfectants[a]

Disinfectant	Concentration Inactivating HBV (10 min, 20°C)	Concentration Inactivating HIV (10 min, 25°C)
Chlorine dioxide	ND[b]	1:200 dilution
Ethyl alcohol	Not effective	50%
Formaldehyde	10%	1% formalin
Glutaraldehyde	2%	2%
Hydrogen peroxide	ND	0.3%
Iodophor	80 ppm	0.25%
Isopropyl alcohol	70%	35%
Phenolic	Not effective	0.5%
Quaternary ammonium	Not effective	0.08%
Sodium hypochlorite	500 ppm (0.1% to 1%)	50 ppm

[a] From Berry AJ. Infection control in anesthesia. Anesth Clin North Am 1989;7:967–981; and du Moulin GC, Hedley-Whyte J. Hospital-associated viral infection and the anesthesiologist. Anesthesiology 1983;59:51–65.
[b] No data.
HBV, hepatitis B virus; HIV, human immunodeficiency virus.

must be routinely used with all patients to prevent exposure when any contact with body fluids is possible. Ninety-eight percent of the anesthesia provider's contacts with patient blood could be prevented by routine use of gloves (227). It reduces the frequency of needle-sticks and percutaneous injury (228). It should be noted that glove's barrier protection is compromised with each activity performed and especially after adhesive tape is torn unless adhesive-sparing moisturizing cream is used (229, 230). It is important to remove or change these barriers immediately after procedures that might contaminate them with blood or saliva, so that these are not spread (231, 160).

Hand Washing

Anesthesia personnel can harbor high bacterial counts on their hands (232). Hands should be washed as soon as possible after removing gloves and immediately if contaminated with blood or other body fluids. Use of gloves does not preclude the need for proper hand-washing techniques.

Prevention of Needle-sticks

Contaminated needles should never be recapped, bent or broken by hand. Puncture-resistant containers for needle disposal must be available in all work locations. If absolutely necessary to recap contaminated needles, a single-handed technique (one in which the needle is never directed toward an unprotected hand) or a mechanical protective device should be used (233).

Emergency Ventilation Devices

When emergency mouth-to-mouth resuscitation is indicated, mouthpieces, resuscitation bags, or other ventilation devices should be used.

Personnel with Cutaneous Lesions

Healthcare workers with breaks in the skin or exudative/weeping lesions should refrain from direct patient contact unless the open area can be protected.

REFERENCES

1. Association for the Advancement of Medical Instrumentation. Guideline for the use of ethylene oxide and steam biological indicators in industrial sterilization processes (ST34-1991). Arlington, VA: AAMI, 1991.
2. Rutala WA. Draft guideline for selection and use of disinfectants. Am J Infect Control 1989;17:24A–38A.
3. Arnold WP, Hug CC. Recommendations for infection control for the practice of anesthesiology. Park Ridge, IL: American Society of Anesthesiologists, 1991.
4. Rendell–Baker L. Maintenance, cleaning, and sterilization of anesthesia equipment. In: Ehrenwerth J, Eisenkraft JB, eds. Anesthesia equipment, principles and applications. St. Louis: CV Mosby, 1992: 492–511.
5. Favero MS. Principles of sterilization and disinfection. Anesth Clin North Am 1989;7:941–949.
6. Chatburn RL. Decontamination of respiratory care equipment. What can be done, what should be done. Respiratory Care 1989;34:98.
7. Rosenquist RW, Stock MC. Decontaminating anesthesia and respiratory therapy equipment. Anesth Clin North Am 1989;7:951–966.
8. Wasse L, Curtis M. Sterilization versus disinfection of anesthesia breathing circuits. Safety and economic considerations. J Am Assoc Nurse Anesth 1982;50: 161–165.
9. Favero MS, Bond WW. Chemical disinfection of medical and surgical materials. In: Block SS, ed. Disinfection, sterilization and preservation. 4th ed. Philadelphia: Lea & Febiger, 1991:617–641.
10. Association for the Advancement of Medical Instrumentation. Selection and use of chemical indicators for steam sterilization monitoring in health care facilities (TIR #3). Arlington, VA: AAMI, 1988.
11. Association for the Advancement of Medical Instrumentation. Safe handling and biological decontamination of medical devices in health care facilities and in nonclinical settings (ST35–1991). Arlington, VA: AAMI, 1996.
12. Garner JS, Favero MS. CDC guidelines for the prevention and control of nosocomial infections. Am J Infect Control 1986;14:110–129.
13. Wilson RD, Traber DL, Allen CR, et al. An evaluation of the Cidematic decontamination system for anesthesia equipment. Anesth Analg 1972;51:658–661.
14. Borick PM, Dondershine FH, Hollis RA. A new automated unit for cleaning and disinfecting anesthesia equipment and other medical instruments. Dev Ind Microbiol 1971;12:266–272.
15. Bennett PJ, Cope DHP, Thompson REM. Decontamination of anaesthetic equipment. Anaesthesia 1968;23:670–675.
16. Nystrom B. New technology for sterilization and disinfection. Am J Med 1991;91:264S–266S.

17. ANSI/AAMI ST46-1993, Good hospital practice: steam sterilization and sterility assurance. Arlington, VA: AAMI, 1993.

18. Detwiler MS. Ultrasonic cleaning in the hospital. J Healthcare Mat Management 1989;7:46–48, 50.

19. Ryan P. Concepts of cleaning technologies and processes. J Healthcare Mat Management 1987;5:20–27.

20. Association for the Advancement of Medical Instrumentation. ANSI/AAMI ST 46:1993. Good hospital practice: steam sterilization and sterility assurance. 3 ed. Arlington, VA: AAMI, 1993.

21. Medical Research Council. Sterilization by steam under increased pressure. Lancet 1959;1:425–435.

22. Rendell–Baker L, Roberts RB. Gas versus steam sterilization: when to use which. Med Surg Rev 1969;5: 10–14.

23. Association for the Advancement of Medical Instrumentation ANSI/AAMI ST37-1996, Flash sterilization: Steam sterilization of patient care items for immediate use. Arlington, VA: AAMI, 1996.

24. Hoyt A, Chaney AL, Cavell K. Studies on steam sterilization and the effects of air in the autoclave. J Bacteriol 1938;36:639–652.

25. Association for the Advancement of Medical Instrumentation. Biological indicators for saturated steam sterilization processes in health care facilities (ST19: 1986). Arlington, VA: AAMI, 1994.

26. Anonymous. Biological sterilization indicators for steam, EtO and radiation developed by NAMSA. Biomedical Safety & Standards 1984;14:31.

27. Rice HM. Testing of air-filters for hospital sterilizers. Lancet 1958;2:1275–1277.

28. Ascenzi JM, Wendt TM, McDowell JW. Important information concerning the reuse of glutaraldehyde-based disinfectants and their tuberculocidal activity. Arlington, TX: Surgikos Inc., Research Division, October 1984.

29. Berry AJ. Infection control in anesthesia. Anesth Clin North Am 1989;7:967–981.

30. Rutala WA. APIC guidelines for infection control practice. Am J Infect Control 1990;18:99–117.

31. U.S. Department of Health, Education and Welfare. Selection and use of disinfectants in health facilities (HEW Publication #HSM 72-4008). Washington, DC: U.S. Government Printing Office, 1967.

32. Hope T. Prepackaging and sterilization of anesthetic equipment. Nurs Times 1964;60:251–252.

33. Padnos E, Horwitz I, Wunder G. Contact dermatitis complicating tracheostomy. Am J Dis Child 1965; 109:90–91.

34. Wahlberg JE. Two cases of hypersensitivity to quaternary ammonium compounds. Acta Derm Venereol (Stockh) 1964;42:230–234.

35. Spaulding EH. Chemical disinfection and antisepsis in the hospital. J Hosp Res 1972;9:7–31.

36. Stark DC. Sterilization by chemical agents in infections and sterilization problems. Int Anesth Clin 1972;10:49–65.

37. Herwick RP, Treweek ON. Burns from anesthesia mask sterilized in compound solution of cresol. JAMA 1933;100:407–408.

38. Kahn G. Depigmentation caused by phenolic detergent germicides. Arch Dermatol 1970;102:177–187.

39. Spaulding EH. Principles and application of chemical disinfection. AORN J 1963;1:36–46.

40. Ayliffe GAJ. Hospital disinfection and antibiotic policies. Chemotherapy 1987;6:228–233.

41. du Moulin GC, Hedley–Whyte J. Hospital-associated viral infection and the anesthesiologist. Anesthesiology 1983;59:51–65.

42. MacDonald E. Rigid endoscopes. Part II. Telescopes, light cables, light sources. AORN J 1984;40:56–63.

43. Spaulding EWH. Alcohol as a surgical disinfectant. AORN J 1964;2:67–71.

44. Kralovic RC, Badertscher DC. Bactericidal and sporicidal efficacy of a peracetic acid based liquid chemical sterilant. Abstract Q114.302. Paper presented at the annual meeting of the American Society of Microbiologists, 1988.

45. Martin LS, McDougal JS, Loskoski SL. Disinfection and inactivation of the human T lymphotrophic virus type III/lymphadenopathy-associated virus. J Infect Dis 1985;152:400–403.

46. Spire B, Barre-Sinoussi F, Montagnier L, et al. Inactivation of lymphadenopathy-associated virus by chemical disinfectants. Lancet 1984;2:899–901.

47. Brown P, Gibbs CJ, Amyx HL, et al. Chemical disinfection of Creutzfeld–Jakob disease virus. N Engl J Med 1982;306:1279–1282.

48. Gajdusek DC, Gibbs CJ, Asher DM, et al. Precautions in medical care of and in handling materials from patients with transmissible virus dementia (Creutzfeldt-Jakob disease). N Engl J Med 1977; 297:1253–1258.

49. Schaeffer AJ, Jones JM, Amundsen SK. Bactericidal effect of hydrogen peroxide on urinary tract pathogens. Appl Environ Microbiol 1980;40:337–340.

50. Mentel R, Schmidt J, Investigations on rhinovirus inactivation by hydrogen peroxide. Acta Virol (Praha) 1973;17:451–454.

51. Wardle MD, Renninger GM. Bactericidal effect of hydrogen peroxide on spacecraft isolates. Appl Microbiol 1975;30:710–711.

52. Turner FJ. Hydrogen peroxide and other oxidant disinfectants. In: Block SS, ed. Disinfection, sterilization and preservation. 3rd ed. Philadelphia: Lea & Febiger, 1983:240–250.

53. Leaper S. Influence of temperature on the synergistic sporicidal effect of peracetic acid plus hydrogen peroxide in *Bacillus subtitis* SA22(NCA 72-52). Food Microbiol 1984;1:199–203.

54. Stonehill AA, Krop S, Borick PM. Buffered glutaraldehyde—a new chemical sterilizing solution. Am J Hosp Pharm 1963;20:458–465.

55. Borick PM, Dondershine FH, Chandler VL. Alkalinized glutaraldehyde, a new antimicrobial agent. J Pharm Sci 1964;53:1273–1275.

56. Borick PM. Chemical sterilizers (chemosterilizers). Adv Appl Microbiol 1968;10:291–312.

57. Borick PM. Antimicrobial agents as liquid chemosterilizers. Biotechnol Bioeng 1965;7:435–443.

58. Kelsey JC, Mackinnon IH, Maurer IM. Sporicidal aspects of hospital disinfectants. J Clin Pathol 1974; 27:632–638.

59. Haselhuhn DH, Brason FW, Borick PM. "In use" study of buffered glutaraldehyde for cold sterilization of anesthesia equipment. Anesth Analg 1967;46:468–474.

60. Pepper RE, Chandler VL. Sporicidal activity of alkaline alcoholic saturated dialdehyde solutions. J Appl Microbiol 1968;11:384–388.

61. Roberts RB. The anaesthetist, cross-infection and sterilization techniques—a review. Anaesthesia and Intensive Care 1973;1:400–406.

62. Richards M, Levitsky S. Outbreak of *Serratia marcescens* infections in a cardiothoracic surgical intensive care unit. Ann Thorac Cardiovasc Surg 1975;19:503–513.

63. Snyder RW. Cheatle EL. Alkaline glutaraldehyde as effective disinfectant. Am J Hosp Pharm 1965;22:321–327.

64. Miner NA, McDowell JW, Willcockson GW, et al. Antimicrobial and other properties of a new stabilized alkaline glutaraldehyde disinfectant/sterilizer. Am J Hosp Pharm 1977;34:376–382.

65. Saitanu K, Lund E. Inactivation of enterovirus by glutaraldehyde. Appl Soc Microbiol 1975;29:571–574.

66. American Hospital Association. Ethylene oxide sterilization (Guideline Report #8, AHA Technology Series). Chicago: AHA, Division of Management and Technology, 1982.

67. Lin KS, Park MK, Baker HA, et al. Disinfection of anesthesia and respiratory therapy equipment with acid glutaraldehyde solution. Respiratory Care 1979; 24:321–327.

68. Masferrer R, Marquez R. Comparison of two activated glutaraldehyde solutions. Cidex solution and Sonacide. Respiratory Care 1977;22:257–262.

69. Collins FM, Montalbine V. Mycobactericidal activity of glutaraldehyde solutions. J Clin Microbiol 1976; 4:408–412.

70. Notarianni GL. Controlling glutaraldehyde exposure: Part II. Infect Control Ster Technol 1995;1:16–25.

71. Iddenden FR. New decontamination procedure cuts costs—reduces staff time. Can Hosp 1972;49:26–28.

72. Belani KG, Priedkalns J. An epidemic of pseudomembranous laryngotracheitis. Anesthesiology 1977;47:530–531.

73. Mostafa SM. Adverse effects of buffered glutaraldehyde on the Heidbrink expiratory valve. Br J Anaesth 1980;52:223–227.

74. Anonymous. Hospitals weigh options and costs in EtO sterilization. Technology for Anesthesia 1995; 15(9):1–4.

75. Association for the Advancement of Medical Instrumentation. Automatic, general-purpose ethylene oxide sterilizers and ethylene oxide sterilant sources intended for use in health care facilities, 2 ed. (ST24: 1992). Arlington, VA: AAMI, 1992.

76. Association for the Advancement of Medical Instrumentation. Selecting airborne ethylene oxide monitoring equipment or services for an EO gas sterilization facility (TIR #1). Arlington, VA: AAMI, 1984.

77. Association for the Advancement of Medical Instrumentation. Good hospital practice: performance evaluation of ethylene oxide sterilizers—ethylene oxide test packs. Arlington, VA: AAMI, 1985.

78. Association for the Advancement of Medical Instrumentation. Good hospital practice: ethylene oxide gas. Ventilation recommendations and safe use, 3 ed. (ANSI/AAMI ST43:1993) Arlington, VA: AAMI, 1993.

79. Association for the Advancement of Medical Instrumentation. Automatic, general-purpose ethylene oxide sterilizers and ethylene oxide sterilant sources intended for use in health care facilities, 2 ed. (ST24: 1992). Arlington, VA: AAMI, 1992.

80. Canadian Standards Association. Ethylene oxide sterilizers for hospitals (CSA Standard Z314.1-M1991). Rexdale, Ontario, Canada: CSA, 1991.

81. Fitzpatrick BG, Reich RR. ETO sterilization monitoring: a performance study. J Healthcare Mat Management 1986;4:32–35.

82. Andersen SR, Halleck F, Kaye S, et al. Technological innovations in sterilizer design. In: AAMI, ed. Inhospital ethylene oxide sterilization. Current issues in EO toxicity and occupational exposure (TAR #8-84). Arlington, VA: AAMI, 1984:21–22.

83. Steenland K, Stayner L, Greife A, et al. Mortality among workers exposed to ethylene oxide. N Engl J Med 1991;324:1402–1407.

84. American National Standards Institute. Biological indicators for ethylene oxide sterilization processes in

health care facilities (ST21-1986). Arlington, VA: Association for the Advancement of Medical Instrumentation, 1986.

85. Rendell–Baker L. Ethylene oxide. II. Aeration. Int Anesthesiol Clin 1972;10(2):101–122.

86. American National Standards Institute Sectional Committee Z-79 and ASA Subcommittee on Standardization. Ethylene oxide sterilization of anesthesia apparatus. Anesthesiology 1970;33:120.

87. Anonymous. Ethylene oxide sterilization. Hospitals 1971;45:99–100.

88. Andersen SR. Ethylene oxide residues in medical materials. Bull Parenteral Drug Assoc 1973;27:49–57.

89. Anonymous. The physician and the law. Anesth Analg 1970;49:889.

90. Lipton B, Gutierrez R, Blaugrund S, et al. Irradiated PVC plastic and gas sterilization in the production of tracheal stenosis following tracheostomy. Anesth Analg 1971;50:578–586.

91. Russell JP. The sterilization dilemma. Where will it end—laboratory aspects. Anesth Analg 1968;47:653–656.

92. Anonymous. Aeration of anesthesia equipment. Hosp Top 1966;44:115.

93. O'Leary RK, Guess WL. The toxicogenic potential of medical plastics sterilized with ethylene oxide vapors. J Biomed Mater Res 1968;2:297–311.

94. Clarke CP, Davidson WL, Johnston JB. Haemolysis of blood following exposure to an Australian manufactured plastic tubing sterilized by means of ethylene oxide gas. Aust N Z J Surg 1966;36:53–56.

95. Hirose T, Goldstein R, Bailey CP. Hemolysis of blood due to exposure to different types of plastic tubing and the influence of ethylene oxide sterilization. J Thorac Cardiovasc Surg 1963;45:245–251.

96. Poothullil J, Shimizu A, Day RP, et al. Anaphylaxis from the product(s) of ethylene oxide gas. Ann Intern Med 1975;82:58–60.

97. Anonymous. Health risk due to EtO residue on sterilized devices is negligible—HIMA. Biomedical Safety & Standards 1988;18:138–139.

98. Glaser ZR. Special occupation hazard review with control recommendations for the use of ethylene oxide as a sterilant in medical facilities (Publication No. 77-200). Washington, DC: U.S. Department of Health, Education, and Welfare (NIOSH), 1977.

99. Roberts RB. Gamma rays + PVC + EO = OK. Respiratory Care 1976;21:223–224.

100. Stetson JB, Whitbourne JE, Eastman C. Ethylene oxide degassing of rubber and plastic materials. Anesthesiology 1976;44:174–180.

101. Bogdansky S, Lehn PJ. Effects of gamma-irradiation on 2-chloro-ethanol formation in ethylene oxide-sterilized polyvinyl chloride. J Pharm Sci 1964;63:802–803.

102. Bryson TK, Saidman LJ, Nelson W. A potential hazard connected with the resterilization and reuse of disposable equipment. Anesthesiology 1979;50:370.

103. Anonymous. Ethylene oxide sterilization. Health Devices 1975;5:27–50.

104. Rendell–Baker L. A hazard alert—reinforced endotracheal tubes. Anesthesiology 1980;53:268–269.

105. Manheimer A. Ethylene oxide: the silent hazard. Respir Ther 1978;8:19–22, 74.

106. Anderson SR. Ethylene oxide toxicity. J Lab Clin Med 1971;77:346–355.

107. Andersen SR. Experimentally produced skin reactions to ethylene oxide. In: AAMI, ed. In-hospital ethylene oxide sterilization. Current issues in EO toxicity and occupational exposure (TAR #8-84). Arlington, VA: AAMI, 1984:21–22.

108. Garry VF. Some thoughts on medical surveillance for ethylene oxide exposure. In: AAMI, ed. In-hospital ethylene oxide sterilization. Current issues in EO toxicity and occupational exposure (TAR #8-84). Arlington, VA: AAMI, 1984:1–3.

109. Marshall C, Dolovitch J. Potential effects on humans of short-term high-dose exposure: allergic reactions to ethylene oxide—clinical data and symptoms. In: AAMI, ed. In-hospital ethylene oxide sterilization. Current issues in EO toxicity and occupational exposure (TAR #8-84). Arlington, VA: AAMI, 1984:26–27.

110. Anonymous. Hospital employees treated after ethylene oxide leak. Biomedical Safety &Standards 1992;22:145, 147.

111. Gross JA, Haas ML, Swift TR. Ethylene oxide neurotoxicity. Report of four cases and review of the literature. Neurology 1979;29:978–983.

112. Morgan TF. Potential effects on humans of short-term high dose exposure. Effects on the nervous system—clinical data and symptoms. In: AAMI, ed. In-hospital ethylene oxide sterilization. Current issues in EO toxicity and occupational exposure (TAR #8-84). Arlington, VA: AAMI, 1984:23–25.

113. Royce A, Moore WKS. Occupational dermatitis caused by ethylene oxide. Br J Ind Med 1955;12:169–171.

114. Lynch DW, Lewis TR, Moorman WJ, et al. Effects on monkeys and rats of long-term inhalation exposure to ethylene oxide. Major findings of the NIOSH Study. In: AAMI, ed. In-hospital ethylene oxide sterilization. Current issues in EO toxicity and occupational exposure (TAR #8-84). Arlington, VA: AAMI, 1984:7–10.

115. Garry VF. Sister chromatid exchange in human lymphocytes following exposure to ethylene oxide. In: AAMI, ed. In-hospital ethylene oxide sterilization. Current issues in EO toxicity and occupational exposure (TAR #8-84). Arlington, VA: AAMI, 1984: 28–30.

116. Hogstedt C, Aringer L, Gukstavsson A. Epidemiologic support for ethylene oxide as a cancer-causing agent. JAMA 1986;255:1575–1578.

117. Hogstedt C, Malmqvist N, Wadman G. Leukemia in workers exposed to ethylene oxide. JAMA 1979;241: 1132–1133.

118. Anonymous. Ethylene oxide exposure. 15-minute "excursion limit" established by OSHA. Biomedical Safety & Standards1988;18:70.

119. Gschwandtner G, Kruger D, Harman P. Compliance with the EtO standard in the US. J Healthcare Mat Management 1986;4:38–41.

120. Anonymous. Revised guidelines for EO sterilization. AORN J 1976;24:1086–1088.

121. Daley WJ, Morse WA, Ridgway MG. Ethylene oxide control in-hospitals. Chicago: American Society of Hospital Central Service Personnel and American Society for Hospital Engineering of the American Hospital Association, 1979.

122. Morford SD. Facility design and engineering controls. In: AAMI, ed. In-hospital ethylene oxide sterilization. Current issues in EO toxicity and occupational exposure (TAR #8-84). Arlington, VA: AAMI, 1984:49–51.

123. Samuels TM. Personnel exposures to ethylene oxide in a central service assembly and sterilization area. Hosp Top 1978;56:27–33.

124. Anonymous. Field evaluation of EtO exposure levels. Health Devices 1982;11:249–52.

125. Meeker MH. In-hospital control of EO residue levels through good aeration practices. In: AAMI, ed. In-hospital ethylene oxide sterilization. Current issues in EO toxicity and occupational exposure (TAR #8-84). Arlington, VA: AAMI, 1984:85–87.

126. Gunther DA, Barron WR, Durnick TJ, Young JH. Sources of environmental ethylene oxide gas contamination in a simulated sterilization facility. Paper presented at the 16th annual meeting of the AAMI, Washington, DC, May 11, 1981.

127. Anonymous. Safe use of EtO sterilizer aided by new ventilation cabinet. Biomedical Safety & Standards 1983;13:44.

128. Ridgeway M. Environmental and employee monitoring. Current techniques. In: AAMI, ed. In-hospital ethylene oxide sterilization. Current issues in EO toxicity and occupational exposure (TAR #8-84). Arlington, VA: AAMI, 1984:795–797.

129. Denny FJ, Jr. Cost-effective EO Monitoring. the experience of the US Veterans Administration. In: AAMI, ed. In-hospital ethylene oxide sterilization. Current issues in EO toxicity and occupational exposure (TAR #8-84). Arlington, VA: AAMI, 1984: 98–101.

130. Reichert M. Cost-effective EO monitoring in a health care facility: the experience of Robinson Memorial Hospital. In: AAMI, ed. In-hospital ethylene oxide sterilization. Current issues in EO toxicity and occupational exposure (TAR #8-84). Arlington, VA: AAMI, 1984:102–104.

131. Loving TJ, Wooter LL. Cost-effective ethylene oxide monitoring: a case study. In: AAMI, ed. In-hospital ethylene oxide sterilization. Current issues in EO toxicity and occupational exposure (TAR #8-84). Arlington, VA: AAMI, 1984:105–107.

132. Anonymous. New passive dosimeter designed for personal and area monitoring for EO gas vapors. Biomedical Safety & Standards 1986;16:21.

133. Anonymous. EtO and formaldehyde exposure measured by personal monitoring badges. Biomedical Safety & Standards 1988;18:110.

134. Anonymous. Passive diffusion monitor detects ethylene oxide. Biomedical Safety & Standards 1988;18: 101.

135. Anonymous. Personal chemical exposure monitor badges developed. Biomedical Safety & Standards 1989;19:29.

136. Anonymous. EtO monitoring analyzer based on crystal growth. Biomedical Safety & Standards 1990;20: 126.

137. Reichert MC. Ethylene oxide environmental monitoring in a health care facility. Med Instrum 1983; 17:113–115.

138. Qazi A, Ketcham NH. A new method for monitoring personal exposure to ethylene oxide in the occupational environment. Am Ind Hyg Assoc J 1977;38: 635–647.

139. McCullough CE. Microcomputer-based system for real-time computation of time-weighted average levels of ethylene oxide and other gases. Med Instrum 1985;19:136–140.

140. Anonymous. ETO. 16 commonly asked questions . . . and their answers. J Healthcare Mat Management 1986;4:42.

141. Loving TJ, Wooter LL. Cost-effective ethylene oxide exposure control: a case study. In: AAMI, ed. In-hospital ethylene oxide sterilization. Current issues in EO toxicity and occupational exposure (TAR #8-84). Arlington, VA: AAMI, 1984:69–73.

142. Reichart M. Reducing occupational exposure in a health care facility: the experience of Robinson Me-

morial Hospital. In: AAMI, ed. In-hospital ethylene oxide sterilization. Current issues in EO toxicity and occupational exposure (TAR #8-84). Arlington, VA: AAMI, 1984:74–77.

143. Anonymous. New pollution control system designed for hospital EtO sterilizers. Biomedical Safety & Standards 1986;16:126.

144. Anonymous. Hazard. Amdek Boekel sterilizer. Health Devices 1975;5:50–51.

145. Anonymous. Hazard. 3M models 100 and 200 sterilizers. Health Devices 1975;5:51.

146. Halleck FE. Hazards of EO sterilization in-hospitals. Hosp Top 1975;53:45–52.

147. Association for the Advancement of Medical Instrumentation. ANSI/AAMI/ISO 11137:1994. Sterilization of healthcare products—Requirements for validation and routine central radiation sterilization. 3rd ed. Arlington, VA: AAMI, 1984.

148. Olander JW. New facilities and equipment for radiation sterilization. Bull Parenteral Drug Assoc 1963; 17:14–21.

149. Artandi C. Sterilization by ionizing radiation. Int Anesthesiol Clin 1972;10(2):123–130.

150. Wilson R. Evaluation of the Plazlyte sterilization system at Richmond Hospital. Richmond, BC. J Healthcare Mat Management 1994; 12:38-40.

151. Thomas ET. The sterilization dilemma. Where will it end? Clinical aspects. Anesth Analg 1968;47: 657–662.

152. Hamilton WK, Feeley TW. A need for aseptic inhalation anesthesia equipment for each case is unproven. In: Eckenhoff JE, ed. Controversy in anesthesiology. Philadelphia: WB Saunders, 1979:84.

153. Dryden GE. Inhalation anesthesia equipment should be aseptic for each use. In: Eckenhoff JE, ed. Controversy in anesthesiology. Philadelphia: WB Saunders, 1979:73–83.

154. Du Moulin GC, Saubermann AJ. The anesthesia machine and circle system are not likely to be sources of bacterial contamination. Anesthesiology 1977;47: 353–358.

155. Feeley TW, Hamilton WK, Xavier B, et al. Sterile anesthesia breathing circuits do not prevent postoperative pulmonary infection. Anesthesiology 1981; 54:369–372.

156. Olds JW, Kisch AL, Eberle BJ, et al. Pseudomonas aeruginosa respiratory tract infection acquired from a contaminated anesthesia machine. Am Rev Respir Dis 1972;105:628–632.

157. Joseph JM. Disease transmission by inefficiently sanitized anesthetizing apparatus. JAMA 1952;149: 1196–1198.

158. Kempen, PM. Avoiding nosocomial infection in anaesthesia. Can J Anaesth 1989;36:254–255.

159. Spengler RF, Greenlough WB III. Hospital costs and mortality attributed to nosocomial bacteremias. JAMA 1978;240:2455–2458.

160. Hall JR. Blood contamination of anesthesia equipment and monitoring equipment. Anesth Analg 1994;78:1136–1139.

161. Ping FC, Oulton JL, Smith JA, et al. Bacterial filters—are they necessary on anaesthetic machines. Can Anaesth Soc J 1979;26:415–419.

162. Garibaldi RA, Britt MR, Webster C, et al. Failure of bacterial filters to reduce the incidence of pneumonia after inhalation anesthesia. Anesthesiology 1981;54: 364–368.

163. Luney SR, Milligan KR, Armstrong MB, et al. The role of bacterial airway filters in the prevention of nosocomial pneumonia in the intensive care unit. Anesth Analg 1993;76:S230.

164. Leigten DTM, Rejger BS, Mouton RT. Bacterial contamination and the effect of filters in anaesthetic circuits in a simulated patient model. J Hosp Infect 1992;21:51–60.

165. Gallagher J, Strangeways JEM, Allt-Graham J. Contamination control in long-term ventilation. A clinical study using a heat-and-moisture-exchanger filter. Anaesthesia 1987; 42:476–481.

166. Grange C. Hepatitis C and anaesthetic breathing systems. Anaesthesia and Intensive Care 1996;24:514.

167. Knoblanche GK. Revision of the anaesthetic aspects of an infection control policy following reporting of hepatitis C nosocomial infection. Anaesthesia and Intensive Care 1996;24:169–172.

168. Lees DE. To reuse or not to reuse, that is the question. ASA Newslett 1992;56:13–15.

169. Walton JR. A new controversy in respiratory equipment management. Reusables versus disposed disposables versus reused disposables. Respir Care 1986;31: 213–217.

170. Canadian Healthcare Association. The reuse of single-use medical devices. Ottawa, Ontario: Canadian Healthcare Association, Ottawa, 1996.

171. Campbell BA, Wells GA, Palmer WN, Martin DL. Reuse of disposable medical devices in Canadian Hospitals. Am J Infect Control 1987;15:196–200.

172. Berry AJ. American Society of Anesthesiologists infection control policy. Anaesthesia and Intensive Care 1996;24:618.

173. Gadalla F, Fong J. Improved infection control in the operating room. Anesthesiology 1990;73:1295.

174. Garner JS, Simmons BP. Guidelines for isolation precautions in-hospitals. Infect Control 1983;4:245–325.

175. Centers for Disease Control. Acquired immune deficiency syndrome (AIDS): precautions for clinical and

laboratory staffs. MMWR Morb Mortal Wkly Rep 1982;31:577–580.

176. Anonymous. Standards for cleaning and processing anesthesia equipment. AORN J 1977;25:1268–1274.

177. Boyce JM, White RL, Spruill EY, et al. Cost-effective application of the Centers for Disease Control guideline for prevention of nosocomial pneumonia. Am J Infect Control 1985;13:228–232.

178. Murphy PM, Fitzgeorge RB, Barrett RF. Viability and distribution of bacteria after passage through a circle anaesthetic system. Br J Anaesth 1991;66: 300–304.

179. Layon AJ, Wathana S, Langevin PB. Further work on ventilator associated infections and their prevention. Anesthesiology 1996;85:A224.

180. du Moulin GC, Hedley–Whyte J. Bacterial interactions between anesthesiologists, their patients, and equipment. Anesthesiology 1982;57:37–41.

181. Chrusciel C, Mayhall CG, Embrey J, et al. A comparative study of bacterial contamination of reusable and disposable soda lime absorbers. Anesth Analg 1988; 67:S31.

182. Browne RA. Infectious diseases and the anaesthetist. Can J Anaesth 1988;35:655–665.

183. Brown RA, Bell R, Pine W, et al. Sterilization of anaesthetic equipment. Can J Anaesth 1989;36:359–361.

184. George RH. A critical look at chemical disinfection of anaesthetic apparatus. Br J Anaesth 1975;47:719–722.

185. Clark R. Sterilization of anaesthetic apparatus. In: Proceedings of the third Asian and Australian congress of anesthesia, 1970. London: Butterworth, 1971.

186. Baker R. Sonic energy cleaning in inhalation therapy. Inhal Ther 1968;13:56.

187. Gurevich I, Tafuro P, Ristuccia P, et al. Disinfection of respirator tubing: a comparison of chemical versus hot water machine-assisted processing. J Hosp Infect 1983;4:199–208.

188. Barry AE, Noble MA, Marrie TJ, et al. Cleaning of anaesthesia breathing circuits and tubings: a Canadian survey. Can Anaesth Soc J 1984;31:572–575.

189. Reference deleted.

190. Reference deleted.

191. Schnierson SS. Sterilization by heat. Int Anesthesiol Clin 1972;10(2):67–83.

192. MacCallum FO, Noble WC. Disinfection of anaesthetic face masks. Anaesthesia 1960;15:307–309.

193. Beeuwkes H, Vijver AED. Disinfection in anaesthesia. Br J Anaesth 1959;31:363–366.

194. Sia-Kho E, Klein R. The use of disposable sleeves on laryngoscopes. Anesth Analg 1997;84:S53.

195. Tobin MJ, Stevenson GW, Hall SC. A simple, cost-

196. effective method of preventing laryngoscope handle contamination. Anesthesiology 1995; 82:790.

196. Morell RC, Ririe D, James RL, et al. A survey of laryngoscope contamination of a university and a community hospital. Anesthesiology 1994;80:960.

197. Neal TJ, Hughes CR, Rothburn MM, et al. The neonatal laryngoscope as a potential source of cross-infection. J Hosp Infect 1995;30:315–317.

198. Foweraker JE. The laryngoscope as a potential source of cross-infection. J Hosp Infect 1995;29:315–6.

199. Sia-Kho E, Klein R, Abalos A, et al. The efficacy of chemical agents versus disposables in cleaning anesthesia laryngoscopes. Anesthesiology 1995;83: A1065.

200. Abramson AL, Gilberto E, Mullooly V, et al. Laryngoscope 1993;103:503–508.

201. Barnette RE, Pietrzak WT, BianRosa JJ. On preventing transmission of viral infections. Anesthesiology 1985;62:845.

202. Frank UK, Daschner FD. Endoscope and device-related infections. Curr Opinion Infect Dis 1992;5; 524–529.

203. Fraser VJ, Jones M, Murray PR, et al. Contamination of flexible fiberoptic bronchoscopes with mycobacterium chelonae linked to an automated bronchoscope disinfection machine. Am Rev Respir Dis 1992;145: 853–855.

204. Gubler JGH, Salfinger M, von Graevenitz A. Pseudo-epidemic of nontuberculous mycobacteria due to a contaminated bronchoscope cleaning machine. Report of an outbreak and review of the literature. Chest 1992;101:1245–1249.

205. Anonymous. Hazard report. Contamination of the modified Olympus EW-10 and EW-20 automatic flexible endoscope reprocessors. Health Devices 1994;23:143–145.

206. Centers for Disease Control. Nosocomial infection and pseudoinfection from contaminated endoscopes and bronchoscopes—Wisconsin and Missouri. MMWR Morb Mortal Wkly Rep 1991; 40:675–682.

207. Cortese DA, Prakash BS. Bronchoscopy in pulmonary infections in bronchoscopy. Prakash, UBS, ed., New York: Raven Press, 1994:183–198.

208. Nicolle LE, McLeod J, Romance L, et al. Pseudo-outbreak of blastomycosis associated with contaminated bronchoscopes. Infect Con Hosp Epidem 1992;13:324.

209. Babb JR, Bradley CR, Deverill CEA, et al. Recent advances in the cleaning and disinfection of fiberscopes. J Hosp Infect 1981;2:329–340.

210. Garcia de Cabo A, Larriba PLM, Pinilla JC, et al. A new method of disinfection of the flexible fiber bronchoscope. Thorax 1978;33:270–272.

211. de Cabo AG, Larriba PLM, Pinila JC, et al. A new method of disinfection of the flexible fibre bronchoscope. Thorax 1978;33:270–272.

212. Moore MW, Bowe EA, Turner JF, et al. Opened endotracheal tubes can be saved. Anesthesiology 1992; 77:A1059.

213. Bosomworth PP, Hamelberg W. Effect of sterilization techniques on safety and durability of endotracheal tubes. Anesth Analg 1965;44:576–584.

214. Bamforth BJ. Questions and answers. Anesth Analg 1963;42:658.

215. Keenleyside HB. Reaction to improperly cleaned endotracheal catheter. Anesthesiology 1957;18: 505–506.

216. Williams OA, Wilcon MH, Nicol CD, et al. Lignocaine spray applicators are a potential source of cross-infection in anaesthetic room. Anaesthesia 1993;48: 61–62.

217. Fierer J, Taylor PM, Gezon HM. *Pseudomonas aeruginosa* epidemic traced to delivery-room resuscitators. N Engl J Med 1967;276:991–996.

218. Thompson AC, Wilder BJ, Powner DJ. Bedside resuscitation bags. A source of bacterial contamination. Infect Cont 1985;6:231–232.

219. Cartwright RY, Hargrove PRJ. Hazard of self-inflating resuscitation bags. Br Med J 1969;4:302.

220. Beard MA, McIntyre A, Rountree PM. Sphygmomanometers as a reservoir of pathogenic bacteria. Med J Aust 1969;2:758–760.

221. Sternlicht AL, VanPoznak A. Significant bacterial colonization occurs on the surface of non-disposable sphygmomanometer cuffs and re-used disposable cuffs. Anesth Analg 1990;70:S450.

222. Anonymous. Blood pressure cuffs designed to protect against infectious agents. Biomedical Safety & Standards 1996;26:142.

223. Wilkins MC. Residual bacterial contamination on reusable pulse oximetry sensors. Respiratory Care 1993;38:1155–1160.

224. Wilkins MC. Are oximeter nondisposable probe disinfection techniques effective? Respiratory Care 1992;37:1347.

225. Peterson GN. CDC sets guidelines for preventing TB transmission in health care facilities. ASA Newsletter 1995;59:24–26.

226. Tait AR. Occupational transmission of tuberculosis: implications for anesthesiologists. Anesth Analg 1997; 85:444–451.

227. Kristensen M, Sloth E, Jensen TK. Relationship between anesthetic procedure and contact of anesthesia personnel with patient body fluids. Anesthesiology 1990;73:619–624.

228. Ben-David B, and Gaitini L. The routine wearing of gloves: impact on the frequency of needle-stick and percutaneous injury and on surface contamination in the operating room. Anesth Analg 1996;83: 623–628.

229. Cork RC, Wood D, Evans B, et al. Leak rate of latex gloves after tearing adhesive tape. Am J Anesth 1995; 22:133–137.

230. Cork R, Wood DD, Mimeles D, et al. Loss of glove barrier protection during anesthesia. Anesthesiology 1995;83:A408.

231. Cullen BF. Yes, put on gloves, but also take them off. Anesth Analg 1995;80:1066.

232. Tessler MJ, Grillas N, Gioseffini S. Bacterial counts on the hands of anesthetists and anesthesia technicians. Anesth Analg 1994; 78:1030–1031.

233. Tait AR, Tuttle DB, Prevention of occupational transmission of human immunodeficiency virus and hepatitis B virus among anesthesiologists: a survey of anesthesiology practice. Anesth Analg 1994;79: 623–628.

QUESTIONS

Each question below contains four suggested answers of which one or more is correct.
Choose the answer:
A if 1, 2, and 3 are correct
B if 1 and 3 are correct
C if 2 and 4 are correct
D if 4 is correct
E if 1, 2, 3 and 4 are correct.

1. Concerning the three levels of disinfection recognized by the Centers for Disease Control and Prevention (CDC),
   1. High level disinfection means that bacterial spores are killed
   2. Semi-critical items can be cleaned with intermediate-level disinfection
   3. The Creutzfeldt-Jakob virus is killed with high level disinfection
   4. Intermediate level disinfection means that mycobacterium tuberculosis is killed

2. Advantages of steam autoclaving include
   1. It is highly effective
   2. Items can be packaged beforehand
   3. It is inexpensive
   4. Absence of toxic residues

3. Factors that affect the effectiveness of liquid chemical disinfection include
   1. Temperature
   2. The use pattern
   3. pH

4. Characteristics of the item to be disinfected

4. Ethylene oxide
   1. Is flammable in concentrations exceeding 5%
   2. Is not useful for items containing petroleum-based lubricant
   3. Is odorless
   4. Cannot be used on items that are wet

5. Concerning the classification of items according to the CDC
   1. Semi-critical items include tracheal tubes
   2. Blood pressure cuffs are noncritical items
   3. High-level disinfection is acceptable for semi-critical items
   4. Phenols are useful for semi-critical items

6. The following statements are correct:
   1. An antiseptic can be safely applied to living tissue
   2. A disinfectant is a germicide to be used solely on inanimate objects
   3. A sanitizer is a low-level disinfectant with no claim for tuberculocidal activity
   4. A sterilant/disinfectant is a germicide that is capable of sterilization or high-level disinfection

ANSWERS

1.	D	4.	C
2.	E	5.	A
3.	E	6.	E

Operating Room Design and Equipment Selection

This chapter is intended to assist anesthesia providers who are involved in construction of and equipment selection for a new facility, or an addition to or renovation of an existing one. It is in the best interest of all to have a member of the anesthesia department play an active role during the early planning stages. Unfortunately, consultation often takes place after the fact or when planning has progressed too far for meaningful input.

When drawing up a plan, it is important to consider both present and future needs. Both available space and its location should be considered. In each section, the flow of patients, staff, and materials should be considered. There should be a method to bring materials into the area and remove trash and soiled linen without coming in contact with the public. Also, physicians and staff should be able to enter and leave without having to encounter patients or their families (1).

PREOPERATIVE EVALUATION CLINICS

Preoperative evaluation clinics may be useful. There is evidence to suggest that they are associated with decreased length of stay, lower costs, a decrease in laboratory tests performed, reduced cancellations on the day of surgery, and improved operating suite efficiency (2).

PREOPERATIVE CARE AREA

The preoperative (holding) area has evolved from a site where patients were left until it was time to enter the operating room into an area where many procedures are performed. These may include preoperative assessment and teaching, consultations, central or arterial line placement, regional blocks, placement of epidural catheters, patient preparation, preoperative marking, venipunctures, starting of intravenous infusions, electrocardiograms (ECGs), X-rays, and premedication. This area must be capable of handling a variety of patients including those admitted to the facility, morning admissions, ambulatory patients and patients admitted from the emergency department.

Location

The preoperative care area should be located near the main entrance to the operating room suite but away from loud activity and the traffic pattern of personnel entering and leaving the operating room suite.

Size

The appropriate size for the area will be determined by the number of operating rooms, the types of cases, and the procedures to be performed in this area. One space per active operating room is the minimum if the area is to hold all the patients at the beginning of the day. The number of spaces can be reduced if the postanesthesia care unit (PACU) can be utilized for some patients. If there are many short cases, it may be necessary to provide more spaces to ensure that there will not be a delay while patients are brought to the unit.

The size needed will vary with the practice. Most patient beds are larger than transport stretchers. If there are to be large orthopedic beds, bigger spaces may be needed. If procedures and preoperative preparations are carried out in the holding area, the spaces may need to be larger or there must be the ability to combine two spaces.

Configuration

The arrangement may involve conflicting requirements. While privacy is of great importance, especially if procedures and examinations are to be performed, it should be possible to view all patient care areas from the nursing station. The nursing station should be located to minimize staff movement.

Most preoperative areas are divided using hanging curtains or partitions. Curtains provide flexibility and allow two spaces to be combined if more space is needed. When privacy is not needed they can be pushed back to allow nursing personnel to better observe the patient.

A separate room may be desirable to isolate patients with transmissible infections or for procedures such as nerve blocks which might bother other patients. It may be desirable to separate patients who are unruly or require guards from the general patient population.

Lighting

It should be possible to vary the lighting for each space. If a patient is simply waiting, the light should be indirect and restful. Increased illumina-

tion will be needed for venipunctures and other procedures. A small spotlight may prove useful.

Pipeline Outlets

Oxygen and suction outlets should be present at each location. If ventilator-dependent patients are to be kept in the holding area, air outlets will be needed.

Electrical and Monitoring Capacity

The minimum monitors for each space include an ECG, noninvasive blood pressure monitor, and pulse oximeter. At least one monitor or module with invasive blood pressure measurement should be available. Adequate electrical outlets for these monitors as well as other uses need to be present.

Storage

Space will be needed to store the supplies needed for the various procedures performed in that area.

Rest Room Facilities

Rest rooms need to be available for patients, staff and visitors.

Administrative Area

There needs to be an administrative area for paperwork, a computer and data management system (Chapter 25, "Electronic Recordkeeping and Perioperative Information Management Systems"). Places to store X-rays, old charts, and reference books will be needed. Intercoms, emergency call capability, and telephones will be required.

Disposal Facilities

Means to dispose of wastes will be needed. There also needs to be an area where dirty linens can be kept until removed from the area.

Changing Rooms

If patients are admitted directly to the holding area, an area for patients to change into hospital attire and lockers for their belongings will be needed.

Pediatric Considerations

If pediatric patients are part of the practice, space to accommodate the family as well as the child should be available. If possible, pediatric holding should be separate from the adult. A portable videocassette recorder with tapes, lap games, toys, rocking chairs, and comfortable seating will help to create a relaxed, nonthreatening environment (3).

OPERATING ROOM SUITE
Location

The operating room suite should be in a cul-de-sac, thereby allowing control of entry and exit. It should be located so that transport between it and the surgical floors is quick and simple. Proximity to the ambulatory and intensive care units is important. An easy route from the emergency department is desirable.

Arrangement

The operating rooms should be arranged in a way that ensures continuous progression from the entrance through zones that increasingly approach sterility. Staff working in the department should be able to move from one clean area to another without having to pass through unprotected zones.

Corridors should be uncluttered. There should be special alcoves or places designated for items which need to be in the hall such as emergency apparatus. The illumination should be diffuse so that patients will not experience glare as they are transported to and from the operating room.

Support Facilities
Storage

There needs to be ample storage space for supplies, equipment, gases, etc. Anesthesia and surgical equipment tends to proliferate so that frequently after a facility has been open a short time, storage space is inadequate.

Laboratory and Radiology Support

Other departments that may need to be accommodated include pathology, blood bank, biochemistry, and x-ray. It may be worthwhile to plan a laboratory for blood-gas analysis close to the rooms for open heart or liver transplant surgery. In-vitro fertilization labs need to be in close proximity to the operating room used for this purpose.

Supply Receiving Area

It is desirable to have a breakout area where items can be removed from shipping containers before being taken into the operating suite. This will protect clean areas from dust and other contaminants that may be present on shipping containers or generated when they are opened.

Communication

The communication systems need to make it possible to locate any member of the operating room staff. An intercom (Fig. 28.1) can provide communication between various operating rooms, the holding area, PACU, anesthesia workroom, frozen section laboratory and x-ray department. Telephones should also be in all these locations. There needs to be a system to alert the operating room staff of an emergency so that the designated team can respond (Fig. 28.2).

Space will be needed for inservicing new equipment, demonstrations of equipment under evaluation, meeting with manufacturer representatives, and ongoing educational activities. This needs to be in the operating room suite since it is not always possible for all personnel to leave the area at the same time.

Anesthesia Induction Rooms

Anesthesia induction rooms can reduce turnover times and make it possible to have a smaller holding area. They are often used for pediatric patients so it is possible for a parent to be present as the child goes to sleep.

Administrative Space

This includes offices for the operating room supervisor, scheduling personnel, purchasing manager, head nurse, and other supervisory personnel. The control area for the operating room needs to be located where the person in charge has the ability to determine the status of the operating rooms, and the holding and recovery areas. It should be located near the entrance in order to regulate the entry of people not directly connected with the operating room.

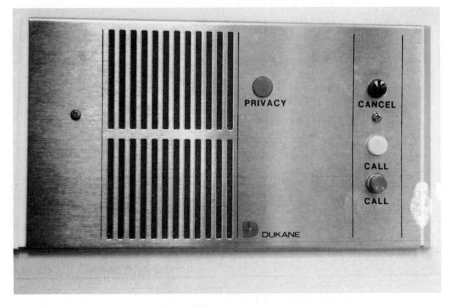

FIGURE **28.1.** Intercom station.

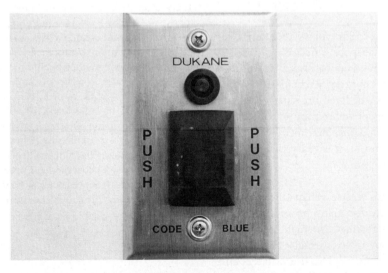

FIGURE **28.2.** Emergency code button.

Personnel Support Space

Locker rooms, showers, rest rooms and changing facilities plus a room where staff members and physicians can relax between cases should be planned. Extra space should allocated for students and visiting personnel.

Operating Rooms
Number

Too few rooms will result in inefficiency in scheduling. On the other hand, if too many rooms are built, they will stay empty and their cost will not be recovered. It is usually relatively easy to determine present needs, but predicting future requirements is more difficult. Factors which must be taken into account include the expected growth of the area, the effects of managed care, and impact of other facilities in the area.

Size

The amount and size of equipment brought into operating rooms are increasing rapidly. Unfortunately space is expensive and the pressure to keep costs down may result in rooms that are smaller than desirable. Small rooms interfere with efficient running of the operating room schedule since small rooms are not suitable for some cases.

Moderate Sized Rooms

An operating room of 400 to 500 sq ft will accommodate many surgical procedures. If large pieces of equipment such as lasers, X-ray machines, or laparoscopic machines are to be used, this size room may entail many logistical problems. Staff may have difficulty moving about the room. As the amount of equipment used increases, this size room may not be adequate.

Large Rooms

A large operating room typically contains over 600 sq. ft. This much space is necessary for many orthopedic, cardiac, and neurosurgical procedures as well as emergency surgery, particularly trauma. Surgical procedures which require laparoscopy, X-ray or video equipment will require a room of this size. With the expected proliferation of specialized equipment in the future, it is likely that this size room will be most common.

Small Rooms

In the past, rooms with less than 400 sq ft were considered adequate for many procedures. Cystoscopy is often performed in small rooms. Because the cystoscopy table is usually fixed to the floor, versatility is limited. The use of lasers and other equipment may strain this size room to its limits. It is unlikely there will be much need for rooms of this size in the future.

Room Arrangement

The room should be designed to optimize the flow of patients, personnel, and supplies. Figure 28.3 shows several features common to most rooms: operating table, anesthesia cart, anesthesia workstation, surgical back table, and ceiling-mounted columns that provide electrical and

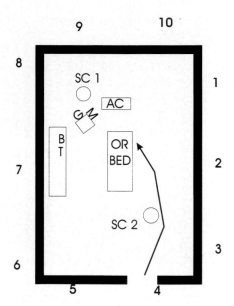

FIGURE 28.3. Operating room with the main components. SC is a service column. GM is gas machine (anesthesia workstation). AC is the anesthesia cart. BT is the (back) instrument table. The main door is at position 4. Locations 1, 2, and 10 are the most suitable locations for the main door. Having it in Positions 3 or 4 would result in the service column's being in the way when the patient is brought into the room. If it were in Positions 5 through 9, entry would be behind the anesthesia space or the back table. Sterile instruments could enter through positions 4, 5, 6, or 8. Personnel could enter through sites 1 through 5 and 10 without contacting the back table or the anesthesia equipment. Locating the pass through to sterile supply in positions 5, 6, or 8 would place sterile instruments in proximity to where they are needed. The sterile field needs to be located away from traffic. It should be near the area where sterile supplies are stored. It should not be near cabinets or doors.

piped gas outlets. The usual arrangement has the workstation, column and anesthesia supply cart at one end of the bed and the sterile back table to one side.

The planning process must take into account the traffic patterns. There is the pattern of the patient entering and exiting the room, the anesthesia and surgical personnel who are not sterile, and sterile personnel and instruments. It is desirable to design the room in a manner which will separate these traffic patterns as much as possible to facilitate movement and minimize compromises in sterility.

Operating Table Orientation

It is usually best to orient the operating table parallel to the long axis of the room. If the table is oriented perpendicular to the long axis, movement from side to side is impeded. Often the rooms are set up to use either end for the head of the table. Usually, however, one setup will be the more efficient.

Doors

The number and locations of the various doors is important because this will determine the traffic flow. A number of possible locations for doors is demonstrated in Figure 28.3.

Main door. The location of the door through which the patient enters and leaves the room will be determined partly by the relationship of the room to the main hallway. It should be wide and high enough to accommodate any bed or equipment that might be needed. It should allow the patient to be brought to the room with as little interference with equipment or the sterile field as possible.

Other door(s). One or more other entrances into the operating room will be needed. If the scrub area is not in the main hall, there will need to be a door to this. A door to a room containing an autoclave and a warming cabinet may be required. A means to move sterile supplies into the room will be needed. A pass-though window (Fig. 28.3) may also be used.

LIGHTING. A number of fluorescent lights in the ceiling is usual. A dimmer will allow the brightness to be varied. Special lighting for anesthesia and circulating nurses during periods of low light should be provided. Lighting along the periphery of the room will be useful for laparoscopic procedures which require low light. Surgical spotlights are usually on articulated arms. Often three of these lights are needed for complicated procedures.

Anesthesia gas services. Supply devices containing the terminal units for the gas pipeline system were discussed in Chapter 2, "Medical Gas Piping Systems."

NUMBER OF OUTLETS. Having more than one supply device will increase the flexibility of the room but can create problems. Gas supply devices are expensive. The second supply device may disturb the traffic patterns in the room. It is difficult to design a room that will allow efficient traffic patterns with opposite orientations. Moving from one supply device to another is increasingly difficult because of the large number of connections. It may be easier to move the operating table than the anesthesia equipment.

TYPES. Another way to gain flexibility is to use different gas supply devices. If the anesthesia machine will be located near a wall and there is no traffic behind it, wall outlets should be considered. Outlets may be incorporated into a single- or double-articulated arm which will allow them to be moved to the most effective location. The arm may be fitted with one or more shelves on which monitors and other equipment may be placed. A column that can be moved up and down will be less of a hindrance to movement of equipment than one that cannot be moved.

SERVICES. At least two (preferably three) oxygen, one nitrous oxide, one air, and one nitrogen outlet per set are recommended. The nitrogen outlet and regulator may be in a separate location. Vacuum will be needed for both surgery and anesthesia and may be used to scavenge excess anesthetic gases. Four outlets will provide two for surgery, one for the anesthesia suctioning, and one for scavenging.

Electrical Service

When considering the electrical needs of the operating room, a number of factors need to be taken into account.

Isolated Power

While isolated power systems were standard in operating rooms when explosive anesthetic agents were employed their use is now optional. In an isolated power system, the grounded power from the power station is converted to ungrounded power using an isolation transformer. If a fault occurs in a piece of equipment, there will not be a shock to personnel or the patient and the equipment will continue to operate. The only way to receive a shock is to contact both the wires of the system.

Figure 28.4 shows an line isolation monitor. It has a meter that gives a continuous indication of the impedance to ground from each side of

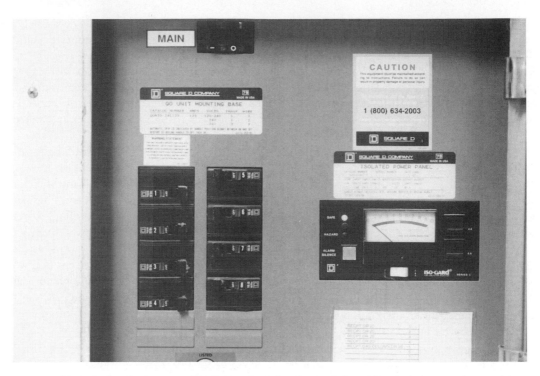

FIGURE 28.4. Isolated power panel showing circuit breakers at left and line isolation monitor at right.

the isolated power system, thus monitoring the integrity of the system (4). When a fault occurs the system will be converted into a grounded one. This will be detected by the line isolation monitor and an alarm will be activated in the operating room (Fig. 28.5)

Grounded Systems

Another type of system is a grounded system similar to that found in homes. It consists of a hot wire, a neutral wire connected to earth, and a ground wire attached to the longer third pin in the plug. The ground wire gives some protection from electrical shock. If the equipment case becomes energized, the ground wire provides a low resistance route to ground.

Ground fault interrupters are used in these systems. They monitor the current in both the hot and neutral sides of the circuit. If the interrupter detects any difference between the two leads it interrupts the system, offering protection from macroshock. The devices being monitored can lose power without warning. This could be a prob-

lem if, for example, a life support machine were in use (4).

Circuit Interrupters

Circuit breakers (interrupters) interrupt the flow of electricity when there is an overload, or, in grounded systems, a ground fault.

Circuits

Most operating rooms will have at least six circuits. They are often divided so that one is on each wall and the remaining two are in the columns. The operating room has many heavy-duty power users and if too many are plugged into one circuit the circuit breaker will be activated.

Outlets

Outlets should be placed on each wall and column. If there are not enough receptacles a block with an outlet strip (Fig. 28.6) can be used. A multitude of wires running across the floor poses a danger to personnel who need to move around the room. In large operating rooms, walls are further from the equipment than in smaller rooms. This causes wires to be stretched (Fig. 28.7).

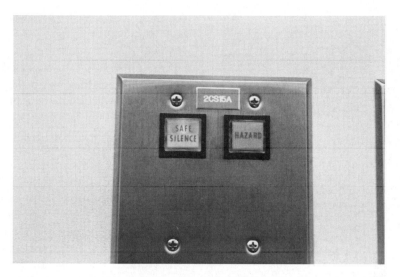

FIGURE **28.5.** Warning panel for isolated power system in the operating room. It indicates when a hazardous situation is present.

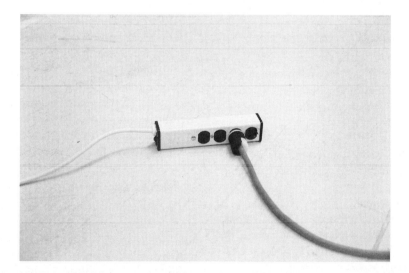

FIGURE **28.6.** An outlet strip may be used to extend the wire to the outlet.

Special Electrical Outlets

Some equipment such as lasers and X-ray machines may require higher voltages or amperages. It is important to have the correct circuits and receptacles for this equipment.

Emergency Power

Healthcare facilities have emergency generators to cover loss of normal power. A special net-

work is created because the entire facility cannot be run from this source. It is important that operating room circuits be connected to the emergency network.

Data Management

Data management systems are discussed in Chapter 25, "Electronic Recordkeeping and Peri-

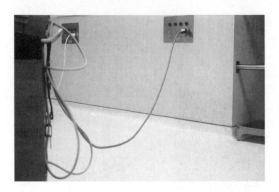

FIGURE 28.7. When the equipment is far from the wall outlet, an extension may be needed to keep the wire on the floor.

operative Information Management Systems." There needs to be a means to connect with the network in each operating room. If it has not been determined what type of connections will be used, a conduit should be installed.

Communications

Telephones

There should be at least one telephone in each operating room. An additional one for the exclusive use of anesthesia personnel should be considered.

Intercom

An intercom is needed to communicate with the control desk, pathology, and other operating rooms.

Code Warning Signal

A signal that when activated signals a cardiac arrest or the need for immediate assistance (Fig. 28.2) should be in each room. This is a legal requirement in many states.

Temperature Control

There needs to be a means of quickly lowering or raising the room temperature. This should be a high priority during the design phase because it is hard to implement as an afterthought. Pediatric operating rooms in particular, need good temperature control.

Ventilation System

There are two types of air-conditioning systems: recirculating and nonrecirculating. A nonre-

circulating system heats or cools the air to the desired temperature and conveys it into the operating room. The air is then exhausted to the outside. These systems are expensive to operate. One advantage is that anesthetic gases dispersed into the room will be automatically removed. The gas disposal tubing from the scavenging system can be connected to the exhaust vent (Chapter 12, "Controlling Trace Gas Lines").

A recirculating system takes some or all the room air, passes it through the temperature controlling mechanism and circulates it back into the operating room. Consideration should be given to designing one operating room to handle patients with tuberculosis. To prevent suspended infectious droplets from leaving the operating room, the operating room should have an anteroom that has a negative pressure in relation to the corridor and operating room (5).

Scavenging System

Consideration should be given to the scavenging system. These are discussed in Chapter 12, "Controlling Trace Gas Lines." The method of scavenging should be determined during the planning stage. If the piped vacuum system is to be used, it is important to have a sufficient number of outlets. Special outlets for use with scavenging systems are available.

Special Use Rooms

Consideration should be given to rooms for intraoperative radiation, stereotactic procedures, and other special uses. When planning these rooms, it is worthwhile if possible to visit a similar room. Another recommended procedure is make a mockup of the room with replicas of the equipment which will be installed. The input of the surgeons and other personnel who will use this room will help in arranging the contents properly.

POSTANESTHESIA CARE UNITS
Location

The PACU should be near the operating rooms to minimize the distance which the patient must travel. Proximity to intensive care units is desirable.

Size

The number of patient spaces needed will vary with the facility and the type of surgery performed. If there are a large number of short surgical cases, the ratio of PACU spaces to operating rooms will need to be higher. If the practice has a high number of monitored anesthesia care patients who do not spend time in the PACU, the number of spaces may be adjusted downward. The availability of critical care spaces should be considered since it affects the duration of stay in the PACU.

Procedures such as electroconvulsive therapy, transesophageal echocardiography, cardioversions, epidural blood patches, vascular line placements, and nerve blocks are often carried out in the PACU. When this is anticipated, the number of spaces needs to be adjusted accordingly. Since these can be performed at nonbusy times such as early in the morning or later in the afternoon, the additional space needed may be less than first imagined. It may be desirable to perform these procedures in an area separate from where patients are recovering from anesthesia.

Configuration

The arrangement of the area should enhance observation of patients. Nursing workspace should be in proximity to the patient locations. Designating a section of the PACU for children and providing some isolation from adults is advantageous for both (3).

The patient may be positioned with the head toward the wall or the aisle. Having the head toward the aisle facilitates maneuvers such as resuscitation and intubation. In addition, a nurse in the aisle will be in close proximity to the heads of four patients. One disadvantage of this position is that monitoring cords, oxygen and suction will need to come over the patient from the wall or from a column at the patient's head. Columns form a barrier that personnel may bump into and sometimes make it hard to observe the patient. Having the patient's head against the wall makes it more difficult to perform airway maneuvers. The bed must be moved away from the wall and the clinician must fight through a maze of wires and tubings to get to the head. An advantage is that cables and tubings can be shorter.

Traffic Flow

If possible, the entrance and exit should be at opposite ends of the area. Patients who are awaiting transportation to their rooms, should be separated from those who are awakening.

Isolation Area

An isolation room is desirable. It should have negative pressure to the surrounding rooms, outside air exhaust, an anteroom to act as an airlock and ultraviolet lights to kill Mycobacterium tuberculosis in infectious droplets (5). The care giver in this area will need to have supplies readily available so it will not be necessary to make many trips into the main recovery area.

Support Space

Sufficient space for storage of equipment, emergency and block carts, hot air warming devices, and blanket warmers and clean and dirty laundry areas, sinks for personnel to wash their hands, a rest room for personnel and patients, dictating and charting areas, and computer terminals will be needed. A separate medication room is desirable. A source of oxygen (either cylinders or portable liquid containers) that can be used if the piped supply fails should be present.

Gas Service

Each patient location should have oxygen, vacuum and air outlets. Vacuum outlets for chest tubes, gastrointestinal suction, etc., should be planned.

Electrical Outlets

There should be at least eight electrical outlets per bed. At least two of these should be connected to emergency power and should be labeled as such. Special outlets for X-ray machines and any other equipment with special electrical supply needs should be included.

Environmental Considerations

The PACU needs to have frequent air changes because patients who are exhaling anesthetic agents will pollute the room with trace amounts of anesthetic gases. At least six exchanges per hour with two of them being fresh are recommended. There needs to be adequate light with separate controls for each patient location. Small spotlights may be desirable if procedures or blocks are to be performed. Soft indirect lighting is desirable if the PACU is to be used for extended care such as overnight stay. Curtains or other methods for privacy need to be available.

ANESTHESIA SUPPORT FACILITIES

The Anesthesia Workroom

This area should be designed so that traffic does not interfere with the technicians' work. It should have reliable two-way communication with each operating room, the control area, the PACU, induction rooms and the holding area.

Storage

Equipment and supplies should be stored in cabinets with transparent doors to allow items to be located easily. Grouping of equipment and supplies (for example, all equipment related to administration of blood products) will facilitate locating them when the technicians are not available.

Disposable Items

The quantity of disposables kept in the anesthesia workroom will depend on the capacity and efficiency of storage areas elsewhere in the facility. If peripheral storage areas can accommodate a large inventory, only a few days' supplies need to be kept in the workroom. If such a peripheral area is not available, the amount stored needs to be enough to cover the lag time in getting orders filled.

Reusable Items

Reusable items such as blood pressure cuffs, laryngoscope blades, and airways which have been cleaned or sterilized need to be stored. The number of these and the time needed for reprocessing will dictate the amount of space required.

Other Equipment

Infrequently used equipment such as Dopplers may be kept in the workroom. It may be a good idea to store backup monitors there, if space permits. There should be plenty of electrical outlets at the back of shelves for equipment utilizing rechargeable batteries. Larger pieces of equipment such as anesthesia machine and electroencephalographic (EEG) machines may be kept in the work room or a more peripheral area. Medical pipeline outlets in this area may be desirable to allow anesthesia machines to be repaired and tested prior to being returned to use.

Portable equipment such as carts for special uses (pediatrics, trauma, malignant hyperthermia, difficult airway) and forced-air patient warming machines may be kept in the workroom.

Medications

In some facilities, it may be necessary to store drugs in the anesthesia workroom. A small refrigerator will be required for certain medications. Space to mix medications such as pentothal may be needed.

Equipment Reprocessing

Reprocessing procedures include disassembly, cleaning, disinfection, and sterilization. How much reprocessing is performed in the anesthesia workroom will depend on how much reprocessing can be carried out by the operating room or central service department for the entire facility. Even if most of the procedures are performed in another area, it may be desirable to disassemble dirty items in the anesthesia workroom, removing gross soil and rendering them safe for handling prior to transport (6).

There should be a receptacle in each operating room into which dirty anesthesia equipment is placed. Transport of soiled equipment should be made on dedicated carts or mechanical conveyances that are clearly marked to indicate that the items are contaminated. These should be placed in a designated area for timely transport to the central processing department or the reprocessing area in the operating room suite. A dedicated soiled cart lift from the operating room to the central supply department is recommended if they are on different floors (7).

In the anesthesia workroom, access to the decontamination area should be restricted. Clean and sterile equipment and supplies MUST be kept separate and protected from contamination. This can be accomplished by facility design (walls or partitions), time and/or traffic patterns (8). Signs showing where dirty equipment should be placed should be prominently displayed. Hand-washing facilities should be conveniently located in or near the decontamination area. They should be separate from sinks used for cleaning or rinsing contaminated items. The ventilation system should be designed to maintain negative air pressure relative to surrounding spaces. Air from this area should be exhausted to the outside or to a filtered partial recirculating system.

The reprocessing area should have adequate space for the intended procedures. It may be desirable to have a machine to wash contaminated items. This will require additional space. Sinks should be large enough that bulky items will fit into them and have attached counters on which soiled and clean items can be placed separately. There should be enough sinks to accommodate concurrent soaking, washing, and rinsing. Racks for drying will be needed.

Rules for care and safe handling of various sterilizing agents must be followed. There are Occupational Safety and Health Administration (OSHA) regulations relating to glutaraldehyde (see Chapter 27, "Cleaning and Sterilization"). It must be used in well-ventilated areas and cannot be in open vessels. Special facilities in a remote location may be needed.

Peracetic acid is used in the Steris system for fiberscopes and other heat-sensitive immersible instruments. This technology is discussed in detail in Chapter 27, "Cleaning and Sterilization." This provides a quick turnaround time and does not present a danger to personnel if properly used. In most facilities the machine is shared with the surgery department. It may be convenient to locate it in the anesthesia workroom if the workload is great enough.

Another relatively new technology for sterilizing items which should be considered is plasma sterilization. Some of these may require special accommodation, such as an exhaust vent to the outside.

Steam sterilization can be used for some anesthesia equipment such as laryngeal mask airways. In the future, more and larger items may be steam autoclavable. These include the canister assembly and parts of the anesthesia ventilator. A steam sterilizer in the anesthesia work area will be useful for these items.

Other Functions

In some facilities it may be necessary to store papers, equipment manuals, records, equipment checklists, and/or equipment incident histories in the anesthesia workroom. There may be a need for mailboxes for anesthesia personnel. A bulletin board may prove useful. Desk or counter space for activities such as filling out forms and adjustment and repair of small equipment should be considered. A desk with a computer connected to the hospital and anesthesia data networks is desirable. This can be used to track inventory, order supplies and keep records.

Gas Storage
Cylinders

The area where cylinders are stored should be well ventilated. They should be stored upright in a rack, preferably metal, which will prevent them from being knocked over. Rules for handling and storage of gas cylinders are covered in Chapter 1, "Compressed Gas Containers."

Liquid Oxygen

Small portable liquid oxygen containers are frequently used for patient transport. Space needs to be provided for a stationary unit from which the portable containers can be filled. Space for storing the portable containers will also be required. Locating these in the PACU will provide an emergency source of oxygen if the pipeline system fails. Rules for safe use and storage of liquid oxygen containers are discussed in Chapter 1, "Compressed Gas Containers."

Medications

Control of medications used in anesthesia can be accomplished in a number of ways. When designing an operating room suite, these methods should be examined and the facility designed to accommodate the one chosen.

There needs to be a way to determine the usage of medications and to charge the patient for those drugs which are not bundled into the anesthesia charges. Unfortunately, because of the nature of anesthesia practice, it is difficult to tightly control all drugs. If an electronic anesthesia data management system is being used, this can be used to augment accountability.

Narcotics and other restricted substances pose special problems (9). Controlled substance abuse is a serious problem among anesthesia personnel

(10–12). Storage, dispensing, and control of narcotics and restricted substances are mandated by law. There needs to be a storage, dispensing, and accounting system that satisfies the legal requirements for documentation and is compatible with efficient patient care. Such a system must be available 24 hours a day to satisfy the requirements of emergency as well as elective surgery. The anesthesia care provider, the amount of drugs dispensed, the patients who received the drugs and dosages, and wasted and unused medications should be recorded. Several bookkeeping/verification forms have been described (13–17).

Pharmacy Control

Satellite Pharmacy

In recent years, increasing numbers of healthcare facilities have recognized the advantages of having a satellite pharmacy in the operating room suite (9, 13, 18–25). Such a unit may be open from 1 to 24 hours per day (26). If it is not open 24 hours, an after-hours system must be established. The on-site pharmacist orders, organizes, and controls drugs stocked in the operating room and checks for outdated medications. Each facility will have its own needs and the pharmaceutical services should be tailored to the practice environment. It may be convenient to have the operating room pharmacy supply drugs and solutions to labor and delivery and/or critical care areas.

Advantages of an on-site pharmacy include improvements in accountability; drug charge capture; inventory control; cost containment; and drug preparation, storage, and labeling. Expedited procurement of drugs not normally stocked in the operating room, waste reduction, on-site information on drugs, and elimination of nursing and anesthesiology staff time spent in gathering and preparing drugs are further benefits. Drugs and intravenous and epidural solutions can be prepared in a laminar hood. The satellite can assemble kits for specific surgical procedures and surgeons as well as for conditions such as malignant hyperthermia; the satellite restock anesthesia trays, individualize patient charges for medications, and dispense controlled substances.

A general review of the surgery and anesthesiology areas should be performed before an operating room satellite pharmacy is set up. If the satellite is shared with adjacent critical care areas, it should be located where access from the outside is convenient. The pharmacy should have a laminar flow hood, a refrigerator, space for drug storage, a locked container (e.g., cabinet, drawer, or cart) for controlled substances, a computer, space for filling out papers, and room for pharmaceutical literature. A locked drop box for return of controlled substances and worksheets after hours should be provided at a convenient location in the operating room suite such as the PACU.

With an operating room pharmacy, a separate supply of controlled drugs can be provided to each anesthesia provider on a daily or case basis (9, 13, 19, 21, 23–25, 27). If the pharmacy is not open 24 hours a day, it may be convenient to prepare kits for after-hours. These can then be dispensed from a locked cabinet by a nurse.

Tray Exchange

Another method for dispensing non-controlled drugs is to use trays or kits which fit into one of the drawers of the anesthesia cart. These can be made up by pharmacy and placed in the anesthesia carts during the night. For efficient cost accounting, each tray should be used for only one case and then returned to the pharmacy with the name of the patient for which it was used. If the tray is used for more than one patient such cost accounting is more difficult.

Each tray or kit should include drugs needed for typical cases plus some emergency medications. There needs to be a method of transporting the trays to the operating room, storing them in a convenient location and securing them against theft. A number of trays for use after hours need to be stocked.

Dispensing Machine (9, 18, 28)

Another way of dispensing medications is a vending machine stocked with drugs. These can be filled with intravenous solutions as well. To obtain items from the machine, a special code or key must be used. If the patient's account number is entered, the drug or intravenous solution can be charged to that patient. A study on these machines found that they saved pharmacy time spent on billing tasks and increased capture of drug and intravenous solution charges (28).

Anesthesia personnel may obtain controlled and noncontrolled substances from a vending machine which is stocked by the pharmacy. This can provide good accountability. To avoid anesthesia personnel leaving a patient, a separate machine must be provided near each anesthetizing location. Unused controlled substances may be wasted or returned to a locked drop box. Disadvantages of this system include the initial purchase price of the machines, difficulty with dispensing large ampoules, and the necessity for providing a mechanism to bypass the system in the event of mechanical breakdown or lost keys.

Prepackaged Drugs

In institutions with many emergency cases, it may be desirable to have a set of emergency drugs set up at all times. Some drugs may be drawn up in syringes and sealed in a container or plastic bag that is kept where it can be easily accessed (29).

In some facilities, individual anesthesia providers have locked containers that contain controlled substances (9, 15). Drugs may be standardized or individually stocked. If the containers are used for more than one case, charges and security between cases can be a problem.

Non-Pharmacy Control

Anesthesia Technicians

In the past it was customary for anesthesia technicians to stock noncontrolled drugs in the anesthesia carts. A major problem with this arrangement is that some anesthesia technicians are not adequately trained to work with medications and could mix up drugs with similar names (e.g., epinephrine and ephedrine) or drugs with similar packaging. Another problem is that some noncontrolled drugs have the potential for abuse (11). Tighter control of these drugs will be necessary in the future.

Dispensing Nurse

Registered nurses may dispense controlled drugs from a locked container. Special prepackaged kits containing groups of controlled substances may be used (13, 17, 30). A disadvantage of this system is that it involves burdensome shift counts.

Biomedical Facilities

Having a biomedical facility in the operating room suite has a number of advantages. The technician is readily available to respond to equipment malfunctions and to observe intermittent problems as they occur. The technician can perform routine preventive maintenance on equipment without removing it from the area. When equipment for evaluation is brought in, the technician is readily available to check its electrical safety. A disadvantage of this system is that the technician may become isolated from the rest of the department in the main facility.

The biomedical workspace needs to be large enough to accommodate a workbench and sufficient storage space for parts. It should have numerous electrical outlets and special outlets required for equipment which is brought in for repair. Pipeline outlets for air, oxygen, nitrous oxide, and nitrogen will be needed. Space must be adequate to allow servicing of large equipment such as anesthesia machines. Space must be provided here or elsewhere in the facility to store equipment awaiting parts.

Storage Space for Bulky Equipment

Storage space will be needed for seldom used or backup equipment and for equipment awaiting servicing or acquisition of parts. This may be part of the biomedical area or in a separate designated area. It may be outside the operating room area, but easy and rapid access is important.

ANESTHESIA EQUIPMENT AND MONITORING NEEDS

Introduction

This section will focus on equipment that should be considered for an operating room. Personal preferences, cost considerations, mandated requirements, and the type of practice will influence the specific devices chosen (8).

Anesthesia Machines

Considerations in purchasing anesthesia machines are discussed in Chapter 4, "Anesthesia Machines." Many departments prefer to have machines from only one manufacturer or even only one model. If a teaching program is in place, it might be the practice to have different machines from various manufacturers to give the trainees more experience.

For small operating rooms such as cystoscopy and local rooms, a smaller machine may be preferable. Machines that have only two gases and two vaporizers can be made smaller than those with a greater number, but this may be unacceptable in certain practices. A small machine may be preferable if it is to be moved from room to room or taken out of the operating room area.

The vast majority of larger infants can be adequately ventilated using a standard anesthesia ventilator. In departments where premature and neonatal patients are frequently anesthetized, consideration should be given to purchasing a ventilator designed for pediatric patients.

Monitors

Monitors for blood pressure (both invasive and noninvasive), ECG, pulse oximetry, central venous pressure, pulmonary artery pressure, temperature, electroencephalogram, cardiac output, and respiratory and anesthetic gases and vapors should be considered.

The choice of monitors will depend on the type and acuity of cases to be performed in a particular room. If cardiac surgery is to be performed or high acuity patients are to be anesthetized, a monitor which includes most of the above parameters would be desirable. If patients are relatively healthy and procedures of low intensity are to be performed, ECG, noninvasive blood pressure, pulse oximetry, inspired oxygen and capnometry will probably be adequate.

It may be desirable to have monitors that are compatible with those in other areas of the facility such as the critical care unit and PACU. This will facilitate transfer of patients. Sensors applied to the patient in the operating room can be used in other areas. Having all monitors in the facility from the same manufacturer may lead to economy in parts and better servicing.

A modular monitor may be advantageous. With this, a basic set of modules including blood pressure, ECG, gas analysis, temperature, and pulse oximetry is kept in each room. Other modules, e.g., invasive pressure and cardiac output, can be added when the situation warrants. Modular equipment may have significant financial advantages, despite higher initial cost. Upgrades can be performed without retiring the entire unit, and modules can be easily swapped if a different monitoring modality is desired.

The use of multivariable integrated monitors is increasing. Some monitors are built into anesthesia machines. This results in economy of space and integration of machine and monitor information and alarms. A disadvantage is that some built-in monitors may not meet all the needs of the user and may be different from monitors in other operating rooms.

Electrocardiogram (31, 32)

American Society of Anesthesiologists' (ASA) standards require that every patient receiving anesthesia have the ECG continuously displayed (33). It is common practice to monitor more than one lead. If a strip recorder is not available, it should be possible to freeze the display. Monitors that can detect ST-T segment displacement may result in increased detection of ischemia. Some of the newer monitors can automatically recognize deviations from sinus rhythm and display them on the screen to be reviewed.

Non-Invasive Blood Pressure Monitors (20, 32)

ASA standards require that every patient receiving anesthesia have blood pressure and heart rate determined at least every 5 minutes (33). Automated sphygmomanometers are reliable and preferable if pressures do not need to be monitored continuously.

Invasive Pressure Monitors (20)

Invasive pressure (central venous, arterial, pulmonary artery) monitoring is frequently used for patients who are very ill or in whom tight control of pressures is necessary.

Pulse Oximetry (21, 22)

ASA standards for basic intraoperative monitoring require that during all anesthetics a quantitative method of assessing oxygenation such as pulse oximetry be employed (33). Pulse oximetry may be incorporated into a multivariable monitor or the anesthesia machine or a dedicated pulse oximeter may be used. For additional information see Chapter 20, "Pulse Oximetry."

Temperature Monitors (23, 24)

ASA standards require that a means to measure the patient's temperature be readily available and the temperature be measured when changes in body temperature are intended, anticipated or suspected (33). A temperature monitor may be part of a multivariable monitor or a stand-alone device. For additional information see Chapter 22, "Temperature Monitoring."

Neuromuscular Transmission Monitors

A variety of neuromuscular transmission monitors is available (25, 34). As yet, these devices are not part of anesthesia workstations or multivariable monitors but may be in the future. It is recommended that there be one in every anesthetizing location. Patterns of stimulation should include twitch, tetanus, train of four, and double burst. There should be a variable output in milliamperes. More complex neuromuscular transmission monitors include the accelerometer and the electromyogram. These are more expensive but have desirable features including the ability to determine the train-of-four ratio accurately. They can be used in cases where the arm is tucked beside the patient. For additional information on these monitors see Chapter 21, "Neuromuscular Transmission Monitoring."

Airway Flow, Volume, and Pressure Monitors (35, 36)

Respirometers are incorporated into all new anesthesia machines. A respirometer may also be part of a multivariable monitor or a separate dedicated monitor. Most anesthesia machines and some multivariable monitors have airway pressure monitoring. Dedicated airway pressure monitors are also available. The pressure may be displayed as a wave. A newer development is pressure-volume and flow-volume loops. For additional information on pressure, volume and flow measurement see Chapter 19, "Airway Pressure, Volume, and Flow Measurements."

Anesthetic and Respiratory Gas Monitors (37, 38)

Gas monitors may measure carbon dioxide, oxygen, helium, nitrogen and/or anesthetic agents. ASA and American Association of Nurse Anesthetists (AANA) practice standards require that during administration of general anesthesia the con-

centration of oxygen in the breathing system be measured by an analyzer with a low oxygen concentration alarm (33). The standards also require that every patient receiving general anesthesia have the adequacy of ventilation continually evaluated. Quantitative monitoring of carbon dioxide is encouraged. When a tracheal tube is used, use of end-tidal carbon dioxide to verify positioning in the tracheobronchial tree is mandated. While anesthetic agent monitoring is not as yet a standard of practice, it is likely that most practitioners will want to use it in the future. When selecting a monitor, consideration should be given to what agents are likely to be used in the future.

A gas monitor can be incorporated into an anesthesia machine or a multivariable monitor, or may be a separate monitor. See Chapter 18, "Anesthesia Gas Monitoring" for more information on gas monitors.

Other Monitors

These include cardiac output, precordial Doppler, transesophageal echocardiography, and the electroencephalograph. The need for these will depend on the type of surgery to be performed in a particular facility.

Breathing Systems (39)

The circle breathing system is the most popular in the United States for adult patients. Completely disposable circle systems are available. These may be especially useful for patients with malignant hyperthermia. Disposable tubes come in a variety of lengths, with and without bacterial filters, and can be stretchable or coaxial. There are a variety of Y-piece configurations. Most disposable breathing tubes are clean but not sterile. If tubes are to be added to the surgical field, sterile ones need to be kept available.

Systems other than the circle, such as one of the Mapleson systems, may be used. These are not commonly used for general anesthesia for adults because they are uneconomical. They may be needed for transport, resuscitation, application of continuous positive airway pressure, and pediatric patients.

Humidification Devices (40)

Disposable heat and moisture exchangers, especially those that are also filters, have become popular. Use of heated humidifiers has decreased with increased use of heat and moisture exchangers, low fresh gas flows and forced-air patient warming machines. Humidification devices are discussed in more detail in Chapter 10, "Humidification Equipment."

Warming Devices

Forced-air warming machines maintain intraoperative normothermia better than circulating-water mattresses (41). However, it is recommended that some circulating-water mattresses be kept for cases where a forced-air machine cannot be used. For pediatric cases, radiant heat warmers may be desirable. Devices for warming fluids are useful if large volumes of cold blood or intravenous fluid are to be administered.

Airway Management Equipment (42, 43)

Tracheal Tubes

Tracheal tubes need to be stocked in sizes commensurate with the practice. Laser tubes, molded tubes for head and neck surgery, double-lumen tubes, wire spiral tubes, and tubes for bronchoscopy or laryngoscopy may be needed for special situations. Tracheal tubes are discussed in more detail in Chapter 17, "Tracheal Tubes."

Double-Lumen Tubes and Blockers

Both right and left double-lumen bronchial tubes with appropriate suction catheters and stylets need to be available if thoracic surgery is to be performed. A means to apply continuous positive airway pressure should be available when a double-lumen tube is used. An alternative to a double-lumen tube is the Univent tube which has a bronchial blocker. Double-lumen tubes and blockers are discussed in greater detail in Chapter 17, "Tracheal Tubes."

Airways

Oral and nasal airways in a variety of sizes need to be available. Special airways for fiberoptic intubation should be available (see Fiberscope and Difficult Intubation Equipment below). This equipment is discussed in more detail in Chapter 14, "Face Masks and Airways."

Airway Accessories

Airway accessories such as forceps, stylets, and adaptors need to be available. The specific items depend on the user's preferences and needs. These are discussed in more detail in Chapter 17, "Tracheal Tubes."

Laryngoscopes

The laryngoscopes needed will depend on the preferences of the user. A variety of shapes and sizes and at least two handles should be kept in each anesthesia cart. Laryngoscopes are discussed in more detail in Chapter 16, "Laryngoscopes."

Fiberscope and Difficult Intubation Equipment

The following equipment may be useful when a difficult intubation is anticipated or when fiberoptic intubation is planned. Some of these items are discussed in Chapters 14 to 17. This list is only an example and should not be considered exhaustive. Examples of arrangement of equipment for fiberoptic intubation are given in several publications (44–47).

Fiberscope	Special Laryngoscopes
Fiberoptic Light	(e.g., Bullard,
Source	WuScope, Upsher
Video Head	Scope)
Videocassette Recorder	Bougies
Defogging Solution	Flexible Suction
Swivel Fiberoptic	Catheters
Adaptors	Yankauer Suction Tips
Local Anesthetic Spray	Laryngeal Mask
Patil-Syracuse	Airways
Endoscopic Mask	Cricothyrotomy Device
Fiberoptic Intubating	Device for
Airways (e.g.,	Transtracheal
Ovassapian, Patil-	Ventilation
Syracuse, Williams,	Combitubes
Berman)	Retrograde Intubation
Fiberoptic Stylet	Kit
Laryngoscope	Tracheostomy Kit
Lighted Intubation	Binasal Airway
Stylet	

Automatic Infusion Devices (48–52)

Automatic infusion pumps are used to administer intravenous fluids, anesthetics, analgesics, vasopressors, and epidural solutions. It is best to have the same type of intravenous fluid pump throughout the facility.

Electronic syringe pumps have become popular. Often standard disposable syringes already stocked by the facility can be used. The selection of a pump depends on several factors, including available features, cost of the pump and infusion sets, the safety and ease of use, and required maintenance. The device should have battery backup so that it will function during transport.

Equipment for Regional Anesthesia

It may be convenient to keep conduction equipment on a cart. A variety of disposable trays are available. It is good practice to keep extra needles to replace ones which become contaminated or damaged without having to open a full tray.

The following should be considered for the cart:

B-Bevel Needles	Various Types of Tape
Extra Long Needles	Scissors
Marking Pen	Nerve Finder and
Insulin Syringe	Special Insulated
Tourniquet	Needles
Prep Pads and Sticks	Sterile Gloves
and Solution	Clear Adhesive
Bactericidal Ointment	Bandage
Double Touniquet for	Control Syringes
Bier Block	Temperature Monitor
Spray Adhesive	Intubation Equipment

Resuscitation Equipment (53)

Each operating room suite should have at least one cart that contains the items needed to deal with a cardiac arrest. A complete supply of drugs needed for emergencies should be present. In addition, the following equipment should be considered:

Spinal Needles 18G, 19G, 20G	Urinary Catheterization Kit
Labels	Nasogastric Tubes
Intravenous Catheters	Wall Suction Setup,
Prep Solutions, Tourniquets, Tape, Gloves	Tubing and Suction Catheters
ECG Pads and Paper	Monitor and Defibrillator
Defibrillator Pads	External Pacemaker

Blood Pressure Cuff	Self-Refilling Bag-Valve-Mask Unit

Pediatric Equipment (54)

While pediatric equipment may be readily available in a healthcare facility which routinely performs pediatric surgery, in one in which pediatric anesthesia is less common it may be preferable to have carts with pediatric equipment. The following should be considered:

Tracheal Tubes in 0.5 mm sizes from 2.5–6.0	Pulse Oximeter Probes in Variety of Shapes of Sizes
Tracheal Tubes 3.5–6.5 Cuffed	Small Temperature Probes
Laryngoscopes Handles and Blades in Pediatric Sizes	Cricothyroid—16- or 1-Ga IV Catheter with 3.0 Tracheal
Bone-Marrow Needle for Interosseous Fluid Administration	Tube Connector Transport System: Mapleson D
Mapleson Breathing Systems (A,D,F)	Breathing System should be considered
Smaller Hoses and Bag to Fit Circle System	Pediatric Urinary Catheters
Pediatric Nasogastric Tubes	Pediatric Self-Refilling Bag-Valve-Mask
Pediatric Ventilator Bellows	Unit Equipment for
Pediatric Airways	Cricothyroid
Precordial Stethoscopes	Puncture 22- and 24-Ga
Pediatric Heat and Moisture Exchangers	Intravenous Catheters
Pediatric Masks	Pediatric Suction Catheters
Automatic Blood Pressure Machine with Pediatric Mode or Capable of Using Small Cuffs	Pediatric Paddles for Cardiac Defibrillator Intravenous—Buretrol Pediatric Arm Boards Pediatric Laryngeal
Pediatric Blood Pressure Cuffs in Assorted Sizes	Mask Airways

Malignant Hyperthermia Cart

The following equipment should be considered for a malignant hyperthermia cart:

Malignant Hyperthermia Protocol and Hot Line Number

Chart for Recording Drugs, Temperatures, Various Interventions

Syringes and Needles

Arterial blood gas (ABG) Kits

Arterial Catheters

Pressure Transducers

Vacutainers for Lab Tests

Central Venous and Swan-Ganz Catheters

Temperature Probes—Esophageal, Rectal, etc., including Pediatric Sizes

Pressure Bags for IV Infusions

Nasogastric Tubes including Pediatric Sizes

Urinary Catheters including Pediatric Sizes

Cold Packs

Trauma Cart

Many departments find it useful to keep a cart designed for handling major trauma cases stocked and ready. The following should be considered for inclusion on such a cart:

Vacutainers for Laboratory Tests

Central Venous and Swan-Ganz Catheters

Pressure Transducers

Arterial Catheters

ABG Kits

Drugs (e.g., Albumin, Hetastatch, Hep-Lock Solution, Heparin)

Blood Filters and Administration Sets

IV Solutions

Fluid Warmers

Pressure Bags for Infusions

Flexible Oximeter Sensors

Urinary Catheters and Urometers

Information Management Systems (53, 55, 56)

Information management systems are discussed in detail in Chapter 25, "Data Management." If such a system is planned there are a number of considerations. Each piece of equipment needs to have an interface. It is important to plan for wiring and cables to connect the various components.

Latex Allergy Cart

Because so many items in operating rooms contain latex, a special latex allergy cart may prove useful. The following should be considered for such a cart:

Glass Syringes

Glass Ampules

Intravenous (IV) Tubing without Ports

Stopcocks for Injections

Needleless IV Systems

Latex-Free Tourniquets (or wrapping for placement under latex tourniquet)

Non-Latex Reservoir Bag

Non-Latex Ventilator Bellows

Plastic Face Masks

Non-Latex Manual Resuscitators

Plastic Nasopharyngeal Airways

Non-Latex gloves

REFERENCES

1. Ehrenwerth J. Operating room design. American Society of Anesthesiologists Newsletter 1994;58:13–16.
2. Lee A, Hillman KM. Anesthesia preoperative evaluation clinic: III. Anesthesiology 1997;86:260–261.
3. Graves SA, Berman LA. Caring for a child in a general postanesthesia care unit. Am J Anesth 1996;6:176–181.
4. Ehrenwerth J. Electrical safety in anesthesia equipment. In: Ehrenwerth J, Eisenkraft JB, eds. Principles and applications. St. Louis: Mosby, 1993;445–469.
5. Peterson GN. CDC sets guidelines for preventing TB transmission in health care facilities. American Society of Anesthesiologists Newsletter 1995;59(5):24–26.
6. Dorsch JA, Dorsch SE. Understanding anesthesia equipment, construction, care and complications, 3rd ed. Baltimore: Williams & Wilkins, 1994;51–147.
7. Eisenkraft JB. The anesthesia machine. In: Ehrenwerth J, Eisenkraft JB, eds. Anesthesia equipment, principles and applications. St. Louis: Mosby, 1993;27–56.
8. Hyndman B, Ream AK. Selection and maintenance of monitoring equipment. In: Saidman LJ, Smith NT, eds. Monitoring in anesthesia, 3rd ed., Boston: Butterworth–Heinemann, 1993;505–514.
9. Moleski RJ, Easley S, Barash PG, et al. Control and accountability of controlled substance administration in the operating room. Anesth Analg 1985;64:989–995.
10. Patt RB. Controlling abuse of drugs from the anesthesia department. JAMA 1985; 254:3180–3181.
11. Ward CF. Substance abuse. Now, and for some time to come. Anesthesiology 1992;77:619–622.
12. Wood PR, Soni N. Anaesthesia and substance abuse. Anaesthesia 1989; 44:672–680.
13. Shafer AL, Lisman SR, Rosenberg MB. Development

of a comprehensive operating room pharmacy. J Clin Anesth 1991;3:156–166.

14. Schmidt KA, Schlesinger MD. A reliable accounting system for controlled substances in the operating room. Anesthesiology 1993;78:184–190.

15. Adler GR, Potts FE, Kirby RR, et al. Narcotics control in anesthesia training. JAMA 1985;253:3133–3136.

16. Davis JL. A practical system for narcotic control within the OR/PACU. J Post Anes Nurs 1989;4:32–35.

17. Maltby JR, Levy DA, Eagle CJ. Simple narcotic kits for controlled-substance dispensing and accountability. Can J Anaesth 1994;41:301–305.

18. Ziter CA, Dennis BW, Shoup LK. Justification of an operating-room satellite pharmacy. Am J Hosp Pharm 1989;46:1353–1361.

19. Donnelly AJ, Shafer AL: ASHP technical assistance bulletin on surgery and anesthesiology pharmaceutical services. Am J Hosp Pharm 1991;48:319–325.

20. Quill TJ. Blood pressure monitoring. In: Ehrenwerth J, Eisenkraft JB, eds. Anesthesia equipment, principles and applications. St. Louis: Mosby, 1993;274–283.

21. Dorsch JA, Dorsch SE. Understanding anesthesia equipment, construction, care and complications, 3rd ed. Baltimore: Williams & Wilkins, 1994;657–686.

22. Barker SJ, Tremper KK. Pulse oximetry. In: Ehrenwerth J, Eisenkraft JB, eds. Anesthesia equipment, principles and applications. St. Louis: Mosby, 1993;249–263.

23. Dorsch JA, Dorsch SE. Understanding anesthesia equipment, construction, care and complications, 3rd ed. Baltimore: Williams & Wilkins, 1994;633–645.

24. Zoll RD. Temperature monitoring. In: Ehrenwerth J, Eisenkraft JB, eds. Anesthesia equipment, principles and applications. St. Louis: Mosby, 1993;264–273.

25. Dorsch JA, Dorsch SE. Understanding anesthesia equipment, construction, care and complications, 3rd ed. Baltimore: Williams & Wilkins, 1994;609–633.

26. Klein RL, Stevens WC, Kingston HGG. Controlled substance dispensing and accountability in United States anesthesiology residency programs. Anesthesiology 1992;77:806–811.

27. Johnson JA, Code WE, Duncan PG. An improved system for narcotic control in the operating room. Can J Anaesth 1990;37:S83.

28. Lee LW, Weldon GS, Birdwell SW, Use of an automated medication storage and distribution system. Am J Hosp Pharm 1992;49:851–855.

29. Bready LL, Orr MD, Mote MA. Drug security for emergency surgical procedures. Anesthesiology 1985; 63:225.

30. Partridge BL, Weinger MB, Sanford TJ. Preventing unauthorized access to narcotics in the operating room. Anesth Analg 1990;71:566–567.

31. Narang J, Thys DM. Electrocardiographic monitoring. In Ehrenwerth J, Eisenkraft JB, eds. Anesthesia equipment, principles and applications. St. Louis: Mosby, 1993;284–296.

32. Perrino AC Jr, Feldman JM, Barash PG. Noninvasive cardiovascular monitoring. In: Saidman LJ, Smith NT, eds. Monitoring in anesthesia, 3rd ed. Boston: Butterworth-Heinemann, 1993;101–143.

33. Standards for Basic Intraoperative Monitoring, American Society of Anesthesiologists, adopted October 6, 1986; amended 1989; effective January 1, 1990.

34. Brul SJ, Silverman DG. Neuromuscular block monitoring. In: Ehrenwerth J, Eisenkraft JB, eds. Anesthesia equipment, principles and applications. St. Louis: Mosby, 1993;297–318.

35. Dorsch JA, Dorsch SE. Understanding anesthesia equipment, construction, care and complications, 3rd ed. Baltimore: Williams & Wilkins, 1994;645–650.

36. Ibid: 650–657.

37. Ibid: 547–607.

38. Eisenkraft JB, Raemer DB. Monitoring gases in the anesthesia delivery system. In: Anesthesia equipment, principles and applications. St. Louis: Mosby, 1993; 201–220.

39. Smith TC. Anesthesia breathing systems. In: Ehrenwerth J, Eisenkraft JB, eds. Anesthesia equipment, principles and applications. St. Louis: Mosby, 1993;89–113.

40. Ramanathan S. Humidification and humidifiers. In: Ehrenwerth J, Eisenkraft JB, eds. Anesthesia equipment, principles and applications. St. Louis: Mosby, 1993;172–197.

41. Kurz A, Kurz M, Poeschl G, et al. Forced-air warming maintains intraoperative normothermia better than circulating-water mattresses. Anesth Analg 1993;77:89–95.

42. Dorsch JA, Dorsch SE. Understanding anesthesia equipment, 3rd ed. Baltimore: Williams & Wilkins, 1994;399–545.

43. Benumof JF. Management of the difficult adult airway with special emphasis on awake tracheal intubation. Anesthesiology 1991;75:1087–1110.

44. Roberts JT, ed. Fiberoptics in anesthesia. Philadelphia: WB Saunders Co., 1991.

45. Ovassapian A, ed. Fiberoptic airway endoscopy in anesthesia and critical care. New York: Raven Press, 1990.

46. Patil V, Stealing L, Exeter H, ed. Fiberoptic endoscopy in anesthesia. Chicago: Year Book Medical Publishers, 1983.

47. Prakash UBS. Bronchscopy. New York, NY: Raven Press, 1994.

48. Zarmsky RF, Parker AJ, Sinatra RS. Infusion pumps.

In: Ehrenwerth J, Eisenkraft JB, eds. Anesthesia equipment, principles and applications. St. Louis: Mosby, 1993;647–673.

49. Emergency Care Research Institute. Infusion controllers. Health Devices 1985;14:219–257.

50. Kwan JW. High-technology i.v. infusion devices. Am J Hosp Pharm 1989;46:320–325.

51. Emergency Care Research Institute. Infusion pumps. Health Devices 1984;13:31–62.

52. Emergency Care Research Institute. Syringe infusion pumps. Health Devices 1987;16:3–30.

53. Smith NT, Gravenstein JS. Manual and automated anesthesia information management systems. In: Saidman LJ, Smith NT, eds. Monitoring in anesthesia, 3rd ed. Boston: Butterworth-Heinemann, 1993;457–474.

54. Hillier SC, McNieve WL. Pediatric anesthesia systems and equipment. In: Ehrenwerth J, Eisenkraft JB, eds. Anesthesia equipment, principles and applications, St. Louis: Mosby, 1993;537–564.

55. Feldman JM, Good ML. Record-keeping and automated record-keepers. In: Ehrenwerth J, Eisenkraft JB, eds. Anesthesia equipment, principles and applications. St. Louis: Mosby, 1993;405–420.

56. Gravenstein JS, Newbower RS, Ream AK, et al. The automated anesthesia record and alarm systems. Boston: Butterworth, 1987.

QUESTIONS

Questions 1 to 9 contains four suggested answers of which one or more is correct. Choose the answer:

A if 1, 2, and 3 are correct
B if 1 and 3 are correct
C if 2 and 4 are correct
D if 4 is correct
E if 1, 2, 3, and 4 are correct.

1. When considering the number of spaces needed for a preoperative care unit
   1. The types of surgical cases to be performed should be considered
   2. The type of procedures performed in that area should be considered
   3. The duration of surgeries should be considered
   4. There should be a minimum of two spaces per active operating room

2. When configuring a preoperative area of the operating room suite
   1. Separate rooms are preferred to allow privacy
   2. Flexible space for procedures is desirable
   3. Patients requiring isolation should not be brought to the area
   4. All spaces must be visible from the nursing station

3. Which outlets are necessary at each bed in the preoperative area?
   1. Oxygen
   2. Air
   3. Vacuum
   4. Nitrous Oxide

4. Which monitoring modalities need to be available at each preoperative bed location?
   1. ECG
   2. Temperature
   3. Noninvasive blood pressure
   4. Invasive blood pressure

5. Flexibility in connections to anesthesia gas services can be achieved by
   1. Having more than one gas supply device

2. Using wall outlets
3. Using articulating arm supply devices
4. Moving the operating table

6. How many of each gas outlet should be available in each supply device in the operating room?
   1. One oxygen
   2. Two air
   3. Two vacuum
   4. One nitrous oxide

7. Concerning isolated power systems
   1. Their use is optional
   2. A faulty piece of equipment will continue to operate
   3. Ground wires are not used in an isolated system.
   4. They need a line isolation monitor

8. In a grounded power system
   1. The ground fault interrupter will cut off power to a device without warning
   2. If the equipment case becomes energized, the ground wire provides a low resistance route to ground
   3. There are three wires to each device
   4. There is protection from microshock

9. Advantages of having a pharmacy located in the operating room suite include
   1. Intravenous drug preparation
   2. Revenue capture
   3. Inventory control
   4. Abuse prevention

10. Which size operating room is likely become most common in the future?
    A. 200–300 sq. ft.
    B. 300–400 sq. ft.
    C. 400–500 sq. ft.
    D. 500–600 sq. ft
    E. over 600 sq. ft.

ANSWERS

1.	A	6.	D
2.	C	7.	E
3.	A	8.	A
4.	B	9.	A
5.	E	10.	E

INDEX

Note: Page numbers in *italics* indicate illustrations; those followed by t indicate tables.